NETTER'S
GASTROENTEROLOGY

NETTER'S GASTROENTEROLOGY

MARTIN H. FLOCH, MD, MACG, AGAF

C. S. PITCHUMONI, MD, MPH, FRCP(C), FRCP(Edin), MACG, MACP, AGAF

NEIL R. FLOCH, MD, FACS

RAUL J. ROSENTHAL, MD, FACS, FASMBS

JAMES S. SCOLAPIO, MD

JOSEPH K. LIM, MD

Illustrations by

Frank H. Netter, MD

Contributing Illustrators

Carlos A. G. Machado, MD

John A. Craig, MD

Kip Carter, MS

David Mascaro, MS

Steven Moon

Kristen Wienandt Marzejon

Mike de la Flor

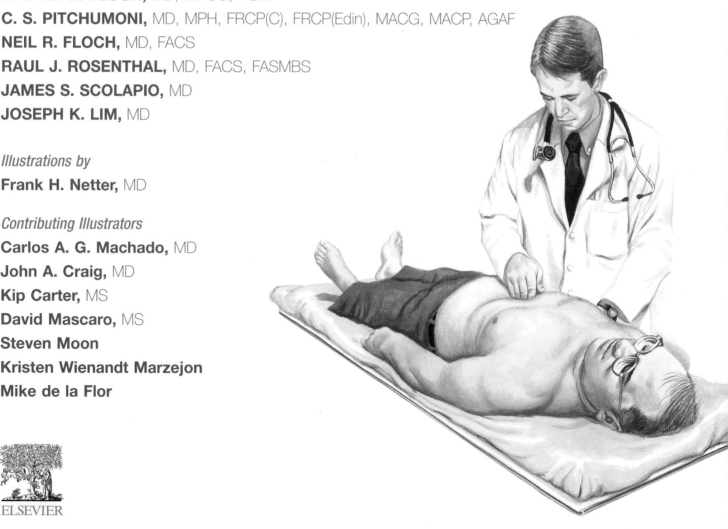

ELSEVIER

NETTER'S GASTROENTEROLOGY, THIRD EDITION

ISBN: 978-0-323-59624-4

Notice

Practitioners and researchers must always rely on their own experience and knowledge in evaluating and using any information, methods, compounds or experiments described herein. Because of rapid advances in the medical sciences, in particular, independent verification of diagnoses and drug dosages should be made. To the fullest extent of the law, no responsibility is assumed by Elsevier, authors, editors or contributors for any injury and/or damage to persons or property as a matter of products liability, negligence or otherwise, or from any use or operation of any methods, products, instructions, or ideas contained in the material herein.

Previous editions copyrighted 2010 and 2005.

International Standard Book Number: 978-0-323-59624-4

Content Strategist: Marybeth Thiel
Publishing Services Manager: Catherine Jackson
Senior Project Manager: Daniel Fitzgerald
Designer: Patrick Ferguson

Printed in China.

Last digit is the print number: 9 8 7 6 5 4 3 2 1

ELSEVIER

1600 John F. Kennedy Blvd.
Ste 1600
Philadelphia, PA 19103-2899

Working together
to grow libraries in
developing countries

www.elsevier.com • www.bookaid.org

*In today's hectic world, writing scientific text takes place during
what most people would consider leisure time. We have forsaken time with
our families to compile this book. Hence, we would like to dedicate it completely
to our wives and children.*

*To our wives—Gladys Floch, Prema Pitchumoni, Robin Floch, Sima Rosenthal,
Elizabeth Scolapio, and Stephanie Lim.*

*To our children—Jeffrey Aaron Floch (in memoriam), Craig Lawrence Floch,
Lisa Susanne Adelmann, Neil Robert Floch, Sheila Pitchumoni,
Shoba Pitchumoni, Suresh Pitchumoni, Noam Rosenthal, Dana Rosenthal,
Julia Scolapio, Anthony Scolapio, Micah Lim,
Vera Lim, and Joshua Lim.*

CONTRIBUTORS

Editors

Martin H. Floch, MD, MACG, AGAF
Clinical Professor of Medicine
Yale University School of Medicine
New Haven, Connecticut
Section II, Stomach and Duodenum; Section IV, Small Intestine; Section V, Colon, Rectum, and Anus

C. S. Pitchumoni, MD, MPH, FRCP(C), FRCP(Edin), MACG, MACP, AGAF
Clinical Professor of Medicine, Rutgers University
Chief, Division of Gastroenterology, Hepatology, and Clinical Nutrition
Saint Peter's University Hospital
New Brunswick, New Jersey
Section VI, Infectious and Parasitic Diseases of the Alimentary Tract; Section VII, Pancreas; Section VIII, Gallbladder and Bile Ducts

Neil R. Floch, MD, FACS
Director of Minimally Invasive Surgery
Director of Bariatric Surgery
Norwalk Hospital
Norwalk, Connecticut
Section I, Esophagus

Raul J. Rosenthal, MD, FACS, FASMBS
Professor of Surgery and Chairman
Department of General Surgery
Director, The Bariatric and Metabolic Institute
President, South Florida Chapter of the American College of Surgeons
President, The Fellowship Council
Cleveland Clinic
Weston, Florida
Section III, Abdominal Wall; Chapter 191, Surgical Treatment of Obesity

James S. Scolapio, MD
Professor
Department of Medicine
Division of Gastroenterology
Associate Chair, Department of Medicine
University of Florida—Jacksonville
Jacksonville, Florida
Section X, Nutrition and Gastrointestinal Disease

Joseph K. Lim, MD
Professor of Medicine
Director, Yale Viral Hepatitis Program
Yale University School of Medicine
New Haven, Connecticut
Section IX, Liver

Contributors

Hira Ahmad, MD
General Surgery Resident
Department of General Surgery and The Bariatric and Metabolic Institute
Cleveland Clinic Florida
Weston, Florida
Chapter 47, Alimentary Tract Obstruction and Intestinal Injuries

Rene Aleman, MD
Research Fellow
Department of General Surgery and The Bariatric and Metabolic Institute
Cleveland Clinic Florida
Weston, Florida
Chapter 49, Abdominal Access

Maria C. Fonseca, MD
Research Fellow
MIS Bariatric Surgery
Cleveland Clinic Florida
Weston, Florida
Chapter 45, Peritoneum and Related Diseases

David R. Funes, MD
Research Fellow
Department of General Surgery
Cleveland Clinic Florida
Weston, Florida
Chapter 46, Mesenteric Ischemia and Other Vascular Lesions

Camila Ortiz Gomez, MD
Research Fellow
Department of General Surgery and The Bariatric and Metabolic Institute
Cleveland Clinic Florida
Miami, Florida
Chapter 48, Abdominal Wall and Abdominal Cavity Hernias

Kandace Kichler, MD
Advanced GI, MIS and Bariatric Surgery Fellow
Cleveland Clinic Florida
Weston, Florida
Chapter 48, Abdominal Wall and Abdominal Cavity Hernias

Kris V. Kowdley, MD, FACP, FACG, AGAF, FAASLD
Gastroenterologist
Swedish Organ Transplant and Liver Center
Seattle, Washington
Chapters 143–151, 153, 155–166, 168–183

Matthew Lange, DO
Advanced GI/MIS Surgery Fellow
Department of General Surgery and The Bariatric and Metabolic Institute
Cleveland Clinic Florida
Weston, Florida
Chapter 44, Abdominal Wall Anatomy

Emanuele Lo Menzo, MD, PhD, FACS, FASMBS
Director, Department of Clinical Research
Staff Surgeon
Digestive Disease Institute
Cleveland Clinic Florida
Weston, Florida
Chapter 44, Abdominal Wall Anatomy; Chapter 45, Peritoneum and Related Diseases; Chapter 46, Mesenteric Ischemia and Other Vascular Lesions; Chapter 47, Alimentary Tract Obstruction and Intestinal Injuries; Chapter 48, Abdominal Wall and Abdominal Cavity Hernias; Chapter 49, Abdominal Access; Chapter 191, Surgical Treatment of Obesity

Cristian Alejandro Milla Matute, MD
Research Fellow
Department of General Surgery and The Bariatric and Metabolic Institute
Cleveland Clinic Florida
Davie, Florida
Chapter 44, Abdominal Wall Anatomy

Savannah Moon, DO
General Surgery Resident
Cleveland Clinic Florida
Davie, Florida
Chapter 45, Peritoneum and Related Diseases

Mobola Oyefule, MD
Department of General Surgery
Cleveland Clinic Florida
Davie, Florida
Chapter 49, Abdominal Access

Mauricio Sarmiento-Cobos, MD
Research Fellow
Minimally Invasive Surgery Department
Cleveland Clinic Florida
Boca Raton, Florida
Chapter 47, Alimentary Tract Obstruction and Intestinal Injuries

Morris Sasson, MD
General Surgery Resident
Department of General Surgery and The
    Bariatric and Metabolic Institute
Cleveland Clinic Florida
Weston, Florida
*Chapter 46, Mesenteric Ischemia and Other
    Vascular Lesions*

Rishabh Shah, MD
General Surgery Resident
Cleveland Clinic Florida
Davie, Florida
Chapter 191, Surgical Treatment of Obesity

Samuel Szomstein, MD, FACS, FASMBS
Director, Advanced MIS and Bariatrics
    Fellowship Training Program
Director, Bariatric Endoscopy
Associate Director, The Bariatric and
    Metabolic Institute and Division of MIS
Department of General and Vascular
    Surgery
Cleveland Clinic Florida
Clinical Associate Professor of Surgery
Florida International University
Weston, Florida
Chapter 191, Surgical Treatment of Obesity

Garrett Wegerif, MD
General Surgery Resident
Cleveland Clinic Florida
Davie, Florida
Chapter 191, Surgical Treatment of Obesity

Luis F. Zorrilla-Nuñez, MD
Professor General Surgery/Bariatric and
    Metabolic Surgery
University Hospital, Autonomous University
    of Nuevo Leon, Mexico
Monterrey, Mexico
Chapter 49, Abdominal Access

PREFACE

Anyone who has studied medicine in the past 25 years knows the tremendous value of the illustrations of the late Dr. Frank H. Netter. Students and teachers alike recognize his illustrations as the criteria by which all others are judged and consider them timeless classics because they "teach rather than intimidate." Perhaps some thus far unimagined technical innovation will one day permit the development of teaching tools that surpass the clarity and educational value of Dr. Netter's illustrations, but even with the present electronic revolution, that day has yet to come, and new generations of students worldwide continue to discover for themselves his remarkable talent.

I have published two previous books in my career—one is among the first texts on the small intestine, and the other is among the first on nutrition in gastrointestinal disease. Although I pledged I would never again undertake such arduous work, the need for a concise yet comprehensive volume covering the basic concepts and the latest developments in the field, along with the opportunity to use the famous Netter collection to illustrate it, overcame my resistance. The result is *Netter's Gastroenterology*. It was a success, and now we have finished the third edition.

My charge from the publisher was to write a text aimed at the generalist, understandable by the student, and of interest to the gastroenterologist. The approach of this book is different from that of traditional textbooks, which rely primarily on the written word. I sought to cover the field of gastroenterology and nutrition and to provide an efficient and meaningful learning experience to my audience by balancing the visual and the verbal, staying true to the philosophy of Dr. Netter by using the power of illustration to teach while providing essential information in the text. I selected approximately 300 of Dr. Netter's best illustrations and, with my coauthors, wrote text to illuminate and expand on the concepts the illustrations present. In a traditional textbook, the text is written first, and illustrations are then created to accompany it. In this case, my coauthors and I wrote with the illustrations before us, and our goal was to forge text and pictures into a seamless whole. In this third edition, we have tried to update the narrative and modify the illustrations where necessary. Because medicine is a constantly advancing science, we called on the talents of medical artists Carlos A. G. Machado, Kip Carter, David Mascaro, Steven Moon, Mike de la Flor, and Kristen Wienandt Marzejon to create new illustrations in the Netter style and to update others where appropriate.

The book is organized into 10 sections that correspond to the organs of the gastrointestinal system and to special topics within that system. These sections have been further divided into concise, condition-oriented chapters, including introductory chapters on anatomy and physiology. The text provides core information about the "clinical picture," diagnosis, treatment and management, course and prognosis, and, when applicable, prevention and control of each condition.

I invited colleagues to undertake areas according to their interests and expertise. Dr. C. S. Pitchumoni, an outstanding scholar in the field of pancreatic diseases working at St. Peter's University Hospital in New Jersey, agreed to write and update the text for the sections on the pancreas and the gallbladder. Dr. Neil Floch, who spent endless hours as a surgeon mastering the techniques of minimally invasive surgery and the Nissan fundoplication procedure and who continues as Head of Minimally Invasive Surgery at Norwalk Hospital in Connecticut, agreed to write and update the section on the esophagus. Dr. Raul Rosenthal, who is so active as a mentor and surgical practitioner at the Cleveland Clinic, in collaboration with his fellows in training, accepted the task of writing the sections on the abdomen. Dr. James Scolapio of the Mayo Clinic in Jacksonville wrote the section on nutrition for this edition. Dr. Joseph Lim, who is Professor of Medicine in the digestive disease section at Yale University and is renowned for his publications and work in hepatitis, joined the team to update the liver section. We are grateful to Dr. Kris V. Kowdley who worked on the liver section in previous editions.

We are grateful to Marybeth Thiel at Elsevier, who advised on chapter changes and helped simplify the tasks, as well as to Candace Peabody, who helped on administrative changes.

We hope this third edition will be educationally stimulating.

Martin H. Floch, MD, MACG, AGAF

Frank H. Netter, MD

Frank H. Netter was born in 1906 in New York City. He studied art at the Art Student's League and the National Academy of Design before entering medical school at New York University, where he received his MD degree in 1931. During his student years, Dr. Netter's notebook sketches attracted the attention of the medical faculty and other physicians, allowing him to augment his income by illustrating articles and textbooks. He continued illustrating as a side-line after establishing a surgical practice in 1933, but he ultimately opted to give up his practice in favor of a full-time commitment to art. After service in the United States Army during World War II, Dr. Netter began his long collaboration with the CIBA Pharmaceutical Company (now Novartis Pharmaceuticals). This 45-year partnership resulted in the production of the extraordinary collection of medical art so familiar to physicians and other medical professionals worldwide.

In 2005, Elsevier, Inc. purchased the Netter Collection and all publications from Icon Learning Systems. There are now over 50 publications featuring the art of Dr. Netter available through Elsevier, Inc. (in the US: www.us.elsevierhealth.com/Netter, and outside the US: www.elsevierhealth.com)

Dr. Netter's works are among the finest examples of the use of illustration in the teaching of medical concepts. The 13-book *Netter Collection of Medical Illustrations,* which includes the greater part of the more than 20,000 paintings created by Dr. Netter, became and remains one of the most famous medical works ever published. *The Netter Atlas of Human Anatomy,* first published in 1989, presents the anatomical paintings from the Netter Collection. Now translated into 16 languages, it is the anatomy atlas of choice among medical and health profession students the world over.

The Netter illustrations are appreciated not only for their aesthetic qualities, but, more important, for their intellectual content. As Dr. Netter wrote in 1949, "…clarification of a subject is the aim and goal of illustration. No matter how beautifully painted, how delicately and subtly rendered a subject may be, it is of little value as a *medical illustration* if it does not serve to make clear some medical point." Dr. Netter's planning, conception, point of view, and approach are what inform his paintings and what makes them so intellectually valuable.

Frank H. Netter, MD, physician and artist, died in 1991.

Learn more about the physician-artist whose work has inspired the Netter Reference collection: https://netterimages.com/artist-frank-h-netter.html.

Carlos A. G. Machado, MD

Carlos Machado was chosen by Novartis to be Dr. Netter's successor. He continues to be the main artist who contributes to the Netter collection of medical illustrations.

Self-taught in medical illustration, cardiologist Carlos Machado has contributed meticulous updates to some of Dr. Netter's original plates and has created many paintings of his own in the style of Netter as an extension of the Netter collection. Dr. Machado's photorealistic expertise and his keen insight into the physician-patient relationship informs his vivid and unforgettable visual style. His dedication to researching each topic and subject he paints places him among the premier medical illustrators at work today.

Learn more about his background and see more of his art at: https://netterimages.com/artist-carlos-a-g-machado.html.

ONLINE CONTENTS

Visit www.ExpertConsult.com for the following:
PRINTABLE PATIENT EDUCATION BROCHURES FROM FERRI'S
NETTER PATIENT ADVISOR, 3rd EDITION

CONTENTS

SECTION I

Esophagus

Neil R. Floch

Anatomy of the Esophagus and the Foregut

Neil R. Floch

TOPOGRAPHIC RELATIONS OF THE ESOPHAGUS

The pharynx ends at the level of the cricoid cartilage and the sixth cervical vertebra (C6) and where the esophagus begins (Figs. 1.1 and 1.2). On average, the esophagus is 40 cm (16 inch) long from the upper incisor teeth to the edge of the cardia of the stomach. The esophagus is divided, with the first part extending 16 cm from the incisors to the lower border of the cricopharyngeus muscle. The remainder is 24 cm long.

The aortic arch crosses behind the esophagus from the left side and is located 23 cm from the incisors and 7 cm below the cricopharyngeus muscle, and 2 cm below this level, the left main bronchus crosses in front of the esophagus. The lower esophageal sphincter (LES) begins 37 to 38 cm from the incisors. The esophageal hiatus is located 1 cm below this point, and the cardia of the stomach is yet lower. In children the dimensions are proportionately smaller. At birth the distance from the incisor teeth to the cardia is approximately 18 cm; at 3 years, 22 cm; and at 10 years, 27 cm.

Like a "good soldier," the esophagus follows a left-right-left path as it marches down the anteroposterior curvature of the vertebral column. It descends anterior to the vertebral column, through the lower portion of the neck and the superior and posterior mediastinum. The esophagus forms two lateral curves that, when viewed anteriorly, appear as a reverse S: the upper esophagus has a convex curve toward the left, and the lower esophagus has a convex curve toward the right. At its origin, the esophagus bends ¼ inch (0.6 cm) to the left of the tracheal margin. It crosses the midline behind the aortic arch at the level of the fourth thoracic vertebra (T4). The esophagus then turns to the right at the seventh thoracic vertebra (T7), after which it turns sharply to the left as it enters the abdomen through the esophageal hiatus of the diaphragm, to join the cardia of the stomach at the gastroesophageal (GE) junction.

The esophagus is composed of three segments: cervical, thoracic, and abdominal. Anterior to the cervical esophagus is the membranous wall of the trachea. Loose areolar tissue and muscular strands connect the esophagus and the trachea, and recurrent laryngeal nerves ascend in the grooves between them. Posterior to the esophagus are the longus colli muscles, the prevertebral fascia, and the vertebral bodies. Although the *cervical esophagus* is positioned between the carotid sheaths, it is closer to the left carotid sheath. The thyroid gland partially overlaps the esophagus on both sides.

The *thoracic esophagus* lies posterior to the trachea. It extends down to the level of the fifth thoracic vertebra (T5), where the trachea bifurcates. The trachea curves to the right as it divides, and thus the left main bronchus crosses in front of the esophagus. Below this, the pericardium separates the esophagus from the left atrium of the heart, which lies anterior and inferior to the esophagus. The lowest portion of the thoracic esophagus passes through the diaphragm into the abdomen.

On the left side of the esophageal wall, in the upper thoracic region, is the ascending portion of the left subclavian artery and the parietal pleura. At approximately the level of T4, the arch of the aorta passes backward and alongside the esophagus. Below this, the descending aorta lies to the left, but when that vessel passes behind the esophagus, the left mediastinal pleura again comes to adjoin the esophageal wall. On the right side, the parietal pleura is intimately applied to the esophagus, except when, at the level of T4, the azygos vein intervenes as it turns forward.

In the upper thorax, the esophagus lies on the longus colli muscle, the prevertebral fascia, and the vertebral bodies. At the eighth thoracic vertebra (T8), the aorta lies behind the esophagus. The azygos vein ascends behind and to the right of the esophagus as far as the level of T4, where it turns forward. The hemiazygos vein and the five upper-right intercostal arteries cross from left to right behind the esophagus. The thoracic duct ascends to the right of the esophagus before turning behind it and to the left at the level of T5. The duct then continues to ascend on the left side of the esophagus.

A small segment of *abdominal esophagus* lies on the crus of the diaphragm and creates an impression in the underside of the liver. Below the tracheal bifurcation, the esophageal nerve plexus and the anterior and posterior vagal trunks adhere to the esophagus.

As the esophagus travels from the neck to the abdomen, it encounters several indentations and constrictions. The first narrowing occurs at the cricopharyngeus muscle and the cricoid cartilage. The aortic arch creates an indentation on the left side of the esophagus, and the pulsations of the aorta may be seen during esophagoscopy. Below this point, the left main bronchus creates an impression on the left anterior aspect of the esophagus. The second narrowing occurs at the LES.

Although the esophagus is described as a "tube," it is oval and has a flat axis anterior to posterior with a wider transverse axis. When the esophagus is at rest, its walls are approximated and its width is 2 cm, but it distends and contracts, depending on its state of tonus.

MUSCULATURE OF THE ESOPHAGUS

The esophagus is composed of outer longitudinal and inner circular muscle layers (Figs. 1.3 and 1.4). On the vertical ridge of the dorsal aspect of the cricoid cartilage, two tendons originate as they diverge and descend downward around the sides of the esophagus to the dorsal aspect. These tendons weave in the midline of the ventral area, creating a V-shaped gap between the two muscles, known as the V-shaped area of Laimer. This gap, or bare area, exposes the underlying circular muscle. Located above this area is the cricopharyngeus muscle. Sparse longitudinal muscles cover the area, as do accessory fibers from the lower aspect of the cricopharyngeus muscle.

In the upper esophagus, longitudinal muscles form bundles of fibers that do not evenly distribute over the surface. The thinnest layers of muscle are anterior and adjacent to the posterior wall of the trachea. The longitudinal muscle of the esophagus receives fibers from an accessory muscle on each side that originates from the posterolateral aspect of the cricoid cartilage and the contralateral side of the deep portion

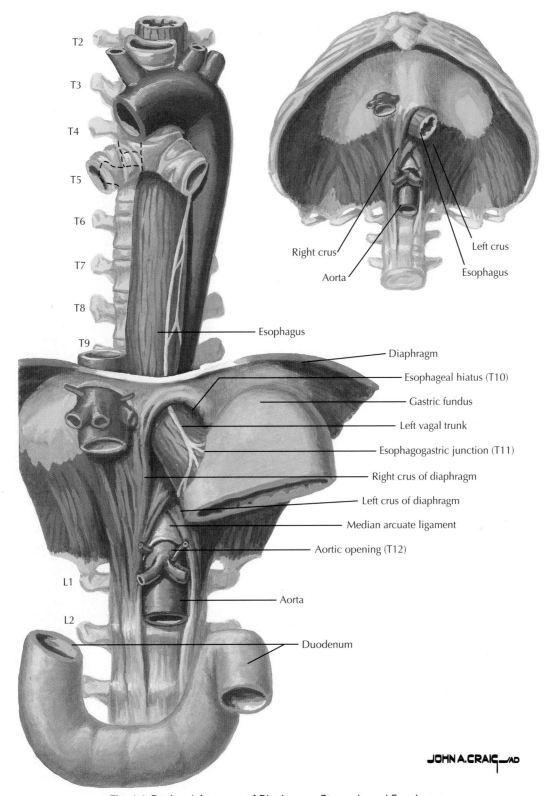

T2

T3

T4

T5

T6

T7

T8

T9

L1

L2

Right crus

Aorta

Left crus

Esophagus

Esophagus

Diaphragm

Esophageal hiatus (T10)

Gastric fundus

Left vagal trunk

Esophagogastric junction (T11)

Right crus of diaphragm

Left crus of diaphragm

Median arcuate ligament

Aortic opening (T12)

Aorta

Duodenum

JOHN A. CRAIG_AD

Fig. 1.1 Regional Anatomy of Diaphragm, Stomach, and Esophagus.

of the cricopharyngeus muscle. As the longitudinal muscle descends, its fibers become equally distributed and completely cover the surface of the esophagus.

The inner, circular, muscle layer is thinner than the outer longitudinal layer. This relationship is reversed in all other parts of the gastrointestinal (GI) tract. In the upper esophagus, the circular muscle closely approximates the encircling lower fibers of the cricopharyngeus muscle. The upper esophageal fibers are not circular but elliptical, with the anterior part of the ellipse at a lower level of the posterior part. The ellipses become more circular as the esophagus descends, until the start of its middle third, where the fibers run in a horizontal plane. In one 1-cm segment, the fibers are truly circular. Below this point, the fibers

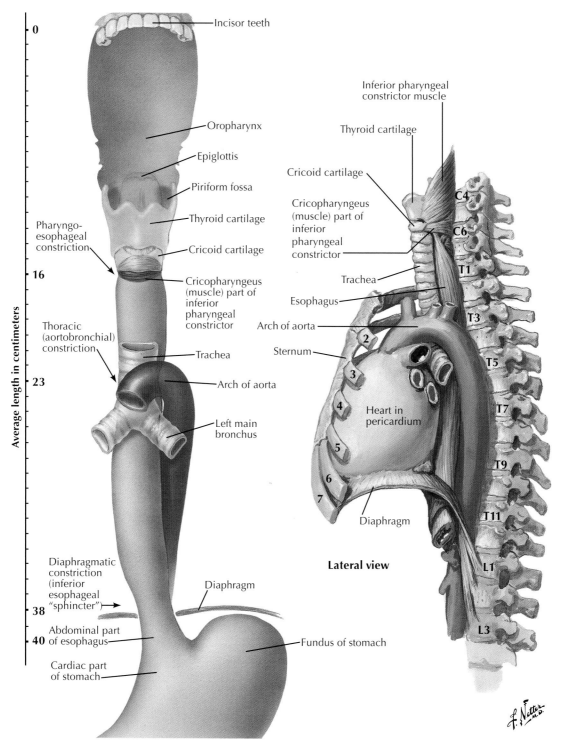

Fig. 1.2 Topography and Constrictions of Esophagus.

become elliptical once again, but they now have a reverse inclination—that is, the posterior part of the ellipse is located at a lower level than the anterior part. In the lower third of the esophagus, the fibers follow a spiral course down the esophagus. The elliptical, circular, and spiral fibers of this layer are not truly uniform and parallel but may overlap and cross, or they may even have clefts between them. Some fibers in the lower two thirds of the esophagus pass diagonally or perpendicularly, up or down, joining fibers at other levels. These branched fibers are 2 to 3 mm wide and 1 to 5 cm long and are not continuous.

The cricopharyngeus muscle marks the transition from pharynx to esophagus. It is the lowest portion of the inferior constrictor of the pharynx and consists of a narrow band of muscle fibers that originate on each side of the posterolateral margin of the cricoid cartilage. The cricopharyngeus then passes slinglike around the dorsal aspect of the pharyngoesophageal (PE) junction. Upper fibers ascend and join the median raphe of the inferior constrictor muscle posteriorly. Lower fibers do not have a median raphe; they pass to the dorsal aspect of the PE junction. A few of these fibers pass down to the esophagus. The

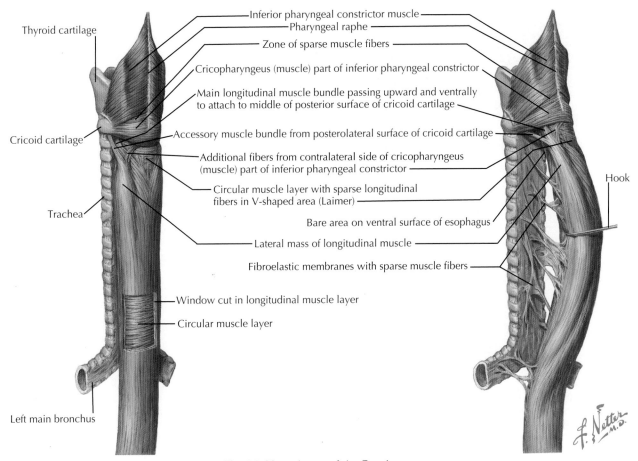

Fig. 1.3 Musculature of the Esophagus.

cricopharyngeus functions as a sphincter of the upper esophagus. Muscle tone of the esophageal lumen is greatest at the level of the cricopharyngeus, and relaxation of this muscle is an integral part of the act of swallowing. There is a weak area between the cricopharyngeus and the main part of the inferior constrictor where Zenker diverticula are thought to develop.

The upper 25% to 33% of the esophagus is composed of striated muscle, whereas the lower or remaining portion is smooth muscle. Within the second fourth of the esophagus is a transitional zone where striated muscle and smooth muscle are present. The lower half contains purely smooth muscle. Between the two muscular coats of the esophagus, a narrow layer of connective tissue is inserted that accommodates the myenteric plexus of Auerbach.

ARTERIAL BLOOD SUPPLY OF THE ESOPHAGUS

The blood supply of the esophagus is variable (Fig. 1.5). The inferior thyroid artery is the primary supplier of the cervical esophagus; esophageal vessels emanate from both side branches of the artery and from the ends of the vessels. Anterior cervical esophageal arteries supply small branches to the esophagus and trachea. Accessory arteries to the cervical esophagus originate in the subclavian, common carotid, vertebral, ascending pharyngeal, superficial cervical, and costocervical trunk.

Arterial branches from the bronchial arteries, the aorta, and the right intercostal vessels supply the thoracic esophagus. Bronchial arteries, especially the left inferior artery, distribute branches at or below the tracheal bifurcation. Bronchial artery branches are variable. The standard—two left and one right—occurs in only about 50% of patients.

Aberrant vessel patterns include one left and one right in 25% of patients, two right and two left in 15%, and one left and two right in 8%. Rarely do three right or three left arteries occur.

At the tracheal bifurcation, the esophagus receives branches from the aorta, aortic arch, uppermost intercostal arteries, internal mammary artery, and carotid artery. Aortic branches to the thoracic esophagus usually consist of two unpaired vessels. The cranial vessel is 3 to 4 cm long and usually arises at the level of the sixth to seventh thoracic vertebrae (T6-T7). The caudal vessel is longer, 6 to 7 cm, and arises at the level of T7 to T8. Both arteries pass behind the esophagus and divide into ascending and descending branches. These branches anastomose along the esophageal border with descending branches from the inferior thyroid and bronchial arteries, as well as with ascending branches from the left gastric and left inferior phrenic arteries. Right intercostal arteries, mainly the fifth, give rise to esophageal branches in approximately 20% of the population.

The abdominal esophagus receives its blood supply from branches of the left gastric artery, the short gastric artery, and a recurrent branch of the left inferior phrenic artery. The left gastric artery supplies cardioesophageal branches either through a single vessel that subdivides or through two to five branches before they divide into anterior and posterior gastric branches. Other arterial sources to the abdominal esophagus are (1) branches from an aberrant left hepatic artery, derived from the left gastric, an accessory left gastric from the left hepatic, or a persistent primitive gastrohepatic arterial arc; (2) cardioesophageal branches from the splenic trunk, its superior polar, terminal divisions (short gastrics), and its occasional large posterior gastric artery; and (3) a direct, slender, cardioesophageal branch from the aorta, celiac, or first part of the splenic artery.

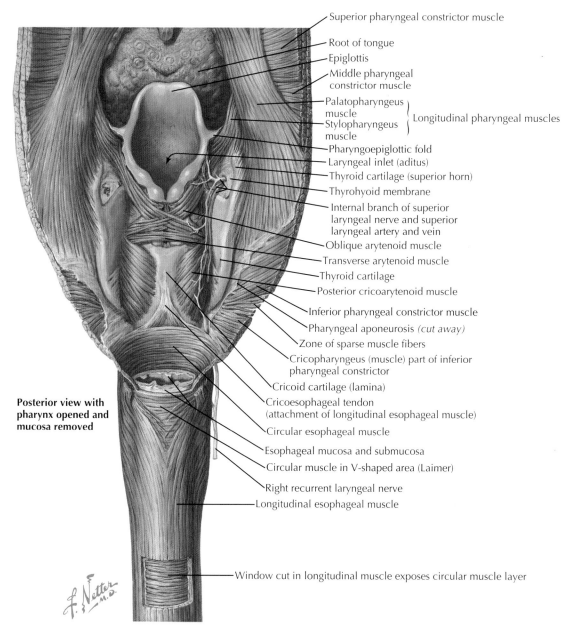

Superior pharyngeal constrictor muscle
Root of tongue
Epiglottis
Middle pharyngeal constrictor muscle
Palatopharyngeus muscle
Stylopharyngeus muscle — Longitudinal pharyngeal muscles
Pharyngoepiglottic fold
Laryngeal inlet (aditus)
Thyroid cartilage (superior horn)
Thyrohyoid membrane
Internal branch of superior laryngeal nerve and superior laryngeal artery and vein
Oblique arytenoid muscle
Transverse arytenoid muscle
Thyroid cartilage
Posterior cricoarytenoid muscle
Inferior pharyngeal constrictor muscle
Pharyngeal aponeurosis *(cut away)*
Zone of sparse muscle fibers
Cricopharyngeus (muscle) part of inferior pharyngeal constrictor
Cricoid cartilage (lamina)
Cricoesophageal tendon (attachment of longitudinal esophageal muscle)
Circular esophageal muscle
Esophageal mucosa and submucosa
Circular muscle in V-shaped area (Laimer)
Right recurrent laryngeal nerve
Longitudinal esophageal muscle

Posterior view with pharynx opened and mucosa removed

Window cut in longitudinal muscle exposes circular muscle layer

Fig. 1.4 Pharyngoesophageal Junction.

With every resection surgery, areas of devascularization may be induced by (1) excessively low resection of the cervical segment, which always has a supply from the inferior thyroid; (2) excessive mobilization of the esophagus at the tracheal bifurcation and laceration of the bronchial artery; and (3) excessive sacrifice of the left gastric artery and the recurrent branch of the inferior phrenic artery to facilitate gastric mobilization. Anastomosis around the abdominal portion of the esophagus is usually copious, but sometimes it is limited.

VENOUS DRAINAGE OF THE ESOPHAGUS

Venous drainage of the esophagus begins in small tributaries that eventually empty into the azygos and hemiazygos veins (Fig. 1.6). Drainage begins in a submucosal venous plexus that exits externally to the surface of the esophagus. Tributaries from the cervical periesophageal venous plexus drain into the inferior thyroid vein, which empties into the right or left brachiocephalic (innominate) vein, or both. Tributaries from

the thoracic periesophageal plexus on the right side join the azygos, the right brachiocephalic, and occasionally the vertebral vein; on the left side, they join the hemiazygos, the accessory hemiazygos, the left brachiocephalic, and occasionally the vertebral vein. Tributaries from the short abdominal esophagus drain into the left gastric (coronary) vein of the stomach. Other tributaries are in continuity with the short gastric, splenic, and left gastroepiploic veins. They may also drain to branches of the left inferior phrenic vein and join the inferior vena cava (IVC) directly or the suprarenal vein before it enters the renal vein.

The composition of the azygos system of veins varies. The *azygos vein* arises in the abdomen from the ascending right lumbar vein, which receives the first and second lumbar and the subcostal veins. The azygos may arise directly from the IVC or may have connections with the right common iliac or renal vein. In the thorax, the azygos vein receives the right posterior intercostal veins from the fourth to eleventh spaces and terminates in the superior vena cava (SVC). The highest intercostal vein drains into the right brachiocephalic vein or into the

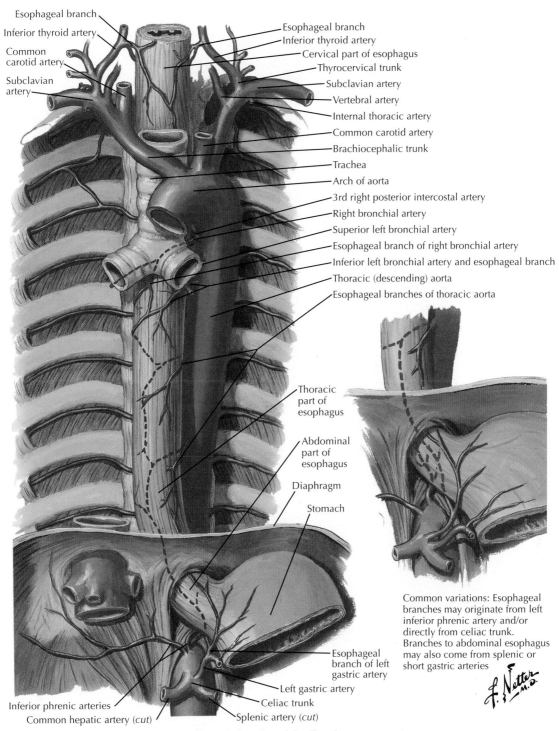

Esophageal branch
Inferior thyroid artery
Common carotid artery
Subclavian artery

Esophageal branch
Inferior thyroid artery
Cervical part of esophagus
Thyrocervical trunk
Subclavian artery
Vertebral artery
Internal thoracic artery
Common carotid artery
Brachiocephalic trunk
Trachea
Arch of aorta
3rd right posterior intercostal artery
Right bronchial artery
Superior left bronchial artery
Esophageal branch of right bronchial artery
Inferior left bronchial artery and esophageal branch
Thoracic (descending) aorta
Esophageal branches of thoracic aorta

Thoracic part of esophagus

Abdominal part of esophagus

Diaphragm

Stomach

Esophageal branch of left gastric artery

Left gastric artery
Celiac trunk
Splenic artery (cut)

Inferior phrenic arteries
Common hepatic artery (cut)

Common variations: Esophageal branches may originate from left inferior phrenic artery and/or directly from celiac trunk. Branches to abdominal esophagus may also come from splenic or short gastric arteries.

f. Netter M.D.

Fig. 1.5 Arteries of the Esophagus.

vertebral vein. Veins from the second and third spaces unite in a common trunk, the right superior intercostal, which ends in the terminal arch of the azygos.

The *hemiazygos vein* arises as a continuation of the left ascending lumbar or from the left renal vein. The hemiazygos receives the left subcostal vein and the intercostal veins from the eighth to the eleventh spaces, and then it crosses the vertebral column posterior to the esophagus to join the azygos vein.

The accessory hemiazygos vein receives intercostal branches from the fourth to the eighth intercostal veins, and it crosses over the spine

and under the esophagus to join the hemiazygos or the azygos vein. Superiorly, the accessory hemiazygos communicates with the left superior intercostal that drains the second and third spaces, and ends in the left brachiocephalic vein. The first space drains into the left brachiocephalic or vertebral vein. Often the hemiazygos, the accessory hemiazygos, and the superior intercostal trunk form a continuous longitudinal channel with no connections to the azygos. There may be three to five connections between the left azygos, in which case a hemiazygos or an accessory hemiazygos is not formed. If the left azygos system is very small, the left venous drainage of the esophagus occurs through its

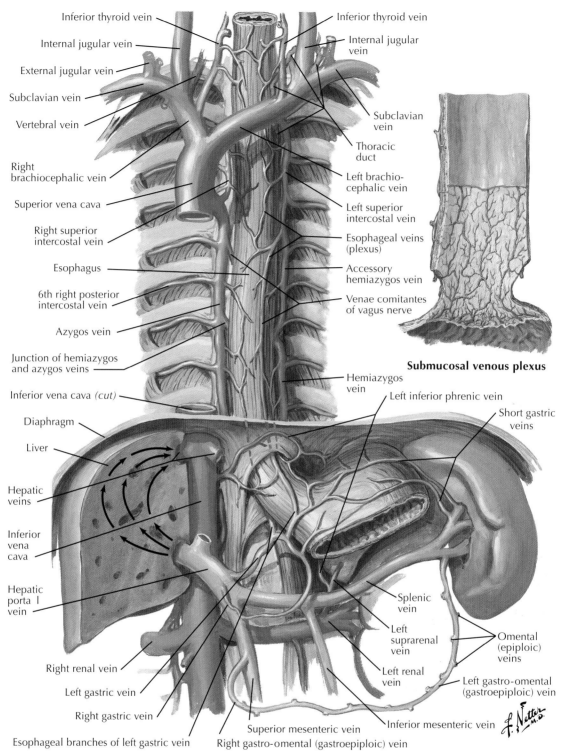

Inferior thyroid vein

Internal jugular vein

External jugular vein

Subclavian vein

Vertebral vein

Right brachiocephalic vein

Superior vena cava

Right superior intercostal vein

Esophagus

6th right posterior intercostal vein

Azygos vein

Junction of hemiazygos and azygos veins

Inferior vena cava *(cut)*

Diaphragm

Liver

Hepatic veins

Inferior vena cava

Hepatic porta l vein

Right renal vein

Left gastric vein

Right gastric vein

Esophageal branches of left gastric vein

Inferior thyroid vein

Internal jugular vein

Subclavian vein

Thoracic duct

Left brachio-cephalic vein

Left superior intercostal vein

Esophageal veins (plexus)

Accessory hemiazygos vein

Venae comitantes of vagus nerve

Hemiazygos vein

Left inferior phrenic vein

Short gastric veins

Splenic vein

Left suprarenal vein

Left renal vein

Omental (epiploic) veins

Left gastro-omental (gastroepiploic) vein

Inferior mesenteric vein

Superior mesenteric vein

Right gastro-omental (gastroepiploic) vein

Submucosal venous plexus

Fig. 1.6 Veins of the Esophagus.

respective intercostal veins. Connections between left and right azygos veins occur between the seventh and ninth intercostal spaces, usually at the eighth.

At the GE junction, branches of the left gastric coronary vein are connected to lower esophageal branches so that blood may be shunted into the SVC from the azygos and hemiazygos veins. At the GE junction, blood may also be shunted into the splenic, retroperitoneal, and inferior phrenic veins to the caval system. Retrograde flow of venous blood through the esophageal veins leads to dilatation and formation of varicosities. Because the short gastric veins lead from the spleen to the GE junction of the stomach, thrombosis of the splenic vein may result in esophageal varices and fatal hemorrhage.

INNERVATION OF THE ESOPHAGUS: PARASYMPATHETIC AND SYMPATHETIC

The esophagus is supplied by a combination of parasympathetic and sympathetic nerves (Fig. 1.7). Constant communication occurs between

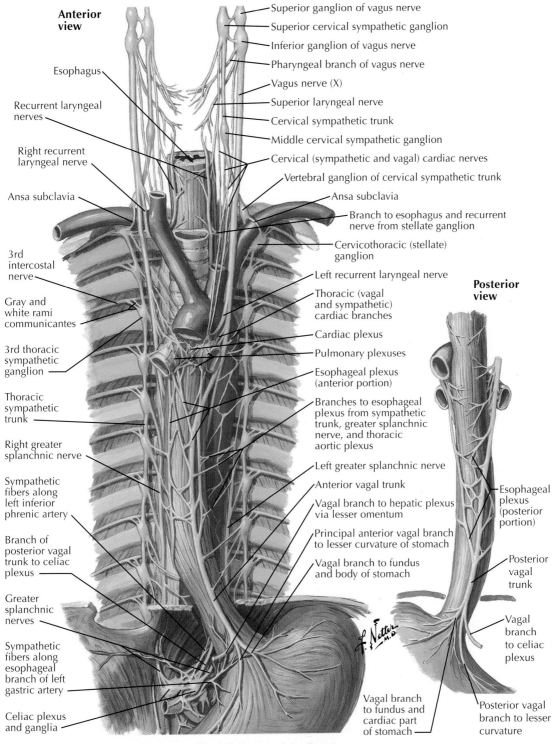

Anterior view

Esophagus

Recurrent laryngeal nerves

Right recurrent laryngeal nerve

Ansa subclavia

3rd intercostal nerve

Gray and white rami communicantes

3rd thoracic sympathetic ganglion

Thoracic sympathetic trunk

Right greater splanchnic nerve

Sympathetic fibers along left inferior phrenic artery

Branch of posterior vagal trunk to celiac plexus

Greater splanchnic nerves

Sympathetic fibers along esophageal branch of left gastric artery

Celiac plexus and ganglia

Superior ganglion of vagus nerve
Superior cervical sympathetic ganglion
Inferior ganglion of vagus nerve
Pharyngeal branch of vagus nerve
Vagus nerve (X)
Superior laryngeal nerve
Cervical sympathetic trunk
Middle cervical sympathetic ganglion
Cervical (sympathetic and vagal) cardiac nerves
Vertebral ganglion of cervical sympathetic trunk
Ansa subclavia
Branch to esophagus and recurrent nerve from stellate ganglion
Cervicothoracic (stellate) ganglion
Left recurrent laryngeal nerve

Posterior view

Thoracic (vagal and sympathetic) cardiac branches
Cardiac plexus
Pulmonary plexuses
Esophageal plexus (anterior portion)
Branches to esophageal plexus from sympathetic trunk, greater splanchnic nerve, and thoracic aortic plexus

Left greater splanchnic nerve
Anterior vagal trunk
Vagal branch to hepatic plexus via lesser omentum
Principal anterior vagal branch to lesser curvature of stomach
Vagal branch to fundus and body of stomach

Esophageal plexus (posterior portion)

Posterior vagal trunk

Vagal branch to celiac plexus

Vagal branch to fundus and cardiac part of stomach

Posterior vagal branch to lesser curvature

Fig. 1.7 Nerves of the Esophagus.

efferent and afferent fibers that transmit impulses to and from the vessels, glands, and mucosa of the esophagus.

Anterior and posterior vagus nerves carry parasympathetic efferent fibers to the esophagus, and afferent fibers carry them from the esophagus. These parasympathetic fibers terminate in the dorsal vagal nucleus, which contains visceral efferent and afferent cells. The striated muscle of the pharynx and upper esophagus is controlled by parasympathetic fibers that emanate from the nucleus ambiguus. Vagus nerves intermingle with nerve fibers from the paravertebral sympathetic trunks and their

branches such that the nerves in and below the neck are a combination of parasympathetic and sympathetic.

In the neck, the esophagus receives fibers from the recurrent laryngeal nerves and variable fibers from the vagus nerves, lying posterior to and between the common carotid artery and the internal jugular vein in the carotid sheath. On the right side, the recurrent laryngeal nerve branches from the vagus nerve and descends, wrapping itself around the right subclavian artery before it ascends in the esophageal-tracheal groove. On the left side, the recurrent laryngeal nerve branches from the left vagus nerve, descends and wraps around the aortic arch, and ascends between the trachea and the esophagus.

In the superior mediastinum, the esophagus receives fibers from the left recurrent laryngeal nerve and both vagus nerves. As the vagus nerves descend, small branches intermingle with fibers from sympathetic trunks to form the smaller anterior and the larger posterior pulmonary plexuses. Below the main-stem bronchi, the vagus nerves divide into two to four branches that become closely adherent to the esophagus in the posterior mediastinum. Branches from the right and left nerves have anterior and posterior components that divide and then intermingle to form a mesh nerve plexus, which also contains small ganglia.

At a variable distance above the esophageal hiatus, the plexus reconstitutes into one or two vagal trunks. As the vagus enters the abdomen, it passes an anterior nerve, which is variably embedded in the esophageal wall, and a posterior nerve, which does not adhere to the esophagus but lies within a layer of adipose tissue. Small branches from the plexus and the main vagus enter the wall of the esophagus. Variations in the vagal nerves and plexuses are important for surgeons performing vagotomy because there may be more than one anterior or posterior vagus nerve.

Sympathetic preganglionic fibers emanate from axons of intermediolateral cornual cells, located in the fourth to sixth thoracic spinal cord segments (T4-T6). Anterior spinal nerve roots correspond to the segments containing their parent cells. They leave the spinal nerves in white or mixed rami communicans and enter the paravertebral sympathetic ganglia. Some fibers synapse with cells in the midthoracic ganglia and travel to higher and lower ganglia in the trunks. Axons of the ganglionic cells have postganglionic fibers that reach the esophagus. Afferent fibers travel the same route in reverse; however, they do not relay on the sympathetic trunks, and they enter the spinal cord through the posterior spinal nerve roots. Afferent nerve perikaryons are located in the posterior spinal nerve root ganglia.

The pharyngeal plexus innervates the upper esophagus. As the esophagus descends, it receives fibers from the cardiac branches of the superior cervical ganglia, but rarely receives them from the middle cervical or vertebral ganglia of the sympathetic trunks. Fibers may also reach the esophagus from the nerve plexus that travels with the arterial supply.

In the upper thorax, the stellate ganglia supply esophageal filaments called ansae subclavia, and the thoracic cardiac nerves may be associated with fibers from the esophagus, trachea, aorta, and pulmonary structures.

In the lower thorax, fibers connect from the greater thoracic splanchnic nerves to the esophageal plexus. The greater splanchnic nerves arise from three to four large pathways, and a variable number of smaller rootlets arise from the fifth to tenth thoracic ganglia and the sympathetic trunks. The roots pass in multiple directions across the sides of the thoracic vertebral bodies and discs to form a large nerve. On both sides, the nerve enters the abdomen through the diaphragm by passing between the lateral margins of the crura and the medial arcuate ligament.

In the abdomen, the nerves branch into the celiac plexus. The lesser and least thoracic splanchnic nerves end primarily in the aortorenal ganglia and the renal plexuses, respectively. Filaments from the terminal part of the greater splanchnic nerve and from the right inferior phrenic plexus reach the abdominal portion of the esophagus.

INTRINSIC INNERVATION OF THE ALIMENTARY TRACT

Enteric plexuses that extend from the esophagus to the rectum control the GI tract (Fig. 1.8). Numerous groups of ganglion cells interconnect in a network of fibers between the muscle layers. Synaptic relays are located in the myenteric plexus of Auerbach and the submucosal plexus of Meissner. The Meissner plexuses are coarse and consist of a mesh of thick, medium, and thin bundles of fiber, which represent the primary, secondary, and tertiary parts. The thin plexus is delicate.

Subsidiary plexuses appear in other areas covered by peritoneum. Enteric plexuses vary in pattern in different parts of the alimentary tract. They are less developed in the esophagus and are more developed from the stomach to the rectum. Ganglion cells also are not uniformly distributed; they are at their lowest levels in the Auerbach plexus and the esophagus, increase in the stomach, and reach their highest levels in the pylorus. Distribution is intermediate throughout the small intestine and increases along the colon and in the rectum. Cell population density in the Meissner plexus parallels that in the Auerbach plexus.

The vagus nerve contains preganglionic parasympathetic fibers that arise in its dorsal nucleus and travel to the esophagus, stomach, and intestinal branches. The proportion of efferent parasympathetic fibers is smaller than that of its sensory fibers. Vagal preganglionic efferent fibers have relays in small ganglia in the visceral walls; the axons are postganglionic parasympathetic fibers. Gastric branches have secretomotor and motor functions to the smooth muscle of the stomach, except for the pyloric sphincter, which is inhibited. Intestinal branches function similarly in the small intestine, cecum, appendix, and colon, where they are secretomotor to the glands and motor to the intestinal smooth muscle, and where they inhibit the ileocecal sphincter.

Enteric plexuses contain postganglionic sympathetic along with preganglionic and postganglionic parasympathetic fibers, afferent fibers, and intrinsic ganglion cells, and their processes. Sympathetic preganglionic fibers have already relayed in paravertebral or prevertebral ganglia; thus the sympathetic fibers in the plexuses are postganglionic and pass through them and their terminations without synaptic interruptions. Afferent fibers from the esophagus, stomach, and duodenum are carried to the brainstem and cord through the vagal and sympathetic nerves, but they form no synaptic connections with the ganglion cells in the enteric plexuses.

Except for interstitial cells of Cajal, two chief forms of nerve cells, types 1 and 2, occur in the enteric plexuses. Interstitial cells of Cajal are pacemaker cells in the smooth muscles of the gut and are associated with the ground plexuses of all autonomic nerves. Type 1 cells are multipolar and confined to Auerbach plexus, and their dendrites branch close to the parent cells. Their axons run for varying distances through the plexuses to establish synapses with type 2 cells, which are more numerous and are found in Auerbach and Meissner plexuses. Most type 2 cells are multipolar, and their longer dendrites proceed in bundles for variable distances before they ramify in other cell clusters. Many other axons pass outwardly to end in the muscle, and others proceed inwardly to supply the muscularis mucosae and to ramify around vessels and between epithelial secretory cells; their distribution suggests that they are motor or secretomotor in nature.

Under experimental conditions, peristaltic movements occur in isolated portions of the gut, indicating the importance of intrinsic neuromuscular mechanisms, but the extrinsic nerves are probably essential for the coordinated regulation of all activities. Local reflex arcs, or axon reflexes, may exist in the enteric plexuses. In addition to types 1 and 2 multipolar cells, much smaller numbers of pseudounipolar and bipolar cells can be detected in the submucosa and may be the afferent links in local reflex arcs.

In megacolon (Hirschsprung disease), and possibly in achalasia, the enteric plexuses apparently are undeveloped or have degenerated over a segment of alimentary tract, although the extrinsic nerves are intact. Peristaltic movements are defective or absent in the affected segment, indicating the importance of the intrinsic neuromuscular mechanism.

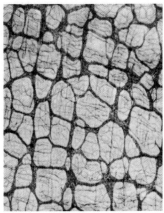

1. Myenteric plexus (Auerbach) lying on longitudinal muscle coat. Fine tertiary bundles crossing meshes (duodenum of guinea pig. Champy-Coujard, osmic stain, ×20)

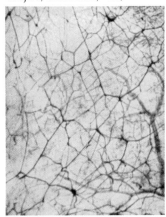

2. Submucous plexus (Meissner) (ascending colon of guinea pig. Stained by gold impregnation, x20)

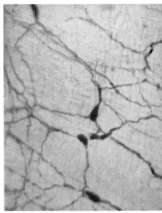

3. Interstitial cells of Cajal forming part of dense network between muscle layers (descending colon of guinea pig. Methylene blue, x375)

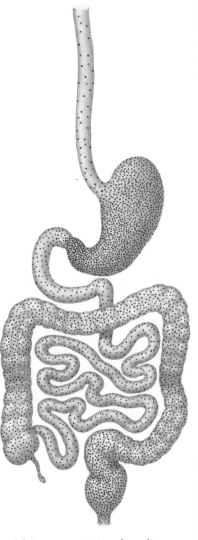

Relative concentration of ganglion cells in myenteric (Auerbach) plexus and in submucous (Meissner) plexus in various parts of alimentary tract (myenteric plexus cells represented by maroon, submucous by blue dots)

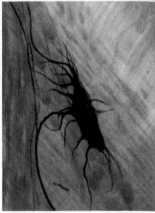

4. Multipolar neuron, type I (Dogiel), lying in ganglion of myenteric (Auerbach) plexus (ileum of monkey. Bielschowsky, silver stain, x375)

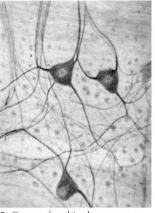

5. Group of multipolar neurons, type II, in ganglion of myenteric (Auerbach) plexus (ileum of cat. Bielschowsky, silver stain, x200)

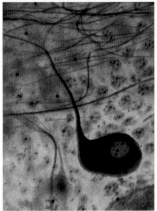

6. Pseudounipolar neuron within ganglion of myenteric plexus (ileum of cat. Bielschowsky, silver stain, x375)

Fig. 1.8 Enteric Plexuses.

HISTOLOGY OF THE ESOPHAGUS

Esophageal layers include the mucosa, submucosa, muscularis externa, and adventitia (Fig. 1.9). The esophageal mucosa ends abruptly at the GE junction, where columnar epithelia with gastric pits and glands are found. The esophageal epithelium is 300 to 500 mm thick, nonkeratinized, stratified, and squamous, and is continuous with the pharyngeal epithelium. Tall papillae rich in blood and nerve fibers assist in anchoring the tissue to its base. The epithelial layer is constantly renewed by mitosis as cuboidal basal cells migrate, flatten, and slough in 2 to 3 weeks.

The barrier wall of the esophagus functions well with the aid of mucus-producing glands that protect against mechanical invasion. However, this protection is limited. Repeated exposure of acid and protease-rich secretions from the stomach may occur during episodes of GE reflux and may cause fibrosis of the esophageal wall. Patients with nonerosive reflux disease (NERD) have evidence of increased cell permeability, which may contribute to their symptoms but does not exhibit visible damage. Exposure may also cause metaplastic epithelial cell changes consistent with Barrett esophagus. In the most serious cases, neoplastic changes may occur. A competent GE sphincter should prevent significant acid exposure.

With its lymphoid aggregates and mucous glands, especially near the GE junction, the lamina propria is supportive. Two types of glands reside in the esophagus. The cardiac glands are at the proximal and distal ends of the esophagus. Their ducts do not penetrate the muscularis mucosae, and their branched and coiled tubules are located in the lamina propria rather than in the submucosa. The other glands, the esophageal glands proper, produce mucus and are located throughout the esophagus.

The muscularis mucosae is composed primarily of sheets of longitudinal muscle that aid in esophageal peristalsis. It loosely adheres to both the mucosa and the muscularis as it invades the longitudinal ridges of the esophagus. Muscularis mucosae contain blood vessels, nerves, and mucous glands. The muscularis externa is approximately 300 mm thick and is composed of an outer longitudinal and an inner circular layer, as described previously.

ANATOMY OF THE GASTROESOPHAGEAL JUNCTION AND DIAPHRAGM

The sphincter mechanism of the GE junction prevents retrograde flow of gastric contents into the lower esophagus while allowing deposition of a food bolus from the esophagus to the stomach (Figs. 1.10 and 1.11). The LES mechanism is a combination of functional contractions of the diaphragm, thickening of the circular and longitudinal muscles of the esophagus, an intraabdominal-esophageal component, gastric sling muscles, and the angle created by the entry of the esophagus into the abdomen through the diaphragm. Proper functioning of the LES mechanism depends on all its muscular components and the complex interaction of autonomic nerve inputs. Failure of this sphincterlike mechanism results in the symptoms of gastroesophageal reflux disease (GERD), with reflux and regurgitation of gastric contents. Physical damage, including esophagitis, ulcers, strictures, Barrett esophagus, and esophageal carcinoma, may develop.

At the GE junction, the Z line, indicating the transition from squamous to columnar gastric mucosa, is easily recognized by the color change from pale to deep red and texture change from smooth to rugose. The Z line is located between the end of the esophagus and the level of the hiatus and diaphragm. In some patients, the gastric mucosa may extend several centimeters proximally, into the esophagus.

Toward the distal esophagus, the circular and longitudinal muscles gradually thicken and reach their greatest width 1 to 2 cm above the hiatus. These characteristics define the location of the LES, which is capable of tonic contraction and neurologically coordinated relaxation. Manometry reveals a high-pressure zone in the distal 3 to 5 cm of the esophagus, with a pressure gradient between 12 and 20 mm Hg.

Pressure magnitude and sphincter length are important for maintaining the competency of the valve. The intraabdominal portion of the esophagus is important for the antireflux mechanism. The intrathoracic esophagus is exposed to −6 mm Hg of pressure during inspiration through 6 mm Hg of pressure within the abdomen, for a pressure difference of 12 mm Hg. *Sliding hiatal hernia* is defined as the lower esophagus migrating into the chest, where the pressure is −6 mm Hg. In this situation, negative pressure resists the LES remaining tonically closed.

The longitudinal muscle of the esophagus continues into the stomach to form the outer longitudinal muscle of the stomach. The inner circular or spiral layer of the esophagus divides at the cardia to become the inner oblique layer and the middle circular layer. Inner oblique fibers create a sling across the cardiac incisura, and the middle circular fibers pass horizontally around the stomach. These two muscle layers cross at an angle and form a muscular ring known as the *collar of Helvetius* and thought to be a component of the complex LES.

Muscle fibers of the hiatus usually arise from the larger right crus of the diaphragm, not from the left crus. Fibers that originate from the right crus ascend and pass to the right of the esophagus as another band, originating deeper than the right crus, ascending and passing to the left of the esophagus. The bands cross scissorlike and insert ventrally to the esophagus, into the central tendon of the diaphragm. Fibers that pass to the right of the esophagus are innervated by the right phrenic nerve, whereas right crural fibers, which pass to the left of the esophageal hiatus, are innervated by a branch of the left phrenic nerve.

In some patients, an anatomic variation may be found by which fibers from the left crus of the diaphragm surround the right side of the esophageal hiatus. Rarely, the muscle to the right of the esophageal hiatus originates entirely from the left crus, and fibers surrounding the left of the hiatus originate from the right crus. The ligament of Treitz originates from the fibers of the right crus of the diaphragm.

The diaphragm independently contributes to sphincter function. As the crura contract, they compress the esophagus. This action is most exaggerated during deep inspiration, when the diaphragm is in strong contraction and the passage of food into the stomach is impeded. The LES mechanism is exaggerated by the angulation of the esophagus as it connects to the stomach at the angle of His. How much this angulation contributes is not clearly defined.

Phrenicoesophageal and diaphragmatic esophageal ligaments connect the multiple components of the sphincter as the esophagus passes through the hiatus. The phrenicoesophageal ligament arises from the inferior fascia of the diaphragm, which is continuous with the transversalis fascia. At the margin of the hiatus, the phrenicoesophageal ligament divides into an ascending leaf and a descending leaf. The ascending leaf passes through the hiatus, climbs 1 to 2 cm, and surrounds the mediastinal esophagus circumferentially. The descending leaf inserts around the cardia deep to the peritoneum. Within the intraabdominal cavity formed by the phrenicoesophageal ligament is a ring of dense fat. The phrenicoesophageal ligament fixates the esophagus while allowing for respiratory excursion, deglutition, and postural changes. Its role in the closure of the sphincteric mechanism is unclear.

Resting LES pressure is maintained by a complex interaction of hormonal, muscular, and neuronal mechanisms. The muscular sphincter component functions with coordinated relaxation and contraction of the LES and the diaphragm. Its action may be observed during deglutition as it relaxes and tonically closes to prevent the symptoms of reflux and regurgitation. As the muscle groups contract externally, the mucosa gathers internally into irregular longitudinal folds.

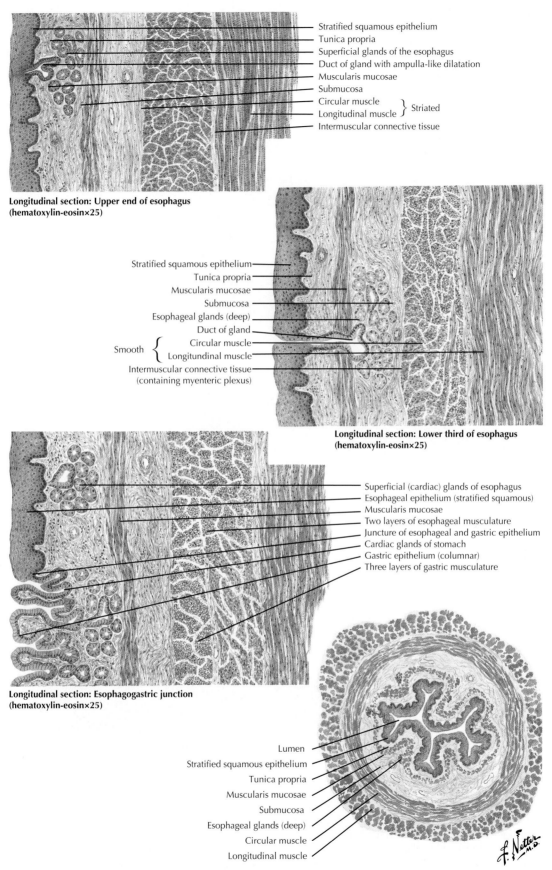

Stratified squamous epithelium
Tunica propria
Superficial glands of the esophagus
Duct of gland with ampulla-like dilatation
Muscularis mucosae
Submucosa
Circular muscle ⎫
Longitudinal muscle ⎬ Striated
Intermuscular connective tissue

Longitudinal section: Upper end of esophagus
(hematoxylin-eosin×25)

Stratified squamous epithelium
Tunica propria
Muscularis mucosae
Submucosa
Esophageal glands (deep)
Duct of gland
Smooth ⎰ Circular muscle
       ⎱ Longitundinal muscle
Intermuscular connective tissue
(containing myenteric plexus)

Longitudinal section: Lower third of esophagus
(hematoxylin-eosin×25)

Superficial (cardiac) glands of esophagus
Esophageal epithelium (stratified squamous)
Muscularis mucosae
Two layers of esophageal musculature
Juncture of esophageal and gastric epithelium
Cardiac glands of stomach
Gastric epithelium (columnar)
Three layers of gastric musculature

Longitudinal section: Esophagogastric junction
(hematoxylin-eosin×25)

Lumen
Stratified squamous epithelium
Tunica propria
Muscularis mucosae
Submucosa
Esophageal glands (deep)
Circular muscle
Longitudinal muscle

Fig. 1.9 Histology of the Esophagus.

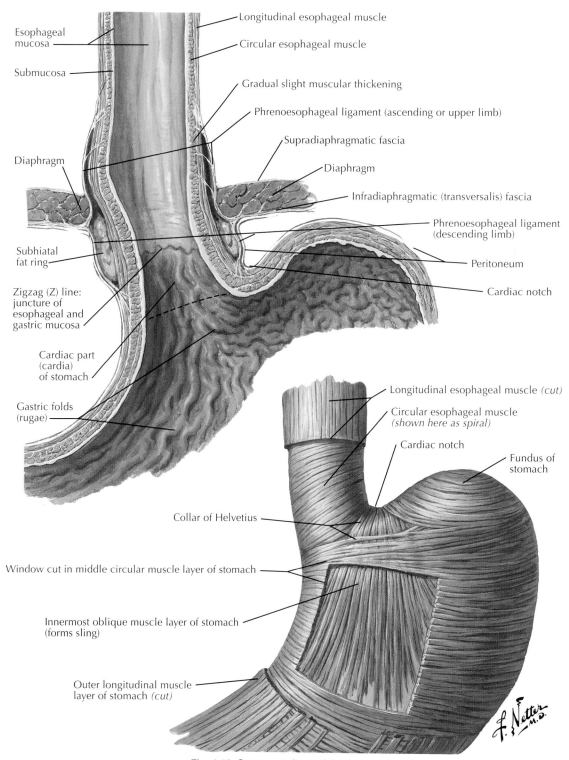

Esophageal mucosa

Submucosa

Diaphragm

Subhiatal fat ring

Zigzag (Z) line: juncture of esophageal and gastric mucosa

Cardiac part (cardia) of stomach

Gastric folds (rugae)

Longitudinal esophageal muscle

Circular esophageal muscle

Gradual slight muscular thickening

Phrenoesophageal ligament (ascending or upper limb)

Supradiaphragmatic fascia

Diaphragm

Infradiaphragmatic (transversalis) fascia

Phrenoesophageal ligament (descending limb)

Peritoneum

Cardiac notch

Longitudinal esophageal muscle (cut)

Circular esophageal muscle (shown here as spiral)

Cardiac notch

Fundus of stomach

Collar of Helvetius

Window cut in middle circular muscle layer of stomach

Innermost oblique muscle layer of stomach (forms sling)

Outer longitudinal muscle layer of stomach (cut)

Fig. 1.10 Gastroesophageal Junction.

When a swallowed bolus of food reaches the LES, it pauses before the sphincter relaxes and enters the stomach. The mechanism depends on the specialized zone of esophageal circular smooth muscle and possibly the gastric sling. At resting state, the LES is under tonic contraction. During swallowing, these muscles relax, the sphincter opens, and the food bolus empties into the stomach. Conversely, during vomiting, the LES relaxes to emit fluid into the esophagus.

The diaphragm contributes an external, sphincterlike function through the right crus of the diaphragm, which is attached by the phrenicoesophageal ligament. Manometry and electromyographic studies reveal that fibers of the crura contract around the esophagus during inspiration and episodes of increased intraabdominal pressure. In patients with hiatal hernia, the diaphragmatic component is no longer functional.

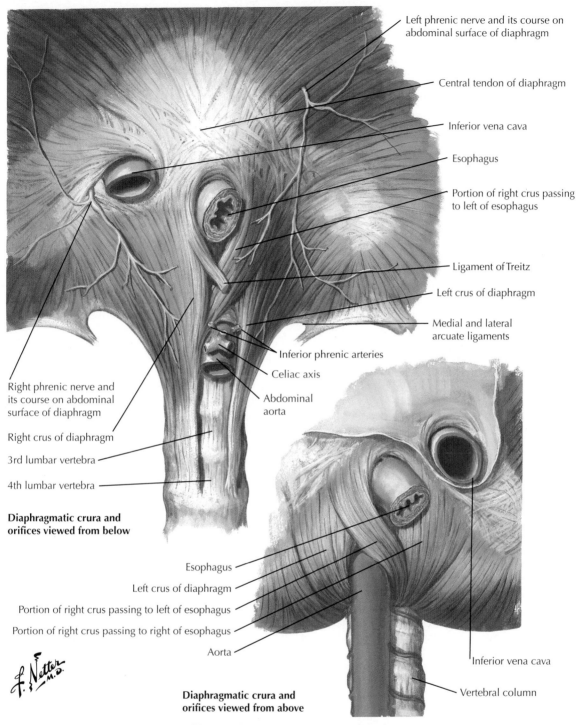

Left phrenic nerve and its course on abdominal surface of diaphragm

Central tendon of diaphragm

Inferior vena cava

Esophagus

Portion of right crus passing to left of esophagus

Ligament of Treitz

Left crus of diaphragm

Medial and lateral arcuate ligaments

Inferior phrenic arteries

Celiac axis

Abdominal aorta

Right phrenic nerve and its course on abdominal surface of diaphragm

Right crus of diaphragm

3rd lumbar vertebra

4th lumbar vertebra

Diaphragmatic crura and orifices viewed from below

Esophagus

Left crus of diaphragm

Portion of right crus passing to left of esophagus

Portion of right crus passing to right of esophagus

Aorta

Diaphragmatic crura and orifices viewed from above

Inferior vena cava

Vertebral column

Fig. 1.11 Diaphragm: Hiatus and Crura.

The muscular component is only partially responsible for the resting LES pressure. Parasympathetic, sympathetic, inhibitory, and excitatory autonomic nerves innervate the intramural plexus of the LES. Resting pressure decreases after administration of atropine, supporting the presence of a cholinergic neural component. Cell bodies of the inhibitory nerves are located in the esophageal plexus, and the vagus nerves supply the preganglionic fibers. These nerves mediate sphincter relaxation in response to swallowing. Evidence suggests that nitric oxide controls relaxation through the enteric nervous system.

ADDITIONAL RESOURCES

Gastroesophageal reflux disease. In Cameron JL, Peters JH, editors: *Current surgical therapy*, ed 6, St Louis, 1998, Mosby, pp 33–46.

Gray H, Bannister LH, Berry MM, Williams PL, editors: *Gray's anatomy: the anatomical basis of medicine and surgery*, New York, 1995, Churchill Livingstone.

Peters JH, DeMeester TR: Esophagus and diaphragmatic hernia. In Schwartz SI, Shires TG, Spencer FC, editors: *Principles of surgery*, ed 7, New York, 1999, McGraw-Hill, pp 1081–1179.

2

Congenital Anomalies of the Esophagus

Neil R. Floch

The most frequently encountered anomaly in the newborn is *esophageal atresia* (EA), which occurs with or without *tracheoesophageal fistula* (TEF). These lesions occur together in 96% of cases except in the case of H-type fistulas (Fig. 2.1). The incidence of EA is 1 in 4500 live births with no gender predilection. Infants born with EA have a 95% chance of survival. TEF and EA occur from an embryonic lung bud that does not branch properly, causing failure of complete separation of the foregut into esophagus and trachea. In 50% of patients there are associated anamolies. These conditions may be present in syndromes such as VACTERL (vertebral abnormalities, anal atresia, cardiac abnormalities, TEF, and/or EA, renal agenesis and dysplasia, and limb defects). Another syndrome is CHARGE (colobama, heart disease, atresia, choanae, retarded growth and development or central nervous system anomalies, genital hypoplasia, ear anomalies, and/or deafness) syndrome, which may involve cardiac or genitourinary abnormalities.

Anatomic classification of EA comprises five categories. The most common category is proximal pouch with distal fistula (A1 and A2), which occurs in 84% of patients. Here the upper esophagus ends at the level of the second thoracic vertebra (T2), leaving a gap of 1 to 2 cm. The lower esophagus enters the trachea at the carina. Over time, the upper esophagus dilates as swallowing ends in a blind pouch. The distal esophagus is of normal caliber but tapers proximally to 3 to 4 mm at its tracheal communication. The second most common EA category is long-gap EA (B), which develops in 8% of patients. In this EA, a fibrous cord connects the proximal and distal parts of the esophagus. Occasionally no cord exists, and the esophagus ends in two pouches. Isolated H-type TEF (D), which can exist anywhere along the posterior wall of the trachea in a normal esophagus, occurs in 4% of patients. EA with distal and proximal fistulas (C) may develop in 6% of patients. Rare variants occur in 2% to 3% of patients; for example, congenital atresia caused by a stenosing web may develop anywhere in the esophagus of a patient with a normal trachea (E).

The pathogenesis of EA remains controversial. In the fetus, the tracheoesophageal septum is a single tube of mesoderm that divides into the esophagus and the lung bud between the fourth and twelfth week of development. The laryngotracheal groove forms the floor of the gut. The esophageal lumen closes as it is filled with epithelium-lining cells. After this, vacuolation occurs, and the lumen is reestablished. An early traumatic event may result in failure of the mesoderm to separate or differentiate during growth of the lung and esophageal components, resulting in reabsorption of a portion of the esophagus. If vacuoles fail to coalesce, a solid core of esophageal cells remains, resulting in atresia. As a result, an abnormal esophagus forms with or without pulmonary communication. Recent evidence indicates that a tracheal fistula may develop as a trifurcation of the trachea that grows and connects to the stomach bud.

Congenital anomalies of the esophagus are frequently associated with organ anomalies. Certain anomalies are incompatible with life unless they are surgically corrected. The most common associated syndrome is the VATER/VACTERL (vertebral, anorectal, cardiac, tracheoesophageal, renal, and limb abnormalities) syndrome, which occurs in 46% of patients; 15% of infants have two or more components of the syndrome.

CLINICAL PICTURE

Polyhydramnios is present in nearly 66% of fetuses with EA, but most are not diagnosed until birth. Shortly after birth, an infant with a congenital abnormality of the esophagus experiences respiratory distress, tachypnea, coughing, and choking, which may result in aspiration and pneumonia. Excessive salivation and drooling occur, along with regurgitation and cyanosis with feedings. H-type TEF presents early in patients with large connections, as choking and aspiration is detected with feeding. Smaller fistulas may not be discovered for up to 4 years, but patients may have recurrent symptoms or respiratory insufficiency and pneumonia. In EA, the obstruction usually occurs 10 to 12 cm from the mouth. The presence of a TEF will result in gastric distention. Cardiac murmur with or without cyanosis may also be present. In newborns, additional findings may relate to VATER/VACTERL.

DIAGNOSIS

Diagnosis of a congenital esophageal anomaly in the prenatal period may be possible with ultrasound. Abdominal radiographs may confirm the diagnosis if air/fluid is found in the mediastinum or if a nasogastric tube in the chest has become curled. TEF may indicate air in the stomach. Barium esophagraphy, upper endoscopy, and bronchoscopy are the best diagnostic tests for TEF. The injection of a small amount of methylene blue into the esophagus may be diagnostic if it appears in the trachea. Three-dimensional computed tomography may also demonstrate the presence of TEF. The VATER syndrome may be detected using radiography, renal ultrasound, or echocardiographic studies.

TREATMENT AND MANAGEMENT

In EA, surgical anastomosis of the esophagus and closure of the TEF is the preferred treatment as soon as the infant is stabilized after birth. Staged procedures may be necessary if defects in the esophageal segment are present, including options of elongation of the esophagus, gastric pull-up, or interposition of colon or jejunum. Staging is preferred in low-birth-weight neonates. Newborns who undergo surgery within the first 48 hours tend to do better, but the timing of repair depends on the individual's condition.

In patients with VATER, the most severe problem is corrected first. Bronchoscopy is performed at surgery, and the incision is made on the side opposite the aortic arch. In patients with dysphagia secondary to webs located at the cricopharyngeal folds, dilation with a bougie may be well tolerated.

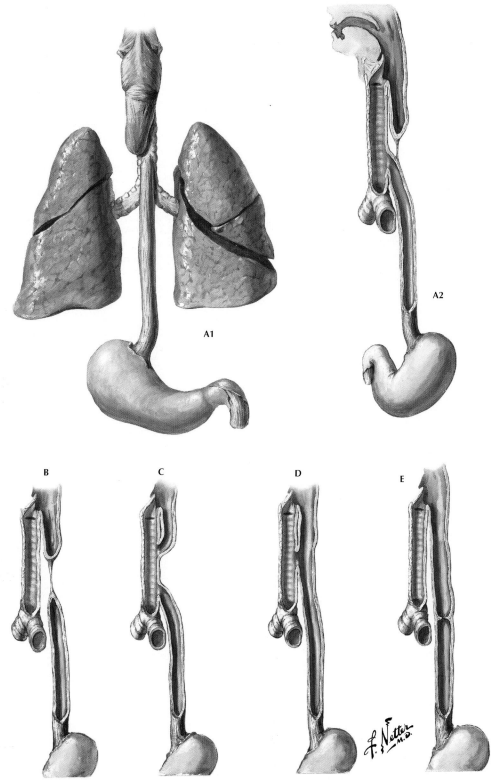

Fig. 2.1 Congenital Anomalies. (A1, A2) Proximal pouch with distal fistula, (B) long-gap esophageal atresia (EA), (C) EA with distal and proximal fistulas, (D) isolated H-type tracheoesophageal fistula, (E) congenital atresia caused by stenosing web.

COURSE AND PROGNOSIS

Although long-term outcomes are favorable, children with EA and TEF encounter many difficulties after initial surgery and later in life. In the first 5 years, patients are treated with proton pump inhibitor (PPI) medications for acid suppression. The PPI medication is usually continued into adulthood. Chronic feeding issues are common. Up to 87% of patients with congenital abnormalities survive. Prognosis depends on birth weight and the length of the esophageal gap if present. The most frequent complications after surgery include an anastomotic leak in 16% and strictures in 35% of patients. Esophageal motility disorders and delayed gastric emptying are common and may account for symptoms of dysphagia and gastroesophageal reflux disease (GERD).

At least 25% of children with EA and TEF contract pulmonary infections. Many experience developmental delays, but these usually resolve as the children grow. Support groups have been successful at helping children mature and helping parents through their children's difficult years.

ADDITIONAL RESOURCES

Karnak I, Senocak ME, Hiçsönmez A, Büyükpamukçu N: The diagnosis and treatment of H-type tracheoesophageal fistula, *J Pediatr Surg* 32:1670, 1997.

Katsura S, Shono T, Yamanouchi T, et al: Esophageal atresia with double tracheoesophageal fistula—a case report and review of the literature, *Eur J Pediatr Surg* 15:354, 2005.

Lautz TB, Mandelia A, Radhakrishnan J: VACTERL associations in children undergoing surgery for esophageal atresia and anorectal malformations: implications for pediatric surgeons, *J Pediatr Surg* 50:1245, 2015.

Little DC, Rescorla FJ, Grosfeld JL, et al: Long-term analysis of children with esophageal atresia and tracheoesophageal fistula, *J Pediatr Surg* 38: 852–856, 2003.

Lupo PJ, Isenburg JL, Salemi JL, et al: Population-based birth defects data in the United States, 2010-2014: A focus on gastrointestinal defects, *Birth Defects Res* 109:1504, 2017.

Spilde TL, Bhatia AM, Marosky JK, et al: Complete discontinuity of the distal fistula tract from the developing gut: direct histologic evidence for the mechanism of tracheoesophageal fistula formation, *Anat Rec* 267:220–224, 2002.

3

Deglutition

Neil R. Floch

Once initiated, swallowing becomes a reflex response that usually occurs hundreds of times a day (Figs. 3.1 and 3.2). It is a complex process involving the coordination of over 30 different muscles. It takes less than a second for food to enter the esophagus and up to 15 seconds to reach the stomach. Although it is continuous, deglutition is divided it into three stages—oral preparatory, pharyngeal, and esophageal: it may be observed by cineradiography and manometry. Deglutition requires the physiologic ability to (1) prepare a bolus of suitable size and consistency, (2) prevent dispersal of this bolus during the phases of swallowing, (3) create differential pressure that propels the bolus in a forward direction, (4) prevent food or liquid from entering the nasopharynx or larynx, (5) pass the bolus rapidly through the pharynx to limit the time respiration is suspended, (6) prevent gastric reflux into the esophagus during free communication between the esophagus and the stomach, and (7) clear residual material from the esophagus. Failure of these mechanisms leads to difficulty with swallowing and may lead to the regurgitation of gastric contents into the esophagus and possibly into the pharynx.

The oral phase of deglutition involves mastication of the food bolus in the mouth as it is broken into smaller pieces with the assistance of saliva. The bolus is shaped into the appropriate size, shape and consistency to pass out of the pharynx. The anterior tongue pushes the bolus to the posterior tongue as the anterior tongue lifts the hard palate and pulls backward, pushing the bolus into the oropharynx as it simultaneously closes the nasopharynx by elevating the tongue with the mylohyoid muscle and—with the help of the soft palate, fauces, and posterior wall of the oropharynx—preventing nasal regurgitation. Afterward, a peristaltic wave propels the bolus distally. Paralysis of the soft palate may occur in patients after a cerebrovascular accident or stroke, causing regurgitation into the nasopharynx.

The pharyngeal phase begins when the bolus enters the oropharynx and the hyoid bone elevates and moves anteriorly. Concomitantly, the larynx elevates, moves forward, and tilts posteriorly, pulling the bolus inward as the anteroposterior diameter of the laryngopharynx increases. This action causes the epiglottis to move under the tongue, tilt backward, and overlap the opening of the larynx to prevent aspiration of the food. Depression of the epiglottis may not completely close the larynx, and small particles of food may infringe on the opening. A liquid bolus may be split by the epiglottis and travel on each side of the larynx through the piriform recesses, rejoining behind the cricoid cartilage. The pharyngeal mechanism of swallowing occurs within 1.5 seconds.

At the same time, the upper esophageal sphincter (UES) closes as the tongue moves backward and the posterior pharyngeal constrictors contract. In the hypopharynx, pressure increases from 15 mm Hg to a closing pressure of 30 to 60 mm Hg. A pressure difference then develops between the hypopharynx and the midesophagus, creating a vacuum effect that, with the help of peristalsis, pulls the food from the hypopharynx into the esophagus during relaxation of the cricopharyngeal muscle. The closing pressure of 30 mm Hg prevents reflux of food back into the pharynx. When the bolus reaches the distal esophagus, the pressure in the UES returns to 15 mm Hg.

Passage of the food bolus beyond the cricopharyngeal muscle signifies the completion of the pharyngeal phase and the beginning of the esophageal phase. Hyoid bone, larynx, and epiglottis return to their original positions, and air reenters the trachea. The peristaltic wave begins in the oropharynx and continues into the esophagus, propelling the food in front of it. Sequential coordinated contractions in the smooth muscles of the middle and distal esophagus function to propel the food down to the lower esophageal sphincter (LES). In its travels, the bolus moves from an area with intrathoracic pressure of −6 mm Hg to an area with intraabdominal pressure of +6 mm Hg.

Peristaltic contractions may range from 30 to 120 mm Hg in a healthy person. The average wave peaks in 1 second, remains at that peak for 0.5 second, and subsides for 1.5 seconds. The total rise and fall of each wave proceeds for 3 to 5 seconds. A primary peristaltic contraction, initiated by swallowing, travels down the esophagus at a rate of 2 to 4 cm/s, reaching the LES approximately 9 seconds after the initiation of swallowing. If swallowing is rapidly repeated, the esophagus remains relaxed; a wave develops only after the ending movement of the pharynx.

Efferent vagal nerves that arise in the medulla control esophageal peristalsis. When the esophagus is distended, a wave is initiated as the UES forcefully closes and contractions commence and then propel down the esophagus. This phenomenon is a secondary contraction that occurs without movement of the mouth or pharynx. Secondary peristalsis is a dependent, local reflex that attempts to remove any food substance that remains in the esophagus after primary contraction is complete. The propulsive force of the esophagus is not very strong. Normal contractions of the esophageal muscles and relaxation of the inferior esophagus are necessary for efficient deglutition. So-called tertiary waves, which occur particularly in elderly persons and in patients with hiatal hernia, are nonperistaltic, repetitive, ringlike contractions at multiple levels in the distal half of the esophagus, usually during stages of incomplete distention. A patient with a large hiatal hernia lacks the ability for distal fixation and adequate food propulsion.

In the resting state, the LES divides the esophagus from the stomach and functions as a pressure barrier with a gradient of 12 mm Hg. The LES comprises thickened muscle fibers that perform a sphincterlike action, although no distinct sphincter exists. Tonically, the LES remains closed, preventing gastroesophageal (GE) reflux. With the onset of swallowing, the peristaltic wave creates a transient peak behind the bolus, which stops in the terminal esophagus. The LES then relaxes through a reflex mechanism. It does not relax completely until the pressure immediately proximal to it is great enough to overcome the LES pressure. The esophagus immediately proximal to the LES functions as a collecting area in which pressure builds after the peristaltic wave and where the bolus is temporarily delayed.

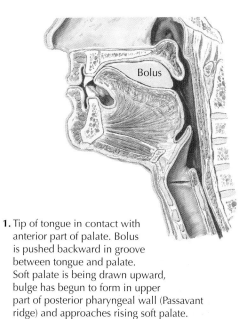

1. Tip of tongue in contact with anterior part of palate. Bolus is pushed backward in groove between tongue and palate. Soft palate is being drawn upward, bulge has begun to form in upper part of posterior pharyngeal wall (Passavant ridge) and approaches rising soft palate.

2. Bolus lying in groove on lingual dorsum formed by contraction of genioglossus and transverse intrinsic musculature of tongue.

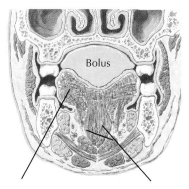

Transverse intrinsic musculature of tongue

Genioglossus muscles

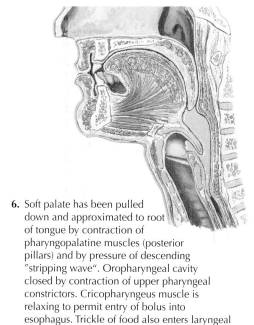

6. Soft palate has been pulled down and approximated to root of tongue by contraction of pharyngopalatine muscles (posterior pillars) and by pressure of descending "stripping wave". Oropharyngeal cavity closed by contraction of upper pharyngeal constrictors. Cricopharyngeus muscle is relaxing to permit entry of bolus into esophagus. Trickle of food also enters laryngeal aditus but is prevented from going farther by closure of ventricular folds.

7. Laryngeal vestibule is closed by approximation of aryepiglottic and ventricular folds, preventing entry of food into larynx (coronal section: AP view).

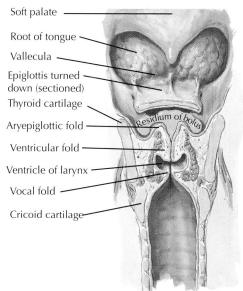

Soft palate

Root of tongue

Vallecula

Epiglottis turned down (sectioned)

Thyroid cartilage

Aryepiglottic fold

Ventricular fold

Ventricle of larynx

Vocal fold

Cricoid cartilage

Residium of bolus

Fig. 3.1 Deglutition: Oral and Pharyngeal.

4. Bolus has reached vallecula; hyoid bone and larynx move upward and forward. Epiglottis is tipped downward. "Stripping wave" on posterior pharyngeal wall moves downward.

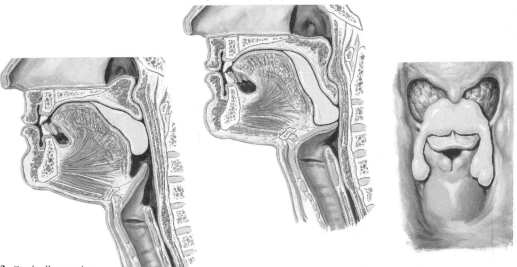

3. Gradually pressing more of its dorsal surface against hard palate, tongue pushes bolus backward into oral pharynx, soft palate is drawn upward to make contact with Passavant ridge, closing off nasopharynx, receptive space in oral pharynx forms by slight forward movement of root of tongue, contraction of stylopharyngeus and upper pharyngeal constrictor muscles draws pharyngeal wall upward over bolus.

5. Epiglottis is tipped down over laryngeal aditus but does not completely close it. Bolus flows in two streams around each side of epiglottis to piriform fossae. Streams will then unite to enter esophagus. Trickle of food may enter laryngeal aditus (viewed from behind).

9. "Stripping wave" has passed pharynx. Epiglottis is beginning to turn up again as hyoid bone and larynx descend. Communication with nasopharynx has been reestablished.

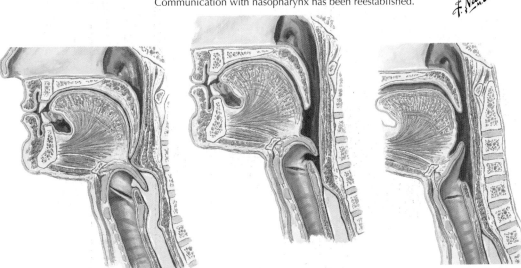

8. "Stripping wave" has reached vallecula and is pressing out last of bolus. Cricopharyngeus muscle has relaxed and bolus has largely passed into esophagus.

10. All structures of pharynx have returned to resting position as "stripping wave" passes down into esophagus, pushing bolus before it.

Fig. 3.1, cont'd

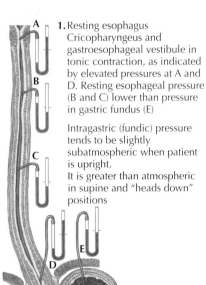

1. Resting esophagus
Cricopharyngeus and gastroesophageal vestibule in tonic contraction, as indicated by elevated pressures at A and D. Resting esophageal pressure (B and C) lower than pressure in gastric fundus (E)

Intragastric (fundic) pressure tends to be slightly subatmospheric when patient is upright.
It is greater than atmospheric in supine and "heads down" positions

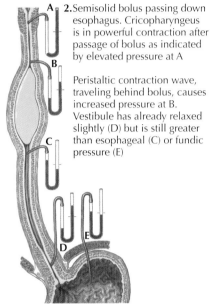

2. Semisolid bolus passing down esophagus. Cricopharyngeus is in powerful contraction after passage of bolus as indicated by elevated pressure at A

Peristaltic contraction wave, traveling behind bolus, causes increased pressure at B. Vestibule has already relaxed slightly (D) but is still greater than esophageal (C) or fundic pressure (E)

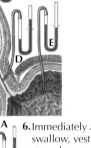

3. Head of bolus has arrived at upper end of vestibule and come to transient arrest. Pressures at cricopharyngeus (A) and in upper esophagus (B) have returned almost to resting levels

Peristaltic contraction wave has reached C, causing elevated pressure

Vestibule is slightly relaxed relative to resting state but pressure here (D) is still great enough to prevent passage of semisolid bolus

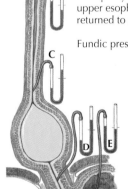

4. Peristaltic wave continues descent, (C) causing bulge (ampulla) in lower esophagus as vestibule (D) has not yet relaxed enough to permit passage of semisolid bolus

Cricopharyngeal pressure (A) and upper esophageal pressure (B) have returned to resting levels

Fundic pressure (E) unchanged

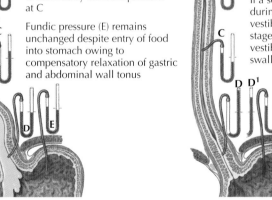

5. Entry of bolus into stomach

Vestibule has fully relaxed as indicated by drop in pressure (D) almost to intragastric (fundic) pressure (E). Bolus is passing into stomach under influence of peristaltic contraction wave, evidenced by elevated pressure at C

Fundic pressure (E) remains unchanged despite entry of food into stomach owing to compensatory relaxation of gastric and abdominal wall tonus

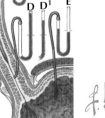

6. Immediately after termination of swallow, vestibule contracts strongly as evidenced by elevated pressure at D. It remains in this state for a few seconds and then gradually returns to resting state (D¹)

If a second swallow takes place during phase of strongly elevated vestibular pressure (refractory stage), bolus may be held up at the vestibule longer than was initial swallow

Fig. 3.2 Deglutition: Esophageal.

After the bolus enters the stomach, LES pressure increases temporarily before it returns to a resting state. The UES returns to its resting pressure. The bolus does not completely clear the esophagus; rather, small amounts may remain, especially if a person consumes thick food or swallows in the recumbent position.

If a pharyngeal swallow does not result in peristalsis of the esophagus, relaxation of the LES results in the reflux of gastric contents that cannot be propelled back into the stomach. Vagal function is responsible for relaxation of the LES. Therefore preventing reflux requires a functioning LES and stomach and an esophagus capable of peristalsis.

NEUROREGULATION OF DEGLUTITION

Swallowing is controlled by the cortical area located in the inferior portion of the precentral gyrus, near the insula (Fig. 3.3). Efferent connections are made by the hypothalamus with the medulla, where a deglutition center is located near the ala cinerea and the nuclei of cranial nerve X. This medullar deglutition center coordinates the nerves and muscles involved in the act of swallowing.

Sensory impulses ready the swallowing center through afferent fibers from the mucosa of the mouth, soft palate, tongue, fauces, pharynx, and esophagus. Stimulation of the anterior and posterior tonsils and of the sides of the hypopharynx may stimulate swallowing as a reflex, but swallowing may also be initiated voluntarily. The glossopharyngeal nerve, the superior laryngeal branches to the vagus, and the pharyngeal branches to the vagus serve as the afferent sensory nerves of the pharynx. These nerves initiate a reflex reaction and regulate the response of the muscle groups that control breathing, positioning of the larynx, and movement of the bolus into the esophagus. The voluntary component of swallowing is completed when sensory nerves on the pharynx detect the food bolus. After this, swallowing is an involuntary process.

Afferent sensory fibers travel through cranial nerves V, IX, and X into their respective nuclei, after which fibers travel to the swallowing center in the medulla. Data are coordinated in the deglutition center and are stimulated by these nerves, which facilitate the act of swallowing by emitting impulses in a delicately timed reflex sequence through cranial nerves V, VII, X, XI, and XII. Fibers from cranial nerves V, X, and XII innervate the levator muscles of the soft palate. Cranial nerve X travels to the constrictor muscles of the pharynx. Cervical and thoracic spinal nerves innervate the diaphragm and intercostal muscles. Cranial nerves V and XII travel to the extrinsic muscles of the larynx. Fibers from cranial nerve X control the intrinsic muscles of the larynx and the musculature of the esophagus. Cranial nerves VII and XI and cervical motor neurons C1 to C3 are also involved. The entire coordinated event occurs over 0.5 second. Swallowing may be initiated by several different impulses. The output, however, always follows the same sequence of coordinated events.

These events may be altered after a cerebrovascular accident or stroke. Efferent nerves through the vagus, cranial nerve X, and recurrent laryngeal nerves activate the cricopharynx and upper esophageal muscles. Innervation is required for the cricopharynx to relax as the pharyngeal constrictors contract concomitantly. Damage to these nerves may result in aspiration.

The bolus is propelled down the esophagus by peristaltic muscle contractions controlled by the vagus nerves. In addition to the recurrent laryngeal nerve, the cervical esophagus receives an additional efferent supply either from a pharyngoesophageal nerve arising proximal to the nodose ganglion or from an esophageal nerve.

Visceral afferent nerves from the upper five or six thoracic sympathetic roots convey nerve stimuli that result from esophageal distention, chemical irritation, spasm, or variations in temperature. These impulses travel to the thalamus and then to the inferior portion of the postcentral gyrus. After this, stimuli are interpreted as sensations of pressure, burning, gas, dull ache, or pain in the tissues innervated by the somatic nerves from the corresponding spinal levels. These connections explain why pain from esophageal disease may be referred to the middle or either side of the chest, to the sides of the neck, or to the jaws, teeth, or ears. The similarity between atypical chest pain and referred pain of cardiac origin is controversial and complicates the differential diagnosis of cardiac and esophageal disease. Distention, hypertonus, or obstruction of the distal esophagus may give rise to difficulty in swallowing and to reflex contraction of the UES, with the resultant sensation of a lump, known as globus, at the level of the suprasternal notch.

ADDITIONAL RESOURCES

Bieger D, Neuhuber W: Neural circuits and mediators regulating swallowing in the brainstem, *GI Motility online* 2006. doi:10.1038/giomo74. Available online at: www.nature.com/gimo/contents/pt1/full/gimo74.html. (Accessed on May 28, 2014).

Corbin-Lewis K, Liss JM, Sciortino KL: *Clinical anatomy and physiology of the swallow mechanism*, New York, 2004, Thomson Delmar Learning.

Gray H, Bannister LH, Berry MM, Williams PL, editors: *Gray's anatomy: the anatomical basis of medicine and surgery*, New York, 1995, Churchill Livingstone.

Massey BT: Physiology of ORal cavity, pharynx and upper esophageal sphincter. Part I ORal cavity, pharynx and esophagus, *GI Motility online* 2006. doi:10.1038/gimo2. Available online at: www.nature.com/gimo/contents/pt1/full/gimo2.html. (Accessed on May 29, 2014).

Shaker R, Hogan WJ: Normal physiology of the aerodigestive tract and its effect on the upper gut, *Am J Med* 115(Suppl 3A):2S, 2003.

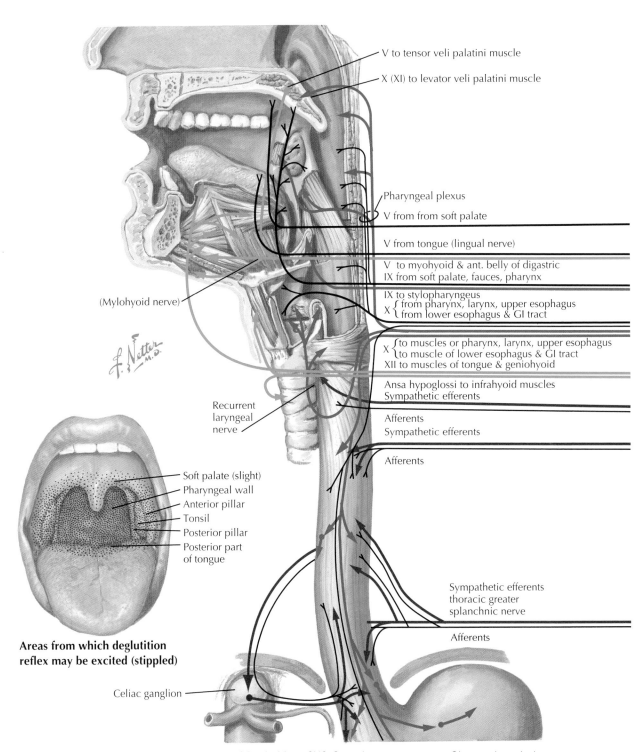

V to tensor veli palatini muscle

X (XI) to levator veli palatini muscle

Pharyngeal plexus
V from from soft palate

V from tongue (lingual nerve)

V to myohyoid & ant. belly of digastric
IX from soft palate, fauces, pharynx

IX to stylopharyngeus
X { from pharynx, larynx, upper esophagus
  { from lower esophagus & GI tract

X { to muscles or pharynx, larynx, upper esophagus
  { to muscle of lower esophagus & GI tract
XII to muscles of tongue & geniohyoid

Ansa hypoglossi to infrahyoid muscles
Sympathetic efferents

Afferents
Sympathetic efferents

Afferents

Sympathetic efferents
thoracic greater
splanchnic nerve

Afferents

(Mylohyoid nerve)

Recurrent
laryngeal
nerve

Soft palate (slight)
Pharyngeal wall
Anterior pillar
Tonsil
Posterior pillar
Posterior part
of tongue

**Areas from which deglutition
reflex may be excited (stippled)**

Celiac ganglion

Fig. 3.3 Neuroregulation of Deglutition. *CNS*, Central nervous system; *GI*, gastrointestinal.

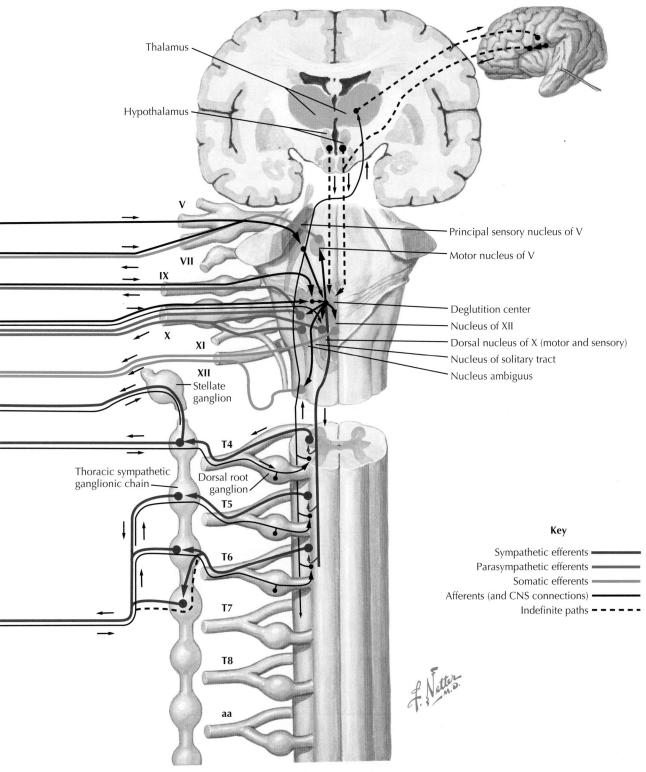

Thalamus

Hypothalamus

V

VII

IX

X

XI

XII

Stellate ganglion

Thoracic sympathetic ganglionic chain

Dorsal root ganglion

T4

T5

T6

T7

T8

aa

Principal sensory nucleus of V

Motor nucleus of V

Deglutition center
Nucleus of XII
Dorsal nucleus of X (motor and sensory)
Nucleus of solitary tract
Nucleus ambiguus

Key

Sympathetic efferents ▬▬▬
Parasympathetic efferents ▬▬▬
Somatic efferents ▬▬▬
Afferents (and CNS connections) ▬▬▬
Indefinite paths ▬ ▬ ▬

Fig. 3.3, cont'd

4

Benign Disease of the Esophagus

Neil R. Floch

ESOPHAGEAL RINGS AND WEBS

Esophageal rings and webs are growths of tissue that partially obstruct the lumen of the esophagus. The prevalence of esophageal rings and webs has not been determined, as most patients are asymptomatic. Most lesions are found incidentally at the time of a radiologic study or endoscopy in 18%. No consensus exists as to the cause, location, or significance of the rings.

Rings are categorized as "A" and "B," formerly known as Shatzki rings (Fig. 4.1). They are most common distally but may occur along the entire length of the esophagus. The structure described as an "A" ring is believed to be a normal smooth muscle contraction of the distal esophagus located at the gastroesophageal junction (GEJ). "A" rings are rare and found mostly in children at the time of a barium swallow or esophagogastroduodenoscopy (EGD). Symptomatic patients present with intermittent dysphagia to solid food.

In 1953, Schatzki first reported a circumferential stricture, or ring, at the GEJ known as a "B" ring. It is composed of the connective tissue and the muscularis mucosa at the squamocolumnar junction and is less than 0.5 cm in length. It has also been attributed to the impression of the diaphragm at the LES. Barium esophagrams performed for symptom of dysphagia demonstrate esophageal "B" rings in 6% to 14% of patients. They are associated with hiatal hernias in 97% patients. Of patients with a Schatzki "B" ring, 65% have reflux, 50% erosive esophagitis, and 25% have a nonspecific dysmotility disorder. It is believed that over time, a ring may progress to form a stricture.

The differential diagnosis of a ring includes a congenital web, gastroesophageal reflux disease, or carcinoma-induced strictures. Eosinophilic esophagitis and reflux may play a role in the development of a Schatzki or "B" ring. Some evidence indicates that a ring may have a protective effect from Barrett esophagus. A Schatzki or "B" ring may be a rare cause of swallow syncope.

An esophageal web is less than 2 mm in diameter and encroaches on the esophageal lumen. It is covered with squamous epithelium and is most commonly found at the cricoid location of the cervical esophagus. The cause of esophageal webs is unknown but they have been thought to be due to chronic GERD. Evidence of reflux as an origin suggests that webs may progress to strictures if reflux is untreated. Congenital development has also been suggested. Webs may be associated with a Zenker diverticulum, iron-deficiency anemia, and chronic graft-versus-host disease following bone marrow transplantation. Webs may also be an extracutaneous manifestation in 14% to 33% of patients with epidermolysis bullosa, bullous pemphigoid, and pemphigus vulgaris.

Clinical Picture

Most patients are asymptomatic, but many have symptoms of dysphagia to solids such as meat, bread, and hard vegetables. Symptoms may be intermittent and patients may modify their eating behavior by increased chewing and the avoidance of certain foods. The severity of the problems depends on the degree of the narrowing. An esophageal lumen of less than 39 Fr or 1.3 cm is likely to result in symptoms of dysphagia. Analysis of the data by Schatzki indicates that decreasing the ring's diameter by 1 mm results in a 46% increase in the incidence of dysphagia. Patients may present with complete obstruction from a pill or a food at the site of a ring or web.

Diagnosis

A Schatzki ring is diagnosed by barium esophagram, which reveals two protrusions of less than 0.3 mm located several centimeters above the diaphragm. The protrusions resemble pencil tips at the GEJ. Muscular rings found on barium esophagram may be transient; they are 0.5 cm wide, multiple, symmetric, indentations. Swallowing a marshmallow bolus results in impaction in 75% of patients during a barium esophagram but this can increase the diagnostic yield from 17% to 100%. Manometry usually reveals high-amplitude contractions. Upper endoscopy is less sensitive in detecting rings and webs and may reveal a web as a smooth, noncircumferential membrane when the esophagus is fully distended. The Shatzki ring is almost always associated with a sliding hiatal hernia. A biopsy performed at endoscopy may reveal a submucosa with basal cell hyperplasia, hyperkeratosis, and eosinophils.

Treatment and Management

Patients should chew food thoroughly to prevent impaction. Esophagoscopy with bolus extraction is the simplest measure to relieve obstruction. Glucagon administration may reduce spasm and allow an obstructed object to pass. Both "A" rings and webs may be torn during upper endoscopy, whereas most other rings are amenable to dilatation. If dilatation is needed, a 50-Fr bougie or 18- to 20-mm balloon dilator may be used. One dilatation is usually all that is needed. Esophageal rings should be biopsied to eliminate the diagnosis of eosinophilic esophagitis, defined by greater than 18 eosinophils per high-power field. Esophageal rings associated with GERD warrant a 6-week treatment with proton-pump inhibitor (PPI) medication. Symptoms recur at 1, 2, and 5 years in 32%, 65%, and 89% of patients, respectively. Repeat dilatation and chronic PPI therapy may be indicated. The ring may be incised if repeat dilatations are ineffective. Dilatation after incision is performed if there is further failure.

PLUMMER-VINSON SYNDROME

This disease was named after two Americans, physician Henry Stanley Plummer and surgeon Porter Paisley Vinson. It usually occurs in edentulous, premenopausal, married women and rarely in men (Fig. 4.2). Plummer-Vinson syndrome (PVS) develops over months to years, manifests in the fourth to fifth decades of life, and is more common in Scandinavian countries than in the United States. It had been

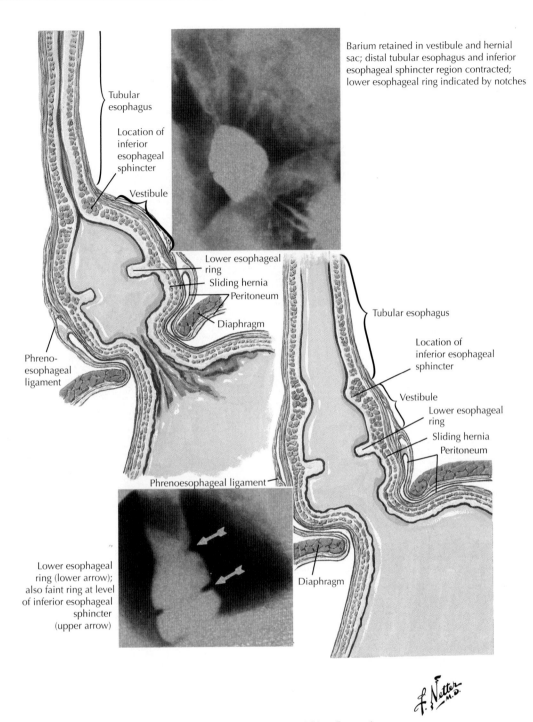

Tubular esophagus

Location of inferior esophageal sphincter

Vestibule

Barium retained in vestibule and hernial sac; distal tubular esophagus and inferior esophageal sphincter region contracted; lower esophageal ring indicated by notches

Lower esophageal ring

Sliding hernia

Peritoneum

Diaphragm

Phreno-esophageal ligament

Phrenoesophageal ligament

Lower esophageal ring (lower arrow); also faint ring at level of inferior esophageal sphincter (upper arrow)

Tubular esophagus

Location of inferior esophageal sphincter

Vestibule

Lower esophageal ring

Sliding hernia

Peritoneum

Diaphragm

Fig. 4.1 Schatzki Esophageal Ring Formation.

attributed to iron-deficiency anemia in northern countries in the past. It has also been found in children and adolescents. PVS is a premalignant process, as it is a risk factor for the development of squamous cell carcinoma of the esophagus and hypopharynx.

The hallmark finding of PVS is a weblike structure that originates on the posterior wall of the cervical esophagus between the hypopharynx, 1 to 2 cm below the cricopharynx. The web is thick at its base and becomes thinner as it protrudes inward, where it has the consistency of paper. The cause of the web is unknown, but genetic factors and nutritional deficiencies may play a role.

Clinical Picture

There is a triad of iron-deficiency anemia, dysphagia, and a cervical esophageal web, although weakness is also one of the most common characteristic symptoms. Dysphagia of solids occurs frequently but dysphagia of liquids is rare. Odynophagia may also be present. Oral symptoms are common, and patients complain of glossitis or burning of the tongue and oral mucosa. Possible atrophy of lingual papillae produces a visually smooth and shiny glossal dorsum. Patients may have stomatitis with painful cracks in the angles of a dry mouth.

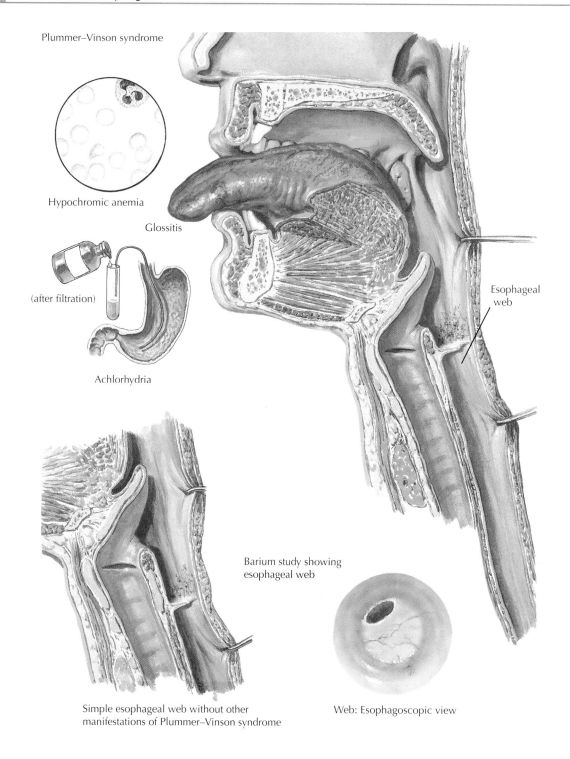

Plummer–Vinson syndrome

Hypochromic anemia

Glossitis

(after filtration)

Achlorhydria

Esophageal web

Barium study showing esophageal web

Simple esophageal web without other manifestations of Plummer–Vinson syndrome

Web: Esophagoscopic view

Fig. 4.2 Plummer-Vinson Syndrome.

Atrophic mucosa may involve the esophagus and the hypopharynx. Patients with PVS may also have achlorhydria, brittle fingernails (which may indicate vitamin deficiency), and splenomegaly (33% of patients). Anemia may result in hemoglobin levels that are 50% of normal values. Other findings include: splenomegaly and an enlarged thyroid.

Diagnosis

Barium esophagraphy reveals a fibrous web under the cricopharyngeus muscle seen as a filling defect below the level of the cricoid cartilage in the esophagus. The web may involve the entire circumference of the esophagus and is thought to be the cause of dysphagia. Serum tests may reveal hypochromic microcytic anemia, consistent with iron-deficiency anemia. Biopsy of mucosa should demonstrate epithelial atrophy and submucosal chronic inflammation as well as possible epithelial atypia or dysplasia.

Treatment and Management

Treatment of PVS is primarily aimed at correcting the iron-deficiency anemia. Patients should receive iron supplementation as well as foods high in iron content, which may lead to resolution of dysphagia prior to resolution of the anemia. With treatment, symptoms such as dysphagia, as well as oral and tongue pain, usually resolve. Iron supplementation usually resolves the anemia.

Dilatation of the esophageal web may be necessary when significant obstruction of the esophageal lumen is present. Only a small amount of pressure ruptures a web, so introducing an endoscope is usually therapeutic because it reestablishes a normal passage through the esophagus. Annual surveillance with upper endoscopy for esophageal squamous cell carcinoma has not been shown to improve patient outcomes.

Course and Prognosis

Iron replacement therapy reverses anemia, and strictures are almost always dilated successfully. Unfortunately malignant lesions of the oral mucosa, hypopharynx, and esophagus may be observed in as many as 100% of patients with PVS on long-term follow-up.

ADDITIONAL RESOURCES

DiSario JA, Pedersen PJ, Bichis-Canoutas C, et al: Incision of recurrent distal esophageal (Schatzki) ring after dilation, *Gastrointest Endosc* 56:244–248, 2002.

Gawrieh S, Carroll T, Hogan WJ, et al: Swallow syncope in association with schatzki ring and hypertensive esophageal peristalsis: report of three cases and review of the literature, *Dysphagia* 20(4):273–277, 2005.

Hoffman RM, Jaffe PE: Plummer-vinson syndrome. A case report and literature review, *Arch Intern Med* 155:2008, 1995.

Johnson AC, Lester PD, Johnson S, et al: Esophagogastric ring: why and when we see it, and what it implies—a radiologic-pathologic correlation, *South Med J* 85:946–952, 1992.

Krishnamurthy C, Hilden K, Peterson KA, et al: Endoscopic findings in patients presenting with dysphagia: analysis of a national endoscopy database, *Dysphagia* 27:101, 2012.

Marshall JB, Kretschmar JM, Diaz-Arias AA: Gastroesophageal reflux as a pathogenic factor in the development of symptomatic lower esophageal rings, *Arch Intern Med* 150:1669–1672, 1990.

Müller M, Gockel I, Hedwig P, et al: Is the schatzki ring a unique esophageal entity?, *World J Gastroenterol* 17:2838, 2011.

Novacek G: Plummer-vinson syndrome, *Orphanet J Rare Dis* 1:36, 2006.

Nurko S, Teitelbaum JE, Husain K, et al: Association of schatzki ring with eosinophilic esophagitis in children, *J Pediatr Gastroenterol Nutr* 39(1):107, 2004.

Pezzullo JC, Lewicki AM: Schatzki ring, statistically reexamined, *Radiology* 228:609–613, 2003.

Plummer HS: Diffuse dilatation of the esophagus without anatomic stenosis (cardiospasm): a report of ninety-one cases, *JAMA* 58:2013–2015, 1912.

Scolapio JS, Pasha TM, Gostout CJ, et al: A randomized prospective study comparing rigid to balloon dilators for benign esophageal strictures and rings, *Gastrointest Endosc* 50:13–17, 1999.

Vinson PP: A case of cardiospasm with dilatation and angulation of the esophagus, *Med Clin North Am* 3:623–627, 1919.

5

Esophageal Diverticula

Neil R. Floch

Based on radiologic and endoscopic studies, esophageal diverticula have a prevalence of up to 3% of individuals. They may be classified according to cause (pulsion or traction), location (pharyngoesophageal, midesophageal, or epiphrenic), or wall component (full thickness [true diverticula] or mucosal/submucosal [pseudodiverticula]) (Fig. 5.1). Zenker diverticula account for 70% of all esophageal diverticula.

CRICOPHARYNGEAL DIVERTICULA

Zenker, or pharyngoesophageal, diverticula occur 10 times more often than other esophageal diverticula; 80% to 90% of cases occur in men, and the average age is 50 years. Predisposing factors may include esophageal dysmotility, a shortened esophagus, as well as dysfunction of the upper esophageal sphincter (UES). Zenker diverticula develop as the mucosa and submucosa of the hypopharynx herniate between the inferior constrictor and the cricopharyngeal muscles in the posterior midline. This area is known as the Killian triangle. The developing sac becomes stretched over time as it protrudes to the left, posterior to the esophagus, and anterior to the prevertebral fascia. Evidence suggests that patients with Zenker diverticula have more scar tissue and that degenerated muscle fibers of the cricopharynx have a smaller opening and increased hypopharyngeal bolus pressure during swallowing. Changes in the morphology of the unique fiber orientation of the cricopharyngeal muscle may impair its dilation and are thought to be caused by progressive denervation of the muscle.

Clinical Picture

Initially patients may have the sensation of a lump in the throat and may accumulate copious amounts of mucus. Patients may report foul-tasting food, halitosis, and nausea. Dysphagia to liquids and eventually dysphagia to solids may occur. Patients may regurgitate undigested food when coughing, and some may develop aspiration pneumonia or a lung abscess. As the disease progresses, obstruction may result in significant weight loss and malnutrition.

Diagnosis

On examination there is usually fullness under the left sternocleidomastoid muscle, with resultant gurgling on compression. Barium esophagraphy may demonstrate the size, location, and degree of distention of the diverticulum. Esophagoscopy reveals a wide mouth pouch that ends blindly as well as two lumens above the cricopharyngeal muscle. The opening of the esophagus may be pushed anteriorly and kinked by the diverticulum. The manometry pattern may demonstrate findings consistent with dysmotility of the UES and may differentiate dysphagia secondary to a recent cerebrovascular accident (stroke).

Treatment, Management, Course, and Prognosis

Treatment for a Zenker diverticulum is surgical, by either an open external cervical or minimally invasive approach. Endoscopic approaches employ either a rigid endoscope and stapler or a flexible endoscope. All techniques to treat Zenker diverticula include a cricopharyngeal myotomy. Minimally invasive approaches depend on the availability of a surgeon skilled in these techniques. Open surgery has been associated with increased morbidity from both its invasive nature and the morbidity of the patient population.

Open surgery for a Zenker diverticulum includes diverticulectomy, invagination, diverticulopexy, and myotomy. Morbidity ranges from 3% for myotomy to 23% for diverticulectomy with myotomy. Significant improvement occurs in 92% of patients; 6% experience recurrence with diverticulectomy, and 21% have recurrence with invagination. Open techniques result in better symptomatic relief than endoscopic staple diverticulostomy (ESD), especially in patients with small diverticula. Resection without myotomy is initially effective but may result in recurrence or fistulas in the long term.

The ESD procedure is a minimally invasive or endoscopic approach. Flexible endoscopy techniques were first reported in 1995. ESD may be performed in up to 85% of patients with Zenker diverticula, although a large diverticulum with redundant mucosa is a risk factor for recurrence. A linear stapler is placed with one blade in the esophagus and the other in the diverticulum as the stapler is fired across the cricopharyngeal muscle. ESD is a safe, effective procedure with a high level of patient satisfaction. The morbidity rate is 2% to 13% with staplers. The recurrence rate is 12%, but it is as high as 64% in some studies.

Flexible endoscopy procedures involve coagulation and cutting of the cricopharyngeal muscle shared by the esophagus and the diverticulum, allowing flow of substances from the diverticulum into the esophagus. The midline of the septum is cut using this technique. The procedure can be performed under light or deep sedation. If bleeding or microperforations occur, they can be treated using endoclips. After more than 2 years, there is a 77% to 95% complete resolution of symptoms. Esophageal microperforation occurs in 3% to 19%, but 82% resolve with conservative treatment. There is a 15% symptom recurrence rate.

Generally patients recover and return to their normal diets quickly, and complication and mortality rates are lower than with open procedures. When ESD is compared with other endoscopic procedures, duration of surgery and mortality rates are similar, but there are fewer complications and a quicker convalescence with ESD.

Small diverticula may be treated by diverticulectomy with or without myotomy. Large diverticula may be treated by any of the mentioned methods. Patients younger than 60 years of age or those with very large diverticula should undergo diverticulectomy. Elderly patients with multiple comorbidities should be treated by ESD.

PULSION DIVERTICULA

Epiphrenic or pulsion diverticula usually occur singly and are located in the distal 10 cm of the esophagus. Multiple diverticula are found in persons with scleroderma. They occur equally on the left and right

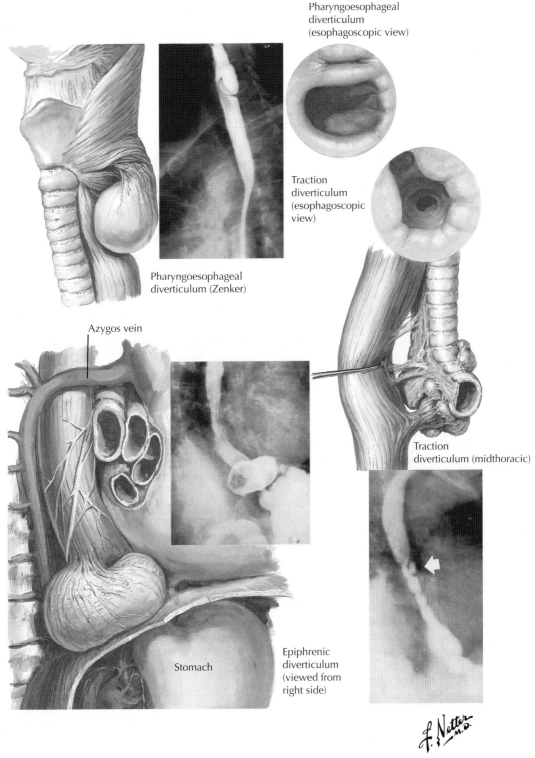

Pharyngoesophageal
diverticulum
(esophagoscopic view)

Traction
diverticulum
(esophagoscopic
view)

Pharyngoesophageal
diverticulum (Zenker)

Azygos vein

Traction
diverticulum (midthoracic)

Stomach

Epiphrenic
diverticulum
(viewed from
right side)

Fig. 5.1 Esophageal Diverticula.

sides at an incidence of less than 1 in 100,000. They usually range in size from 3 to 10 cm.

There is a high prevalence (up to 100% of patients) of primary motility disorders in patients with epiphrenic diverticula. Diverticula may be associated with achalasia, diffuse esophageal spasm (DES), nutcracker esophagus (NE), hypertensive lower esophageal sphincter (HLES), and other nonspecific dysmotility disorders (see Chapter 14). They are believed to occur secondary to dyscoordination of muscular contractions that cause the inner mucosa to protrude through the outer esophageal muscle and to a high resting lower esophageal sphincter (LES) pressure with resultant increased intraluminal pressure. Patients usually have associated hiatal hernia with reflux, which may result from poor esophageal clearance due to dysmotility. Histologic abnormalities of the esophageal myenteric plexus were found in 80% of patients without motility disorders. Distal esophageal diverticula have also been associated with reflux strictures and other lesions. Earlier literature categorized diverticula according to location and not by cause. Midesophageal diverticula are usually pulsion diverticula that develop secondary to motility disorders.

Clinical Picture

In the largest Cochrane analysis, symptoms usually related to the size of the diverticula, with a median size of 5 cm and a range of 1 to 16 cm. Primary symptoms were dysphagia in approximately 81% of patients, regurgitation in 71%, and pulmonary symptoms in 25%. The usual duration of the primary symptoms before presentation was 10 years. In more than one-third of patients, these symptoms were severe, making lethal aspiration a risk. Halitosis may occur from the retention of food contents in the lesion, and chest pain may result from an associated motility disorder. If the contents of the pouch become infected, the pouch can rupture, resulting in bronchopulmonary complications such as bleeding or sepsis. Symptoms of midesophageal diverticula are similar to those of epiphrenic diverticula except that reflux is usually not present.

Diagnosis

An esophageal diverticulum is easily visualized during barium esophagraphy. Videoesophagraphy may add further benefit. Endoscopy should be performed to evaluate any coexistent abnormalities or to obtain a biopsy specimen. Manometry has been traditionally performed in only 80% of operative patients and is used to determine the function of the esophageal body and LES pressure; it usually indicates that the diverticula result from a motility disorder. An esophageal motor disorder is diagnosed through motility testing in approximately 70% to 90% of patients. When diagnosis is difficult, 24-hour ambulatory motility testing may be used and can clarify the diagnosis in almost 100% of patients. Underlying disorders are achalasia in 17% to 43%, HLES in 14%, DES in 24%, NE in 10%, and nonspecific motor disorder in 10% to 66% of patients.

Treatment and Management

Esophageal diverticula are surgical problems and 50% to 75% of patients undergo surgery. Treatment is indicated for diverticula that are 5 cm or larger in size. Surgery must include treatment of the underlying motor disorder, which may be the cause of the diverticula. Although 89% of diverticula are removed, other options include performing a diverticulopexy in 3% or leaving the diverticulum alone and performing only a myotomy in 7%. The surgical approach is by thoracotomy in over 50%, with the remaining procedures being treated with minimally invasive, thoracoscopic, or laparoscopic techniques. Leak rates are lower than with open left thoracotomy. Length of stay is shorter with minimally invasive techniques. Concomitant endoscopy can test for leaks and confirm repair. If a diverticulum is excised at its base, muscle is closed over the area, and myotomy is performed on the opposite side at the same level.

Small diverticula are inverted and oversewn. Whether the diverticulum should be surgically resected or suspended depends on its size and proximity to the vertebral body. Usually midesophageal diverticula are those adjacent to the spine and may be suspended. Patients improve or symptoms resolve in 85% with diverticulectomy compared with 65% of those who underwent a diverticulopexy or only a myotomy. Diverticulectomy should be performed when symptoms such as regurgitation can be directly correlated with the presence of the diverticulum.

A myotomy is performed in 85% of patients. This is done from the neck of the diverticulum to below the LES. Long myotomy is performed for patients with motility disorders, and its length is tailored according to manometry results. Myotomy of the LES should be performed to prevent breakdown of the staple line and rupture of the esophagus, which may be caused by the same intraluminal pressure that initially gave rise to the diverticulum. If the underlying motility disorder is not treated, leak is likely to occur. In a major Cochrane analysis, myotomy significantly reduced staple-line leak rates from 26% to 12%.

The need for an antireflux procedure in diverticular patients remains controversial, but 66% of patients undergo a procedure that is most commonly a partial fundoplication. Postoperative leak and reflux rates are the same; they are 19% with or 21% without the addition of a fundoplication procedure. The types of procedures performed are Dor, 40%; Belsey Mark IV, 25%; Toupet, 20%; and Nissen, 15%.

Midesophageal diverticula are treated with thoracotomy or thoracoscopy. Patients with moderate to severe symptoms undergo surgery. Diverticula are removed, and myotomy is performed. Because the LES is not divided, fundoplication is not performed.

Course and Prognosis

Results are good to excellent in 90% to 100% of surgical patients that are followed long-term after resection or imbrication of the diverticula. The most common morbidity is caused by staple-line leak in 13%. Good results are indicated by resolution of symptoms, weight gain, and no clinical recurrence. Approximately 50% of patients who do not undergo myotomy have less favorable results. Results for thoracoscopy and laparoscopy approach those for open techniques, but with less morbidity. The overall morbidity is 21%, with 26% for open surgery and 17% for minimally invasive surgery. There is an overall reoperation rate of 9% and an in-hospital mortality rate of 6%. Diverticulectomy resulted in better symptom resolution and lower rates of staple-line leak. Leak rates are reduced by routine myotomy. Both open and minimally invasive approaches have resulted in similar outcomes. The addition of an antireflux procedure does not significantly improve postoperative reflux symptoms. Approximately 66% of patients who do not undergo surgery remain symptomatic or become symptomatic.

TRACTION DIVERTICULA

Traction diverticula were first discovered in patients with tuberculosis and mediastinal lymph nodes. Currently tuberculosis and histoplasmosis are the usual causes, although other etiologies, such as sarcoidosis, have been reported.

Traction diverticula result from inflammation of paratracheal and subcarinal lymph nodes that adhere to and scar the esophagus. Adhesion pulling results in a diverticulum, usually in the midesophagus. Traction diverticula are an outpouching of all the esophageal layers and differ from pulsion diverticula that occur in the midesophagus but are caused by dysmotility.

Clinical Picture

Most midesophageal diverticula are asymptomatic and discovered incidentally. Symptomatic patients report chest pain, odynophagia, and regurgitation. Evaluation should be conducted to determine the presence of an esophageal motility disorder to distinguish it from pulsion diverticula. If dysmotility is not present, a traction or congenital diverticulum should be suspected. Rarely, a young infant will be born with a bronchoesophageal fistula with symptoms of coughing and aspiration of food.

Diagnosis

Traction diverticula of the midesophagus are usually incidental findings on barium swallow or upper endoscopy. Barium esophagraphy reveals poorly demarcated diverticula. Endoscopy may also be helpful in the diagnosis.

Treatment and Management

Most patients with traction diverticula are not treated. If symptoms are severe, thoracotomy is performed, the diverticulum is removed, and the opening is sewn. No myotomy is necessary.

Course and Prognosis

If left untreated, some lesions may erode or extend into the adjacent lung or bronchial arteries and may cause clinical symptoms such as pneumonia or gastrointestinal bleeding.

ADDITIONAL RESOURCES

Anselmino M, Hinder RA, Filipi CJ, Wilson P: Laparoscopic heller cardiomyotomy and thoroscopic esophageal long myotomy for the treatment of primary esophageal motor disorders, *Surg Laprosc Endosc* 3:437–441, 1993.

Evrard S, Le Moine O, Hassid S, Deviere J: Zenker's diverticulum: a new endoscopic treatment with a soft diverticuloscope, *Gastrointest Endosc* 58:116–120, 2003.

Guirguis S, Azeez S, Amer S: Sarcoidosis causing mid-esophageal traction diverticulum, *ACG Case Rep J* 3(4):e175, 2016. Published online 2016 Dec 7.

Klaus A, Hinder RA, Swain J, Achem SR: Management of epiphrenic diverticula, *J Gastrointest Surg* 7:906–911, 2003.

Lewis A, Clark WG, Blackshaw GWB: Systematic review and meta-analysis of surgical treatment of non-zenker's oesophageal diverticula, *J Gastrointest Surg* 21:1067–1075, 2017.

Melman L, Quinlan J, Robertson B, et al: Esophageal manometric characteristics and outcomes for laparoscopic esophageal diverticulectomy, myotomy, and partial fundoplication for epiphrenic diverticula, *Surg Endosc* 23:1337–1341, 2009.

Nehra D, Lord RV, DeMeester TR, et al: Physiologic basis for the treatment of epiphrenic diverticulum, *Ann Surg* 235:346–354, 2002.

Schima W, Schober E, Stacher G, et al: Association of midoesophageal diverticula with oesophageal motor disorders: videofluoroscopy and manometry, *Acta Radiol* 38:108–114, 1997.

Zaninotto G, Portale G, Costantini M, et al: Long-term outcome of operated and unoperated epiphrenic diverticula, *J Gastrointest Surg* 12(9):1485–1490, 2008.

6

Foreign Bodies in the Esophagus

Neil R. Floch

More than 100,000 cases of ingested foreign bodies occur in the pediatric population each year. Although most are accidental, intentional ingestion starts in adolescence. Children under 5 years of age are often exposed to random household objects, and they often swallow coins; such cases were as high as 76% in one large study. Children also swallow toy parts, jewels, batteries, sharp objects (needles, pins, fish or chicken bones), metal objects, food, seeds, plastic material, magnets, buttons, nuts, hard candy, and jewelry, which can become lodged in the esophagus. Sharp objects such as a safety pin can become impacted in the esophagus of an infant or small child. Batteries represent less than 2% of foreign bodies ingested by children. Ingestion of multiple magnets can cause esophageal obstruction and perforation.

Foreign bodies become entrapped as frequently in adults as in children (Fig. 6.1). Psychiatric patients and prisoners may intentionally swallow objects for ulterior motives. In adults, the foreign body most often entrapped is food, usually meat (33%). Hasty eating may result in the swallowing of chicken or fish bones. Tacks, pins, and nails held between the lips may be swallowed and may attach to the esophageal wall or descend into the stomach and beyond. Pill ingestion may also be a cause of impaction.

In the esophagus, obstruction typically occurs at the three narrowest areas, including the upper esophageal sphincter, compression by the aortic arch in the esophagus, and at the lower esophageal sphincter. Of the 40% to 60% that become lodged in the esophagus, ingested objects are found above the cricopharynx in 57% to 89% of patients, at the level of the thoracic esophagus in approximately 26% of patients, and at the gastroesophageal junction in 17% of patients. A large proportion (30%–38%) of these people may have an underlying esophageal disease. Along their way, foreign bodies can cause destruction in the form of impactions, ulcerations, and perforations. The presence of other lesions in the esophagus—such as rings, strictures, diverticula, and tumors—may form a nidus for impaction. Impaction is also more likely in the presence of a dysmotility disorder such as achalasia. Most foreign bodies, or 80%, will migrate through the intestine and into the stool without incident. The remaining 20% will have to be extracted surgically.

CLINICAL PICTURE

Symptoms caused by foreign bodies lodged in the esophagus depend on the object's size, shape, consistency, and location. Many children will have had only transient symptoms or may be asymptomatic. About 50% of patients have symptoms at the time of ingestion, such as retrosternal pain, choking, gagging, or cyanosis. They may drool; dysphagia may occur in up to 70% and vomiting in 24%. Patients also report odynophagia, chest pain, and intrascapular pain. Children or adults with long-standing esophageal foreign bodies reveal signs such as weight loss, aspiration pneumonia, and fever. If esophageal perforation is the eventual presentation, there will be crepitus, pneumomediastinum, or gastrointestinal bleeding.

Infants are unable to express their discomfort or locate the sensation of pain; they may have vague symptoms, making diagnosis difficult. Retching, difficulty swallowing, and localized cervical tenderness may be the only ways in which the obstruction can be confirmed.

DIAGNOSIS

Radiopaque substances, such as metallic objects, chicken or fish bones, or clumps of meat can readily be recognized on x-ray film. Therefore an anteroposterior and lateral x-ray of the neck, chest, and abdomen should be performed. Nonradiopaque objects, such as cartilaginous and thin fish bones, may be seen on computed tomography (CT) or during esophagoscopy if other modalities are not diagnostic.

TREATMENT AND MANAGEMENT

Treatment of foreign bodies depends on the type of object, its location, and the patient's age and size. Emergent removal of foreign bodies of the esophagus may be necessary because of the risk of respiratory complications and esophageal erosion or perforation.

Objects that are long and sharp, magnets, and those that contain superabsorbent polymers as well as disk batteries should always be removed because of their ability to cause a caustic injury and perforation. If the object is causing obstruction of the trachea or airway compromise, removal is imperative. Esophageal obstruction requires urgent removal; symptoms of fever, abdominal pain, or vomiting may be indicative. If the time since ingestion is unknown or more than 24 hours, earlier removal has a better prognosis. Ingestion of a single magnet may be treated observantly; however, multiple magnets can attract in the bowel and cause necrosis and perforation and should be promptly removed.

Patients who are capable of tolerating their own secretions can delay treatment for a day. Objects such as food, coins, or blunt objects may have time to pass through the bowel spontaneously. Passage occurs naturally in 50% of all foreign body ingestions. Small, smooth objects and all objects that have passed the duodenal sweep should be managed conservatively by radiographic surveillance and stool inspection.

Spontaneous passage of coins in children occurs in 25% to 30% of cases without complications; therefore these patients should be observed for 24 hours, especially with distally located coins. Spontaneous passage of coins is more likely in older, male patients, especially when the coins become lodged in the distal third of the esophagus. If coins do not pass, esophageal bougienage or endoscopic removal may be required. For most objects, esophageal bougienage entails the lowest complication rate and the lowest cost.

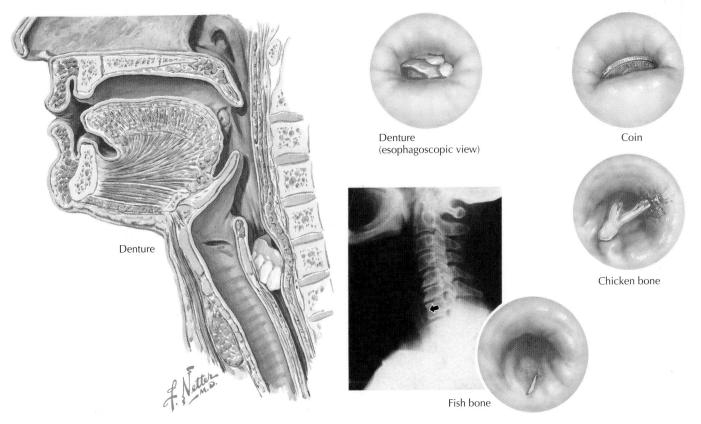

Denture

Denture
(esophagoscopic view)

Coin

Chicken bone

Fish bone

Fig. 6.1 Foreign Bodies in the Esophagus.

When foreign bodies are trapped in the upper esophagus or hypopharynx, rigid endoscopy or Magill forceps are most successful at extracting objects. Esophagoscopy is used for most foreign body extractions in the middle to lower esophagus because it is both diagnostic and therapeutic. Endoscopy can be adapted to extract multiple different types of objects in the esophagus as well as the stomach and duodenum. It can also assess for damage to the intestinal lining. It is successful in 95% to 98% of patients and results in minimal morbidity. Innovative methods such as a loop basket, suction retrieval, suture technique, double-snare technique, and combined forceps/snare technique for long, large, and sharp foreign bodies, along with newer equipment such as retrieval nets and specialized forceps, may be necessary if removal is difficult.

Management of blunt objects have a less than 1% complication rate. Sharp foreign bodies have a complication rate between 15% to 35% but straight pins cause less problems unless multiple are ingested. Ingested batteries that lodge in the esophagus require urgent endoscopic removal even in the asymptomatic patient because of the high risk of burns and possible death. Batteries that are 2 cm or larger in size are especially likely to become lodged. Patients must be anesthetized. Approximately 90% can tolerate conscious sedation; the rest require general anesthesia. The pressure from a large mass in the esophagus against the trachea may cause asphyxia, necessitating tracheotomy before the object can be removed, especially in children.

Food often accumulates above an entrapped object and must be removed by forceps. Food boluses can be removed using grasper devices, polypectomy snares, or retrieval nets; friction-fit adaptors can be used to break up the food or retrieve it in total or piecemeal. Small pieces of food may be pushed into the stomach. Maximal dilatation of the esophageal wall will allow visualization of the foreign body. Sharp or pointed objects (e.g., nails, pins, bristles) may become embedded in the esophageal wall with only their tips visible; they must be retrieved using endoscopic forceps.

On occasion, magnets are used to localize a metallic foreign body and position it so that it can be removed. Magill forceps enable quick, uncomplicated removal of coins in children, especially coins lodged at or immediately below the level of the cricopharyngeal muscle. Proximal dilatation using an oral side balloon is safe and effective for removing sharp foreign bodies from the esophagus, thus avoiding surgery and possible perforation; it is successful in 95% of patients.

Surgical treatment is unavoidable for the 1% of patients from whom an object cannot be retrieved by endoscopy and therefore the risk of perforation arises. These objects are usually lodged in the cervical esophagus. Surgical treatment of perforation includes cervical mediastinotomy or thoracotomy and drainage. Success of surgery depends on the size of the injury, its location, the time elapsed between rupture and diagnosis, the patient's underlying medical condition, and whether sepsis has developed. Ultimately poor conditions in esophageal perforation may result in mortality.

Conservative treatment is successful in patients with perforation but no abscess or significant contamination. These patients are treated immediately with broad-spectrum antibiotics and are not permitted food or liquids, receiving either enteral feeding or total parenteral nutrition until healing is documented by meglumine diatrizoate (Gastrografin) swallow. If the patient develops a cervical abscess or mediastinitis, he or she should undergo exploratory surgery with surgical drainage.

ADDITIONAL RESOURCES

Athanassiadi K, Gerazounis M, Metaxas E: Management of esophageal foreign bodies: a retrospective review of 400 cases, *Eur J Cardiothorac Surg* 21:653–656, 2002.

Janik JE, Janik JS: Magill forceps extraction of upper esophageal coins, *J Pediatr Surg* 38:227–229, 2003.

Jeen YT, Chun HJ, Song CW, et al: Endoscopic removal of sharp foreign bodies impacted in the esophagus, *Endoscopy* 33:518–522, 2001.

Kay M, Wyllie R: Pediatric foreign bodies and their management, *Curr Gastroenterol Rep* 7(3):212–218, 2005.

Kramer RE, Lerner DG, Lin T, et al: Management of ingested foreign bodies in children: a clinical report of the NASPGHAN Endoscopy Committee, *J Pediatr Gastroenterol Nutr* 60:562–574, 2015.

Lam HC, Woo JK, van Hasselt CA: Esophageal perforation and neck abscess from ingested foreign bodies: treatment and outcomes, *Ear Nose Throat J* 82:786, 789–794, 2003.

Mosca S, Manes C, Martino R, et al: Endoscopic management of foreign bodies in the upper gastrointestinal tract: report on a series of 414 adult patients, *Endoscopy* 33:692–696, 2001.

Waltzman ML, Baskin M, Wypij D, et al: A randomized clinical trial of the management of esophageal coins in children, *Pediatrics* 116(3):614–619, 2005.

Yardeni D, Yardeni H, Coran AG, et al: Severe esophageal damage due to button battery ingestion: can it be prevented?, *Pediatr Surg Int* 20(7):496–501, 2004.

7

Caustic Injury of the Esophagus

Neil R. Floch

Each year in the United States, 34,000 people ingest caustic substances (Fig. 7.1), leading to tissue destruction through liquefaction or coagulation reactions. The severity of destruction depends on the type, concentration, and amount of substance; whether it is in solid or liquid form; and the duration of contact with the esophageal mucosa. Ingestion of a caustic substance is the most common toxic exposure in children and is almost always accidental. In all patients, 60% of cases of caustic substance ingestion is suicidal, and in 40% it is accidental. Adults usually ingest caustic substances in attempts at suicide and are likely to have more severe injuries.

The most commonly ingested substances with suicidal intent are strong alkali composed of lye with sodium or potassium hydroxide. Solid crystal lye was most often used for suicide attempts until 1960, when liquid oven cleaners became most common. Liquid oven cleaners cause more distal esophageal burns that are more severe than those caused by lye. Household products such as drain cleaners and other house cleaning products are also common. Highly concentrated acids such as hydrochloric, sulfuric, and phosphoric acid used in toilet bowl or swimming pool cleaners are less common. Bleach, which is 5% sodium hypochlorite, rarely causes a severe esophageal injury. Batteries containing highly concentrated alkaline solutions can cause burns and perforations and should be removed emergently with endoscopy.

Alkali ingestion is more caustic to the esophagus compared with the more distal stomach and bowel, but acid such as glacial acetic acid results in a worse outcome. Acid victims were more likely to have severe mucosal injury, be in an intensive care unit, have perforation, and suffer higher mortality. Ingestion of alkali such as ammonia or sodium hydroxide results in a full-thickness injury to the esophageal wall, causing liquefactive necrosis at a pH greater than 11; this may result in perforation and mortality. The liquefactive process progresses over 4 days, leading to mucosal inflammation, thrombosis of vessels, and ulceration of the esophageal lumen. Cell death is complete by 4 days, and 80% of scars are formed within 60 days. The natural areas of esophageal approximation include the cricopharyngeus, aortic arch, and lower esophageal sphincter and are most commonly involved.

Over 2 weeks the wall becomes thin; fibrosis and regrowth occur, but this process is not complete for 3 months. The development of strictures depends on the depth of damage and degree of collagen deposition. The ingestion of alkali leads to esophageal stricture formation more often than exposure to acid. Morbidity and mortality result most often from severe second- and third-degree burns. Compared with alkali injury, acid-induced injury creates a superficial coagulation necrosis where the mucosal blood vessels thrombose and the connective tissue forms a protective eschar. Acid injury is also limited as it causes pain on contact, thus limiting intake, and moves quickly into the stomach.

CLINICAL PICTURE

Signs and/or symptoms of caustic injury may be misleading, as they may not correlate with the extent or severity of injury. Common symptoms include oropharyngeal, retrosternal, and epigastric pain, dysphagia/odynophagia, and/or an increase drooling and saliva production. The presence of additional symptoms and signs suggests a more severe injury, which warrants more aggressive management. Severe retrosternal or back pain may be a sign of the mediastinitis found in esophageal perforation. Airway injury may present with hoarseness, stridor, aphonia, and respiratory insufficiency. Hoarseness and stridor may indicate a need for intubation.

DIAGNOSIS

Before any diagnostic examination can be conducted, a detailed history of the type and quantity of ingested material must be taken. Plain radiographs of the abdomen will reveal a pneumothorax, pneumomediastinum, perforated viscus, or pleural effusion.

Patients may have significant esophageal injury despite the lack of oropharyngeal involvement. Once the patient has been stabilized, the clinician performs laryngoscopy to examine the vocal cords. Upper endoscopy should be performed, regardless of the presence or absence of symptoms, in the first 24 hours to evaluate for the presence of injury and determine the treatment and prognosis. Patients must be hemodynamically stable to proceed and may have to be intubated if there is respiratory instability.

Caustic injuries to the gastrointestinal tract and esophagus are classified similarly to burns. The following grading system is used to assess the level of caustic injury to the esophagus: grade 0, normal; grade 1, superficial mucosal damage with diffuse erythema, edema, and hemorrhage; grade 2A, both mucosal and submucosal damage with ulcers, exudates, and vesicles; grade 2B, deep focal or circumferential ulcers; grade 3A, transmural injury with ulceration; grade 3B, extensive necrosis.

Patients with grades 1 and 2A injuries usually have an excellent outcome without stricture formation. From 70% to 100% of patients with grades 2B and 3A will eventually develop strictures. Early mortality occurs in 65% of grade 3B patients. Another grading system is based on computed tomography (CT) findings of esophageal wall edema and surrounding tissue damage; this modality may be able to predict the future occurrence of strictures.

TREATMENT AND MANAGEMENT

Patients who are asymptomatic and have accidentally ingested a small amount of dilute acid or alkali do not need endoscopy and can be

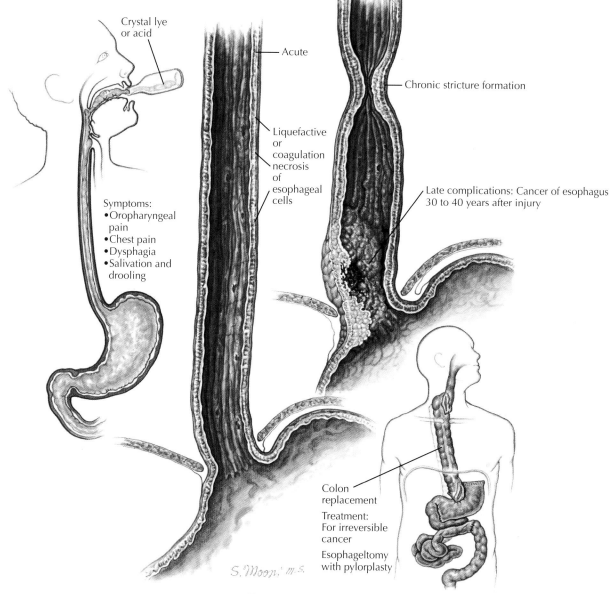

Crystal lye or acid

Acute

Chronic stricture formation

Liquefactive or coagulation necrosis of esophageal cells

Symptoms:
• Oropharyngeal pain
• Chest pain
• Dysphagia
• Salivation and drooling

Late complications: Cancer of esophagus 30 to 40 years after injury

Colon replacement

Treatment: For irreversible cancer

Esophageltomy with pylorplasty

S. Moon, M.S.

Fig. 7.1 Caustic Injury.

followed as outpatients. Signs and symptoms are not reliable guides to direct treatment, so endoscopy is performed in the first 24 hours. If endoscopy is normal, patients may be discharged home. Patients with grade 2A injuries or less may be started on a liquid diet and advanced to a regular diet in 2 days. All other patients are admitted, receive no food by mouth (are kept NPO), receive intravenous fluids, and are followed with repeated chest x-rays to check for complications. With minor burns, high-dose corticosteroids may improve the prognosis and prevent the formation of esophageal strictures. Overall, however, corticosteroids have no other benefit in treating caustic injuries or preventing strictures but tend instead to increase the risk for other complications.

Patients with a grade 2B or greater injury are severely ill and are treated in an intensive care unit. These patients should receive nasogastric feeding after 24 hours; liquids may be begun after 2 days of observation. If oral or nasogastric intake is restricted, high-protein and high-calorie feedings are given via a jejunostomy tube. Grade 3 injuries are observed for perforation for 1 week. Proton pump inhibitors (PPIs)

for ulcer prevention and narcotics for pain are given. Broad-spectrum antibiotics are given for grade 3 burns. If respiratory distress is present, laryngoscopy is performed, and patients are intubated if necessary. Antiemetics should be used to prevent vomiting of the caustic agent and reexposing the esophagus to the caustic agent. Neutralizing agents such as weakly acidic or basic substances should not be given as they may also damage the mucosa. Nasogastric tube placement may also lead to vomiting and should thus be avoided.

The findings on CT of esophageal wall blurring, periesophageal fat blurring, and the absence of esophageal wall enhancement are indicators for emergent surgery. A technique of endoscopic vacuum therapy with sponges in and on the esophagus combined with dilation may be used. Decreased tension and adequate vascular flow are the best indicators of anastomotic healing. The prognosis depends on the extent of esophageal injury and the patient's overall medical condition at the time of surgical intervention. Perforation and leaks lead to mediastinitis, which accounts for sepsis and most deaths.

Surgical esophagectomy is performed for patients with severe strictures as well as acutely for perforation, mediastinitis, or peritonitis. The need for surgery is a negative survival factor. Esophagectomy with colon interposition is usually performed, although gastric tube pull-up and small-bowel interposition are alternative options. In experienced hands, minimally invasive combined laparoscopic and thoracoscopic esophagectomy is the procedure of choice. It is associated with a faster recovery, quicker return to work, and shorter hospital stay. Despite these advantages, there are higher rates of anastomotic stenosis with minimally invasive procedures. Early complications of surgery include graft ischemia (10%), anastomotic leak (6%–10%), proximal strictures (5%), small-bowel obstruction (2%), and death (1%). Late complications include stenosis requiring dilation (50%), graft stenosis (1%), and bile reflux requiring surgical diversion (2%). Swallowing function postsurgery is excellent in 24% of patients, good in 66%, and poor in 10%. Surgical revision is required in 4%. Overall mortality is 4%, which is predicted by increased age, the ingestion of a strong acid, and an elevated white blood cell count.

COURSE AND PROGNOSIS

After resolution of the initial injury, patients are at risk for developing esophageal strictures, which occur in 33% and are associated with severe esophagitis. Most strictures occur after grade 2B or 3 injuries. Severe endoscopic lesions, involvement of the entire length of the esophagus, hematemesis, and increased levels of serum lactate dehydrogenase (LDH) are risk factors for stricture formation. Strictures are mild in approximately 15% of patients, moderate in 60%, and severe in 25%. Dysphagia may ensue from 2 weeks to many years after ingestion. Dysphagia from caustic strictures may be due to esophageal dysmotility where long waves of low amplitude occur in a damaged esophagus. Barium swallow may reveal strictures but is less sensitive than endoscopy.

Strictures are treated with dilations that are repeated, gradually increasing the diameter to avoid perforation. Earlier treatment results in better outcomes. Dilation is started 3 to 6 weeks after the initial injury, with the goal of dilating to 15 mm and thus relieving dysphagia. Some patients require repeated dilation to maintain an adequate lumen diameter.

With severe strictures, the lumen may be restricted to 2 to 3 mm. Temporary placement of self-expanding stents has been used; they are left in place for 2 to 13 months. Self-dilation can be performed with 45- to 60-Fr dilators. Mitomycin C may be used in conjunction with stents as it is an antifibroblastic substance. Patients treated with mitomycin C and dilation required fewer dilations to achieve success. Temporary esophageal stenting has been used to prevent stricture formation with some success, but prophylactic bougienage does not prevent stricture formation. Perforation occurs in approximately 0.5% of procedures. Dilation is successful in 60% to 80% of patients. Severe strictures may require esophagectomy. If the patient's condition deteriorates, surgery may be indicated.

Pharyngoesophageal strictures may be associated with a laryngeal injury. If these are present, a retrograde approach with a minilaparotomy

and gastrostomy may be necessary. If antegrade dilation is not technically possible, retrograde dilation may be attempted. Therapy depends on the location of the stricture, its length, the time of presentation after injury, proximity to the larynx, condition of the airway, presence of a cervical esophageal lumen, and presence or other strictures. Surgical options include colonic interposition or myocutaneous flaps with or without a tracheostomy. Satisfactory swallowing may be restored in 88% of cases.

After caustic ingestion, progression to cancer of the esophagus occurs in 2% of patients. Esophageal squamous cell carcinoma occurs 1000 times more frequently in individuals who have been exposed to lye ingestion compared with the general public. Carcinoma develops on average 41 years after the inciting event, more commonly with alkali exposure than acid exposure. Carcinoma in a lye scar presents at earlier stages and responds better to surgery and radiation. The prognosis is better because the scar causes dysphagia and is discovered early. Scar also blocks the lymphatic spread of the malignancy.

There is no proven benefit of screening, and the American Society for Gastrointestinal Endoscopy (ASGE) established guidelines only recently. Although there is no proven benefit, surveillance beginning 15 to 20 years after the ingestion and continuing every 1 to 3 years thereafter is suggested.

ADDITIONAL RESOURCES

Ananthakrishnan N, Kate V, Parthasarathy G: Therapeutic options for management of pharyngoesophageal corrosive strictures, *J Gastrointest Surg* 15:566, 2011.

ASGE Standards of Practice Committee, Lightdale JR, Acosta R, et al: Modifications in endoscopic practice for pediatric patients, *Gastrointest Endosc* 79:699, 2014.

Cabral C, Chirica M, de Chaisemartin C, et al: Caustic injuries of the upper digestive tract: a population observational study, *Surg Endosc* 26:214, 2012.

Chirica M, Resche-Rigon M, Bongrand NM, et al: Surgery for caustic injuries of the upper gastrointestinal tract, *Ann Surg* 256:994, 2012.

El-Asmar KM, Hassan MA, Abdelkader HM, Hamza AF: Topical mitomycin C application is effective in management of localized caustic esophageal stricture: a double-blinded, randomized, placebo-controlled trial, *J Pediatr Surg* 48:1621, 2013.

Hamza AF, Abdelhay S, Sherif H, et al: Caustic esophageal strictures in children: 30 years' experience, *J Pediatr Surg* 38:828–833, 2003.

Katzka DA: Caustic injury to the esophagus, *Curr Treat Options Gastroenterol* 4:59–66, 2001.

Kuehn F, Klar E, Schwandner F, et al: Endoscopic continuity-preserving therapy for esophageal stenosis and perforation following colliquative necrosis, *Endoscopy* 46(Suppl 1 UCTN):E361, 2014.

Nijhawan S, Udawat HP, Nagar P: Aggressive bougie dilatation and intralesional steroids is effective in refractory benign esophageal strictures secondary to corrosive ingestion, *Dis Esophagus* 29:1027, 2016.

Ryu HH, Jeung KW, Lee BK, et al: Caustic injury: can CT grading system enable prediction of esophageal stricture?, *Clin Toxicol (Phila)* 48:137, 2010.

Usta M, Erkan T, Cokugras FC, et al: High doses of methylprednisolone in the management of caustic esophageal burns, *Pediatrics* 133:E1518, 2014.

8

Esophageal Rupture and Perforation

Neil R. Floch

Esophageal perforation and rupture may occur from small penetrations after endoscopy; full-thickness ruptures may follow from a tear or penetration. Presentation, diagnosis, and treatment are variable. The rarity of the diagnosis and variability in clinical presentation often lead to diagnostic and treatment delays. This is especially true of spontaneous perforation, where the clinical suspicion is low. Evaluation for more common medical conditions—such as myocardial infarction, pneumonia, and peptic ulcer disease—usually occurs first. The most severe, traumatic perforations represent 75% of esophageal injuries, with spontaneous rupture of the esophagus less common; however, both are surgical emergencies (Fig. 8.1).

Greater than 50% of esophageal perforations are iatrogenic, most occurring during endoscopy with dilation, ablation, resection, or endoscopic antireflux procedures. Major causes include barotrauma in 15% from seizure, weightlifting, or Boerhaave syndrome. Foreign body ingestion occurs in 12% of patients and includes objects (e.g., coins, pins) and food (e.g., fish or chicken bones). Trauma may be the cause in 9% and can result from penetration and blunt injury. Intraoperative injury may occur in 2% due to the placement of nasogastric tubes, endotracheal or Sengstaken-Blakemore tubes, and bougies; it may also occur in the course of neck or chest surgery and laparoscopic foregut surgery.

Perforation may result from malignancies in 1% or from inflammatory processes such as Crohn disease and gastroesophageal reflux with ulcers. Infection is always a possibility as well. Caustic alkaline or acid injury may also cause esophageal damage, as may peptic ulcers, pill esophagitis, or esophageal diseases such eosinophilic esophagitis. Approximately 70% of perforations occur on the left side of the esophagus, 20% occur on the right side, and 10% are bilateral.

Esophageal perforation usually occurs at the narrowest areas of the esophagus: the cricopharyngeal muscle, the bronchoaortic constriction, and the esophagogastric junction. Increased intraluminal pressure at these sites along with predisposing conditions of a malignancy, foreign body, or physiologic dysfunction are more likely to lead to rupture of the esophagus.

Perforation of the cervical esophagus through endoscopy is likely in areas of blind pouches, such as a Zenker diverticulum or the pyriform sinus. It is common in elderly persons who have kyphosis and are unable to open their mouths completely because of muscle contracture. The endoscopist is usually immediately aware of the perforation because bleeding occurs, and the anatomy is difficult to discern. Overall, the distal third of the esophagus is the most common site of perforation because it is also the most frequent location for tumors and inflammation. Patients with evidence of a malignancy at the time of esophagogastroduodenoscopy may have as high as a 10% incidence of perforation.

Boerhaave syndrome, or spontaneous rupture of the esophagus, occurs from barotrauma due to violent coughing, vomiting, or weightlifting or from the Heimlich maneuver. A sudden pressure transfer of 150 to 200 mm Hg across the gastroesophageal junction causes damage. Spontaneous rupture occurs in the distal or lower third of the esophagus on the posterolateral wall and results in a 2- to 3-mm linear tear, frequently on the left side of the chest and in alcoholic patients. Penetrating trauma is more likely to cause rupture than blunt trauma. Tearing may occur during misidentification of the retroesophageal space during laparoscopy or with improper passage of a bougie.

With only a sparse connective tissue barrier and no adventitia, the esophagus has limited defenses. Once it is ruptured, infection migrates diffusely and rapidly. The mortality rate from perforation is high because the anatomy of the esophagus enables direct communication with the mediastinum, allowing the entry of bacteria and digestive enzymes and leading to sepsis, mediastinitis, empyema, and multiorgan failure.

CLINICAL PICTURE

Symptoms are determined by the location and size of the perforation and by the interval between injury and discovery. Diagnosis is difficult in most patients because 50% have atypical histories. Often, however, patients with esophageal injury have an acute attack or "ripping" chest, back, and epigastric pain. Crepitus may be palpated, and hematemesis, fever, and leukocytosis may develop. Patients with cervical injuries frequently have dysphagia and odynophagia, which increases with neck flexion. Thoracic perforations cause not only substernal chest pain but also epigastric pain. Substernal pain, cervical crepitus, and vomiting affect 60% of patients with spontaneous rupture from barotrauma. Patients with abdominal perforations have epigastric, shoulder, and back pain. Fever, dyspnea, cyanosis, sepsis, shock, and eventually multiorgan failure may develop with increasing contamination of the mediastinum and chest.

DIAGNOSIS

Chest radiographs are obtained first in patients with esophageal injury but have limited sensitivity and specificity. An hour after the incident, the chest radiograph may show air under the diaphragm or subcutaneous/mediastinal emphysema in 40% of patients. Pneumothorax may be seen in 77% of patients, in which case the pleura must also have been injured. Pleural effusion then develops.

Meglumine diatrizoate (Gastrografin) esophagraphy is performed next because the material used is better tolerated if leaked into the mediastinum. If no leak is found, a barium study is performed because it has 90% sensitivity for finding a small leak. Patients at risk for aspiration should have a barium swallow, given that meglumine diatrizoate may cause pulmonary edema. Studies are performed in the right lateral decubitus position. Computed tomography can confirm the diagnosis by revealing extraluminal air, periesophageal fluid, esophageal thickening, or extraluminal contrast. Esophagoscopy may demonstrate small

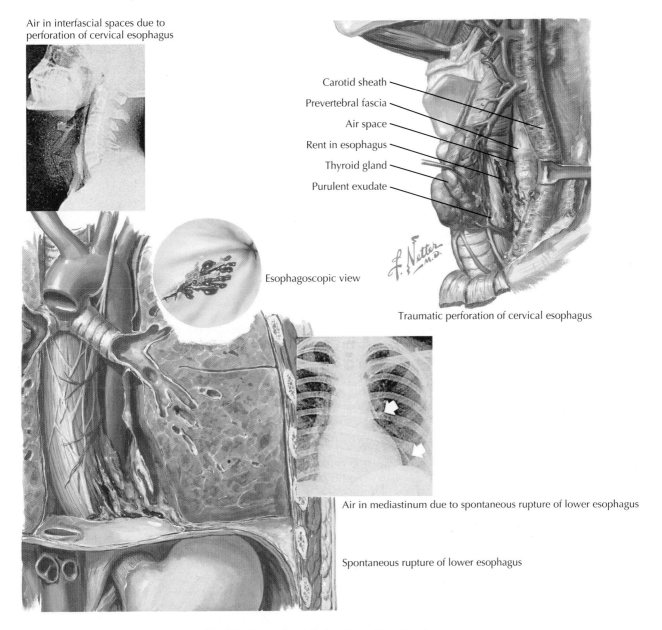

Air in interfascial spaces due to perforation of cervical esophagus

Carotid sheath
Prevertebral fascia
Air space
Rent in esophagus
Thyroid gland
Purulent exudate

Esophagoscopic view

Traumatic perforation of cervical esophagus

Air in mediastinum due to spontaneous rupture of lower esophagus

Spontaneous rupture of lower esophagus

Fig. 8.1 Rupture and Perforation of the Esophagus.

bruises or tears and is most diagnostic in penetrating trauma. The use of an endoscope has not been shown to worsen the clinical situation.

TREATMENT AND MANAGEMENT

In most instances esophageal perforation is a surgical emergency. The diagnosis should be rapid, and treatment should begin with hemodynamic monitoring in the intensive care unit (ICU). Patients should be optimized for surgery with the intention to close the defect with control of infection. Nutrition must also be maintained. All treatment begins with intravenous fluids and broad-spectrum antibiotics as well as an antifungal, especially for those on proton pump inhibitor (PPI) medications. Treatment depends on the location of the injury and presence of any underlying disease.

The simplest injuries to the esophagus, such as an enterotomy in the operating room with minimal to no contamination, may be closed primarily with drainage and possible nasogastric tube placement. For major perforations, primary repair remains the preferred treatment up to 24 hours after the incident. Exceptions to this treatment include cervical perforations that cannot be visualized, mediastinal necrosis, defects that are too large to repair, malignancy, achalasia, or an unstable patient. Devitalized tissue is removed, then the muscular layer is opened longitudinally to expose the complete perforation. The mucosa is then closed with absorbable interrupted sutures with a second interrupted layer of the muscularis with nonabsorbable sutures. Muscular flaps are optional for improved healing when there is significant contamination. An intercostal muscle flap is the first choice, followed by serratus, latissimus dorsi, diaphragm, parietal pleura, and omentum. The lower esophageal injuries are buttressed by placing the gastroesophageal junction in the abdomen to prevent reflux and performing either a posterior Nissen or an anterior Dor fundoplication depending on the location of the injury.

Cervical perforations may be repaired primarily if they are visualized and have no distal obstruction. Otherwise, irrigation and external drainage is performed. Alternatives include applying dressings to an open wound or using a wound vac. A feeding tube is used in the case of significant malnutrition. Perforations of the thoracic esophagus are treated with a thoracotomy. A right thoracotomy at the sixth or seventh intercostal space is used for a midesophageal perforation, whereas a distal esophageal perforation is performed through a left thoracotomy at the seventh or eighth intercostal space. A posterior intercostal muscle flap or pedicled flap is used to reinforce a primary repair. Pulmonary decortication, irrigation, and drainage with large 28- to 32-Fr chest tubes, a nasogastric tube, and a feeding jejunostomy are used. Abdominal perforations are treated with the same principles as cervical and thoracic perforations. The hiatus is closed posteriorly and a Dor partial anterior fundoplication or a Nissen complete posterior fundoplication is used depending on the location of the perforation and history of dysphagia. Drains and a feeding jejunostomy are used as well.

Alternatives to primary repair may be necessary when there is either hemodynamic instability or minimal contamination. In the presence of severe mediastinitis, friability, and necrosis, only drainage and/or diversion are used. Surgical drainage alone is used when a cervical esophageal perforation is not visualized and is not obstructed. Drainage alone is not recommended in the thoracic or intraabdominal esophagus because leakage will not be controlled.

In severe mediastinal sepsis, significant comorbid illness, and large thoracic esophageal perforations, multiple techniques may be used together, such as debridement, drainage, muscle flap, and endoscopic stent placement performed to control sepsis and prevent the need for a second operation. A T-tube can be inserted into the perforation proximally and distally to create a controlled fistula in an unstable patient.

A diversion is performed in the left neck in unstable patients where the defect is difficult to repair because of its large size, friability, or the presence of preexisting disease. Diversion includes resection of the distal esophagus, control of leakage, drainage, a cervical esophagostomy, gastrostomy, and feeding jejunostomy. If the patient is severely unstable, the distal esophagus can be stapled and a cervical esophagostomy, a gastric feeding tube, and drains in the mediastinum are placed, with the remaining esophagus removed later. Reconstruction is performed 6 to 12 months later, after recovery, and may entail a colonic interposition.

Metallic stents are being used with success for esophageal perforations, avoiding open surgery, as they may be inserted and removed endoscopically. Stents cover the area of perforation and halt leakage and contamination into the mediastinum. A covered stent with a 2-cm or greater overlap proximally and distally is preferred. Potential complications of stents include bleeding and fistulization. Despite the skill of the endoscopist, the stent may kink or cause an erosion. Patients may become intolerant to the symptoms of gastroesophageal reflux disease, especially reflux. Stent migration is the greatest problem, occurring in 33% of patients. The stents are monitored with repeat abdominal x-rays to follow their location.

The four risk factors for stent failure include perforations that are in the proximal cervical area, that traverse the gastroesophageal junction, that are longer than 6 cm, and that include anastomotic and distal leaks. A percutaneous endoscopic gastrostomy (PEG) should be placed before a stent is inserted. The stent must completely cover the area of leakage. Debridement and drainage of extraluminal contamination, if significant, must be also performed. Esophagography with oral contrast is used to assess placement of the stent and ensure exclusion. Oral intake is started once leakage has been controlled.

Endoscopic clipping can close an esophageal mucosal defect in clinically appropriate patients. Endoscopists experienced with peroral endoscopic myotomy (POEM) for the treatment of achalasia may be capable of performing this procedure. Clipping works best for iatrogenic injuries with limited contamination that can be drained or small defects with healthy surrounding tissue that is pliable. Management is the same as for stents, and barium esophagraphy is used to make sure that closure is maintained.

An esophagectomy is performed at the time of a perforation in stable patients with minimal contamination who have a malignancy, extensive esophageal damage that cannot be repaired, or severe benign disease such as achalasia or a stricture that cannot be dilated.

COURSE AND PROGNOSIS

Morbidity occurs in 38% of patients; the most common complications include continued leak, fistulization, mediastinitis, empyema, stricture, pneumonia, abscess, mediastinitis, and sepsis. Treatment outcome depends on comorbidities, the interval between diagnosis and treatment, the cause and location of injury, and the presence of esophageal disease. Mortality from an esophageal perforation is dependent on the cause of the perforation, the type of repair, the location of perforation, and the length of delay in diagnosis. Patients commonly will die of sepsis causing multiorgan failure. Mortality rates are dependent on the cause and location of the perforation. The cause of mortality in ruptured esophagus is spontaneous in 39%, iatrogenic in 19%, and traumatic in 19%. Location dictates mortality with cervical (6%), thoracic (34%), and intraabdominal lesions (29%). The overall mortality for diagnosis within 24 hours was 14% versus 27% if there was greater than a 24-hour delay.

ADDITIONAL RESOURCES

Boumitri C, Kumta NA, Patel M, Kahaleh M: Closing perforations and postperforation management in endoscopy: duodenal, biliary, and colorectal, *Gastrointest Endosc Clin N Am* 25:47, 2015.

Cooke DT, Lau CL: Primary repair of esophageal perforation, *Oper Tech Thorac Cardiovasc Surg* 13:126, 2008.

Duncan M, Wong RK: Esophageal emergencies: things that will wake you from a sound sleep, *Gastroenterol Clin North Am* 32:1035–1052, 2003.

Guirguis S, Sulaiman A, Sarwat A: Sarcoidosis causing Mid-esophageal traction diverticulum, *ACG Case Rep J.* 3(4):e175, 2016. Published online 2016 Dec 7.

Gupta NM, Kaman L: Personal management of 57 consecutive patients with esophageal perforation, *Am J Surg* 187:58–63, 2004.

Kollmar O, Lindemann W, Richter S, et al: Boerhaave's syndrome: primary repair vs. esophageal resection—case reports and meta-analysis of the literature, *J Gastrointest Surg* 7:726–734, 2003.

Port JL, Kent MS, Korst RJ, et al: Thoracic esophageal perforations: a decade of experience, *Ann Thorac Surg* 75:1071–1074, 2003.

Rubesin SE, Levine MS: Radiologic diagnosis of gastrointestinal perforation, *Radiol Clin North Am* 41:1095–1115, 2003.

Sharma P, Kozarek R, Practice Parameters Committee of American College of Gastroenterology: Role of esophageal stents in benign and malignant diseases, *Am J Gastroenterol* 105:258, 2010.

Zubarik R, Eisen G, Mastropietro C, et al: Prospective analysis of complications 30 days after outpatient upper endoscopy, *Am J Gastroenterol* 94:1539–1545, 1999.

Zumbro GL, Anstadt MP, Mawulawde K, et al: Surgical management of esophageal perforation: role of esophageal conservation in delayed perforation, *Am Surg* 68:36–40, 2002.

9

Esophageal Varicosities

Neil R. Floch

Esophageal varices are diagnosed in almost one-third of compensated cases and almost two-thirds of decompensated cases of cirrhosis. Bleeding may occur in one-third of cases and is related to the size of the varix and the severity of the liver disease. There is a 1 in 8 chance of bleeding annually if varices are present. Each bleed has up to a 20% risk of resulting in death.

Varicosities occur secondary to portal hypertension and are defined as dilatations of various alternative pathways when cirrhosis obstructs the portal return of blood (Fig. 9.1). Varicosities occur most often in the distal third but may occur throughout the esophagus. *Acute variceal hemorrhage* is the most lethal complication of portal hypertension. The median age of these patients is 52 years, and 73% are men.

The most common cause of portal hypertension, affecting 94% of patients, is cirrhosis. The most common causes of cirrhosis are alcoholism (57%), hepatitis C virus (30%), and hepatitis B virus (10%).

Mortality rates from the initial episode of variceal hemorrhage range from 17% to 57%. Larger vessels bleed more frequently. Hospitalizations for acute bleeding from esophageal varices have been declining in recent years; this is believed to be a result of more active primary and secondary prophylaxis. Bleeding occurs when the tension in the venous wall leads to rupture, and shock may follow. Occasionally the bleeding may stop spontaneously, but more often it will recur. Thrombocytopenia and impaired hepatic synthesis of coagulation factors both interfere with hemostasis.

CLINICAL PICTURE

Cardinal symptoms of esophageal varicosities are recurrent hematemesis and melena. Patients with acute variceal bleeding have hemodynamic instability (61%), tachycardia (22%), hypotension (29%), and orthostatic hypotension (10%).

DIAGNOSIS

To prevent a first variceal hemorrhage, patients with cirrhosis should undergo upper endoscopy to screen for esophageal varices and, if present, characterize them. Endoscopy should be performed when the patient's condition is stable. The risk of initiating bleeding from the varices is negligible. Endoscopy should also be performed for any patient who has hemorrhage of unexplained cause. In 25% of patients with varices that present with upper intestinal bleeding, the diagnosis hemorrhage from a source other than the varices. Esophageal varices are believed to be the cause of bleeding if no other source of the bleeding is found. Other causes include gastric or duodenal ulcers, gastritis, a Mallory-Weiss tear, and gastric varices.

At endoscopy, the varices are blue, round, and surrounded by congested mucosa as they protrude into the lumen of the distal esophagus. They are soft and compressible, and an esophagoscope can easily be passed beyond them. Erosion of the superficial mucosa with an adherent blood clot signifies the site of a recent hemorrhage. On establishing the presence of esophageal varices, the clinician should also search for gastric varicosities, because the surgical treatment may have to be modified if these have developed.

Imaging is not part of the screening process. Only 40% of varicosities can be seen on radiographs. A typical finding is a "honeycomb" formation produced by a thin layer of barium surrounding the venous protrusion that does not constrict the lumen. Endoscopic color Doppler ultrasonography is a useful modality for obtaining color-flow images of esophageal varices and their hemodynamics. Capsule endoscopy is now being studied as a possible screening tool for esophageal varices; it has a sensitivity and specificity of 84% and 88%, respectively. Recently, 64-row multidetector computed tomography (CT) portal venography reliably displayed the location, morphology, origin, and collateral types of esophageal varices, showing promise as a diagnostic tool. CT was found to have 90% sensitivity and 50% specificity in finding esophageal varices. It also has the benefit of detecting extraluminal pathology that cannot be seen by endoscopy.

TREATMENT AND MANAGEMENT

Variceal management encompasses three phases: (1) prevention of initial bleeding, (2) management of active bleeding, and (3) prevention of rebleeding. Treatment includes pharmacology, endoscopy, radiologic shunting, and surgery. Preprimary prophylaxis attempts to prevent varices from developing in patient with portal hypertension. In these individuals, liver disease should be treated, but nonselective beta blockers have not proven to be beneficial. The goal of primary prophylaxis is to prevent hemorrhage from occurring in patients with known esophageal varices. There are two acceptable treatments that have been shown to be better than observation. Endoscopic variceal ligation (EVL) has been demonstrated in studies to prevent an initial bleed; however, it does not ensure a lower mortality risk, and EVL carries potential complications. When beta-blockers are used and tolerated, they may result in a low incidence of side effects and may be beneficial in reducing the development of both ascites and spontaneous bacterial peritonitis. Secondary prophylaxis aims to prevent individuals with a history of bleeding varices from having another variceal bleed.

Prophylaxis can then be instituted according to categorization. Low-risk patients with hepatitis C are found to have platelet counts ≥150,000/μL and liver stiffness below 20 kPa on transient elastography; such individuals may avoid endoscopy as long as these parameters are not exceeded. In other patients who, on screening, do not have varices and compensated cirrhosis, endoscopy can be repeated every 2 to 3 years. If small varices are found, esophagogastroduodenoscopy (EGD) should be performed every 1 to 2 years. Those with decompensated cirrhosis should have yearly endoscopies.

Although many endoscopists categorize them simply as small or large, the North Italian Endoscopic Club has categorized esophageal varices as follows:

- F1: Small varices, straight in appearance
- F2: Large tortuous varices involving less than 33% of the esophagus

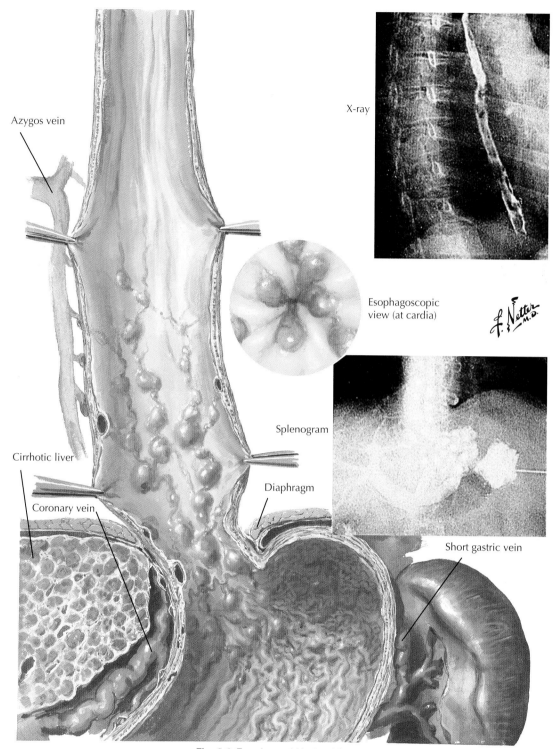

Azygos vein

X-ray

Esophagoscopic
view (at cardia)

Splenogram

Cirrhotic liver

Diaphragm

Coronary vein

Short gastric vein

Fig. 9.1 Esophageal Varicosities.

- F3: Large coiled varices involving more than 33% of the esophageal lumen

The Child-Pugh classification is a predictor of surgical risk in patients with cirrhosis. It has been modified from the Child-Turcotte classification, which was based on the variables of serum albumin, bilirubin, ascites, encephalopathy, and nutritional status. Nutritional status was replaced with the prothrombin time in the new classification. A score of 5 or 6 is Child-Pugh class A cirrhosis with a 10% mortality risk, 7 to 9 is class B cirrhosis with a 30% mortality risk, and 10 to 15 is class C cirrhosis with an 82% mortality risk after undergoing nonshunting abdominal surgery.

Prophylaxis is started with nonselective beta blockers, of which nadolol 40 mg/day is the treatment of choice. It reduces portal pressure and variceal blood flow and decreases the risk of bleeding by 50%. The medication can be adjusted according to the patient's response. Carvedilol may be used as an alternative. The goal of beta blockade is to reduce the HVPG (hepatic venous portal gradient). "Red signs" are the appearance of varices on endoscopy that appear as red wale marks or long red marks, red, flat spots known as cherry-red spots, red, raised spots or hematocystic spots or the presence of diffuse erythema. Prophylaxis is given to patients who have small varices with red signs or Child B or C cirrhosis and those with medium or large varices. Other patients with Child A and small varices do not receive prophylactic treatment and are followed by endoscopy. Patients with small varices with red signs or Child B or C cirrhosis are treated with a nonselective beta blocker. Those who cannot tolerate this are treated with EVL. In individuals with medium or large varices, either a nonselective beta blocker or EVL is used, but EVL may be more effective with larger varices.

Measurements of hepatic venous pressure are used to monitor the success of pharmacologic therapy, which has been shown to be superior to sclerotherapy and possibly superior to band ligation. A recent meta-analysis showed that a combination of endoscopic and pharmacologic therapy reduces overall and variceal rebleeding in cirrhosis more than either therapy alone.

If beta blockers are not tolerated or contraindicated or if patients are at high risk for bleeding, endoscopic band ligation is preferred. The surveillance of varices, with potential rebanding, should be repeated every 6 months.

Acute bleeding requires simultaneous control, resuscitation, and prevention/treatment of complications. Medical treatment of bleeding with vasopressin, terlipressin, somatostatin, or octreotide is started. These medications stop the bleeding in 65% to 75% of patients, but 50% will bleed again within a week. Vasopressin is a posterior pituitary hormone that constricts splanchnic arterioles and reduces portal flow and pressure. Prophylactic intravenous antibiotics should also be started. Endoscopy is performed to diagnose and treat hemorrhage.

Definitive therapy is first performed with sclerotherapy or band ligation, which is successful in 90% of patients. Varices are injected with sclerosing solutions to stop acute bleeding. Repeated injections will cause variceal obliteration and may prevent recurrent bleeding. However, recurrence is common before complete obliteration, and esophageal strictures typically develop.

Endoscopic band ligation results in fewer strictures and ulcers than sclerotherapy and faster eradication. Rebleeding is less frequent with ligation than with sclerotherapy (26% vs. 44%), but the number of blood transfusions, duration of hospital stay, and mortality risk are comparable.

When bleeding is under control, endoscopic ligation and sclerotherapy are repeated every 1 to 2 weeks until the varices are eradicated. This technique has the fewest complications and the lowest incidence of recurrence. Surveillance is performed at 3- to 6-month intervals to detect and treat any recurrence. Patients who have two or more rebleeding episodes should be considered for surgery or transplantation.

Balloon tamponade is used as a bridge to definitive therapy in 6% of patients when hemostasis is not achieved. Connected balloons in the stomach and the esophagus compress the varices. Bleeding stops in 80% to 90% of patients but, unfortunately, 60% have recurrences. Complications such as aspiration and esophageal rupture may also occur. A new method involves the use of a self-expanding stent to stop acute variceal bleeding, and initial studies reveal no method-related mortality or complications.

If medical and endoscopic therapies fail, transjugular intrahepatic portosystemic shunt (TIPS) is the procedure of choice in case of emergency. TIPS should be reserved for patients who have poor liver function. It can be performed in 90% of patients but is used in only 7%. The mortality rate with TIPS is low. Bleeding may recur in 15% to 20% of patients over 2 years. Patients must be followed closely because the shunt may occlude in up to 50% of cases within 18 months.

Shunt procedures are not the modality of choice because they result in a high rate of complications compared with medical therapy. Shunts are now used in less than 1% of patients. Emergency bleeding may be controlled with a central portocaval shunt or with combined esophageal transection, gastric devascularization, and splenectomy in patients hoping for liver transplantation. Emergency shunt surgery carries a 50% mortality risk and is rarely undertaken.

Surgical shunts should be used to prevent rebleeding in patients who do not tolerate or who are noncompliant with medical therapy and who have relatively preserved liver function. Portal decompression procedures create a connection between the high-pressure portal and low-pressure systemic venous systems. Nonselective shunts include portacaval anastomoses and TIPS, which decompress the entire portal system. Selective shunts, such as the distal splenorenal shunt, decompress only esophageal varices. Shunt surgery does not improve survival and may result in hepatic encephalopathy. Elective shunt procedures are avoided in candidates for liver transplantation but may be performed in those with Child A and B cirrhosis. Liver transplantation is the best therapy for patients with Child C cirrhosis and is performed in only 1% of patients.

COURSE AND PROGNOSIS

Acute variceal hemorrhage occurs more often in patients with Child B and C cirrhosis. Endoscopic banding is the most common single endoscopic intervention. Early rebleeding occurs in 13% of patients within a week. Although medical therapy, banding, and sclerotherapy are still used frequently for rebleeding, balloon tamponade is necessary in 17%, TIPS in 15%, and surgical shunting in 3% of patients. Early complications after acute variceal bleeding include esophageal ulceration (2%–3% of patients), aspiration (2%–3%), medication adverse effects (0%–1%), dysphagia and odynophagia (0%–2%), encephalopathy (13%–17%), and hepatorenal syndrome (2%). The prognosis for patients with bleeding esophageal varices depends directly on liver function. Overall short-term mortality rates after acute bleeding are 10% to 15%. However, in patients with cirrhosis who have variceal bleeding, mortality risk is as high as 60% at 1 year.

Maintenance screening depends on the presence of varices and whether the patient's disease is chronic. Those with chronic disease should have endoscopy every 1 to 2 years. Patients with compensated cirrhosis but no varices should have endoscopy every 2 years, and those with compensated cirrhosis and small varices should have yearly surveillance. In patients where the liver injury has subsided, such as former alcoholics and those cured of hepatitis C, an EGD every 2 to 3 years is appropriate. Prophylactic treatment is started if varices increase in size or red signs develop. Decompensation at any time warrants an endoscopy. Patients with larger varices who are on beta blocker treatment need endoscopy only if there is bleeding.

Patients who receive variceal banding should have a repeat EGD every 1 to 2 weeks or until all the varices have been treated. Thereafter, an endoscopy is repeated at 1 to 3 months and every 6 to 12 months thereafter to rule out recurrences.

ADDITIONAL RESOURCES

Comar KM, Sanyal AJ: Portal hypertensive bleeding, *Gastroenterol Clin North Am* 32:1079–1105, 2003.

De Franchis R, Eisen GM, Laine L, et al: Esophageal capsule endoscopy for screening and surveillance of esophageal varices in patients with portal hypertension, *Hepatology* 47(5):1595–1603, 2008.

Jamal MM, Samarasena JB, Hashemzadeh M, et al: Declining hospitalization rate of esophageal variceal bleeding in the United States, *Clin Gastroenterol Hepatol* 6(6):689–695, quiz 605, 2008.

Laine L, el-Newihi HM, Migikovsky B, et al: Endoscopic ligation compared with sclerotherapy for the treatment of bleeding esophageal varices, *Ann Intern Med* 119:1–7, 1993.

Perri RE, Chiorean MV, Fidler JL, et al: A prospective evaluation of computerized tomographic (CT) scanning as a screening modality for esophageal varices, *Hepatology* 47(5):1587–1594, 2008.

Sorbi D, Gostout CJ, Peura D, et al: An assessment of the management of acute bleeding varices: a multicenter prospective member-based study, *Am J Gastroenterol* 98:2424–2434, 2003.

Zaman A: Current management of esophageal varices, *Curr Treat Options Gastroenterol* 6:499–507, 2003.

Zehetner J, Shamiyeh A, Wayand W, et al: Results of a new method to stop acute bleeding from esophageal varices: implantation of a self-expanding stent, *Surg Endosc* 22(10):2149–2152, 2008.

10

Eosinophilic Esophagitis

Neil R. Floch

Eosinophilic esophagitis (EOE) is a chronic inflammatory disorder propagated by interleukin-5 (IL-5); it is unrelated to gastroesophageal reflux disease (GERD). Formerly a rare disease initially described in children and young men, EOE has been diagnosed more frequently in the past 10 years. According to current estimates, EOE has an annual incidence of 10 per 100,000 in children and teenagers and 30 per 100,000 in the adult population. EOE has a male:female ratio of 3:1. It leads to structural esophageal alterations but does not affect the nutritional state and has no malignant potential. EOE is distinguished by the presence of eosinophilic infiltration of the esophageal mucosa of at least 15 eosinophils per high-power field (hpf) in a patient without a previously identified cause of eosinophilia.

The pathogenesis of EOE is not completely understood, but clinical evidence and basic science support that it is an immune-mediated disease initiated by allergens that are inhaled or consumed. Exposure to the allergens with resultant sensitization may be a genetically acquired predisposition. The foods that are most allergenic include corn, chicken, wheat, beef, soy, eggs, and milk. The pathologic process may entail the activation of eosinophils, mast cells, and lymphocytes with the resultant release of molecules that trigger the onset of symptoms.

CLINICAL PICTURE

EOE is suspected in adults with symptoms of progressive and persistent dysphagia, food impaction, or GERD that fail to respond to proton pump inhibitor (PPI) therapy. EOE should also be suspected in children with feeding intolerance, vomiting, abdominal pain, dysphagia, food impaction, and GERD symptoms. Patients with EOE may have signs and symptoms similar to those of GERD, but EOE often continues despite prolonged treatment with PPIs. The diagnosis is more suspicious in younger males with a history of food and environmental allergies and/or asthma.

A recent analysis of 24 studies revealed the presence of dysphagia in 93% of EOE patients, food impaction in 62%, heartburn in 24%, and peripheral eosinophilia in 31%. Other symptoms include chest pain, dyspepsia, nausea, vomiting, odynophagia, abdominal pain, and weight loss.

DIAGNOSIS

The diagnosis of EOE necessitates the presence of both symptoms and histologic findings. Upper endoscopy is performed to visualize the esophagus and obtain biopsy results. Biopsies should be performed following 2 months of treatment with a twice-daily PPI or a negative DeMeester score on 24-hour pH monitoring. Two to four biopsies should be obtained from the distal esophagus 5 cm above the gastroesophageal junction (GEJ) as well as two to four more from either the middle or proximal esophagus at least 15 cm above the GEJ. The results of four

biopsies have a sensitivity approaching 100%. Patients should also undergo gastric and duodenal biopsies to rule out eosinophilic gastroenteritis. Although endoscopy is normal in 7% of patients, other endoscopic features consistent with EOE include stacked circular rings in 55%. strictures in 38%. attenuation of the subepithelial vascular pattern and linear furrowing that may extend the entire length of the esophagus in 33%, eosinophilic microabscesses in 16%, and a small-diameter esophagus in 10% (Fig. 10.1).

Diagnosis is established by the finding of 15 or more eosinophils/hpf on microscopy of a mucosal biopsy. Histologic findings include eosinophilic microabscesses, superficial layering of eosinophils, sheets of eosinophils, extracellular eosinophilic granules, subepithelial and lamina propria fibrosis and inflammation, basal cell hyperplasia, and papillary lengthening. Although not diagnostic, radiographic findings of strictures and a ringed esophagus as well as laboratory findings such as IgE levels greater than 114,000 U/L may also support the diagnosis of EOE. Esophageal manometry is not a diagnostic modality for EOE but will reveal evidence of a concomitant esophageal motility disorder in 40% of patients.

TREATMENT AND MANAGEMENT

The management of EOE includes pharmacologic, endoscopic, and dietary interventions. Both adults and children should be evaluated by a food allergist, as active environmental and food allergens should be identified and avoided. A six-food elimination diet is now being used as a primary treatment. This diet can improve symptoms of EOE while also helping to identify foods that may be causative. Nutritionists must closely monitor patients on elimination diets, as a reduction of nutrients and calories may be detrimental. Dietary changes may lead to complete healing and resolution of symptoms in patients with EOE, but the reintroduction of foods may bring about a return of symptoms. Treatment must be based on a balance between food exclusion, patient tolerance, and compliance with diet.

After skin and patch tests, three options exist: removal of foods that react to the skin test, removal of foods most often responsible, or use of an elemental or elimination diet. The patient is instructed to follow the diet for 2 months, after which endoscopy is repeated with biopsy. If the biopsy is normal, foods are reintroduced. If abnormal, an elemental or elimination diet is once again implemented. Reintroduction of food starts with the least allergenic foods, then slow introduction of more allergenic foods. If foods are associated with symptoms, they are stopped. This method has resulted in a socially acceptable diet in almost 70% of patients.

Medical treatment includes swallowed fluticasone using a metered-dose inhaler without a spacer. The medication is first sprayed into the mouth and then swallowed. Patients should not eat or drink for 30 minutes after taking this medication. Treatment starts for 6 to 8 weeks

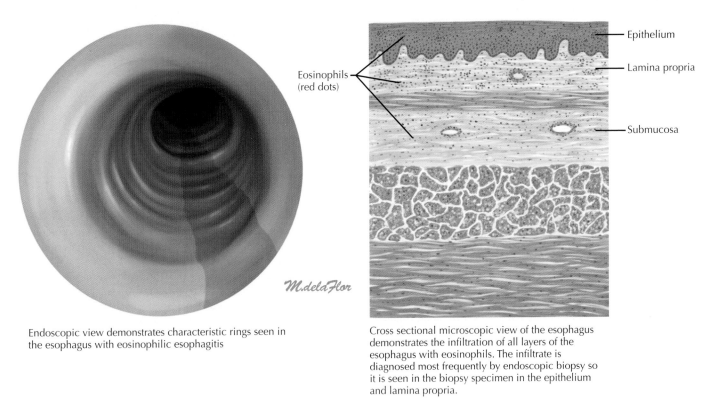

Endoscopic view demonstrates characteristic rings seen in the esophagus with eosinophilic esophagitis

Cross sectional microscopic view of the esophagus demonstrates the infiltration of all layers of the esophagus with eosinophils. The infiltrate is diagnosed most frequently by endoscopic biopsy so it is seen in the biopsy specimen in the epithelium and lamina propria.

Fig. 10.1 Eosinophilic Esophagitis.

and may be continued indefinitely, as eosinophilia will return once the medication is discontinued. The administration of corticosteroids results in symptomatic improvement in more than 95% of patients with EOE. Strategies include treatment on a symptomatic basis and using the lowest effective dosage that eliminates symptoms. When dysphagia becomes more severe, the presence of a candida esophagitis must be entertained. When fluticasone therapy fails, budesonide or an elimination diet is recommended. Adverse effects include growth retardation, bone abnormalities, and adrenal suppression.

Adult patients with strictures or rings who may need dilatation should receive fluticasone prior to attempting dilation for symptom relief. This is a safe therapy that rarely results in perforation, although superficial mucosal tears can occur in one-third of dilatations. Most patients will need two dilatations to achieve symptomatic relief.

COURSE AND PROGNOSIS

The diagnosis of EOE is made in individuals who fail twice-daily PPI therapy and undergo esophagogastroduodenoscopy (EGD) with positive biopsies. Long-term PPI therapy is recommended only when reflux is suspected. Endoscopic surveillance is usually not routine but repeat EGD is performed when symptoms change. The long-term treatment of EOE focuses on symptomatic control and mucosal healing. Currently topical and inhaled fluticasone and an elimination diet are the most successful options to achieve this goal.

ADDITIONAL RESOURCES

Dellon ES, Gonsalves N, Hirano I, et al: ACG clinical guideline: evidenced based approach to the diagnosis and management of esophageal eosinophilia and eosinophilic esophagitis (EoE), *Am J Gastroenterol* 108:679, 2013.

Furuta GT, Katzka DA: Eosinophilic esophagitis, *N Engl J Med* 373:1640, 2015.

Furuta GT, Lightdale CJ: Eosinophilic esophagitis, *Gastrointest Endosc Clin North Am* 18:1, 2008.

Helou EF, Simonson J, Arora A: Three-year follow-up of topical corticosteroid treatment for eosinophilic esophagitis in adults, *Am J Gastroenterol* 103:2194–2199, 2008.

Lucendo AJ, Castillo P, Martín-Chávarri S, et al: Manometric findings in adult eosinophilic oesophagitis: a study of 12 cases, *Eur J Gastroenterol Hepatol* 19(5):417–424, 2007.

Sgouros SN, Bergele C, Mantides A: Eosinophilic esophagitis in adults: a systematic review, *Eur J Gastroenterol Hepatol* 18(2):211–217, 2006.

11

Gastroesophageal Reflux Disease

Neil R. Floch

GASTROESOPHAGEAL REFLUX DISEASE

Gastroesophageal reflux is a normal occurrence involving the movement of gastric contents through the lower esophageal sphincter (LES) into the esophagus. Physiologic reflux is usually harmless until the process causes symptoms and physical changes in the esophagus; then typical reflux becomes a disease.

Gastroesophageal reflux disease (GERD) is a common condition that may require long-term treatment. It accounts for 75% of diseases that occur in the esophagus. GERD cannot be diagnosed by symptoms alone because patients with a similar presentation may have other conditions—such as achalasia, diffuse esophageal spasm, gastritis, cholecystitis, duodenal ulcer, esophageal cancer, or coronary artery disease—that share similar symptoms. Patients may also have atypical symptoms and may initially be misdiagnosed.

Esophagogastroduodenoscopy (EGD) is used to distinguish between the two types of GERD: erosive esophagitis (EE) with physical changes in the esophageal mucosa and nonerosive reflux disease (NERD) where no changes are visible and there is no endoscopic evidence of esophagitis. EGD may reveal esophagitis, of which only 90% is secondary to reflux. Ambulatory 24-hour pH testing or capsule based ambulatory pH testing may be diagnostic for acid or nonacid reflux. (Fig. 11.1).

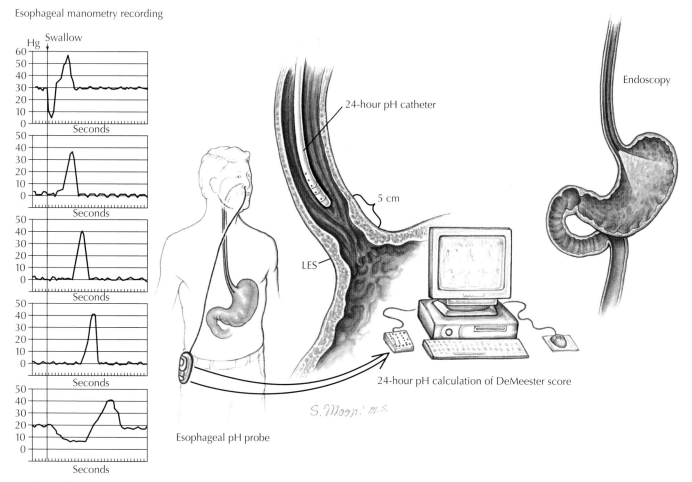

Esophageal manometry recording

Intraluminal esophageal pressures in response to swallowing.

Esophageal pH probe

24-hour pH catheter

5 cm

LES

24-hour pH calculation of DeMeester score

Endoscopy

S. Moon, M.S.

Fig. 11.1 Esophageal Tests. *LES,* Lower esophageal sphincter. (Graph from Waters PF, DeMeester TR: Foregut motor disorders and their surgical management, *Med Clin North Am* 65:1238, 1981.)

The pathophysiology of GERD is complex and not completely understood. The antireflux mechanism depends on proper function of the esophageal muscle, LES, and stomach. Reflux develops when LES pressure drops with gastric distention and the LES length shortens. Over time, transient lower esophageal sphincter relaxations (TLESRs) become more common and the valve becomes permanently damaged, resulting in manifestations of GERD. The esophageal muscle works to clear the lumen to both acid and duodenal contents. Poor luminal clearance increases the exposure time, allowing previously healthy epithelium to become damaged. The composition of the reflux fluid and the susceptibility of the esophagus, oropharynx, and respiratory structures to damage may lead to complications or extraintestinal manifestations of the disease.

NERD is the most common type of GERD; it is characterized by typical reflux symptoms but there are no visible mucosal changes on endoscopy. Only 50% of patients with NERD have abnormal 24-hour pH monitoring. The histopathologic feature found in NERD patients is dilated intercellular spaces within the squamous cell epithelium. This ultrastructural abnormality is detected on transmission electron microscopy and light microscopy.

Although GERD is chronic and usually nonprogressive, complications may include esophageal erosions, ulceration, stricture, Barrett's esophagus, and esophageal adenocarcinoma (as discussed elsewhere). Progression from one condition to another is not clearly established across the GERD continuum, although there is a clear progression from Barrett's esophagus to esophageal adenocarcinoma. Evidence suggests that patients with NERD may be less susceptible to complications. Recent studies reveal that *Helicobacter pylori* eradication leads to more resilient GERD.

There are 120 million Americans with GERD symptoms, 19 million of whom suffer from nonacid reflux symptoms, or *duodenogastroesophageal reflux* (DGER). Patients who have GERD-like symptoms despite maximum proton pump inhibitor (PPI) therapy and lack evidence of acid reflux may be diagnosed with nonacid reflux. The presence of bile, pepsin, and pancreatic enzymes in addition to acid indicates a more destructive environment and therefore more severe disease.

Clinical Picture

Heartburn is the main symptom of GERD. It is a burning sensation in the chest or epigastrium caused by stomach acid that has risen into the esophagus. Among American adults, 44% experience heartburn monthly, 18% weekly, and 5% to 10% daily. Typical symptoms of GERD also include reflux of acid, regurgitation of food, epigastric abdominal pain, dysphagia, odynophagia, nausea, bloating, and belching. Recent data support that being overweight or even moderate weight gain among persons of normal weight may cause or exacerbate symptoms of reflux. The severity of symptoms is not a reliable indicator of the severity of EE. Chronic abnormal gastric reflux results in EE in 50% of patients, but GERD patients may also be asymptomatic.

Atypical or extraesophageal symptoms include noncardiac chest pain, choking, laryngitis, coughing, wheezing, difficulty breathing, sore throat, hoarseness, asthma, and dental erosions. GERD is present in the 50% of patients who have atypical chest pain and negative results on coronary angiography. GERD is linked to asthma and chronic cough, and it is found in 80% of persons with asthma. Increasing vagal output, bronchoconstriction, and microaspiration are believed to be the mechanisms that lead to asthma in patients with GERD.

Reflux symptoms are responsible for almost 33% of otolaryngologic disorders. Patients with extraesophageal reflux (EER) have increased amounts of laryngeal reflux despite an adequate esophageal clearance mechanism. Chronic laryngitis may occur from laryngopharyngeal reflux (LPR), as acid can irritate the larynx, resulting in voice changes. Other symptoms include coughing, choking, clearing of the throat, and airway spasm. Patients with LPR may develop laryngeal and tracheal stenosis. They may present with symptoms of airway obstruction such as shortness of breath, coughing, wheezing, and hemoptysis. Increased TSLERs may cause the problem. The ciliated epithelium of otolaryngologic structures is more susceptible to damage from gastric reflux, and upper airway damage may occur from fewer and briefer episodes. The active pepsin in EER disease contributes to laryngeal lesions and eustachian tube dysfunction.

Symptomatic patients with nonacid reflux complain of heartburn and regurgitation most frequently while actively taking PPI medications. Extraesophageal symptoms of GERD are not often believed to be associated with nonacid reflux. Episodes of nonacid reflux occur most frequently after meals as the LES muscle relaxes transiently at a higher frequency. These episodes are triggered by a meal that stretches the stomach. Nonacid refluxate is composed of consumed food and liquid that is nonacid and dilutes the gastric stomach acid. PPI treatment decreases the acidity of the stomach contents but does not alter the physiologic mechanisms that cause fluid to come up through the LES owing to the presence of a hiatal hernia, a weak LES, or transient relaxation. It is unclear how nonacid material irritates the lower esophagus and causes symptoms.

Diagnosis

In patients presenting with classic GERD symptoms such as heartburn and/or regurgitation, a diagnosis may be established. These individuals will have a 40% to 90% symptomatic response to treatment with PPIs; however, as a meta-analysis of reflux testing confirms, a medical response does not confirm a GERD diagnosis. Diagnosis of GERD, its complications and future treatment depends on a combination of radiologic, pathologic, physiologic, and endoscopic findings. Tests are selected based on the information needed and may include esophageal pH monitoring, impedance testing, acid provocation tests, modified barium swallow, and endoscopy.

Simple barium esophagraphy is the easiest test to order and perform; therefore it may be completed first in any workup. It may reveal esophageal disease, but it is not as sensitive as cineradiography because it cannot detect spontaneous reflux in 60% of patients. However, when reflux is found on barium swallow, it is specific and is almost always confirmed by 24-hour pH testing. Video radiography records the act of swallowing, which may then be observed at several speeds. This technique is helpful during the pharyngeal phase of swallowing by identifying structural abnormalities of the esophagus, such as ulcers, strictures, paraesophageal hernia, masses, reflux, and obstruction.

In most patients with newly suspected problems, endoscopy is the preferred method to diagnose reflux or hiatal hernia, grade esophagitis, and obtain a biopsy. EGD is not recommended for patients who have only typical symptoms of GERD. Diagnostic testing in the form of upper endoscopy should be performed in patients who have alarm features or symptoms on clinical presentation. Alarm features are symptoms or clinical findings that suggest the presence of malignancy and include the following: a first episode of dyspepsia when in a patient 60 years of age or older, any new onset of upper or lower gastrointestinal (GI) bleeding or guaiac positivity, iron-deficiency anemia, anorexia, unattempted weight loss, difficulty swallowing or pain on swallowing, dysphagia, continued vomiting, or a history of a GI cancer in a first degree relative.

If a patient has had GERD for over 5 to 10 years and not had an endoscopy, EGD should be performed to rule Barrett's esophagus. Other risk factors that should warrant screening for Barrett include age over 50, Caucasian ethnicity, presence of a hiatal hernia, body mass index (BMI) greater than 30, nighttime reflux symptoms, present tobacco use or history of same, or a first-degree relative with either Barrett's esophagus or adenocarcinoma of the esophagus. Upper endoscopy should also be performed in patients who have persistent symptoms despite having initially been treated with medication for 4 to 8 weeks. Repeat EGD is performed for those at risk for complications of esophagitis with Los Angeles classification C and D (see esophagitis section) or after 2 months of treatment with PPI medication.

The Los Angeles Classification is the most widely accepted of the classification systems used to grade disease severity. Up to 50% of patients with GERD have NERD. Compared with patients who have EE (75%) and Barrett's esophagus (93%), patients with NERD (45%) were significantly less likely to have abnormal pH findings.

With respect to the treatment of GERD, esophageal pressure topography (EPT) analysis of high resolution manometry (HRM) and the Chicago Classification have greatly improved the diagnosis of motility disorders. HRM establishes the diagnosis of esophageal motility disorder and the LES pressure in consideration of performing surgery as an option to treat GERD. A decreased LES pressure confirms the presence of a weak valve consistent with GERD. HRM can establish the diagnosis of esophageal gastric outlet obstruction (EGJOO) and achalasia, where valve pressure is too high. Manometry may also diagnose the absence of peristalsis and ineffective esophageal motility (IEM). A complete absence of peristalsis and a hypotensive LES are characteristic of scleroderma. In diagnoses of poor esophageal motility, a Toupet (partial) fundoplication is required instead of a full fundoplication in order to avert postoperative obstruction.

In 24-hour pH testing for GERD, a probe is placed 5 cm above the LES to obtain pH readings. This test measures real-time acid exposure and the ability of acid to clear the esophagus, correlating symptoms with acid exposure. Six determinants are used to calculate a DeMeester score: total time of reflux, upright time, supine time, number of episodes, number of episodes longer than 5 minutes, and longest episode. Any patient with a score greater than 14.72 is considered positive; the sensitivity and specificity of the test is 96%. Although 24-hour pH monitoring is the most sensitive and specific test for GERD, 25% of patients with GERD-compatible symptoms have a normal pH test. This test must be performed before surgery if the patient has no signs of GERD on EGD (i.e., the patient has NERD). The capsule based ambulatory pH testing system (Medtronic, Minneapolis, MN) is an endoscopically placed device that measures 24-hour pH without the need for a nasogastric tube. It is a more comfortable option for patients.

The standard acid reflux test, formerly the Bernstein test, is performed by placing a pH probe 5 cm above the LES and injecting 300 mL of 0.1 M hydrochloric solution into the stomach with a manometry probe. Four maneuvers are performed in four different positions, giving 16 recordings. More than two reflux episodes is a positive finding. This test is helpful for patients receiving long-term PPI therapy whose 24-hour pH values may be inaccurate. In several studies, PPIs were found 40 days after the dose was taken.

Multichannel intraluminal impedance (MII) is a new technique to assess the movement of substances in the esophagus based on differences in their conductivity to an alternating current. MII reacts to the electrical charges within the esophageal mucosal, submucosal, and muscular layers and to any other material within the esophagus that produces a charge. Electrical *impedance* is the converse of conductivity and decreases from air to mucosal lining, to saliva, to swallowed material, and finally to refluxed gastric contents (lowest impedance). Impedance increases and decreases depending on the material encountered. The use of multiple impedance detection sites on a single catheter reveals the direction of bolus movement. Combining MII with esophageal manometry or 24-hour pH on the same catheter expands the diagnostic tools for evaluation of esophageal function. Combined MII-pH

allows for the detection of all types of gastroesophageal refluxate: acid, nonacid, liquid, mixed, and air. In combined MII-pH, the pH sensor is used simply to characterize whether the refluxate is acid- or nonacid-based. The MII technology is not a replacement for current manometry or pH techniques but rather a complementary procedure that expands the diagnostic potential of esophageal function testing.

Recent studies reveal that 60% of reflux episodes are not conventional and can be detected only by impedance changes, not by 24-hour pH testing. More than 98% of reflux events detected by a decrease in pH to less than 4 were detected by impedance changes. Liquid-only reflux occurs in approximately 35% of patients, mixed liquid and gas reflux in 36%, and gas reflux in 27%. Liquid is confined to the distal esophagus in approximately 30% of patients, reaches the midesophagus in 60%, and reaches the proximal esophagus in 11%. Additional information provided by impedance technology is likely to have a major impact on the clinical management of patients with GERD.

The diagnosis of nonacid reflux or DGER is established in patients with breakthrough GERD symptoms while taking maximal PPI medication. Confirmation can be performed by combined multichannel intraluminal impedance and pH (MII-pH) testing indicating a pH of less than 4 in the refluxed fluid. This technique has mostly replaced 24-hour ambulatory bile monitoring. Bile served as a marker for duodenal substances and was detected by its light wavelength using an indwelling spectrophotometer probe. The presence of acid reflux may be confirmed by pH testing and is measured above 4.0, weakly acidic between 4.0 and 7.0 and below 7.0 as nonacid reflux. Most consider the criteria as above and below 4.0 to differentiate acid from nonacid reflux. MII-pH testing in a patient who is on PPI therapy can determine whether symptoms occur when all acid is eliminated, thus establishing the diagnosis of nonacid reflux.

Alternative diagnoses for reflux other than nonacid reflux may be reflux of gastric contents from poor gastric emptying, a hypersensitive esophagus, or functional heartburn. Impedance pH testing is needed to differentiate these diseases. Gastric emptying as measured with a radionucleotide-tagged meal is helpful in determining delayed emptying. Solids and liquids may be measured simultaneously with different markers. Pictures are taken at 5-minute intervals for 2 hours.

In the setting of a normal level of esophageal acid exposure but a positive correlation with episodic reflux of acid or weakly acid fluid, the diagnosis of a hypertensive esophagus is made. Functional heartburn is found when the pH testing demonstrates normal acid exposure with no symptom correlation. Dysphagia and reflux symptoms can indicate eosinophilic esophagitis (EOE) or an esophageal motility disorder.

Treatment and Management
Medical Treatment

Medical therapy cannot resolve abnormal LES function. Therefore the medical treatment of GERD centers on the suppression of intragastric acid secretion. Goals of treatment are to provide effective symptomatic relief, prevent symptom relapse, heal esophageal damage, and prevent complications of GERD.

Lifestyle and dietary changes are the first steps in treatment because of their low cost and simplicity; these changes include elevating the head of the bed, modifying the size and composition of meals, consuming low-fat foods, and avoiding coffee, wine, tomato, chocolate, and peppermint. An analysis of 16 randomized trials revealed that of all lifestyle changes, only weight loss and head-of-bed elevation improved esophageal pH and GERD-associated symptoms.

Medical treatment may begin with a step-up approach. In patients with fewer than two episodes per week, a systematic increase in the minimal dose of medication necessary to resolve symptoms is appropriate. Changes in dosage may be altered every 2 to 4 weeks. Patients who present with GERD for the first time are recommended to change their lifestyle and diet; but if these measures do not change symptoms, an H2 blocker is started at the lowest dosage. An antacid or sodium alginate may be taken for breakthrough if symptoms occur on a weekly basis or less. Breakthrough symptoms warrant twice-daily therapy with an H2 blocker at a normal dose. This is continued for 2 weeks, at which point, if breakthrough symptoms are present, a once-daily PPI is instituted. This dosage may be doubled if needed. Therapy continues for 2 months prior to reevaluation.

Antacids do not prevent GERD; their role is limited to intermittent (on demand) use for relief of mild GERD symptoms that occur less than once a week. Antacid medications are composed of either magnesium trisilicate, aluminum hydroxide, or calcium carbonate. These compounds neutralize gastric pH, causing refluxed gastric contents to be less irritating to the esophageal lining. They have a 5-minute onset of action but last less than 1 hour.

Histamine two-receptor antagonists (H2RAs) are the second most effective medication for GERD. They reduce acid secretion by blocking the H2RA receptor on the gastric parietal cells. In up to 6 weeks of continued use, patients will develop a decreased response to the same dosage of medication. Whereas antacids begin effectiveness in 5 minutes, it takes 2.5 hours for H2RAs to start to be effective, but H2RAs last up to 10 hours and are more effective than antacids.

PPI medications are the strongest antacids. They stop acid production by binding irreversibly to the parietal cell hydrogen-potassium (H-K) ATPase pump. They work most effectively when exposed to the highest amount of H-K-ATPase, which is 30 minutes before the first meal of the day. PPIs are prescribed for patients who have failed twice-daily H2RA therapy, who have EE, twice or more weekly heartburn, or have experienced quality-of-life impairment from GERD. PPIs are most effective at symptom relief and healing when taken once a day. Despite numerous studies, there remains no significant difference in efficacy of PPI medications when varied for dose and frequency when symptom relief or healing are being considered. However, with regard to the different types of PPI medications, esomeprazole at 40 mg once daily is more effective than standard doses of lansoprazole (30 mg PO qday), omeprazole (20 mg PO qday), pantoprazole (40 mg PO qday), or rabeprazole (20 mg PO qday) in patients with symptoms of GERD. Numerous meta-analyses have confirmed that the use of PPIs leads to faster and more effective resolution of heartburn and other symptoms than H2RAs.

There is little evidence of clinically effective therapies for the treatment of nonacid reflux. These patients should modify their lifestyle and diet. PPI medication should be taken half an hour before the biggest meal. Weight loss should be encouraged, the head of the bed elevated, patients should sit upright after meals, and the last meal should occur 3 hours before sleep is anticipated. The addition of the gamma-aminobutyric acid (GABA) receptor agonist baclofen may be beneficial as the medication may reduce the quantity of TSLERs. The addition of baclofen to PPI therapy can reduce both acid and nonacid reflux in the presence of a hiatal hernia. Baclofen 5 to 10 mg twice daily is started before meals up to a maximum dose of 20 mg three times a day. Side effects may include sleepiness, fogginess, dizziness, weakness, and shaking. Treatment is attempted for 2 months before stopping. Prokinetic agents may also alleviate symptoms by promoting increased gastric emptying. In patients with refractory disease, a Roux-en-Y diversion or duodenal-switch procedure may be helpful.

PPI have a higher cost and have recently been associated with more and significant side effects. PPI use has been associated with an increased risk of *Clostridium difficile* and enteric infections and reinfections with or without antibiotic use. Microscopic, lymphocytic, and collagenous colitis has also been associated with PPIs. Malabsorption of minerals and vitamins such as magnesium, calcium, chloride, iron, and vitamin B-12 have all been associated. Long-term PPI treatment poses an increased risk of chronic atrophic gastritis but has rare sequalae. Hypergastrinemia after PPI treatment is associated with gastric carcinoid tumors in rats. Humans treated with omeprazole for over 11 years have developed enterochromaffin-like cell hyperplasia, but no neoplastic changes have occurred.

PPIs may incite acute interstitial nephritis (AIN), increased risk of chronic kidney disease (CKD), and end-stage renal disease. PPIs may induce cutaneous and systemic lupus erythematosus (SLE) and increasing severity of existing disease. There are conflicting data on the development of dementia, pneumonia, and overall life span by PPI medication, as some studies have confounding variables.

Surgical Treatment

Antireflux surgery, including open and laparoscopic versions of Nissen and Toupet fundoplication, is as effective as PPI therapy and should be offered to patients with DGER as an alternative to medication for patients with chronic reflux, DGER, and recalcitrant symptoms. Surgery should be performed if symptoms fail to resolve while the patient is taking medication or if symptoms develop during drug therapy or recur after medication is stopped. Similarly, surgery should be performed if the patient is noncompliant, has lifelong PPI dependence, has experienced complications despite medication, or has recurrent strictures, pulmonary symptoms, severe esophagitis, symptomatic Barrett's esophagus, or symptomatic paraesophageal hernia. Best results from surgery occur in patients who are young, have typical GERD symptoms, have abnormal pH study findings, and show a good response to PPI therapy. However, these patients are the best candidates for medical therapy, as well.

The Nissen fundoplication is the most successful and popular antireflux procedure. It is most commonly performed laparoscopically but had been developed as an open operation. Laparoscopy results in less pain and a faster recovery, but otherwise the results of the two procedures are similar and there is symptomatic improvement in 85% to 90% of patients. Nissen or laparoscopic antireflux surgery (LARS) involves reduction of a hiatal hernia if present, mobilization of the esophagus, crural closure, short gastric division, and a 360-degree posterior fundoplication. The Belsey Mark IV is a transthoracic partial fundoplication that allows full esophageal mobilization for patients with poor esophageal motility. The Hill gastropexy involves imbrication of the anterior and posterior lesser gastric curve around the esophagus, suturing to the median arcuate ligament, and closing the crura. Intraoperative manometry is used to calibrate the LES pressure. The Roux-en-Y gastric bypass (RYGB) is now considered an antireflux surgery and may be the procedure of choice for the treatment of GERD in the morbidly obese.

The laparoscopic anterior fundoplication (LAF) or Dor procedure is a 90- to 180-degree wrap. When it is compared with the laparoscopic posterior fundoplication, LPF, or Toupet procedure 180- to 360-degree wrap, it results in less postfundoplication symptoms but higher rates of recurrence of reflux. Patients undergoing LPF experience less acid exposure (0.8% versus 3.3%), less heartburn (8% versus 21%), and a lower reoperation rate (4% versus 8%) when compared with those who have had LAF. Optimal PPI treatment with esomeprazole 20 to 40 mg/day and LARS provide similar 5-year remission rates, 85% for PPI versus 92% for LARS for controlling GERD symptoms.

When patients treated with a partial wrap were compared with those who have undergone a total fundoplication, there were similar rates of bloating, flatulence, and dysphagia in both. Patients undergoing a partial fundoplication experience less dysphagia; but greater esophageal acid exposure, esophagitis, and need for reoperation than patients undergoing total fundoplication.

After Nissen fundoplication, the most common complications, which occur infrequently, are gastric or esophageal injury, splenic injury, pneumothorax, bleeding, pneumonia, fever, and wound infections. Side effects include bloating (21%), diarrhea (12%), regurgitation (6%), heartburn (6%), and chest pain (4%); 28% of patients reported dysphagia and 7% required dilation.

Postoperative symptoms are dependent upon the tightness of the fundoplication. Dysphagia occurs in 8% to 12% of all LARS patients. Dysphagia occurs more frequently with the laparoscopic Rosetti-Nissen variation, where the short gastric vessels are left intact (11%), than with the laparoscopic Nissen (2%) and the Toupet (2%).

Postoperative dysphagia is expected in most patients and may last up to 12 weeks, after which it should be evaluated first with a barium swallow. If the wrap is visually tight or the patient is unable to swallow a barium tablet, dilatation should be performed. Approximately 6% to 12% of LARS patients required dilation. Conversion to a partial fundoplication is an option for individuals who fail multiple dilatations.

Gas bloat syndrome is a sensation of intestinal gas with the inability to belch that occurs after fundoplication procedures. It is more common after a tight fundoplication and may be due to delayed gastric emptying, aerophagia, or vagal dysfunction. Treatment begins with simethicone or charcoal tablets and advances to the use of metoclopramide 10 to 15 mg PO q6 hours. Other options that may help are domperidone (10 mg PO tid to 20 mg tid and bedtime) and erythromycin (3 mg/kg IV q8 hours over 45 minutes or erythromycin 250 mg to 800 mg q6 hours). Symptoms subside over time and revisional surgery is rarely needed.

Approximately 5% to 10% of patients will need a revision for recurrent heartburn or severe dysphagia after laparoscopic fundoplication. Recurrence of the hiatal hernia and migration of the fundoplication may occur from incomplete esophageal mobilization in the posterior mediastinum or an unrecognized shortened esophagus. Most common reasons to perform a revision are dysphagia (48%), recurrent reflux (33%), paraesophageal herniation (15%), and atypical symptoms (4%). The success rate for revisional surgery is lower, as 10% of patients will continue to be symptomatic from reflux or dysphagia, leaving medical treatment the only option.

Long-term studies of laparoscopic fundoplication by experienced surgeons point to a 90% to 95% satisfaction rate. Failure is considered to be continued use of antacid medications, although some patients are instructed to remain on medication for gastric or Barrett treatment. Post-LARS, 18% of patients require antacids for symptom relief and 16% will need revisional surgery at 5 years.

The sphincter augmentation procedure with the LINX device achieves results similar to those of a Nissen fundoplication. Placement of the device increases the LES pressure, keeping it closed with a ring of 12 to 18 magnets. Swallowing will overcome the resting pressure, open the magnets, and allow the passage of food. At 5 years after LINX placement, GERD-related quality of life was improved, only 12% of patients complained of heartburn, 1% of regurgitation, and 8% of gas bloat; daily PPI use was 15%. After the procedure, patients return to normal eating after several days and are able to belch and vomit when needed. Early dysphagia is frequent with the LINX but usually resolves after some weeks. Long-term dysphagia is 6%. The results and complications of the procedure are comparable to those of the laparoscopic Nissen with the advantage of less gas bloating. Rarely have there been explanations for dysphagia and erosions.

Endoluminal transoral procedures offer an outpatient therapy option that is less invasive than laparoscopic fundoplication. The Stretta system uses radiofrequency energy to cauterize the gastroesophageal junction (GEJ) in five locations and causes thickening of the muscle and therefore reduced compliance of the sphincter. It is effective in patients with a LES pressure of at least 8 mm Hg and hiatal hernia less than 3 cm in size. Transoral incisionless fundoplication (TIF) is an endoscopic procedure that creates a 3- to 5-cm partial fundoplication with a full-thickness serosa-to-serosa contact. It is an option for patients that have typical GERD, grade A and/or B esophagitis, and a hiatal hernia up to 2 cm. TIF results in less gas bloating and dysphagia than a Nissen fundoplication but a significantly lower success rate and a 69% satisfaction rate at 6 months. Long-term studies have not been promising. Although these procedures are less invasive and induce fewer complications than antireflux surgery, their success rates are significantly lower. The role of these procedures in the treatment of reflux is secondary; they remain an option for those who want a less invasive procedure but are willing to accept less significant results.

Course and Prognosis
Medical Course

Antacids result in symptom relief in only 20% of GERD patients; they have minimal effect on pH and no effect on healing esophagitis. H_2RA therapy results in symptom relief in 40% to 70% of patients and healing in 20% to 50%. Remission is maintained in only 25% to 40%. Higher and more frequent doses may improve symptoms minimally. All H_2RAs are similar in efficacy, and adverse effects are uncommon and mild.

PPIs have the best acid-blocking effect, alleviating symptoms in 90% of patients and promoting healing in 80% to 90%. Once-daily omeprazole (20 mg) has a greater acid-blocking effect than twice-daily ranitidine (150 mg). An estimated 30% of all GERD patients who require a PPI once daily will fail treatment. Up to 70% of patients do not have adequate nocturnal control of gastric acid secretion with omeprazole (20 mg) twice daily. GERD is a chronic, relapsing disease; long-term maintenance therapy is necessary to relieve symptoms, prevent complications, and prevent recurrence in 40% to 50% patients.

Suggested mechanisms of failure include weakly acidic reflux, duodenal gastric reflux (DDGR), visceral hyperalgesia, delayed gastric emptying, psychologic comorbidity, and functional bowel disease. If symptom control fails or symptoms return after medication is discontinued, endoscopy may establish the diagnosis.

Most often patients who fail have NERD, 66% of whom will have recurrent symptoms when medications are stopped. When this occurs, the previous effective dosage should be reinstituted and an endoscopy performed if less than 3 months have passed and long-term maintenance therapy is continued. If greater than 3 months have passed, the previous dose alone is started. Increasing dosage may be instituted as previously described.

For patients who have EE, as identified on endoscopy, a PPI is the initial treatment of choice. These patients should undergo 24-hour pH testing and bile probe testing in selected centers to determine the severity of reflux. Patients who have supine reflux, poor esophageal contractility, EE, Barrett's esophagus, or defective LES are predicted to do poorly with medication and are at high risk for complications of GERD. These patients should be offered the option of surgery.

Unfortunately pH testing cannot pinpoint a causative relationship between GERD and extraesophageal symptoms. Effective treatment resulting in significant symptom improvement or resolution is the best evidence that extraesophageal symptoms are caused by GERD. Treatment for extraesophageal symptoms relies on higher doses of PPIs, as is typical GERD. Patients who fail to respond to medication, require long-term maintenance, or request to discontinue medication may be candidates for surgical therapy.

Long-term management of nonacid reflux depends on the response to treatment. Patients who respond to baclofen may remain on the drug and have their PPI dosage lowered or stopped. Patients who do not respond to medical therapy may be considered for surgical treatment such as a Nissen fundoplication.

Surgical Course

Since its advent in 1991, laparoscopic Nissen fundoplication has become the gold standard for the treatment of severe GERD. Results after 10 years reveal at least a 90% success rate. Although 14% of patients continue receiving PPI therapy, 79% of these patients are treated for vague abdominal or chest symptoms with unclear indications. Multiple trials comparing surgical fundoplication and PPI therapy reveal similar effectiveness in controlling GERD and its symptoms. Longer studies reveal an advantage of surgery that is eliminated when PPI dosage is increased.

ESOPHAGITIS: ACUTE AND CHRONIC

Acute esophagitis may have numerous causes, of which GERD is the most common (Fig. 11.2). *Chronic* esophagitis occurs more frequently and results from multiple episodes of acute inflammation. Of patients undergoing EGD, 14% have esophagitis and most are men. Hiatal hernia is present in 79% to 88% of patients with active reflux esophagitis. The

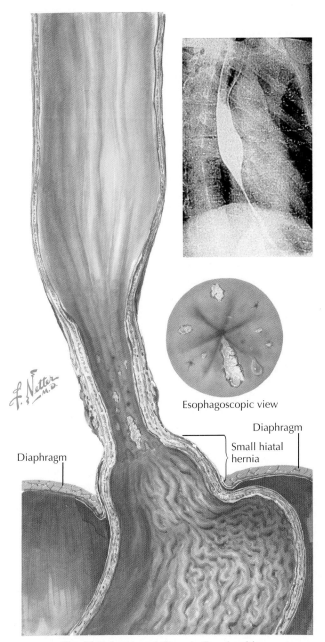

Esophagoscopic view

Diaphragm

Small hiatal hernia

Diaphragm

Fig. 11.2 Acute and Chronic Esophagitis.

incidence of reflux esophagitis is rapidly increasing; in one study, it had doubled over 10 years. In Belgium the incidence of EE rose dramatically and then stabilized with a sixfold increase in the use of PPIs.

Esophagitis is believed to be caused not only by acid but also by the reflux of bile, enzymes, pepsin, and pancreatic juices. Acid-induced esophagitis may induce hyperresponsive longitudinal smooth muscle contraction and impairment of circular smooth muscle contractility, which may lead to chronic complications.

Esophagitis may occur from pills that remain in the esophagus for an extended period, causing irritation. Opportunistic infections of the esophagus are a common cause of morbidity in patients with human immunodeficiency virus (HIV) infection and may reflect the severity of the underlying disease. Less frequent causes of esophagitis include swallowing acid or basic household materials, severe vomiting, irritation by feeding tubes or suction catheters, and candida or other infectious diseases.

Clinical Picture

Only 50% of patients with endoscopic evidence of esophagitis have typical reflux symptoms of GERD. Heartburn, the most common symptom in patients with esophagitis, is present in only 28% of those with endoscopic evidence. Other symptoms are dysphagia (19%), acid regurgitation (18%), odynophagia (6%), nausea, vomiting, and belching. Older age, male gender, severe symptoms, and presence of a hiatal hernia are independent risk factors for severe esophagitis. Patients with HIV-related diseases have symptoms associated with the specific etiology.

Diagnosis

Esophagogastroduodenoscopy (EGD) allows for the direct visualization of the esophageal mucosa and is best for diagnosing esophagitis. Untreated GERD patients have a 30% prevalence of esophagitis. EGD may reveal congestion, erythema, and edema of the mucosa as well as pinpoint hemorrhages. Infectious and medication-induced esophagitis is usually found in the proximal esophagus. Acid reflux esophagitis is usually found in the distal esophagus. Histologic findings of biopsies reveal epithelial necrosis, erosions, small cell infiltration, and hypertrophy of muscle fibers. Esophagitis is usually located between the GE junction and 10 cm above it.

Historically the most widely used grading system for esophagitis has been the Savary-Miller classification. This system has been largely replaced because grade IV has become overly inclusive of several complications such stenosis, ulcers, and Barrett esophagitis.
- Grade I: One or more nonconfluent reddish spots with or without exudate
- Grade II: Erosive and exudative lesions in the distal esophagus that may be confluent but not circumferential
- Grade III: Circumferential erosions in the distal esophagus covered by hemorrhagic and pseudomembranous exudate
- Grade IV: Chronic complications such as deep ulcers, stenosis, or scarring with Barrett metaplasia

The most widely used grading system for esophagitis as determined by upper endoscopy is the Los Angeles classification. It grades esophagitis according to characteristics found on the mucosa. Mucosal breaks are sloughing of the mucosa adjacent to normal squamous epithelium independent of the presence of exudate.
- Grade A: One or more mucosal breaks each up to 5 mm in length
- Grade B: At least one mucosal break more than 5 mm long but not continuous between the tops of adjacent mucosal folds
- Grade C: At least one mucosal break that is continuous between the tops of adjacent mucosal folds but that is not circumferential
- Grade D: A mucosal break that involves at least three-fourths of the luminal circumference

Treatment and Management

Goals of treatment for EE are to heal lesions, relieve symptoms, and prevent relapse. Patients with severe esophagitis with symptoms affecting their quality of life should be started on maximum therapy and tapered down to the least dose to resolve symptoms of GERD and heal esophagitis. Patients should be started on a maximum dose of PPI once a day along with diet and lifestyle changes for a total of 8 weeks. EE is resolved in 86% of patients treated with this therapy. Specifically, multiple prospective trials indicate that esomeprazole has a higher rate of action, lower interpatient variability, and more prolonged action in achieving esophageal healing in the subset of patients with esophagitis. Numerous PPI studies show no difference in effectiveness with intravenous versus oral treatment or with the intake of pills versus oral an granular suspension in treatment of EE.

In the past, short-term treatment with both PPIs and H_2 blockers was effective in healing EE, but PPIs have proved to be better; therefore H_2 blockers are no longer used as a primary treatment. However, after the initial period of PPI treatment the dosage should be decreased to a normal level or, when patients only have mild symptoms, to H-2 blockers.

Patients with Los Angeles grade C and D esophagitis should undergo a repeat upper endoscopy after 8 weeks of PPI treatment to confirm healing and rule out the development of Barrett's esophagus. A third endoscopy is necessary only if Barrett is discovered, there is bleeding, dysphagia develops, of symptoms dramatically change while the patient is on maintenance medical PPI therapy. In the presence of severe EE or Barrett's esophagus, patients should be maintained on a daily dose of PPI.

Course and Prognosis

PPIs consistently reduce symptoms, the incidence, and the interval to relapse, making them the recommended medical therapy for the long-term management of EE. Maintenance success at 6 to 12 months varies from 82% to 93% with most PPIs and is cost-effective. If maintenance therapy is not initiated, most patients relapse within 1 year. Relapse increases the severity of esophagitis and the risk for complications such as Barrett's esophagus and adenocarcinoma. Poor compliance is the main reason for failure and relapse, followed by nonacid reflux, especially in patients with regurgitation or cough that persists despite treatment.

LARS is effective in relieving symptoms and healing EE. It is performed after medical treatment has failed or as an alternative to long-term maintenance. The effectiveness of newer modalities of endoscopic treatment is not yet known. Multiple studies show at least similar effectiveness of long-term continuous medical therapy and surgery, although data at up to 7 years suggest a benefit to surgery. Long-term surgical problems include increased gas bloat and use of PPIs. Patients may become poorly compliant or may have nonacid reflux.

ESOPHAGEAL ULCERS

Esophageal ulcers are mucosal defects that have distinct margins (Fig. 11.3). They are found in 1% of patients undergoing EGD. In 66% of patients, the cause is GERD usually associated with a hiatal hernia, resulting from prolonged contact between squamous epithelial cells and gastric refluxate containing acid, pepsin, bile, and pancreatic juices. Drug-induced ulcers account for 23% of all esophageal ulcers and are usually caused by nonsteroidal antiinflammatory drugs (NSAIDs) that have prolonged direct contact with the esophageal mucosa. Ulcers may also be a complication of medications such as bisphosphonates and some antibiotics, one of which is doxycycline. Foods containing acid,

caffeinated drinks, alcohol, and cigarette smoking may all contribute to more severe ulcer formation.

Infectious causes of esophageal ulcer, which are less prevalent, include *Candida, Mycobacterium tuberculosis, Actinomyces,* herpes simplex virus (HSV), and cytomegalovirus (CMV). Infections may result from caustic injury, marginal ulceration, foreign bodies, variceal banding, repeat vomiting with bulimia nervosa, as well as unknown etiologies. Patients with HIV have a higher incidence of infectious ulcers from CMV (45%), idiopathic causes (40%), *Candida* esophagitis (27%), and HSV (5%).

Esophageal ulcers may be complicated by hemorrhage, perforation, and fistulization into the airway. Ulcers may lead to the formation of fibrous tissue and collagen production (strictures). Healing may occur with intestinal epithelium. This metaplastic process results in Barrett's esophagus; ulceration occurs in 46% of patients with Barrett's esophagus. Since the advent of PPI therapy, esophageal ulcers occur less frequently.

Clinical Picture

Symptoms are rarely different from those in patients with GERD. Most patients have heartburn, regurgitation, substernal chest pain, dysphagia, odynophagia, globus, nausea, and vomiting; others may be asymptomatic. The most common sign of esophageal ulcer is anemia; one-third of patients may present with acute GI bleeding. Patients with a bleeding ulcer may have hemetesis, coffee ground emesis, and substernal chest pain radiating to the back. Of patients with Barrett's esophagus and ulcers, 24% present with active GI bleeding. Melena occurs in 40% of patients, and melena and hematemesis occur concomitantly in another 40%. Fifty percent of patients have orthostatic hypotension, and 8 in 10 patients require blood transfusion.

Bleeding ulcers are associated with NSAIDs in 50% of patients, hiatal hernia in 60%, and esophagitis in 40%. Drug-induced ulcers are usually located in the midesophagus, near the aortic arch, at an area of natural esophageal tapering where pills may become temporarily lodged. Only 13% of ulcers occur in the distal esophagus. Midesophageal ulcers have a greater tendency to hemorrhage than ulcers at the GE junction; this may reflect the cause. Strictures occur in 12.5% and esophageal perforation in 3.4% of patients.

Diagnosis

Barium esophagraphy or endoscopy establishes the diagnosis of esophageal ulcer. Both studies may show evidence of GERD, such as overt reflux. Barium esophagraphy may reveal the position of the ulcer, which may be posterior in 69% of patients, lateral in 17%, and anterior in 14%. Nine of 10 ulcers are within 4 cm of the LES. Esophagraphy may also reveal hiatal hernias, mucosal nodularity, and strictures, each in 40% of cases. Esophagraphy can make optimal determinations at an average depth of 5 mm.

Endoscopy is the best study to establish a diagnosis. Location, visual characteristics, and biopsy results at esophagoscopy elucidate the cause of the ulcer. A chronic GERD ulcer may be well demarcated, may have undetermined edges and a crater of granulation tissue, and may be covered with a yellow-gray membrane. Esophagitis is usually adjacent to the GERD ulcer and has signs of inflammation, congestion, edema, and superficial erosions. At the site of these changes is a narrowing secondary to segmental spasms. NSAID ulcers have normal surrounding mucosa. Drug-induced ulcers are larger and shallower than GERD-induced ulcers, but both range from 2.75 to 3.0 cm. Biopsy should be performed to exclude the presence of Barrett's esophagus and malignancy. Biopsy during EGD is integral to the diagnosis of ulcers in patients with HIV. Bleeding ulcers may be diagnosed by upper endoscopy.

Endoscopic views

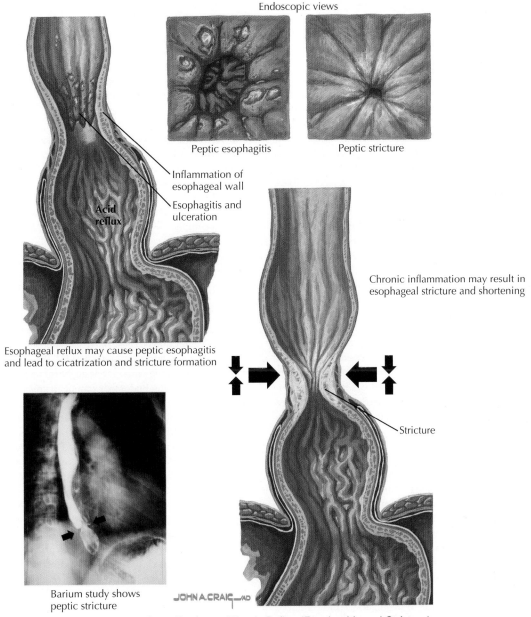

Peptic esophagitis

Peptic stricture

Inflammation of esophageal wall

Esophagitis and ulceration

Acid reflux

Esophageal reflux may cause peptic esophagitis and lead to cicatrization and stricture formation

Chronic inflammation may result in esophageal stricture and shortening

Stricture

Barium study shows peptic stricture

JOHN A. CRAIG—AD

Fig. 11.3 Complications of Peptic Reflux (Esophagitis and Stricture).

Treatment and Management

Determining the cause of esophageal ulcer is most important in order to dictate the most appropriate treatment. In patients with GERD, uncomplicated, previously untreated esophageal ulcers should be treated with PPI therapy. Currently the most clinically effective medication for healing EE and later maintenance therapy is esomeprazole. With a drug-induced esophageal ulcer, healing occurs if the ulcer is recognized early. The medication should then be discontinued and the patient instructed to swallow pills in the upright position in the future and to drink a glass of water each time. Antacids and H$_2$ blockers are the fastest-acting therapy, and PPIs allow optimal acid blockade. In patients with HIV, medical therapy focuses on the specific cause of the ulcer. Infectious causes are treated by eradication with the appropriate antimicrobial agent. CMV infection is treated with ganciclovir and fluconazole is used to treat esophageal candidiasis.

Although acute bleeding frequently necessitates blood transfusion, most bleeding stops without endoscopic therapy. Endoscopic hemostasis for esophageal bleeding from ulcers may be required as emergency therapy in 4% of patients, including the techniques of argon plasma coagulation epinephrine injection and endoscopic clip placement. Interventional radiology is rarely used to stop bleeding. Emergency surgery is rare, occurring in 0.6% of cases, but more common for complications such as esophageal stricture and perforation in 8% of patients. Elective laparoscopic fundoplication may be necessary for patients whose ulcers fail to heal over the long term.

Course and Prognosis

Nonsurgical therapy is successful in 92% of patients with GERD- and drug-induced ulcers. Follow-up endoscopy indicates that NSAID-induced ulcers heal in 3 to 4 weeks. The healing rate in treated HIV patients is 98%. Strictures complicate GERD-induced but not drug-induced esophageal ulcers. Esophageal dilation is an effective treatment for most strictures associated with esophageal ulcers. Death from ulcers is rare, but 2% of patients die from acute hemorrhage or perforation.

BENIGN ESOPHAGEAL STRICTURE

Strictures occur more frequently in men and are most common in elderly white patients. Esophageal strictures develop in 10% to 15% of patients with GERD (Fig. 11.4) and in 13% of patients with esophageal ulcers. GERD accounts for almost 70% of all esophageal strictures. Less common causes of strictures include ingestion of caustic substances, Barrett's esophagus, mediastinal irradiation, ingestion of drugs, malignancy, surgical resection line, congenital esophageal stenosis, skin diseases, and pseudo diverticulosis.

In reflux esophagitis, acid and pepsin secretions eventually erode the mucosa of the esophagus, causing replacement with fibrous tissue, which eventually contracts and results in a lumen as narrow as 2 to 3 mm. Severe strictures form less frequently since the advent of PPI therapy. In general, GERD strictures are associated with severe esophagitis or Barrett's esophagus. They occur at the squamocolumnar (SC) junction. As intestinal metaplasia (IM) advances to the proximal esophagus in Barrett, the stricture follows.

Clinical Picture

Patients report varying symptoms of dysphagia, odynophagia, regurgitation, and chest pain. Dysphagia begins with solid foods and advances to liquids as the stenosis becomes severe. Painful swallowing (odynophagia) develops as food irritates the mucosa overlying the strictured area. The patient's inability to ingest proper amounts of food results in weight loss and poor nutrition.

Diagnosis

Clinical history suggests the diagnosis, and a combination of endoscopy and barium esophagraphy confirms stricture. Usually barium esophagraphy shows a variable segment of narrowed esophagus. The margins are smoothly tapered and not jagged, as found in patients with malignancy. EGD allows direct visualization, and biopsy confirms a benign stricture. The esophagus is rigid, and the endoscope may meet resistance as it advances. In severe cases, a pediatric endoscope may be used to pass through the lumen. In GERD, the active reflux of acid may be observed above the level of the lesion. Twenty-four-hour pH monitoring should be performed to distinguish GERD-induced strictures from drug-induced strictures in 45% of patients. Peptic strictures must also be differentiated with a Schatzki ring, or weblike narrowing, thought to be related to reflux and found at the SC junction (see Chapter 4).

Treatment and Management

Repeated bougie dilatation with either rigid dilators or balloons is the treatment of choice for strictures. Bougie dilatation of GERD-related strictures results in resolution of symptoms in 75% of patients. Multiple topical post dilatation applications of mitomycin C show promise in decreasing dilatations and increasing their intervals, with overall improved results; however, further trials are needed. The underlying cause of reflux must be treated chronically with aggressive PPI therapy.

Surgery is indicated when recurring strictures require frequent dilatations or medical therapy fails or is impractical. Surgical fundoplication should be performed within 2 years of diagnosis to resolve the underlying cause of reflux. Laparoscopic repair may be performed with good results and minimal complications. A recent study of 200 medical and surgical patients concluded that the resection of peptic strictures is rarely indicated.

Course and Prognosis

In 30% to 40% of patients with benign strictures, symptoms will recur within 1 year. Patients with nonpeptic and narrow strictures have the highest rates of recurrence. In GERD-related strictures, continued heartburn and hiatal hernia are the strongest predictors for failure of PPI therapy. When drug-induced strictures are resolved, heartburn does not have to be treated. Drug-induced injury may occur in a patient with an underlying GERD-induced stricture, causing pills to become lodged and resulting in further injury. These strictures may not respond to dilatation.

In a Mayo Clinic study, dilatations decreased from 5.3 per patient 26 months before surgery to 1.8 per patient 25 months after surgery. After laparoscopic fundoplication for dysphagia and strictures, the overall satisfaction rate was 88% to 91%, with a 10% recurrence rate for dysphagia. Laparoscopic surgery results in a good clinical outcome with minimal complications and a good quality of life.

BARRETT'S ESOPHAGUS

Barrett's esophagus is defined as metaplasia occurring in any length of epithelium at any location above the GEJ that is identified at endoscopy and confirmed by biopsy and that does not include metaplasia of the gastric cardia (Fig. 11.5). Squamous epithelium is replaced by columnar epithelium with goblet cells. Barrett's esophagus originally included gastric fundic type, junctional type, and IM. Fundic-type epithelium has minimal malignant potential and is no longer included in the definition of Barrett's esophagus. Endoscopy cannot accurately distinguish between IM and gastric-type epithelium, so biopsy is necessary for diagnosis.

Evidence supports a strong correlation between Barrett's esophagus and chronic GERD. Abnormal pH study findings are present in 93% of Barrett's esophagus patients compared with 45% to 75% of all other GERD patients. Barrett's esophagus is twice as prevalent in men as in women. The men are usually white, have chronic heartburn, and are older than 50. Barrett's esophagus is present in 10% to 20% of patients undergoing endoscopy for GERD. It occurs in 3% of patients with weekly heartburn, 5% of patients with daily heartburn, and 0.5% to 2% of asymptomatic adults in the United States.

Barrett's esophagus has the potential to progress to *adenocarcinoma*, the incidence of which has increased dramatically over the past 20 to 30 years, making it the most rapidly increasing cancer in the United States. Barrett's esophagus develops in the presence of persistent GERD, which is an independent risk factor for adenocarcinoma. Patients with GERD have a risk for esophageal adenocarcinoma that is 30 to 60 times greater, at an incidence rate more than 100 times greater, than that of the general population. The prevalence of Barrett's esophagus and adenocarcinoma increases with age and severity of symptoms. A surgical series of esophageal resections shows that adenocarcinoma predominates in older white men.

Carcinoma is the final step in the progression from squamous cells, to IM, to *low-grade dysplasia* (LGD), to *high-grade dysplasia* (HGD), and then to invasive disease. All stages may coexist. Other risk factors for adenocarcinoma in patients with Barrett's esophagus include length of Barrett epithelium, LGD, and HGD.

IM is the most important risk factor for the development of dysplasia and cancer, and most adenocarcinomas of the esophagus and GE junction are accompanied by IM. Short-segment Barrett's esophagus carries a lower risk for dysplasia. Patients with long-segment Barrett's esophagus have greater pH exposure and LES pressure than those with short-segment disease. Recently attempts were made to differentiate short-segment Barrett's esophagus from IM of the gastric cardia. The distinction between short- and long-segment Barrett's esophagus has been poorly defined.

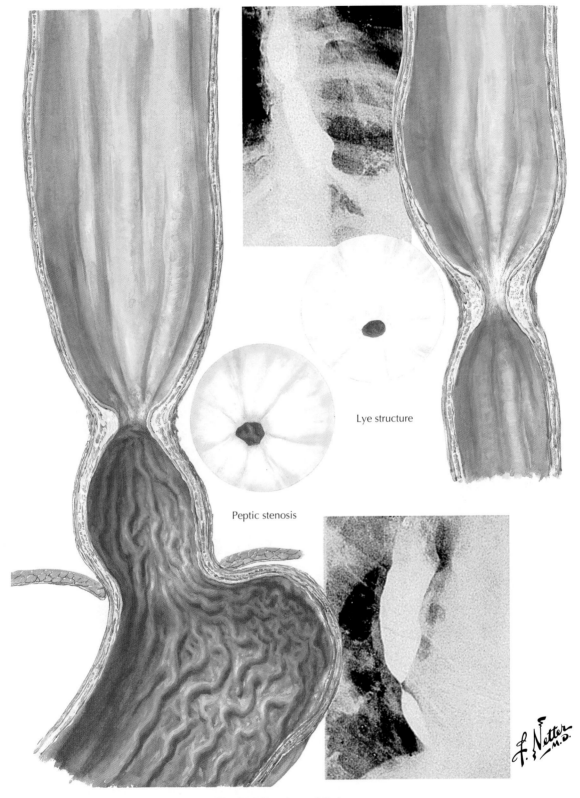

Lye structure

Peptic stenosis

Fig. 11.4 Esophageal Stricture.

Reflux of acid and duodenal contents may contribute to the development of Barrett's esophagus. Bile, in conjunction with acid and pepsin, disrupts the mucosal barrier of the esophagus and causes esophagitis. Acid exposure is associated with the development of columnar mucosa, and bile exposure has been deemed an independent predictor of Barrett's esophagus. Severe DGER occurs after subtotal esophagectomy and pyloroplasty and provides an environment for development of Barrett metaplasia through a sequence that begins with cardiac epithelium and eventually transforms into IM. In this human model of severe DGER, 33% of patients have esophagitis, 23% have Barrett's esophagus,

GE junction   **Esophageal epithelium**

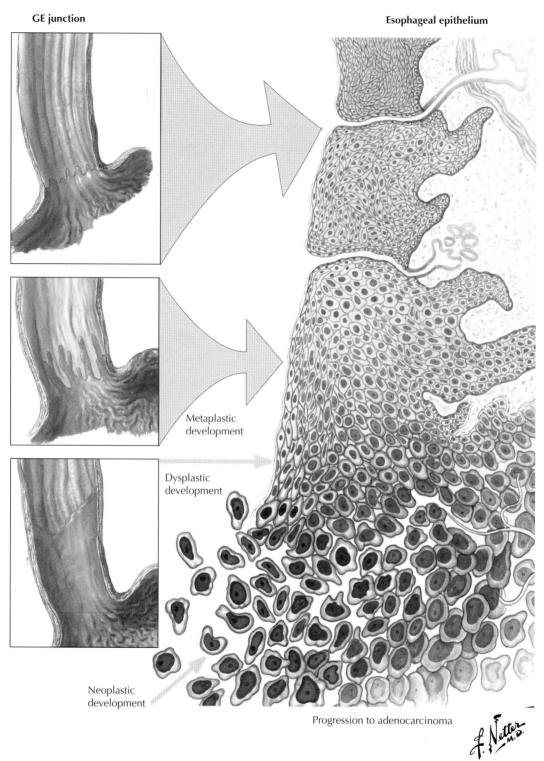

Metaplastic
development

Dysplastic
development

Neoplastic
development

Progression to adenocarcinoma

Fig. 11.5 Barrett's Esophagus.

and another 18% progress from cardiac mucosa to Barrett's esophagus over time. Clearly acid is not the only cause.

Clinical Picture

No symptoms or signs distinguish patients with Barrett metaplasia from those without it. Signs and symptoms of GERD are the same as those for Barrett's esophagus.

Diagnosis

Patients with an extensive history of GERD symptoms are more likely to have Barrett's esophagus and should undergo EGD. Patients at higher risk may be male and may have abnormal bile reflux, hiatal hernia larger than 4 cm, defective LES, distal esophageal dysmotility, reflux episodes longer than 5 minutes, and GERD symptoms for more than 5 years.

The diagnosis of Barrett's esophagus requires biopsy of abnormal-appearing mucosa to determine the presence of IM and dysplasia. SC and GE junctions should be specified. When the SC junction is displaced cranial to the GE junction, Barrett's esophagus is suspected. Gastric folds define the beginning of the stomach. It is difficult to distinguish gastric mucosa and esophagitis from Barrett's esophagus by visualization, but Barrett is typically described as salmon-colored. Guidelines suggest that biopsies be taken in four quadrants, beginning 1 cm below the GE junction and extending 1 cm above the SC junction at 2-cm intervals. Endoscopic staining with methylene blue may assist in locating cells with IM in the esophagus.

Treatment and Management

Management includes controlling reflux, healing esophagitis, and detecting dysplasia early. The principles and treatment for Barrett's esophagus are the same as those for GERD, although patients with Barrett's esophagus have worse responses because of more severe disease. How to prevent Barrett's esophagus or stop its progression has not been determined. Treatment involves a combination of endoscopy, medical therapy, surgery, and possibly ablative therapies.

Surveillance is based on the increasing risk for adenocarcinoma, and dysplasia is the most sensitive indicator of the risk for cancer. Surveillance endoscopy is recommended in all patients with Barrett's esophagus to detect dysplasia and to initiate early intervention. These measures attempt to decrease the incidence of esophageal adenocarcinoma and improve patient survival. The result has been detection of adenocarcinoma at an earlier stage compared with cancer detected after symptoms such as dysphagia have appeared, but these surveillance measures have not yet affected survival.

Unfortunately most patients with Barrett cancer were not found to have a premalignant condition such as dysplasia and were not under surveillance. Asymptomatic patients still account for most patients with adenocarcinoma. Therefore all patients undergoing EGD should undergo careful examination of the distal esophagus. The goal is to detect dysplasia, which occurs on top of IM. Any level of dysplasia may be located adjacent to frank carcinoma.

Unfortunately evidence-based data to determine the timing of surveillance endoscopy intervals for screening remain to be defined. The interval at which endoscopy is performed depends on the grade of dysplasia. Any nodule or ulcer on the epithelial surface should undergo careful biopsy. Endoscopy for surveillance may be performed every 3 years if there is no evidence of dysplasia on two consecutive endoscopies.

If LGD is found at endoscopy, patients should be treated intensively with high-dose PPI therapy for 3 to 12 weeks, after which repeat biopsy should be performed. Esophagitis will resolve but dysplasia will not, eliminating confusion regarding the diagnosis at repeat biopsy. If LGD is found after repeat biopsy, repeat endoscopy should be performed at 6-month intervals for 1 year. If LGD has not progressed, annual endoscopy should be performed. The presence of HGD should be confirmed by a second pathologist and warrants aggressive treatment.

In patients with Barrett's esophagus, medical and surgical therapies are effective in controlling reflux symptoms. However, more than 60% of patients continue to have pathologic GERD and abnormally low esophageal pH despite doses of esomeprazole that control reflux symptoms. Higher doses of PPIs must be used to prevent the development of esophageal adenocarcinoma. Treatment success can be measured only by repeat pH monitoring. Although aggressive PPI therapy is the first-line treatment, no significant clinical evidence supports that acid suppression prevents adenocarcinoma or the progression of IM to dysplasia. PPI treatment entails titration of medication dosage to a level that controls symptoms and heals esophagitis.

Heartburn is alleviated in 96% and resolves in 70% of patients with Barrett's esophagus after LARS. No differences occur in medication use or symptom control after LARS, but the failure rate is higher in patients with Barrett's esophagus (12%) than in those without it (5%). In 89% of patients with Barrett's esophagus, LARS provides excellent control of esophageal acid exposure.

Antireflux surgery is superior to medical therapy for inhibiting the progression of Barrett's esophagus and preventing the development of Barrett's carcinoma. A meta-analysis reports that the risk for adenocarcinoma in patients with Barrett's esophagus is low and decreases by 1.5 cancers per 1000 patient-years, more after antireflux surgery than after medical treatment; however, these findings are not significant. Regression of Barrett's esophagus depends on the length of the columnar-lined esophagus and the time of follow-up after antireflux surgery. Endoscopy and pathology findings reveal complete regression of IM in 33% to 55% of patients with short-segment Barrett's esophagus after LARS. In patients with segments of Barrett's esophagus longer than 3 cm, 20% have disease regression, but 20% have disease progression from IM to dysplasia.

If HGD is found at endoscopy, there are three options for treatment: esophagectomy, intense surveillance, and ablation therapy. Intense surveillance for up to 46 months results in the development of adenocarcinoma in approximately 25% of patients, regression in 25% of patients, and stability in the remaining 50% of patients. The chance for concomitant esophageal cancer is 47% in all patients.

Esophagectomy is the most conservative approach but has high morbidity and mortality rates (3%–10%). Endoscopic therapy may be performed with multiple techniques, including thermal, chemical, and mechanical methods. The goal is to remove all dysplastic epithelium to allow the regrowth of squamous epithelium. Argon beam, laser, electrocautery, and photodynamic therapy have been used. Photodynamic therapy results in a downgrading of dysplasia in 90% of patients, but residual Barrett's esophagus may be found in 58% of patients. Complications of chest pain, nausea, and esophageal strictures may develop.

ADDITIONAL RESOURCES

GERD

Bammer T, Hinder RA, Klaus A, Klingler PJ: Five- to eight-year outcome of the first laparoscopic nissen fundoplications, *J Gastrointest Surg* 5:42–48, 2001.

Fass R: Proton-pump inhibitor therapy in patients with gastro-oesophageal reflux disease: putative mechanisms of failure, *Drugs* 67(11):1521–1530, 2007.

Frazzoni M, Piccoli M, Conigliaro R, et al: Refractory gastroesophageal reflux disease as diagnosed by impedance-pH monitoring can be cured by laparoscopic fundoplication, *Surg Endosc* 27:2940, 2013.

Jacobson BC, Somers SC, Fuchs CS, et al: Body-mass index and symptoms of gastroesophageal reflux in women, *N Engl J Med* 354(22):2340–2348, 2006.

Kahrilas PJ: GERD pathogenesis, pathophysiology, and clinical manifestations, *Cleve Clin J Med* 70(Suppl 5):S4–S19, 2003.

Li S, Shi S, Chen F, Lin J: The effects of baclofen for the treatment of gastroesophageal reflux disease: a meta-analysis of randomized controlled trials, *Gastroenterol Res Pract* 2014:307805, 2014.

Lundell L, Attwood S, Ell C, et al: Comparing laparoscopic antireflux surgery with esomeprazole in the management of patients with chronic gastro-oesophageal reflux disease: a 3-year interim analysis of the LOTUS trial, *Gut* 57(9):1207–1213, 2008.

Martinez SD, Malagon IB, Garewal HS, et al: Non-erosive reflux disease (NERD)–acid reflux and symptom patterns, *Aliment Pharmacol Ther* 17:537–545, 2003.

Napierkowski J, Wong RK: Extraesophageal manifestations of GERD, *Am J Med Sci* 326:285–299, 2003.

Richter JE: Diagnostic tests for gastroesophageal reflux disease, *Am J Med Sci* 326:300–308, 2003.

Richter JE: Duodenogastric reflux–induced (alkaline) esophagitis, *Curr Treat Options Gastroenterol* 7:53–58, 2004.

Sifrim D, Castell D, Dent J, Kahrilas PJ: Gastro-oesophageal reflux monitoring: review and consensus report on detection and definitions of acid, non-acid, and gas reflux, *Gut* 53:1024, 2004.

Spechler SJ: Clinical manifestations and esophageal complications of GERD, *Am J Med Sci* 326:279–284, 2003.

Tutuian R, Castell DO: Management of gastroesophageal reflux disease, *Am J Med Sci* 326:309–318, 2003.

Xie Y, Bowe B, Li T, et al: Risk of death among users of proton pump inhibitors: a longitudinal observational cohort study of United States veterans, *BMJ Open* 7:e015735, 2017.

Esophagitis: Acute and Chronic

Coron E, Hatlebakk JG, Galmiche JP: Medical therapy of gastroesophageal reflux disease, *Curr Opin Gastroenterol* 23(4):434–439, 2007.

Edwards SJ, Lind T, Lundell L: Systematic review: proton pump inhibitors (PPIs) for the healing of reflux oesophagitis—a comparison of esomeprazole with other PPIs, *Aliment Pharmacol Ther* 24(5):743–750, 2006.

Fornari F, Callegari-Jacques SM, Scussel PJ, et al: Is ineffective oesophageal motility associated with reflux oesophagitis?, *Eur J Gastroenterol Hepatol* 19(9):783–787, 2007.

Kahrilas PJ, Hughes N, Howden CW: Response of unexplained chest pain to proton pump inhibitor treatment in patients with and without objective evidence of gastro-oesophageal reflux disease, *Gut* 60:1473, 2011.

Katz PO, Ginsberg GG, Hoyle PE, et al: Relationship between intragastric acid control and healing status in the treatment of moderate to severe erosive oesophagitis, *Aliment Pharmacol Ther* 25(5):617–628, 2007.

Lundell L, Miettinen P, Myrvold HE, et al: Seven-year follow-up of a randomized clinical trial comparing proton-pump inhibition with surgical therapy for reflux oesophagitis, *Br J Surg* 94(2):198–203, 2007.

Okamoto K, Iwakiri R, Mori M, et al: Clinical symptoms in endoscopic reflux esophagitis: evaluation in 8031 adult subjects, *Dig Dis Sci* 48:2237–2241, 2003.

Pandolfino JE: Gastroesophageal reflux disease and its complications, including Barrett's metaplasia. In Feldman M, Friedman LS, Sleisenger MH, editors: *Gastrointesinal and liver disease*, ed 7, Philadelphia, 2002, Saunders, pp 599–622.

Wells RW, Morris GP, Blennerhassett MG, Paterson WG: Effects of acid-induced esophagitis on esophageal smooth muscle, *Can J Physiol Pharmacol* 81:451–458, 2003.

Esophageal Ulcers

Higuchi D, Sugawa C, Shah SH, et al: Etiology, treatment, and outcome of esophageal ulcers: a 10-year experience in an urban emergency hospital, *J Gastrointest Surg* 7:836–842, 2003.

Murphy PP, Ballinger PJ, Massey BT, et al: Discrete ulcers in Barrett's esophagus: relationship to acute gastrointestinal bleeding, *Endoscopy* 30:367–370, 1998.

Raghunath AS, Green JR, Edwards SJ: A review of the clinical and economic impact of using esomeprazole or lansoprazole for the treatment of erosive esophagitis, *Clin Ther* 25:2088–2101, 2003.

Spechler SJ: Clinical manifestations and esophageal complications of GERD, *Am J Med Sci* 326:279–284, 2003.

Sugawa C, Takekuma Y, Lucas CE, Amamoto H: Bleeding esophageal ulcers caused by NSAIDs, *Surg Endosc* 11:143–146, 1997.

Tarnawski AS: Cellular and molecular mechanisms of gastrointestinal ulcer healing, *Dig Dis Sci* 50(Suppl 1):S24–S33, 2005.

Wander P, Castaneda D, D'Souza L, et al: Single center experience of a new endoscopic clip in managing nonvariceal upper gastrointestinal bleeding, *J Clin Gastroenterol* 52(4):307–312, 2018.

Wolfsen HC, Wang KK: Etiology and course of acute bleeding esophageal ulcers, *J Clin Gastroenterol* 14:342–346, 1992.

Benign Esophageal Stricture

Bonavina L, DeMeester TR, McChesney L, et al: Drug-induced esophageal strictures, *Ann Surg* 206:173–183, 1987.

Kelly KA, Sare MG, Hinder RA: *Mayo Clinic gastrointestinal surgery*, Philadelphia, 2004, Saunders, p 49.

Klingler PJ, Hinder RA, Cina RA, et al: Laparoscopic antireflux surgery for the treatment of esophageal strictures refractory to medical therapy, *Am J Gastroenterol* 94:632–636, 1999.

Olson JS, Lieberman DA, Sonnenberg A: Practice patterns in the management of patients with esophageal strictures and rings, *Gastrointest Endosc* 66(4):670–675, quiz 767, 770, 2007.

Rosseneu S, Afzal N, Yerushalmi B, et al: Topical application of mitomycin C in oesophageal strictures, *J Pediatr Gastroenterol Nutr* 44(3):336–341, 2007.

Said A, Brust DJ, Gaumnitz EA, Reichelderfer M: Predictors of early recurrence of benign esophageal strictures, *Am J Gastroenterol* 98:1252–1256, 2003.

Barrett's Esophagus

Bammer T, Hinder RA, Klaus A, et al: Rationale for surgical therapy of Barrett's esophagus, *Mayo Clin Proc* 76:335–342, 2001.

Cossentino MJ, Wong RK: Barrett's esophagus and risk of esophageal adenocarcinoma, *Semin Gastrointest Dis* 14:128–135, 2003.

Dresner SM, Griffin SM, Wayman J, et al: Human model of duodenogastro-oesophageal reflux in the development of Barrett's metaplasia, *Br J Surg* 90:1120–1128, 2003.

Fass R, Sampliner RE: Barrett's oesophagus: optimal strategies for prevention and treatment, *Drugs* 63:555–564, 2003.

Gurski RR, Peters JH, Hagen JA, et al: Barrett's esophagus can and does regress after antireflux surgery: a study of prevalence and predictive features, *J Am Coll Surg* 196:706–712, discussion 712–713, 2003.

Lee TJ, Kahrilas PJ: Medical management of Barrett's esophagus, *Gastrointest Endosc Clin North Am* 13:405–418, 2003.

Morales TG, Camargo E, Bhattacharyya A, Sampliner RE: Long-term follow-up of intestinal metaplasia of the gastric cardia, *Am J Gastroenterol* 95:1677–1680, 2000.

Peters JH, DeMeester TR: Esophagus and diaphragmatic hernia. In Schwartz SI, Shires TG, Spencer FC, editors: *Principles of surgery*, ed 7, New York, 1999, McGraw-Hill, pp 1081–1179.

12

Sliding and Paraesophageal Hiatal Hernias Types 1, 2, and 3

Neil R. Floch

Hiatal hernias develop in 10% to 50% of the population with an average age of 48 for patients with a sliding hernia and 65 to 75 for a paraesophageal hernia. There are four types of hiatal hernias. Type 1, accounting for over 90% of all hernias, develops when the gastroesophageal junction (GEJ) slides above the diaphragm. The remaining hernias, 10%, are either type 3 or mixed type 2, which is a pure paraesophageal hernia. Type 2 hernias develop when the gastric fundus herniates into the chest, lateral to the esophagus, but the GE junction remains fixed in the abdomen; these account for 14% of the remaining 14% of hernias. Type 3, or mixed paraesophageal hernias, account for 86% of the remaining 14% of hernias. They develop with movement of the lower esophageal sphincter (LES) and the fundus into the chest (Figs. 12.1 and 12.2). The type 4 hernia is a subset of type 3 and contains not only the entire stomach but also other viscera, such as the omentum, colon (13%), spleen (6%), and small bowel. *Parahiatal hernia* is movement of the stomach through a diaphragmatic defect separate from the hiatus and accounts for less than 1% of all hiatal hernias.

A hiatal hernia forms as the phrenoesophageal membrane, preaortic fascia, and median arcuate ligament become attenuated over time. The pressure differential between the abdomen and the chest creates a vacuum effect during inspiration that pulls on the stomach. The degree of herniation into the posterior mediastinum and the type of volvulus that occurs may depend on the relative laxity of the gastrosplenic, gastrocolic, and gastrohepatic ligaments. As the hiatal hernia becomes larger, two types of volvulus may develop. *Organoaxial* volvulus (longitudinal axis) occurs with movement of the greater curvature of the stomach anterior to the lesser curvature. *Mesenteric axial* volvulus is less common and occurs when the stomach rotates along its transverse axis.

When the GEJ cannot be reduced below the diaphragm, despite extensive dissection in the mediastinum, then a shortened esophagus is present. This phenomenon is believed to occur in patients with chronic gastroesophageal reflux disease (GERD), with resultant transmural inflammation and contraction of the esophageal tube.

CLINICAL PICTURE

Although small type 1 hiatal hernias may be asymptomatic, most patients complain of typical and atypical symptoms of GERD. Heartburn is the main symptom of GERD, but patients may also complain of acid reflux, regurgitation of food, epigastric abdominal pain, dysphagia, odynophagia, nausea, bloating, and belching. Atypical or extraesophageal symptoms include noncardiac chest pain, choking, laryngitis, coughing, wheezing, difficulty breathing, sore throat, hoarseness, asthma, and dental erosions.

Symptoms of type 2 and 3 paraesophageal hernias differ from GERD symptoms. Although the symptoms vary, most series describe dysphagia, chest pain, and regurgitation as the most common. One series defined the symptoms as regurgitation (77%), heartburn (60%), dysphagia (60%), chest pain (52%), pulmonary problems (44%), nausea, and vomiting (35%), hematemesis or hematochezia (17%), and early satiety (8%). Asymptomatic patients may constitute 11% of the population, and the hernia may be discovered on routine chest radiography or endoscopy. Questioning may reveal the presence of symptoms in most patients.

Dysphagia may result from twisting of the esophagus by a herniated stomach. Chest pain may be confused with angina, resulting in emergency cardiac evaluation with negative results. Dyspnea may be secondary to loss of intrathoracic volume. Coughing may be a sign of aspiration, which can develop into pneumonia or bronchitis.

Iron-deficiency anemia occurs in 38% of patients. Usually but rarely is there evidence of gastrointestinal (GI) bleeding. Cameron ulcers or mucosal ulcerations of the stomach, found in 5.2%, are a cause of anemia. Ischemia and mucosal injury occur secondary to the friction of the stomach moving through the esophageal hiatus during respiration.

Postprandial distress—defined as chest pain, shortness of breath, nausea, and vomiting—occurs in 66% of patients. Eventually, as the hernia enlarges, most patients have these symptoms. Conversely, as a hernia enlarges, heartburn decreases. Heartburn is less common in type 3 than in type 1 hernias.

As many as 30% of patients will need emergency surgery for bleeding, acute strangulation, gastric volvulus, or total obstruction. Surgery is performed to treat perforation after strangulation with peritonitis, but mortality is 17%. If gastric necrosis has developed, mortality may reach 50%.

DIAGNOSIS

Most type 1 hiatal hernias are detected either by barium esophagraphy or by upper endoscopy. Computed tomography (CT) may also detect a hiatal hernia. Preferentially all patients should undergo esophageal manometry to determine the presence of an associated motility disorder before any surgical intervention. Specifically, achalasia should be ruled out. Patients with ineffective esophageal motility (IEM) or scleroderma may benefit from surgery but should undergo a partial fundoplication. Determination of the presence of acid or bile reflux can be performed with classic 24-hour pH testing, impedance testing, or the Bravo technique.

Upright chest radiography may reveal an air-fluid level behind the heart in 95% of patients. Nasogastric tube placement in the intrathoracic stomach confirms the diagnosis. Paraesophageal hernia can also easily be detected on CT. An upper GI series can establish the type of hiatal hernia. In a series of 65 patients, 56 (86%) were found on barium swallow or esophagogastroduodenoscopy (EGD) to have a type 3 paraesophageal hernia. EGD will reveal a hiatal hernia best on retroflexion. Nine (14%) had type 2 paraesophageal hernia. More than half of the stomach was in the chest in 21% of patients.

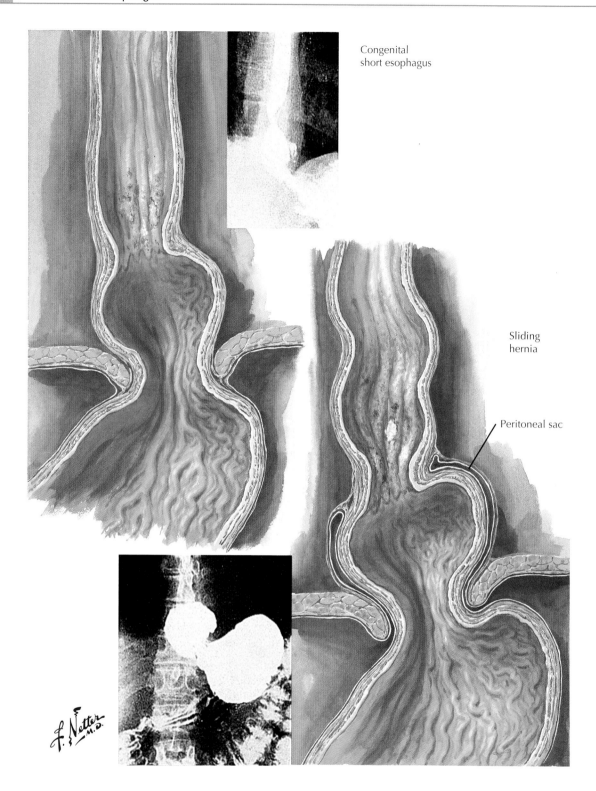

Congenital
short esophagus

Sliding
hernia

Peritoneal sac

Fig. 12.1 Type I: Sliding Hiatal Hernia.

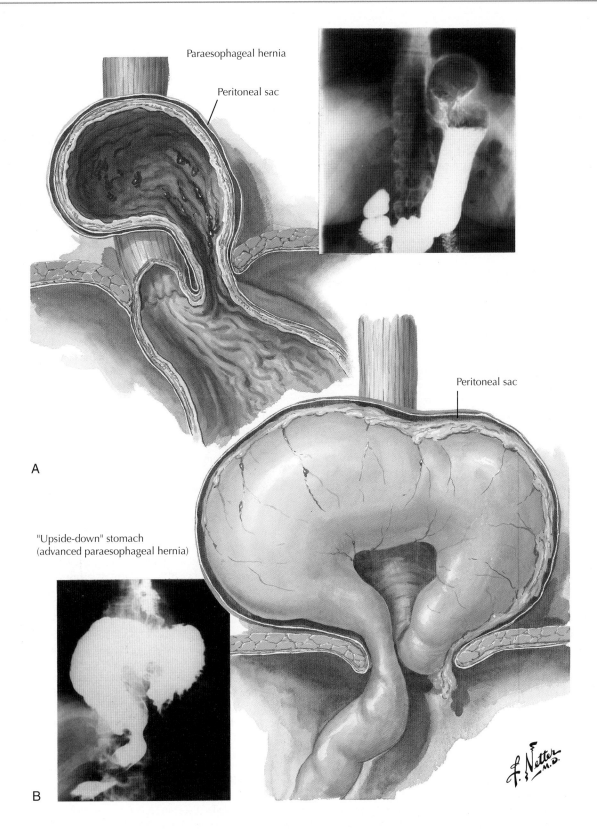

Paraesophageal hernia

Peritoneal sac

Peritoneal sac

A

"Upside-down" stomach
(advanced paraesophageal hernia)

B

Fig. 12.2 Paraesophageal Hernias. (A) Type II. (B) Type III.

A herniated stomach can be intubated only by using EGD, a nasogastric tube, or manometry. When possible, manometry can assess esophageal body motility, LES pressure, LES length, and total esophageal length. Manometry may be possible in only approximately 50% of patients. (Traditional manometry has been replaced by high-resolution manometry [HRM] with esophageal pressure topography [EPT], as described in Chapter 13.) At least 50% of patients with paraesophageal hernias have a hypotensive LES. An incompetent LES was found in 56% to 67% of patients, with an average pressure of less than 6 mm Hg. Short intraabdominal length of the LES combined with a sliding hernia may also contribute to reflux.

The amplitude of peristaltic waves is reduced in 52% to 58% of patients. Poor body motility can result in the delayed clearance of refluxed acid; this requires partial fundoplication, although some authors advocate the floppy Nissen procedure in this situation. A short esophagus may be related to a mixed, or type 3, paraesophageal hernia and is believed to result from injury to the esophageal wall secondary to stricturing and fibrosis from reflux. Whether the short esophagus is a result or the cause of paraesophageal herniation has yet to be determined.

Twenty-four-hour esophageal pH testing is not a diagnostic test for a paraesophageal hernia but may be helpful in identifying associated gastroesophageal reflux in 50% to 65% of patients.

TREATMENT AND MANAGEMENT

Repair of a small type 1 sliding hiatal hernia entails reduction of the hernia sac from the chest and performing either a partial (Toupet) or total (Nissen) fundoplication. If the fundus moves alongside the esophagus, the hernia is then classified as paraesophageal. The most difficult type 1 sliding hernias involve a shortened esophagus. When the GEJ cannot be reduced easily 3 to 4 cm below the diaphragm, the technique of extensive mediastinal dissection must be used. This involves dissecting all lateral, anterior, and posterior attachments of the esophagus to the mediastinum, taking care to avoid entering the pleura or disturbing major vessels. Dissection may be necessary up to the level of the aortic arch. GERD treatment or type 1 hiatal hernia repair results in at least 90% patient satisfaction rate.

Observation of paraesophageal hernias can result in emergency complications such as incarceration, strangulation, perforation, splenic vessel bleeding, and acute dilation of the herniated stomach in 20% of patients. A cohort study concluded that watchful waiting is reasonable for the initial management of patients with asymptomatic or minimally symptomatic paraesophageal hernias. Asymptomatic patients at high risk for morbidity after surgery may be observed. Nonsurgical management resulted in 29% mortality, but this rate is now believed to be lower. Asymptomatic patients have a lower risk for complications. Symptoms indicate the need for elective repair. Elective surgery carries a zero to 3% mortality rate. In comparison, emergency surgery results in up to a 40% mortality rate.

Studies are indeterminate as to the best technique for repairing paraesophageal hernias. Patients with comorbidities who undergo laparoscopy may experience the low complication rate, short recovery, and long-term results seen after open surgery.

Paraesophageal hernia is a surgical disease that cannot be adequately treated medically. Symptoms of reflux may be reduced with H$_2$ blockers and PPIs, but the hernia cannot be fixed without surgery. Paraesophageal hernia repair (PEHR) may, at the discretion of an experienced foregut surgeon, be performed by any of the following three approaches: laparoscopic, open transabdominal, or transthoracic. It can be accomplished with low mortality and morbidity with any of these approaches. All three procedures are equal in resolving symptoms such as acid reflux and dysphagia. Open PEHR has average morbidity of

14%, an average mortality of 3%, and length of hospital stay of 3 to 10 days. Major complications include bowel obstruction and splenectomy. The recurrence rate after laparotomy is 11%. Transthoracic PEHR is advocated by some surgeons for patients who are obese, have shortened esophagus, have large or complex hiatal hernias, or have recurrent hernias. The procedure has a higher morbidity and should therefore be performed only for recurrences or in those patients who cannot be approached through the abdomen. Thoracotomy results in 19% morbidity and up to 25% mortality. Reoperation may be necessary in 5% of patients.

Laparoscopy involves significantly lower rates of blood loss, intensive care unit stay, ileus, hospital stay, and overall morbidity. Laparoscopy is beneficial in the elderly population.

Failure to perform concomitant antireflux surgery results in postoperative reflux in 20% to 40% of patients. Antireflux surgery may improve motility in 50% of patients. Concomitant antireflux surgery should be performed for the following reasons: (1) especially when positive findings on 24-hour pH testing are found; (2) because destruction of the LES after surgical dissection of the hiatus predisposes to the development of GERD if not already present; (3) because incompetence of the LES is no longer masked by the paraesophageal hernia after it is reduced; (4) because the fundoplication secures the stomach into the abdominal cavity; (5) because there is minimal morbidity added to the procedure; and (6) because emergency surgery may need to be performed and thus preoperative testing cannot be performed.

Short esophagus has an overall incidence of 1.5%. Among patients with paraesophageal hernias, 15% to 20% have short esophagus. The diagnosis of short esophagus is made at surgery if the LES is 5 cm above the hiatus or if the esophagus is difficult to mobilize from the mediastinum.

In the past, the Collis-Belsey procedure has been recommended to treat short esophagus in patients with type 3 paraesophageal hernias. Newer techniques rely on more aggressive dissection. First, the hernia sac is reduced. Extensive dissection enables the esophagus to be mobilized from the chest into the abdomen. Patients with short esophagus who undergo laparoscopic transmediastinal dissection have a 90% success rate for fundoplication, almost equal the rate for patients with normal esophageal length (89%). The advent of laparoscopic transmediastinal dissection has rendered the Collis gastroplasty less necessary.

Gastrostomy and anterior gastropexy should be considered for elderly and debilitated patients who have many comorbidities and cannot tolerate extensive surgery. Both procedures secure the stomach to the abdominal wall, thus preventing future herniation. Disadvantages are the discomfort and inconvenience of a gastrostomy tube.

Alternatively, for severely debilitated patients, an endoscopic hernia reduction with or without laparoscopy can be performed with a double percutaneous endoscopic gastrostomy (PEG) tube placement to secure the stomach in the abdomen temporarily. A formal laparoscopic PEHR can be performed at a later time if the patient's medical condition improves.

If a primary crural closure is not possible, a tension-free mesh repair may be indicated. Most recent reports promote a primary suture closure of the muscle reinforced with an onlay of mesh that has a keyhole opening stapled to the crura. A defect larger than 5 cm is usually reported when mesh is used. Various prosthetic materials—including polyester (Mersilene), polytetrafluoroethylene (PTFE), and polypropylene—have been used for mesh. Along with these permanent mesh materials, multiple biologic materials have been used. All types of mesh have been effective in randomized trials. A meta-analysis of four randomized trials comparing mesh over primary repair with primary repair with sutures alone demonstrated a 2% versus 9% reoperation rate and a 16% versus 27% recurrence rate with equal complications at 10%.

COURSE AND PROGNOSIS

Immediately after surgery, patients should be treated with antiemetics to prevent the tearing of sutures. A swallow of diatrizoate (Gastrografin) is performed routinely on postoperative day one to confirm no leakage and the stability and location of the fundoplication.

Complications may be divided into intraoperative, postoperative, and late sequelae. Intraoperative complications occur in up to 17% of patients. Esophageal and gastric perforations related to bougie usage, tears, and lacerations occur in 11% of patients. Excessive bleeding may occur after dissection, tearing of the short gastric vessels, or liver retraction. Vagal nerve injury is rare but may lead to gastric atony, delayed gastric emptying, and bezoar formation.

Pleural entry and pneumothorax may occur in 14% of patients. Rarely of clinical significance is pneumomediastinum or crepitus, which resolves with no sequelae other than respiratory acidosis secondary to carbon dioxide exposure or, rarely, pulmonary embolus.

The 3% conversion rate frequently reflects the inability to decrease mediastinal contents caused by mediastinal scarring of a shortened esophagus. Traumatic vessel injury is a common reason for conversion, but other causes may be adhesions and difficulty with exposure. Exposure may be limited in patients who are obese or who have hepatomegaly.

Postoperative complications occur in 3% to 28% of patients. The most serious postoperative complications are pulmonary embolism, myocardial infarction (heart attack), cardiac dysrhythmias, cerebrovascular accident (stroke), and respiratory failure. Other conditions that may develop are pneumonia or pleural effusion, congestive heart failure, deep venous thrombosis, urinary retention, and superficial wound infections. Dysphagia is the most frequent postoperative problem. Dilation may be required in 6% of patients. Over time, some fundoplications slip, become undone, or migrate to the mediastinum. Postoperative pain is usually limited to incisions, but patients may have left shoulder pain caused by diaphragmatic irritation.

Reoperation rates range from zero to 9%. Early reoperation may be necessary for recurrence of a hernia, fundoplication slippage, esophageal or stomach perforation, or small-bowel obstruction. Dilation may be necessary for patients with dysphagia after surgery.

Mortality rates range from zero to 5%. Frequently, patients have gas-bloat syndrome, which includes bloating, abdominal gas, increased flatus, uncontrolled flatus, belching, and abdominal discomfort. Patients may also experience early satiety, pain after meals, and weight loss.

Operative time averages from 1 to 3 hours. Most patients stay in the hospital for 1 to 2 days. On average, patients return to normal activities within 1 to 3 weeks. Displacement of the paraesophageal hernia from the chest results in improved (15%–20%) pulmonary function. On average follow-up at 1.5 years, 92% of patients are satisfied with the surgical result.

Asymptomatic recurrence rates may be very high, but they range only from zero to 32% when barium esophagraphy is used. Clinically symptomatic recurrences are much lower, as indicated by the zero to 9% reoperation rate. Most patients with recurrences undergo surgery only if they have symptoms. Evaluation usually reveals a sliding herniation of the wrap in about 80% of patients. Although a recurrent paraesophageal hernia may occur, reoperation is not usually necessary.

ADDITIONAL RESOURCES

Floch NR: Paraesophageal hernias: current concepts, *J Clin Gastroenterol* 29:6–7, 1999.

Kohn GP, Price RR, DeMeester SR, et al: Guidelines for the management of hiatal hernia, *Surg Endosc* 27:4409, 2013.

Lidor AO, Steele KE, Stem M, et al: Long-term quality of life and risk factors for recurrence after laparoscopic repair of paraesophageal hernia, *JAMA Surg* 150:424, 2015.

Mattioli S, Lugaresi M, Ruffato A, et al: Collis-nissen gastroplasty for short oesophagus, *Multimed Man Cardiothorac Surg* 2015, 2015.

Memon MA, Memon B, Yunus RM, Khan S: Suture cruroplasty versus prosthetic hiatal herniorrhaphy for large hiatal hernia: a meta-analysis and systematic review of randomized controlled trials, *Ann Surg* 263:258, 2016.

Paul S, Nasar A, Port JL, et al: Comparative analysis of diaphragmatic hernia repair outcomes using the nationwide inpatient sample database, *Arch Surg* 147:607, 2012.

Perdikis G, Hinder RA, Filipi CJ, et al: Laparoscopic paraesophageal hernia repair, *Arch Surg* 132:586–589, 1997.

Rathore MA, Andrabi SI, Bhatti MI, et al: Metaanalysis of recurrence after laparoscopic repair of paraesophageal hernia, *JSLS* 11:456, 2007.

Stylopoulos N, Gazelle GS, Rattner DW: Paraesophageal hernias: operation or observation?, *Ann Surg* 236(4):492–500, 2002.

White BC, Jeansonne LO, Morgenthal CB, et al: Do recurrences after paraesophageal hernia repair matter? Ten-year follow-up after laparoscopic repair, *Surg Endosc* 22:1107–1111, 2008.

13

Esophageal Motility Disorders and Diagnosis

Neil R. Floch

ESOPHAGEAL MOTILITY DISORDERS

The connection between unexplained chest pain and esophageal spasm was first discovered by William Osler in 1892. Since then, multiple esophageal motility disorders have been encountered in clinical practice, with a wide range of symptoms, manometric findings, and responses (Fig. 13.1). These disorders vary from minimal changes to extensive radiologic and manometric abnormalities. The etiology of motility disorders has yet to be clearly defined.

Esophageal pressure topography (EPT) analysis of high-resolution manometry (HRM) and analysis by the Chicago Classification (CC) has clarified the diagnosis of esophageal motility disorders by first determining the lower esophageal sphincter (LES) pressures and then defining peristalsis of the esophageal body. Motility disorders fall into four categories: (1) achalasia, (2) esophagogastric junction outflow obstruction (EGJOO), (3) major disorders of peristalsis, and (4) minor disorders of peristalsis. (Achalasia is discussed further on.) Esophageal dysmotility may occur primarily or secondary to other diseases.

EGJOO may be a precursor to achalasia or to benign or malignant infiltrative disorders. EGJOO has the same pathophysiology as achalasia. In these patients the LES cannot relax and there is an elevated LES pressure. It is an uncommon manometric abnormality found in patients with dysphagia and chest pain that is sometimes associated with gastroesophageal reflux disease (GERD). Absent contractility occurs most often with GERD and collagen vascular diseases such as scleroderma. Failed peristalsis may result from a 360-degree fundoplication that is "too tight."

Diffuse esophageal spasm (DES) is a disease of the esophageal body characterized by rapid wave progression down the esophagus. It has an incidence of 1 in 100,000 individuals per year and is found in 4% of patients undergoing manometry. DES is unique in that it is distinguished by a nonperistaltic response to swallowing and may be closely related to achalasia in that 33% of individuals have an elevated LES pressure with poor relaxation.

Hypercontractile (jackhammer) esophagus or nutcracker esophagus (NE) was first diagnosed in the 1970s. It is found in 12% of individuals undergoing manometry. Patients are symptomatic with dysphagia. It is believed to occur from overexcitation of the esophageal smooth muscle or as a response to esophagogastric junction outflow obstruction (EGJOO).

Ineffective esophageal motility (IEM) is a monometrically defined disorder associated with severe GERD, obesity, respiratory symptoms, delayed acid clearance, and mucosal injury. IEM may occur secondary to other diseases, including alcoholism, diabetes mellitus, multiple sclerosis, rheumatoid arthritis, scleroderma, and systemic lupus erythematosus. Fragmented esophageal muscle segments may indicate the presence of hypomotility, which can lead to the inability to clear refluxed acid from the distal esophagus.

Unfortunately pathologic distinction between these disorders is usually not helpful because muscles and neural plexuses cannot be properly biopsied. The degree of increase in muscle mass may be an important determinant of the type and severity of esophageal motor dysfunction. The LES and esophageal muscles are thickest in patients with achalasia, thicker in patients with esophageal spasm disorders, and least thick in patients with DES and NE. In some studies no specific change in ganglion cells, vagus nerve, or disease progression has been found. However, a nerve defect is suspected because many patients may be sensitive to cholinergic stimulation.

Clinical Picture

Classic symptoms of esophageal motility disorders include chest pain (80%–90% of patients), dysphagia (30%), and heartburn (20%). Dysphagia of liquids and solids indicates a functional disorder of the esophagus; dysphagia of solids alone indicates a physical lesion. Very hot or cold liquids and stress may exacerbate dysphagia. The pain is usually retrosternal and frequently radiates to the back. Patients describe a pain more severe than angina that is intermittent and variable from day to day. It may last from minutes to hours. Usually a disparity exists between symptoms and manometric findings, and the chest pain may be unrelated to the dysmotility. Anxiety and depression are common in these patients. Stress, loud noises, and ergonovine maleate may stimulate muscular contractions. The cause may be a sensory abnormality, and psychiatric illness may alter patients' sensory perceptions.

Patients with EGJOO have dysphagia (71%) and chest pain (49%). Other common symptoms are regurgitation (75%) and heartburn (71%). Patients with absent contractility complain of dysphagia to liquids and solids. Patients with a low LES pressure and aperistalsis have severe GERD and its complications.

Patients with DES complain of chest pain and dysphagia. The pain may be associated with eating quickly or drinking hot, cold, or carbonated beverages. Anxiety is common. Patients with jackhammer esophagus or NE usually present with chest pain; dysphagia is present in only 10%. There is a 30% incidence of associated psychiatric disorders.

Patients with IEM present with typical symptoms of heartburn and reflux and rarely have nonobstructive dysphagia with impaired bolus transit through the esophagus. Patients with fragmented peristalsis are likely to complain of coughing and have reflux symptoms due to hypomotility and poor acid clearance.

Diagnosis

Several tests may be helpful with the diagnosis of motility disorders. Barium esophagraphy may detect nonpropulsive contractions with

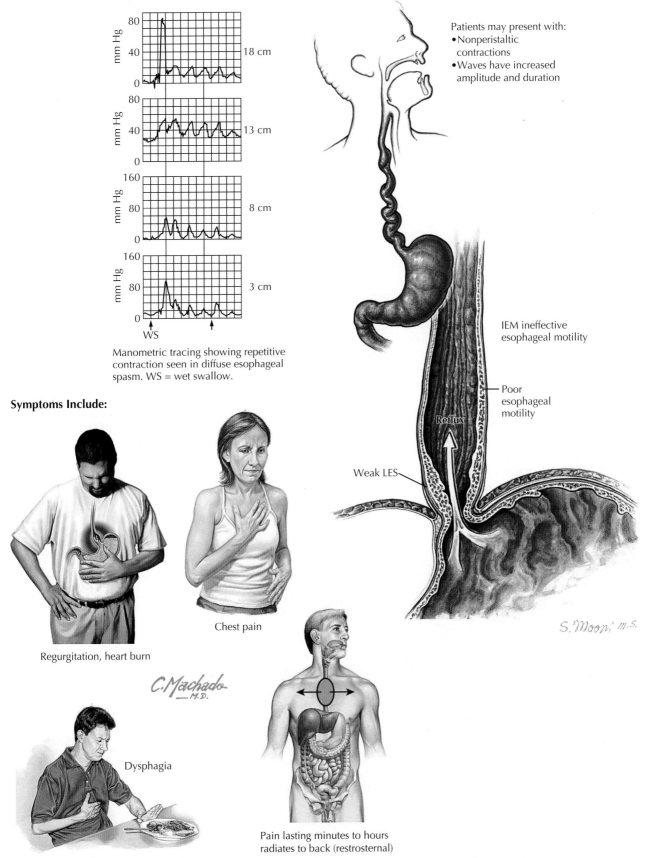

Manometric tracing showing repetitive contraction seen in diffuse esophageal spasm. WS = wet swallow.

Patients may present with:
• Nonperistaltic contractions
• Waves have increased amplitude and duration

IEM ineffective esophageal motility

Poor esophageal motility

Reflux

Weak LES

Symptoms Include:

Regurgitation, heart burn

Chest pain

Dysphagia

Pain lasting minutes to hours radiates to back (restrosternal)

Fig. 13.1 Esophageal Spasm Syndromes. *IEM,* Ineffective esophageal motility; *LES,* lower esophageal sphincter.

segmentation, which are diagnostic for "corkscrew" esophagus or DES. NE and other spastic disorders may present with minimal findings. Endoscopy is not diagnostic but should be performed to exclude malignancy or associated disorders such as hiatal hernia, reflux esophagitis, and strictures. Degeneration of esophageal vagal branches may be seen on biopsy in DES.

Of patients with GERD and respiratory symptoms, 30% to 50% have IEM, and 75% of IEM patients and 25% of EGJOO patients have an abnormal DeMeester score on 24-hour pH monitoring. In DES patients, computed tomography (CT) has been found to be sensitive in detecting esophageal wall thickening in the distal 5 cm of the esophagus; thus CT shows promise as a diagnostic test.

In the past most esophageal motility disorders have been diagnostically nonspecific.

Manometry is the definitive test for evaluating esophageal motility disorders, but symptoms correlate poorly with findings. Traditionally classic manometry has been used. HRM with EPT differs from traditional manometry; it has 36 sensors, each 1 cm apart, compared with 3 to 5 cm apart in traditional manometry (Fig. 13.2). Indications for usage, transnasal placement, and the number of swallows needed are the same, but HRM is more tolerable as only one placement of the catheter is needed. In HRM, sensors are located longitudinally and radially and pressure values between the sensors are extrapolated by software to create a complete pressure continuum, which is converted into a color three-dimensional graph. The red color tones indicate high pressures and blue color tones indicate low pressures. A topographic plot combining both the anatomy and physiology of the esophagus is developed from the data. The graph plots time and location on one axis and pressure as color on the other axis, creating an isobaric contour (IBC) map. The map demonstrates physiologic changes in the variables of space, contraction, and velocity, tracking the movement along the esophageal anatomy.

HRM and EPT both define esophageal motor function but EPT is more sensitive in determining peristalsis and LES function. EPT plots demonstrate the anatomy, physiology, and pathophysiology of the esophagus. The UES, LES, and passage through the crura are indicated by sudden increases in pressure along the EPT map, indicating tightness in the esophageal lumen. The LES is categorized as a type I at the LES, type II slightly separate, and type III, complete separation defined only by a respiratory inversion point (RIP).

Esophageal peristalsis comprises three contractile segments. The first is the UES, second the tubular esophagus in two places, and third the LES. There is a transition zone, a pressure trough between the first and second zones of the esophagus, where control of peristalsis shifts from the central nervous system to the enteric nervous system (myenteric plexus).

The contractile deceleration point (CDP) is measured on EPT by the slope of the IBC at 30 mm Hg. In the esophagus, conduction occurs faster proximally, correlating with the presence of a transient phrenic ampulla distally, which stretches, then the LES valve is elevated and is responsible for the slower emptying. The CDP is located within 3 cm of the upper aspect of the LES. Integrated relaxation pressure (IRP) measures the ability of the LES to relax. Manometry cannot differentiate between LES abnormalities of stenosis versus compression, which can cause outflow obstruction. The e-sleeve is a 10-second period, averaging 10 to 20 mm Hg at the LES, which includes crural contraction pressures. The IRP is the average pressure measured during the 4 seconds when the e-sleeve value is lowest. Distal latency (DL)—median 6.2 seconds and minimum of 4.6 seconds—measures the time at the end of a swallow between UES relaxation and the CDP.

The distal contractile integral (DCI) combines distal esophageal length, time of contraction, and mean amplitude of contraction. DCI measures the distance from the proximal to the distal pressure troughs excluding the first 20 mm Hg. According to the CC, contractile vigor relies on the DCI. Lower than 100 mm Hg/s/cm indicates failed peristalsis, whereas between 100 and 450 mm Hg/s/cm indicates weak peristalsis; however, both are ineffective. Normal is between 450 and 8000 mm Hg/s/cm, whereas hypercontractility is defined as above 8000 mm Hg/s/cm. Fragmented peristalsis is defined as a large break (>5 cm) in the 20 mm Hg IBC and is commonly found in patients with dysphagia. A premature contraction has a DL less than 4.5 seconds and a DCI greater than 450 mm Hg/s/cm.

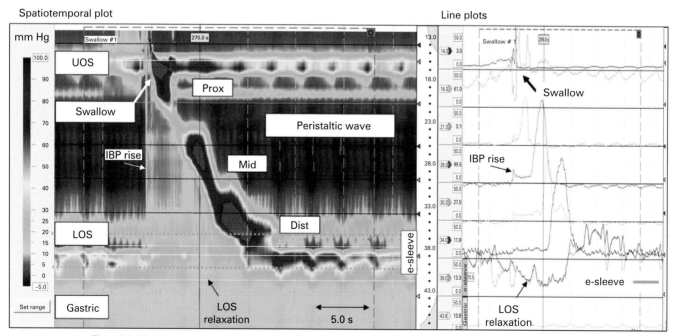

Fig. 13.2 High-Resolution Manometry. *IBP,* Isobaric pressure; *LOS,* lower oesophageal sphincter; *UOS,* upper oesophageal sphincter. (Reused with permission from Fox MR, Bredenoord AJ: Oesophageal high-resolution manometry: moving from research into clinical practice, *Gut* 57:405-423, 2008, F2.)

Esophageal contraction and pressurization differ in that a contraction must squeeze the muscle and close the lumen whereas pressurization occurs with the UES, LES, and esophageal lumen all open. Pressurization is visualized on EPT with vertical lines indicating increased pressure obstructed at both ends by a greater pressure. Pressure along the entire length of the esophagus is termed *panesophageal pressurization* and is diagnostic of type II achalasia. Compartmentalized pressurization can be found in postsurgical patients after a fundoplication surgery, hiatal hernia repair, or bariatric surgery.

The CC, version 3.0, enables the diagnosis of dysmotility disorders using EPT. The prevalence of esophageal dysmotility disorders is 5% of the general population. HRM has been used to characterize EPT findings in motility disorders. (Achalasia is explained further on.) EGJOO is defined by HRM as having a median IRP above the upper limit of normal with evidence of weak peristalsis, not meeting the threshold of severity of achalasia. The treatment for both may be similar. Initial therapy is botulinum toxin (Botox) injection and dilation, reserving surgical myotomy or peroral endoscopic myotomy (POEM) for cases where less invasive treatments have failed.

The first of the major motility disorders, absent contractility, occurs with a normal average IRP and 100% failed peristalsis. Distal esophageal spasm (DES) is defined as a normal median IRP with greater than 20% percent premature contractions and a DL less than 4.5 seconds. HRM has defined DES more accurately than traditional manometry. Diagnostically, DL is specific for DES. When DL is reduced, which is rarely found, symptoms of dysphagia or chest pain are almost always present and are consistent with either DES or type III achalasia. Hypercontractile (jackhammer) esophagus was previously called NE with diagnosis by traditional manometry. It is defined as two swallows or more with a DCI greater than 8000 mm Hg/s/cmin conjunction with single-peaked or multipeaked contraction. When hypercontractile esophagus is present with EGJ outflow obstruction, the motility resolves when the obstruction is corrected.

The minor disorders of peristalsis include IEM and fragmented peristalsis. IEM is defined by an average IRP less than 15 mm Hg and ≥50% ineffective swallows. IEM is associated with GERD. Nontransmitted contractions are present and ineffective at propelling food through a normal LES. Promotility drugs are recommended for IEM, but there is little evidence that they resolve symptoms. Fragmented peristalsis is defined as an average IRP less than 15 mm Hg with a normal DL, ≥50% fragmented contractions, and a DCI above 450 mm Hg/s/cm. Large breaks, defined as greater than 5 cm in the 20 mm Hg IBC, are significantly more common in patients complaining of dysphagia. The evidence of normal DL, or contraction vigor, distinguishes "fragmented peristalsis" from IEM.

Treatment and Management

Despite the categorization of motility disorders into separate entities based on HRM and EPT, disorders involving different pathophysiologic mechanisms and manometric findings do not always correlate with symptoms. The advancement of HRM and EPT has been extremely beneficial in diagnosis, but there remains few successful therapies with which to treat motility disorders. Treatment focuses on symptom reduction and begins with reassurance, because many disorders may have a psychiatric component. Patients' most frequent complaint is pain, which may be related to GERD and not the motor disorder; therefore treatment should also include proton pump inhibitors (PPIs). It is unknown whether IEM is the cause or the effect of GERD, but resolving reflux helps to improve IEM. Unfortunately effective motility medications for IEM, such as cisapride, are no longer available.

Besides PPI medications for associated acid reflux, limited treatments have been developed to address the symptoms and not the specific diseases. If dysphagia is the initial complaint, patients are initially treated with a calcium channel blocker such as diltiazem 80 to 240 mg/day. If chest pain is the primary complaint, treatment should be initiated with diltiazem. In NE, diltiazem, 60 to 90 mg four times daily significantly reduces chest pain more than a placebo. In DES, diltiazem reduces both chest pain and dysphagia.

Tricyclic antidepressants such as imipramine 25 to 50 mg/day or trazadone, 100 to 150 mg/day administered at bedtime may also be used for chest pain symptoms. Tricyclic antidepressants have not been demonstrated to improve dysmotility but are believed to improve the visceral sensory perception to chest pain. Tricyclic antidepressants, which have proven benefit for chest pain, have produced the most success with motility disorders. A 70% incidence of concomitant psychiatric disorders has been observed with motility disorders.

In patients who fail to respond to primary treatments, secondary options for NE, DES, and EGJOO include botulinum toxin injection above the EGJ, which relieves dysphagia but not chest pain, regurgitation, or heartburn. The effects last 6 months and therefore the injection must be repeated. Other options to reduce LES pressure include: a nitric oxide–contributing drug such as isosorbide 10 mg or sildenafil 50 mg, which is given for chest pain. Bougie dilation may also be used and may be beneficial in 40% of patients with severe manometric abnormalities. In DES, peppermint oil, as in Altoids, can improve manometric abnormalities and chest pain.

Surgical therapy is reserved for patients who have failed medical treatment with severe dysphagia and/or chest pain. Surgical options include a long myotomy from the arch of the aorta across the LES, with an added antireflux procedure to address severe esophageal dysmotility. Thoracoscopy is the preferred technique for long myotomy and a viable alternative to open surgery. Myotomy with partial fundoplication for isolated EGJOO relieves dysphagia and chest pain, suggesting a primary sphincter dysfunction. Some data support POEM for patients with NE and DES, but long-term results are not documented and patients can develop recurrent dysphagia and reflux. Because medication for IEM is used only to treat associated reflux, patients may be offered partial fundoplication to treat GERD, with expected relief of reflux in 79% of patients.

Course and Prognosis

Motility disorders rarely progress and are not known to be fatal. Time alone has demonstrated improvement in DES symptoms and manometry findings. Up to 75% of patients treated with tricyclic antidepressants for chest pain may experience prolonged remission of symptoms. Achalasia with worsening dysphagia and regurgitation develops in 5% of patients. Open surgical therapy has been successful in 50% of patients when dysmotility is associated with dysphagia. Thoracoscopic myotomy for NE and DES has resulted in a good or excellent result in 80% of patients, compared with only 26% of patients treated with medication or dilation. Minimally invasive surgery offers patients with NE and DES the best opportunity to become asymptomatic. Patients with IEM should undergo laparoscopic partial fundoplication for relief of reflux.

ACHALASIA

With an incidence of 1 to 6 per 100,000 population in North America, achalasia is the most common motor disorder of the esophagus (Fig. 13.3). It affects both genders equally and most commonly occurs in people 25 to 60 years of age. With the advent of HRM and EPT findings in motility disorders, normal and vigorous achalasia subtypes have now been more specifically classified into three subtypes. The traditional form, characterized by extensive esophageal dilatation, aperistalsis,

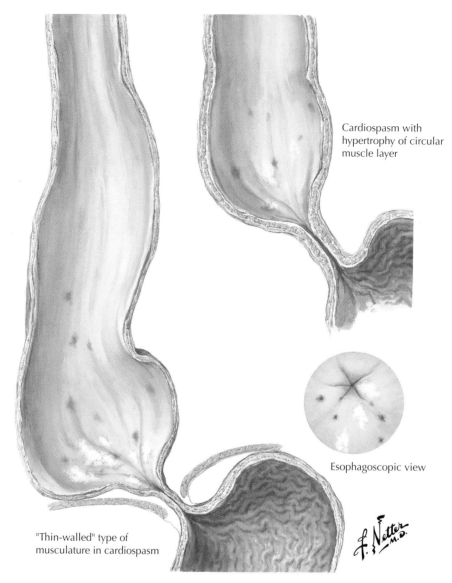

Cardiospasm with hypertrophy of circular muscle layer

Esophagoscopic view

"Thin-walled" type of musculature in cardiospasm

Fig. 13.3 Achalasia (Cardiospasm or Achalasia Cardiae).

and a thickened LES that does not relax to baseline pressure affects 75% of patients with achalasia. The remaining 25% have "vigorous" achalasia. Compared with patients with traditional achalasia, those with vigorous achalasia seek treatment at an earlier stage of disease and have higher muscle contraction amplitude, minimal esophageal dilatation, higher LES pressure, and prominent tertiary contractions. Patients with achalasia lack ganglion cells in the myenteric plexus of Auerbach in the distal esophagus. Degeneration of the vagal motor dorsal nucleus and destruction of the vagal nerve branches have been observed.

The etiology of primary or idiopathic achalasia remains unknown. Achalasia may be an immune-mediated inflammatory disease in which esophageal neurons are destroyed by herpes simplex virus type 1 (HSV-1) reactive T cells present in the LES muscles. Myenteric antiplexus antibodies are present in 100% of women and 67% of men with achalasia. The response occurs after HSV-1 infection and is believed to have a genetic predisposition.

Secondary achalasia results from diseases that cause esophageal motor abnormalities that are similar to achalasia. These diseases include amy-loidosis, chronic idiopathic intestinal pseudo-obstruction, eosinophilic esophagitis, Fabry disease, juvenile Sjögren syndrome, sarcoidosis, multiple endocrine neoplasia type 2B, and neurofibromatosis.

Clinical Picture

Almost all patients with achalasia have dysphagia of solids, and 66% to 85% have dysphagia of liquids. Patients initially feel heaviness or constriction in the chest when under stress. Food itself causes some stress, eventually resulting in obstruction. Retrosternal chest pain may occur in 40% to 60% of patients but improves over time. Patients eventually become afraid to eat as symptoms of dysphagia, chest pain, and regurgitation of food develop. Regurgitation of undigested food occurs in 60% to 90% of patients. Difficulty belching occurs in up to 85% of patients due to poor relaxation of the UES. Most patients maintain their nutritional status with little weight loss. Pneumonia is common in elderly patients, approximately 8%, from the regurgitation and aspiration of food.

Neither the severity nor the total number of achalasia-related symptoms correlates with the severity of radiographic findings. Although it is the most common symptom, dysphagia is the initial symptom in only 39% of patients. Heartburn occurs in 25% to 75%. Slow eating occurs in 79% of patients, regurgitation occurs in 76%, and 60% engage in characteristic movements such as arching the neck and shoulders, raising the arms, standing and sitting straight, and walking to assist in swallowing food. Rapid progression of weight loss may be a sign of pseudoachalasia from a malignancy.

Diagnosis

Barium esophagraphy shows dilatation of the distal esophagus, aperistalsis, and poor relaxation of the LES. There is a classic bird-beak appearance as a dilated portion of the LES esophagus tapers to a point. Fluoroscopy may visualize spasms in the esophagus as it attempts to empty its contents through the LES. Epiphrenic diverticula are often associated with achalasia. Esophagraphy is not sensitive and may appear normal in 33% of patients.

Despite its unique visual appearance, the diagnosis of achalasia is made through manometric evaluation. Traditional manometry has revealed simultaneous low-amplitude contractions of the esophageal body that do not propagate. The LES narrows to 2 cm, and the LES relaxes incompletely.

HRM has become the standard as it is able to more specifically characterize motility disorders by the EPT findings. As a result, achalasia may now be diagnosed and described in thee subtypes by this technology. Type I achalasia has a median IRP that is greater than the upper limit of normal, 100% failed peristalsis with a DCI less than 100 mm Hg/s/cm, and minimal pressurization within the lumen of the esophagus. Type II achalasia has a median IRP that is greater than the upper limit of normal, there is no normal peristalsis, and panesophageal pressurization is seen with ≥20% of swallows. Type III achalasia has a median IRP that is greater than the upper limit of normal, there is no normal peristalsis, preserved fragments of nonpropagating distal peristalsis or premature contractions with a DCI greater than 450 mm Hg/s/cm with ≥20% of swallows.

In the past, achalasia and vigorous achalasia had no measurable diagnostic definitions. HRM and EPT have provided a measurable technique to categorize the subtypes, thus allowing for different therapeutic options and resultant outcome results.

Esophagoscopy is performed to rule out malignancy and other diseases that are a part of the differential diagnosis and to evaluate the mucosa before any procedure is undertaken. Endoscopic findings may include dilatation and atony of the esophageal body and LES closing that is difficult to open; a pop may be detected as the scope passes through the LES. Small particles of food may be retained early and large amounts retained late in the disease process. Inspissated food particles may adhere to the thickened mucosa, causing leukoplakia, and there may be resultant erythema, inflammation, or ulceration. The esophagus may also become elongated before dilatation.

Endoscopic ultrasound (EUS) may reveal a LES with a thickened circular muscle layer at the LES and along the esophagus. It may also detect a distal esophageal or gastric cardia tumor which then may be biopsied; 10 mm thick or greater is suspicious. The differential diagnosis of achalasia includes GERD, pseudoachalasia from a malignancy, or other esophageal dilation disorders such as DES and jackhammer or NE.

Treatment and Management

Therapy consists of medications, local injections, pneumatic dilatation, and surgery and is directed at palliation of symptoms and prevention of complications. Medications have had limited success in relieving achalasia symptoms and are a last resort if botulinum toxin does not relieve symptoms.

Sublingual medications that relieve some symptoms of achalasia include nifedipine 10 to 30 mg, isosorbide dinitrate 5 mg, and nitroglycerin 0.4 mg; nifedipine is taken 30 minutes before meals; isosorbide dinitrate and nitroglycerin are taken 15 minutes before meals. These medications relax the smooth muscle of the LES. Oral calcium channel blockers have resulted in some symptom improvement, as has sublingual nitroglycerin, in 53% to 87%.

Botulinum toxin A (Botox) inhibits acetylcholine release from the nerve endings within the myenteric plexus and at the nerve-muscle junction. It decreases LES pressure in patients with achalasia and has limited adverse effects. It is successful in 30% to 75% of patients but the results last only 6 to 9 months so the injection must be repeated. Only 50% of patients respond for more than 1 year, and 70% experience relapse at 2 years. Long-term success is highest in elderly patients and in those with LES pressure that exceeds normal by only 50%. Botulinum toxin injection is a good option for elderly, debilitated patients who are not candidates for more invasive procedures as well as for patients who prefer this option.

Pneumatic dilatation is another option that is less invasive than surgery. Dilatation with a 50-Fr dilator provides temporary relief for only 3 days. Forceful dilatation with a balloon is more successful because the circular muscles must be torn to achieve long-term relief. The balloon creates pressure to 300 mm Hg for 1 to 3 minutes and distention to a diameter of 3 cm. After dilatation, a meglumine diatrizoate (Gastrografin) swallow is performed and the patient is observed for 6 hours before discharge. The most severe complication after dilatation is esophageal perforation, which occurs in 3% of patients. Small tears with free flow of contrast back into the esophagus may be treated conservatively. If there is free flow into the mediastinum, emergency thoracotomy is indicated. Surgery is usually necessary for 50% of perforations. Symptom relief is successful in 55% to 70% of achalasia patients with an initial dilatation and up to 93% with multiple dilatations. Symptom relief is the traditional measure used to assess treatment success. The timed barium study (TBS) is also used to assess esophageal emptying and correlates with a successful outcome in patients undergoing pneumatic dilatation. Poor esophageal emptying can be seen on barium esophagraphy in almost 30% of achalasia patients reporting complete symptom relief after pneumatic dilatation; 90% of these patients experience failed treatment within 1 year.

Laparoscopic Heller myotomy is the procedure of choice for patients with achalasia. It results in all the same benefits as thoracoscopy with less dysphagia and less reflux. Surgery is indicated in patients younger than 40 years or in those who have recurrent symptoms after botulinum type A treatment or pneumatic dilatation. It is also indicated in those who are at high risk for perforation from dilatation because of diverticula, previous GEJ surgery, or a tortuous or dilated esophagus.

Myotomy involves the division of all layers of muscle down to the mucosa with extension of at least 1 cm onto the stomach. A postoperative esophagram is performed to indicate adequate esophageal clearance and exclude a leak. Resting pressures of the esophageal body and LES are lower after surgery. Esophageal transit improves in postoperative patients but is still slower than in healthy controls. Persistent postoperative dysphagia may occur in up to 5% and may be treated with dilatation or repeat surgery.

A partial fundoplication, Toupet or Dor, should be performed to prevent reflux. Median hospital stay is only 2 days. The incidence of GE reflux in patients who had undergone esophageal myotomy alone was 64%, but 27% in those who had myotomy and antireflux procedure. At 15 years after surgery, 11% of patients will develop esophagitis and more than 40% will have reflux with a partial fundoplication. Good to excellent long-term results were seen in approximately 90% of patients at 3-year follow-up and in 75% to 85% after 15 years. Approximately 2% of patients develop esophageal cancer after surgery.

Thoracoscopic myotomy without fundoplication produces an excellent response in 80% to 90% of patients. Compared with thoracotomy, surgery is shorter, there is less blood loss and less need for a narcotic, and recovery to normal activity is faster. Median hospital stay is 3 days, compared with 2 days after laparoscopic Heller myotomy. GERD may develop in 60% of patients after thoracoscopic myotomy, and dysphagia persists in approximately 10%.

POEM is a technique that uses endoscopy to perform an esophageal myotomy and division of the LES sphincter. The mucosa is divided to gain access to the underlying muscle; the endoscope is then inserted down the plane to the gastric cardia, where the muscularis propria of the LES is divided by cautery. An antireflux procedure is not performed. Postoperative GERD occurs in 17% to 21% of patients at 2 months and 3 years, respectively. Small studies have not reported mortality, but complications of pneumothorax, bleeding, mucosal perforation, and pleural effusions in 3% of patients have been reported. Results reveal decreased LES pressures and marked symptomatic improvement. Unique to POEM are the surprisingly good results in patients with type III "end stage" achalasia, who usually fail all other treatments.

Course and Prognosis

Achalasia can now be more specifically classified. Type II patients are most likely to respond to all therapies—such as botulinum toxin with a response in 71%, pneumatic dilatation with a response in 91%, and Heller myotomy with a response in 100%—compared with only a 56% overall response in type I patients and 29% in type III patients. If left untreated, esophagitis may develop from stasis of retained food; 30% of patients may aspirate esophageal contents. Coughing attacks and pulmonary infections may also occur. Carcinoma may develop in 2% to 7% of patients. Currently there is no recommended surveillance program for malignancy.

In the primary treatment of achalasia, dilatation is superior to botulinum type A treatment in the short term; clinical remission rates at 4 months are approximately 90% (dilatation) versus 40% (Botox). Also, myotomy is more reliable in reducing LES pressure than pneumatic dilatation. Good or excellent relief of dysphagia is obtained in 90% of myotomy patients (85% after thoracoscopic myotomy, 90% after laparoscopic myotomy). Mortality is rare. After documentation that laparoscopic treatment outperforms balloon dilatation and botulinum type A injection, the laparoscopic Heller myotomy is the preferred treatment for the appropriately indicated patients diagnosed with achalasia.

Surgery for achalasia can fail in 10% to 15% of patients, more frequently in those who have had previous endoscopic procedures, a longer duration of symptoms, severely dilated esophagus, and very low LES pressure. Recurrent dysphagia after myotomy should first be treated with pneumatic dilatation. If this fails, laparoscopic reoperation for achalasia is safe and feasible and is the procedure of choice. It is performed in approximately 5% of patients with recurrent or persistent dysphagia. Repeat surgery improves symptoms in more than 85% of patients. The surgeon's experience and recognition of the cause for failure of the original surgery are the most important factors in predicting outcome.

The future role of POEM has yet to be defined, as the procedure is being performed only in centers with significant experience, and the development of GERD postprocedure remains a potential problem. Patients with type III achalasia may preferentially benefit from this procedure.

Over their lifetimes, patients with achalasia develop many complications that warrant therapy, but their life expectancy and eventual cause of death do not differ from those in the average population.

ADDITIONAL RESOURCES

Achem SR: Treatment of spastic esophageal motility disorders, *Gastroenterol Clin North Am* 33(1):107–124, 2004.

Balaji NS, Peters JH: Minimally invasive surgery for esophageal motility disorders, *Surg Clin North Am* 82:763–782, 2002.

D'Onofrio V, Annese V, Miletto P, et al: Long-term follow-up of achalasic patients treated with botulinum toxin, *Dis Esophagus* 13:96–101, (discussion 102–103), 2000.

Ghosh SK, Pandolfino JE, Zhang Q, et al: Quantifying esophageal peristalsis with high-resolution manometry: a study of 75 asymptomatic volunteers, *Am J Physiol Gastrointest Liver Physiol* 290:G988, 2006.

Gorecki PJ, Hinder RA, Libbey JS, et al: Redo laparoscopic surgery for achalasia, *Surg Endosc* 16:772–776, 2002.

Inoue H, Sato H, Ikeda H, et al: Per-oral endoscopic myotomy: A series of 500 patients, *J Am Coll Surg* 221:256, 2015.

Kahrilas PJ: Treating achalasia; more than just flipping a coin, *Gut* 65:726, 2016.

Kahrilas PJ, Bredenoord AJ, Fox M, et al: The Chicago classification of esophageal motility disorders, v3.0, *Neurogastroenterol Motil* 27:160, 2015.

Lin Z, Kahrilas PJ, Roman S, et al: Improving the integrated relaxation pressure (IRP) cutoff value for the diagnosis of achalasia using a classification and regression tree (CART) model (abstract), *Gastroenterology* 142(Suppl 1):S281, 2012.

Ortiz A, de Haro LF, Parrilla P, et al: Very long-term objective evaluation of Heller myotomy plus posterior partial fundoplication in patients with achalasia of the cardia, *Ann Surg* 247(2):258–264, 2008.

Pandolfino JE, Kwiatek MA, Nealis T, et al: Achalasia: a new clinically relevant classification by high-resolution manometry, *Gastroenterology* 135:1526, 2008.

Rohof WO, Salvador R, Annese V, et al: Outcomes of treatment for achalasia depend on manometric subtype, *Gastroenterology* 144:718, 2013.

Roman S, Lin Z, Pandolfino JE, Kahrilas PJ: Distal contraction latency: a measure of propagation velocity optimized for esophageal pressure topography studies, *Am J Gastroenterol* 106:443, 2011.

Schuchert MJ, Luketich JD, Landreneau RJ, et al: Minimally invasive esophagomyotomy in 200 consecutive patients: factors influencing postoperative outcomes, *Ann Thorac Surg* 85(5):1729–1734, 2008.

Smout AJ: Advances in esophageal motor disorders, *Curr Opin Gastroenterol* 24(4):485–489, 2008.

Sweis R, Anggiansah A, Wong T, et al: Normative values and inter-observer agreement for liquid and solid bolus swallows in upright and supine positions as assessed by esophageal high-resolution manometry, *Neurogastroenterol Motil* 23:509, 2011.

Watson DI, Jamieson GG, Bessell JR, et al: Laparoscopic fundoplication in patients with an aperistaltic esophagus and gastroesophageal reflux, *Dis Esophagus* 19(2):94–98, 2006.

14

Neoplastic Disease of the Esophagus

Neil R. Floch

BENIGN LESIONS OF THE ESOPHAGUS

Benign tumors of the esophagus are rare, accounting for less than 10% of all esophageal tumors and occurring with a prevalence of 0.5%. However, autopsy studies indicate that benign lesions occur in 8% of the adult population and may account for the higher frequency of individuals that remain undiagnosed and asymptomatic. Esophageal carcinoma is 50 times more prevalent than benign lesions. Since the advent of computed tomography (CT), tumors have been discovered more frequently (Fig. 14.1). Benign esophageal lesions can be classified either histologically according to their involvement in the epithelial or subepithelial tissue layers or by endoscopically visualized characteristics such as flat, raised, or cystic features.

The histologic frequency of epithelial lesions occurs most commonly to least, including glycogenic acanthosis, heterotopic gastric mucosa, squamous papilloma, hyperplastic polyp, ectopic sebaceous gland, and xanthoma. Subepithelial lesions occur most frequently with hemangioma, leiomyoma, and granular cell tumor. (Leiomyomas are the most common subepithelial lesions and are described in another section). (Gastrointestinal stromal tumors [GISTs] are benign and malignant and leiomyosarcomas are malignant; these subepithelial lesions are described in rare malignant lesions of the esophagus.) The benign lesions in this section are categorized by endoscopic features.

Clinical Picture

Benign lesions of the esophagus are rarely symptomatic. They are usually found incidentally at the time of upper endoscopy or barium esophagraphy that is performed for another reason. They are unlikely to be malignant or a precursor to malignancy. They have been classified as raised, flat, or cystic.

Diagnosis, Treatment, and Management by Lesion

Benign esophageal lesions can be classified as raised, flat, or cystic. Most can be diagnosed based upon their endoscopic appearance, findings on routine biopsy, and, in the case of submucosal lesions, by endoscopic ultrasound (EUS).

Raised Lesions

Schwannomas are rare benign tumors derived from Schwann cells in the peripheral nerves. Microscopically, they are diagnosed by lymphoid cuffing, nuclear atypia, and the presence of spindle-shaped cells. Rarely do they cause dysphagia, and malignant schwannomas are highly unusual. Small lesions may be enucleated and larger ones may be surgically resected.

Lymphangiomas arise from lymphatic tissue malformations. They are rare in the esophagus, occurring most frequently in patients younger than 2 years of age. Endoscopy reveals translucent yellow compressible mass structures less than 0.5 cm. Biopsy may be negative, as they are submucosal, but EUS is diagnostic. Histology reveals dilated endothelial cavities with eosinophilic material lined by flat endothelial cells. Treatment is with observation unless they grow to 4 to 5 cm. They are resected by band-assisted mucosectomy, endoscopic submucosal dissection (ESD), or by using a CO_2 laser.

Esophageal hemangiomas occur in 0.04% of autopsies. Most are cavernous and rarely involve capillary lesions. Usually they occur alone, but multiple lesions are seen in disorders such as Osler-Weber-Rendu disease, Klippel-Trénaunay syndrome, or congenital blue rubber bleb nevus syndrome. They are found incidentally on endoscopy and are nodular, soft, and bluish-red; they blanch when compressed. These lesions have been confused with Kaposi sarcoma. Rarely, they may bleed or cause dysphagia, which is the only reason to resect them endoscopically or surgically.

Fibrovascular polyps arise from nodular mucosa and take up 0.5% to 1.0% of all benign esophageal lesions; most are located proximally and 75% occur in men. They are most common in the upper esophagus and are usually attached to the cricopharyngeus. They are a conglomerate of fibrous, vascular, and adipose tissues with a squamous epithelium. Histologically they are inclusive of different fibromas, fibrolipomas, myomas, and lipomas. They are rare, accounting for 0.5% to 1% of all benign esophageal lesions. Fibrovascular polyps rarely cause symptoms of dysphagia, chronic cough, nausea, and vomiting. They can grow to 20 cm and prolapse into the larynx, causing airway obstruction. Gastric prolapse can result in ulceration and bleeding. If fibrovascular polyps are symptomatic, they are removed. They usually have stalks that are vascular and can be detected by EUS. Lesions can be removed endoscopically if an Endoloop is used to ligate the nutrient vessels.

Approximately 10% of granular cell tumors arise in the gastrointestinal (GI) tract; the esophagus is involved in 65% of such cases. Granular cell tumors of the esophagus are rare, occurring in 0.033% of all individuals at endoscopy and composing 1% of benign esophageal tumors. Approximately 60% of those affected are men. Endoscopic exam reveals sessile yellowish-white lesions with normal mucosa with a thick consistency. Of all, 90% are solitary with histologically large polygonal cells containing eosinophilic granules. They are believed to be of neural origin, as they resemble Schwann cells under electron microscopy and are positive for S100 protein. Deeper tunneling biopsies are needed to diagnose these deeper lesions. The larger the lesion, the faster the growth and the higher the malignant potential. Lesions of 4 cm and greater compose all of the 4% of malignant lesions that demonstrate infiltrative growth. These lesions must therefore be removed, which is usually possible with the techniques of classic biopsy, endoscopic mucosal resection or submucosal tunnel endoscopic.

Esophageal adenomas usually arise in segments of Barrett esophagus. They are dysplastic, polypoid, or nodular lesions that may reach 1.5 cm and may be multiple. They may be found in conjunction with esophageal adenocarcinoma; therefore adjacent areas must be biopsied along with

Pedunculated lipoma in esophagus

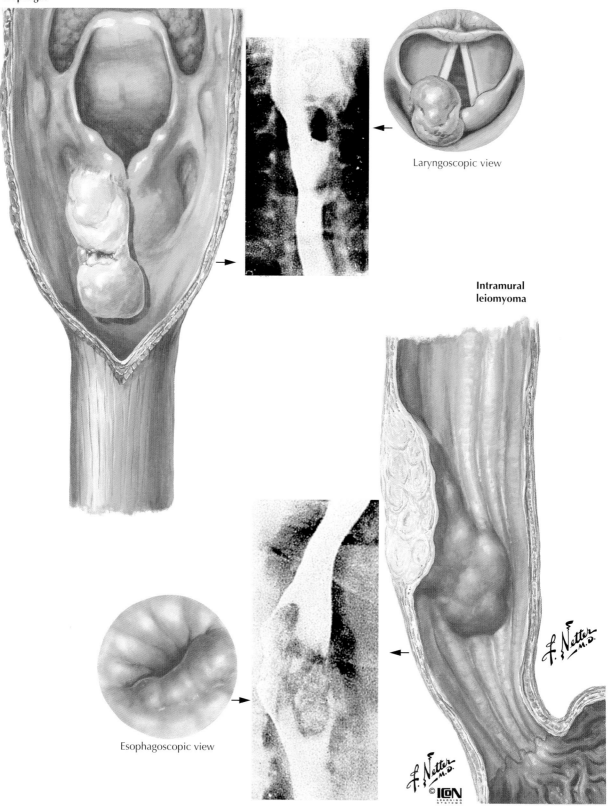

Laryngoscopic view

Intramural leiomyoma

Esophagoscopic view

Fig. 14.1 Benign Neoplasms.

narrow-band imaging and chromoendoscopy. If surrounding Barrett is detected, patients are treated as having Barrett esophagus with dysplasia. If there is no Barrett, lesions smaller than 1 cm are removed endoscopically and those greater than 1 cm with high-grade dysplasia (HGD) undergo mucosal resection or surgery.

Inflammatory fibroid polyps are composed of many lesions with reactive blood vessels, fibroblasts, and inflammatory cells such as hamartomas, inflammatory pseudopolyps, and eosinophilic granulomas. They are extremely rare, at 3 per million cases, and less likely to be found in the esophagus than any other section of the intestine. They are believed to be caused by acid reflux.

Inflammatory fibroid polyps are benign, incidentally found, reactive and inflammatory, with a connective tissue stroma and eosinophilic infiltrate. They occasionally cause dysphagia and hemorrhage and may grow to 9 cm, at which point endoscopic snare removal or surgery is warranted.

Esophageal papillomas are rare, with an incidence up to 0.04%, benign epithelial with microscopic fingerlike projections of squamous cells, connective tissue, and blood vessels. The cause of these lesions is unknown but believed to be an underlying inflammatory condition. Approximately 70% are located in the distal third of the esophagus and associated with reflux, esophagitis, or mechanical manipulation. Substances such as benzopyrene and nitrosamines may be a cause as well. Human papillomavirus (HPV) is associated in up 5% to 46% of cases and may be a cause. Sexual transmission may be the route of spread, as serotypes 6 and 11 are commonly found in the human oropharynx and genital tract. HPV is documented to be associated with cancer of the larynx and cervix. HPV is also involved with esophageal squamous cell carcinoma, along with papillomas. Malignant transformation related to HPV infection has not been proven.

Esophageal papilloma is most common in individuals in their 50s, with a mostly equal gender frequency. Most lesions are solitary, but rarely up to 10 are found. Endoscopy reveals small whitish-pink wart-like exophytic projections with a differential diagnosis of verrucous squamous cell carcinoma, granulation tissue, and papillary leukoplakia. Papillomas are found more frequently in patients with tylosis, acanthosis nigricans, and Goltz syndrome. Large lesions can cause dysphagia, but most may be endoscopically resected with forceps when they are 1 cm or less in size; mucosal resection can be performed when they are larger.

Flat Lesions

Heterotopic sebaceous glands are found in ectodermal tissues such as the genitalia, parotid gland, palms, soles, eyelashes, lips, mouth, and tongue; they are rare in the esophagus. They are unlikely congenital, resulting from heterotopic mucosa or reactive metaplasia of the esophagus. Endoscopy reveals yellowish-gray plaquelike lesions occurring in clusters of up to 100 in one area. Histology reveals groups of sebaceous cells in the lamina propria. Lesions may be observed as they have no malignant potential.

Glycogen acanthosis occurs in 3.5% to 15% of all endoscopies and 30% of barium esophagrams. There are multiple round protrusions 2 to 15 mm in size in the midesophagus. The pathogenesis is unclear but has been associated with Cowden disease. Most lesions present in patients in their 40s and 50s, mainly in men, and increase in number and frequency with age. Endoscopic mucosal biopsies reveal plaques of hyperplastic squamous epithelium with glycogen in the cells.

Esophageal parakeratosis on endoscopy appears as whitish membranous linear plaques. Histologically they manifest epithelial acanthosis, basal hyperplasia, and parakeratosis covered by nonnucleated squamous cells. Esophageal parakeratosis has been associated with esophageal and head and neck carcinoma but is not premalignant and represents 40%

of new squamous cell cancers (SCCs) of the head and neck. It is also associated with submucosal fibrosis in smokers and betel nut chewers.

Esophagitis dissecans superficialis is a rare condition involving sloughing of mucosal epithelium and characterized by tubular casts within the esophageal lumen. It occurs with pemphigus vulgaris in 5% of patients or as a complication of rigid endoscopy with esophageal dilation, ingestion of oral bisphosphonates, and celiac disease.

An esophageal inlet patch is heterotopic gastric mucosa of the upper esophagus (HGMUE) occurring with a prevalence of 5% of adults by autopsy and 11% at endoscopy. These lesions are most commonly found in individuals their 50s and are most often located in the proximal 3 cm of the esophagus. Patches range from 2 mm to 4.5 cm in size and can occur alone or be multiple. They are red, velvety, and flat but rarely raised or polypoid. Microscopically they have fundic-type of gastric mucosa with some parietal cells and evidence of an inflammatory infiltrate.

The origin of the esophageal inlet patch is unclear; it is unknown whether they develop from "heterotopic" gastric mucosa or are embryonic. They are frequently found in children and their prevalence does not increase with age. Immunohistochemical analysis reveals that the cells are reactive to glucagon, which is an embryonic finding that is not noted in mature gastric cells. Controversy exists as to their origin, which may be the failure to replace the columnar lining of the esophagus with squamous epithelium during maturation as well as the belief that inlet patches are more similar to Barrett mucosa, which has been believed to be an acquired lesion. Trauma to the lining with rehealing by squamous mucosa has also been suggested.

Clinical problems have been attributed to the inlet patches by association. Tracheoesophageal fistula has occurred at the site of an inlet patch secondary to acid production with perforation. Patients with strictures, rings, and webs that have a patch frequently have dysphagia. Patches have been suggested as a cause of Plummer-Vinson syndrome. *Helicobacter pylori* grows in the patch in 19% to 73% of those that are *H. pylori*–positive in the stomach, indicating that the esophagus may be a reservoir. Barrett esophagus has been found in the distal esophagus of 20% of individuals with a patch. Esophageal and laryngeal adenocarcinoma has been found arising from inlet patches in the upper esophagus. Symptoms of globus, cough, and laryngopharyngeal reflux have been associated with patches, and improvement in globus symptoms has occurred after argon plasma ablation. Diagnosis is made on endoscopic visualization and confirmed by biopsy. Patches are benign and are treated only if symptomatic. Risk factors for malignancy are unclear. Endoscopic ablation and treatment a PPI can result in replacement with squamous mucosa.

Cystic Lesions

Cystic lesions of the esophagus occur in 1 in 8200 patients and most commonly are bronchogenic or originate from the GI tract. Bronchogenic cysts are lined by columnar cells and contain a milky-white substance, smooth muscle, hyaline cartilage, and seromucous glands. Enterogenous cysts are lined with columnar, bowel, or cuboidal cells or gastric mucosa and contain green mucus. They occur secondary to abnormal embryonal budding; they are located periesophageally or may be intrapulmonary and average 4 cm in size. Endoscopy and barium esophagraphy reveal protruding masses with normal mucosa, but EUS must be performed to confirm their presence. If dysphagia is present from a large cyst, surgical resection is indicated. These lesions do not have malignant potential.

Duplication cysts are congenital and are found in 1 in 8000 live births. They are rarely found in the esophagus, where they are located within the esophageal wall and are covered by two muscle layers covered by squamous epithelium. The cysts contain gastric mucosa in 33% of cases but they may also contain pancreatic mucosa. They are usually located to the right side of the esophagus. There is no cyst-esophageal communication in 80%, but 20% are parallel with esophagus and do communicate. They usually cause symptoms, resulting in 80% being diagnosed in patients younger than 2 years of age. Compression of adjacent structures causes dysphagia in 70%, epigastric pain in 20%, and mediastinal pain in 10% as well as respiratory symptoms and occasional hematemesis. Symptoms are an indication for surgical resection. Malignancy is rare.

Course and Prognosis

Benign lesions of the esophagus are rarely malignant or have malignant potential. Only in rare instances do lesions transform; therefore most patients have a normal life expectancy with minimal symptoms. Management of benign lesions is dependent on accurate diagnosis to rule out other potentially malignant lesions. Symptomatic lesions may warrant resection, but most benign lesions can be observed. Few lesions have the potential to progress to malignancy, although they may be markers for an increased risk of malignancy. In themselves, however, they do not have malignant potential.

Esophageal schwannomas have a low risk, but symptomatic lesions should be enucleated or removed by partial esophagectomy. When esophageal parakeratosis is found, patients should be referred to a head and neck specialist for a careful exam of the proximal esophagus, mouth, and pharyngeal structures because the findings can be associated with head and neck malignancies. Esophageal papilloma should be removed because of their association with esophageal squamous cell carcinoma. Esophageal adenomas are almost always found in areas of Barrett esophagus, and such patients should be treated similarly to any other individual with Barrett esophagus. Granular cell tumors have a malignant potential, and all lesions larger than 1 cm should be resected either with biopsy forceps or endoscopic mucosal resection. Inlet patches and duplication cysts have a low likelihood of malignant transformation and do not warrant treatment or surveillance.

BENIGN NEOPLASMS OF THE ESOPHAGUS: LEIOMYOMAS

Esophageal leiomyomas account for 0.6% of all esophageal neoplasms. Leiomyomas are the most common benign tumor of the esophagus, accounting for two-thirds of all benign esophageal tumors. They typically occur in individuals aged 20 to 50 years; 80% are intramural, 33% occur in the middle, and 56% are found in the distal third of the esophagus. In 13% of patients, intraluminal leiomyomas are annular or completely encircle the esophagus. Leiomyomas may extend into the stomach as well. Half the tumors are smaller than 5 cm. They are usually firm, encapsulated, rubbery, and elastic and typically are not pedunculated because they are muscular in origin and are covered by the mucosa. They are usually isolated but may appear in multiples in 5% of such cases. Malignant degeneration of leiomyomas is extremely rare. Pathologic examination of cells reveals a positivity for smooth muscle actin and negativity for the proteins CD34 and CD117. Leiomyomatosis with multiple leiomyomas along the entire esophagus is associated with Alport syndrome. Esophageal leiomyomas are also associated with multiple endocrine neoplasia (MEN) type 1.

Clinical Picture

Esophageal leiomyomas rarely cause symptoms in those with an average tumor size of 0.4 cm. The majority of leiomyomas have been discovered incidentally during evaluation for dysphagia or in the course of autopsy. Large tumors that average 5.2 cm may be symptomatic. The most common presenting symptoms for these leiomyomas are dysphagia (71%), pain (50%), weight loss (15%), and nausea or vomiting (12%).

Other symptoms include odynophagia, reflux, regurgitation, respiratory symptoms, shoulder pain, chest pain, hiccups, and anorexia. Larger pedunculated tumors may occlude the esophageal lumen, causing dysphagia, or may be aspirated into the trachea. Bleeding into the lumen may occur from ulceration of lesions such as angiomas.

Diagnosis

A large endoluminal tumor may be visualized on barium esophagraphy as a concave mass with smooth borders. CT is 91% sensitive and excellent for the visualization of smaller lesions. If obstruction has occurred, proximal dilation of the esophagus may be detected. Endoscopy is most sensitive and may determine the presence, location, and integrity of the mucosa. The lesions are identified as mobile submucosal masses. Endoscopy should be performed to rule out malignancy. Normal mucosa over a leiomyoma frequently rules out malignancy. In patients with leiomyoma, biopsy is contraindicated because it may cause infection, bleeding, or perforation. It also increases the risk for a mucosal tear at surgical excision. Brush cytology should be performed to establish a diagnosis. If an ulcer is identified on endoscopy, biopsy should be performed.

The best method of classification is EUS, which is capable of delineating five layers of the esophageal wall. These layers are detected by alternating hyperechoic and hypoechoic transmissions. The superficial or inner, layer is hyperechoic and the remaining layers alternate as described; deep mucosa (second layer), submucosa (third layer), and muscularis propria (fourth layer). Periesophageal tissue is seen as the fifth layer. Ultrasound is limited in determining the nature of the tumor and whether it is malignant.

Treatment and Management

Most patients without symptoms can be managed periodically with barium swallow because of the benign nature of the lesions. Surgical excision should be performed for symptomatic lesions, those greater than 5 cm, those increasing in size, or lesions with mucosal ulceration. Resection is the definitive method to confirm that a tumor is benign or malignant.

Traditionally transthoracic excision by thoracotomy was the most common approach, as lesions of the middle third of the esophagus are accessed through a right thoracotomy whereas those in the distal third are addressed with a left thoracotomy. Enucleation of the mass with primary closure is the preferred technique. Benign tumors larger than 8 cm may require esophagectomy with gastric pull-up, using thoracotomy, thoracoscopy, or laparoscopy.

Lesions may preferably be removed by combined esophagoscopy and thoracoscopy or laparoscopy. Endoscopic removal is being performed but remains experimental. Initial studies indicate that endoscopic submucosal tunnel dissection (ESTD) is safe and effective and has advantages over ESD, such as shorter operating times, hospital stays, and time needed for healing. There is no significant difference in the incidence of complications when both techniques are compared.

Course and Prognosis

Results of leiomyoma enucleation are excellent, and recurrence is rarely reported. Symptoms resolve with tumor excision. Overall the prognosis is excellent because the lesions are benign. Minimally invasive techniques result in minimal morbidity and rare mortality.

MALIGNANT NEOPLASMS: UPPER AND MIDDLE PORTIONS OF THE ESOPHAGUS

Both carcinomas and SCCs occur in the upper third of the esophagus. Carcinomas are more common in women (Fig. 14.2), but the upper

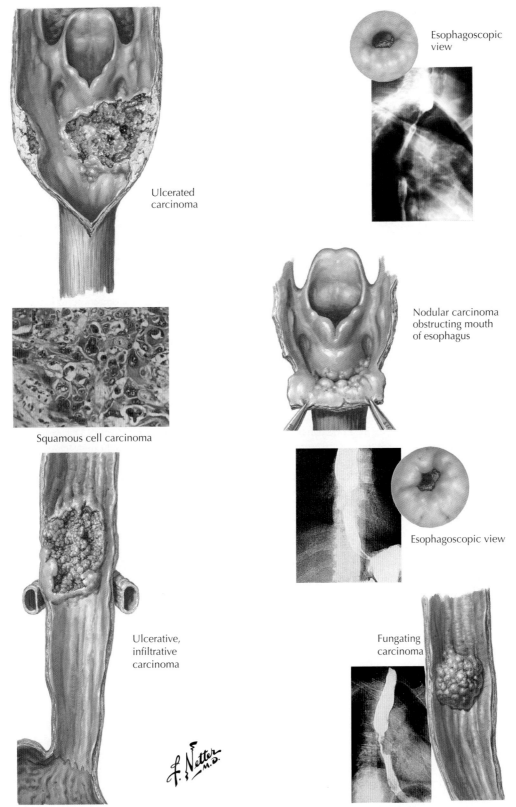

Ulcerated carcinoma

Squamous cell carcinoma

Ulcerative, infiltrative carcinoma

Esophagoscopic view

Nodular carcinoma obstructing mouth of esophagus

Esophagoscopic view

Fungating carcinoma

Fig. 14.2 Malignant Tumors: Upper and Middle Portions of the Esophagus.

third of the esophagus is the *least* common site for them to occur, as 5% to 6% of esophageal cancers arise in the cervical portion. Anatomically, this area is 6 to 8 cm long, beginning at the hypopharynx and commencing at the thoracic inlet or suprasternal notch. At the time of diagnosis, most patients with cancer of the cervical esophagus have locally advanced disease with extension to the hypopharynx. There is an association in up to 14% between SCC of the head and neck located in the oral cavity, oropharynx, hypopharynx, larynx, lung, or esophagus with synchronous or metachronous SCC of the esophagus. Cervical esophageal adenocarcinoma and SCC share common risk factors of smoking and/or alcohol usage.

Clinical Picture

Most commonly patients with cervical esophageal cancer will present with weight loss and dysphagia. Up to 24% will have hoarseness at the time of presentation which results from recurrent laryngeal nerve involvement by the tumor. Dysphagia may be the first symptom, and its presence should initiate a thorough evaluation. Aspiration may be a late symptom.

Diagnosis

Evaluation should include flexible laryngoscopy and esophagoscopy to evaluate the upper respiratory and GI tracts and to determine the location of the lesion and local disease spread and to exclude a synchronous malignancy of the head and neck. If a lesion is encountered, biopsy should be performed. CT or magnetic resonance imaging (MRI) may show the soft tissue lesion more accurately. Determination of the need for resection or radiation therapy (RT) may be made on the basis of this test. Preoperative bronchoscopy with biopsy and brush cytology may be performed as the last procedure in the staging workup in patients with locally advanced nonmetastatic disease of the cervical esophagus. Bronchoscopy is superior to CT in that it may reveal airway invasion in up to 10% of patients, excluding surgery as the most appropriate treatment option.

Treatment and Management

Treatment of SCC of the esophagus is similar to treatment of SCC of the head and neck. Locally advanced malignancy of both SCC and adenocarcinoma is usually treated with a combination of radiation and chemotherapy with the advantage of organ preservation with the same overall survival, local failure-free survival (FFS), and distant FFS as proximal esophageal surgical excision. Major morbidity is avoided without surgery. The recommended treatment is usually cisplatin chemotherapy given with RT.

Surgery is an option for individuals found to have a malignancy at an early stage of the disease or for patients who fail chemotherapy and radiation. Cervical esophageal SCCs are usually difficult to resect and often require removal of part or all of the pharynx, larynx, and thyroid as well as the proximal esophagus. The most aggressive resection is a complete pharyngo-laryngo-esophagectomy (PLE) requiring cervical, abdominal, and thoracic incisions and a tracheostomy. A gastric pull-up or jejunal interposition with a pharyngeal anastomosis reestablishes GI continuity. Myocutaneous flaps or skin grafts may be necessary to close the resected areas and spaces. Bilateral radical dissections are performed to remove lymph nodes in the neck and superior mediastinum. Surgical resection is contraindicated if there is involvement of the prevertebral fascia, posterior larynx, membranous trachea or encasement of major neurovascular structures.

Course and Prognosis

The 2-year results of cervical esophageal cancer treated primarily with RT versus surgery with or without follow-up treatment with chemo-therapy or surgery for local FFS, distant FFS, and overall survival were 70% versus 69%, 74% versus 63%, and 49% versus 51%, respectively. Although results were similar, the mortality of RT versus surgery was significantly better, 4% versus 13% for surgery. Patients who undergo complete resection usually succumb to metastatic disease. Unfortunately 80% of patients fail after radiation, and 20% require palliation to control local disease.

MALIGNANT NEOPLASMS: LOWER END OF THE ESOPHAGUS

Malignancy of the esophagus accounts for 5% of all GI cancers (Fig. 14.3). *Squamous cell carcinoma* is the most common esophageal malignancy worldwide. *Adenocarcinoma* is the most common malignancy in Western countries and has continued its 20-year increase in incidence, especially in white men in the sixth decade of life. The black/white male ratio is 3:0 for adenocarcinoma; the reverse is true for SCC. The incidence of superficial esophageal cancers limited to the mucosa or submucosa has increased globally; this be attributed to more aggressive endoscopic surveillance in patients with Barrett esophagus. It is not surprising that now 85% of cancers occur in the middle to distal esophagus. Recommendations of routine surveillance and aggressive surgical treatment for patients with HGD have been instituted to discover and treat esophageal cancer early.

Patients with achalasia, caustic strictures, Barrett esophagus, or gastroesophageal reflux disease (GERD) are predisposed to adenocarcinoma; those who drink alcohol, smoke, or have tylosis or Plummer-Vinson syndrome are predisposed to SCC. Unfortunately, despite best attempts, only 5% of patients seek treatment while they have local disease. Five-year survival ranges from 16% to 32% of patients.

Adenocarcinoma is thought to develop from metaplastic columnar mucosa or Barrett esophagus, which occurs in the distal esophagus in patients with GERD. Distal esophageal and proximal gastric malignancies are similar. Bile, pancreatic juice, pepsin, and gastric acid may cause a transformation of squamous cells to columnar cells. In time, metaplastic cells may be transformed from dysplastic to malignant. Barrett mucosa is almost always present in those with adenocarcinoma. *Helicobacter pylori* infection may be protective for adenocarcinoma but can cause gastritis, ulcers, and lymphoid tumors. Adenocarcinomas and SCCs invade the mucosa and submucosa, spreading quickly up the length of the esophagus. Other uncommon lower-end esophageal malignancies include adenosquamous carcinoma, small cell cancer, and lymphoma.

Clinical Picture

Early adenocarcinomas that develop from Barrett esophagus in the distal esophagus may be completely asymptomatic and be discovered only at the time of endoscopy. Most patients with tumors have initial symptoms of dysphagia, odynophagia, and weight loss. Presentation with luminal obstruction indicates a poor prognosis, as does progressive dysphagia. As a tumor invades, there may be pain, hoarseness from recurrent laryngeal nerve involvement, superior vena cava syndrome, malignant pleural effusions, hematemesis, or bronchotracheoesophageal fistulas.

Diagnosis

Diagnosis is not limited to determining the presence of malignancy and must include determination of its extent. History and physical examination suggest the disease, but diagnosis is usually made by upper endoscopy with biopsy. Early lesions include plaques, nodules, or ulcerations. The visual characteristics of more advanced tumors are usually highly suspicious and include: ulcerated or circumferential masses of

Adenocarcinoma of cardiac end of stomach infiltrating esophagus submucosally

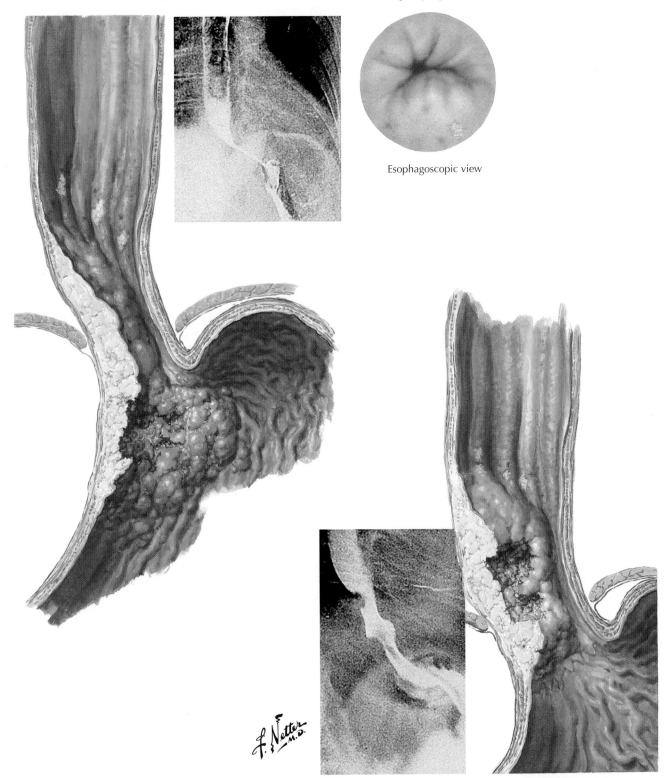

Esophagoscopic view

Primary carcinoma of lower end of esophagus

Fig. 14.3 Malignant Tumors: Lower End of the Esophagus.

very large ulcers of the esophagus. The biopsy is diagnostic in over 90% of cases.

Investigations may include barium esophagraphy to determine mucosal extent, EUS with or without fine-needle aspiration (FNA) to determine depth of invasion, CT or MRI to determine local invasion and lymph node involvement, bronchoscopy to determine invasion of the airway, and positron emission tomography (PET) to detect distant metastases. Diagnostic mediastinoscopy, laparoscopy, or thoracoscopy may determine metastasis to the lymph nodes.

Once the diagnosis of esophageal cancer has been established, staging is performed, as it is the best predictor of survival. The *tumor-node-metastasis* (TNM) classification of the American Joint Committee on Cancer (AJCC) and the Union for International Cancer Control (UICC) for esophageal cancer is used universally (eighth edition, 2017). These are the most current staging systems. (Visit http://www.annalscts.com/article/view/14237/14430 [Accessed August 2018].)

Local and distant disease presence must be assessed. Local disease assessment is performed best with the use of EUS as it is superior to CT for determining depth of tumor wall invasion, lymph node involvement, and characteristics of adjacent structures. US has the added benefit of facilitating endoscopic-guided FNA of lymph nodes and mediastinal lesions. US is capable of delineating four layers of the esophageal wall and has 90% and 85% accuracy, respectively, for measuring tumor and lymph node status. Assessment of distant metastases is performed by obtaining a contrast-enhanced CT of the neck, chest, and abdomen. Whole-body integrated fluorodeoxyglucose (FDG) PET/CT may also be used as well as EUS, and exploratory laparoscopy. FDG-PET/CT scans are more sensitive than CT scans and more successful at detecting metastases. EUS with needle biopsy of the liver or aspiration of abdominal ascites may also be performed. Laparoscopy and laparoscopic US may be superior to CT and EUS and can avoid noncurative laparotomies in 11% to 48% of patients. However, it is usually reserved for suspected clinical T3/T4 adenocarcinoma in the abdominal esophagus when the lesion is potentially resectable or metastatic disease cannot otherwise be ruled out.

Treatment and Management

Over the past several decades the incidence of adenocarcinoma of the distal esophagus has increased as squamous cell carcinoma has decreased, but the operative treatment of both has remained the same. Esophageal cancer tends to spread early and rapidly, as two-thirds of patients have lymph node metastases at presentation. Aggressive multimodal therapy is necessary to achieve control. If cure is not possible, palliation with attempts at maintaining nourishment and quality of life is paramount. The TNM classification aids in determining the feasibility of surgical resection and treatment options.

Use of the two major treatment options for early esophageal cancer—surgical esophagectomy and endoscopic resection (ER)—is dependent on procedural risk. Choice depends on submucosa or muscularis mucosa invasion (M3 tumors) and lymphovascular invasion, which increase the risk for lymph node metastases. Signs of submucosal growth include poor lifting and inability to suction during ER. Determining factors in treatment include lesion size, lymphovascular invasion, histologic grade, Barrett mucosa, varices, comorbidities, age, treatment availability, and patient desire.

Cure is maximized in submucosal (T1b) cancers treated with esophagectomy. In otherwise healthy patients with M1 or M2 tumors and well-differentiated M3 tumors without lymphovascular invasion, esophagectomy is best. ER is an alternative in poor surgical candidates in experienced centers. If lymphatic invasion is present, PDT or radiofrequency ablation (RFA) therapy may be used in conjunction with ER. Esophagectomy should be performed for persistent positive margins after ER, recurrence, and long lesions not amenable to ER. RT and/or chemoradiotherapy is performed for otherwise ER candidates who have varices, had previous perforation, or have severe cervical spine disease that make them poor candidates.

Other than superficial early esophageal cancers, total esophagectomy to obtain free margins and to clear all mediastinal lymph nodes is the standard first line of therapy and may be the only modality necessary for those with T1-2 N0 M0 disease. More recently, surgical resection has been extended to localized T1 to T3 lesions and certain T4a lesions that may have invaded structures such as pleura, pericardium, or the diaphragm. The mortality rate associated with surgery is 3%.

Lesions of the thoracic esophagus are usually removed by a total thoracic esophagectomy with cervical esophagogastrostomy. A radical two-field lymph node dissection is performed with placement of a feeding jejunostomy. The tri-incisional approach consists of a right posterolateral thoracotomy or thoracoscopy with a laparotomy or laparoscopy. An en bloc excision with gastric dissection and mobilization is performed. There is complete dissection of abdominal and mediastinal lymph nodes and a left neck incision and cervical anastomosis. Cancers of the GEJ are approached by total esophagectomy with cervical esophagogastrostomy with a partial gastrectomy or a minimally invasive Ivor-Lewis procedure, with a thoracic esophagogastrostomy. Randomized trials do not support any one technique over another.

In patients with T1N0 esophageal or GEJ adenocarcinoma or SCC, surgery alone is strongly supported as the only treatment needed, but chemoradiotherapy is an alternate option for patients who are not surgical candidates. The type of chemotherapy remains low-dose weekly carboplatin plus paclitaxel. An alternate option is two treatments of cisplatin plus fluorouracil (FU). Neoadjuvant chemoradiotherapy, combined with surgery for patients with clinical stage T2N0 tumors demonstrated a survival benefit in three clinical trials in patients with adenocarcinoma. Resection alone is considered for those with 2N0 SCCs.

In patients with surgically resected T2N0 adenocarcinomas that are poorly differentiated, have lymphovascular or perineural invasion, arising in patients at or younger than 50 years of age, adjuvant chemotherapy or chemoradiotherapy are options. These options are considered only in SCC if the margins are positive. In resected T3 or pT4 adenocarcinomas, independent of node status, in patients who are not treated with neoadjuvant therapy, postoperative adjuvant therapy is recommended. Chemoradiotherapy is given for nonsurgical candidates. Chemoradiation alone for complete responders with SCC is an option but is known to have a higher rate of locoregional control.

For patients who are potential surgical candidates who have SCC and an endoscopically documented complete response, definitive chemoradiotherapy is also an option, but surgery is recommended if the patient remains a candidate. In the similar situation with adenocarcinoma, surgical resection remains recommended.

Palliation of metastatic disease is reserved for those with any T, any N, M1 disease. Chemotherapy is the treatment of choice, but radiation may be added. Endoscopic metal stents, photodynamic tumor ablation with laser, metalloporphyrin, and brachytherapy may be used for palliation of obstruction. Radical surgery to bypass obstruction is rarely performed.

Other tumors of the esophagus are usually treated by surgery. Most patients with small cell carcinoma have metastatic disease at presentation and rarely survive a year. Therapy is palliative, but surgery and chemoradiation may result in a rare cure. Melanomas of the esophagus have a worse prognosis than cutaneous disease because they are discovered late. Surgery is performed but rarely helpful. Results after surgical excision of salivary tumors are worse than after excision of head and neck tumors. Lymphomas develop after direct spread from other organs. Primary lymphomas usually develop in patients with immune disorders.

Sarcomas may develop, but not from the degeneration of benign tumors and are removed by surgery. Metastatic lesions of the breast and lung and melanomas are most common and are treated by palliation.

Course and Prognosis

Patient survival depends directly on disease stage. Five-year survival rates for esophageal cancer are 78.9% for stage I, 37.9% for stage IIA, 27.3% for stage IIB, 13.7% for stage III, and 0% for stage IV.

RARE MALIGNANCIES OF THE ESOPHAGUS: GASTROINTESTINAL STROMAL TUMORS AND LEIOMYOSARCOMAS

The two most common types of malignancies of the esophagus are squamous cell carcinoma and adenocarcinoma. Less commonly, esophageal leiomyosarcoma accounts for less than 1% of all malignant esophageal tumors, and only 165 cases have been reported. Leiomyosarcomas grow slowly and metastases occur late, giving them a better prognosis than squamous cell tumors and carcinoma. Esophageal GISTs are the most common mesenchymal neoplasms in the digestive tract, but esophageal GISTs are extremely rare. GISTs develop from the interstitial cells of Cajal, which are located in the muscle layer. The cells overexpress the tyrosine kinase receptor KIT.

Clinical Picture

Esophageal GISTs accounts for only 1% of all neoplasms found in the GI tract. Their clinical, endoscopic, and radiographic appearance is similar to that of leiomyomas. The esophagus lacks a serosa layer and has a limited blood supply, making GISTs in this location more difficult treat with surgical resection. Mesenchymal tumors are most commonly located from the middle to the distal esophagus. They are usually asymptomatic until they grow to a large size and cause dysphagia. The majority of mesenchymal tumors located in the esophagus are leiomyomas and occur most commonly in men. Leiomyosarcomas are significantly less common. The treatment of GISTs and leiomyosarcomas of the esophagus depends upon the preoperative diagnosis, tumor location, size, presence of metastases, and complications such as obstruction, perforation, or hemorrhage.

Diagnosis

Diagnosis of leiomyosarcoma is usually made incidentally at the time of a barium esophagram or endoscopy. The lesions are round and submucosal, with intact mucosa. They have a rubberlike consistency and do not ulcerate or bleed. A TNM classification system is used for soft tissue sarcomas of the abdominal viscera, but there are no prognostic stage groupings.

GISTs enhance more than leiomyomas on contrast CT and FDG-PET. Definitive diagnosis is made and differentiated from leiomyomas by EUS-guided FNA with immunohistochemical staining for KIT. Lesions that are well circumscribed, submucosal, larger than 2 cm, enlarging, or FDG-enhancing are suspicious for a GIST. Preoperative biopsies may preclude surgery for chemotherapy treatment or nonresectable, metastatic disease.

Treatment and Management

ER of leiomyosarcoma submucosal lesions is recommended as it is difficult to distinguish between a well-differentiated leiomyosarcoma and leiomyoma histologically. Resection by endoscopic snare polypectomy is performed on lesions less than 2 cm in size that are polypoid, have a round protrusion, and are elevated. Larger or flat lesions must be enucleated with an electrocautery snare and coagulated after removal

of the overlying mucosa. Small lesions are rarely found to be malignant. Alternatively, small asymptomatic lesions may be followed with EUS at 6 months, 1 year, and less frequently if no changes are found. Surgical excision is reserved for lesions that become symptomatic, grow bigger than 1 cm, develop structural changes, or when there is suspicion of a malignancy. Despite stability, lesions greater than 2 cm should be excised. Local excision is usually adequate to remove all lesions. Total or partial esophagectomy may be required.

An algorithmic approach to management of gastric GISTs based upon size and EUS appearance has been proposed, but one does not exist for esophageal lesions. The recommended treatment is surgical resection, including the pseudocapsule with negative margins preceded by neoadjuvant treatment with imatinib. Neoadjuvant imatinib is given to decrease the size of the tumor and prevent locoregional recurrence. Patients with locally advanced tumors that may not be completely resected are good candidates for neoadjuvant imatinib. GISTs of the esophagus, especially located at the LES may undergo imatinib treatment in order to reduce the tumor burden and allow for a segmental resection instead of total esophagectomy. Patients are treated for 6 to 12 months with periodic barium esophagram or CT to evaluate changes in tumor size.

Despite the very small risk of metastases, controversy exists as to whether GISTs less than 2 cm in size should be observed, resected, or resected only if they increase in size. Follow-up with EUS is recommended for nonoperative lesions. Canadian guidelines, for example, recommend excision of all GISTs irrespective of size because of metastatic risk. GISTs 2 cm or greater in size are surgically excised. Lesions greater than 2 cm or located near the GEJ despite imatinib may require esophagectomy. ER or enucleation may result in positive margins, tumor spillage, and perforation and is therefore not recommended. The prognosis for negative margins of lesions larger than 10 cm has an uncertain benefit. Although positive margins may lead to increased locoregional recurrence, factors such as size and tumor grade are more significant. GIST prognosis is influenced by size, mitotic rate, tumor site, and the completeness of resection. Lymphadenectomy is unnecessary because nodal metastases are rare. The abdomen, peritoneum, and liver should be examined for possible metastases. Rupture of the tumor yields a worse prognosis. Recurrences may be treated with imatinib with or without a reexcision. Most GISTs are completely excised but only 50% remain recurrence-free at 5 years.

Tyrosine kinase inhibitors (TKIs) of which imatinib is the first line therapy, are used to help decrease the growth of GIST cells after surgery. imatinib is indicated for use as adjuvant therapy for primary GISTs 3 cm or larger. Patients with very low/low-risk GISTs do not need to receive it. One year of imatinib reduces GIST recurrence in the first year, but the best results occur after 3 years of treatment. The longest studies reveal a median survival of advanced GISTs of 60 months. The median time that tumors progress is 2 years, and the most common sites for metastasis to occur are the peritoneum and liver, which is the most common site in 67% of patients with recurrent disease. Despite an 80% control rate of tumor growth, metastatic GISTs are treated with imatinib because complete responses are rare. Imatinib treatment reduces the tumor bulk in order to prevent resistance to the drug from mutations in the KIT gene.

Metastases resection is best after 3 to 9 months of imatinib treatment as there is little tumor reduction seen thereafter. Up to 30% of patients may have resectable disease. Surgical resection of metastases is beneficial for patients who have localized progression, stable disease, or partial responses. Patients with multifocal disease progression are poor surgical candidates. Five-year survival is 27% to 34% when only the lesion is resected. Resection combined with imatinib results in the longest survival. It is less important for the tumor to shrink in size than to reduce its density and vascularity. The National Comprehensive Cancer Network (NCCN) and European Society for Medical Oncology (ESMO) both recommend continual lifelong treatment with imatinib after metastases are resected.

Course and Prognosis

Patients with a surgically resected leiomyosarcoma have a 5-year survival of 30% to 40%, which is influenced by tumor grade and size. Generally outcomes for leiomyosarcomas of the GI tract are less favorable than for GISTs arising in similar locations.

No consensus exists on the follow-up treatment of GISTs. Regular follow-up may detect recurrences at an earlier stage and may lead to improved postrecurrence progression-free and overall survival. NCCN guidelines are as follows: For patients with a completely resected GIST tumor, history and physical every 3 to 6 months for 5 years, then yearly. Also a CT scan every 3 to 6 months for 3 to 5 years, then yearly. For patients with locally advanced or metastatic disease, receiving imatinib, history and physical and abdominal/pelvic CT scan every 3 to 6 months. Very low risk GISTs do not need routine follow-up, although recurrence may rarely be seen. MRI is a reasonable alternative to CT scans when there is concern for x-ray exposure in low-risk lesions.

Follow-up for a completely resected leiomyosarcoma includes a physical examination with an abdominal/pelvic CT or MRI scan every 3 to 6 months for 3 years and then every year. For patients with positive margins, CT or MRI should be continued every 6 months for 2 more years. Some centers recommend including a chest CT as well as one of the abdomen/pelvis to rule out lung metastases, which are a high risk.

ADDITIONAL RESOURCES

Affleck DG, Karwande SV, Bull DA, et al: Functional outcome and survival after pharyngolaryngoesophagectomy for cancer, *Am J Surg* 180:546, 2000.

Akbayir N, Alkim C, Erdem L, et al: Heterotopic gastric mucosa in the cervical esophagus (inlet patch): endoscopic prevalence, histological and clinical characteristics, *J Gastroenterol Hepatol* 19:891, 2004.

Azar C, Jamali F, Tamim H, et al: Prevalence of endoscopically identified heterotopic gastric mucosa in the proximal esophagus: endoscopist dependent?, *J Clin Gastroenterol* 41:468, 2007.

Blum MG, Bilimoria KY, Wayne JD, et al: Surgical considerations for the management and resection of esophageal gastrointestinal stromal tumors, *Ann Thorac Surg* 84:1717, 2007.

Burt BM, Groth SS, Sada YH, et al: Utility of adjuvant chemotherapy after neoadjuvant chemoradiation and esophagectomy for esophageal cancer, *Ann Surg* 266:297, 2017.

Chen WS, Zheng XL, Jin L, et al: Novel diagnosis and treatment of esophageal granular cell tumor: report of 14 cases and review of the literature, *Ann Thorac Surg* 97:296, 2014.

Choong CK, Meyers BF: Benign esophageal tumors: introduction, incidence, classification, and clinical features, *Semin Thorac Cardiovasc Surg* 15:3–8, 2003.

Collin CF, Spiro RH: Carcinoma of the cervical esophagus: changing therapeutic trends, *Am J Surg* 148:460, 1984.

Daiko H, Hayashi R, Saikawa M, et al: Surgical management of carcinoma of the cervical esophagus, *J Surg Oncol* 96:166, 2007.

Demetri GD, Benjamin RS, Blanke CD, et al: NCCN task force report: optimal management of patients with gastrointestinal stromal tumor (GIST)—update of NCCN clinical practice guidelines, *J Natl Compr Canc Netw* 5(2 Suppl):S1–S29, 2007.

Gamboa AM, Kim S, Force SD, et al: Treatment allocation in patients with early-stage esophageal adenocarcinoma: prevalence and predictors of lymph node involvement, *Cancer* 122:2150, 2016.

Godey SK, Diggory RT: Inflammatory fibroid polyp of the oesophagus, *World J Surg Oncol* 3:30, 2005.

Gronchi A, Raut CP: The combination of surgery and imatinib in GIST: a reality for localized tumors at high risk, an open issue for metastatic ones, *Ann Surg Oncol* 19:1051, 2012.

Hihara J, Mukaida H, Hirabayashi N: Gastrointestinal stromal tumor of the esophagus: current issues of diagnosis, surgery and drug therapy, *Transl Gastroenterol Hepatol* 3:6, 2018.

Jiang W, Rice TW, Goldblum JR: Esophageal leiomyoma: experience from a single institution, *Dis Esophagus* 26:167–174, 2013.

Joensuu H, Martin-Broto J, Nishida T, et al: Follow-up strategies for patients with gastrointestinal stromal tumour treated with or without adjuvant imatinib after surgery, *Eur J Cancer* 51:1611, 2015.

Kelly KA, Sarr MG, Hinder RA: *Mayo clinic gastrointestinal surgery*, Philadelphia, 2004, Saunders, p 49.

Lordick F, Mariette C, Haustermans K, et al: Oesophageal cancer: ESMO clinical practice guidelines for diagnosis, treatment and follow-up, *Ann Oncol* 27:v50, 2016.

Luh SP, Hou SM, Fang CC, Chen CY: Video-thoracoscopic enucleation of esophageal leiomyoma, *World J Surg Oncol* 10:52, 2012.

Mandard AM, Marnay J, Gignoux M, et al: Cancer of the esophagus and associated lesions: detailed pathologic study of 100 esophagectomy specimens, *Hum Pathol* 15:660, 1984.

Manner H, Pech O, Heldmann Y, et al: Efficacy, safety, and long-term results of endoscopic treatment for early stage adenocarcinoma of the esophagus with low-risk sm1 invasion, *Clin Gastroenterol Hepatol* 11:630, 2013.

McGarrity TJ, Wagner Baker MJ, Ruggiero FM, et al: GI polyposis and glycogenic acanthosis of the esophagus associated with PTEN mutation positive cowden syndrome in the absence of cutaneous manifestations, *Am J Gastroenterol* 98:1429, 2003.

Mendenhall WM, Sombeck MD, Parsons JT, et al: Management of cervical esophageal carcinoma, *Semin Radiat Oncol* 4:179, 1994.

Miettinen M, Sarlomo-Rikala M, Sobin LH, Lasota J: Esophageal stromal tumors: a clinicopathologic, immunohistochemical, and molecular genetic study of 17 cases and comparison with esophageal leiomyomas and leiomyosarcomas, *Am J Surg Pathol* 24:211, 2000.

Park SJ, Ryu MH, Ryoo BY, et al: The role of surgical resection following imatinib treatment in patients with recurrent or metastatic gastrointestinal stromal tumors: results of propensity score analyses, *Ann Surg Oncol* 21:4211, 2014.

Seremetis MG, Lyons WS, deGuzman VC, et al: Leiomyomata of the esophagus. An analysis of 838 cases, *Cancer* 38:2166–2177, 1976.

Triboulet JP, Mariette C, Chevalier D, Amrouni H: Surgical management of carcinoma of the hypopharynx and cervical esophagus: analysis of 209 cases, *Arch Surg* 136:1164, 2001.

Tsai S, Lin C, Chang C, et al: Benign esophageal lesions: endoscopic and pathologic features, *World J Gastroenterol* 21(4):1091–1098, 2015.

Uppal P, Kaur J, Agarwala S, et al: Communicating oesophageal duplication cyst with heterotopic pancreatic tissue—an unusual cause of recurrent pneumonia in an infant, *Acta Paediatr* 99:1432, 2010.

Van Dam J: Endosonographic evaluation of the patient with esophageal cancer, *Chest* 112(Suppl):184S–190S, 1997.

Wang HW, Chu PY, Kuo KT, et al: A reappraisal of surgical management for squamous cell carcinoma in the pharyngoesophageal junction, *J Surg Oncol* 93:468, 2006.

Wang L, Ren W, Zhang Z, et al: Retrospective study of endoscopic submucosal tunnel dissection (ESTD) for surgical resection of esophageal leiomyoma, *Surg Endosc* 27(11):4259–4266, 2013.

Xu GQ, Qian JJ, Chen MH, et al: Endoscopic ultrasonography for the diagnosis and selecting treatment of esophageal leiomyoma, *J Gastroenterol Hepatol* 27:521–525, 2012.

Zenda S, Kojima T, Kato K, et al: Multicenter phase 2 study of cisplatin and 5-fluorouracil with concurrent radiation therapy as an organ preservation approach in patients with squamous cell carcinoma of the cervical esophagus, *Int J Radiat Oncol Biol Phys* 96:976, 2016.

SECTION II

Stomach and Duodenum

Martin H. Floch

15

Anatomy of the Stomach and Duodenum

Martin H. Floch

ANATOMY OF THE STOMACH: NORMAL VARIATIONS AND RELATIONS

The stomach is a J-shaped reservoir of the digestive tract in which ingested food is soaked in gastric juice containing enzymes and hydrochloric acid and then is released spasmodically into the duodenum by gastric peristalsis. The form and size of the stomach vary considerably, depending on the position of the body and the degree of filling. Special functional configurations of the stomach are of interest to the clinician and radiologist (Fig. 15.1).

The stomach has a ventral surface and a dorsal surface that may be vaulted or flattened and that almost make contact when the organ is empty. The stomach also has two borders, the concave *lesser curvature* above on the right and the convex *greater curvature* below on the left. The two join at the *cardia*, where the esophagus enters. The poorly defined cardia is the point of demarcation between both curvatures, whereas on the right the esophagus continues smoothly into the lesser curvature. On the left there is a definite indentation, the incisura cardialis (cardial or cardiac incisure, or notch), that becomes most obvious when the uppermost, hoodlike portion of the stomach (fundus, or fornix) is full and bulges upward. The major portion of the stomach (body, or corpus) blends imperceptibly into the pyloric portion, except along the lesser curvature, where a notch, the incisura angularis (angular incisure), marks the boundary between the corpus and the pyloric portion. The pylorus consists of the pyloric antrum, or vestibule, which narrows into the pyloric canal and terminates at the pyloric valve. External landmarks of the pylorus form a circular ridge of sphincter muscle and the subserosal pyloric vein.

During esophagogastroduodenoscopy, selective views can evaluate almost all these areas. For example, retroflexion of the endoscope permits visualization of the scope entering the stomach. The endoscopist can see the normal mucosa of the gastroesophageal junction as it hugs the scope, forming a fold or flap at the cardiac incisure. The pyloric channel is usually closed, and waves of contractions move aborally from the pylorus and end at the angular incisure of the pyloric antrum.

The stomach is entirely covered with peritoneum. A double layer of peritoneum, deriving from the embryonal ventral mesogastrium, extends on the lesser curvature beyond the stomach, known as the *lesser omentum*. It passes over to the porta hepatis and may be divided into a larger, thinner, proximal portion (hepatogastric ligament) and a smaller, thicker, distal portion (hepatoduodenal ligament), which attaches to the pyloric region and to the upper horizontal portion of the duodenum. The free edge of the hepatoduodenal ligament, through which run the portal vein, hepatic artery, and common bile duct, forms the ventral margin of the epiploic foramen of Winslow, which gives access to the lesser peritoneal sac (bursa omentalis). The *greater omentum*, a derivative of the embryonal dorsal mesogastrium, passes caudally from the greater curvature and contains, between its two frontal and two dorsal sheets, the inferior recess of the bursa omentalis.

The anterior surface of the stomach abuts the anterior abdominal wall, against the inferior surface of the left lobe of the liver and, to some extent in the pyloric region, against the quadrate lobe of the liver and the gallbladder. Its posterior surface is in apposition with retroperitoneal structures (pancreas, splenic vessels, left kidney, and adrenal gland) from which, however, it is separated by the bursa omentalis. The fundus bulges against the left diaphragmatic dome. On the left, adjacent to the fundus, is the spleen, which is connected to the stomach by the gastrosplenic ligament (also derived from the dorsal mesogastrium).

The four recognized principal functional types of stomach are known as *orthotonic, hypertonic, hypotonic,* and *atonic.* In the hypotonic and atonic types, the axis of the stomach is more longitudinal, whereas in the orthotonic and particularly the hypertonic types, it is more transverse.

ANATOMY AND RELATIONS OF THE DUODENUM

The duodenum, the first part of the small intestine, has a total length of approximately 25 to 30 cm (10–12 inches). It is horseshoe shaped, with the open end facing left, and is divided into four parts (Fig. 15.2).

The first part of the duodenum, or the *pars superior,* lies at the level of the first lumbar vertebra (L1) and extends almost horizontally from the pylorus to the first flexure. As a result of its intraperitoneal position, this first duodenal portion is freely movable and can adapt its course according to the filling condition of the stomach. The anterior and superior surfaces of the first half of this duodenal segment are in close relation to the inferior surface of the liver (lobus quadratus) and the gallbladder. The radiographic designation *duodenal bulb* refers to the most proximal end of the pars superior duodeni, which is slightly dilated when the organ is filled and then is more sharply separated from the stomach because of pyloric contraction.

The two layers of peritoneum, which cover the anterosuperior and the posteroinferior surfaces, join together on the upper border of the superior portion of the duodenum and move as the hepatoduodenal ligament cranially toward the liver, forming the right, free edge of the lesser omentum. This ligament contains the important triad of the portal vein, hepatic artery, and common bile duct.

The second part of the duodenum, the descending portion, extends vertically from the first to the second duodenal flexure, the latter lying approximately at the level of the third lumbar vertebra (L3). The upper area of this portion rests laterally on the structures of the hilus of the right kidney; medially, its whole length is attached by connective tissue to the duodenal margin of the caput pancreatis (head of pancreas). Approximately halfway its length, the descending portion is crossed anteriorly by the parietal line of attachment of the transverse mesocolon.

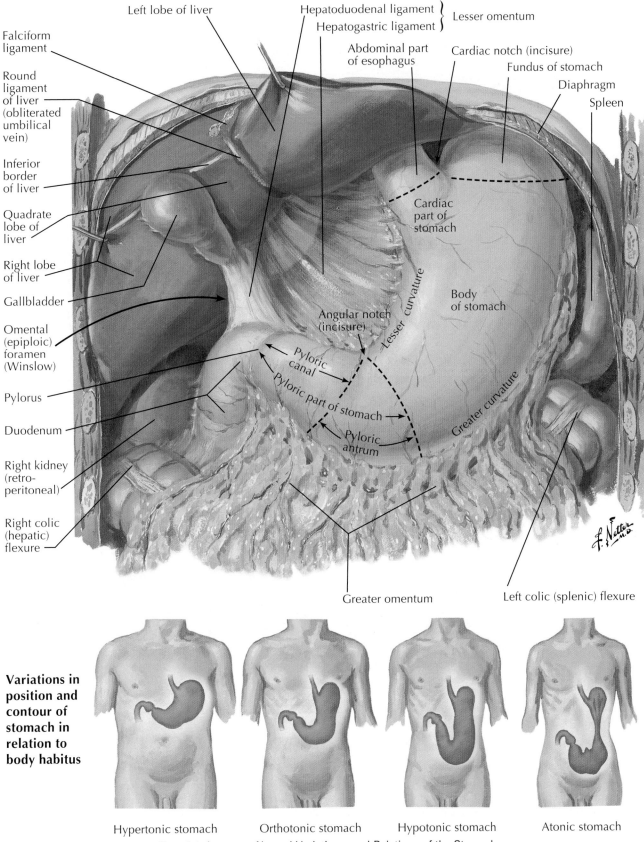

Left lobe of liver

Hepatoduodenal ligament } Lesser omentum
Hepatogastric ligament }

Abdominal part
of esophagus

Cardiac notch (incisure)

Fundus of stomach

Diaphragm

Spleen

Falciform
ligament

Round
ligament
of liver
(obliterated
umbilical
vein)

Inferior
border
of liver

Quadrate
lobe of
liver

Right lobe
of liver

Gallbladder

Omental
(epiploic)
foramen
(Winslow)

Pylorus

Duodenum

Right kidney
(retro-
peritoneal)

Right colic
(hepatic)
flexure

Cardiac
part of
stomach

Body
of stomach

Lesser curvature

Angular notch
(incisure)

Pyloric
canal

Pyloric part of stomach

Pyloric
antrum

Greater curvature

Greater omentum

Left colic (splenic) flexure

**Variations in
position and
contour of
stomach in
relation to
body habitus**

Hypertonic stomach

Orthotonic stomach

Hypotonic stomach

Atonic stomach

Fig. 15.1 Anatomy, Normal Variations, and Relations of the Stomach.

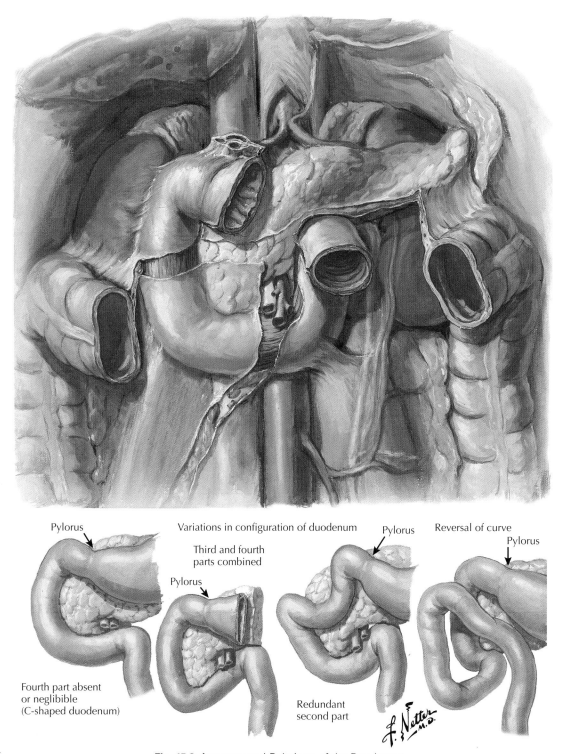

Pylorus

Variations in configuration of duodenum

Pylorus

Reversal of curve

Pylorus

Third and fourth
parts combined

Pylorus

Fourth part absent
or neglibible
(C-shaped duodenum)

Redundant
second part

Fig. 15.2 Anatomy and Relations of the Duodenum.

The common bile duct, together with the portal vein, occupies the start of the hepatoduodenal ligament, a position dorsal to the superior duodenal portion, and continues its course between the descending portion and the pancreatic head to its opening at the major duodenal papilla (Vater).

The third part of the duodenum, the inferior portion, begins at the second flexure. It begins almost horizontally (horizontal part) or sometimes in a slightly ascending direction, until it reaches the region of the left border of the aorta, where it changes direction and curves cranially to pass into the terminal duodenal segment (ascending part). Although the caudal part of the second portion and the second flexure lie over the psoas major of the right side of the body, the third duodenal portion, with its horizontal segment, passes over the vena cava and the abdominal aorta. The superior mesenteric vessels, before entering the root of the mesentery, cross over the horizontal part of the third portion near its transition to the ascending part. During its course, the third portion is increasingly covered by the peritoneum, and a complete intraperitoneal configuration is attained at the duodenojejunal flexure, which is located caudal to the mesocolon transversum at the level of the second lumbar vertebra (L2) or of the disk between L1 and L2.

As the third part of the duodenum courses up to the left of the aorta to reach the border of the pancreas, it is frequently referred to as the fourth part of the duodenum. This fourth part joins the jejunum and is fixed posteriorly by the *ligament of Treitz*, a suspensory muscle of the duodenum. The fourth part of the duodenum then leaves the retroperitoneal area to join the intraperitoneal jejunum. On radiographs, the duodenum usually takes the form of a C, although it may show

individual variations, such as a redundant second part or a reversal of curve (see Fig. 15.2).

MUCOSA OF THE STOMACH

The reddish gray mucous membrane of the stomach, composed of a single surface layer of epithelial cells (tunica propria) and the submucosa, begins at the cardia along an irregular or zigzag line, often referred to as the Z line (Fig. 15.3). The mucosa appears as a more or less marked

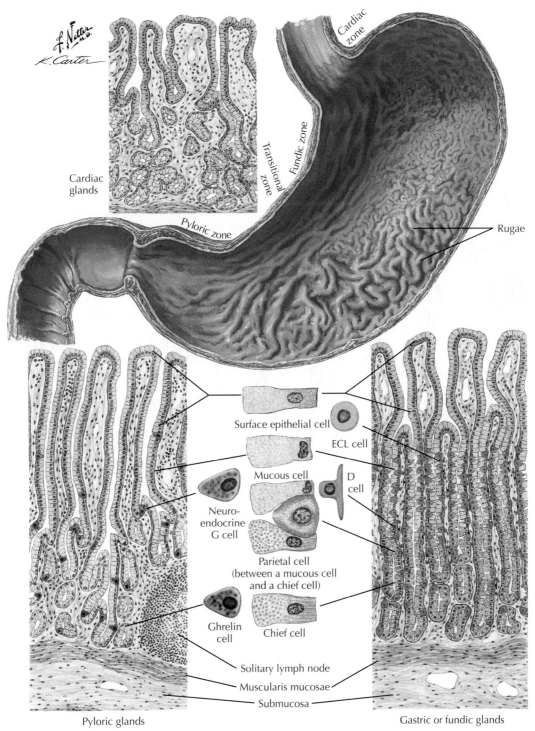

Fig. 15.3 Mucosa of the Stomach. *ECL,* Enterochromaffin-like.

relief of folds, or *rugae,* which flatten considerably when the stomach is distended. In the region of the lesser curvature, where the mucosa is more strongly fixed to the muscular layer, the folds take a longitudinal course, forming what has been called the *magenstrasse* ("stomach street," canalis gastricus). The rugae are generally smaller in the fundus and become larger as they approach the antrum, where they tend to run diagonally across the stomach toward the greater curvature. In addition to these broad folds, the gastric mucosa is further characterized by numerous shallow invaginations, which divide the mucosal surface into a mosaic of elevated areas varying in shape. When viewed under magnification with a lens, these *areae gastricae* reveal several delicate ledges and depressions, the latter known as gastric pits, or *foveolae gastricae.* The glands of the stomach open into the depth of these pits, which have varying widths and lengths.

The gastric epithelium, a single layer of columnar cells at the gastroesophageal junction, is sharply demarcated from the stratified and thicker esophageal mucosa. The *epithelial cells* are mucoid type and contain mucigen granules in their outer portions and an ovoid nucleus at their base.

The glands of the stomach are tubular; three types can be differentiated. The *cardiac glands* are confined to a narrow 0.5- to 4-cm zone in width around the cardiac orifice. They are coiled and are lined by mucus-producing cells. The *gastric, oxyntic,* or *fundic glands* are located in the fundus and over the greater part of the body of the stomach. They are fairly straight, simply branched tubules, with a narrow lumen reaching down almost to the muscularis mucosae. They are lined largely by three types of cells. *Mucoid cells* are present in the neck and differ from the cells of the surface epithelium in that their mucigen granules have slightly different staining qualities and their nuclei tend to be flattened or concave at the cell base. *Chief cells,* or *zymogenic cells,* line the lower half of glandular tubules. They have spheric nuclei and contain strongly light-refracting granules and a Golgi apparatus, the size and form of which vary with the state of secretory activity. Chief cells produce pepsinogen, the precursor of pepsin (see Chapter 18). *Parietal cells* are larger than chief cells and are usually crowded away from the lumen, to which they connect by extracellular capillaries stemming from intracellular canaliculi. Their intraplasmatic granules are strongly eosinophilic and less light refracting than those of the chief cells. Parietal cells produce hydrochloric acid. Histochemical and electron microscope studies have shown the elaborate molecular mechanisms by which hydrogen chloride forms and is secreted as hydrochloric acid within parietal cells and reacts to hormonal, chemical, and neurologic stimuli.

Pyloric glands, the third type of stomach gland, are located in the pyloric region but also spread to a transitional zone, where gastric and pyloric glands are found and which extends diagonally and distally from the lesser to the greater curvature. Tubes of the pyloric glands are shorter, more tortuous, and less densely packed and their ends more branched than in fundic glands. Pits are much deeper in the region of the pyloric glands. These glands are lined by a single type of cell, which resembles, or may be identical to, the mucoid neck cells of the fundic glands.

Specialized endocrine-secreting cells have been identified and are scattered through gastric glands, in the antrum, and in the pylorus. They are fewer in number than chief or parietal cells but are significant in their endocrine and physiologic functions. They secrete into the lumen to affect other endocrine cells or into the circulation for a distal endocrine effect. The *D (delta) cells* secrete somatostatin, which may have a paraendocrine or an endocrine effect. *Enterochromaffin-like* (ECL) cells, or *argentaffin cells* that stain with silver, secrete histamine. Other argentaffin cells that stain with potassium dichromate are called *enterochromaffin* (EC) *cells,* and these contain serotonin. The pylorus also contains a small but significant number of gastrin-secreting cells, called

C cells. The role of gastrin is discussed in Chapters 16 and 19. *Ghrelin* is secreted by endocrine cells of the pylorus and has a significant effect on appetite and eating behavior.

DUODENAL MUCOSA AND DUODENAL STRUCTURES

The mucosa of the widened first portion of the duodenum, also known as the bulbus duodeni (duodenal bulb), is flat and smooth, in contrast to the more distal duodenal part, which displays the mucosal *Kerckring folds,* as does the entire small intestine (Fig. 15.4). These circular folds (plicae), which augment the absorption surface of the intestine, begin in the region of the first flexure and increase in number and elevation in the more distal parts of the duodenum. Kerckring folds do not always form complete circles along the entire intestinal wall; some are semicircular, and others branch out to connect with adjacent folds. Both the mucosa and the submucosa participate in the structure of these plicae, whereas all the other layers of the small intestine, including its two muscular coats, are flat and smooth.

Approximately halfway down the posteromedial aspect of the descending portion of the duodenum, at a distance of 8.5 to 10 cm from the pylorus, is the *papilla of Vater.* The papilla and its relationship to the local anatomy and the anatomic variations are essential to the investigating endoscopist for interpretation of endoscopic retrograde cholangiopancreatography (ERCP) and endoscopic ultrasound of the area. Here the common bile duct (ductus choledochus) and the major pancreatic duct, or duct of Wirsung, open into the duodenum. The common bile duct approaches the duodenum within the enfolding hepatoduodenal ligament of the lesser omentum and continues caudally in the groove between the descending portion of the duodenum and the pancreas (see Section VII). In the posteromedial duodenal wall, the terminal part of the ductus choledochus produces a slight but perceptible longitudinal impression known as the plica longitudinalis duodeni. This fold usually ends at the papilla but occasionally may continue for a short distance beyond the papilla in the form of the so-called frenulum. Small, hood-like folds at the top of the papilla protect the mouth of the combined bile duct and pancreatic duct.

Numerous variations occur in the types of union of the bile and pancreatic ducts, as illustrated and discussed in Section VII. A small, wartlike, and generally less distinct second papilla, the papilla duodeni minor, is situated approximately 2.5 cm above, and slightly farther medially from, the major papilla. It serves as an opening for the minor pancreatic duct, or duct of Santorini, which is almost always present, despite great variations in development (see also Section VIII).

Except for the first portion of the duodenum, the mucosal surface, which is red in living patients, is lined with villi (see Section IV); these account for its typical velvetlike appearance. The high magnification of videoendoscopes enables endoscopists to determine when villi are flattened. A biopsy specimen is still needed to be certain of villous atrophy.

The duodenal bulb, varying in form, size, position, and orientation, appears in the anteroposterior radiographic projection as a triangle, with its base at the pylorus and its tip pointing toward the superior flexure or the transitional region of the first and second parts of the duodenum. As with the wall of the whole intestinal tract, the wall of the duodenum comprises one mucosal, one submucosal, and two muscular layers and an adventitia, or a subserosa and a serosa, wherever the duodenum is covered by peritoneum. Embryologically, morphologically, and functionally, the duodenum is an especially differentiated part of the small intestine. The epithelium of the duodenal mucosa consists of a single layer of high columnar cells with a marked cuticular border. In the fundus of the crypts, there are cells filled with eosinophilic granules (cells of Paneth) and some cells filled with yellow granules,

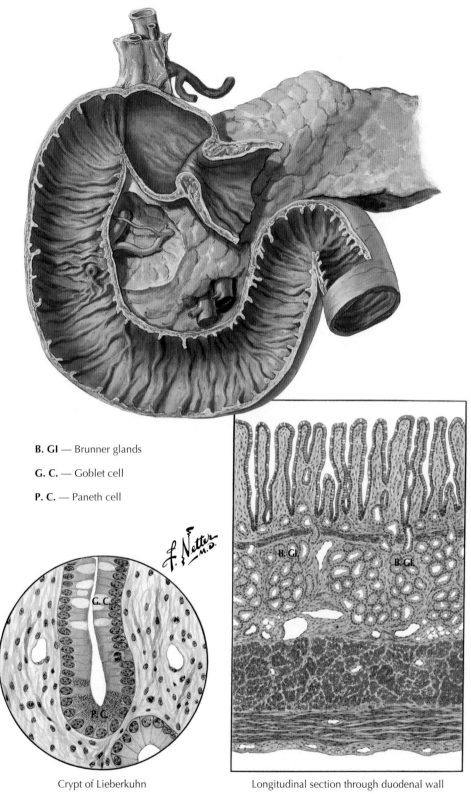

B. Gl — Brunner glands

G. C. — Goblet cell

P. C. — Paneth cell

Crypt of Lieberkuhn   Longitudinal section through duodenal wall

Fig. 15.4 Duodenal Bulb and the Mucosal Surface of the Duodenum.

which have a strong affinity to chromates. The tunica or lamina propria of the mucosa consists of loose connective tissue. Between the mucosa and the submucosa lies a double layer of smooth muscle cells, the fibers of which enter the tunica propria and continue to the tips of villi, enabling the villi to perform a sucking and pumping function.

The submucosa, lying between the mucosal and the muscular layers, allows these two layers to shift in relation to each other. It is made up of collagenous connective tissue, the fibers of which are arranged in the form of a mesh. In this network are embedded the duodenal *glands of Brunner,* characteristic of the duodenum. These are tortuous, acinotubular glands with multiple branches at their ends; breaking through the muscularis mucosae, they open into the crypts. Brunner glands are more numerous and denser in the proximal parts of the duodenum, diminishing in size and density as the duodenum approaches the duodenojejunal junction, although their extension and density vary greatly among individuals.

BLOOD SUPPLY AND COLLATERAL CIRCULATION OF UPPER ABDOMINAL ORGANS

Conventional textbook descriptions of the blood supply of the stomach and duodenum and associated organs (e.g., spleen, pancreas) present the misleading concept that the vascular pattern of these organs is relatively simple and uniform. On the contrary, these vascular patterns are always unpredictable and vary in almost all cases. Clinicians should remember this when interpreting angiography and imaging. It is important for the student of gastroenterology to understand the rich collateral circulation in this area of the body. The following are classic descriptions.

Typically, the entire blood supply of the liver, gallbladder, stomach, duodenum, pancreas, and spleen is derived from the *celiac artery;* a small, supplementary portion is supplied by the superior mesenteric artery, inferior pancreoduodenal branch. The celiac varies from 8 to 40 mm in width. When typical and complete, it gives off three branches—hepatic, splenic, and left gastric—constituting a complete trunk, frequently in the form of a tripod.

This conventional description of the celiac artery, with its three branches, occurs in only 55% of the population. In the other 45%, numerous variations occur; the interested reader is referred to classic anatomy texts. Observing a bleeding vessel through endoscopy, surgery, or angiography can be frustrating but requires an open mind and an understanding of the variations in the vascular anatomy.

No other region in the body presents more diversified collateral pathways of blood supply than the supracolonic organs (stomach, duodenum, pancreas, spleen, liver, and gallbladder). Michels identified at least 26 possible collateral routes to the liver alone (Fig. 15.5). Because of its many blood vessels and loose arrangement of its extensive connective tissue network, the great omentum is exceptionally well adapted as an area of compensatory circulation, especially for the liver and the spleen, when either the hepatic or the splenic artery is occluded. Through interlocking arteries, the stomach may receive its blood supply from six primary and six secondary sources: the pancreas from the hepatic, splenic, and superior mesenteric arteries; and the liver from three primary sources—celiac, superior mesenteric, and left gastric arteries—and, secondarily, from communications with at least 23 other arterial pathways. In view of the relational anatomy of the splenic artery, it is obvious that most of the collateral pathways to the upper abdominal organs can be initiated through this vessel and its branches and can be completed through communications established by the gastroduodenal and superior mesenteric arteries.

The most important collateral pathways in the upper abdominal organs are as follows:

- *Arcus arteriosus ventriculi inferior.* This infragastric omental pathway is made by the right and left gastroepiploics (RGEs and LGEs) as they anastomose along the greater curvature of the stomach. The arc gives off ascending gastric and descending epiploic (omental) arteries.
- *Arcus arteriosus ventriculi superior.* This supragastric pathway, with branches to both surfaces of the stomach, is made by the right and left gastrics anastomosing along the lesser curvature. Branches of the right gastric may unite with branches from the gastroduodenal, supraduodenal, retroduodenal superior pancreaticoduodenal, or

RGE. Branches of the left gastric may anastomose with the short gastrics from the splenic terminals or the LGE or with branches from the recurrent cardioesophageal branch of the left inferior phrenic or with those of an accessory left hepatic, derived from the left gastric.
- *Arcus epiploicus magnus.* This epiploic (omental pathway) is situated in the posterior layer of the great omentum below the transverse colon. Its right limb is made by the right epiploic from the RGE; its left limb is made by the left epiploic from the LGE. Arteries involved in this collateral route include hepatic, gastroduodenal, RGE, right epiploic, left epiploic, LGE, and interior terminal of the splenic.
- *Circulus transpancreaticus longus.* This important collateral pathway is affected by the inferior transverse pancreatic artery coursing along the inferior surface of the pancreas. By way of the superior or the dorsal pancreatic, of which it is the main left branch, it may communicate with the first part of the splenic, hepatic, celiac, or superior mesenteric, depending on which artery gives rise to the dorsal pancreatic. At the tail end of the pancreas, it communicates with the splenic terminals through the large pancreatic and the caudal pancreatic and at the head of the pancreas with the gastroduodenal, superior pancreaticoduodenal, or RGE.
- *Circulus hepatogastricus.* This is a derivative of the primitive, embryonic, arched anastomosis between the left gastric and the left hepatic. In the adult, the arc may persist in its entirety; the upper half may give rise to an accessory left gastric, the lower half to a so-called accessory left hepatic from the left gastric (25%).
- *Circulus hepatolienalis.* An aberrant right hepatic or the entire hepatic, arising from the superior mesenteric, may communicate with the splenic through a branch of the dorsal pancreatic or gastroduodenal or through the transverse pancreatic and caudal pancreatic.
- *Circulus celiacomesentericus.* Through the inferior pancreaticoduodenal, blood may be routed through the anterior and posterior pancreaticoduodenal arcades to enter the gastroduodenal, from which, through the right and LGEs, it reaches the splenic, or, through the common hepatic, it reaches the celiac.
- *Circulus gastrolienophrenicus.* This pathway may be affected by a communication between the short gastrics from the splenic terminals and the recurrent cardioesophageal branches of the left inferior phrenic or by a communication between the latter and the cardioesophageal branches given off by the left gastric, its aberrant left hepatic branch, or an accessory left gastric from the left hepatic.

For venous drainage, see Section IX.

LYMPHATIC DRAINAGE OF THE STOMACH

Lymph from the gastric wall collects in lymphatic vessels, which form a dense subperitoneal plexus on the anterior and posterior surfaces of the stomach (Fig. 15.6). The lymph flows in the direction of the greater and lesser curvatures, where the first regional lymph nodes are situated.

On the upper half of the lesser curvature (i.e., portion near cardia) are situated the *lower left gastric* (LLG) *nodes* (lymphonodi gastrici superiores), which are connected with the *paracardial nodes* surrounding the cardia. Above the pylorus is a small group of suprapyloric nodes (not labeled). On the greater curvature, following the trunk of the RGE artery and distributed in a chainlike fashion within the gastrocolic ligament, are the *RGE nodes* (lymphonodi gastrici inferiores). From these nodes the lymph flows to the right toward the *subpyloric* (S'pyl) *nodes,* which are situated in front of the head of the pancreas,

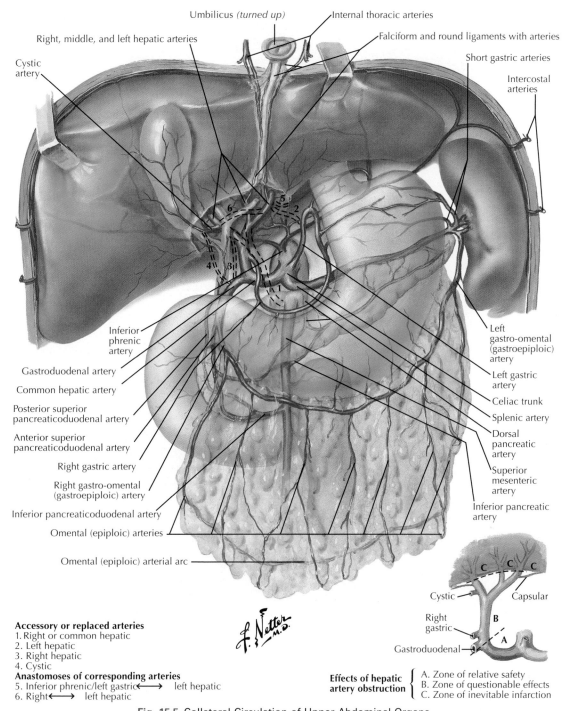

Umbilicus *(turned up)*

Internal thoracic arteries

Right, middle, and left hepatic arteries

Falciform and round ligaments with arteries

Cystic artery

Short gastric arteries

Intercostal arteries

Inferior phrenic artery

Left gastro-omental (gastroepiploic) artery

Gastroduodenal artery

Left gastric artery

Common hepatic artery

Celiac trunk

Posterior superior pancreaticoduodenal artery

Splenic artery

Anterior superior pancreaticoduodenal artery

Dorsal pancreatic artery

Right gastric artery

Superior mesenteric artery

Right gastro-omental (gastroepiploic) artery

Inferior pancreatic artery

Inferior pancreaticoduodenal artery

Omental (epiploic) arteries

Omental (epiploic) arterial arc

Cystic

Capsular

Right gastric

Gastroduodenal

Accessory or replaced arteries
1. Right or common hepatic
2. Left hepatic
3. Right hepatic
4. Cystic
Anastomoses of corresponding arteries
5. Inferior phrenic/left gastric ⟷ left hepatic
6. Right ⟷ left hepatic

Effects of hepatic artery obstruction { A. Zone of relative safety
B. Zone of questionable effects
C. Zone of inevitable infarction

Fig. 15.5 Collateral Circulation of Upper Abdominal Organs.

below the pylorus and the first part of the duodenum. There are a few smaller *LGE nodes* in the part of the greater curvature nearest the spleen.

For purposes of simplification, a distinction can be made among four different draining areas into which the gastric lymph flows, although, in fact, these areas cannot be so clearly separated. The lymph from the upper left anterior and posterior walls of the stomach (region I in the diagram) drains through the LLG and paracardial nodes. From here, the lymphatics follow the left gastric artery and the coronary vein toward the vascular bed of the celiac artery. Included in this system are the *upper left gastric* (ULG) *nodes,* which lie on the left crus of the diaphragm.

The LLG nodes, paracardial nodes, and ULG nodes are known collectively as the left gastric nodes.

The pyloric segment of the stomach, in the region of the lesser curvature (region II), discharges its lymph into the *right suprapancreatic* (RS'p) *nodes,* directly and indirectly, through the small suprapyloric nodes. The lymph from the region of the fundus facing the greater curvature (i.e., adjacent to spleen) flows along lymphatic vessels running within the gastrosplenic ligament. Some of these lymphatics lead directly to the *left suprapancreatic* (LS'p; pancreaticolienal) *nodes,* and others lead indirectly through the small *LGE nodes* and through the splenic nodes lying within the hilus of the spleen.

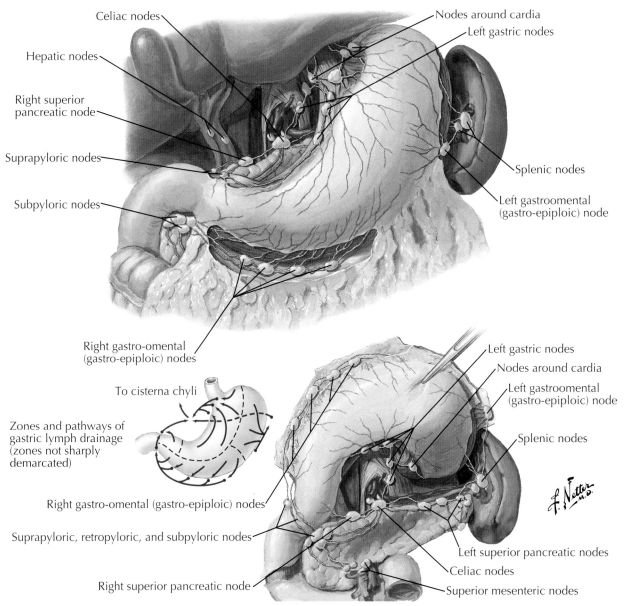

Fig. 15.6 Lymphatic Drainage of the Stomach.

Lymph from the distal portion of the corpus facing the greater curvature and from the pyloric region (region IV) collects in the RGE nodes. From here, the lymph flows to the subpyloric nodes, which lie in front of the head of the pancreas. From the ULG nodes (region 1), RS'p nodes (regions 2 and 4), and LS'p (pancreaticolienal) nodes (region III), the lymph stream leads to the celiac (middle suprapancreatic [MS'p]) nodes, which are situated above the pancreas and around the celiac artery and its branches. From the celiac lymph nodes, the lymph flows through the gastrointestinal (GI) lymphatic trunk to the thoracic duct, in the initial segment of which (i.e., where it arises from various trunks) there is generally a more or less pronounced expansion in the form of the cisterna chyli.

In the region where the thorax borders on the neck, the thoracic duct—before opening into the angle formed by the left subclavian and left jugular veins—receives, among other things, the left subclavian lymphatic trunk. In cases of gastric tumor, palpable metastases may develop in the left supraclavicular nodes (also known as Virchow or

Troisier nodes). The lymphatics of the duodenum drain into the nodes that also serve the pancreas.

INNERVATION OF THE STOMACH AND DUODENUM

This description of the innervation of the stomach and duodenum, although complex and detailed, is important to those who want to understand the common motility disorders of the stomach, such as gastroparesis and dyspepsia.

Sympathetic and parasympathetic nerves that contain efferent and afferent fibers innervate the stomach and the duodenum (Fig. 15.7). The sympathetic supply emerges in the anterior spinal nerve roots as *preganglionic fibers,* which are axons of lateral cornual cells located at approximately the sixth to ninth or tenth thoracic segments. These fibers are carried from the spinal nerves in rami communicantes, which pass to the adjacent parts of the sympathetic ganglionated trunks, then

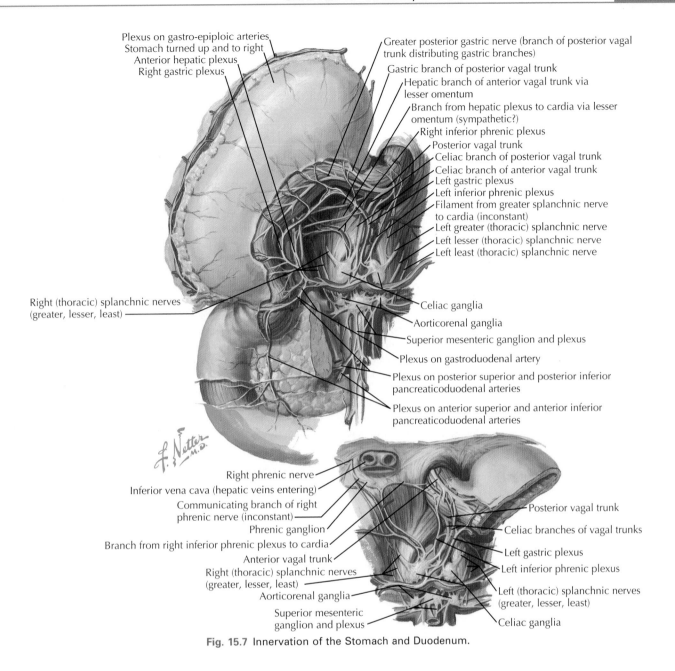

Plexus on gastro-epiploic arteries
Stomach turned up and to right
Anterior hepatic plexus
Right gastric plexus

Greater posterior gastric nerve (branch of posterior vagal trunk distributing gastric branches)
Gastric branch of posterior vagal trunk
Hepatic branch of anterior vagal trunk via lesser omentum
Branch from hepatic plexus to cardia via lesser omentum (sympathetic?)
Right inferior phrenic plexus
Posterior vagal trunk
Celiac branch of posterior vagal trunk
Celiac branch of anterior vagal trunk
Left gastric plexus
Left inferior phrenic plexus
Filament from greater splanchnic nerve to cardia (inconstant)
Left greater (thoracic) splanchnic nerve
Left lesser (thoracic) splanchnic nerve
Left least (thoracic) splanchnic nerve

Right (thoracic) splanchnic nerves (greater, lesser, least)

Celiac ganglia
Aorticorenal ganglia
Superior mesenteric ganglion and plexus
Plexus on gastroduodenal artery
Plexus on posterior superior and posterior inferior pancreaticoduodenal arteries
Plexus on anterior superior and anterior inferior pancreaticoduodenal arteries

Right phrenic nerve
Inferior vena cava (hepatic veins entering)
Communicating branch of right phrenic nerve (inconstant)
Phrenic ganglion
Branch from right inferior phrenic plexus to cardia
Anterior vagal trunk
Right (thoracic) splanchnic nerves (greater, lesser, least)
Aorticorenal ganglia
Superior mesenteric ganglion and plexus

Posterior vagal trunk
Celiac branches of vagal trunks
Left gastric plexus
Left inferior phrenic plexus
Left (thoracic) splanchnic nerves (greater, lesser, least)
Celiac ganglia

Fig. 15.7 Innervation of the Stomach and Duodenum.

into the thoracic splanchnic nerves to the celiac plexus and ganglia. Some fibers form synapses in the sympathetic trunk ganglia, but most form synapses with cells in the celiac and superior mesenteric ganglia. The axons of these cells, the *postganglionic fibers*, are conveyed to the stomach and duodenum in the nerve plexuses alongside the various branches of the celiac and superior mesenteric arteries. These arterial plexuses are composed mainly of sympathetic fibers but also contain some parasympathetic fibers, which reach the celiac plexus through the celiac branches of the vagal trunks.

Afferent impulses are carried in fibers that pursue the reverse route of that just described. However, afferent impulses do not form synapses in the sympathetic trunks; their cytons (perikaryons) are located in the posterior spinal root ganglia and enter the cord through the posterior spinal nerve roots.

The *celiac plexus* is the largest of the autonomic plexuses and surrounds the celiac arterial trunk and the root of the superior mesenteric artery. It consists of right and left halves, each containing one larger

celiac ganglion, a smaller aorticorenal ganglion, and a superior mesenteric ganglion, which is often unpaired. These and other, even smaller ganglia are united by numerous nervous interconnections to form the celiac plexus. It receives sympathetic contributions through the greater (superior), lesser (middle), and least (inferior) thoracic splanchnic nerves and through filaments from the first lumbar ganglia of the sympathetic trunks. Its parasympathetic roots are derived from the celiac division of the posterior vagal trunk and from smaller celiac branches of the anterior vagal trunk.

The celiac plexus sends direct filaments to some adjacent viscera, but most of its branches accompany the arteries from the upper part of the abdominal aorta. Numerous filaments from the celiac plexus unite to form open-meshed nerve plexuses around the celiac trunk and the left gastric, hepatic, and splenic arteries. Subsidiary plexuses from the hepatic arterial plexus are continued along the right gastric and gastroduodenal arteries and from the latter along the RGE and anterior and posterior superior pancreaticoduodenal arteries. The splenic arterial plexus sends offshoots along the short gastric and LGE arteries.

The *superior mesenteric plexus* is the largest derivative of the celiac plexus and contains the superior mesenteric ganglion or ganglia. The main superior mesenteric plexus divides into secondary plexuses, which surround and accompany the inferior pancreaticoduodenal, jejunal, and other branches of the artery.

The *left gastric plexus* consists of one to four nervelets connected by oblique filaments that accompany the artery and supply "twigs" to the cardiac end of the stomach, communicating with offshoots from the left phrenic plexus. Other filaments follow the artery along the lesser curvature between the layers of the lesser omentum to supply adjacent parts of the stomach. They communicate with the *right gastric plexus* and with gastric branches of the vagus.

The *hepatic plexus* also contains sympathetic and parasympathetic efferent and afferent fibers and gives off subsidiary plexuses along all its branches. Following the right gastric artery, these branches supply the pyloric region, and the gastroduodenal plexus accompanies the artery between the first part of the duodenum and the head of the pancreas, supplying fibers to both structures and to the adjacent parts of the common bile duct. When the artery divides into its anterosuperior pancreaticoduodenal and RGE branches, the nerves also subdivide and are distributed to the second part of the duodenum, terminations of the common bile and pancreatic ducts, head of the pancreas, and parts of the stomach. The part of the hepatic plexus lying in the free margin of the lesser omentum gives off one or more hepatogastric branches, which pass to the left between the layers of the lesser omentum, to the cardiac end and lesser curvature of the stomach; they unite with and reinforce the left gastric plexus.

The *splenic plexus* gives off subsidiary nerve plexuses around its pancreatic, short gastric, and LGE branches, which supply the structures indicated by their names. A filament may curve upward to supply the fundus of the stomach.

The *phrenic plexuses* assist in supplying the cardiac end of the stomach. A filament from the *right* phrenic plexus sometimes turns to the left, posteroinferior to the vena caval hiatus in the diaphragm, and passes to the region of the cardiac orifice. The *left* phrenic plexus supplies a constant twig to the cardiac orifice. A delicate branch from the left phrenic nerve (not illustrated) supplies the cardia.

The parasympathetic supply for the stomach and duodenum arises in the dorsal vagal nucleus in the floor of the fourth ventricle. The afferent fibers also end in the dorsal vagal nucleus, which is a mixture of visceral efferent and afferent cells. The fibers are conveyed to and from the abdomen through the vagus nerves, esophageal plexus, and vagal trunks. The vagal trunks give off gastric, pyloric, hepatic, and celiac branches.

The *anterior vagal trunk* gives off gastric branches that run downward along the lesser curvature, supplying the anterior surface of the stomach almost as far as the pylorus. The pyloric branches (not illustrated) arise from the anterior vagal trunk or from the greater anterior gastric nerve and run to the right between the layers of the lesser omentum, before turning downward through or close to the hepatic plexus to reach the pyloric antrum, pylorus, and proximal part of the duodenum. Small celiac branches run alongside the left gastric artery to the celiac plexus, often uniting with corresponding branches of the posterior vagal trunk.

The *posterior vagal trunk* gives off gastric branches that radiate to the posterior surface of the stomach, supplying it from the fundus to the pyloric antrum. One branch, the *greater posterior gastric nerve*, is usually larger than the others. As on the anterior aspect, these branches communicate with adjacent gastric nerves, although no true posterior gastric plexus exists. The celiac branch is large and reaches the celiac plexus alongside the left gastric artery. Vagal fibers from this celiac branch are distributed to the pylorus, duodenum, pancreas, and so on, through the vascular plexuses derived from the celiac plexus.

ADDITIONAL RESOURCES

Reynolds J: *The netter collection of medical illustrations* (vol 9), Digestive System, Part II, Cambridge, MA, 2016, Elsevier.

Semrin MG, Russo MA: Anatomy, histology, and developmental anomalies of the stomach and duodenum. In Feldman M, Friedman LS, Brandt LJ, editors: *Gastrointestinal and liver disease*, ed 10, Philadelphia, 2016, Saunders-Elsevier, pp 795–809.

16

Gastric Secretion

Martin H. Floch

Gastrin, the main stimulus of acid secretion, is produced by G cells of the duodenum and in the pyloric antrum of the stomach. Gastrin is synthesized as a large molecule of 101 amino acids. It is converted to progastrin and then further processed to yield peptides with C gaminocyclicine of G34 or G17. Gastric physiology is complex, with the key factor in stimulation being histamine and production of acid.

The early history of gastric secretion studies indicated that there were lasting active gastric and intestinal phases. Although there is truth to this, it is far more complex as we now understand the hormone involvement.

The stomach produces endocrine and exocrine secretions. The *endocrine* secretions are somatostatin, histamine, gastrin, neuropeptides (gastrin-releasing peptide [GRP]), calcitonin, pituitary adenylate cyclase–activating polypeptide, and ghrelin. The *exocrine* secretions are water, electrolytes (hydrogen, potassium, sodium, chlorate, bicarbonate), pepsinogen, lipase, intrinsic factor, and mucins. Small amounts of zinc, iron, calcium, and magnesium are also secreted. (Pepsinogen and lipase are activated in acid media to assist in digestion.)

The anatomy and the cells involved in gastric secretion are described in Chapter 15, the influences on secretion are described here, and the role in digestion in Chapter 18. Gastric secretion varies greatly during the day, from resting periods to active periods while eating (Fig. 16.1). Actual secretion is integrated and includes many stimulatory and inhibitory factors. Basal secretion does have a circadian variation. Observations on gastric secretion clearly identify an interdigestive period and a digestive period. The *interdigestive* phase includes the basic secretion and is influenced heavily by emotional factors. Although most experiments have been on animals, human experiments have shown that anger, resentment, hostility, and fear can influence the volume and content of secretion. Secretions clearly are influenced by vagus and neurohumoral stimuli.

The *digestive* period can be divided into three phases: cephalic, gastric, and intestinal. The *cephalic* phase includes the secretory response to all stimuli acting in the region of the brain. These may be unconditional (unlearned) reflexes, such as the secretion to sham feeding in a decorticate animal or the conditioned (learned) reflexes exemplified by the secretory effect of the thought, odor, sight, or taste of food. Conditioned or psychic secretion (Pavlov) is the principal component of the cephalic phase; the copious flow of gastric juice that occurs when appetizing food is masticated amounts to almost half the volume output of the gastric glands. Its presence contributes to the effective initiation and the subsequent efficiency of gastric digestion. The cephalic phase is mediated primarily through the vagus nerve and hormonal stimuli as gastrin release from the antrum.

The *gastric* (second) phase is so named because effective stimuli are within the stomach and are of two types: *mechanical,* from distension of the stomach as a result of the meal, and *chemical,* from secretagogues in foods or hormones that are released in the process of digestion. Hormonal stimulation of the secretion occurs by humoral and paraendocrine methods through receptors and intracellular signal transduction. The most potent stimulators are gastrin, acetylcholine, neurotransmitters such as GRP, and histamine.

The *intestinal* phase begins when chyme enters the duodenum and humoral effects occur. By the time a significant amount of the gastric content has been delivered to the intestine, regulatory mechanisms are already in operation to terminate the digestive period of gastric secretion. When the stomach is filled and absorption begins, satiety sets in, eating ceases, and psychic stimuli are withdrawn. Acidity of pH 1.5 or less acts on the antral mucosa to inhibit the release of gastrin. The production of secretoinhibitory hormones from the antrum results in the withdrawal of humoral and mechanical stimuli of the gastric phase. The main inhibitors of secretion are somatostatin, secretin, and a host of peptides that include corticotropin-releasing factor, b-endorphin, bombesin, neurotensin, calcitonin, calcitonin gene–related peptide, and interleukin-1 (IL-1). Other polypeptides, such as tropin-releasing hormone, peptide-y, and peptide-yy, have action, but their roles are unclear.

The relationship between secretions and food is discussed in Chapter 18. Importantly, a viscous layer of mucus is secreted. The mucous layer, consisting of a glycoprotein, coats the stomach and measures approximately 0.2 to 0.6 mm. Transport occurs across this mucous barrier of hydrogen ions (H^+), which is constantly being digested by pepsin and then replaced as it acts as an interface between the passage of H^+ and the neutralization by bicarbonate. This mucous barrier presumably prevents autodigestion of the stomach.

The role of prostaglandins has some importance in gastric physiology, but their exact effect is not clear. Similarly, the role of ghrelin in secretion has not been fully explained.

ADDITIONAL RESOURCES

Schubert ML, Kaunitz JD: Gastric secretion. In Podolsky DK, Camilleri M, Fitz JG, et al, editors: *Yamada's Textbook of Gastroenterology*, ed 6, West Sussex England, 2015, Wiley-Blackwell, pp 839–853.

Interdigestive period

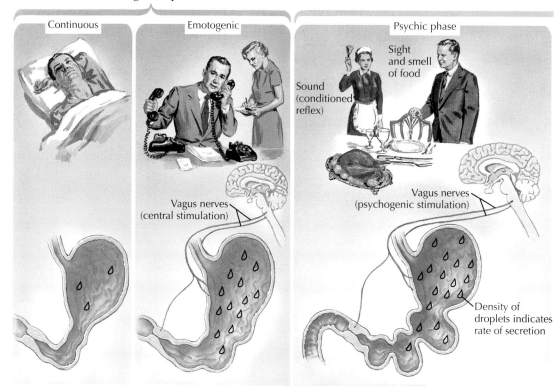

Digestive period

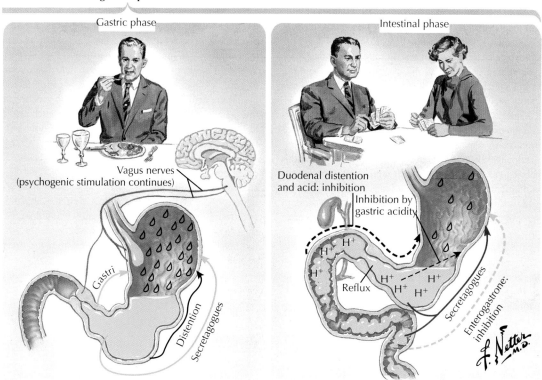

Fig. 16.1 Mechanisms of Gastric Secretion.

17

Factors Influencing Gastric Activity

Martin H. Floch

Stomach activity is modified by the factors that stimulate and inhibit gastric secretion (Fig. 17.1). Emptying of the stomach is affected by many factors; the types of food eaten and the environment in which they are eaten play major roles through direct nerve and hormonal influences. Factors that modify motor and secretory activities of the stomach, usually simultaneously and in the same direction, include the following:

1. *Tonus of the stomach.* The hypertonic, or "steerhorn," stomach is hypermotile and empties relatively rapidly compared with the hypotonic, or "fishhook," type. In addition, the hypertonic stomach secretes more hydrochloric acid (HCl) and, as a corollary, experiences accelerated secretion and diminished intragastric stasis. Barium residue in the stomach 4 or 5 hours after upper gastrointestinal (GI) x-ray examination must be interpreted with consideration that the stomach's inherent tonicity is a factor in its emptying rate.

2. *Character of the food.* A meal sufficiently high in fat to yield an intragastric fat content in excess of approximately 10% empties more slowly and stimulates considerably less acid secretion than does a meal consisting predominantly of protein. The inhibitory effect of fat on gastric secretion is not local but is a primarily a result of enterogastric neural reflexes and hormones, primarily cholecystokinin, after fat has entered the upper intestine.

3. *Starch and protein.* A meal consisting exclusively or mainly of starch tends to empty more rapidly, although stimulating less secretion, than does a protein meal. Thus, other factors being equal, a person may expect to be hungry sooner after a breakfast of fruit juice, cereal, toast, and tea than after bacon, eggs, and milk. The amount of total secretion and of acid content is highest with the ingestion of proteins. However, the relationship of quantity and rate of secretion to its acid or pepsin concentration varies greatly among individuals and in a single person under different conditions. Numerous GI hormones and neural mechanisms are involved in feedback to the stomach. The so-called ileal break occurs when fat enters the ileum.

4. *Consistency of the food.* Liquids, whether ingested separately or with solid food, leave the stomach more rapidly than do semisolids or solids. This does not apply to liquids such as milk, from which solid material is precipitated on contact with gastric juice. With any foods requiring mastication, the consistency of the material reaching the stomach should normally be semisolid, thereby facilitating gastric secretion, digestion, and evacuation. Important exceptions to the general rule that liquids are weak stimulants of gastric secretion are (1) the broth of meat or fish, because of their high secretagogue content, and (2) coffee, which derives its secretory potency from its content of caffeine and of the secretagogues formed in the roasting process.

5. *Mixed meals.* In a mixed meal, liquids empty first and solids empty in two phases. An initial lag phase is followed by linear emptying.

6. *Hunger.* A meal eaten at a time of intense hunger tends to be evacuated more rapidly than normal, apparently in consequence of the heightened gastric tonus. Because hunger results from the depletion of body nutrient stores (see Section X), it is understandable on teleologic grounds that in the hunger state, the body should have some mechanism for hastening the delivery of ingested nutrients into the intestine.

7. *Exercise.* Mild exercise, particularly just after eating, shortens the emptying time of the meal. With strenuous exercise, gastric contractions are temporarily inhibited, then augmented, so that final emptying is not significantly delayed. Secretory activity does not appear to be materially influenced by exercise.

8. *Position.* In some persons, gastric emptying is facilitated when the position of the body is such that the pylorus and the duodenum are in a dependent position (i.e., with the person lying on the right side). In the supine position, particularly in infants and adults with cascade stomach, the gastric content pools in the dependent fundic portion, and emptying is delayed. No evidence suggests that secretion is affected by position.

9. *Emotion.* The impairing effect of emotional states on gastric motility and secretion has been well documented by clinical and experimental observations. Evidence indicates that the influence of emotions on gastric activity may be augmentative or inhibitory, depending on whether the emotional experience is of an aggressive (hostility, resentment) or a depressive (sorrow, fear) type, respectively. One point of view holds that it is not the manifest or conscious emotion that determines whether the stomach is stimulated or inhibited, but rather the unconscious or symbolic content of the emotional state, and furthermore, that certain emotions may be accompanied by dissociation in the response among the various components of the gastric secretions.

10. *Pain.* Severe or sustained pain in any part of the body (e.g., kidney stones or gallstones, migraine, sciatica, neuritis) inhibits gastric motility and evacuation by nervous reflex pathways.

Factors Affecting Gastric Emptying

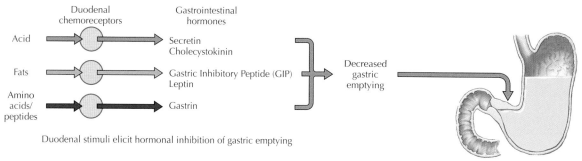

Duodenal stimuli elicit hormonal inhibition of gastric emptying

Sequence of Gastric Motility

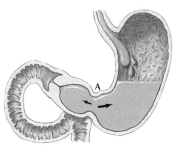

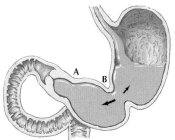

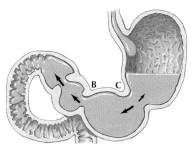

1. Stomach is filling. A mild peristaltic wave (A) has started in antrum and is passing toward pylorus. Gastric contents are churned and largely pushed back into body of stomach

2. Wave (A) fading out as pylorus fails to open. A stronger wave (B) is originating at incisure and is again squeezing gastric contents in both directions

3. Pylorus opens as wave (B) approaches it. Duodenal bulb is filled, and some contents pass into second portion of duodenum. Wave (C) starting just above incisure

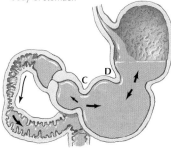

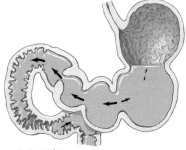

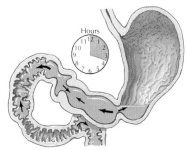

4. Pylorus again closed. Wave (C) fails to evacuate contents. Wave (D) starts higher on body of stomach. Duodenal bulb may contract or may remain filled as peristaltic wave originating just beyond it empties second portion

5. Peristaltic waves are now originating higher on body of stomach. Gastric contents are evacuated intermittently. Contents of duodenal bulb area pushed passively into second portion as more gastric contents emerge

6. 3 to 4 hours later, stomach is almost empty. Small peristaltic wave empties duodenal bulb with some reflux into stomach. Reverse and antegrade peristalsis present in duodenum

Fig. 17.1 Factors Influencing Gastric Activity.

ADDITIONAL RESOURCES

Collins PJ, Houghton LA: Nutrients and the control of liquid gastric emptying, *Am J Physiol* 276:997, 1999.

Collins PJ, Houghton LA, Read NW, et al: Role of the proximal and distal stomach in mixed solid and liquid meal emptying, *Gut* 32:615–619, 1991.

Moran TH, Wirth JB, Schwartz GS, et al: Interactions between gastric volume and duodenal nutrients and the control of liquid gastric emptying, *Am J Physiol* 276:R997, 1999.

Schubert ML, Kaunitz JD: Gastric secretion. In Podolsky DK, Camilleri M, Fitz JG, et al, editors: *Yamada's textbook of gastroenterology*, ed 6, West Sussex England, 2015, Wiley-Blackwell, pp 839–853.

18

Role of the Stomach in Digestion

Martin H. Floch

The stomach plays an important role in nutrition; maintaining adequate weight and nutrient intake would be difficult without a stomach. When adequately chewed, food arrives in the stomach, where the motility enables churning and the initial digestive processes (see Chapters 17 and 24). Regulating cephalic, gastric, and intestinal phases of gastric secretion is complicated (see Chapter 16).

Normal gastric secretion is essential for the normal digestion of foods (Fig. 18.1). Hydrochloric acid (HCl) is secreted from the parietal cell in a concentration of 0.16 N, but this maximal concentration is quickly diluted by the metabolic activity in the mucus layer and with food. In addition to the normal physiologic regulator mechanisms of gastric secretion, a number of systemic and local effects are unique to HCl secretion. The stimulating effect of the oral administration of sodium bicarbonate ($NaHCO_3$), popularly called "acid rebound," probably results from a combination of factors, including a direct stimulating action on the gastric mucosa, annulment of the antral acid-inhibitory influence, and acceleration of gastric emptying. The "alkaline tide," or decrease in urinary acidity that may occur after a meal, is generally attributed to increased alkalinity of the blood resulting from the secretion of HCl. An alkaline tide is not predictable and is influenced by (1) relative rate of HCl formation and alkaline digestive secretions, mainly pancreatic, with the high $NaHCO_3$ content in the pancreas; (2) rate of absorption of HCl from the gut; (3) neutralizing capacity of the food; (4) respiratory adjustments after the meal; and (5) diuretic effect of the meal.

Pepsin, the principal enzyme of gastric juice, is preformed and is stored in the chief cells as *pepsinogen.* At pH less than 6, pepsinogen is converted to pepsin, a reaction that then proceeds autocatalytically. Pepsin exerts its proteolytic activity by attacking peptide linkages containing the amino groups of the aromatic amino acids, with the liberation principally of intermediate protein moieties and a few polypeptides and amino acids. An accessory digestive function of pepsin is the clotting of milk, which serves to improve its use by preventing too rapid passage, rendering it more susceptible to enzymatic hydrolysis. Anything that mobilizes vagal impulses for the stomach serves as a powerful stimulus for pepsin secretion. Thus a gastric juice rich in pepsin content is evoked by sham feeding; by hypoglycemia, which stimulates the vagal centers; and by direct electrical stimulation of the vagus nerves.

The mucoid component of gastric juice consists of at least two distinct mucoproteins. The "visible mucus" has a gelatinous consistency and, in the presence of HCl, forms a white coagulum; evidence indicates that it is secreted by the surface epithelium. The "soluble mucus" or "dissolved mucus" appears to be a product of the neck's chief cells and the mucoid cells of the pyloric and cardiac glands. The secretion of soluble mucus is activated primarily by vagal impulses, whereas the secretion of visible mucus occurs principally in response to direct chemical and mechanical irritation of the surface epithelium. Because of its adherent and metabolic properties and its resistance to penetration by pepsin, mucus secretion protects the mucosa of the stomach against damage by various irritating agents, including its own acid, pepsin.

A normal constituent of the gastric juice, but characteristically deficient or absent in patients with pernicious anemia, is *intrinsic factor.* It interacts with vitamin B_{12} to prepare it for absorption in the intestine. An R factor from saliva mixes and binds with vitamin B_{12}. The R factor is cleaved by pancreatic enzyme action when the combined B_{12}–R factor enters the duodenum, and the intrinsic factor from the stomach binds to B_{12} to enable absorption by receptors in the proximal intestine. Large amounts of intrinsic factor usually are secreted to enable adequate amounts to bind with the B_{12} in the intestine.

Salivary amylases may mix with the starch in foods and may have an initial digestive effect, but major carbohydrate digestion occurs in the intestine from the action of pancreatic enzymes. The degree of salivary enzyme activity in the stomach depends on how long the food is masticated and how fast it is swallowed, because salivary amylases are inactivated rapidly in the stomach by peptic action.

Gastric lipases may begin the process of fat digestion and may account for as much as 25% of intraluminal fat digestion. Again, however, this depends on how fast the stomach empties, as well as other factors that affect emptying. Because of the pH and molar-sensitive receptors in the duodenum, a delay in gastric emptying results when the chyme is too acid or hypertonic at the beginning of the intestinal phase of digestion.

In summary, the major digestive activity in the stomach is proteolytic and prepares chyme to pass into the duodenum for orderly digestion and absorption.

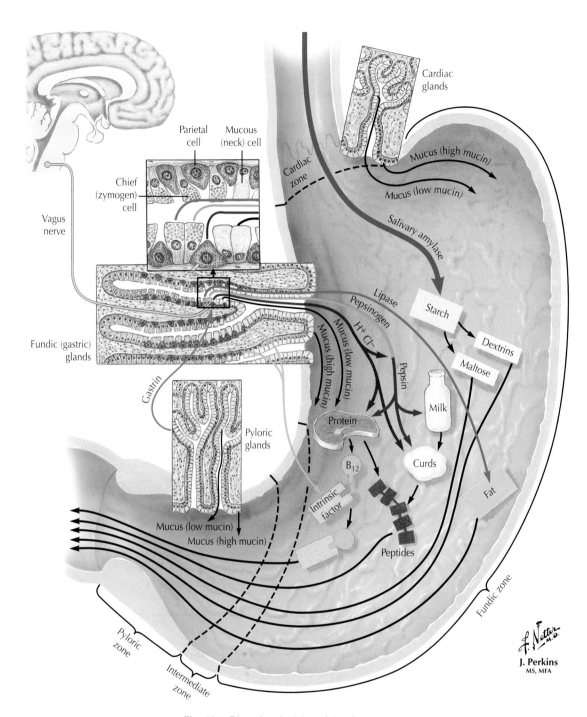

Fig. 18.1 Digestive Activity of the Stomach.

ADDITIONAL RESOURCES

Camilleri M: Integrated upper gastrointestinal response to food intake, *Gastroenterology* 131:640–658, 2006.

Schubert ML, Kaunitz JD: Gastric secretion. In Podolsky DK, Camilleri M, Fitz JG, et al, editors: *Yamada's textbook of gastroenterology*, ed 6, West Sussex England, 2015, Wiley-Blackwell, pp 839–853.

19

Gastric Acid Secretion Tests: Hydrochloric Acid and Gastrin

Martin H. Floch

Fasting serum gastrin levels can vary greatly. The normal range is 0 to 200 pg/mL. However, medications and other suppressants or stimulants can widen the normal range to as high as 400 pg/mL. Greater than 1000 pg/mL is usually considered diagnostic of Zollinger-Ellison syndrome (ZES). In some cases, there may be uncertainty because of chronic severe gastritis. Prolonged use of proton pump inhibitors may also create uncertainty in combination of very high fasting gastrin level and high levels of gastrin acid secretion usually confirm the diagnosis of ZES. However, renal failure can also result in high serum gastrin levels because of poor clearance. Therefore the secretin provocative test was designed to confirm the diagnosis of ZES. It is used when the serum gastrin level is less than 1000 or whenever the diagnosis is uncertain. A fasting serum gastrin level is obtained; secretin (2 U/kg) is rapidly injected; and serum gastrin blood levels are obtained at 2, 5, and 10 minutes after injection. In ZES, serum gastrin levels usually rise rapidly after 5 minutes. A 200 pg/mL or greater elevation in gastrin level confirms the diagnosis. The secretin provocative test has a sensitivity of 90% for ZES.

Gastric analysis is now rarely used; it was a major test before the development of significant medical therapy for duodenal and gastric ulcer. *Qualitative* gastric analysis is used only in the differential diagnosis of pernicious anemia and gastric atrophy. However, *quantitative* gastric analysis (the classic method is illustrated in Fig. 19.1) is still important in the diagnosis and monitoring of ZES and the multiple endocrine neoplasm syndrome.

The technique seeks to determine, by 1-hour monitoring of basal secretion, the amount of hydrochloric acid (HCl) secreted by the stomach. After an overnight fast, the patient is intubated with a radiopaque tube, and the position is checked by fluoroscopy. The tip of the tube should be in the gastric antrum. Studies have revealed that no more than 5% to 10% of acid secretion is lost by aspirating continually when the tube is positioned correctly. After the tube is placed, the residuum in the stomach is emptied, and then collections are made in separate tubes every 15 minutes. The amount in each tube is measured. Topfer reagent is used to check quickly for acid. Any device that maintains negative pressure can be used to aspirate all the secretions. The patency of the tube should be checked with air every 5 minutes to make sure it is not plugged. The amount of HCl in each tube is calculated using one of two methods: titration with sodium hydroxide or by pH electrode, which measures hydrogen activity. The hydrogen chloride secreted is then calculated and reported as milliequivalents per liter (mEq/L). The total quantity of acid (volume × concentration) can then be reported as milliequivalents per hour. Basal acid output may be zero in approximately one of three people, but the upper limit of normal for the basal acid output is approximately 10 mmol/h in men and 5 mmol/h in women. It varies from hour to hour and certainly varies greatly during various phases of gastric activity.

"Maximal acid output" and "peak acid output" are no longer used. They represented the amount of acid after either pentagastrin or histamine stimulation. Neither drug is available in the United States.

Functionally, *gastrin* is the most potent stimulant of acid secretion. The stimulation of acid secretion and the role of gastrin are complex (see Chapters 15, 16, and 18). Specialized G cells of the stomach, along with pyloric and duodenal glands, produce gastrin. It is secreted as preprogastrin, and then by enzymatic action, all the active forms are produced. The two main gastrins are G_{17} and G_{34} (chain lengths of 17 and 34 amino acids). Gastrin stimulates enterochromaffin-like (ECL) cells to release histamine. Histamine stimulates acid secretion by parietal cells and release of other neurotransmitters, such as acetylcholine and gastrin-releasing peptide. Major inhibitors of parietal cell secretion are somatostatin and cholecystokinin. Secretin and other peptides also enter in the inhibitory process, but their roles are less well understood.

ADDITIONAL RESOURCES

Gregory RA, Tracy J: The constitution and properties of two gastrins extracted from hog antral mucosa, *Gut* 5:103–117, 1964.

Pisegna JR: The effect of Zollinger-Ellison syndrome and neuropeptide secreting tumors on the stomach, *Curr Gastroenterol Rep* 1:511–517, 1999.

Schubert ML, Kaunitz JD: Gastric secretion. In Podolsky DK, Camilleri M, Fitz JG, et al, editors: *Yamada's textbook of gastroenterology*, ed 6, West Sussex England, 2015, Wiley-Blackwell, pp 839–853.

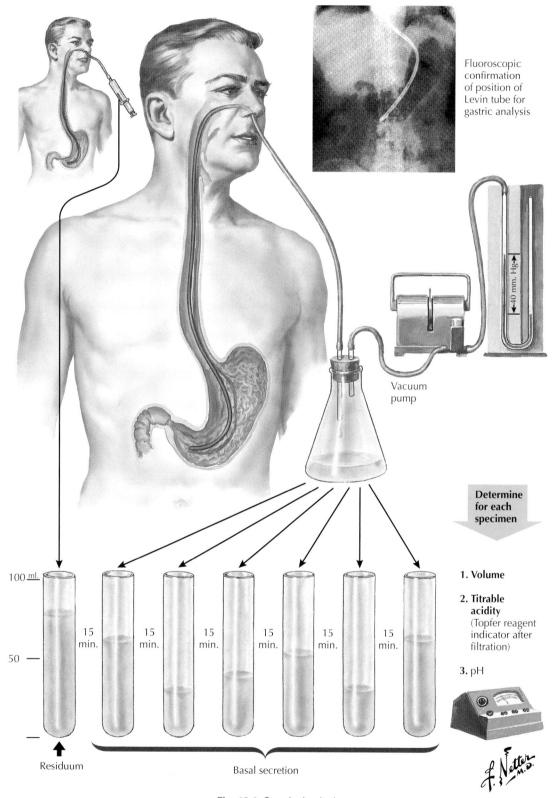

Fluoroscopic
confirmation
of position of
Levin tube for
gastric analysis

40 mm. Hg

Vacuum
pump

**Determine
for each
specimen**

1. **Volume**

2. **Titrable
acidity**
(Topfer reagent
indicator after
filtration)

3. pH

100 ml.

50

15
min.

Residuum

Basal secretion

Fig. 19.1 Gastric Analysis.

20

Effects of Drugs on Gastric Function

Martin H. Floch

Many of the pharmacologic agents widely used in medical therapy adversely affect the upper gastrointestinal (GI) tract (Fig. 20.1). Therefore every patient with symptoms referable to the esophagus, stomach, or duodenum should be questioned carefully regarding the recent use of drugs. Drugs may also adversely affect the liver (see Section IX), pancreas (see Section VII), and other organs. This chapter discusses specific agents and drug categories often implicated in gastric disorders.

SALICYLATES

The primary offenders are salicylates, alone or in combination with other analgesics, antacids, opiates, or steroids. The inflammatory action of salicylates in the stomach of susceptible persons can result in mild dyspepsia to massive hemorrhage. Aspirin is widely used to prevent cardiac disease and polyp formation in the GI tract. The potential for bleeding is dose related, but in some persons, even small doses (81 mg) may lead to bleeding tendencies.

CAFFEINE

Although it is a common component of headache remedies and is responsible for the widespread use of coffee and tea, caffeine is a gastric irritant and a stimulant of gastric secretion and gastric motility. Beverages containing caffeine, which also include most sodas containing cola, have the same effect as the pure xanthine preparation. A cup of coffee contains 100 to 150 mg of caffeine. Teas have even larger amounts. The amount of caffeine in the beverage varies with the brewing process and amount ingested.

Theophylline and its water-soluble salt aminophylline are closely related to caffeine and have similar effects but are used effectively in bronchospasm.

NONSTEROIDAL ANTIINFLAMMATORY DRUGS

Nonsteroidal antiinflammatory drugs (NSAIDs) are prescribed more frequently worldwide than any other group of medicines. Approximately 25 different NSAIDs are available in the United States. They cause significant rates of morbidity and mortality because of the adverse effects on the GI tract. The most serious complications are bleeding and perforation, which account for almost all associated deaths. The major damage occurs in the stomach and duodenum, but NSAIDs may also affect the small and large intestines. Significant endoscopic evidence indicates that NSAIDs and aspirin directly injure the GI mucosa. However, damage has been observed even when medications are administered intravenously and in enteric-coated preparations, questioning whether the effect is topical or systemic.

The benefit of NSAIDs is decreased cyclooxygenase (COX-1 and COX-2) activity, which in turn decreases the cascade of cytokine formation in inflammation, although NSAIDs also decrease the prostaglandin protection of the GI mucosa. COX-2 appears to cause less, but still significant, GI damage. Common COX-1 inhibitors are diclofenac, ibuprofen, indomethacin, naproxen, and sulindac. Common COX-2 inhibitors are celecoxib and rofecoxib and are used to decrease the side effects of COX-1 agents.

ISONICOTINIC ACID HYDRAZIDE

Isonicotinic acid hydrazide (isonicotinylhydrazine) is used in to treat tuberculosis. When administered in large doses, isonicotine hydrazine and the related drug isoniazid (INH) are gastric secretory stimulants associated with gastric irritation and liver disease.

ANTIBIOTICS

Antibiotics may cause local irritant effects (tetracyclines) or greatly increased motility (erythromycin and clarithromycin). The tetracycline drugs often cause esophageal ulceration. Care must be taken in administration and make sure they are swallowed with adequate amounts of fluid.

CARDIOVASCULAR DRUGS

Digitalis and antihypertensive medications may cause gastric hyperemia. Some may have a central nervous system effect and may cause significant nausea. α-Blockers and β-blockers may be associated with GI disturbances.

ANTICOAGULANTS AND VASODILATORS

Anticoagulants and vasodilators frequently are used to prevent thromboembolism in cardiac and neurologic disease. However, they may dilate blood vessels in the stomach and the upper GI tract, and they may decrease clotting and result in significant GI hemorrhage. An occult ulcer or tumor of the GI tract may start to bleed when anticoagulation is administered. Once bleeding occurs in a patient taking anticoagulants, the clinician must search for a previously hidden lesion.

ANTICHOLINERGICS

Anticholinergic drugs, both the naturally occurring and the synthetic forms, are used primarily for effects on the GI tract to reduce motility and secretion. Evidence indicates that large doses are needed to decrease gastric secretion, but therapeutic doses can decrease motility and consequently help in some hyperactive states.

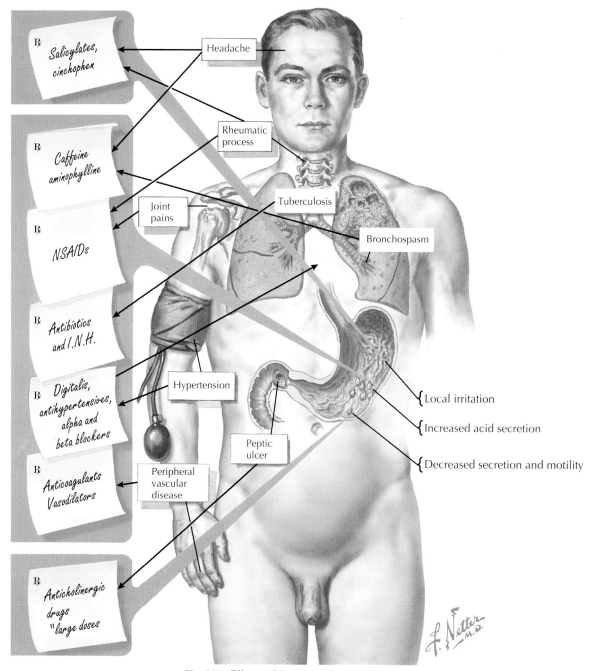

Fig. 20.1 Effects of Drugs on Gastric Function.

ADDITIONAL RESOURCES

Chan FKL, Lau JYN: Peptic ulcer disease. In Feldman M, Friedman LS, Brandt LJ, editors: *Gastrointestinal and liver disease*, ed 10, Philadelphia, 2016, Saunders-Elsevier, pp 884–900.

Lanza FL, Royer CL, Nelson RS: Endoscopic evaluation of the effects of aspirin, buffered aspirin, and enteric-coated aspirin on gastrointestinal duodenal mucosa, *N Engl J Med* 303:136–138, 1980.

Physicians' desk reference, ed 53/54, Montvale, NJ, 2003, Medical Economics Data Production.

Talley NJ, Evans JM, Fleming KC: Nonsteroidal anti-inflammatory drugs and dyspepsia in the elderly, *Dig Dis Sci* 40:1345–1350, 1995.

21

Upper Gastrointestinal Endoscopy: Esophagogastroduodenoscopy

Martin H. Floch

Endoscopic visualization of the esophagus, stomach, or proximal duodenum is an essential procedure in the diagnosis and treatment of diseases of the esophagus, stomach, and duodenum (Fig. 21.1). Examining the esophagus and stomach has evolved from using rigid and semirigid instruments to using flexible instruments, first fiberoptic and now videoendoscopic. During the past decade, all endoscopic laboratories converted to videoendoscopy and are adding *endoscopic ultrasound* (EUS) to evaluate the full thickness of the esophagus, stomach, or duodenum and adjacent structures, as well as for direct visualization and histology of the mucosal surface. Further advances in technology now include confocal imaging of the mucosa and staining of mucosa to identify neoplasia. This chapter describes techniques and normal findings; abnormal findings are described in Section I.

Although many variations exist, most videoendoscopes now use a color chip that gathers the image at the tip of the endoscope and transmits it through a videoprocessor into a monitor. The image can be preserved and then transmitted to computerized recording systems. Images can be stored easily for reports or archival records.

Most endoscopes include a portal for a biopsy channel. Very thin instruments can be passed transnasally but may not have biopsy capability. Instruments usually are 8 to 10 mm wide, but transnasal instruments may be only 2 to 3 mm wide.

The EUS instruments are wider than other endoscopes but are still easily passable, and they allow direct imaging, biopsy, and ultrasound (US) imaging. There are two types of EUS instruments, and each has a US device built into the tip. The more common type has a US device and an imaging endoscope, but a thin US device can be passed through a large endoscope channel. EUS is a complicated procedure, but it enables better submucosal and full–wall thickness images. It is especially useful for evaluating large folds, submucosal nodules, tumor extensions through the wall, lymph nodes, and associated structures (e.g., pancreas).

Upper endoscopy is used for numerous indications, including dysphasia, gastroesophageal reflux disease (GERD), esophageal (Barrett) or gastric metaplasia, dyspepsia, gastric ulcers, duodenal ulcers, upper gastrointestinal tract bleeding, infection in the esophagus, removal of foreign bodies, caustic injuries, drug-induced injuries; evaluation for esophageal cancer and for all possible premalignant lesions, including mass lesions, esophageal metaplasia (Barrett), achalasia, atrophic gastritis, pernicious anemia; and follow-up after surgery for all malignant lesions.

Although useful for many of these indications, EUS is more complicated, with fewer trained ultrasonographers, than the major screening and diagnostic procedure, video *esophagogastroduodenoscopy* (EGD). After an appropriate indication is identified and the procedure scheduled, EGD usually begins with a local anesthetic throat spray or gargle, followed by injection for sedation. Although drugs used for sedation vary widely worldwide, most protocols include a drug to reduce pain and a drug to induce sedation and produce an amnesic effect. Common drugs include meperidine (50–100 mg) or hydromorphone (2–4 mg) in combination with diazepam or midazolam (titrated at 1–10 mg). Endoscopists may choose to use fentanyl citrate (Sublimaze; 75–100 mg) alone or in combination with midazolam.

Once the patient is appropriately sedated, the endoscope can be passed in several ways through the pharynx. Some endoscopists prefer passing it blindly over the base of the tongue into the upper esophagus. Others insist on passage by direct visualization. Direct visualization permits an examination of the epiglottis and a "peek" at the vocal cords. Once the pharynx is passed, the endoscopist evaluates the esophagus. The upper esophagus, midesophagus, and distal esophagus can be visualized with an injection of air, as in a tubular structure. Contractions are often starlike. Ringlike contractions indicate a motility disturbance. Fixed rings, strictures, polypoid masses, and varices are all described under the particular pathologic condition in other chapters.

After passing through the gastroesophageal (GE) junction (see Section I), the endoscope enters the stomach, and the clinician notes whether any food or significant bilious secretions are retained from duodenal reflux. An injection of air permits evaluation of the fundus, body, and antrum. Normal contractions are seen radiating from the pylorus into the antrum and back in the opposite direction. By retroflexing the instrument along the lesser curvature, the endoscopist can fully evaluate the fundus and the GE junction from below. Hiatal hernias and gastric lesions of this area can be identified.

Staining of the mucosa to differentiate neoplasia is used in some centers but has not gained wide acceptance. Obtaining biopsy specimens from the visualized lesions remains the procedure of choice.

The endoscopist then observes the pyloric channel and, with mild pressure, passes the instrument into the duodenal bulb and then into the second and as far into the third part of the duodenum as needed. The ampulla of Vater can be seen with direct-viewing instruments but is best examined with a lateral-viewing instrument. However, masses, abnormal mucosa, and bleeding sites can be thoroughly evaluated with a direct-viewing instrument.

Biopsy specimens can be obtained from any location in the esophagus, stomach, or duodenum. Specimens are usually processed in a fixative medium to be sent for evaluation.

EUS has rapidly developed into an important technique in the differential diagnosis of benign and malignant disease. Upper endoscopes are now made for several types of US probes at the end of the scope that provide clear endoscopic and US images. The US image delineates normal layers of the wall of the mucosa, enlarged nodes outside the wall, and extent and type of tumor. Therapeutic and diagnostic EUS has evolved to allow both biopsy of nodes and lesions and drainage of cysts through US guidance.

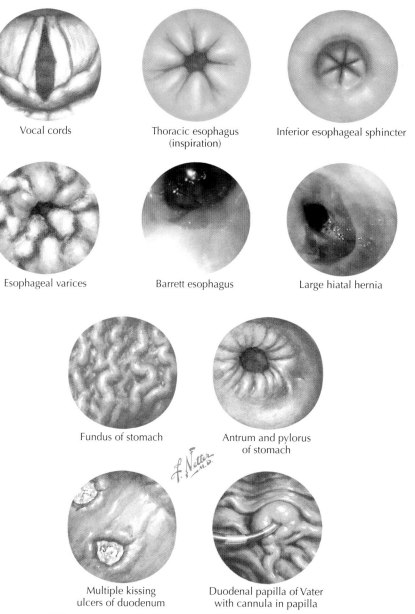

Vocal cords

Thoracic esophagus
(inspiration)

Inferior esophageal sphincter

Esophageal varices

Barrett esophagus

Large hiatal hernia

Fundus of stomach

Antrum and pylorus
of stomach

Multiple kissing
ulcers of duodenum

Duodenal papilla of Vater
with cannula in papilla

Fig. 21.1 Esophagogastroduodenoscopy and Endoscopic Ultrasound.

ADDITIONAL RESOURCES

Canard J, Letard J-C, Palazzo L, et al, editors: *Gastrointestinal Endoscopy in Practice*, London England, 2011, Churchill Livingstone.

Chun HJ, Yang S-K, Choi M-G, editors: *Clinical Gastrointestinal Endoscopy: A Comprehensive Atlas*, Berlin Heidelberg, 2014, Springer.

Pech O, Rabenstein T, Manner H, et al: Confocal laser endomicroscopy for in vivo diagnosis of early squamous cell carcinoma in the esophagus, *Clin Gastroenterol Hepatol* 6(1):89–94, 2008.

Rogart JN, Nagata J, Loeser CS, et al: Multiphoton imaging can be used for microscopic examination of intact human gastrointestinal mucosa ex vivo, *J Gastroenterol Hepatol* 6(1):95–101, 2008.

Wilcox CM, Munoz-Navas M, Sung JJ, editors: *Atlas of Clinical Gastrointestinal Endoscopy*, 3rd ed, Philadelphia, 2012, Saunders.

22

Coated Tongue, Halitosis, and Thrush

Martin H. Floch

The tongue is kept clean and normally colored by the cleansing action of saliva, the mechanical action of mastication, the customary oral flora, and adequate nutrition. Consequently, when salivary secretion is insufficient, when the dietary regimen eliminates chewing, when the bacterial flora is altered, or when certain vitamins necessary for the preservation of the normal epithelium are deficient, the normal appearance of the tongue may change. It may become coated with food particles, sloughed epithelial cells, and inflammatory exudates (Fig. 22.1). Fungal growths may be deposited on its surface.

Patients at risk for abnormal conditions of the tongue are those whose saliva is diminished by mouth breathing, dehydration, or anticholinergic drugs; those who are comatose and are unable to eat, drink, or rinse the mouth; and those with impaired mobility of the tongue caused by cranial nerve XII paralysis. An exudative oral or pharyngeal inflammatory process or antibiotic therapy that destroys the normal flora may result in an overgrowth of fungi. Hypertrophy of the papillae may give the appearance of a black or hairy tongue, especially in smokers.

Geographic tongue (benign migratory glossitis) is a migratory lesion of unknown cause. It may occur intermittently. Lesions are often irregular and appear as denuded, grayish patches. If lesions persist or any uncertainty exists in the diagnosis, an otolaryngologist should evaluate and biopsy the lesions if necessary. Other tongue lesions of uncertain identity should also prompt a full evaluation.

Fissured tongue is a benign lesion with longitudinal grooves usually considered congenital lingual defects. Again, if the diagnosis is uncertain, otolaryngologic evaluation is indicated.

In patients with pernicious anemia, a varicolored appearance caused by patchy loss of papillae may evolve into geographic tongue, but this does not denote a diagnosis of pernicious anemia. In allergic reactions in the mouth, usually a manifestation of sensitivity to an ingested food, the tongue may swell, and epithelial elements may desquamate and coat the surface.

Unpleasant breath, sometimes imagined, is reported by people who conclude that their sensations of unpleasant taste must be a reflection of, or must be reflected in, breath odor. *Halitosis* is often present, however, brought to a patient's attention by a spouse or other family member. Common causes include infection or neoplasm in the oronasopharyngeal structures, poor oral hygiene, bronchiectasis or lung abscess, cirrhosis with hepatic fetor, gastric stasis inducing aerophagia and eructation, gastroesophageal reflux, and diabetes. Halitosis may also result from absorption of intestinal products and their excretion through the lungs.

The odor of garlic remains on the breath for many hours because garlic is absorbed into the portal circulation and passes through the liver into the general circulation. Volatile oils applied to denuded or even intact skin surfaces are also recognizable on the breath. Enzymatic processes in the intestine in some persons liberate absorbable gases of offensive odor. When introduced rectally, material not normally found in the upper gastrointestinal tract may be recovered from the stomach, which supports the possibility that retrograde passage of odoriferous substances reaches the mouth through the intestine. In a patient with pyloric obstruction, the breath is typically offensive only at eructation. It has also been postulated that substances such as fats, fatty acids, and some end products of fat digestion may cause halitosis, for which a low-fat diet is indicated.

Often, the diligent search for the cause of halitosis uncovers no clues, and recourse must be made to frequent mouth rinsing with antiseptic solutions that contain pleasant-smelling ingredients. Diet manipulation may be helpful in select patients but necessitates individual trials. Manipulation of the enteric flora and use of probiotics may be attempted as well.

Thrush may develop after the use of antibiotics. White or red fibrous lesions appear on the tongue. Thrush is also referred to as *mucocutaneous candidiasis* because of its association with *Candida* species, primarily *Candida albicans*. This organism is part of the normal flora of the tongue but can be disrupted and become infectious after antibiotic therapy or after long-term glucocorticoid therapy. Thrush occurs more frequently in elderly persons, in patients with metabolic disturbances, and in those with autoimmune suppression. Treatment with nystatin, in liquid form or as tablets in 100,000-U doses, is usually effective. Holding the liquid in the mouth or slowly dissolving the tablets three or four times daily for 1 to 2 weeks usually resolves the immediate infection.

Treatment of recurrent Aphthous ulcers is complex. Vitamin deficiencies should be corrected. The patient should avoid very spicy or very salty foods. Analgesics and topical anesthesia, such as bismuth subsalicylate (Kaopectate), and sucralfate may be helpful. Topical glucocorticoid, such as fluocinonide or clobetasol ointment, can also help. Second-line therapy includes colchicine, 0.6 mg three times daily; tetracycline, 250 mg four times daily, cimetidine, 400 to 800 mg daily, azathioprine, 50 mg daily, or thalidomide, 200 mg daily. Short courses of systemic prednisone, 20 to 60 mg daily, may be effective when more conservative approaches are not working. Diets may be attempted with antiallergic approaches. Certainly, a gluten-free diet is necessary in patients with celiac disease.

ADDITIONAL RESOURCES

Mirowski GM, Leblank J, Mark LA: Oral disease and oral-cutaneous manifestations of gastrointestinal and liver disease. In Feldman M, Friedman LS, Brandt LJ, editors: *Gastrointestinal and Liver Disease*, ed 10, Philadelphia, 2016, Sanders-Elsevier, pp 377–396.

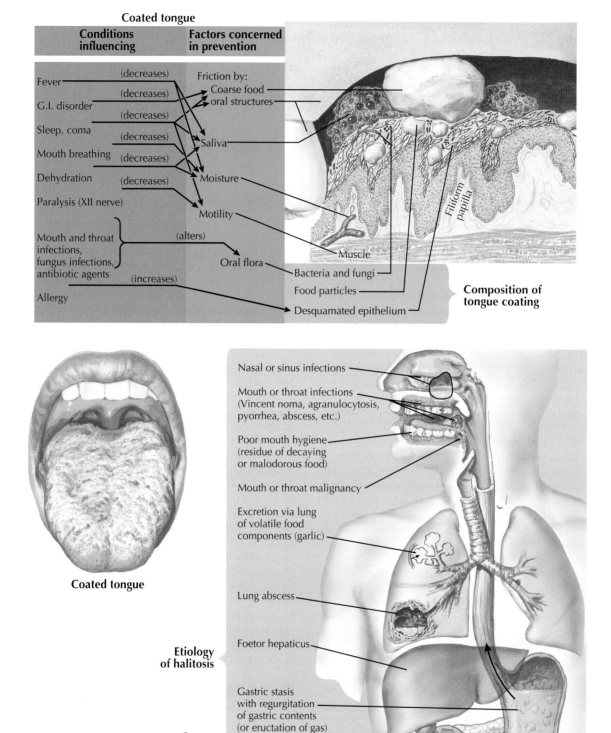

Coated tongue

Conditions influencing		Factors concerned in prevention
Fever	(decreases)	Friction by:
	(decreases)	Coarse food
G.I. disorder		oral structures
	(decreases)	
Sleep, coma	(decreases)	Saliva
Mouth breathing	(decreases)	
Dehydration	(decreases)	Moisture
Paralysis (XII nerve)		Motility
Mouth and throat infections, fungus infections, antibiotic agents	(alters)	Oral flora — Bacteria and fungi — Food particles
	(increases)	
Allergy		Desquamated epithelium

Composition of tongue coating

Filiform papilla

Muscle

Coated tongue

Etiology of halitosis

Nasal or sinus infections

Mouth or throat infections (Vincent noma, agranulocytosis, pyorrhea, abscess, etc.)

Poor mouth hygiene (residue of decaying or malodorous food)

Mouth or throat malignancy

Excretion via lung of volatile food components (garlic)

Lung abscess

Foetor hepaticus

Gastric stasis with regurgitation of gastric contents (or eructation of gas)

Diabetes mellitus (acetone breath)

Fig. 22.1 Coated Tongue and Halitosis.

23

Aerophagia and Eructation

Martin H. Floch

Aerophagia is characterized by excessive swallowing of air that results in repeated belching. Air may be swallowed unconsciously by the patient; when it results in repeated eructation, it becomes a clinical problem (Fig. 23.1).

Patients with aerophagia report frequent, uncontrollable belching, or eructation, which often is loud and disturbs family or coworkers. The condition may be acute in onset, but careful history usually reveals it is slow in developing but increases in severity until the patient seeks medical attention. It has been noted in children and may occur at any age. To fulfill the criteria of a functional gastrointestinal (GI) disorder, the condition should have been noted for at least 12 weeks in the year preceding the onset of troublesome, repetitive belching.

PATHOPHYSIOLOGY AND DIAGNOSIS

Eructation is normal during or after a meal, occurring two to six times without significance. Early in life, infants are made to burp with a change of position and then are able to resume a meal interrupted because of stomach distention caused by air swallowed during feeding. Frequent eructation by adults may become a habit.

In the act of belching, the glottis is closed, and the diaphragm and thoracic muscles contract. When the increased intraabdominal pressure transmitted to the stomach is sufficient to overcome the resistance of the lower esophageal sphincter, the swallowed air is eructated.

No diagnostic tests demonstrate normal or abnormal belching. However, in a patient with any symptom associated with belching, the history might indicate that the esophagus or stomach should be evaluated. Patients who are uncomfortable from mild upper abdominal distress may swallow a great amount of air and may have frequent eructation. Upper endoscopy to evaluate for organic disease is important with this symptom complex. The diagnosis is established by observing either the air swallowing or the frequent belching.

DIFFERENTIAL DIAGNOSIS

Aerophagia is now classified as a functional GI disorder. Once the diagnosis is established, the differential is minimal. However, the clinician must be certain that aerophagia is not secondary to upper abdominal discomfort from disease. Esophageal reflux with significant esophagitis, peptic ulcer of the stomach or duodenum, or discomfort from pancreatic or biliary disease in rare cases may cause mild aerophagia. However, other symptoms are apparent, and disease of upper GI organs can easily be evaluated. Often, the classic picture of aerophagia and loud belching confirms the diagnosis.

Persons who consume bicarbonate and patients with aerophagia are basically similar, unless the bicarbonate was taken to relieve the gas pains of peptic ulcer, in which case the carbon dioxide (CO_2) generated in the stomach is belched. The patient obtains relief from the antacid that is not obtained by belching the swallowed air. The relief that follows the ingestion of soda is explained not by deflation of the distended stomach with belching, but rather by neutralization of the acid. Also, some patients buy large amounts of soda or sodium bicarbonate to help them belch not because of aerophagia, but because they are chronic belchers.

Instead of swallowing air, some people are able to suck it in through a relaxed superior esophageal sphincter. This may occur in a patient with emphysema who is "pulling for air," or it may occur deliberately in an accomplished belcher. The same principle of using swallowed air is put to practical use in the development of so-called esophageal speech in patients who have undergone laryngectomy.

TREATMENT AND MANAGEMENT

The rational management of aerophagia and loud belching depends on correction of the underlying disturbance, whether organic or psychologic. Aerophagia is a functional disorder, and its management includes reassurance of the patient, education into the process of air swallowing and eructation, and treatment of any psychiatric component, such as anxiety or depression. Patients with aerophagia are always in some distress, and the physician must reassure them that they have no organic disease, then use pharmacologic therapy or recommend psychologic assistance. The family is frequently upset, so the social situation must be carefully assessed, and family or partners must be involved in the therapeutic regimen of reassurance and therapy.

Although no specific pharmacologic therapy exists, some clinicians have used tranquilizers, whereas others have used antidepressants. Simethicone and activated charcoal are usually ineffective. Again, reassurance, psychotherapy, and behavioral modification may be needed.

ADDITIONAL RESOURCES

Azpiroz F: Intestinal Gas. In Feldman M, Friedman LS, Brandt LJ, editors: *Gastrointestinal and liver disease*, ed 10, Philadelphia, 2016, Saunders-Elsevier, pp 242–250.

Bredenoord AJ, Smout AJ: Physiologic and pathologic belching, *Clin Gastroenterol Hepatol* 5:772–775, 2007.

Bredenoord AJ, Weusten BL, Timmer R, Smout AJ: Psychological factors affect the frequency of belching in patients with aerophagia, *Am J Gastroenterol* 101:2777–2781, 2006.

Drossman DA: *The functional gastrointestinal disorders*, ed 2, Lawrence, Kan, 2000, Allan Press, pp 328–330, 556–557.

Hasler WL: Nausea, gastroparesis and aerophagia, *J Clin Gastroenterol* 39:S223–S229, 2005.

Tack J, Talley NJ, Camilleri M, et al: Functional gastroduodenal disorders, *Gastroenterology* 130:1666–1679, 2006.

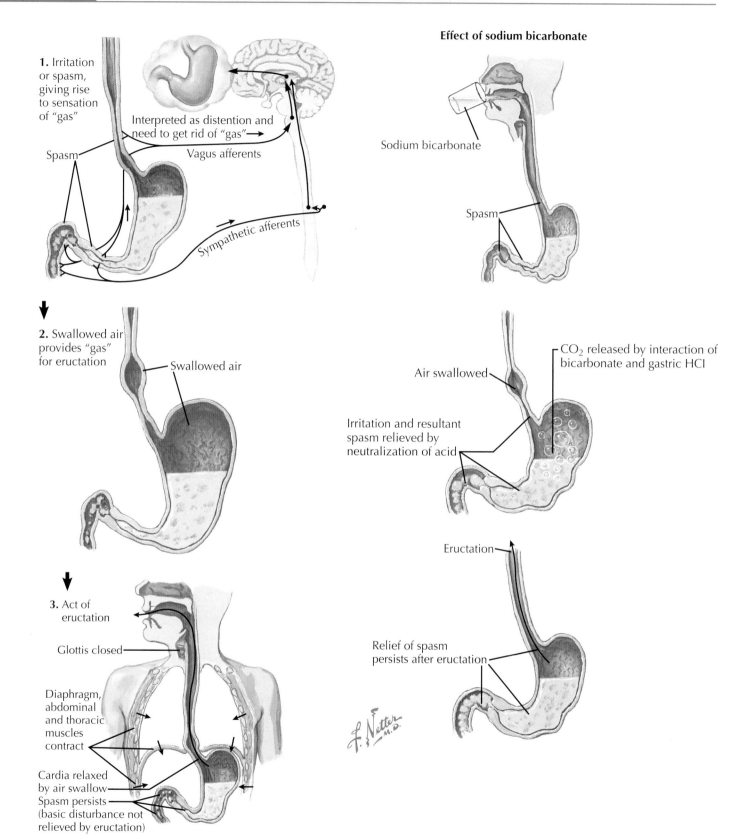

Effect of sodium bicarbonate

1. Irritation or spasm, giving rise to sensation of "gas"

Spasm

Interpreted as distention and need to get rid of "gas" →

Vagus afferents

Sympathetic afferents

Sodium bicarbonate

Spasm

2. Swallowed air provides "gas" for eructation

Swallowed air

CO_2 released by interaction of bicarbonate and gastric HCl

Air swallowed

Irritation and resultant spasm relieved by neutralization of acid

3. Act of eructation

Glottis closed

Diaphragm, abdominal and thoracic muscles contract

Cardia relaxed by air swallow

Spasm persists (basic disturbance not relieved by eructation)

Eructation

Relief of spasm persists after eructation

Fig. 23.1 Aerophagia and Eructation.

24

Motility of the Stomach

Martin H. Floch

Peristalsis usually commences minutes after food reaches the stomach through vagal and splanchnic nerve stimuli. It is first noted in the pyloric portion because of the greater thickness of its musculature, which gives it the strongest triturating (grinding) power (Fig. 24.1).

The contractions originate in shallow indentations in the region of the incisura angularis and deepen as they move toward the pylorus. After 5 to 10 minutes, the contractions increase in strength and become progressively more vigorous. The pylorus opens incompletely and intermittently as the waves advance toward it. Most of the material reaching the pyloric portion is forced back into the fundus.

This process continues until some of the content has been reduced to a fluid or semifluid consistency suitable for passing into the small intestine. Evacuation is regulated by the influence of the gastrointestinal (GI) hormones secreted by the stomach and duodenum. Adverse mechanical or physiochemical properties of the chyme (e.g., hypertonicity) or large particles of food give rise to intrinsic or extrinsic nervous and hormonal influences that modify the tone of the pyloric sphincter and the motor activity of the pylorus. Large volumes of food, increased acidity, hypertonicity, large amounts of fat, and concentrated nutrients all slow motility and emptying. Reflexes slow because of fat in the ileum, the so-called ileal brake, and distention of the rectum and colon. The pylorus provides constant resistance to the passage of chyme and blocks the exit of solid particles. By maintaining a narrow orifice, the pylorus filters the gastric contents and helps prevent duodenal reflux.

Antral and duodenal contractions are well synchronized by nerve and hormone influences. Electrophysiologic patterns of gastric motor activity are based on a constant slow-wave pattern. They occur in the stomach at approximately three cycles per minute but do not cause contractions. It is believed that slow waves originate on the greater curvature approximately in the middle of its body. This area is now referred to as the "gastric pacemaker." Electrical signals do not pass the pylorus. Slow waves in the duodenum occur at about 11 to 12 cycles per minute. Electrical impulses of the stomach and the duodenum are clearly separated.

The interstitial cells of Cajal, commonly known as the pacemaker, and muscle cells form a sophisticated network that initiate action potentials and begin the process of muscle contraction and peristaltic activity. Muscle activity of the fundus appears to be separate from muscle activity of the antrum and the pylorus. The churning of the chyme occurs during these contractions and relaxations.

The fasting stomach has a basic migrating motor complex that tends to begin and end simultaneously at all sides, whereas in the duodenum and the small bowel, the motor complexes become progressive and migrate aborally. When food swallowing begins, the vagus nerve induces relaxation of the stomach, changing the balance of excitatory and inhibitory tone. Once food enters the stomach, the migrating motor complex pattern is replaced by the fed pattern, which may last anywhere from 2 to 8 hours. The entire feeding process is under the influence of the vagus nerve and parasympathetic pathways, as well as corticotropin-releasing peptide, cholecystokinin, and other hormonal substances (e.g., vasoactive intestinal peptide, gastrin, somatostatin, dopamine, glucagon, bombesin).

Liquids are usually disbursed rapidly and have a slower lag period than solids. Solids empty in two phases. First, there is a lag period with slow emptying. Second, as the churning continues, emptying of the mixed chyme that has been exposed to acid and enzymes becomes more rapid. The lag phase for solids usually lasts anywhere up to 60 minutes.

The pylorus and the coordinated antral pyloric and duodenal activity regulate emptying of the stomach. Once emptying is complete, electrophysiologic activity of the stomach returns to the basic migrating motor complex, awaiting the next feeding.

ADDITIONAL RESOURCES

Koch KL: Gastric neuromuscular function and neuromuscular disorders. In Feldman M, Friedman LS, Brandt LJ, editors: *Gastrointestinal and liver disease*, ed 10, Philadelphia, 2016, Saunders-Elsevier, pp 811–838.

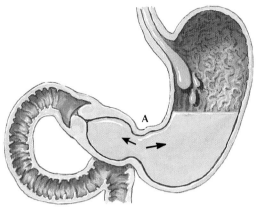

1. Stomach is filling, a mild peristaltic wave (A) has started in antrum and is passing toward pylorus. Gastric contents are churned and largely pushed back into body of stomach

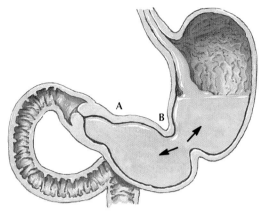

2. Wave (A) fading out as pylorus fails to open. A stronger wave (B) is originating at incisure and is again squeezing gastric contents in both directions

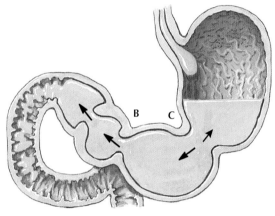

3. Pylorus opens as wave (B) approaches it. Duodenal bulb is filled and some contents pass into second portion of duodenum. Wave (C) starting just above incisure

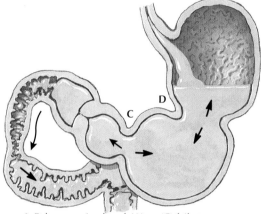

4. Pylorus again closed. Wave (C) fails to evacuate contents. Wave (D) starting higher on body of stomach. Duodenal bulb may contract or may remain filled, as peristaltic wave originating just beyond it empties second portion

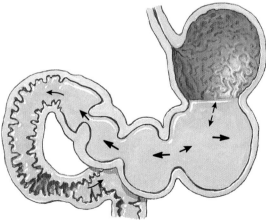

5. Peristaltic waves are now originating higher on body of stomach, gastric contents are evacuated intermittently. Contents of duodenal bulb area pushed passively into second portion as more gastric contents emerge

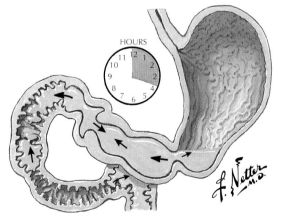

6. 3 to 4 hours later stomach almost empty, small peristaltic wave emptying duodenal bulb with some reflux into stomach. Reverse and antegrade peristalsis present in duodenum

Fig. 24.1 Motility of the Stomach.

Gastroparesis and Gastric Motility Disorders

Martin H. Floch

Gastroparesis is defined as delayed emptying of the stomach. The most common causes of this motility disturbance of the stomach encountered in clinical practice are the association with diabetes mellitus and idiopathic forms (Fig. 25.1 and Box 25.1). Gastroparesis affects persons of almost any age, with no gender predilection.

CLINICAL PICTURE

The presenting symptom of gastroparesis may be bloating, abdominal pain or distention, nausea, or vomiting. The patient may report a history of continued postprandial fullness. Nausea can be persistent and unexplained as the initial symptom. Vomiting may or may not accompany the nausea. The patient may vomit undigested fluid or may experience mild regurgitation of undigested fluid. Anorexia and weight loss may occur when the symptom complex persists over time. There are no

---

BOX 25.1 Causes of Gastroparesis

Metabolic
Diabetes mellitus
Hypothyroidism
Pregnancy
Uremia

Associated Gastric/Esophageal Disease
Gastroesophageal reflux
Gastritis
Atrophic gastritis
Peptic ulcer disease of stomach
Acute gastroenteritis

Associated Diseases
Muscular dystrophy
Parkinson disease
Scleroderma
Amyloidosis
Chronic liver disease
Idiopathic pseudo-obstruction
Anorexia nervosa
Postsurgical and other trauma
Vagotomy

Roux-en-Y Surgery
Head injuries
Spinal cord injuries
Medications
Idiopathic causes

---

hallmark physical findings other than the weight loss if the symptom has persisted.

Acute infectious diseases cause poor gastric emptying but resolve; the diagnosis of gastroparesis is based on chronicity. If gastroparesis symptoms are associated with postsurgical or other trauma or with neurologic disease, the findings of the primary disorder are significant. Patients with diabetes may be unable to control glycemia because of many factors, but irregular gastric emptying may play a role, as well as insulin secretion. In addition, associated findings in diabetes, such as neuropathy or enteropathy, may be present.

DIAGNOSIS

Of the many ways to document gastric emptying, the most common currently used is scintigraphy. Radioactive tracers are added to liquid and solid foods. Indium-111–diethylenetriamine pentaacetic acid (DTPA)-labeled water or technetium-99m–labeled egg or egg salad is most frequently used for liquid and solid phases. Many institutions use both; others have success using only the labeled solid food.

Breath tests with carbon 13 (^{13}C)–octanoic acid or ^{13}C–acetic acid are used in some institutions, but these require more time than the 1- or 2-hour testing with scintigraphy. Tests vary greatly from institution to institution and require the availability of an accredited nuclear medicine laboratory. Ultrasonography has also been used but requires specialized operator expertise.

Regardless of the method used to diagnose delayed emptying, the finding then must be correlated with a list of associated diseases or deemed "idiopathic" (unknown cause or spontaneous condition). Therefore it is essential to document any related diseases before treatment. Again, the most common associations are diabetes and idiopathic causes. Diabetes may be subtle and must be discerned; gastroparesis may be the first presentation. The patient who does not have diabetes must be carefully evaluated to rule out associated neurologic disorders before the condition is called idiopathic.

TREATMENT AND MANAGEMENT

Controlling diabetes, if present, is essential. Careful history taking is done to uncover any medication-related cause. Substances that can delay gastric emptying include alcohol, aluminum hydroxide antacids, atropine, β-adrenergic antagonists, calcitonin, calcium channel blockers, dexfenfluramine, diphenylhydromine, glucagon, H_2-receptor antagonists, interleukin-1 (IL-1), L-dopa, lithium, octreotide, opiates, phenothiazine, progesterone, propantheline bromide, sucralfate, synthetic estrogens, tetrahydrocannabinol, tobacco, and tricyclic antidepressants. For patients with idiopathic causes and associated diseases, several medications can be prescribed. However, when the diagnosis points to an idiopathic condition, the clinician must keep in mind that it may become a

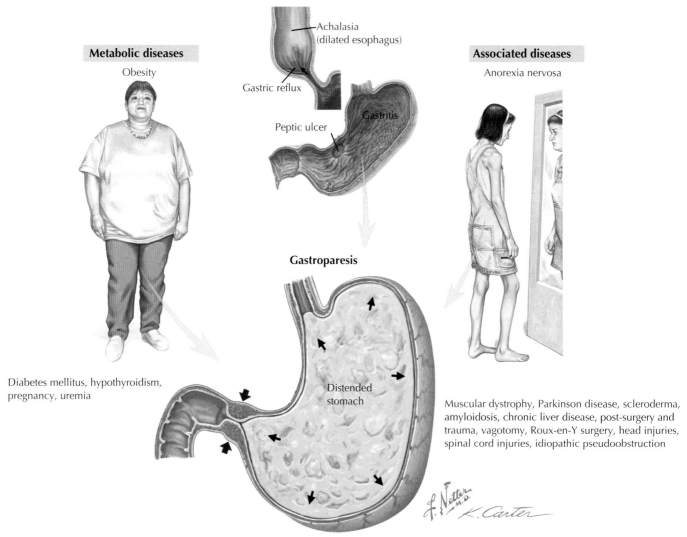

Associated gastric/esophageal disease

Metabolic diseases

Obesity

Achalasia
(dilated esophagus)

Gastric reflux

Peptic ulcer

Gastritis

Associated diseases

Anorexia nervosa

Diabetes mellitus, hypothyroidism, pregnancy, uremia

Gastroparesis

Distended stomach

Muscular dystrophy, Parkinson disease, scleroderma, amyloidosis, chronic liver disease, post-surgery and trauma, vagotomy, Roux-en-Y surgery, head injuries, spinal cord injuries, idiopathic pseudoobstruction

Fig. 25.1 Gastroparesis and Gastric Motility Disorders.

functional disorder and that all forms of therapy used in functional disorders (e.g., reassurance, antianxiety/antidepressant drugs) may be needed.

With recent progress in drug therapy and research into prokinetic agents, the following four categories of drugs are now used in patients with gastroparesis:

1. *Dopamine antagonists.* Domperidone (10–30 mg four times daily) and metoclopramide (5–20 mg four times daily) are dopamine antagonists. Unfortunately, domperidone is available in the United States only in special situations, and metoclopramide, although used frequently, can cause neurologic symptoms with long-term use.
2. *Substituted benzamides.* Cisapride (5–20 mg twice daily) is effective but is unavailable in the United States.
3. *Macrolides.* Erythromycin (50–200 mg four times daily) often may cause pain in women.
4. *Cholinergic agonists.* The use of bethanechol (5–25 mg four times daily) is controversial, but the drug may be helpful in some patients.

Ghrelin, the gastrointestinal hormone that stimulates eating, also has a positive effect on gastric emptying. Although only a few studies have used ghrelin in subjects with gastroparesis, results are promising, and there are research advocates for its use in these patients.

Careful descriptions of therapies also differ in references by Koch and Camilleri. Although Cisapride is not available in many countries, there is now a new addition in the drug armory. Relamorelin has shown to be affective in diabetic gastroparesis. Investigators at the Mayo Clinic have shown that this synthetic pentapeptide ghrelin receptor antagonist has potent prokinetic properties. In their initial study, they used anywhere from 10 μg b.i.d. to 30 μg or 100 subcutaneously b.i.d., which was effective.

COURSE AND PROGNOSIS

It is important to monitor the patient with gastroparesis and to repeat the gastric-emptying study while the patient is taking medication, to determine if the drug is effective. Often, the clinician can correlate the decrease in symptoms with increased gastric emptying. Gastroparesis is chronic but may vary in severity; thus therapy can be modulated depending on the symptom phase.

Mild cases of gastroparesis may be controlled by prokinetic medication, but patients with severe gastroparesis may require nutrition support and possibly jejunostomy feeding. Weight must be monitored, and when the patient is losing weight and cannot eat sufficiently, nutrition support must be started. Supplemental feedings may control weight loss, but enteral feeding may be necessary in some patients.

Recent experimental therapeutic methods include electronic devices that are wired to the gastric mucosa, with gastric electrical pacing. These techniques have been instituted only in research centers but hold promise for patients who require long-term therapy.

OTHER DISORDERS

Other gastric motility disorders are rare and mainly involve disturbances that can be identified in gastric muscle activity. To identify these abnormalities, sophisticated electrogastrography is necessary. Although available only at a few large university centers, this procedure can identify disturbances in gastric motility and gastric pacing that can cause nausea, vomiting, abdominal pain, anorexia, and weight loss. Gastric pacing disturbances are now experimentally treated with gastric electrical pacing. The dumping syndrome occurs rarely but particularly in patients who have had a gastrectomy and pyloroplasty or gastrojejunostomy. Because of poor relaxation of the stomach, foods do no empty normally and therefore liquid and solid nutrients rapidly empty into the duodenum or jejunum. Symptoms of the syndrome include abdominal pain, bloating, and nausea and vomiting. Some patients may only have light headedness or perspiration, and symptoms of diarrhea can occur hours after food intake. This may be followed by diarrhea. When patients have been tested and if positive diagnosis is made, dietary monitoring is necessary.

ADDITIONAL RESOURCES

Camilleri M, Acosta A: Emerging treatments in neurogastroenterology: relamorelin: a novel gastrocolokinetic synthetic ghrelin agonist, *Neurogastroenterol Motil* 27:324–332, 2015.

Camilleri M, Parkman HP, Shafi MA, et al: Clinical guideline: management of gastroparesis, *Am J Gastroenterol* 108:18–38, 2013.

Koch KL: Gastric neuromuscular function and neuromuscular disorders. In Feldman M, Friedman LS, Brandt LJ, editors: *Gastrointestinal and liver disease*, ed 10, Philadelphia, 2016, Saunders-Elsevier, pp 811–838.

Parkman HP, Yates KP, Hasler WL, et al: Dietary intake and nutritional deficiencies in patients with diabetic or idiopathic gastroparesis, *Gastroenterology* 141:486–498, 2011.

Parkman HP, Yates K, Hasler WL, et al: Similarities and differences between diabetic and idiopathic gastroparesis, *Clin Gastroenterol Hepatol* 9:1056–1064, 2011.

Szarka LA, Camilleri N, Vella A, et al: A stable isotope breath test with a standard meal for abnormal gastric emptying of solids in the clinic and in research, *Clin Gastroenterol Hepatol* 6:635–643, 2008.

26

Pyloric Obstruction and the Effects of Vomiting

Martin H. Floch

Pyloric obstruction occurs when the outlet of the stomach narrows to the point of serious interference with gastric emptying (Fig. 26.1). In Western countries, tumors are the most common cause of pyloric obstruction in adults. Duodenal ulcer was once a common cause but is now rarely encountered because of the high cure rate of *Helicobacter pylori* and the use of H_2-antagonist and proton pump inhibitor (PPI) therapy for peptic ulcer. It is important to understand the effect of pyloric obstruction, which is vomiting.

Infantile hypertrophic pyloric stenosis is the most common cause of abdominal surgery in the first 6 months of life. The incidence in the United States is approximately 3 in 1000 births. Although rare in adults, hypertrophic pyloric stenosis does occur when missed early in life or when symptoms were not severe in childhood and progressed to diagnosis later in life (see Chapter 28).

CLINICAL PICTURE

When the outlet of the stomach becomes narrowed to the point of interference with gastric emptying, the gastric musculature responds at first with increased peristalsis in an effort to build up sufficient pressure to overcome the resistance at its pyloric end. At this stage, the patient may experience a sensation, or burning, in the epigastrium or left hypochondrium. With persisting obstruction and further stagnation of ingested food and gastric secretion, the stomach begins to dilate; the musculature becomes atonic, and peristaltic activity is minimal. At this stage, the patient reports fullness, vomiting of undigested food consumed many hours earlier, and foul-smelling eructation. If the obstruction is unrelieved, vomiting becomes more frequent and more copious. With so little gastric content now passing into the intestine because of the profound gastric atony, the patient is powerless to keep up with the fluid and electrolytes lost in the vomitus. Dehydration, hypochloremia, hypokalemia, and alkalosis supervene, which in turn affect renal function, with development of oliguria, azotemia, and retention of other electrolytes. Clinically, the patient is weak, anorexic, and drowsy. Unless measures are instituted to correct the metabolic disorder and to relieve the obstruction, the condition progresses to irreversible tissue damage and death.

Pyloric obstruction is not the only cause of vomiting (see Chapter 27), but the diagnosis may be suspected because of the history just described, the pattern of the emesis, and the appearance of the vomitus. In duodenal ulcer, which is the most common cause of pyloric obstruction, the patient usually gives a history of ulcer symptoms. The vomiting is at first intermittent, perhaps 2 or 3 days apart, and the vomitus often contains recognizable particles of food eaten the previous day.

As with excessive vomiting from any cause, the patient has appreciable losses of fluids and hydrogen (H^+), chloride (Cl^-), and potassium (K^+) ions. Because the gastric juice is poor in sodium (Na^+), usually no sodium deficiency occurs, and although Na^+ remains in the blood, bicarbonate (HCO_3^-) substitutes for Cl^-. Loss of K^+ occurs because parietal cells secrete significant amounts of this ion.

Vomiting does not usually occur in uncomplicated ulcer disease, except when the ulcer is located in the pyloric canal. However, many patients with ulcers empty the stomach through vomiting to obtain pain relief.

DIAGNOSIS

Barium contrast imaging or computed tomography can provide a diagnosis of pyloric obstruction, and endoscopic visualization of the pylorus and mucosal biopsy can clarify the cause. The differential diagnosis, as previously indicated, includes benign or malignant tumor and scarring resulting from chronic peptic disease. Rare causes, such as polyp intussusception, usually are more acute in presentation than a chronic obstructive process.

TREATMENT AND MANAGEMENT

Managing the consequences of repeated or excessive vomiting consists of fluid and electrolyte replacement, evacuation of the stomach with adequate drainage, and continuous gastric aspiration with a nasogastric tube for 48 to 72 hours. If the obstruction itself is not relieved, surgery is necessary to reestablish gastrointestinal passage, but only after fluid and electrolyte balance has been restored. The cause of the obstruction is treated after the effects of vomiting are managed. Treatment of tumor obstruction is discussed in Chapter 39, and treatment of peptic disease is discussed in Chapters 33 and 34. Medical treatments depend on the cause, but surgical relief of the obstruction is invariable. In incurable malignant obstruction, stents may be placed to gain temporary relief.

A clinical and physiologic disturbance similar to pyloric obstruction, known as *milk-alkali* (Burnett) *syndrome,* may result from excessive ingestion of a soluble alkali and a rich source of calcium.

COURSE AND PROGNOSIS

Immediate treatment of the vomiting and its metabolic disturbance are usually successful. The long-term course and prognosis for pyloric obstruction and vomiting depend on the cause. If the vomiting was caused by a benign tumor or by scarring from chronic ulcer, the prognosis is usually excellent. If cancer was the cause, the prognosis depends on its type and extent and on the effectiveness of other treatments. However, if cancer causes pyloric obstruction, the prognosis is usually poor.

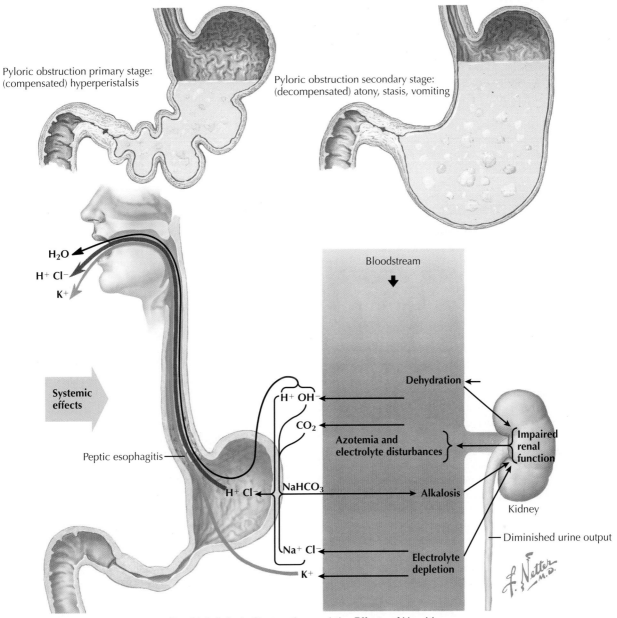

Pyloric obstruction primary stage: (compensated) hyperperistalsis

Pyloric obstruction secondary stage: (decompensated) atony, stasis, vomiting

H_2O

H^+ Cl^-

K^+

Systemic effects

Bloodstream

Peptic esophagitis

H^+ OH^-

CO_2

Azotemia and electrolyte disturbances

H^+ Cl ← $NaHCO_3$ → Alkalosis

Na^+ Cl

K^+

Dehydration

Impaired renal function

Kidney

Diminished urine output

Electrolyte depletion

Fig. 26.1 Pyloric Obstruction and the Effects of Vomiting.

ADDITIONAL RESOURCES

Malagelada JR, Malagelada C: Nausea and vomiting. In Feldman M, Friedman LS, Brandt LJ, editors: *Gastrointestinal and liver disease*, ed 10, Philadelphia, 2016, Saunders-Elsevier, p 107.

Semrin MG, Russo MA: Anatomy, histology and developmental anomalies of the stomach and duodenum. In Feldman M, Friedman LS, Brandt JS, editors: *Gastrointestinal and liver disease*, ed 8, Philadelphia, 2006, Saunders-Elsevier, p 795.

27

Nausea and Vomiting

Martin H. Floch

Nausea and vomiting are nonspecific but clinically important symptoms associated with numerous causes. Nausea is variously described as a sick feeling, a tightness in the throat, a sinking sensation, or a feeling of imminent vomiting. It generally precedes vomiting and may be associated with retching when the stomach is empty. Although associated with any disease, acute nausea and vomiting are most often associated with infectious disease, pregnancy, medications (including chemotherapy), postoperative status, and motion sickness. Other common causes include radiation sickness, gastrointestinal (GI) obstruction, hepatitis, metabolic disturbances (e.g., diabetes mellitus, thyroid disease), systemic diseases (e.g., myocardial infarction, renal failure, asthma), Addison disease, and central nervous system (CNS) causes (e.g., brain tumors, stroke, hemorrhage, meningitis). This wide list of associated diseases and causes makes it necessary to understand the nausea/vomiting process and its treatment.

Furthermore, many patients have nausea and vomiting associated with gastric motility disorders or with anorexia nervosa or psychogenic causes, in which the inciting disease or cause is not apparent or diagnosable. Some of these may be considered functional disorders.

CLINICAL PICTURE AND PHYSIOLOGY

Salivation, pallor, tachycardia, faintness, weakness, and dizziness frequently occur concomitantly. Nausea and vomiting may result from disturbances throughout the body and may be precipitated by the following:

- Emotional disturbances
- Intracranial vasomotor and pressure changes
- Unpleasant olfactory, visceral, or gustatory stimuli
- Functional or anatomic alterations in the thoracic and abdominal viscera, including the urogenital tract
- Intense pain in somatic parts
- Exogenous or endogenous toxins
- Drugs (notably opiates)
- Stimulation of the vestibular apparatus (usually by motion)

Impulses from all these sources reach the CNS through the corresponding sensory nerves (Fig. 27.1).

The CNS control of vomiting is based in two areas: (1) the *vomiting center,* located in the lateral reticular formation of the medulla, among cell groups governing such related activities as salivation and respiration, and (2) the *chemoreceptor trigger zone,* in a narrow strip along the floor of the fourth ventricle, close to the vomiting center. Functions of these two areas are distinct, although not independent. The vomiting center is activated by impulses from the GI tract and other peripheral structures. The chemoreceptor trigger zone is stimulated by circulating toxic agents and by impulses from the cerebellum; this zone's influence on the vomiting center results in the emetic action.

After irritation in any somatic or visceral area or in any sense organ, impulses travel through their respective sensory nerves to reach the medulla, where they activate the vomiting center. Toxic agents, whether introduced into the body or accumulated endogenously, act on the chemoreceptor trigger zone, through which impulses reach and activate the nearby vomiting center. Before the vomiting threshold is exceeded, impulses passing to the cortex lead to the sensation of nausea. The vomiting center coordinates the discharge of impulses from adjacent neural components to the various structures that participate in the act of vomiting. Salivation, which almost invariably precedes the actual ejection of the vomitus, is stimulated by impulses from the salivary nuclei. Contraction of the intercostal muscles and the diaphragm produces a sharp inspiratory movement and increased intraabdominal pressure, facilitated by contraction of the abdominal muscles. Closure of the glottis forestalls aspiration into the respiratory passages. The pyloric portion of the stomach contracts; the body of the stomach, cardia, esophagus, and cricopharyngeus muscle relax, and the gastric contents are forced out through the mouth and, in vigorous emesis, also through the nose.

Nausea and vomiting brought on by motion do not require a vertical component; some persons develop the symptoms merely from being rotated. Attempts to resolve the visual disorientation through eye and head movements may result in stimulation of the labyrinth, either directly or by decreased gastric tonus. Visual stimuli are not essential for the development of motion sickness; even blind persons may be susceptible.

Rapid downward motion that comes to a sudden stop, or that is followed by upward motion, causes the abdominal viscera to sag and pull on their attachments. This is the origin of the sinking feeling experienced at the end of a rapid descent in an elevator, or a sudden steep decline in a plane. The sensation does not occur if the subject stands on his head in the elevator, and it is reduced if the subject assumes a horizontal position when the plane is bouncing up and down, because the viscera cannot be displaced as far in the anteroposterior direction as in the craniocaudal direction. Nausea and retching may be induced in a patient under spinal anesthesia by downward traction on the exposed stomach.

Nausea may be difficult to relieve and becomes a serious clinical problem if sufficiently prolonged to interfere with nutrition. *Primary nausea,* or nausea occurring in the postabsorptive state, occasionally accompanies eye strain, myocardial infarction, azotemia, or visceral neoplastic disease, but it is usually of psychologic origin. Protracted vomiting is detrimental not only because of nutrition concerns but also because of electrolyte depletion (see Chapter 26).

If vomiting does not respond to antiemetic drugs, nasogastric suction should be instituted. Correction of a gastric hypotonus may be the factor that brings the condition under control.

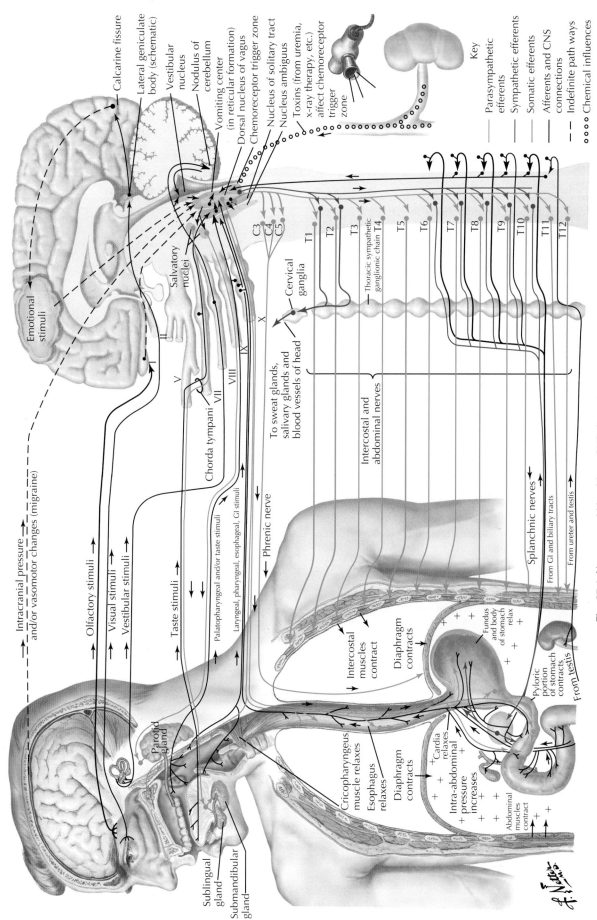

Fig. 27.1 Nausea and Vomiting. *CNS,* Central nervous system.

DIAGNOSIS

Thorough evaluation must include all possible causes of nausea and vomiting. In the pregnant patient, the pregnancy may be the paramount cause, but GI conditions during pregnancy, such as cholecystitis and appendicitis, must be explored. The large number of causes must therefore be considered in the workup. Once established, the specific cause must be evaluated to determine correct therapy and prognosis. When no cause is found and the nausea and vomiting fall into the category of "psychogenic" or cyclic vomiting, therapy must include not only pharmacologic but also psychiatric modalities.

Cyclic vomiting syndrome (CVS) is much more common than previously believed. CVS is most often seen in children but now is recognized in adolescents, as well as young and older adults. The classic presentation involves sudden attacks of severe vomiting and retching that subside with acute treatment, often in the emergency room. Migraine headache and abdominal migraine are often associated with CVS. In addition, prodromal symptoms may be identified. The cause and frequency of attacks vary. There are no good evidence-based treatment protocols, and many drugs are used. Specific treatment for CVS, as well as those listed next, in the acute phase includes preventing shock and dehydration and electrolyte loss. Ondansetrone is tried, hydromorphone for pain and, if needed, sedative agents. Removal to a dark area may be helpful and removal of any stimulating actions that are known to precipitate an attack. Prevention of attacks has been tried with cyproheptadine, propranolol, tricyclic antidepressants, and 5-HT$_{1d}$ agonists such as sumatriptan and eletriptan if the patient has migraine symptoms. Management requires an aggressive approach to prevention, and most patients can be helped to live with the disorder.

TREATMENT AND MANAGEMENT

Severe acute vomiting and protracted vomiting may cause significant metabolic and electrolyte disturbances, usually necessitating intravenous treatment for replacement of potassium, sodium, and other electrolytes. Prolonged nausea and vomiting also cause nutritional deficiencies, which must be treated according to duration of the illness (see Section X).

Many drugs are available for pharmacologic therapy (Table 27.1). Dosage and frequency of administration depend on the disease process (e.g., motion sickness vs. illness caused by acute disease vs. chemotherapy).

Chemotherapy can cause intensive nausea and recurrent vomiting. Often, oncologists use a combination of drugs, such as the selective 5-HT$_3$ receptor antagonists ondansetron and granisetron, although these are expensive, or tetrahydrocannabinol, the active ingredient of marijuana. Treating nausea and vomiting during chemotherapy is challenging because it includes nutrition support and symptom relief.

TABLE 27.1	**Drugs for Therapy of Nausea and Vomiting**
Drug Class	**Medications**
Antihistamine	Meclizine Promethazine Dimenhydrinate
Anticholinergic	Scopolamine Hyoscyamine
Antidopaminergic	Prochlorperazine Chlorpromazine
Prokinetic	Metoclopramide Cisapride Erythromycin Domperidone Bethanechol Octreotide Trimethobenzamide

If vomiting is persistent and does not respond to the administration of antiemetic drugs, nasogastric suction should be instituted. Again, correcting gastric hypotonia may be the factor that brings the condition under control.

COURSE AND PROGNOSIS

Course and prognosis depend on the cause of the nausea and vomiting. If the cause is idiopathic, the symptoms can be frustrating and challenging to the patient and physician. However, if the cause is benign and idiopathic, the course is usually benign. Progress may be intermittent, however, and both patient and physician can become frustrated. Psychotherapeutic drugs may be helpful, as well as psychiatric treatment, if necessary.

ADDITIONAL RESOURCES

Basch E, Prestrud AA, Hesketh PJ, et al: Antiemetics: American society of clinical oncology clinical practice guideline update, *J Clin Oncol* 29:4189–4198, 2011.

Camilleri M, Parkman HP, Shafi MA, et al: Clinical guideline: management of gastroparesis, *Am J Gastroenterol* 108:18–38, 2013.

Malagelada JR, Malagelada C: Nausea and vomiting. In Feldman M, Friedman LS, Brandt JS, editors: *Gastrointestinal and liver disease*, ed 10, Philadelphia, 2016, Saunders-Elsevier, p 107.

28

Hypertrophic Pyloric Stenosis

Martin H. Floch

Hypertrophic pyloric stenosis is an obstruction in the pylorus caused by hyperplasia of the circular muscle surrounding the pyloric outlet channel (Fig. 28.1). It is more common in infants than adults and actually is rare in adults. The incidence is approximately 3 in 1000 live births; boys are affected more often than girls by a ratio of 4:1 to 5:1. The disorder is more common among white persons of northern European descent than among persons of African or Asian descent.

The cause of hypertrophic pyloric stenosis is unknown, but a deficiency of nitric oxide synthetase is suspected. In addition, interstitial cells of Cajal are not seen throughout the pylorus. Fifty percent of identical twins are affected, but the disorder does not follow Mendelian inheritance patterns. Both genetic and environmental factors are thought to be important.

CLINICAL PICTURE

The clinical presentation of hypertrophic pyloric stenosis is different in infants than in adults. The classic infant presentation is vomiting that occurs in the second to sixth weeks of life. Vomiting increases in frequency and severity and is characterized early as occurring suddenly with great force (projectile vomiting). The infant cries, indicating hunger. Because less food is able to pass the pylorus, the infant becomes dehydrated and loses weight. At this stage, metabolic acidosis may become a serious problem. On examination of the infant, the classic "olive" might be felt in the area of the pylorus, and strong peristaltic movements in the stomach may be observed on inspection of the abdomen.

In adults, nausea, vomiting, satiety, and epigastric pain after eating are major symptoms. Physical examination is not helpful because the condition is chronic and the pyloric mass is not easy to palpate. Patients may lose weight if symptoms persist.

DIAGNOSIS

Hypertrophic pyloric stenosis is diagnosed in children based on timing of the presentation and physical examination findings. X-ray examination is important before surgery. The large, dilated stomach is evident; if further evidence is needed, careful barium study can be performed to visualize the narrowed pylorus. Ultrasonography is important because the classic 3-mm sonolucent "doughnut" can be seen in children.

In adults, the clinician first must consider the possibility of stenosis. Ultrasonography is then helpful, but barium contrast reveals the classic narrowed segment. Upper endoscopy is recommended to rule out chronic peptic or malignant disease.

TREATMENT AND MANAGEMENT

In the past, some clinicians preferred a trial of medical treatment with anticholinergic therapy and very soft food for patients with hypertrophic pyloric stenosis. However, the medical therapy had a high failure rate. Pyloromyotomy is the treatment of choice. Ramstedt pyloromyotomy includes a longitudinal incision through the hyperplastic pyloric muscle. Some surgeons prefer resection of the adult pylorus, to rule out malignancy. Although endoscopy can dilate the pylorus, these procedures have failed in as many as 80% of patients within the first 6 months of therapy.

PROGNOSIS

The prognosis is excellent, and once the correct therapy has been applied for hypertrophic pyloric stenosis, patients go on to lead normal lives.

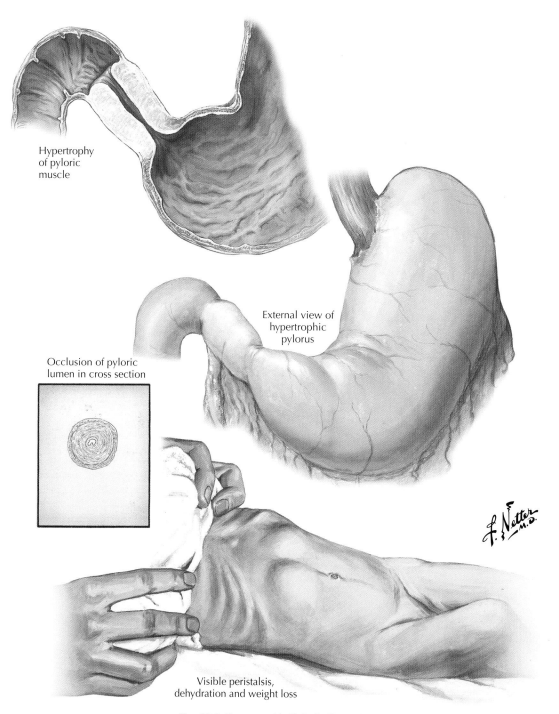

Hypertrophy
of pyloric
muscle

External view of
hypertrophic
pylorus

Occlusion of pyloric
lumen in cross section

Visible peristalsis,
dehydration and weight loss

Fig. 28.1 Hypertrophic Pyloric Stenosis.

ADDITIONAL RESOURCES

Graadt Van Roggen JF, Van Krieken JH: Adult hypertrophic pyloric stenosis: case report and review, *J Clin Pathol* 51:479–480, 1998.

Safford SD, Pietrobon R, Safford KM, et al: A study of 11,003 patients with hypertrophic pyloric stenosis and the association between surgeon and hospital volume and outcomes, *J Pediatr Surg* 40:967–972, 2005.

Vandiwinden JM, Liu H, de Laet MH, et al: Study of interstitial cells of Cajal in infantile pyloric stenosis, *Gastroenterology* 111:279–288, 1996.

Yamataka A, Tsukada K, Yokoyama-Laws Y, et al: Pyloromyotomy vs. atropine sulfate for infantile hypotrophy pyloric stenosis, *J Pediatr Surg* 35: 338–341, (discussion 342), 2000.

29

Diverticula of the Stomach and Gastrointestinal Prolapse

Martin H. Floch

Gastric diverticula are rare and are found in 0.02% of autopsy specimens. Almost all are located on the posterior wall of the cardia and to the left of the esophagus (Fig. 29.1). They are thought to be congenital but occur at the structural weakness of the longitudinal muscles on the posterior surface. Usually, the diverticula contain all layers of the muscle wall and are 2 to 3 cm long and 1.2 cm in diameter. Openings are wide, permit free communication with gastric contents, and may be seen endoscopically. Gastric diverticula are best visualized on a retroflexion view. On barium radiography, they can be missed when the stomach is distended but often are seen on the lesser curvature, and they fill and empty regularly.

CLINICAL PICTURE

Diverticula of the stomach are asymptomatic. However, complications have been reported and resulted in resection. Laparoscopic techniques are used effectively to resect the diverticula.

TREATMENT AND PROGNOSIS

No treatment is needed for diverticula unless the infrequent complication occurs. When bleeding, perforation from the manipulation, or the rare associated malignancy occurs, resection is performed laparoscopically. Small and most other diverticula are asymptomatic, and prognosis is excellent.

GASTRODUODENAL PROLAPSE

Prolapse of the gastric mucosa into the duodenum probably results from extreme mobility of the antral mucosa and submucosa. The mucosa of the antrum, which normally is thicker than the mucosa of other parts of the stomach and sometimes assumes a cushionlike quality, is pushed through the pyloric ring to lie like a turned-back cuff of a sleeve within the duodenum (see Fig. 29.1). Although a fully developed prolapse is rare, partial prolapse is common but of little or no clinical significance.

Gastroduodenal prolapse is most often a radiologic curiosity, and the duodenal bulb can appear to be filled with a tuberous mass with irregular contours. Diagnosis is easy to make. Occasionally, however, it is difficult to differentiate a prolapse from a polyp or an acute ulcer from marked mucosal edema of the surrounding area. Endoscopists rarely report gastroduodenal prolapse.

The literature contains a report of a rare episode of strangulation of the mucosa with subsequent signs of pyloric obstruction or gastrointestinal bleeding that required surgical correction.

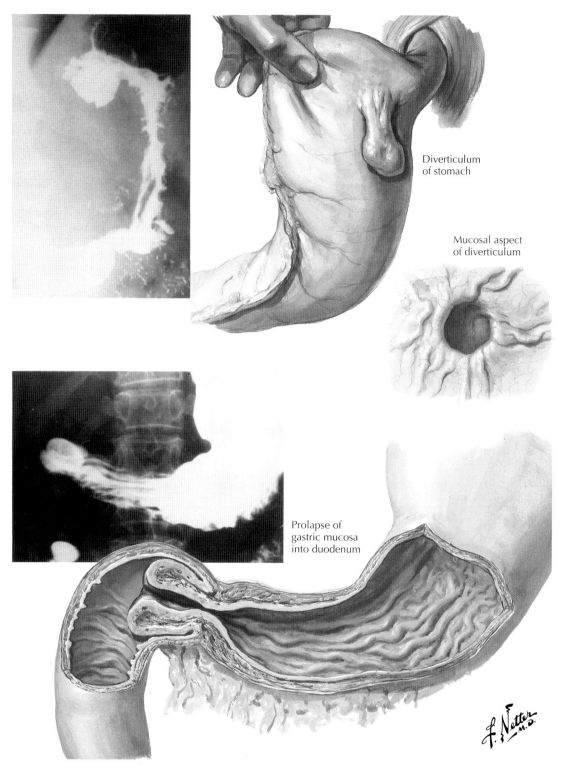

Diverticulum
of stomach

Mucosal aspect
of diverticulum

Prolapse of
gastric mucosa
into duodenum

Fig. 29.1 Gastric Diverticula and Gastroduodenal Prolapse.

ADDITIONAL RESOURCES

Dickenson RJ, Freeman AH: Gastric diverticula: radiologic and endoscopic features in six patients, *Gut* 27:954–957, 1986.

Fine A: Laparoscopic resection of a large proximal gastric diverticulum, *Gastrointest Endosc* 48:93–95, 1998.

Fork FT, Toth E, Lindstrom C: Early gastric cancer in a fundic diverticulum, *Endoscopy* 30:S2, 1998.

Kim SH, Lee SW, Choi WJ, et al: Laparoscopic resection of gastric diverticulum, *J Laparoendosc Surg Tech* 9:87–91, 1999.

30

Diverticula of the Duodenum

Martin H. Floch

Asaccular "true" diverticulum can originate from any part of the duodenum (Fig. 30.1). It is rare in the first part and usually develops in the second part in the region of the ampulla of Vater. Diverticula have been reported in approximately 6% of barium studies but in as many as 27% of endoscopy studies and in 23% of autopsy evaluations. They have been noted close to the ampulla, and in some cases the ampulla enters the diverticulum.

EXTRALUMINAL DIVERTICULA

Extraluminal duodenal diverticula are common with an interesting etiology, but debate is ongoing concerning congenital weakness in the duodenal wall and increased internal pressure. In rare cases, diverticula may be multiple. They usually develop on the inner or concave border of the duodenal curve and rarely on the outer border.

Clinical Picture

Approximately 10% of patients with extraluminal diverticula have symptoms. Abdominal discomfort may result when the diverticulum becomes inflamed, particularly from prolonged retention of duodenal content. The resultant diverticulitis can cause pain that radiates the epigastrium or back. Pancreatitis may occur when the ampulla is involved. Diverticula on the lateral wall have been reported to perforate (see Section VII).

Although there is a high incidence of extraluminal diverticula, most patients are asymptomatic. When diverticula are multiple, they can be associated with a malabsorption or bacterial overgrowth syndrome (see Section IV).

Diagnosis

Diagnosis of extraluminal duodenal diverticulum is easily made on barium study or endoscopy. Computed tomography may also make the diagnosis. A simple x-ray film of the abdomen may reveal an air-fluid level in the area of the duodenal sweep that is explained by a diverticulum. When the diverticulum is associated with pancreatic disease, endoscopic retrograde cholangiopancreatography (ERCP) is necessary for full evaluation (see Section VII).

Treatment and Management

Bleeding from the extraluminal diverticulum may be treated endoscopically, but in rare situations, surgical intervention may be necessary. In associated pancreatitis, the ampulla must be evaluated using ERCP, followed by appropriate intervention. Surgery is difficult; pancreatic or biliary surgical intervention may be needed. Therefore medical and endoscopic treatment is preferred for these patients. Surgery should be performed only in emergencies and only under controlled conditions.

Prognosis

Complications rarely occur, and duodenal surgery is rarely necessary. The prognosis for extraluminal duodenal diverticula is usually excellent unless a severe complication necessitates surgery.

INTRALUMINAL DUODENAL DIVERTICULA

Unlike the prevalent extraluminal type, intraluminal duodenal diverticula are rare. They are congenital abnormalities in which the diverticulum develops within the duodenal wall; occasionally, clinical problems surface in adulthood. They may cause obstruction in the duodenum, with loculation of food particles, and are reportedly associated with pancreatitis.

When patients with intraluminal diverticula present with clinical syndromes, intervention is usually required. Surgical and endoscopic techniques have been successful in opening the intraluminal wall so that there is free passage through the duodenum.

ADDITIONAL RESOURCES

Goelho J, Sousa GS, Lobo DN: Laparoscopic treatment of duodenal diverticula, *Surg Laparosc Endosc* 9:74–77, 1999.

Gore RM, Ghahremani GG, Kirsch MD: Diverticulitis of the duodenum: clinical and radiological manifestations of seven cases, *Am J Gastroenterol* 86:981–985, 1991.

Lobo DN, Balfour TW, Iftikhar SY, et al: Periampullary diverticula and pancreaticobiliary disease, *Br J Surg* 86:588–597, 1999.

Lotveit T, Skar V, Osnes M: Juxtapapillary duodenal diverticula, *Endoscopy* 20:175–178, 1988.

Uomo G, Manes G, Ragozzino A, et al: Periampullary extraluminal duodenal diverticula and acute pancreatitis: estimated etiological association, *Am J Gastroenterol* 91:1186–1188, 1996.

Periampullary diverticulum

Multiple diverticula

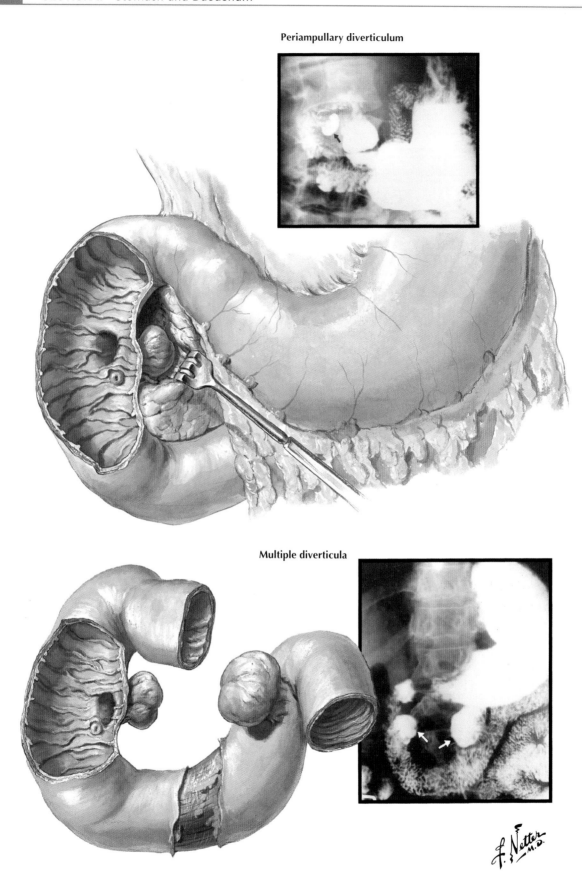

Fig. 30.1 Diverticula of the Duodenum.

31

Dyspepsia, Functional Dyspepsia, and Nonulcer Dyspepsia

Martin H. Floch

Dyspepsia is pain or discomfort centered in the upper abdomen. Associated disease may cause the symptom. As a *functional* disorder, the term *dyspepsia* is used when the discomfort or pain is chronic, lasts at least 12 weeks during the preceding 12 months, and is accompanied by no evidence of biochemical, metabolic, or organic disease.

Dyspepsia is common. Approximately 25% of adults experience such discomfort, but only 5% seek medical attention. Fewer than half the patients with this type of centered epigastric discomfort have any associated organic disease. Dyspepsia of no organic cause is called *functional dyspepsia.* Therefore the cause of dyspepsia may be true organic disease, which, when treated, cures the dyspepsia. Without some identifiable pathophysiology, it becomes functional dyspepsia. Patients with associated abnormality usually are also classified as having functional dyspepsia when the abnormality is considered irrelevant.

CLINICAL PICTURE

Patients of all ages have epigastric discomfort. Medical attention is usually sought after the discomfort becomes chronic. Often, the patient has some initial therapy and evaluation, but the treatment is unsuccessful, and it becomes apparent that the discomfort will persist. There may be associated early satiety and loss of appetite, a feeling of fullness, bloating in the upper abdomen, mild nausea, and sometimes even retching without vomiting of food. The degree of associated symptoms varies greatly.

DIAGNOSIS

Because of the discomfort and chronicity of dyspepsia, a work-up must ensue. Screening for gastric lesions is essential. Upper endoscopy esophagogastroduodenoscopy (EGD) is preferred, and during the procedure the patient should be evaluated for *Helicobacter pylori.* Because interpretation at endoscopy can vary, it is wise to perform mucosal biopsies of the esophagus and the stomach. Other pertinent evaluation includes a study for gastric emptying, especially if any food is retained in the stomach. If the EGD and biopsy results are negative, ultrasonography should be performed to rule out gallbladder, liver, and pancreatic disease. Depending on the findings, computed tomography may be necessary to rule out gross lesions in the pancreas. Full serum screening should be performed to rule out liver or metabolic disease.

As indicated, 50% of patients will have definite disease, and thus their dyspepsia is caused by disease and is *not* functional. Patients with an identified physiologic abnormality should be treated and the abnormality evaluated. Unfortunately, many of these symptoms persist, and it becomes clear that the abnormality is not the cause. These patients then fall into the category of functional dyspepsia.

Because *H. pylori* is ubiquitous in most societies and because it can cause peptic disease, the recommendation is to treat it before making a diagnosis of functional dyspepsia. Data and studies clearly reveal that as many as 50% of patients may be cured of symptoms after the *H. pylori* infection is treated. However, symptoms persist in many patients, who then fall into the category of functional dyspepsia.

The accompanying algorithm (Fig. 31.1) outlines the diagnosis and management of functional dyspepsia.

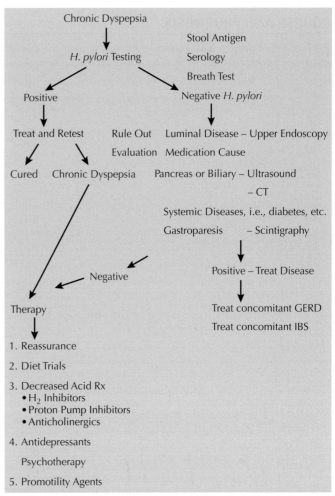

Fig. 31.1 Diagnosis and Treatment of Functional Dyspepsia. *CT,* Computed tomography; *GERD,* gastroesophageal reflux disease; *IBS,* irritable bowel syndrome.

TREATMENT AND MANAGEMENT

If the cause of the dyspepsia is found and treated, the treatment of that particular entity solves the problem. However, if the diagnosis is functional dyspepsia, the treatment becomes challenging and includes the following:

- *Strong reassurance.* Make sure the patient with dyspepsia understands that he or she has a functional disorder, probably with visceral hypersensitivity. Carefully continue to evaluate dietary stress factors that may aggravate the symptoms, such as caffeine, coffee, alcohol, and spices. Drug therapy may include trials of antisecretory, promotility, and antidepressant agents.
- *Antisecretory agents.* Some patients report some relief using H_2-receptor antagonists or proton pump inhibitors (PPIs). However, it is now agreed from long-term studies using PPIs that patients should not be left on this group of medications long term. The course should be limited and certainly, if necessary, only intermittent.
- *Promotility agents.* Domperidone is available only in some parts of the world. Metoclopramide is more readily available, but long-term use is generally discouraged. These drugs can be effective intermittently in some patients.
- *Antidepressant therapy.* Many dyspeptic patients experience symptom relief once an appropriate antidepressant is used in adequate dosage.

Treating functional dyspepsia is challenging. It requires reassurance and working closely with patients to maintain their confidence.

COURSE AND PROGNOSIS

Patients with dyspepsia have an excellent prognosis, but the disease course varies with periods of increasing and decreasing symptoms.

Frequently, patients are satisfied with one or the other forms of therapy: H_2 inhibitor, PPI, or antidepressant. Many require more intensive work and even psychotherapy to manage severe symptoms.

Concomitant disease often includes gastroesophageal reflux disease (GERD), as confirmed on upper endoscopy and other studies. Treating GERD is often helpful. Similarly, some dyspeptic patients have irritable bowel syndrome (IBS) accompanied by recurrent diarrhea or constipation, and treatment for those symptoms often helps their epigastric distress. It is essential that concomitant disease, such as GERD or IBS, be treated simultaneously. This often helps in dyspeptic patients' long-term management.

ADDITIONAL RESOURCES

Camilleri M: Functional dyspepsia: mechanisms of symptom generation and appropriate management of patients, *Gastroenterol Clin North Am* 36: 649–664, 2007.

Moayyedi P, Soo S, Deeks J, et al: Eradication of *Helicobacter pylori* for non-ulcer dyspepsia, *Cochrane Database Syst Rev* (1):CD002096, 2003.

Tack J: Dyspepsia. In Feldman M, Friedman LS, Brandt LJ, editors: *Gastrointestinal and liver disease*, ed 10, Philadelphia, 2016, Saunders-Elsevier, pp 194–206.

Talley NJ: The role of endoscopy in dyspepsia (clinical update), *Am Soc Gastrointest Endosc* 15:1–4, 2007.

Talley NJ, Stanghellini V, Heading RC, et al: Functional gastrointestinal disorders. In Drossman DA, editor: *The functional gastrointestinal disorders*, McLean, Va, 2000, Degnon Associates, pp 302–327.

Talley NJ, Vakil N, Moayyedi P: AGA Technical Review on the evaluation of dyspepsia, *Gastroenterology* 129:1756–1780, 2005.

32

Helicobacter pylori Infection

Martin H. Floch

Helicobacter pylori is a gram-negative, spiral, flagellated bacterium that inhabits the mucous layer of the stomach. Warren and Marshall first described *H. pylori* as a pathogen in humans and clearly documented and correlated the organism's association with gastritis and peptic ulceration.

The prevalence of *H. pylori* varies greatly. Approximately 40% of persons in developed countries are affected, and as many as 85% are affected in underdeveloped countries. In all areas, prevalence is associated with low socioeconomic status and advanced age. Most people remain infected for life unless they are treated. Marriage does not appear to be a strong risk factor for acquiring the infection.

Data on how the organism is acquired are controversial, although crowded living conditions and poor hygiene are associated with higher infection rates. Transmission does appear to be based on person-to-person spread (Fig. 32.1). However, the exact mode of transmission remains unclear. *Helicobacter heilmanii* colonizes both animals and humans. Although it may be pathogenic, *H. heilmanii* has not been shown to be as prevalent a pathogen as *H. pylori*.

CLINICAL PICTURE

It is now clear that *H. pylori* is a major risk factor for gastritis, peptic ulcer, gastric adenocarcinoma, and gastric lymphoma. Consequently, patients may have epigastric pain and ulceration, bleeding from gastritis or ulceration, or pain, nausea, vomiting, and weight loss from malignancy. It is not clear why *H. pylori* rarely causes diarrhea. Anemia from chronic blood loss may be the only symptom in those who feel little pain. The picture of chronic dyspepsia may unfold over the years.

H. pylori has been known to cause acute gastritis. In these patients, it may actually cause severe acute achlorhydria, which appears to be self-limiting. Not only can prolonged disease cause ulceration, but it also has been known to cause gastric atrophy and, in association with any metaplasia, appears to result in a high risk for adenocarcinoma.

DIAGNOSIS

The diagnosis of *H. pylori* infection can be made using histologic, serologic, breath, or stool testing.

Histology

Histologic examination is made through endoscopy with biopsy material of the gastric mucosa and appropriate histologic and staining evaluation. Because it is difficult to grow *H. pylori* in culture, cultures are no longer used for the diagnosis of gastric aspirants or gastric tissue. Instead, the rapid urease test (CLO test) can be used by placing gastric biopsy material into a urease medium that changes color when urease from the bacteria metabolizes the urea.

Serology

Serologic tests are sensitive and as specific as histologic biopsy evaluation. Many have been adopted for whole-blood, rapid use in the office. However, only immunoglobulin G (IgG) antibody is reliable. IgA and IgM antibodies are unreliable. Serologic tests are useful because they establish that the patient has had *H. pylori* infection. However, controversy surrounds the rapidity with which the antibody disappears after treatment, and consequently, serology is not a good test to determine whether treatment is effective.

Breath Test

The urea breath test with either carbon 13 or 14 (C_{13} or C_{14}) is accurate. The subject ingests the carbon label, and the test determines whether the carbon is freed by urease activity from the bacteria in the stomach and absorbed, then measures it in expired breath.

Stool Test

The stool antigen test is the latest noninvasive method for diagnosing *H. pylori* infection. Evaluations are as accurate as histologic methods. The stool test can be used easily for monitoring the effectiveness of therapy.

TREATMENT AND MANAGEMENT

Once a diagnosis of a *H. pylori* infection is made, treatment must follow. Many treatment regimens use combinations of bismuth sulfate and numerous antibiotics, including metronidazole, tetracycline, amoxicillin, and clarithromycin. The course varies from 7 to 14 days. The literature attests to the effectiveness of the different regimens, which can be categorized into three types of therapy; double, triple, and quadruple.

Most often used and recommended is *triple therapy,* which includes a proton pump inhibitor (PPI) twice daily, plus amoxicillin (1000 mg) twice daily, plus clarithromycin (500 mg) or metronidazole (500 mg) twice daily. Triple or quadruple therapy using bismuth is equally effective. Triple therapy administers two bismuth tablets four times daily plus tetracycline (500 mg) four times daily and metronidazole (250 mg) three times daily; quadruple therapy uses bismuth and includes a PPI twice daily in addition to the two antibiotics. In trials, clinicians have used variations of these antibiotics with reported success. If a patient develops an allergy or intolerance to one of the drugs, other options are available.

With resistant cases always present and unsuccessful therapy reported in the 20% range, new regimens are constantly being tested. Sequential therapy is new, but initial analysis reveals it may be effective and possibly better than previous therapies. The initial effective regimen consisted of 5 days of amoxicillin (1 g) plus a PPI twice daily, followed by 5 days of triple therapy with a PPI, clarithromycin (500 mg), and tinidazole

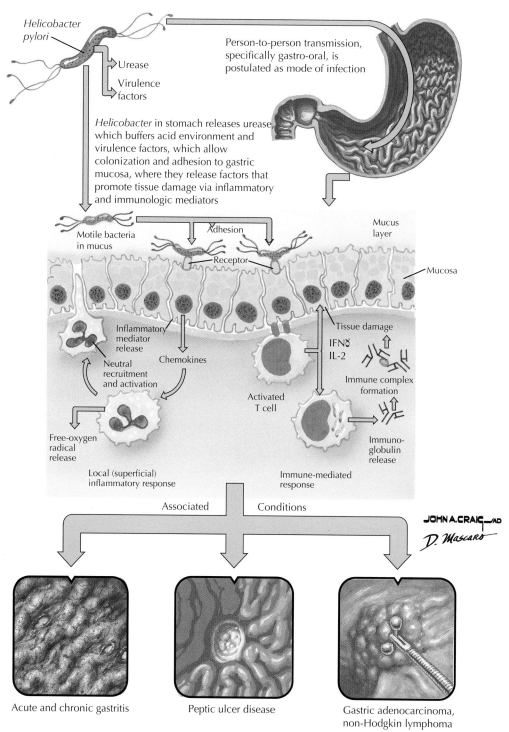

Helicobacter pylori

Urease

Virulence factors

Person-to-person transmission, specifically gastro-oral, is postulated as mode of infection

Helicobacter in stomach releases urease, which buffers acid environment and virulence factors, which allow colonization and adhesion to gastric mucosa, where they release factors that promote tissue damage via inflammatory and immunologic mediators

Motile bacteria in mucus

Adhesion

Mucus layer

Receptor

Mucosa

Inflammatory mediator release

Chemokines

Neutral recruitment and activation

Tissue damage

IFNγ IL-2

Immune complex formation

Free-oxygen radical release

Activated T cell

Immuno-globulin release

Local (superficial) inflammatory response

Immune-mediated response

Associated Conditions

JOHN A. CRAIG—AD
D. Mascaro

Acute and chronic gastritis

Peptic ulcer disease

Gastric adenocarcinoma, non-Hodgkin lymphoma

Fig. 32.1 Etiology and Pathogenesis of *Helicobacter pylori* Infection.

(500 mg), all twice daily. These sequential therapies are now in meta-analysis and appear to be more effective than 14 days of triple therapy.

If a patient has carcinoma, treatment of the malignancy is paramount. However, when a lymphoma or mucosa-associated lymphoid tissue (MALT) lesion develops, remission of the lymphoma has been reported if *H. pylori* has been eradicated. Those lesions must be treated in a specific manner (see Chapter 38).

Some organisms are resistant, and failure occurs. It must be emphasized that *H. pylori* requires acid for reproduction; thus most microbi-

ologists and clinicians believe acid suppression should be part of therapy. Failed therapy occurs in 5% to 10% of treated patients. Failure may result from resistant strains or may be associated with smoking or dense colonization with the *cag*-negative strain. Repeat therapy is often successful, but resistant strains do grow.

Table 32.1 demonstrates the many options for treating *H. pylori*. Option 1 is the most recommended as a beginning, but the other options vary worldwide, with options 3, 6, and 7 often used in repeat therapies. These are the older regimens but are still widely used; newer antibiotics

TABLE 32.1 Treatment and Retreatment Options/Preferences for *Helicobacter pylori* Infection

Option	Treatment
1	P-A-C
2	P-M-C
3	O-B-M-T
4	O-B-F-T
5	P-A-R
6	P3-A3
7	P3-A3-CF

Clinical Program[a]	Treatment Preference
SVZ	$1 \leftrightarrow 2 \rightarrow 3$
LL	$6 \rightarrow 5 \rightarrow 7$
DG	$3 \rightarrow 4$
AA	$1 \leftrightarrow 2 \rightarrow 3 \rightarrow 6$
BM	$1 \leftrightarrow 2 \rightarrow 7$

Treatment Code	Drug/Dose
A	Amoxicillin, 1 g bid
A3	Amoxicillin, 1 g tid
M	Metronidazole, 500 mg tid
C	Clarithromycin, 500 mg bid
P or O	Any PPI (omeprazole, 20 mg bid, or equivalent)
P3	Triple-dose PPI (omeprazole, 40 mg tid, or equivalent)
R	Rifabutin, 300 mg bid
F	Furazolidone, 100 mg qid
CF	Ciprofloxacin, 500 mg bid
B	Bismuth citrate, 120 mg qid (De Nol) *or* Bismuth subsalicylate, 250 mg qid (2 Pepto-Bismol tablets qid)
T	Tetracycline, 500 mg qid

[a]Clinical programs at five academic centers.
bid, Twice daily; *PPI,* Proton pump inhibitor; *qid,* four times daily; *tid,* three times daily.
Modified from Megraud F, Marshall BJ: How to treat *Helicobacter pylori.* First-line, second-line and future therapies, *Gastroenterol Clin North Am* 29:759-773, 2000.

such as levoquin and rifabutin are also used. Most agree that at least 7 days of therapy is required, although some are using shorter courses and others require 14 days.

COURSE AND PROGNOSIS

Effective therapy for *H. pylori* infection is rewarding when patients with chronic gastritis or peptic ulceration are cured of their symptoms and disease. Initial therapy is effective in 70% to 95% of patients, depending on the patient and the regimen. When a strain is resistant, treatment of the associated disease must be continued until rescue therapy can be implemented to eradicate the organism. Attempts to eradicate *H. pylori* should continue, even if it takes years with different antibiotics and extended treatment; to do otherwise is now considered a risk factor for adenocarcinoma.

If a patient has an associated malignancy, course and prognosis depend on the extent of the cancer. *H. pylori* definitely causes MALT lesions, which may respond to, and may be cured by, *H. pylori* eradication (see Chapter 35).

ADDITIONAL RESOURCES

Blaser MJ: *Helicobacter pylori* and other gastric *Helicobacter* species. In Mandell GL, Bennett JE, Dolin R, editors: *Principles and Practice of Infectious Diseases,* ed 6, Philadelphia, 2005, Churchill Livingstone–Elsevier, pp 2557–2566.

Chey WD, Wong CY: American College of Gastroenterology guideline on the management of *Helicobacter pylori* infection, *Am J Gastroenterol* 102:1808–1825, 2007.

Gisbert JP, Gisbert JL, Marcos S, et al: Empirical rescue therapy after *Helicobacter pylori* treatment failure: a 10-year single-centre study of 500 patients, *Aliment Pharmacol Ther* 27:346–354, 2008.

Graham DY, Malaty HM, Evans DG, et al: Epidemiology of *Helicobacter pylori* in an asymptomatic population in the United States: effective age, race, and socioeconomic status, *Gastroenterology* 100:1495–1501, 1991.

Jafri NS, Hornung CA, Howden CW: Meta-analysis: sequential therapy appears superior to standard therapy for *Helicobacter pylori* infection in patients naïve to treatment, *Ann Intern Med* 148:923–931, 2008.

Megraud F, Marshall BJ: How to treat *Helicobacter pylori:* first-line, second-line, and future therapies, *Gastroenterol Clin North Am* 29:759–773, 2000.

Suerbaum S, Michetti P: *Helicobacter pylori* infection, *N Engl J Med* 347:1175–1186, 2002.

Warren J, Marshall B: Unidentified curved bacilli in gastric epithelium and acute and chronic gastritis, *Lancet* 1:1273–1275, 1983.

Zullo A, De Francesco V, Hassen C, et al: The sequential therapy regimen for *Helicobacter pylori* eradication: a pooled-data analysis, *Gut* 56:1353–1357, 2007.

33

Gastritis: General, Erosive, and Acute

Martin H. Floch

GASTRITIS

Gastritis is inflammation of the gastric mucosa, submucosa, or muscularis (Fig. 33.1). A gastritis classification proposed in 1991 by an international convention in Sydney, Australia, has not gained support in the past two decades, reflecting the clinical confusion in this area. However, the basic pathologic entity of "inflammation in the mucosa" is considered gastritis. It may be acute or chronic, or it may result in atrophy. Each condition is associated with a clear endoscopic clinical picture.

Gastritis may be chronic, may be associated with disease (e.g., *Helicobacter pylori,* autoimmune), or may be a progressive atrophic form. It may be associated with all forms of infectious disease (viral, bacterial, parasitic, fungal), or it may be granulomatous and associated with chronic disease (e.g., Crohn, tumors). Gastritis may be erosive (often referred to as *reactive*) because of foreign agents such as aspirin, nonsteroidal antiinflammatory drugs (NSAIDs), bile reflux, alcohol, and caffeine. It may be classified as rare entities such as collagenous, lymphocytic, and eosinophilic gastritis (referred to as *distinctive*). A hypertrophic form is known as *Ménétrier disease,* and a postgastric surgery form is known as *gastritis cystica profunda.* A form now appearing in patients who have had grafts or transplants is known as *graft-versus-host disease,* in which the stomach and other parts of the gastrointestinal (GI) tract are involved.

Recent attempts to classify gastritis according to topography, morphology, and etiology have not changed clinical practice. In the most recent consensus, gastritis was categorized into *nonatrophic, atrophic,* and special forms. *H. pylori* gastritis is classified as nonatrophic.

Clinical Picture

The clinical picture of gastritis can be specific in that patients have abdominal pain, nausea, and anorexia. Patients may report bloating or a burning discomfort in the epigastrium. In severe acute gastritis, patients may vomit and have food intolerance. In chronic gastritis, patients may have anorexia with weight loss. Many academicians believe that gastritis can exist without symptoms; therefore symptoms often will not be attributed to the mucosal inflammation. Nevertheless, if a cause such as *H. pylori* or an associated disease can be identified and treated, symptoms can be resolved. Gastritis is often part of another disease process.

Diagnosis

The history of onset of symptoms is important. When symptoms are acute and the gastritis is associated with infection, symptoms usually subside within days, and evaluation is unnecessary. The use of NSAIDs must be evaluated. However, when symptoms persist longer than 7 to 14 days, an investigation is necessary. The standard evaluation includes upper GI endoscopy with biopsy to determine the disease process.

When atrophy is present, a test for parietal cell antibodies is indicated. Serum gastrin levels may be elevated if atrophy is diffuse. Evaluation for vitamin B_{12} is necessary.

The most common cause of gastritis is *H. pylori* (see Chapter 32). Finding the organism through endoscopy and biopsy confirms the diagnosis. When present, other organisms can be identified on biopsy, but careful histologic staining must be done to identify chronic infections, such as tuberculosis and fungi. Anisakiasis can be diagnosed on endoscopy; with the increased ingestion of raw fish, *Anisakis* infection should be considered in patients with an appropriate history. Other parasites also may be identified in the stomach.

Treatment and Management

When an infectious agent is identified, such as *H. pylori* or any parasite, treatment for that infectious agent cures the gastritis. Autoimmune diseases and nonspecific gastric diseases are treated symptomatically.

When another disease involving the gastric mucosa is identified, such as Crohn disease or sarcoid, it must be treated. Erosive gastritis is treated by removing its cause, whether alcohol, drugs, or other agents.

During the healing phase of gastritis therapy, acidic and spice-containing foods could further irritate the mucosa and must be removed from the patient's diet. Neutralizing acid is also recommended because the mucosa has many breaks in its barrier and can be invaded by acid. Therefore it is advisable to use acid suppression therapy (H_2 inhibitors, proton pump inhibitors [PPIs], antacids) as tolerated.

Course and Prognosis

The course of gastritis depends on the cause. It can be chronic, troublesome, and difficult to treat. Most acute forms resolve rapidly. An association with NSAID use must be considered and may be treated by changing the NSAID or adding a PPI to alleviate symptoms if the NSAID is essential therapy. Chronic forms are related to the natural history of an associated disease and must be treated by diet restrictions and antacid therapy. A true atrophic gastritis may be associated with vitamin B_{12} deficiency, which should be evaluated.

EROSIVE GASTRITIS: ACUTE GASTRIC ULCERS

Erosive gastritis consists of small, acute gastric ulcers that occur in the body or antrum of the stomach. The cause may be an infectious organism or damage to the mucosa from numerous possible agents. The ulcers may range in size from a few millimeters to a centimeter. They often appear as multiple lesions.

Clinical Picture

Clinical findings in patients with acute gastric ulcers vary greatly. If associated with a simple streptococcal infection, the ulcer may last for

Gastritis

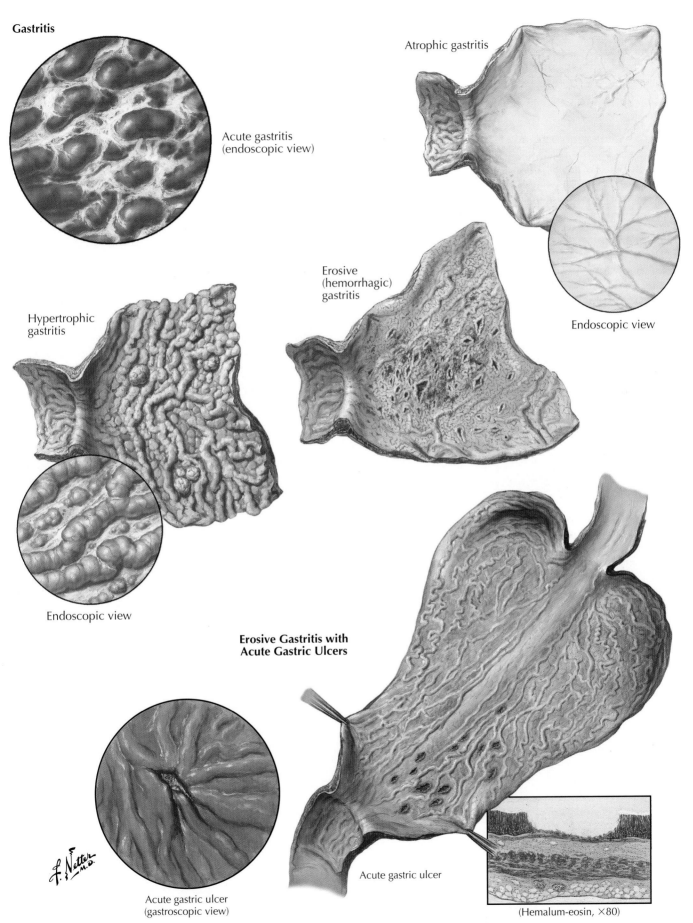

Acute gastritis
(endoscopic view)

Atrophic gastritis

Endoscopic view

Erosive
(hemorrhagic)
gastritis

Hypertrophic
gastritis

Endoscopic view

**Erosive Gastritis with
Acute Gastric Ulcers**

Acute gastric ulcer
(gastroscopic view)

Acute gastric ulcer

(Hemalum-eosin, ×80)

Fig. 33.1 Gastritis and Erosive Gastritis With Acute Gastric Ulcers.

a few days and cause nausea, vomiting, and mild abdominal pain. The ulcer also may be asymptomatic or may cause severe bleeding and hematemesis. If the symptoms are short term, endoscopy is not necessary; if bleeding occurs or symptoms persist, endoscopy confirms the diagnosis.

Diagnosis

Erosive ulcers are small. *H. pylori* must be ruled out as a cause. If serologic, breath test, stool antigen, or histologic findings are negative, the cause must be determined by history. Microscopically, the erosions reveal acute and perhaps mild chronic inflammation in the superficial mucosa, which can extend down to the muscularis. Endoscopy may reveal very small ulcers. A brown or a black spot indicates recent bleeding. The ulcers rarely may be chronic. The greatest danger from these ulcers is massive bleeding.

It is surprising that these small ulcers can cause great pain or bleed excessively. If they are duodenal and caused by *H. pylori,* therapy for the infection relieves the symptoms. If they result from NSAID therapy, the ulcers can become chronic in patients who continue using NSAIDs to relieve osteoarthritic pain (see Chapter 20).

Treatment and Management

For effective long-term management of erosive gastritis, it is best to determine the cause of the ulcers. Any patient in the acute state should receive a PPI. If the ulcer is bleeding, the PPI can be administered intravenously. If the erosions are caused by a drug or by an infectious agent, or if they are of peptic origin, they invariably heal. Follow-up endoscopy is usually not needed, but if symptoms persist or there is any sign of continued disease, such as prolonged nausea, occasional vomiting, or mild pain, repeat endoscopy is essential to rule out an underlying malignancy. If a drug is the cause, eliminating the drug is the only therapy required. If an infection is the cause, eliminating the infection will cure the small ulcers. If the cause is unknown, the patient may require long-term antacid therapy.

Course and Prognosis

The course of erosive gastritis is usually short, with an excellent prognosis. Bleeding stops with treatment, and symptoms subside. Rarely, the bleeding may be massive, and the diagnosis is usually associated with another gastropathy or ischemia; emergency surgery is needed.

ADDITIONAL RESOURCES

Carr NJ, Leadbetter H, Marriott A: Correlation between the endoscopic and histologic diagnosis of gastritis, *Ann Diagn Pathol* 16:13–15, 2012.

Feldman M, Lee EL: Gastritis. In Feldman M, Friedman LS, Brandt LJ, editors: *Gastrointestinal and Liver Disease*, ed 10, Philadelphia, 2016, Saunders-Elsevier, pp 868–883.

Graham DH, Genta RM, Dixon MF: *Gastritis*, Philadelphia, 1999, Lippincott Williams & Wilkins.

Nordenstedt H, Graham DY, Kramer JR, et al: Helicobacter pylori-negative gastritis: Prevalence and risk factors, *Am J Gastroenterol* 108:65–71, 2013.

Petersson F, Franzen LE, Borch K: Characterization of the gastric cardia in volunteers from the general population, *Dig Dis Sci* 55:46–53, 2010.

34

Peptic Ulcer Disease

Martin H. Floch

Peptic ulcer disease is a term used to refer to ulceration of the gastric or duodenal mucosa aggravated by penetration of the mucosal barrier by acid and pepsin (Figs. 34.1 and 34.2). The natural history of peptic ulcer disease was dramatically revised with the discovery of H_2 inhibition of acid secretion and then proton pump acid inhibition. The discovery that *Helicobacter pylori* is a major factor in all ulcer disease led to its treatment and to the cure of peptic ulcer when associated with *H. pylori* infection. The identification of iatrogenic causes (e.g., nonsteroidal antiinflammatory drugs [NSAIDs]) further defined the nature and causes of peptic ulceration.

Before the advent of these findings, peptic ulcer had been considered an acute and chronic disease that required long-term diet, psychotherapy, and surgical therapy. However, these approaches have changed greatly, as have descriptions of the causes, ulcerations, and complications.

Surgical removal has become a rarity, and the diagnosis of peptic ulcer disease is most often made endoscopically. Therefore referring to "superficial" ulcers that do not penetrate is not clinically practical. Acute and chronic ulcers are currently difficult to define and no longer fit their historical definitions.

PATHOPHYSIOLOGY

The gastric and duodenal epithelium is protected by a mucous coat, which in turn is usually covered by an unstirred, bicarbonate-rich layer of water. Mucus and bicarbonate are secreted by gastric epithelial cells, as well as duodenal Brunner glands. Whenever acid and pepsin break these layers, cells may be injured. Minor injuries from irritants are usually rapidly healed. However, when the injury is prolonged by any

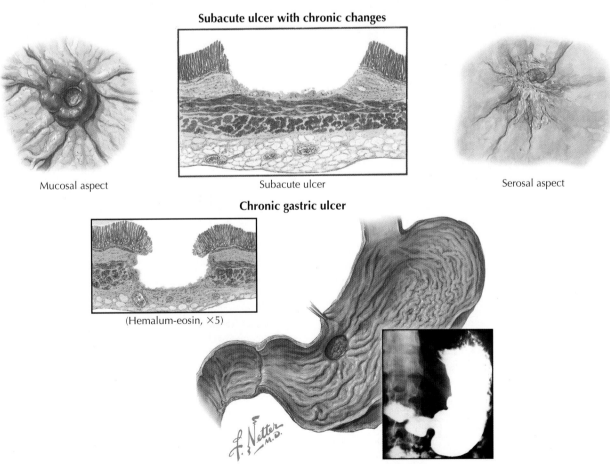

Subacute ulcer with chronic changes

Mucosal aspect   Subacute ulcer   Serosal aspect

Chronic gastric ulcer

(Hemalum-eosin, ×5)

Fig. 34.1 Subacute and Chronic Gastric Ulcers.

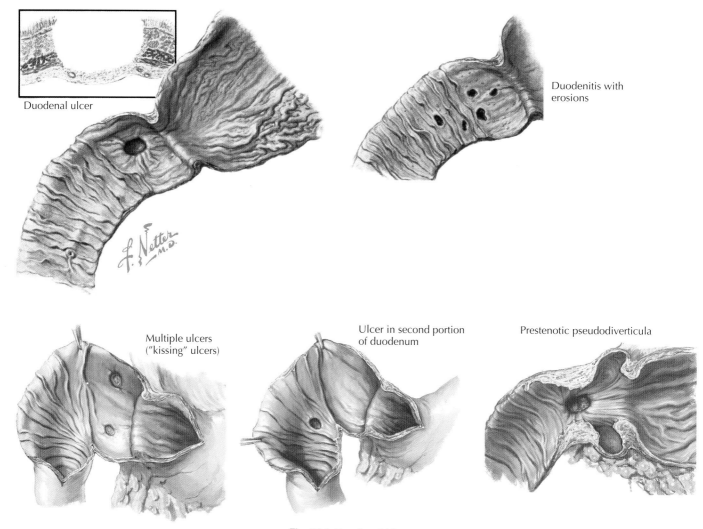

Duodenal ulcer

Duodenitis with erosions

Multiple ulcers ("kissing" ulcers)

Ulcer in second portion of duodenum

Prestenotic pseudodiverticula

Fig. 34.2 Duodenal Ulcers.

of the causes elaborated here, ulceration may occur. Acid and pepsin overrun the defensive and regenerative processes to break down the mucosa.

CAUSES AND ASSOCIATIONS

Causes and associations of peptic ulceration can be classified in four categories: infectious *(H. pylori)*, drug related (NSAIDs), hypersecretory, and miscellaneous.

Infectious Causes

H. pylori is probably the most common cause of peptic ulceration, depending on the prevalence in a particular area. As discussed in Chapter 32, *H. pylori* infection penetrates the mucous layer. It requires acid for its survival but can protect itself from acid destruction by an alkaline material that it secretes.

Because *H. pylori* affects approximately half the world's population, people with the bacterium are susceptible to peptic ulceration. Once the bacterium is present, its effects range from mild degrees of inflammation to ulceration. In the gastric mucosa, *H. pylori* causes inflammation, and in the duodenal mucosa, it causes metaplasia to gastric epithelium and then the resultant damage. Approximately 60% of patients

with gastric ulcer and 80% of those with duodenal ulcer have chronic *H. pylori* infection. It is estimated that only 20% of those infected ever acquire peptic ulcer. Whether ulceration develops depends on several factors, including the strain of *H. pylori* and other risk factors in the host. Regardless, treating the *H. pylori* infection dramatically decreases the occurrence of ulcer.

Drug-Related Causes

Worldwide use of NSAIDs for the relief of pain and neurologic disorders has made these drugs the first or second most common cause of peptic ulceration, depending on the extent of their use. NSAIDs injure the gastrointestinal (GI) mucosa topically and systemically. Again, when the mucosal barrier is broken in the stomach or the duodenum, peptic ulceration develops. Attempts to decrease the harmful topical effects of NSAIDs have included applying enteric coating, but the systemic effects persist, resulting in simple, superficial petechiae becoming deep ulcerations. Careful endoscopic studies have revealed that mucosal petechiae or small erosions develop in 15% to 30% of patients who use NSAIDs. However, serious pain or bleeding is still relatively rare and is estimated to affect less than 1% of patients. Certain risk factors, including smoking, old age, and concomitant *H. pylori* infection, increase the chances of peptic ulceration or bleeding. It also appears that selective cyclooxygenase-2 (COX-2) inhibitors produce less damage than the standard COX-1 NSAIDs. Given all these facts, the physician still must consider NSAIDs as one of the most common causes of peptic ulceration.

Two other ulcerogenic drugs, alendronate and risedronate, are frequently used to treat osteoporosis. As newer and more potent drugs become available, clinicians must be aware that they are potential ulcerogenic agents.

Hypersecretory Causes

With regard to the third category, hypersecretory states, it is well known that patients with duodenal ulcer appear to produce higher amounts of gastric acid, but this fact is less important now that *H. pylori* is known to be a major cause of ulcer. *H. pylori* itself may stimulate acid production and may increase gastrin levels. Studies in acid production since the contribution of *H. pylori* became known are not readily available.

In *Zollinger-Ellison syndrome* (ZES), the gastrinoma secretes gastrin, and there is an associated proliferation of enterochromaffin-like (ECL) cells in the stomach, stimulating hypersecretion of acid (see Chapter 19). With this high level of acid secretion, the mucosal barrier becomes overwhelmed, and breaks occur in the gastric and duodenal mucosa to cause ulceration. Treating gastrinomas may simply require proton pump inhibitors (PPIs) in high doses, to combat hypersecretion, or chemotherapy, embolization, or surgical resection, depending on the patient and the extent of the lesion.

Another cause of acid hypersecretion is *systemic mastocytosis*, in which proliferating numbers of mast cells produce large amounts of histamine that affect gastric secretion and have systemic effects on the skin, liver, and bone marrow. In patients with systemic mastocytosis, treatment with H_1-receptor and H_2-receptor antagonists, anticholinergics, oral disodium chromoglycate, and even corticosteroids, with or without cyclophosphamide, may be helpful.

Massive resection of the small bowel in patients with short-bowel syndrome is often associated with hypergastrinemia and hypersecretion. These patients require selective therapy because of absorption problems. In addition, antral G-cell hyperfunction syndrome may be confused with ZES and is usually treated medically.

Miscellaneous Causes

All clinicians encounter patients whose ulcers do not fit any of the categories just described. Since the discovery of *H. pylori*'s role, there is always suspicion that other infectious agents may cause chronic ulceration. Stress is no longer considered a major factor. However, results from Pavlov's experiments on stress ulceration still hold true. There is no question that psychologic stress can stimulate hormonal release, and peptic ulceration certainly may be caused by severe environmental or psychologic stress. However, the stress must be severe to be a factor in ulceration. Similarly, as indicated, cigarette smoking, alcohol, and consumption of hot spices or high amounts of caffeine (coffee, tea, colas) may be factors in the production of peptic ulceration.

DUODENITIS AND ULCER OF THE DUODENAL BULB

Peptic ulcer occurs when the duodenal bulb or the first or second part of the duodenum becomes ulcerated because of severe focal inflammation. The inflammation may be in areas of the bulb or proximal duodenum, referred to as *duodenitis*. As discussed in Chapter 33, frequently the causes of this phenomenon are *H. pylori* infection or NSAIDs. This discussion is limited to duodenitis and disease of the bulb and the first and second parts of the duodenum. Duodenitis from other origins and affecting the entire duodenum is discussed in Section IV.

Clinical Picture

The most common symptom of duodenal ulcer or duodenitis is *epigastric pain*. However, nausea, recurrent vomiting, and occult or gross bleeding may be the presenting symptoms and the reason patients seek treatment. It is surprising how often (almost 50% of patients) duodenal ulcers and duodenitis manifest as bleeding. The bleeding may be in the form of chronic anemia or massive upper GI hemorrhage (see Chapter 34).

Diagnosis

The most common cause of duodenal ulcer and duodenitis is *H. pylori* infection. Therefore some clinicians diagnose *H. pylori* infection noninvasively and treat the patient. Symptoms may completely resolve without endoscopic evaluation. However, if the patient has anemia or acute bleeding, endoscopy is essential even with a noninvasive diagnosis of *H. pylori* infection.

During endoscopy, the duodenal bulb is often swollen and difficult to distend. Consequently, the endoscopist will observe the duodenitis but may miss the ulcer bed.

More common, and clinically important, is *chronic duodenal ulcer*. With few exceptions, this lesion is seated within the duodenal bulb. It develops with essentially the same frequency on the anterior or posterior wall. The average size of a duodenal ulcer is 0.5 cm, but ulcers on the posterior wall are usually larger than those on the anterior wall, primarily because the posterior wall ulcers, separated by the pancreas lying below the ulcer, can enlarge without free perforation.

Duodenal peptic ulcer is usually round and has a punched-out appearance. When small, the ulcer may be slitlike, crescent shaped, or triangular. Unlike acute ulcers, which stop at the submucosa, chronic ulcers involve all layers, penetrating to the muscular coat and beyond. An ulcer on the anterior wall may show a moderate amount of proliferation, but an ulcer on the posterior wall shows evidence of considerable edema and fibrosis. Healing may proceed as with a gastric ulcer—with the disappearance of the crater and bridging of the gap through the formation of fibrous tissue covered by new mucous membrane—but healing becomes more difficult once the destruction of the muscular layer has gone too far.

Symptoms of chronic ulcer are typical and are characterized by periodic episodes of gnawing pain, usually located in the epigastrium. The pain occurs 1 to 2 hours after meals and may be relieved by food.

Peptic ulcers in a region distal to the duodenal bulb occur infrequently (<5% of all duodenal ulcers), decreasing in frequency with their distance from the pylorus. Ulcers in the second portion of the duodenum cause the same symptoms and complications as ulcers of the duodenal bulb. However, the clinical picture and later the clinical significance of acute ulcers may be much more complex because of the functional and anatomic implications for the adjoining structures. Because of the edema of their margins and surroundings and because of penetration or shrinkage, acute ulcers may cause obstruction and eventually stenosis of the papilla of Vater or the lower part of the common bile duct, along with one or both of the pancreatic ducts, so that chronic pancreatitis or biliary obstruction with jaundice, or even both, may result. Deep penetration may give rise to choledochoduodenal fistula.

Multiple chronic ulcers of the duodenum are common, occurring in 11% to 45% of autopsy cases. Rarely have more than two been found. Ulcers developing on both the anterior and the posterior wall are referred to as *kissing ulcers*.

Only a small percentage of patients with active duodenal ulcer also have active gastric ulcer. One of the most typical duodenal deformities occurring with the ulcerative process is the *prestenotic pseudodiverticulum*. Seen from the lumen, it represents a relatively flat, sinuslike indentation, usually between the pylorus and the site of the ulcer or proximal to a duodenal stricture resulting from a cicatricial remnant of an ulcer. Although all layers of the duodenal wall participate in the formation of such a pouch, this differs from a true duodenal diverticulum (see Chapter 32) in that the mucosa has not evaginated through a small muscular gap.

Treatment and Prognosis

Treatment for duodenitis and duodenal ulcer is similar to (or the same as) treatment for acute gastric ulcers (see Chapter 33) and depends on the cause. Once again, if infectious (*H. pylori*), eradication of the organism is curative. If the cause is an irritating agent or a metabolic disease, treatment varies and is discussed according to conditions in Chapter 33, for which the cause must be identified and then the appropriate therapy used. In the acute phase, H_2 or PPIs will usually relieve pain until specific therapy is available, and certainly until the ulcer heals, which may take 2 to 4 weeks. Antacids and sucralfate can also be helpful.

COMPLICATIONS

Numerous complications can occur from acute or chronic ulceration of the stomach or duodenum. These include perforation, bleeding, scarring stenosis and obstruction, and various forms of malabsorption (Fig. 34.3).

Acute Perforation
Clinical Picture and Pathophysiology
Perforation of an ulcer may be free and may extend into the peritoneal cavity or into an adjacent organ. Free perforation is an acute, life-threatening complication. It appears to be more common in smokers and elderly persons.

The duration of an ulcer (stomach or duodenum) does not seem to affect how quickly the ulcerative and inflammatory processes penetrate the muscular and serous layers. Acute peptic ulcer may penetrate the gastric or intestinal wall so rapidly that 10% to 25% of patients may have no history of previous symptoms. On the other hand, chronic ulcers may exist for years without progressing so deep as to implicate the serosa, although chronic ulcers that cause severe, persistent symptoms and recurrent or calloused ulcers can always cause perforation. The rapidity with which the digestive effect of the strongly acid gastric juice destroys the wall layers and approaches the serosa cannot be anticipated.

Once perforation has taken place, the location of the ulcer plays a dominant role in subsequent events. Ulcers of the anterior wall of the stomach and the duodenum have a greater access to the so-called free peritoneal cavity than those on the posterior wall. Ulcers of the posterior wall may penetrate the underlying organs, such as the left lobe of the liver, the pancreas, or the gastrohepatic ligament. These may block the ulcer and prevent the entry of gastric or duodenal contents into the peritoneal cavity. This blocked perforation, in which a new floor for the ulcer has been organized outside the visceral wall, is called *chronic perforation* or *penetration,* whereas the term *subacute perforation* is reserved for certain tiny ruptures in the serosa that occur only with the relatively slowly advancing penetration of a chronic gastric ulcer. In such cases, fibrous adhesions to contiguous parenchymal organs or peritoneal attachments result from periinflammatory tissue reactions, long before the ulcer has permeated the serosal layer. Adhesions intercept the small amount of gastric content that might escape through the usually tiny apertures, thus enveloping the fluid, which may lead to the development of localized abscesses.

Free perforation occurs most frequently with ulcers of the anterior wall of the duodenal bulb. The hole resulting from an acute perforation is usually round, varying in diameter from 2 to 4 mm. One of the characteristic features of these holes is their sharp edge, which makes them appear to have been punched out. Surrounding tissue may fail to show any signs of chronic induration, edema, or inflammation.

Acute and free perforations, whether in the stomach or duodenum, are dramatic episodes. Perforation causes sudden, excruciating, explosive pain throughout the abdomen that may radiate to the chest and shoulder. The patient becomes pale and often breaks into a cold sweat. To reduce the abdominal pain, the patient may flex the thighs toward the abdomen, which is extremely rigid and tender. This early phase may last 10 minutes to a few hours, and depending in part on the amount and type of GI content released into the peritoneal cavity, the patient's body temperature becomes subnormal, but the pulse rate and blood pressure remain within normal ranges (pulse rate may even be rather slow). Breathing may become superficial and panting. Within a short time, sometimes introduced by a period of apparent subjective improvement, all the typical signs (nausea, vomiting, dry tongue, rapid pulse, fever, leukocytosis) of severe, acute, diffuse peritonitis appear. The tenderness, in the early phase confined mostly to the upper part of the abdomen, has spread over the total abdominal area. It may be excessive in the lower-right quadrant if, with a perforated duodenal ulcer, the intestinal material dissipates into the right lumbar gutter along the ascending colon.

Diagnosis

The differential diagnosis between a perforated gastric or duodenal ulcer and pancreatitis or mesenteric thrombosis may be difficult, but these signs are seldom encountered with a ruptured appendix. Other conditions, such as ectopic pregnancy, ruptured diverticulum, renal colic, acute episodes of biliary tract disease, acute intestinal obstruction or volvulus, and sometimes coronary thrombosis, must be considered.

The most helpful sign to confirm a suspected diagnosis of ulcer perforation is the presence of free air in the peritoneal cavity, particularly in the subphrenic space, demonstrable by upright x-ray examination. If the patient can sit or stand, the air will accumulate under the diaphragm. Escaped air is rarely present only under the left diaphragm and may be detected under both diaphragmatic leaves, but usually, air is found only under the right diaphragm. Computed tomography (CT) assists in making the correct diagnosis when there is clinical uncertainty or no free air is present.

Treatment and Prognosis

If escaped air is found, emergency surgery is indicated. The prognosis for the patient with a perforated gastric or duodenal ulcer is better when surgery is performed early. At present, the procedure of choice is closure of the perforation. If the facilities are suboptimal and the patient is in poor general condition, efforts to treat conservatively with suction through an indwelling catheter in the stomach, massive antibiotics, and supportive therapy entail greater risk and are less successful than surgery. Closing the perforation, irrigating the peritoneum, and administering antibiotics currently represent the usual treatment. In some patients, more definitive ulcer surgery, such as vagotomy with or without resection, may be considered.

Chronic Perforation
Clinical Picture and Pathophysiology
Erosion of the serosal layer by a chronic peptic ulcer on the posterior walls of the stomach and duodenum and its penetration into a contiguous organ is a slow process; the patient may not even feel the actual perforation. Typical ulcer pains, associated with and relieved by eating, gradually become continuous, gnawing, boring pain that no longer responds to the ingestion of food. The pain may radiate to the back, shoulder, clavicular areas, or umbilicus or down to the

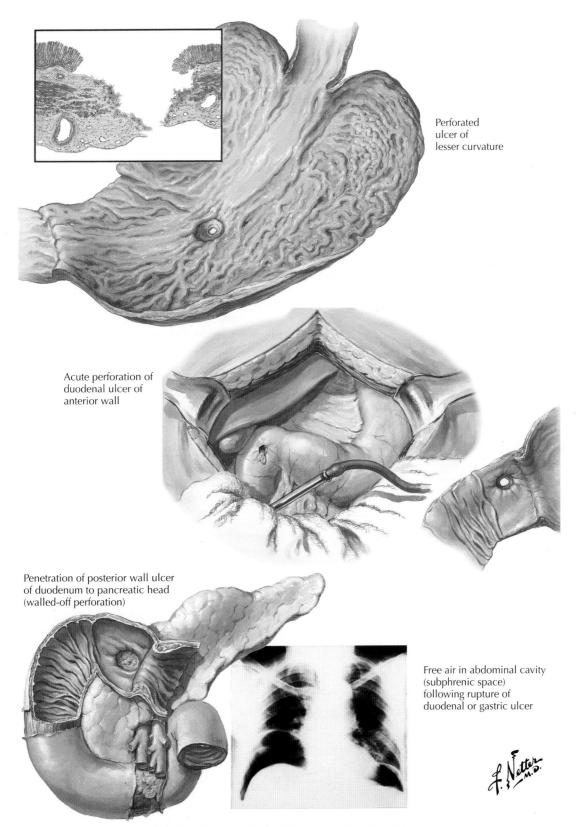

Perforated ulcer of lesser curvature

Acute perforation of duodenal ulcer of anterior wall

Penetration of posterior wall ulcer of duodenum to pancreatic head (walled-off perforation)

Free air in abdominal cavity (subphrenic space) following rupture of duodenal or gastric ulcer

Fig. 34.3 Complications of Gastric and Duodenal Ulcers.

lumbar vertebrae and the pubic or inguinal regions. A classic example of chronic perforation is the ulcer of the posterior wall of the duodenal bulb, penetrating into and walled off by the pancreas. During surgery for this condition, while attempting to remove the entire ulcer with its floor in the pancreatic tissue, the surgeon risks producing a pancreatic lesion that may open accessory pancreatic ducts. Therefore it may be advisable to leave the ulcer floor untouched after careful dissection of the ulcer from the duodenal wall.

Ulcers located in the upper parts of the posterior duodenal wall tend to penetrate the hepatoduodenal ligament. This process is usually accompanied by the development of extensive, fibrous, and thickened adhesions, to which the greater omentum may contribute. The supraduodenal and retroduodenal portions of the common bile duct, coursing within the leaves of the ligament, may become compromised in these adhesions. As a result of a constriction or distortion of the common duct, mild obstructive icterus may confuse the clinical picture. Fortunately, perforation into the duct with subsequent cholangitis is rare. Acute, perforated ulcers of the posterior gastric wall seldom release chyme into the bursa omentalis, only producing signs of localized peritonitis without free air in the abdominal cavity.

Diagnosis

Endoscopy is invariably performed when the symptoms are chronic. The presence or absence of *H. pylori* is established and the degree of damage assessed. CT is essential to further determine the damage caused by scarring and to assess whether surgery is needed. If bile or pancreatic ducts are involved, magnetic resonance imaging (MRI) or endoscopic retrograde cholangiopancreatography (ERCP) may be needed.

Treatment and Prognosis

Each patient must be evaluated carefully to decide whether medical treatment with eradication of any infection and PPI therapy will enable healing or whether surgical intervention is necessary. The location of the perforated area will influence the choice of surgical approach. Again, the course will depend on these factors. If the pancreas or bile ducts require revision, the course will be prolonged, and morbidity and mortality will be higher.

Obstruction
Clinical Picture and Pathophysiology

Another typical complication of chronic relapsing duodenal or juxtapyloric ulcer is *stenosis of the pylorus*, which develops as the result of the gradual thickening of the duodenal wall and the progressive fibrotic narrowing of the lumen. The incidence of complete pyloric stenosis as

a sequela to ulcer has decreased in recent decades because of improved medical management of this type of ulcer and prompt recognition of its initial phases. When the pyloric lumen begins to narrow, the stomach tries to overcome the impediment by increased peristalsis, and its muscular wall becomes hypertrophic. This stage is called *compensated pyloric stenosis* because, with these adaptation phenomena, the stomach succeeds in expelling its contents with only mild degrees of gastric retention. Later, when the lumen is appreciably narrowed, the expulsive efforts of the stomach fail, and the clinical picture is dominated by incessant vomiting and distress resulting from progressive dilation of the stomach, which at times may be massive.

Treatment

Decompensated pyloric stenosis, resulting in the retention of ingested material and the products of gastric secretion, is irreversible and is an unequivocal indication for surgical intervention.

Hemorrhage

Minor bleeding occurs in most patients with acute or chronic peptic ulcer. Occult blood can be found in the stools or gastric juice of most ulcer patients, the result of the oozing characteristic of ulcerative lesions. Along with perforation, massive hemorrhage is the most dangerous ulcer complication, but fortunately, it occurs much less often than minor bleeding. It has been estimated that of all massive hemorrhages of the GI tract, 50% stem from peptic ulcer.

The diagnosis, course, and treatment of acute and chronic bleeding are discussed in Chapter 34.

ADDITIONAL RESOURCES

Brunicardi FC: *Schwartz's principles of surgery*, ed 10, New York, 2015, McGraw-Hill Education.

Chan FFL, Lan JYN: Peptic ulcer disease. In Feldman M, Friedman LS, Brandt LJ, editors: *Gastrointestinal and liver disease*, ed 8, Philadelphia, 2006, Saunders-Elsevier, pp 864–899.

Gisbert JP, Calvet X: *Helicobacter pylori* "test-and-treat" strategy for management of dyspepsia: a comprehensive review, *Clin Transl Gastroenterol* 4e32, 2013.

Kelly KA, Sarr MG, Hinder RA: *Mayo clinic gastrointestinal surgery*, Philadelphia, 2004, Saunders.

Laine L, Takeuchi K, Tarnawski A: Gastric mucosal defense and cytoprotection: Bench to bedside, *Gastroenterology* 135:41–60, 2008.

Malfertheiner P, Megraud F, O'Morain CA, et al: Management of Helicobacter pylori infection-The Maastricht IV/Florence Consensus Report, *Gut* 61: 646–664, 2012.

35

Upper Gastrointestinal Bleeding

Martin H. Floch

Gastrointestinal (GI) bleeding may indicate acute or chronic loss of blood from the GI tract. It may originate in the upper or the lower part of the tract. Acute bleeding may be life threatening; chronic bleeding is slow or even occult (Fig. 35.1). The GI tract can lose as much as 50 mL of blood per day, which is replaced, without anemia, but it is a signal of a GI lesion. This chapter discusses upper GI bleeding; Chapter 82 describes lower intestinal bleeding.

The incidence of bleeding from the upper GI tract is approximately 100 cases per 100,000 population. The most common cause of upper GI hemorrhage is peptic ulceration of the stomach or duodenum, with or without aspirin or nonsteroidal antiinflammatory drug (NSAID) use. Approximately 50% of duodenal ulcers are silent. Clacerations from excessive vomiting with trauma, and then simple erosive disease of the stomach or duodenum. Less common causes are vascular ectasia, Dieulafoy vascular malformation, upper GI neoplasm, severe esophagitis, and rare causes of severe bleeding such fistula, hemobilia, and esophageal ulceration or lesion. Age appears to be a major factor; elderly persons are at increased risk and make up 30% to 45% of the population with upper GI bleeding. Portal hypotension and esophagogastric variceal bleeding are discussed in Section IX.

CLINICAL PICTURE

Patients with massive upper GI bleeding may also have hematochezia (blood in feces), causing them to quickly seek treatment. Other patients bleed slowly and seek treatment after significant anemia and paleness have developed. Often, patients with slow bleeding report weakness, but the paleness is apparent on first examination. In patients with acute bleeding, the massive loss of blood may manifest as sudden syncope or, in emergency situations, as hypovolemia with significant hypotension and occasionally shock.

The patient with slow GI bleeding may seek treatment for anemia, with findings of paleness and weakness. In other patients, the bleeding may truly be occult, and stool samples will be positive for occult blood at routine examination.

Syncope, hematochezia, melena, and hypotension are emergencies requiring hospitalization and circulatory stabilization.

If the bleeding is occult and the presentation is iron-deficiency anemia, the presentation may merely be of a patient seeking a cause for the iron loss. The workup and differential diagnosis may follow on an outpatient basis.

DIAGNOSIS

It is rare that a patient bleeds so heavily that he or she is brought to the operating room without a diagnostic evaluation; endoscopy is readily available in most emergency situations. Endoscopy is performed with or without prior cleansing lavage of the stomach, depending on the patient's condition and the endoscopist's preference. Identifying gastric or duodenal peptic disease may be simple but is often obscured by blood coating or clots in the stomach. Varices usually are easily identified, as are vascular lesions, which can include vascular ectasia, arteriovenous malformation, hereditary hemorrhagic telangiectasia, and angioma. Vascular lesions are difficult to identify and may not become apparent until the bleeding slows and the stomach is emptied. Upper endoscopy is the best procedure for diagnosing GI bleeding. However, occasionally, it is difficult to establish the exact source, and angiography may be helpful. When direct endoscopy is nondiagnostic, wireless capsule endoscopy should be performed as soon as possible to identify the bleeding site or lesion.

For patients with occult bleeding, or when it is unclear from endoscopy whether a small lesion is causing the bleeding, the diagnostic tools available are angiography and capsule endoscopy. Enteroscopy with a longer upper endoscope may be helpful, but full-length, small-bowel enteroscopy of the ileum is difficult to perform and is used less often than wireless capsule endoscopy, which is simple and has become the procedure of choice when the diagnosis is uncertain. Double-balloon enteroscopy to visualize the small bowel is another choice when a lesion is suspected on capsule evaluation, but it is a difficult technique and is not used in many institutions. Whenever a patient has occult bleeding, the small bowel must be considered; thus capsule endoscopy, enteroscopy, or computed enterography is used. Vascular malformations account for almost 70% to 80% of bleeding in the small bowel and can be diagnosed using capsule endoscopy. Tumors of the small bowel are visualized with capsule endoscopy or other imaging techniques (see Section IV).

TREATMENT AND MANAGEMENT

Approximately 85% of massive upper GI bleeding is controlled by transfusion and by proton pump inhibitor (PPI) or significant antacid therapy. When the endoscopist identifies a bleeding vessel, endoscopic therapy has proven extremely successful. Epinephrine injections, cauterization, and heater-probe cautery have been successful in controlling most lesions. Nevertheless, approximately 10% to 15% of patients with severe bleeding require surgical intervention. The criterion is usually lack of control of the bleeding, as evidenced by the need for a transfusion of more than 4 to 6 units of blood. When surgery is required, the options (simple sewing vs. resection) depend on the patient's age, anatomy, and clinical status.

In patients with occult bleeding and rare lesions, the final therapy usually involves surgical intervention. However, ectasias are a major problem. When ectasias are numerous or cannot be cauterized, therapy is frustrating; if localized, surgical resection is possible; if diffuse, various modalities are attempted. Estrogen therapy has been used in different trials but has not been universally successful. For the 5% to 10% of

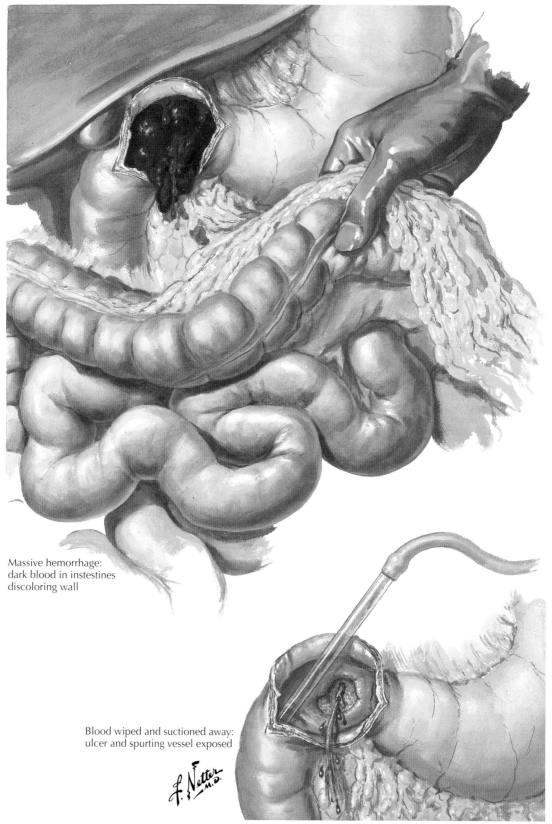

Massive hemorrhage:
dark blood in instestines
discoloring wall

Blood wiped and suctioned away:
ulcer and spurting vessel exposed

Fig. 35.1 Gastrointestinal Hemorrhage.

patients with unidentified GI bleeding, therapy becomes supportive, with intermittent blood replacement and continuing diagnostic efforts.

COURSE AND PROGNOSIS

Most GI bleeding is successfully controlled by medical therapy, and the difficult cases are controlled by surgery. The prognosis in these patients is excellent. However, mortality from acute GI bleeding ranges from 5% to 12%. When the bleeding is stopped, the prognosis for the patient is good. Inability to stop the bleeding leads to a failed outcome. It is estimated that more than 20,000 deaths occur annually in the United States because of GI bleeding. Even during surgery, it may be difficult to identify the bleeding site. Intraoperative endoscopy has been helpful, but if the cause of the bleeding cannot be found, the prognosis is guarded, especially for the elderly patient.

If the cause of occult bleeding cannot be determined, patient and physician are similarly frustrated. Slow bleeds are easily handled with transfusion and iron replacement, but prognoses vary. Prognoses for specific lesions are discussed under the appropriate disease chapters (e.g., neoplasms, varices, lower GI bleeding).

ADDITIONAL RESOURCES

Gralnek IM, Barkun AN, Bardou M: Management of acute bleeding from a peptic ulcer, *N Engl J Med* 359:928–937, 2008.

Savides TJ, Jensen DM: Gastrointetinal bleeding. In Feldman M, Friedman LS, Brandt LJ, editors: *Gastrointestinal and liver disease*, ed 10, Philadelphia, 2016, Saunders-Elsevier, pp 297–335.

Villaneuva C, Colomo A, Bosch A, et al: Transfusion strategies for acute upper gastrointestinal bleeding, *N Engl J Med* 368:11–21, 2013.

36

Therapeutic Gastrointestinal Endoscopy

Martin H. Floch

Visualization of the proximal gastrointestinal (GI) tract began in 1868 with Adolfe Kussmaul, who was able to visualize the stomach using a rigid tube. Later, Rudolf Schindler used lenses to make the lower half of the "gastroscope" flexible. By 1960, Basel Hirskowitz helped to develop and popularize the use of fiberoptics with a flexible "fiberscope" that permitted intubation of the duodenum. Videoendoscopes were introduced in 1983, using a chip, a charge-coupled device, of a photosensitive silicon grid to produce current by means of photoactivation. Many revisions and technologic advances followed, and videoscopes are now standard equipment for all endoscopists. Additional developments enabled use of therapeutic techniques in the esophagus, stomach, and duodenum. Attaching an ultrasound receiver to the tip of the scope has further developed endoscopy as a diagnostic tool by combining endoscopy with ultrasound (EUS).

STANDARD PROCEDURE

Upper endoscopy, or esophagogastroduodenoscopy (EGD), is now performed as an ambulatory procedure. After appropriate consent is obtained, the patient is sedated. The type of sedation used varies greatly across countries and institutions. Some still use simple topical anesthesia, whereas others choose sedation or general anesthesia. The most common sedation is often referred to as "conscious" sedation and consists of pain relief and some form of sleep induction that may have an amnesic effect. Meperidine or fentanyl plus diazepam or midazolam is frequently used.

Standard endoscopy is used for diagnostic purposes and has channels that permit biopsy specimens to be obtained for histologic evaluation. The development of flexible videoscopes with larger channels and various angulations created a revolution in instrumentation and enhanced the development of therapeutic procedures (Fig. 36.1).

THERAPEUTIC PROCEDURES

In *pneumatic dilatation* for achalasia, guidewires are placed through an endoscope into the stomach. A pneumatic, dilating hydrostatic balloon is passed over the guidewire and positioned across the lower esophageal sphincter (LES). The balloon is then inflated, and the increased hydrostatic pressure tears the sphincter. Although most gastroenterologists recommend pneumatic dilatation, many prefer *surgical splitting* of the sphincter. *Clostridium botulinum* toxin (botulinum toxin A, Botox) administration is usually reserved for patients unable to undergo surgery or vigorous pneumatic dilatation.

Monopolar and *bipolar electrocoagulation* and *heater probe* are used to coagulate mucosa. They are especially helpful in treating bleeding ulcers. The tip of the probe is placed directly on the bleeding side or on the four quadrants surrounding it. Coagulation occurs, and the bleeding usually stops.

In *laser treatment,* the flexible quartz probe is passed through the endoscopic channel and can conduct either an argon or an Nd:YAG laser so that the light beam "hits" tissue. This may be used to coagulate or ablate bleeding sites, ectasias, or tumors. It has been a useful procedure but has not gained wide acceptance. Laser treatment for esophageal cancer is a palliative procedure, but the principle is the same as that used for bleeding.

Injection therapy to control bleeding requires a thin flexible catheter with a retractable needle at the tip. An agent is injected into the mucosa to occlude vessels around a bleeding site, including ethanol, diluted epinephrine, and other sclerosing agents. This is often used to stop bleeding vessels. Saline injection is also used to raise a small lesion from the wall so that it can be more easily snared. (This technique is used in the colon to remove flat polyps.)

The use of *injection and banding* for sclerosis of esophageal varices is described in Section IX. Both techniques are important and have been successful in controlling and treating variceal bleeding.

Once a stricture is identified in the esophagus, it is customary to dilate. *Esophageal dilatation* techniques include (1) "blind" passage with weighted catheters; (2) *savory dilatation,* in which a guidewire is passed into the stomach and successively larger catheters are passed over the guidewire through the stricture; and (3) *balloon dilatation,* in which a collapsed balloon is passed through the endoscope and, once placed at the stricture site, is inflated to stretch or tear the stricture. Metal dilators (Eder-Puestow) are available. Savory dilators are hard plastic, and hydrostatic balloon dilators consist of plastic polymers. Weighted bougies can be passed with no sedation or local sedation, whereas savory dilators and hydrostatic balloons require endoscopy.

Plastic or metal *stents* are passed through a large port channel of an endoscope and used to bridge malignant lesions in the esophagus. The stents are temporary but provide effective palliation for short periods.

With *polypectomy,* polyps in the esophagus, stomach, and colon can be removed by passing a snare through the endoscope. The endoscopist loops the snare around the base of the polyp, then applies cautery to cut the base. The polyp is removed through suction or, if too large, is retrieved by removing the scope with the polyp held by the snare's loop or by suction. The same technique can be used in any of the hollow organs. At times, the snare is flat. When the base can be lifted by saline injection, the mucosa can be snared and the tissue retrieved.

Endoscopic retrograde cholangiopancreatography is described in detail in Section VII. Using a lateral-viewing scope, the endoscopist can cut the sphincter in the ampulla with electric cautery, permitting removal of stones, passage of stents to dilate strictures in the common duct, and passage of special scopes to visualize the common duct or pancreatic ducts.

Esophageal and gastric foreign bodies (boluses) can be removed through an endoscope using loops, snares, and baskets. If the bolus is soft, it can be broken up and pushed into the stomach. If the bolus

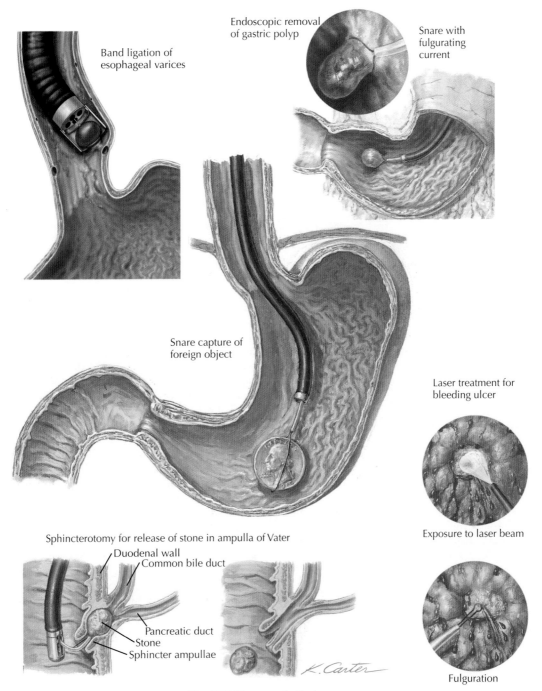

Band ligation of esophageal varices

Endoscopic removal of gastric polyp

Snare with fulgurating current

Snare capture of foreign object

Laser treatment for bleeding ulcer

Exposure to laser beam

Sphincterotomy for release of stone in ampulla of Vater

Duodenal wall
Common bile duct
Pancreatic duct
Stone
Sphincter ampullae

Fulguration

K. Carter

Fig. 36.1 Therapeutic Endoscopy.

is firm or hard, it can be snared for retrieval. The technique used varies with the size and type of bolus and the patient's condition. Some endoscopists use an *overtube* to remove parts of the obstructing bolus with the scope and then pass the scope again to continue to remove the bolus. Boluses in the stomach can be large, and surgery may be needed if they cannot be broken up or removed. After a bolus is removed from the esophagus, follow-up endoscopy is usually performed when the traumatized area has healed, to ensure that the patient does not have a chronic disease and to establish the cause of the obstructing event.

ADDITIONAL RESOURCES

ASGE Standards of Practice Committee, Faulx AL, Lightdale JR, et al: Guidelines for privileging, credentialing, and proctoring to perform GI endoscopy, *Gastrointest Endosc* 85:273–281, 2017.

Dam JV: *Gastrointestinal endoscopy*, Boston, 2004, Landes Bioscience.

Ginsberg GG, Kochman ML, Norton I, Gustout CJ: *Clinical gastrointestinal endoscopy*, Philadelphia, 2005, Saunders-Elsevier.

Policy and Procedure Manual for Gastrointestinal Endoscopy: Guidelines for Training and Practice, Manchester, Mass, 2002, American Society for Gastrointestinal Endoscopy.

37

Benign Tumors of the Stomach and Gastrointestinal Stromal Tumors

Martin H. Floch

Benign tumors of the stomach are relatively rare. Numerous autopsy studies reveal that gastric polyps are present in approximately 0.1% of gastric specimens. However, with the advent of endoscopy, small tumors have been more readily identified (Fig. 37.1). These tumors can be classified as epithelial, submucosal, and ectopic.

Benign tumors of epithelial origin include hyperplastic, fundic gland, and adenomatous polyps. Submucosal lesions include leiomyomas, lipomas, fibromas, hamartomas, hemangiomas, neurofibromas, gastrointestinal stromal tumors (GISTs), eosinophilic granulomas, and inflammatory polyps. Ectopic tissue, such as pancreatic rests or Brunner gland hyperplasia, may result in apparently benign tumors.

CLINICAL PICTURE

In general, benign tumors are asymptomatic and are identified on radiography or endoscopy. Although benign, these tumors may be associated with bleeding or obstructive phenomena. Severe, acute bleeding may occur with a lipoma that has surface erosion and an active bleeding vessel on the surface. Chronic bleeding and anemia may develop from an intermittent or slow leak from the polyp. A rare presentation is gastric outlet obstruction caused by prolapse of a large polyp into the duodenum.

DIAGNOSIS

If the lesion is identified using radiography, barium contrast, or computed tomography (CT), endoscopy is required for biopsy and further evaluation. Endoscopic ultrasound (EUS) is helpful to evaluate the depth of the lesion, and characteristic findings of various benign lesions confirm diagnosis. Initial endoscopy with biopsy is often preferred. It may be possible to remove the entire lesion endoscopically; therefore the procedure is therapeutic.

TREATMENT AND COURSE

Small lesions may be hyperplastic polyps, fundic gland polyps, or adenomas. All are benign and of epithelial origin. Once histologic diagnosis is made, these require no further therapy. Dilated, distorted fundic glands are usually very small polyps, smaller than 1 cm, but they may develop in large numbers. *Fundic gland polyps* are usually asymptomatic and are not associated with bleeding. Frequently, the polyps are hyperplastic and consist of a proliferation of epithelial elements without atypia. *Hyperplastic polyps* also are very small and are not premalignant or associated with bleeding. *Adenomatous polyps* (adenomas) may be larger than fundic gland or hyperplastic polyps. Adenomas have the potential for malignancy and may be associated with adenocarcinoma.

The risk for carcinoma, once adenomatous polyps are identified, may be as high as 10%. Once the lesion is larger than 2 cm, it is associated with malignancy. These polyps should be removed, and patients with adenomas should be enrolled in a surveillance program once the adenomatous histology is identified.

GISTs, also referred to as *mesenchymal stromal tumors,* are derived from smooth muscle. GISTs make up to 70% of all GI mesenchymal tumors. They tend to be slow growing and often are not diagnosed until the fifth or sixth decade of life. However, they may be associated with bleeding and upper GI distress. Unfortunately, a certain percentage is malignant and does metastasize. When GISTs are identified at endoscopy but are too deep for histologic examination, EUS can help to define the depth and identify possible lymph node involvement. The tumors must be surgically removed. At surgery, the specimen can be graded, depending on the number of mitoses. If the mitotic rate is greater than 2 per 10 high-power fields, the lesions are more likely to metastasize and spread (see Chapter 34). GIST is augmented, and it will require ongoing oncologic therapy.

Very small lesions (<1 cm), identified as stromal on EUS, may be monitored. However, if they become larger than 2 to 3 cm, they should be removed so that the histology and aggressiveness of the tumor can be determined and metastasis can be prevented.

Gastric tumors may develop as part of hereditary *gastrointestinal polyposis syndromes.* Gastric lesions are seen in conjunction with familial adenomatous polyposis. Although they are invariably benign, severe dysplasia has been reported in some patients. Given that these patients often undergo colectomy, their stomachs and their duodenums have to be monitored carefully.

Patients with *Peutz-Jeghers syndrome* have formation of *hamartomatous polyps* (hamartomas) in the small intestine and may have stomach hamartomas (24% in one series). These polyps are invariably benign, but malignancy has been reported; therefore these patients must have their stomachs and their small bowels monitored. Patients with *juvenile polyposis* also have multiple hamartomas. Although the syndrome can occur rarely in the stomach, it is more often associated with colonic lesions. As in Peutz-Jeghers syndrome, potential malignancy is a concern; therefore patients with juvenile polyposis should also be monitored.

PROGNOSIS

Simple polyps of the stomach that reveal no other risk factors or familial syndromes usually imply a benign prognosis. However, if a GIST is suspected or if the polyps are associated with familial syndromes, patients should be monitored carefully for potential malignancy (see Chapter 34).

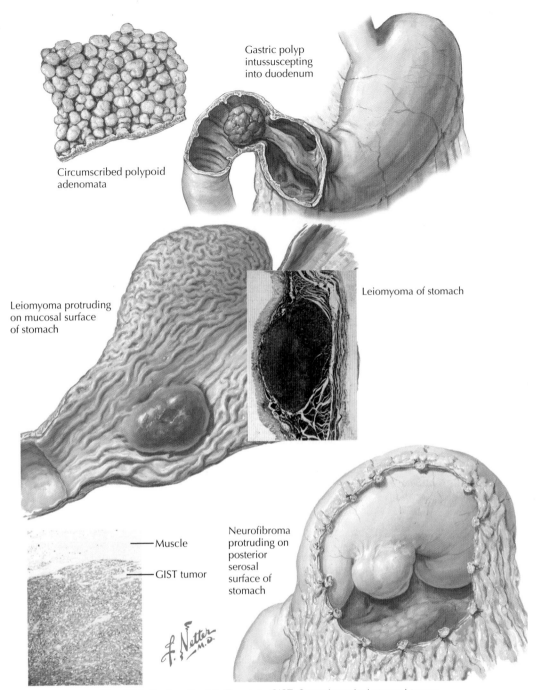

Gastric polyp intussuscepting into duodenum

Circumscribed polypoid adenomata

Leiomyoma protruding on mucosal surface of stomach

Leiomyoma of stomach

Muscle

GIST tumor

Neurofibroma protruding on posterior serosal surface of stomach

Fig. 37.1 Benign Gastric Tumors. *GIST,* Gastrointestinal stromal tumor.

ADDITIONAL RESOURCES

Burt RW: Gastric fundic gland polyps, *Gastroenterology* 125:1462–1469, 2003.

El-Omar EM, McLean MH: Tumors of the stomach. In Podolsky DK, Camilleri M, Fitz JG, et al, editors: *Yamada's textbook of gastroenterology,* ed 6, West Sussex England, 2015, Wiley-Blackwell, pp 1121–1140.

Feldman M: Gastrointestinal stromal tumors (GISTs). In Feldman M, Friedman LS, Brandt LJ, editors: *Gastrointestinal and liver disease,* ed 10, Philadelphia, 2016, Saunders-Elsevier, pp 487–500.

He Z, Sun C, Zheng Z, et al: Endoscopic submucosal dissection of large gastrointestinal stromal tumors in the esophagus and stomach, *J Gastroenterol Hepatol* 28:262–267, 2013.

Perez DR, Baser RE, Cavnar MJ, et al: Blood neutrophil-to-lymphocyte ratio is prognostic in gastrointestinal stromal tumor, *Ann Surg Oncol* 20:593–599, 2013.

38

Gastrointestinal Lymphoma and Mucosa-Associated Lymphoid Tissue

Martin H. Floch

Lymphomas of the stomach are of two types, both of B-lymphocyte origin: marginal zone B-cell lymphoma of the mucosa-associated lymphoid tissue (MALT) type and diffuse, large B-cell lymphoma (Fig. 38.1).

MUCOSA-ASSOCIATED LYMPHOID TISSUE TUMOR

The stomach is the most common site of lymphoma in Western societies. The MALT type arises from malignant transformation of B cells that exist normally in the gut but that proliferate in the inflammatory process. Gastric tissue acquires MALT in the pathologic response to *Helicobacter pylori* infection. The MALT type represents 40% of gastric lymphomas.

Because MALT tumor is related to *H. pylori* infection, the incidence is higher where there is a greater incidence of chronic infection. Evidence has established that *H. pylori* has a key role in the development of MALT lymphoma. It is believed that the disease starts with *H. pylori* infection, which causes gastritis and initiates the immune response of T and B cells. In this tissue, MALT is formed. *H. pylori*–reactive T cells drive B-cell proliferation, which eventually leads to genetic abnormalities that result in aggressive tumor activity.

Tumors are often located in the antrum, but they can be multifocal in as many as 33% of patients. MALT lymphomas may appear as erosions, erythema, or ulcers. Histologically, there is invasion and partial destruction of gastric glands by tumor cells. Cells are usually small and infiltrate the lamina propria. Often, it is difficult to make the diagnosis of lymphoma when the lesions are small. However, invasion and distortion of the tissue clarify the diagnosis. MALT lymphomas are usually staged as follows:

- Stage I: tumors are confined to the mucosa.
- Stage II: tumors extend into the abdomen.
- Stage III (II$_E$): tumors penetrate the serosa to involve adjacent organs.
- Stage IV: tumors are disseminated to nodal tissue and beyond, or they are supradiaphragmatic.

Clinical Picture

Patients with MALT tumors usually have epigastric pain or dyspepsia. However, some may present with nausea, bleeding, or weight loss.

Diagnosis

Diagnosis of MALT tumors is made by endoscopic visualization and tissue biopsy. Thorough evaluation must include computed tomography (CT) of the abdomen, pelvis, and chest, evaluation of bone marrow, and measurement of serum lactate dehydrogenase (LDH) concentration, which is usually normal in MALT and elevated in other lymphomas. Endoscopic ultrasound (EUS) is important to assess the extent through the wall and to assess nodal involvement. After the histologic diagnosis, staging is essential.

Treatment, Course, and Prognosis

During stage I, MALT is treated with antibiotic eradication of *H. pylori*; the recommended regimens are listed in Chapter 32. Monitoring and follow-up are essential. At 1 to 2 months, eradication must be established, with tumor regression recorded at endoscopy. When the tumor is eradicated, follow-up endoscopy must be performed at 6-month intervals for 2 years. Complete remission is reported in 70% of patients. Remissions occur rapidly but may take as long as 18 months.

Reinfection and relapse have been reported; incomplete remission or removal is always a concern. Controversy surrounds the use of surgery, which some believe is indicated for all MALT tumors.

In stage II or II$_E$ (III), antibiotic eradication of *H. pylori* has been attempted, with reports of complete remission. However, most oncologists agree that chemotherapy should be added for these patients, and some recommend surgery with or without radiation. This vigorous regimen has resulted in an 82% survival rate.

Stage IV disease requires chemotherapy and evaluation for local radiation with or without surgery; prognosis is guarded.

DIFFUSE LARGE B-CELL LYMPHOMA

Diffuse, large B-cell lymphoma tumors make up 45% to 50% of gastric lymphomas, but their cause is not clear. Although associated, *H. pylori* infection has not been implicated as causing large B-cell lymphoma of the stomach. Therefore eradicating *H. pylori* is not considered adequate therapy when diffuse, large B-cell lymphoma is identified. Lesions occur in the body and in the antrum of the stomach and tend to be multifocal. They typically invade the tunica muscularis, and histology reveals clusters or sheets of large cells. As many as 40% of these patients show evidence of MALT association, but once it evolves, a large B-cell mass is the primary diagnosis and concern.

Clinical Picture

These lesions are ulcerating and therefore may present with bleeding. Some lesions are large enough to cause symptoms of obstruction. Patients may have pain and associated nausea or anorexia. An elevated LDH concentration sometimes occurs.

Diagnosis

Evaluation must include upper endoscopy and CT evaluation of the chest, abdomen, and pelvis. EUS is helpful for assessing the full depth of the lesion in the wall of the stomach and the surrounding nodes.

Treatment, Course, and Prognosis

Approximately 70% of patients with stage I disease have no recurrence for 5 years with surgical therapy. However, some investigators believe that with adequate endoscopic diagnosis, patients can be treated with

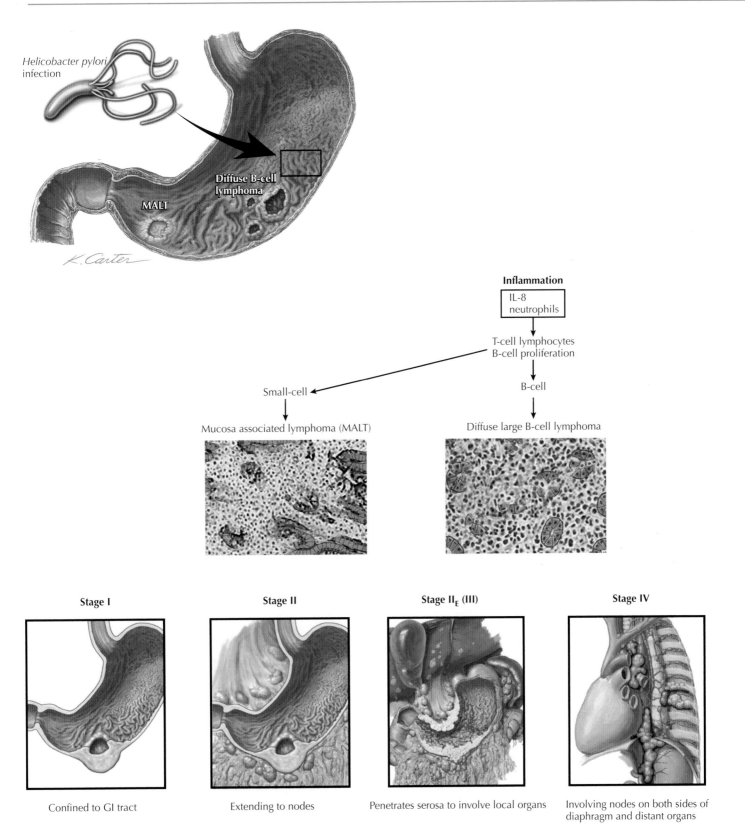

Fig. 38.1 Gastric Lymphoma and Mucosa-Associated Lymphoid Tissue *(MALT)* Tumor. *GI,* Gastrointestinal; *IL-8,* interleukin-8.

multiple chemotherapy regimens and radiation without surgery, providing there is thorough EUS evaluation. Large B-cell lymphoma appears to be responsive to radiation and to chemotherapy. Therefore controversy surrounds the role of surgery and the relative roles of chemotherapy and radiation. Many oncologists think that radiation results in relapses and that chemotherapy thus should be combined with radiation, which has become the standard of care when nodes are involved. There is a large study in which the authors feel that rituximad produces superior event-free survival in the treatment of patients with extranodal marginal zone B-cell lymphoma. Surgery should be considered in all these patients in combination with radiation and chemotherapy. One series reported survival at 40%.

When *H. pylori* infection is identified and treated, diffuse large B-cell lymphoma has responded to antibiotic therapy in rare cases, but such unimodal treatment is not recommended.

ADDITIONAL RESOURCES

Bautista-Quach MA, Ake CD, Chen M, et al: Gastrointestinal lymphomas: morphology, immunophenotyped and molecular features, *J Gastrointest Oncol* 3:209–225, 2012.

Ferreri AJ, Govi S, Raderer M, et al: *Helicobacter pylori* eradication as exclusive treatment for limited-stage gastric diffuse large B-cell lymphomas. Results of a multicenter phase 2 trial, *Blood* 120:3858–3860, 2012.

Fischbach W, Al-Taie O: Staging role of EUS, *Best Pract Res Clin Gastroenterol* 24:13–17, 2010.

Li HC, Collins RH: Gastrointestinal lymphomas. In Feldman M, Friedman LS, Brandt LJ, editors: *Gastrointestinal and liver disease*, ed 10, Philadelphia, 2016, Saunders-Elsevier, pp 471–486.

Ruskone-Fourmestraux A, Fischbach W, Aleman BM, et al: Egils consensus report. Gastric extranodal marginal zone B-cell lymphoma of MALT, *Gut* 60:747–758, 2011.

Zinzani PL: The many faces of marginal zone lymphoma, *Hematology Am Soc Hematol Educ Program* 2012:426–432, 2012.

Zucca E, Conconi A, Laszlo D, et al: Addition of rituximab to chlorambucil produces superior event-free survival in the treatment of patients with extranodal marginal zone B-cell lymphoma: 5-year analysis of the IELSC-19 randomized study, *J Clin Oncol* 31:565–572, 2013.

39

Cancers of the Stomach

Martin H. Floch

Cancer involving the stomach is the second most common cancer in the world. Although it is decreasing in North America, stomach cancer continues to increase throughout the rest of the world. The incidence of adenocarcinoma has increased only in lesions at the cardioesophageal junction (Fig. 39.1).

The etiology of stomach cancer remains complex, and multiple factors are involved. Tobacco, alcohol, dietary nitrates, nitrites, and nitrosamines have all been implicated. High intake of salt has also been implicated in certain parts of the world, whereas increased refrigeration has been associated with a decrease in cancer. Epidemiologic studies show that *Helicobacter pylori* plays a role in gastric carcinogenesis. Chronic inflammation associated with *H. pylori* gastritis is the presumed mechanism. Atrophy of the gastric mucosa (as in pernicious anemia) and intestinal metaplasia are predisposing factors (see Chapter 33).

Most stomach cancers conform to one or two types: the *intestinal form,* which contains glandlike tubular structures, and the *diffuse form,* which contains poorly differentiated cells. The intestinal form is thought to involve steplike development, with the predisposing atrophic gastritis and intestinal metaplasia progressing to dysplasia and finally to cancer.

Genetic changes include loss of heterogenicity and loss of the effectiveness of P53G suppression and, in some patients, mutation of the APC/β-catenin pathway; expression of P16 and P27 is also decreased. Decreased expression of the epithelial cadherin gene in patients with diffuse gastric cancer may account for the morphologic differences between intestinal and diffuse gastric lesions. Families with hereditary diffuse gastric cancer have mutations in epithelial cadherin. Geneticists are beginning to understand the effect of environmental factors on the development of stomach cancer.

CLINICAL PICTURE

The clinical picture of stomach cancer varies greatly depending on the site of the cancer. Lesions at the cardioesophageal junction, which are increasing in incidence in North America, tend to manifest early; they cause dysphagia or early dyspepsia and are diagnosed at endoscopy in the work-up. Larger lesions in the fundus and body or ulcerating lesions may cause dyspeptic symptoms, anemia, or frank bleeding. Many are associated with anorexia and weight loss and manifest at a later stage. Of particular interest is *linitis plastica,* which diffusely involves the stomach, with a fibrotic-type histology that results in anorexia and weight loss.

DIAGNOSIS

As endoscopy becomes more effective, the diagnosis of stomach cancer is frequently made on visualization and biopsy of the lesion. Radiographic studies, still used in many parts of the world, show the classic lesions, from a bottleneck linitis plastica to an ulceration that requires endoscopic evaluation and biopsy. It is still difficult to differentiate between a benign and a malignant ulcer. Differentiating gastric ulcer requires biopsy, as well as healing. Reevaluation is done in 3 to 6 weeks to ensure the ulcer has healed; if not, vigorous repeat biopsy evaluation is necessary.

Once the lesion has been identified on histologic evaluation, endoscopic ultrasound (EUS) can be helpful in determining the extent of the lesion through the stomach wall and whether lymph nodes are involved. Small nodes can still contain malignant cells and therefore can be diagnosed only during surgical exploration. Computed tomography (CT) can assist in identifying nodes missed on EUS and should be used for full evaluation. Endoscopy, EUS, and CT enable classification and staging of the disease.

TREATMENT AND MANAGEMENT

The only curative treatment for stomach cancer is surgery to remove the lesion. Surgery also provides important palliation for patients with large or obstructing lesions. Surgery is *not* used when there is extensive linitis plastica or when the lesions have metastasized and carcinomatosis is present and resection or palliation would be useless.

The extent of surgery and lymph node resection varies, as decided by the patient and surgeon. Use of adjuvant chemotherapy or chemotherapy plus radiation is becoming more common. Depending on the center and experience of the staff, adjuvant therapy may be used before or after surgical resection. The benefits of vigorous chemotherapy and radiation after surgical resection also depend on the patient's clinical status.

Endoscopic mucosal resection of very small lesions is used in Japan. Endoscopic resection has been reserved for the intestinal histology in which EUS has demonstrated no lymph node involvement. The maximum size of the tumors has been less than 2 cm.

COURSE AND PROGNOSIS

Five-year survival rates of patients with stomach cancer range from 18% to 25% in the United States to as high as 50% in Japan. Survival may be higher in patients with very small lesions that are identified early. The intensive screening programs in Japan seem to be effective. Survival rates vary with the extent of the surgery and with the extent of the disease. Naturally, carcinoma in situ has the best prognosis. T1 lesions that involve the mucosa or submucosa have a better prognosis than T2 lesions that invade the tunica muscularis, T3 lesions that go beyond the serosa, or T4 lesions that invade adjacent organs. The stratification of lesions is further delineated by nodal involvement, which has a poor prognosis, as does any sign of metastasis.

Early gastric carcinoma, which involves T1 lesions, has up to an 85% to 90% cure rate. Because of early detection techniques, more

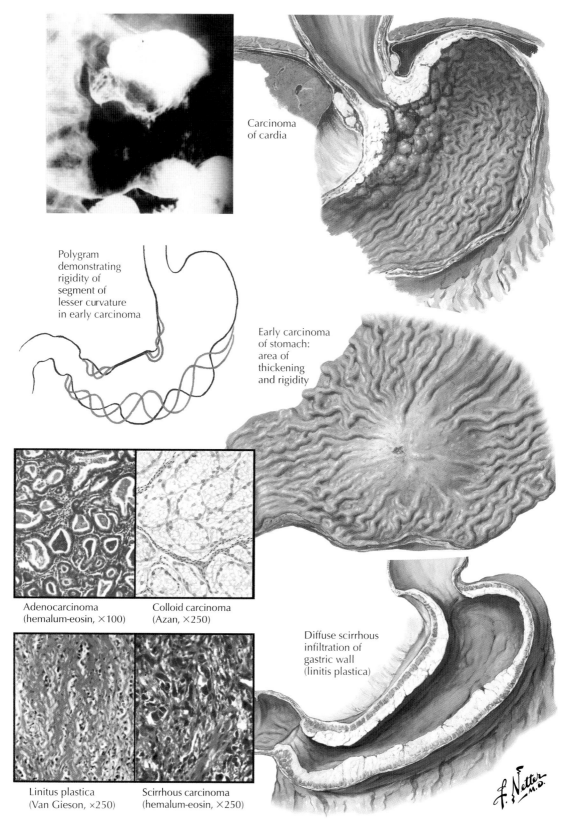

Carcinoma
of cardia

Polygram
demonstrating
rigidity of
segment of
lesser curvature
in early carcinoma

Early carcinoma
of stomach:
area of
thickening
and rigidity

Adenocarcinoma
(hemalum-eosin, ×100)

Colloid carcinoma
(Azan, ×250)

Diffuse scirrhous
infiltration of
gastric wall
(linitis plastica)

Linitus plastica
(Van Gieson, ×250)

Scirrhous carcinoma
(hemalum-eosin, ×250)

Fig. 39.1 Cancers of the Stomach.

lesions of early gastric cancer are discovered, and the prognosis has improved. Recent advances in chemotherapy have improved outcomes. Oral fluoropyrimidine S-1 has improved 3-year survival from 70% to 80% in East Asian patients who had a D2 dissection for locally advanced lesions.

GASTROINTESTINAL STROMAL TUMORS

Gastrointestinal stromal tumors (GISTs), also called *leiomyomas* or *leiomyosarcomas,* are rare (see also Chapter 33). Approximately 70% occur in the stomach, but they may also occur in other parts of the GI tract. Their phenotypic feature is that of tumors originating from smooth muscle, neural elements, or both. GISTs appear to be relatively benign lesions, but when the pathologist can count more than five mitoses per 50 high-power fields, they are considered aggressive and can be of higher risk.

Clinically, GISTs often present with bleeding or as endoscopic findings on evaluation for dyspepsia. Endoscopically, GISTs may appear thimble shaped, and on EUS, they clearly arise from the stromal cell element. When larger than 4 cm, they are considered malignant.

Treatment is surgical removal. However, if the tumors are malignant and have metastasized, GISTs may respond to the tyrosine kinase inhibitor imatinib mesylate (Gleevec), used widely as adjuvant therapy. There are imatinib-resistant GISTs, and newer agents are being developed that appear effective. Therefore an aggressive diagnostic and therapeutic approach is indicated to provide the appropriate therapy.

CARCINOID TUMORS

Approximately 2% to 3% of all carcinoid tumors arise in the stomach. They may be poorly differentiated or well differentiated, but carcinoids are thought to arise from neuroendocrine cells. They rarely have metabolic activity, unlike small-bowel carcinoids (see Chapter 68).

Carcinoid tumors are usually small and produce incidental findings when they originate in the stomach. However, there are rare reports of malignancy and spread, and these patients can have all the symptoms described for adenocarcinoma of the stomach. If the tumors are metabolically active, patients will present with the clinical picture of the small-bowel variety.

During endoscopy, carcinoid tumors may be seen as small ulcers, polyps, or tumors. They develop more frequently in patients with atrophic gastritis. The treatment of choice is removal of the lesion, but true *carcinoid syndrome* often metastasizes, and then the treatment is chemotherapy. Somatostatin has been used to control symptoms, although rarely in gastric carcinoid and primarily in the active, small-bowel lesions.

ADDITIONAL RESOURCES

Abrams JA, Quante M: Adenocarcinoma of the stomach and other gastric tumors. In Feldman M, Friedman LS, Brandt LJ, editors: *Gastrointestinal and liver disease,* ed 10, Philadelphia, 2016, Saunders-Elsevier, pp 901–920.

Bang YJ, Van Cutsem E, Feyereislova A, et al: Trastuzumab alone for treatment of HER2-posivite advanced gastric or gastro-oesophageal junction cancer (toga): a phase 3 open-label, randommised controlled trial, *Lancet* 376:687–697, 2010.

De Vries AC, van Grieken NC, Looman CW, et al: Gastric cancer risk in patients with premalignant gastric lesions: a nationwide cohort study in the Netherlands, *Gastroenterology* 134:945–952, 2008.

Dulak AM, Schumacher SE, van Lieshout J, et al: Gastrointestinal adenocarcinoma of the esophagus, stomach, and colon exhibit distinct patterns of genome instability and oncogenesis, *Cancer Res* 72:4383–4393, 2012.

Fuccio L, Zagari RM, Eusebi LH, et al: Meta-analysis: can Helicobacter pylori eradication treatement reduce the risk for gastric cancer?, *Ann Intern Med* 151:121–128, 2009.

Gupta P, Tewari M, Shukia HS: Gastrointestinal stromal tumor, *Surg Oncol* 17:129–138, 2008.

Katz SC, Dematteo RP: Gastrointestinal stromal tumors and leiomyosarcomas, *Surg Oncol* 97:350–359, 2008.

Kaurah P, MacMillan A, Boyd N, et al: Founder and recurrent CDHI mutations in families with hereditary diffuse gastric cancer, *JAMA* 297:2360–2372, 2007.

Wang C, Yuan Y, Hunt RH: The association between *Helicobacter pylori* infection and early gastric cancer: a meta-analysis, *Am J Gastroenterol* 102:1789–1798, 2007.

40

Tumors of the Duodenum

Martin H. Floch

Tumors of the duodenum are rare. The *benign* neoplasms that may be encountered are Brunner gland hyperplasia, polypoid adenomas, lipomas, leiomyomas, neurofibromas, hemangiomas, and aberrant pancreatic tissue. All benign tumors are rare and often only slightly elevated. A polyp may be on a pedicle and then appear mobile, shifting back and forth by peristaltic motion, and occasionally prolapsing into the pylorus (Fig. 40.1).

Carcinoma of the duodenum is also rare, but it is the most common site of primary small-bowel adenocarcinoma. The incidence of 0.35%, based on autopsy studies, is postulated to be a result of the rapid transit of material through the duodenum, lower bacterial load, neutralizing pH, and benzopyrene hydrolase, which is present in much higher concentrations and appears to detoxify benzopyrene, a carcinogen found in various foods. High-risk situations for adenocarcinoma are celiac sprue and familial adenomatous polyposis. Adenomas occur infrequently in patients with duodenal tumors, and the transition to malignancy does occur (see Chapter 70). Tumors of the ampulla are described in Chapter 141.

CLINICAL PICTURE

In sporadic reports, obstruction symptoms have occurred when a large polyp on a pedicle prolapsed into the pylorus, acting as a ball valve. However, the usual presentation of duodenal tumors is bleeding, anemia, or jaundice. Unfortunately, by the time of diagnosis, the lesions have frequently spread: In one series, as many as 70% were beyond the local site at presentation.

DIAGNOSIS

Endoscopy is the main tool for diagnosing duodenal tumors. Computed tomography may be helpful, and endoscopic ultrasound can assist in staging the disease. In some cases, barium contrast studies can help determine the extent of the lesion and evaluate the anatomy at surgery.

TREATMENT, COURSE, AND PROGNOSIS

Treatment is primarily surgical resection and removal of regional lymph nodes. Radical resection, including pancreaticoduodenectomy, may be of little help once node metastasis occurs. Chemotherapy is usually adjunctive or palliative.

Five-year survival rate for adenocarcinoma ranges from 10% to 20%. The presence of positive nodes reduces 5-year survival of 55% to 12%.

ADDITIONAL RESOURCES

Ferreira MR, Jung BLL: Tumors of the small intestine. In Podolsky DK, Camilleri M, Fitz JG, et al, editors: *Yamada's textbook of gastroenterology*, ed 6, Hoboken NJ, 2016, Wiley-Blackwell, pp 1324–1345.

Gill SS, Heuman DM, Mihas AA: Small intestine neoplasm, *J Clin Gastroenterol* 33:267–282, 2001.

Howe JR, Karnell LH, Menck HR, Scott-Conner C: Adenocarcinoma of the small bowel: review of the National Cancer Data Base, 1985-1995, *Cancer* 86:2693–2706, 1999.

Paski SC, Semrad CE: Small bowel tumors, *Gastrointest Endosc Clin N Am* 19:461–479, 2009.

Schottenfeld D, Beebe-Dimmer JL, Vigneau FD: The epidemiology and pathogenesis of neoplasia in the small intestine, *Ann Epidemiol* 19:58–69, 2009.

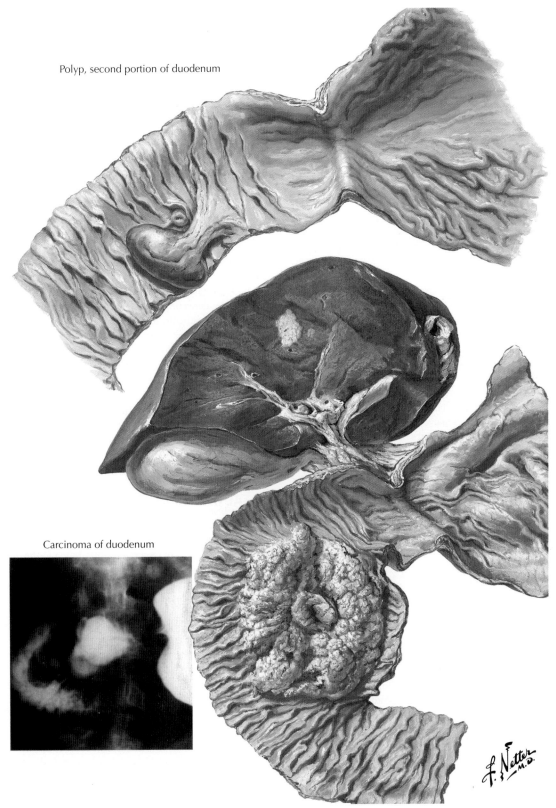

Polyp, second portion of duodenum

Carcinoma of duodenum

Fig. 40.1 Tumors of the Duodenum.

41

Principles of Gastric Surgery

Martin H. Floch

With the advent of H_2 inhibitors and proton pump inhibitors (PPIs) and treatment of *Helicobacter pylori,* gastric surgery has declined significantly. Previously, the primary indication for gastric surgery was control of peptic ulcer disease, but the success of medical therapy greatly decreased the need for gastric surgery.

Indications for gastric surgery have not changed: uncontrollable gastrointestinal (GI) bleeding, perforation, or obstruction. A recent indication for gastric surgery is control of morbid obesity (see Chapter 191).

PEPTIC ULCER SURGERY AND VAGOTOMY

The procedure of choice for the surgical treatment of gastroduodenal ulcer is *subtotal gastrectomy* (Fig. 41.1). Two thirds to three quarters of the distal portion of the stomach is removed, to reduce the acid-secreting mucosa to such a degree that the gastric juice becomes *anacidic* (achlorhydric), or at least hypoacidic. Complete removal of the entire antrum is necessary. Several procedures have been developed, but only a few have stood the test of time.

The Viennese surgeon Billroth was the first to perform partial gastrectomy, which included the pylorus and connected the distal end of the remaining stomach with the open end of the duodenum (Billroth I). In some cases, however, because of technical difficulties, a sufficiently wide duodenal cuff is not available, or fibrosis in the area or anatomic restrictions may make the procedure difficult. Therefore, Billroth developed another type of gastrectomy (Billroth II), in which the duodenal stump is closed, and the stump of the stomach is connected to a loop of jejunum. Such a gastrojejunostomy can be constructed in front of the transverse colon or in retrocolic fashion. In the antecolic procedure, surgeons are careful to ensure that the afferent loop is free from the colon, and a side-to-side anastomosis of the afferent and efferent loops is created.

Vagotomies were performed before the development of PPIs and the excellent drugs that reduce acid secretion. Although now rarely used, vagotomy may be performed during a procedure for bleeding or may be necessary during radical surgery for cancer.

Surgery for peptic ulcer disease is rarely performed. Occasionally, however, it is performed after intractable bleeding or when a patient has difficulty using medications. For these patients, truncal vagotomy with drainage, highly selective vagotomy, or truncal vagotomy and antrectomy may be selected, depending on the surgical experience and the patient. Truncal vagotomy requires identification and destruction of the anterior and posterior vagi at the level of the distal esophagus. Highly selective vagotomy attempts to preserve other functions of the vagus but eliminates vagal innervation to the acid-producing stomach by dissecting the vagal distribution along the stomach. This procedure is difficult, and risk of ulcer recurrence depends on the surgical experience. When vagotomy is performed, complementary surgery—either gastrojejunostomy, to increase drainage through the pylorus, or antrectomy—is also usually performed to ensure the stomach can empty.

ROUX-EN-Y GASTROJEJUNOSTOMY

Previously reserved for complications of gastric surgery or as part of pancreatic resection for carcinoma, Roux-en-Y gastrojejunostomy is now used for obesity surgery.

TOTAL GASTRECTOMY

Total gastrectomy is usually performed with a resultant esophagojejunostomy or colon segment interposition to preserve food transit. These radical procedures are reserved for carcinoma of the upper part of the stomach or for unusual trauma to the upper abdomen. These patients become very difficult to treat. Consequently, alternates for most types of therapy may be needed.

ADDITIONAL RESOURCES

Hass DJ: Complementary and alternative medicine. In Feldman M, Friedman LS, Brandt LJ, editors: *Gastrointestinal and liver disease,* ed 10, Philadelphia, 2016, Saunders-Elsevier, pp 244–259.

Kelly KA, Sarr MG, Hinder RA: *Mayo clinic gastroenterology surgery,* Philadelphia, 2004, Saunders.

Periyakoil VS: Palliative care for patients with gastrointestinal and hepatic disease. In Feldman M, Friedman LS, Brandt LJ, editors: *Gastrointestinal and liver disease,* ed 10, Philadelphia, 2016, Saunders-Elsevier, pp 2359–2369.

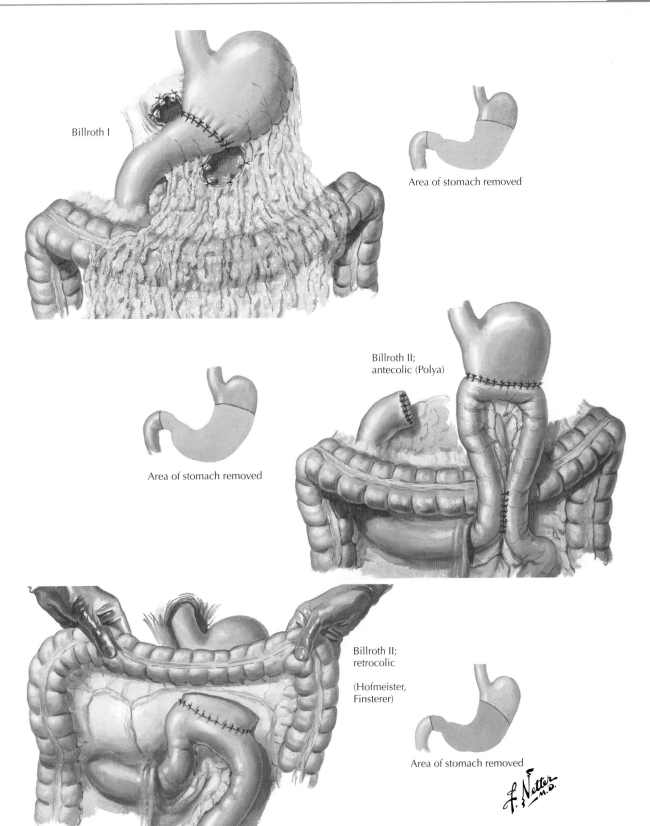

Billroth I

Area of stomach removed

Area of stomach removed

Billroth II; antecolic (Polya)

Billroth II; retrocolic

(Hofmeister, Finsterer)

Area of stomach removed

Fig. 41.1 Principles of Gastric Surgery.

42

Postgastrectomy Complications: Partial Gastrectomy

Martin H. Floch

Complications in the postgastrectomy period occur with both open and laparoscopic surgical techniques and may occur after complete healing. These include recurrent ulceration, gastroparesis (delayed gastric emptying), afferent loop syndrome, dumping syndrome and postvagotomy diarrhea, bile reflux gastritis, and gastric adenocarcinoma. Symptoms vary depending on the complication and are briefly described here.

RECURRENT ULCERATION

Marginal ulcers, or *jejunal ulcers*, are rare and may occur in less than 1% of postgastrectomy patients. These ulcers usually are caused by inadequate acid suppression, which is highly unlikely since the advent of proton pump inhibitors (PPIs), and Zollinger-Ellison syndrome is always suspected. Taking nonsteroidal antiinflammatory drugs (NSAIDs) can cause ulceration. The presenting symptom is most frequently pain, although occult bleeding and anemia have been reported. Endoscopic evaluation provides the diagnosis. Endoscopy and biopsy are essential to rule out early malignant carcinoma. These lesions can be controlled by removal of irritating drugs and PPI acid suppression. Although rarely required as treatment, if carcinoma is present, surgical resection is paramount.

GASTROPARESIS (DELAYED GASTRIC EMPTYING)

Gastroparesis is most often associated with truncal vagotomy or basic motility disturbance, as occurs in diabetes. The symptom usually is nausea or inability to eat and occasionally, vomiting of feedings. Attempts at medical treatment with prokinetic agents, such as metoclopramide or erythromycin, may be of help. Some patients have gastroparesis before their surgery, and treatment is complicated (see Chapter 4).

AFFERENT LOOP SYNDROME

Afferent loop syndrome occurs only in patients who have undergone gastrojejunostomy. The loop from the duodenum running to the gastrojejunostomy may become obstructed. The obstruction is partial and intermittent. It often creates the symptom of epigastric fullness or upper abdominal pain, which is relieved only by vomiting. The vomitus is most often bile colored to relieve the obstruction. The obstruction can be caused by scarring or adhesions or by a twisting of the intestinal loop. Diagnosis is made when the dilated loop is demonstrated on radiographic study. Endoscopy may or may not be helpful but is needed to evaluate for the presence of strictures or malignancy. However, demonstration of the dilated loop is essential, often achieved through imaging. The treatment for afferent loop syndrome is invariably surgery, with conversion of the gastrojejunostomy to either a Billroth I or a Roux-en-Y configuration. At times, the surgeon is able to reconform the gastrojejunostomy.

DUMPING SYNDROME AND POSTVAGOTOMY DIARRHEA

Dumping syndrome and postvagotomy diarrhea may be the most common complications of gastrojejunostomy, occurring in as many as 5% to 10% of procedures. Symptoms occur immediately after eating, and even during eating in some patients. Symptoms vary from epigastric discomfort and a vague feeling of oppression to sudden episodes of profuse sweating, tachycardia, tremor, and a tendency to syncope. Often, patients may deny their symptoms, but they feel relieved by eating or lying in a supine position. Some patients can adjust to the symptoms, but others cannot overcome the lightheadedness and tachycardia that may occur immediately on eating to 30 minutes after meals.

Dumping is usually triggered by jejunal distention as hypertonic gastric contents rapidly enter the small bowel (Fig. 42.1). Symptoms are usually caused by the shift in volume of fluid into the jejunum. Symptoms occurring later may be caused by hyperglycemia, which can occur 1 to 2 hours after meals. Intestinal and vasomotor symptoms develop after rapid passage of a hyperosmolar meal from the stomach pouch to the intestine. A concomitant drop in plasma volume occurs with symptoms, although this can also be demonstrated in healthy persons. The type of gastric resection is not related to the syndrome. Large quantities of hypertonic solution produce the syndrome in all patients after gastrectomy.

In the typical sequence of events, a susceptible patient eats a meal of hyperosmolar food (usually concentrated, simple carbohydrates), which rapidly enters the jejunum, where it causes a sudden shift in fluid so that a measurable fall occurs in plasma volume. Bloating, diarrhea, and varying degrees of weakness, dizziness, sweating, pallor, and tachycardia may develop. At this stage, the patient is usually hyperglycemic, but rebound hypoglycemia and hypokalemia have been recorded. Hypoglycemia is often referred to as the "late aspect" of the dumping syndrome and results from a rapid increase in blood sugar, followed by a rapid decrease that may cause symptoms.

Treatment is careful dietary management, which includes the elimination of simple-carbohydrate foods and fluid. It is usually successful in 80% of patients. Consuming high-fiber foods may also be helpful. It has been shown that guar (10 g) can prevent the syndrome. Five-gram sachets of pectin twice daily are usually effective. If all measures fail, surgical correction is needed, but this is rare.

After gastrectomy, all patients are advised to consume smaller meals, ideally six small feedings daily, and to restrict their intake of simple carbohydrates. It is best to increase the protein and fat content of the food. Most patients will learn to accommodate. Less than 1% acquire debilitating symptoms and may require conversion to a Roux-en-Y procedure. Before conversion surgery, a trial of somatostatin may be helpful now that daily injections can be decreased by depot injections.

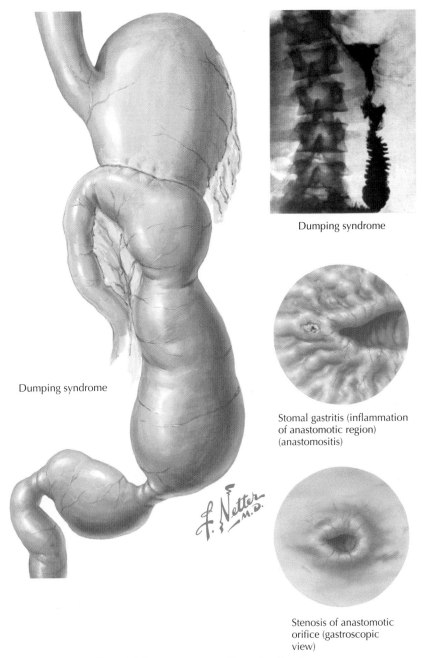

Dumping syndrome

Dumping syndrome

Stomal gastritis (inflammation of anastomotic region) (anastomositis)

Stenosis of anastomotic orifice (gastroscopic view)

Fig. 42.1 Postgastrectomy Dumping Syndrome.

Somatostatin slows emptying and delays the onset of glucose and insulin release. However, if long-term somatostatin treatment if needed, conversion to Roux-en-Y may be preferred.

Because vagotomy is rarely performed, the complication rate is low. However, many patients experience diarrhea after vagotomy. Often, patients adjust, and treatment with antidiarrheal agents, such as codeine or loperamide, helps them during the period of adjustment. Again, somatostatin may be tried if symptoms are severe.

BILE REFLUX GASTRITIS

When bile easily refluxes from the gastrojejunostomy into the gastric stump, it can cause significant inflammation of the remaining gastric lining. Patients may become symptomatic and experience pain or occasional vomiting. Although an infrequent complication, bile reflux gastritis may rarely require revision of the procedure to a Roux-en-Y. Trials of therapy with coating agents, such as sucralfate, may be helpful in selected patients. Trials to increase gastric emptying that may be delayed by the use of prokinetic agents are also suggested. To make this diagnosis, gastritis must be demonstrated by endoscopy, and it must be clearly demonstrated that the bile is causing the gastritis. This is difficult to prove; thus, trials of therapy and finally surgical recorrection may be needed.

GASTRIC ADENOCARCINOMA

Patients who have undergone subtotal gastrectomy have been reported to have a twofold increase in cancer risk after 15 years. However, these epidemiologic data are controversial, and it is unclear how subtotal gastrectomy is related to *Helicobacter pylori* infection or reflux of duodenal content. Nevertheless, many clinicians believe that after gastrectomy, patients should be surveyed by endoscopy every 2 to 3 years. Again, this is controversial. At this point, the surveillance recommendations are not clearly defined and depend on physician and patient in each case.

ADDITIONAL RESOURCES

Kelly KA, Sarr MC, Hinder RA: *Mayo clinic gastroenterology surgery*, Philadelphia, 2004, Saunders.

Tanimura S, Higashino M, Fukunaga Y, et al: Laparoscopic gastrectomy for gastric cancer: experience with more than 600 cases, *Surg Endosc* 22: 1161–1164, 2008.

43

Effects of Total Gastrectomy

Martin H. Floch

Total gastrectomy almost always results in nutritional problems (Fig. 43.1). Usually performed to attempt a curative procedure for carcinoma, total gastrectomy also may be done to treat trauma.

CLINICAL PICTURE

After total gastrectomy, patients have great difficulty gaining weight, and most never regain their preoperative weight. Others may develop selected deficiencies. The clinical picture is a patient having difficulty gaining weight after surgery who may report postprandial fullness, anorexia, and nausea (rarely vomiting, with or without diarrhea).

DIAGNOSIS

The diagnosis is clear from the patient's history, but when the presentation is of a selected deficiency, a more detailed workup is necessary. After barium study to demonstrate the anatomy, a full biochemical workup establishes immunologic status, electrolyte findings, and mineral levels.

Loss of the reservoir function of the stomach deprives the patient of the capacity to hold a normal meal, which necessitates the ingestion of frequent, small feedings and careful deglutition and chewing. The triturating (grinding) action of the stomach is lost; therefore, mastication is essential. Intestinal transit is frequently accelerated. Resultant problems include dumping syndrome and weight loss.

Selected deficiencies are caused by absorptive defects such as steatorrhea, protein malnutrition, osteoporosis and osteomalacia, anemia secondary to vitamin B_{12} deficiency or iron deficiency, hypoglycemia, and vitamin A deficiency.

Postoperative complications such as anastomotic ulcers, afferent loop syndrome, and intussusception may occur. Loss of the bacteriostatic function of the stomach results in altered microecology or bacterial overgrowth in the small intestine.

A diagnostic workup may also include a study of transit time to help in the therapeutic management. Selective absorptive studies may also be helpful to determine the function of the small bowel, such as a xylose absorption test for carbohydrates, quantitative stool studies to determine the degree of steatorrhea, and vitamin blood levels.

TREATMENT AND MANAGEMENT

Treatment is clear. Any complication such as the dumping syndrome must be treated, and the patient must have adequate caloric and nutrient intake. Weight should be monitored carefully. Patients must be encouraged to eat a high-protein, high-fat diet and to avoid simple carbohydrates. Usually, frequent feedings with snacks between meals and at bedtime can help maintain the body weight at a stable level. Patients should be reassured that they are not going to gain large amounts of weight and that maintaining a normal but low body mass index is adequate. In patients with steatorrhea, consuming too much fat compounds the problem; more readily absorbed fats, such as medium-chain triglycerides, may be helpful.

These patients need vitamin B_{12} injections for life to maintain adequate B_{12} stores. With any suggestion of osteoporosis, adequate calcium and vitamin D are essential for maintaining bone health. In one study, 50% of patients developed iron deficiency after subtotal gastrectomy; therefore, supplements are frequently needed. Vitamin A stores may become depleted after total gastrectomy and are absorbed poorly after subtotal gastrectomy. These patients frequently require vitamin A supplementation.

Nutrition supplementation may be necessary with liquid formulas when patients cannot tolerate or consume enough food. However, tube feeding through a jejunostomy or total parenteral nutrition should not be required and is rarely indicated.

COURSE AND PROGNOSIS

If gastrectomy is performed to remove a malignant tumor, the prognosis depends on the status of the cancer. If the cancer is curable, or if the gastrectomy was performed for trauma, patients can do fairly well and maintain normal life status. Weight will always be a problem, and patients will require frequent feedings with nutrition supplements, as previously described. All postgastrectomy patients should take at least one vitamin tablet daily and select nutrition replacement as indicated.

ADDITIONAL RESOURCES

Floch MH: *Nutrition and Diet Therapy in Gastrointestinal Disease*, New York, 1981, Plenum.

Hoffman WA, Spiro H: Afferent loop syndromes, *Gastroenterology* 40: 201–209, 1961.

Jenkins DJA, Gassull MA, Leeds AR, et al: Effect of dietary fiber on complications of gastric surgery: prevention of postprandial hypoglycemia by pectin, *Gastroenterology* 72:215–220, 1977.

Kiefer ED: Life with a subtotal gastrectomy: a follow-up study 10 or more years after operation, *Gastroenterology* 37:434–440, 1959.

Lundh G: Intestinal digestion absorption after gastrectomy, *Acta Chir Scand* 114(Suppl 231):1–83, 1958.

Metz G, Gassull MA, Drasar BS, et al: Breath hydrogen test for small intestinal bacterial colonization, *Lancet* 1:668–670, 1976.

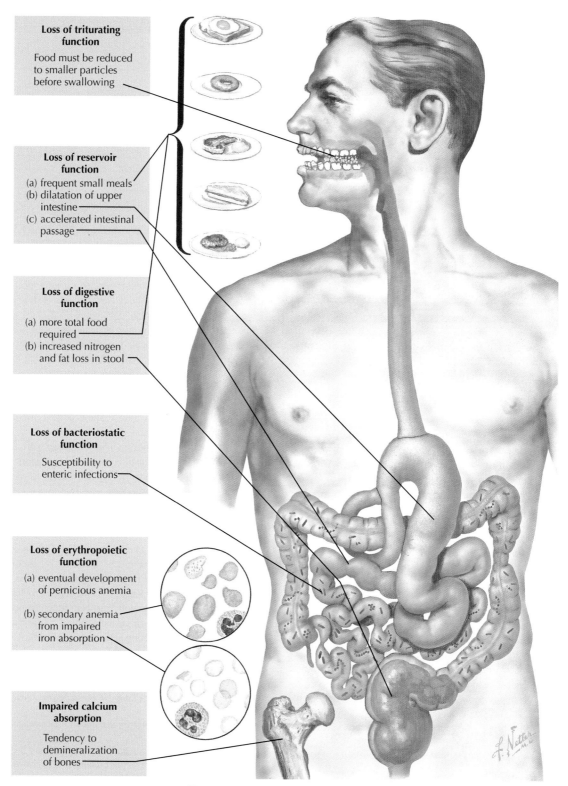

Loss of triturating function

Food must be reduced to smaller particles before swallowing

Loss of reservoir function

(a) frequent small meals
(b) dilatation of upper intestine
(c) accelerated intestinal passage

Loss of digestive function

(a) more total food required
(b) increased nitrogen and fat loss in stool

Loss of bacteriostatic function

Susceptibility to enteric infections

Loss of erythropoietic function

(a) eventual development of pernicious anemia

(b) secondary anemia from impaired iron absorption

Impaired calcium absorption

Tendency to demineralization of bones

Fig. 43.1 Effects of Total Gastrectomy.

SECTION III

Abdominal Wall

Raul J. Rosenthal

44

Abdominal Wall Anatomy

Cristian Alejandro Milla Matute, Matthew Lange,
Emanuele Lo Menzo, Raul J. Rosenthal

ANTEROLATERAL ABDOMINAL WALL

Before describing the abdominal *parietes (wall),* it is important to define the anatomic limits of the abdomen. For the purpose of a specific description, the abdomen is the area of the body that limits with the diaphragm superiorly and the pelvic cavity inferiorly. The *parietes* of the abdomen can be divided into four general parts: anterolateral abdominal wall; posterior abdominal wall; diaphragm (roof of the abdominal cavity); and *parietes* of the pelvis (floor of the abdominal cavity).

The *anterolateral abdominal wall* fills in the bony cartilaginous frame between the costal margin above and the hipbones below (Fig. 44.1). This wall can contract and relax, which helps accommodate the size of the abdominopelvic cavity to changes in the volume of contained viscera, regulating the intraabdominal pressure. Surgical approach to the abdominopelvic cavity is usually made through this wall.

General layers of the anterolateral abdominal wall from the outside in are skin, subcutaneous tissue, superficial fascia, muscles with their related fascia, transversalis fascia, extraperitoneal fascia, and parietal peritoneum.

The abdominal skin is of an average thickness, usually thicker dorsally, and loosely attached to the underlying layers except in the umbilical area. The *superficial fascia (tela subcutanea)* is soft and mobile and contains a variable amount and distribution of fat, depending on the patient's nutritional status. At the area inferior to the level of the umbilicus, the superficial fascia is classically described as having a superficial fatty layer (Camper fascia) and a deep membranous layer (Scarpa fascia). *Camper fascia* is continuous with the fatty layer of surrounding areas, as seen in the fatty layer of the thigh. *Scarpa fascia* merges with the fascia lata in a parallel line to and below the inguinal ligament and is adherent to the linea alba in the midline. Medial to the pubic tubercle, both layers continue into the urogenital region. In males, the two layers merge into the scrotum and blend into a single smooth muscle-containing layer; at this point, the layers begin to form the scrotum. Cephalad to the symphysis pubis, additional closely set strong bands of Scarpa fascia form the fundiform ligament of the penis, extending down into the dorsum and the sides of the penis.

The outer investing layer of the *deep fascia* is not readily distinguishable from the muscular fascia on the external surface of the external abdominal oblique muscle and its aponeurosis. It is easily demonstrated over the fleshy portion of the muscle; however, separating this from the aponeurotic portion of the muscle can be difficult. This layer is attached to the inguinal ligament and merges with the fascia emerging from the ligament to form the *fascia lata.* In addition, it joins the fascia on the inner surface of the external oblique at the subcutaneous inguinal ring to form the external spermatic fascia. External to the lower end of the linea alba, the outer investing layer thickens into the suspensory ligament of the penis, anchoring the penis to the symphysis and the arcuate ligament of the pubis. It is also continuous with the deep investing fascia.

The nerve supply of the external abdominal oblique muscle is derived from the anterior primary division of the 6th to 12th thoracic (T6–T12) spinal nerves. T7 to T11 are intercostal nerves that continue from the intercostal spaces into the anterolateral abdominal wall, to lie in the plane between the internal oblique and transversus muscles. T12 is the subcostal nerve and follows a similar course. The iliohypogastric nerve, from T12 and first lumbar (L1), also contributes to the nerve supply.

The *cremaster muscle,* which is variably developed only in males, represents an extension of the lower border of the internal oblique, and possibly the transversus abdominus, over the testis and the spermatic cord. Laterally, the cremaster is thicker and fleshier and attaches to the middle of the turned-under edge of the external oblique aponeurosis and to the inferior edge of the internal oblique. From here, the scattered fibers, interspersed with connective tissue (cremasteric fascia), spread in loops over the spermatic cord and testis to end at the pubic tubercle and the anterior layer of the rectus sheath. The cremaster's nerve supply is from the genital (external spermatic) branch of the genitofemoral nerve and, generally, a branch from the ileo-inguinal nerve. The action of the cremaster muscle is to lift the testis toward the external inguinal ring.

The rectus abdominis muscle generally acts in conjunction with the external oblique, internal oblique, and transversus abdominis muscles, but it is specifically involved in producing forced expiration and flexion of the vertebral column. With a fixed pelvis and thoracic cavity, the rectus abdominus serves to constrict the contents of the abdominal cavity and increase intraabdominal pressure to aid in things such as defecation and vomiting.

ABDOMINAL REGIONS AND PLANES

The abdomen can be divided into *areas* or *regions* (Fig. 44.2). A simple view shows two imaginary planes passing through the umbilicus, one vertically and the other horizontally. The abdomen is thus divided into four quadrants: a right and a left upper quadrant and a right and a left lower quadrant.

Another division of the abdomen for descriptive purposes uses two vertical and two horizontal planes that divide the abdomen into nine regions. The zone above the upper of the two horizontal planes is divided by the two vertical planes into a centrally placed *epigastric region.* The middle portion is called epigastrium and the lateral parts are called hypochondric regions (hypochondrium). The zone between the two horizontal planes is divided into a centrally placed *umbilical region,* with a specified left and right *lumbar* or *lateral abdominal* region. The zone below the lower of the two horizontal planes has a centrally placed *hypogastric* or *pubic* (suprapubic) *region,* with a specified left and right *inguinal* or *iliac* region on either side.

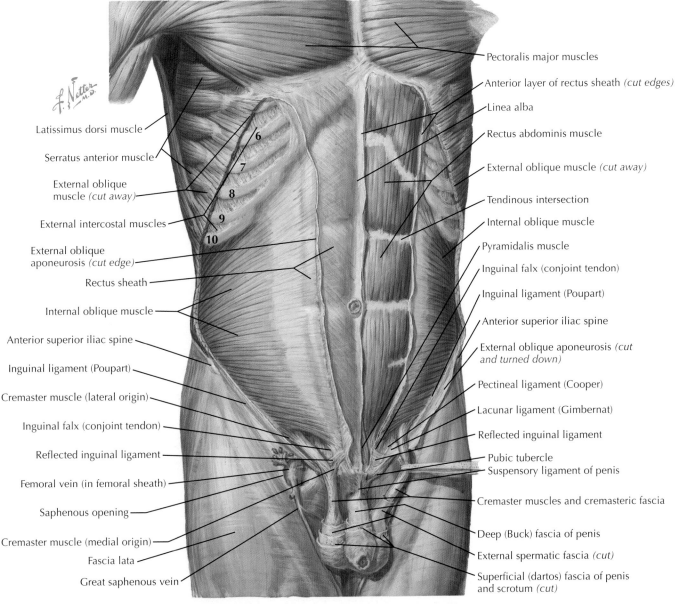

Fig. 44.1 Anterior Abdominal Wall: Intermediate Dissection.

Pectoralis major muscles

Anterior layer of rectus sheath *(cut edges)*

Linea alba

Rectus abdominis muscle

External oblique muscle *(cut away)*

Tendinous intersection

Internal oblique muscle

Pyramidalis muscle

Inguinal falx (conjoint tendon)

Inguinal ligament (Poupart)

Anterior superior iliac spine

External oblique aponeurosis *(cut and turned down)*

Pectineal ligament (Cooper)

Lacunar ligament (Gimbernat)

Reflected inguinal ligament

Pubic tubercle

Suspensory ligament of penis

Cremaster muscles and cremasteric fascia

Deep (Buck) fascia of penis

External spermatic fascia *(cut)*

Superficial (dartos) fascia of penis and scrotum *(cut)*

Latissimus dorsi muscle

Serratus anterior muscle

External oblique muscle *(cut away)*

External intercostal muscles

External oblique aponeurosis *(cut edge)*

Rectus sheath

Internal oblique muscle

Anterior superior iliac spine

Inguinal ligament (Poupart)

Cremaster muscle (lateral origin)

Inguinal falx (conjoint tendon)

Reflected inguinal ligament

Femoral vein (in femoral sheath)

Saphenous opening

Cremaster muscle (medial origin)

Fascia lata

Great saphenous vein

6
7
8
9
10

Although localization using these nine regions is more specific than with the four quadrants, localization is still general. The upper horizontal (superior transverse) line, or plane, may be drawn midway between the upper border of the sternum and the upper border of the symphysis pubis. This plane passes through the pylorus and consequently is named the *transpyloric plane.* It has also been described as midway between the xiphisternal junction and the umbilicus, passing through the tip of the ninth costal cartilage, the fundus of the gallbladder, and the lower part of the body of the first lumbar vertebra. The most caudal part of the costal margin is an important landmark called the *subcostal plane.*

Two vertical planes, one on either side, may be located halfway between the median plane and the anterior superior spine of the ilium. Vertical planes on each side may also be identified by using the lateral border of the rectus abdominis muscle or the semilunar line, which, if followed inferiorly and medially toward the pubic tubercle, brings the entire inguinal canal into the inguinal region.

INGUINAL CANAL

The inguinal canal is an oblique tunnel, 3 to 5 cm long, through the muscular and deep fascial layers of the anterior abdominal wall, parallel to and superior to the inguinal ligament (Fig. 44.3). The canal extends between the internal inguinal ring, located in the transversalis fascia halfway between the anterior superior spine of the ilium and the pubic symphysis, and the external inguinal ring, located in the aponeurosis of the external abdominal oblique muscle just superior and lateral to the pubic tubercle. In the male, the canal conveys the spermatic cord, comprising the vas deferens and the vessels and nerves of the testes (Fig. 44.4). The anatomy of the inguinal canal is similar in the female but is somewhat less well developed. It contains the round ligament of the uterus as it travels toward the labia majora.

The *internal inguinal ring,* a funnel-shaped opening in the transversalis fascia, is the site at which the transversalis fascia becomes the

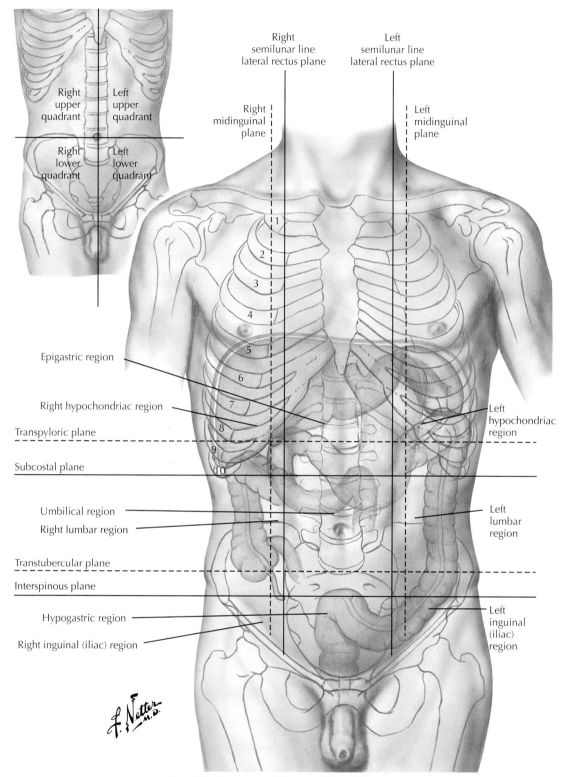

Fig. 44.2 Regions and Planes of the Abdomen.

innermost covering of the spermatic cord, the internal spermatic fascia. Inferior epigastric vessels are just medial to the internal inguinal ring. The external inguinal ring is formed by fibers of the external abdominal oblique aponeurosis that pass superomedial to the ring attaching to the pubic symphysis. This portion of the external oblique aponeurosis is called the *superior crus* of the external (superficial) ring. Fibers of

the external oblique aponeurosis that pass inferolateral to the superficial inguinal ring are called the *inferior crura* of the ring.

The lower border of the external oblique *aponeurosis* is folded under itself, with the edge of the fold forming the inguinal ligament. The fascia lata on the anterior aspect of the thigh is closely blended to the full length of the ligament, and its lateral half is fused with the iliac

Anterior view

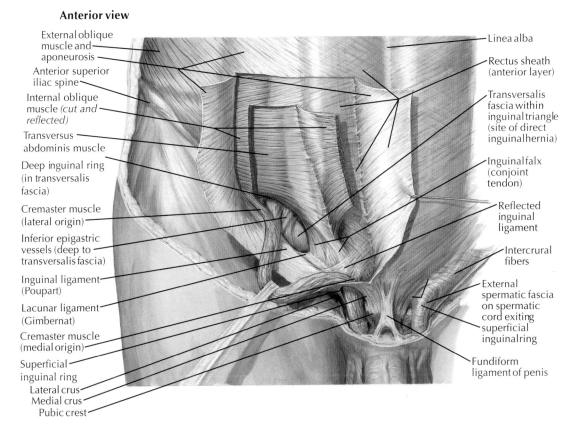

External oblique muscle and aponeurosis

Anterior superior iliac spine

Internal oblique muscle *(cut and reflected)*

Transversus abdominis muscle

Deep inguinal ring (in transversalis fascia)

Cremaster muscle (lateral origin)

Inferior epigastric vessels (deep to transversalis fascia)

Inguinal ligament (Poupart)

Lacunar ligament (Gimbernat)

Cremaster muscle (medial origin)

Superficial inguinal ring

Lateral crus

Medial crus

Pubic crest

Linea alba

Rectus sheath (anterior layer)

Transversalis fascia within inguinal triangle (site of direct inguinal hernia)

Inguinal falx (conjoint tendon)

Reflected inguinal ligament

Intercrural fibers

External spermatic fascia on spermatic cord exiting superficial inguinal ring

Fundiform ligament of penis

Posterior (internal) view

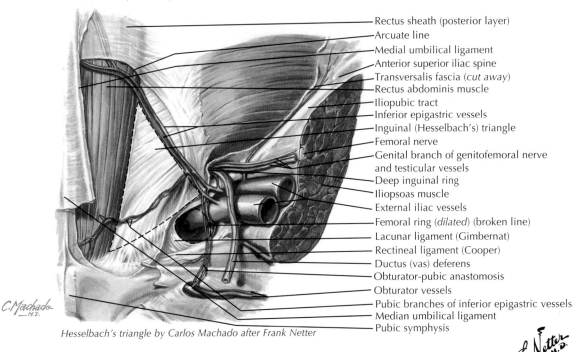

Rectus sheath (posterior layer)

Arcuate line

Medial umbilical ligament

Anterior superior iliac spine

Transversalis fascia *(cut away)*

Rectus abdominis muscle

Iliopubic tract

Inferior epigastric vessels

Inguinal (Hesselbach's) triangle

Femoral nerve

Genital branch of genitofemoral nerve and testicular vessels

Deep inguinal ring

Iliopsoas muscle

External iliac vessels

Femoral ring *(dilated)* (broken line)

Lacunar ligament (Gimbernat)

Rectineal ligament (Cooper)

Ductus (vas) deferens

Obturator-pubic anastomosis

Obturator vessels

Pubic branches of inferior epigastric vessels

Median umbilical ligament

Pubic symphysis

Hesselbach's triangle by Carlos Machado after Frank Netter

Fig. 44.3 Inguinal Region: Dissections.

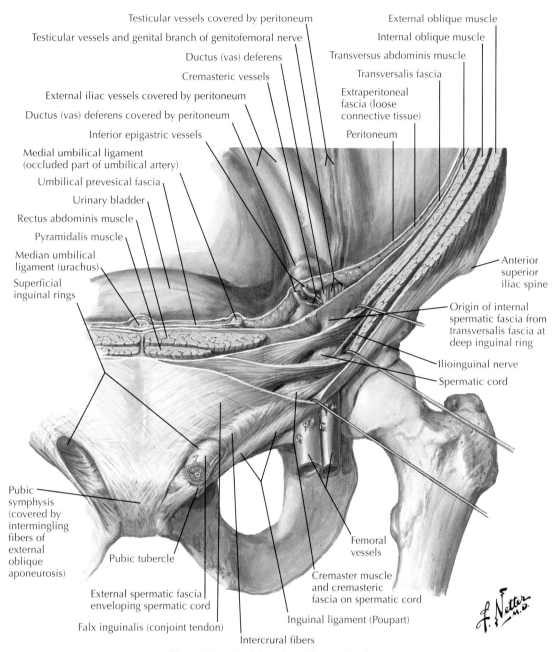

Testicular vessels covered by peritoneum

Testicular vessels and genital branch of genitofemoral nerve

Ductus (vas) deferens

Cremasteric vessels

External iliac vessels covered by peritoneum

Ductus (vas) deferens covered by peritoneum

Inferior epigastric vessels

Medial umbilical ligament (occluded part of umbilical artery)

Umbilical prevesical fascia

Urinary bladder

Rectus abdominis muscle

Pyramidalis muscle

Median umbilical ligament (urachus)

Superficial inguinal rings

External oblique muscle

Internal oblique muscle

Transversus abdominis muscle

Transversalis fascia

Extraperitoneal fascia (loose connective tissue)

Peritoneum

Anterior superior iliac spine

Origin of internal spermatic fascia from transversalis fascia at deep inguinal ring

Ilioinguinal nerve

Spermatic cord

Pubic symphysis (covered by intermingling fibers of external oblique aponeurosis)

Pubic tubercle

External spermatic fascia enveloping spermatic cord

Falx inguinalis (conjoint tendon)

Intercrural fibers

Femoral vessels

Cremaster muscle and cremasteric fascia on spermatic cord

Inguinal ligament (Poupart)

Fig. 44.4 Inguinal Canal and Spermatic Cord.

fascia as the iliacus muscle passes into the thigh. The lowest fibers in the aponeurosis attach the farthest laterally on the pecten. The portion of the aponeurosis that runs posteriorly and superiorly from the folded edge of the ligament to the pecten pubis is called the pectineal part of the inguinal ligament, or the *lacunar ligament.*

The inguinal canal can be viewed as a tubular tunnel having a roof, a floor, and anterior and posterior walls. The two openings are the deep inguinal ring in the transversalis fascia at the internal (lateral) end of the canal and the superficial inguinal ring in the aponeurosis of the external oblique muscle at the external (medial) end of the canal. The external oblique aponeurosis, strengthened by the intercrural fibers, is present in the entire length of the anterior wall of the canal. For approximately the lateral one third of the canal, fibers of the internal oblique muscle, which arise from the inguinal ligament and the related iliac fascia, form

the anterior wall of the canal deep to the external oblique aponeurosis. The floor of the canal is formed in its medial two thirds by the rolled-under portion of the external oblique aponeurosis, together with the lacunar ligament, forming a shelf on which the spermatic cord rests.

The *transversalis fascia* is present for the entire length of the posterior wall of the inguinal canal. Toward the medial end of the canal, reinforcing the part of this wall posterior to the superficial inguinal ring, is the reflected inguinal ligament. The tendon of the rectus abdominis muscle fuses with the posterior aspect of the conjoined tendon. All the reinforcing structures are anterior to the transversalis fascia. The subserous fascia and the peritoneum are posterior to the transversalis fascia and continue behind the deep inguinal ring. At the lateral end of the canal, the inferior epigastric artery and vein are posterior to the canal in the subperitoneal fascia.

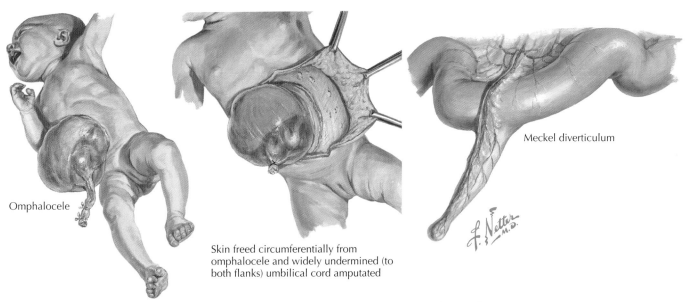

Omphalocele

Skin freed circumferentially from
omphalocele and widely undermined (to
both flanks) umbilical cord amputated

Meckel diverticulum

Fig. 44.5 Abdominal Wall and Cavity: Congenital Abnormalities.

The roof of the inguinal canal is formed by the most inferior fasciculi of the internal oblique muscle as they gradually pass in a slightly arched fashion, from a position at their origin anterior to the canal to a position at their insertion posterior to the canal. At the lateral end of the canal, the lower fasciculi of the transversus abdominis arch similarly cover the canal.

The weakest area in the anterolateral wall in relation to the inguinal canal is the area of the superficial inguinal ring. This generally weakened area is through which direct inguinal hernias pass. It is often described as a triangle, bounded superolaterally by the inferior epigastric vessels, superomedially by the lateral margin of the rectus, and inferiorly by the inguinal ligament, known as the *inguinal (Hesselbach) triangle.*

The *preperitoneal space* is bordered posteriorly by the peritoneum and anteriorly by the transversalis fascia. This space contains connective tissue along with vascular structures and nerves. Vascular structures of the preperitoneal space include the iliac vessels. External iliac vessels run on the medial aspect of the psoas muscle before passing under the iliopubic tract and the inguinal ligament and becoming the femoral vessels. Five major nerves in the preperitoneal space are responsible for innervation of the lower abdominal wall, inguinal, and genital regions: the iliohypogastric, hypogastric, ilioinguinal, genitofemoral, and lateral femoral cutaneous nerves.

CONGENITAL ABNORMALITIES

The most common variant of the abdominal wall and congenital abnormality is the *diastasis recti.* This consists of an upper midline protrusion of the abdominal wall between the right and left rectus abdominis muscles. This is a weakness of the linea alba and does not require treatment unless an epigastric hernia develops in association with the diastasis recti.

Omphalocele may be seen in neonates and represents a defect in the closure of the umbilical ring (Fig. 44.5). The herniated viscera are usually covered with an amniotic sac.

Gastroschisis, a defect in the abdominal wall lateral to the umbilicus, is caused by failure of the body wall to close. The abdominal viscera protrude through the defect, and no sac is present to cover the herniated intestine.

Omphalomesenteric vitelline duct remnants may present as abnormalities related to the abdominal wall. In the fetus, the omphalomesenteric duct connects the fetal midgut to the yolk sac. This normally obliterates and disappears completely. However, any part of or the entire fetal duct may persist and give rise to symptoms.

Meckel diverticulum results when the intestinal end of the omphalomesenteric duct persists (see Fig. 44.5). This is a true diverticulum of the intestine, with all layers of the intestinal wall represented.

Anomalies of the urachus, a fetal structure that connects the developing bladder to the umbilicus, can occur. The urachus is normally obliterated at birth. It may persist in toto, resulting in a vesicoumbilical fistula manifested by the drainage of urine from the umbilicus. Proper treatment is excision of the fistula after distal urinary obstruction has been excluded.

Urachal sinus results when the umbilical end of the urachus does not obliterate normally. Such sinuses present as the chronic drainage of small amounts of urine from the umbilicus.

ADDITIONAL RESOURCES

Annibali R, Fitzgibbons RJ: Laparoscopic anatomy of the abdominal wall. In Phillips EH, Rosenthal RJ, editors: *Operative strategies in laparoscopic surgery,* Berlin, 1995, Springer, pp 75–82.

Annibali R, Quinn TH, Fitzgibbons RJ: Surgical anatomy of the inguinal region and the lower abdominal wall: the laparoscopic perspective. In Bendavid R, editor: *Prostheses and abdominal wall hernias,* Austin, Texas, 1994, Landes Medical, pp 82–103.

Chung BI, Sommer G, Brooks JD: 68. *Campbell-walsh urology: surgical, radiographic, and endoscopic anatomy of the male pelvis,* 2015, Campbell-Walsh Urology, pp 1611–1630.

Drake RL, Vogl AW, Mitchell AWM: 4. *Gray's atlas of anatomy,* 2012, pp 133–209.

Sabiston A: Abdominal wall, umbilicus, peritoneum, mesenteries, omentum and retroperitoneum. In Sabiston A, editor: *Textbook of surgery: the biological basis of the modern surgical practice,* ed 15, Philadelphia, 1997.

45

Peritoneum and Related Diseases

Savannah Moon, Maria C. Fonseca, Emanuele Lo Menzo, Raul J. Rosenthal

PERITONEUM

Peritoneum is derived from Greek origins, *peri* meaning "around" and *tonos* meaning "stretching." The peritoneum is the extensive serous membrane that lines the innermost surface of the abdominal wall and abdominal organs. The serous layer consists of dense mesothelial cells and encompasses a surface area of 1.8 m². The peritoneum is divided into parietal and visceral peritoneum. The parietal peritoneum is attached to the innermost surface of the abdominal wall, the lining of the abdominal diaphragm, and the pelvis. The visceral peritoneum covers the intraperitoneal organs and anterior aspect of the retroperitoneal organs. In men the peritoneum is enclosed, while in women the peritoneal cavity is open through the ostia of the Fallopian tubes (Figs. 45.1 and 45.2).

Embryology

The peritoneum development begins in the fifth week of gestation at the gastrulation stage, during which a trilaminar layer of endoderm, mesoderm, and ectoderm develops. The future parietal peritoneum will originate from the lateral parietal plate of the mesoderm and the ectoderm, as with the visceral peritoneum from the visceral plate of the mesoderm and the endoderm. Between this, two layers of the mesothelial membrane will form and its visceral portion will cover most of the surface of intraperitoneal organs and anterior aspect of retroperitoneal organs. The peritoneal cavity contains approximately 100 mL of sterile fluid, which lines the visceral organs and aids in defense. The intraperitoneal organs are suspended by peritoneal ligaments. Meyers et al. describe 11 peritoneal ligaments and mesenteries; these allow continuity of anatomic planes and direct the circulation of fluid within the peritoneal cavity. This leads to the spread of infection or malignancy between intraperitoneal and extraperitoneal compartments.

Anatomy and Physiology

The omentum is a protective vascular peritoneal fold, walling off inflammatory processes, infection, or malignancy. The greater omentum (gastrocolic omentum, or ligament) is the largest peritoneal fold; it drapes over from the greater curvature of the stomach overlying the abdominal viscera. The upper end of the left border is continuous with the gastrosplenic ligament, and the upper end of the right border extends to the first portion of the duodenum. The *greater omentum* is usually a thin, delicate layer of fibroelastic tissue; it usually also contains some adipose tissue and may accumulate a large amount of fat in an obese patient.

The *lesser sac* peritoneum on the posteroinferior surface of the stomach and the *greater sac* peritoneum on the anterosuperior surface meet at the greater curvature of the stomach and course inferiorly to the free border of the greater omentum, where they turn superiorly to the transverse colon.

The *lesser omentum* (gastrohepatic omentum, or ligament), hepatogastric ligaments, and hepatoduodenal ligaments extend from the posteroinferior surface of the liver to the lesser curvature of the stomach and the beginning of the duodenum. The lesser omentum is extremely thin, on the left portion, and sometimes fenestrated, while the right is thicker and ends in a free, rounded margin that contains the common bile duct to the right, the hepatic artery to the left, and the portal vein posterior to these; it then forms the anterior border of the epiploic foramen. In addition to these structures, the lesser omentum contains the right and left gastric arteries close to the lesser curvature of the stomach and the accompanying veins, lymphatics, and autonomic nerve plexuses. The peritoneum forming the anterior layer of this omentum and continuing onto the anterosuperior surface of the stomach is the *greater sac* peritoneum, and that forming the posterior layer and continuing onto the posteroinferior surface of the stomach is the *lesser sac* peritoneum. The lesser omentum reaches the liver at the porta, and to the left of the porta it extends to the bottom of the fossa for the ligamentum venosum.

The blood supply and innervation of the peritoneum is distinct from the visceral and parietal. The parietal peritoneum receives its blood supply from intercostal, lumbar, and iliac vessels while the visceral blood supply is from the splanchnic vasculature. The visceral peritoneum is supplied by nonsomatic nerves and parietal supplied by somatic nerves. Visceral pain will be vague and generalized, stimulated by irritation of splanchnic nerves. Parietal pain is sharp and localized due to direct stimulation of phrenic, thoracoabdominal, subcostal, or lumbar sacral nerves. This distinction is critical for clinical assessment.

ACUTE ABDOMEN: ACUTE PERITONITIS

The assessment and management of an acute abdomen depends on the clinician's ability to obtain a detailed history and physical examination, establish differential diagnoses, and obtain the appropriate studies to determine if the patient requires operative intervention (Fig. 45.3).

The etiology of an acute abdomen, or abdominal peritonitis, can result from any local trigger of inflammation, usually an infection process (Fig. 45.4). However, infection may not be present at the earliest stage of peritonitis and inflammation of the peritoneum may be caused by various etiologies, including bacterial, fungal, viral, chemical irritants, or foreign bodies. The peritoneal cavity's circulation allows absorption of bacteria, endotoxins, and inflammatory cytokines.

Primary peritonitis is defined as a monomicrobial infection of previously sterile ascitic fluid without intraabdominal source. *Secondary peritonitis* is inflammation of the peritoneum due to infection or perforation of gastrointestinal or genitourinary origin. *Tertiary peritonitis* develops after the treatment of secondary peritonitis resulting from failure of the inflammatory response.

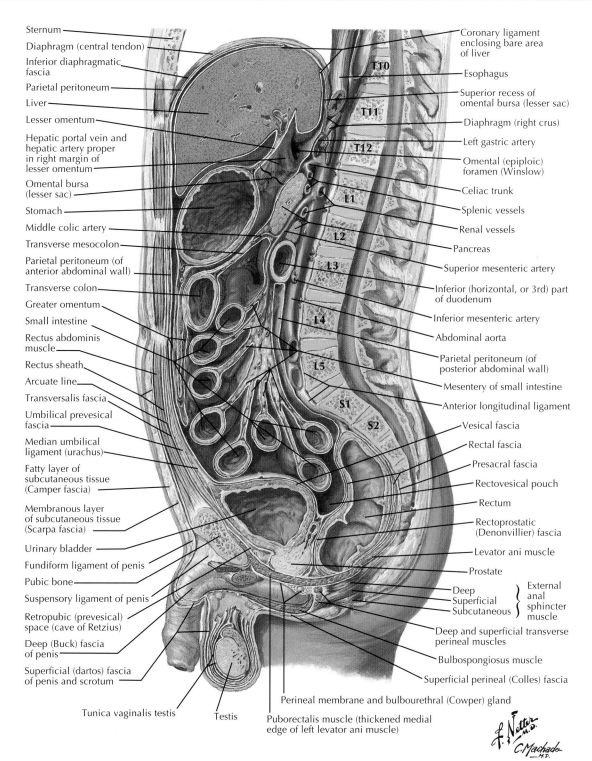

Fig. 45.1 Abdominal Wall and Viscera: Median (Sagittal) Section.

Diagnosis

The diagnosis of peritonitis depends on history, examination, and laboratory and radiologic findings. Early features depend on the severity and extent of the peritonitis. Clinically, pain may be localized or generalized. Extensive peritonitis that involves subdiaphragmatic abscess or collection may be accompanied by shoulder pain. Vomiting often occurs early in the disease course, as well malaise and fevers. As disease process progresses, abdomen may become more distended.

The differential diagnosis for acute peritonitis includes appendicitis, perforated peptic ulcers, pelvic inflammatory disease or ruptured ovarian cyst, diverticulitis, ischemic bowel and perforation, gangrenous cholecystitis, or necrotizing pancreatitis.

Abdominal radiography reveals free subdiaphragmatic gas from hollow viscus perforation. Abdominal ultrasound and computed tomography (CT) should be reserved for cases requiring further confirmation to obtain an accurate diagnosis. Ultrasound is an effective tool to evaluate the acute abdomen and to rapidly assess multiple organs. Doppler

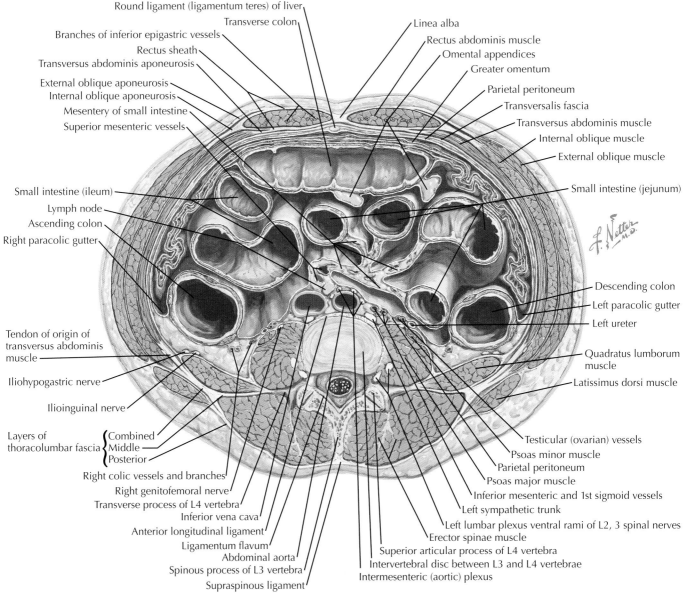

Round ligament (ligamentum teres) of liver
Transverse colon
Branches of inferior epigastric vessels
Rectus sheath
Transversus abdominis aponeurosis
External oblique aponeurosis
Internal oblique aponeurosis
Mesentery of small intestine
Superior mesenteric vessels

Linea alba
Rectus abdominis muscle
Omental appendices
Greater omentum
Parietal peritoneum
Transversalis fascia
Transversus abdominis muscle
Internal oblique muscle
External oblique muscle

Small intestine (ileum)
Lymph node
Ascending colon
Right paracolic gutter

Small intestine (jejunum)

Descending colon
Left paracolic gutter
Left ureter

Tendon of origin of
transversus abdominis
muscle

Quadratus lumborum
muscle
Latissimus dorsi muscle

Iliohypogastric nerve

Ilioinguinal nerve

Layers of
thoracolumbar fascia { Combined
Middle
Posterior

Testicular (ovarian) vessels
Psoas minor muscle
Parietal peritoneum
Psoas major muscle
Inferior mesenteric and 1st sigmoid vessels
Left sympathetic trunk
Left lumbar plexus ventral rami of L2, 3 spinal nerves
Erector spinae muscle
Superior articular process of L4 vertebra
Intervertebral disc between L3 and L4 vertebrae
Intermesenteric (aortic) plexus

Right colic vessels and branches
Right genitofemoral nerve
Transverse process of L4 vertebra
Inferior vena cava
Anterior longitudinal ligament
Ligamentum flavum
Abdominal aorta
Spinous process of L3 vertebra
Supraspinous ligament

Fig. 45.2 Peritoneum.

imaging reveals any vascular abnormalities, including embolic or thrombotic site, aortic and visceral arterial aneurysm, or arteriovenous fistula.

CT is a safe, noninvasive, and efficient method that provides sensitive detection of free air, abscesses, calcifications, and collections of intraperitoneal fluid, as well as detailed information of the bowel wall, mesentery, and retroperitoneum—in particular, kidneys, pancreas, duodenum, and the aorta. Use of intravenous and oral contrast materials is recommended to delineate obstruction, collections, and vasculature. Special attention must be given to patients with impaired renal function and/or contrast allergy. In addition, CT magnetic resonance imaging (MRI) requires more time and is generally less useful than CT.

CHRONIC PERITONITIS: PERITONEAL TUBERCULOSIS

While uncommon in Western countries, 10,000 new cases of tuberculous peritonitis in the United States were reported in 2012. The populations most at risk of developing tuberculous peritonitis are immunocompromised patients, especially with human immunodeficiency virus (HIV), incarcerated patients, and the homeless. Peritoneal tuberculosis (TB) is the sixth most common site of extrapulmonary TB, after lymphatic, small intestine, bone, joint, military, and meningeal. It occurs from hematogenous spread from the lungs to the peritoneum or transmitted mycobacterium from small bowel TB.

Diagnosis

Tuberculous peritonitis has an insidious onset, persisting from weeks to months (Fig. 45.5). Patients present with progressive ascites, abdominal pain, fever, night sweats, malaise, and anorexia. The diagnosis of tuberculous peritonitis should be suspected with patients with a known history of TB. Patients will have a positive tuberculin skin test. Peritoneal fluid will show elevated white blood cell count with lymphocytes. Laparoscopic visualization of the lesions and peritoneal biopsy will confirm the diagnosis. The pathology will reveal caseating granulomas.

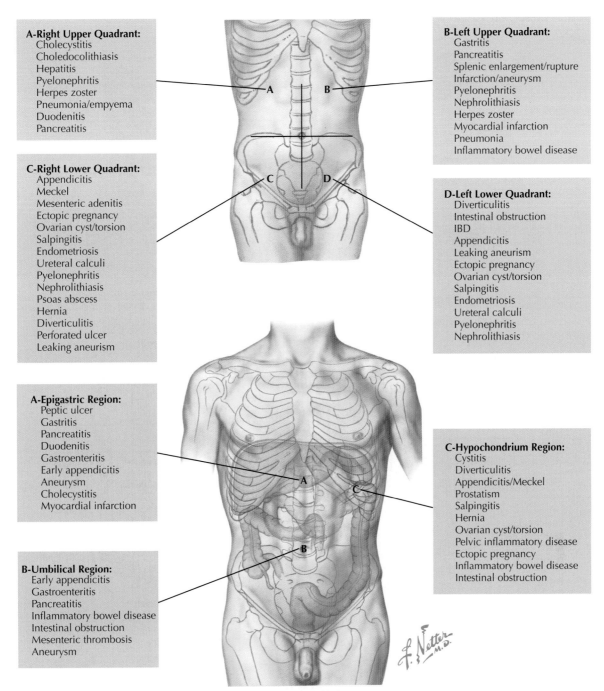

A-Right Upper Quadrant:
Cholecystitis
Choledocolithiasis
Hepatitis
Pyelonephritis
Herpes zoster
Pneumonia/empyema
Duodenitis
Pancreatitis

B-Left Upper Quadrant:
Gastritis
Pancreatitis
Splenic enlargement/rupture
Infarction/aneurysm
Pyelonephritis
Nephrolithiasis
Herpes zoster
Myocardial infarction
Pneumonia
Inflammatory bowel disease

C-Right Lower Quadrant:
Appendicitis
Meckel
Mesenteric adenitis
Ectopic pregnancy
Ovarian cyst/torsion
Salpingitis
Endometriosis
Ureteral calculi
Pyelonephritis
Nephrolithiasis
Psoas abscess
Hernia
Diverticulitis
Perforated ulcer
Leaking aneurism

D-Left Lower Quadrant:
Diverticulitis
Intestinal obstruction
IBD
Appendicitis
Leaking aneurism
Ectopic pregnancy
Ovarian cyst/torsion
Salpingitis
Endometriosis
Ureteral calculi
Pyelonephritis
Nephrolithiasis

A-Epigastric Region:
Peptic ulcer
Gastritis
Pancreatitis
Duodenitis
Gastroenteritis
Early appendicitis
Aneurysm
Cholecystitis
Myocardial infarction

C-Hypochondrium Region:
Cystitis
Diverticulitis
Appendicitis/Meckel
Prostatism
Salpingitis
Hernia
Ovarian cyst/torsion
Pelvic inflammatory disease
Ectopic pregnancy
Inflammatory bowel disease
Intestinal obstruction

B-Umbilical Region:
Early appendicitis
Gastroenteritis
Pancreatitis
Inflammatory bowel disease
Intestinal obstruction
Mesenteric thrombosis
Aneurysm

Fig. 45.3 Acute Abdomen.

Treatment

The treatment approach is the same as pulmonary TB, with a 6- to 9-month course of isoniazid, rifampin, and pyrazinamide. With medical management, symptoms resolve within the first few weeks. Surgery is indicated for perforation, abscess, fistula formation or obstruction, or failure of medical management.

BENIGN PAROXYSMAL PERITONITIS (FAMILIAL MEDITERRANEAN FEVER)

Familial Mediterranean fever (FMF) is an autoinflammatory auto-recessive disorder characterized by recurrent episodes of fevers and peritonitis. (Fig. 45.6) FMF is most prevalent in patients from Medi-terranean background, including Greeks, Italians, Armenian, Turkish, North African, and Jewish.

FMF develops from a mutation in the Mediterranean fever (MEFV) gene on the short arm of chromosome 16. The MEFV gene codes for the *Pyrin* protein; when expressed, it blocks an antiinflammatory response. Mutation in MEFV causes exaggerated inflammatory response through uncontrolled production of interleukin 1. Heterogeneity among the disease-modifying proteins may contribute to the variable phenotypes seen in patients with FMF. The triggering mechanism for acute attacks of FMF is unknown.

Clinical Picture

The presentation of FMF is recurrent fevers, as high at 103°F (39.4°C), accompanied by signs of peritonitis, pleuritis, or acute monoarticular

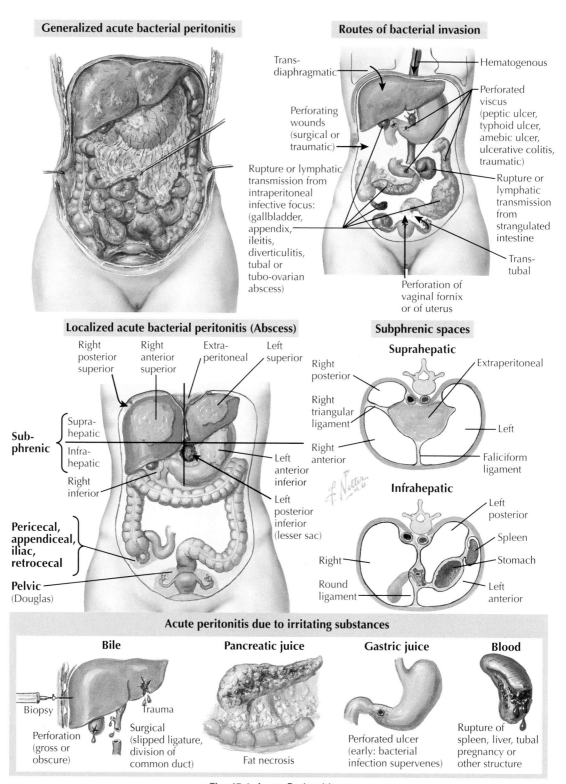

Fig. 45.4 Acute Peritonitis.

synovitis, lasting 24 to 72 hours, and resolves spontaneously. For the clinician, FMF peritonitis is indistinguishable from an acute surgical abdomen and consequently may lead one to the operating room. Other manifestations of FMF include erysipelas-like erythema, aseptic meningitis, febrile myalgia, and vasculitis.

The most significant complication is amyloidosis and development of end-stage renal disease due to amyloid deposition to the kidneys.

FMF may cause infertility or spontaneous abortion due to pelvic adhesions.

Diagnosis

FMF is a clinical diagnosis and may be confirmed with genetic testing. The diagnosis is considered in patients with recurrent, self-limited fevers and serositis. The *Livneh criterion* includes major criteria: peritonitis

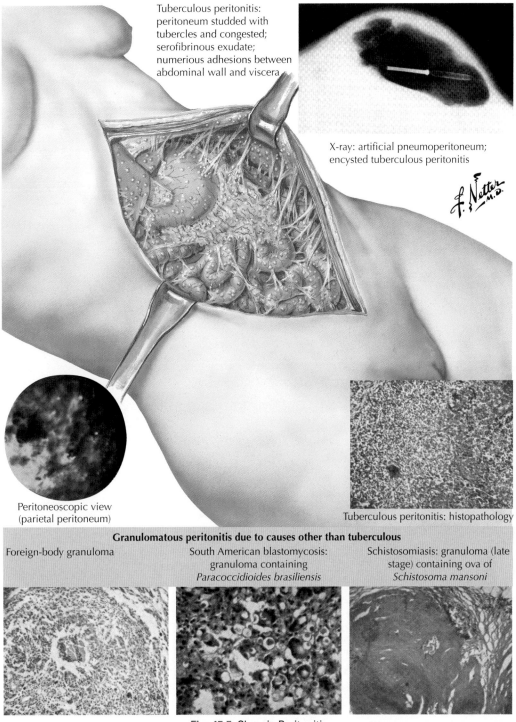

Tuberculous peritonitis: peritoneum studded with tubercles and congested; serofibrinous exudate; numerious adhesions between abdominal wall and viscera

X-ray: artificial pneumoperitoneum; encysted tuberculous peritonitis

Peritoneoscopic view (parietal peritoneum)

Tuberculous peritonitis: histopathology

Granulomatous peritonitis due to causes other than tuberculous

Foreign-body granuloma

South American blastomycosis: granuloma containing *Paracoccidioides brasiliensis*

Schistosomiasis: granuloma (late stage) containing ova of *Schistosoma mansoni*

Fig. 45.5 Chronic Peritonitis.

(generalized), pleuritis (unilateral) or pericarditis, monoarthritis (hip, knee, ankle), or fever alone as well as minor criteria (incomplete attacks) involving the chest, joints, and extremities.

Genetic analysis is used to support the diagnosis in cases with significant family history of FMF or amyloidosis. Conversely, the carriage of *MEFV* variants is not always accompanied by clinical symptoms. Levels of acute-phase reactants, such as erythrocyte sedimentation rate, C-reactive protein, and fibrinogen, are almost always elevated during these attacks.

Treatment

The management of FMF focuses on the prevention of acute attacks and progression to amyloidosis. Colchicine is the prophylactic treatment of choice. Colchicine inhibits neutrophils and interferes with inflammatory response. It prevents febrile attacks in 60% of patients, induces remission up to 35%, and reduces renal disease from amyloid deposition. High-dose colchicine may be used in acute attacks. In patients who do not show response to colchicine, antiinterleukin (IL)-1 therapy has shown to be a safe alternative.

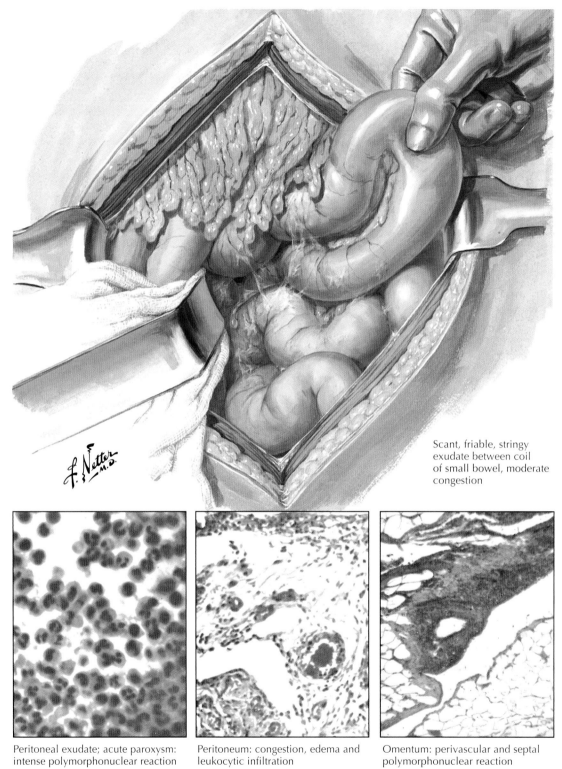

Scant, friable, stringy
exudate between coil
of small bowel, moderate
congestion

Peritoneal exudate; acute paroxysm:
intense polymorphonuclear reaction

Peritoneum: congestion, edema and
leukocytic infiltration

Omentum: perivascular and septal
polymorphonuclear reaction

Fig. 45.6 Benign Paroxysmal Peritonitis, or Familial Mediterranean Fever.

TUMORS OF THE PERITONEUM

Desmoid Tumors

Discovered in 1832, *desmoid tumors* are primary peritoneal tumors. They are soft tissue tumors, arising from connective tissue. They can occur in trunk/extremity, abdominal wall, or intraabdominally, within bowel and mesentery. They do not have metastatic potential but are locally aggressive. Desmoid tumors are rare, approximately 3% of all soft tissue neoplasms, and occur sporadically, while 5% to 15% are associated with familial adenomatous polyposis (FAP). Most patients are young males. Typically asymptomatic, these tumors are slow growing, and will eventually cause symptoms with local invasion. Diagnosis is confirmed with biopsy; histological examination will demonstrate spindle cells and stain for nuclear beta-catenin and vimentin and smooth muscle actin.

The treatment of choice for desmoid tumors is surgical resection with negative margins. Intraabdominal desmoid tumors may present at the root of the mesentery and present as a challenging surgical resection. If deemed unresectable, a multimodality approach is utilized, including noncytotoxic therapy, including nonsteroidal antiinflammatory drugs (NSAIDs) and antiestrogen agents (tamoxifen), radiation therapy, or targeted chemotherapy (imatinib).

Peritoneal Mesothelioma

First described in 1908, malignant peritoneal mesothelioma is a rare disease, accounting for 10% to 20% of all mesotheliomas. In the United States, there are approximately 400 new cases annually of peritoneal mesothelioma. Most are directly linked to asbestos exposure. This tumor is aggressive, arising from mesothelial cells of the peritoneum (Fig. 45.7). More common in middle-age men, patients present with abdominal distention, increased abdominal girth, anorexia, and weight loss. CT imaging will show peritoneal and omental thickening, masses or nodules, and typically widespread involvement of the peritoneum. Percutaneous

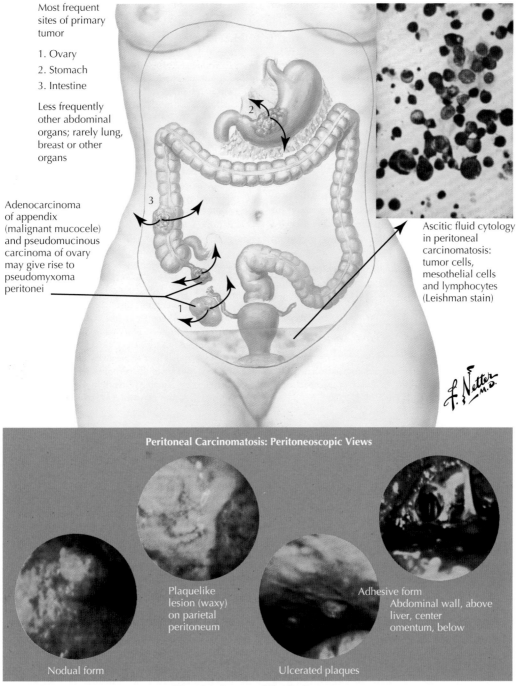

Most frequent sites of primary tumor

1. Ovary
2. Stomach
3. Intestine

Less frequently other abdominal organs; rarely lung, breast or other organs

Adenocarcinoma of appendix (malignant mucocele) and pseudomucinous carcinoma of ovary may give rise to pseudomyxoma peritonei

Ascitic fluid cytology in peritoneal carcinomatosis: tumor cells, mesothelial cells and lymphocytes (Leishman stain)

Peritoneal Carcinomatosis: Peritoneoscopic Views

Plaquelike lesion (waxy) on parietal peritoneum

Adhesive form Abdominal wall, above liver, center omentum, below

Nodual form

Ulcerated plaques

Fig. 45.7 Cancer of the Peritoneum.

biopsy or diagnostic laparoscopy can provide diagnosis. Due to its rarity, there is no standard of care for treatment modality. The literature supports treatment with cytoreductive surgery and hyperthermic intraperitoneal chemotherapy (HIPEC).

Peritoneal Carcinomatosis

Primary peritoneal malignancy is rare; most neoplasms of the peritoneum are metastatic, originating from seeding of gastrointestinal cancers, ovarian carcinoma, or abdominopelvic sarcomas. Clinically, patients will present with increased abdominal girth, anorexia, weight loss, and ascites. Palliative paracentesis may provide some relief in patients. Carcinomatosis may cause obstructive symptoms, with increased tumor burden. Peritoneal carcinomatosis carries a poor prognosis, with median survival in colorectal patients of 5 to 8 months without treatment. Treatment with cytoreductive surgery and HIPEC may be an option in selected patients with limited disease.

Pseudomyxoma Peritonei

Pseudomyxoma peritonei (PMP) is characterized by diffuse mucinous gelatinous implants to the peritoneum and mucinous ascites, referred to as "jelly belly." PMP may be caused by low-grade mucinous cystadenocarcinoma of appendix or ovary, secreting large amounts of mucuscontaining epithelial cells, or from diffuse peritoneal adenomucinosis (DPAM), which consists of proliferative mucinous epithelium. PMP is rare; incidence is 1 per 1,000,000. Histology is a prognostic factor; survival for DPAM is 75% at 5 years, with peritoneal mucinous carcinomatosis 14% at 5 years.

PMP is more common in females and presentation is usually progressive abdominal girth. The circulation of peritoneal fluid allows for PMP to disseminate and is seen in two areas in the abdominal cavity, at sites of absorption: the undersurface of the diaphragm and omentum and dependent areas and abdominal and pelvic gutter. CT imaging will show classic peritoneal scalloping of liver, calcified plaque, ascites, and possibly low-density mass. Treatment includes symptomatic debulking. Sugarbaker et al. described treatment with aggressive surgical debulking and HIPEC, with improved overall survival rates.

ADDITIONAL RESOURCES

Chow KM, Chow VC, Hung LC, et al: Tuberculous peritonitis-associated mortality is high among patients waiting for the results of mycobacterial cultures of ascitic fluid samples, *Clin Infect Dis* 35:409, 2002.

Chua TC, Moran BJ, Sugarbaker PH, et al: Early- and long-term outcome data of patients with pseudomyxoma peritonei from appendiceal origin treated by a strategy of cytoreductive surgery and hyperthermic intraperitoneal chemotherapy, *J Clin Oncol* 30:2449, 2012.

Evans R, Mouras M, Dvorkin L, Bramhall S: Hepatic and intra-abdominal tuberculosis: 2016 update, *Curr Infect Dis Rep* 18:45, 2016.

Eviatar T, Zaks N, Kukuy OL, et al: The effect of pregnancy on disease course in FMF, *Pediatr Rheumatol Online J* 11(Suppl 1):A63, 2013.

Giancane G, Ter Haar N, Wulffraat N, et al: Evidence-based recommendations for genetic diagnosis of familial mediterranean fever, *Ann Rheum Dis* 74:635–641, 2015.

Hall JC, Heel KA, Papadimitrou JM, Platell C: The pathobiology of peritonitis, *Gastroenterology* 114:185–196, 1998.

Kim J, Bhagwandin S, Labow DM: Malignant peritoneal mesothelioma: a review, *Ann Transl Med* 5(11):236, 2017.

Koskenvuo L, Peltomäki P, Renkonen-Sinisalo L, et al: Desmoid tumor patients carry an elevated risk of familial adenomatous polyposis, *J Surg Oncol* 113:209, 2016.

Lidar M, Yaqubov M, Zaks N, et al: The prodrome: a prominent yet overlooked pre-attack manifestation of familial mediterranean fever, *J Rheumatol* 33:1089, 2006.

Livneh A, Langevitz P, Zemer D, et al: Criteria for the diagnosis of familial mediterranean fever, *Arthritis Rheum* 40:1879, 1997.

Lopez N, Kobayashi L, Coimbra R: A comprehensive review of abdominal infections, *World J Emerg Surg* 6:7, 2011.

Low RN, Barone RM, Gurney JM, Muller WD: Mucinous appendiceal neoplasms: preoperative MR staging and classification compared with surgical and histopathologic findings, *AJR Am J Roentgenol* 190:656, 2008.

Nieuwenhuis MH, Casparie M, Mathus-Vliegen LM, et al: A nation-wide study comparing sporadic and familial adenomatous polyposis-related desmoid-type fibromatoses, *Int J Cancer* 129:256, 2011.

Padeha S, Berkun Y: Familial mediterranean fever, *Curr Opin Rheumatol* 28(5):523–529, 2016.

Sohar E, Gafni J, Pras M, Heller H: Familial mediterranean fever. A survey of 470 cases and review of the literature, *Am J Med* 43:227, 1967.

Sugarbaker PH: Management of peritoneal surface malignancy: the surgeon's role, *Arch Surg* 384:576–587, 1999.

Sugarbaker PH: Managing the peritoneal surface component of gastrointestinal cancer. Part 2. Perioperative intraperitoneal chemotherapy, *Oncology (Williston Park)* 18:207, 2004.

Sugarbaker PH, Ronnett BM, Archer A, et al: Pseudomyxoma peritonei syndrome, *Adv Surg* 30:233, 1996.

Van Baal J, Van de Vijver K, Nieuwland R, et al: The histophysiology and pathophysiology of the peritoneum, *Tissue Cell* 49:95–105, 2017.

van der Hilst JC, Simon A, Drenth JP: Hereditary periodic fever and reactive amyloidosis, *Clin Exp Med* 5:87, 2005.

46

Mesenteric Ischemia and Other Vascular Lesions

Morris Sasson, David R. Funes, Emanuele Lo Menzo, Raul J. Rosenthal

MESENTERIC ISCHEMIA

The mesenteric circulation receives approximately 25% of cardiac output under resting conditions. *Mesenteric ischemia* results from inadequate blood flow to the intestine and it is commonly classified as an acute episode or as a chronic disease. It can be segmental, with localized areas of bowel ischemia, or extensive, where most of the bowel is affected (Fig. 46.1):

1. Acute mesenteric ischemia is due to intestinal hypoperfusion resulting from occlusive or nonocclusive reduction of the arterial blood supply or venous outflow of the intestine.
2. Chronic mesenteric ischemia results from progressive and longstanding mesenteric atherosclerosis with subsequent episodic intestinal hypoperfusion related to eating.

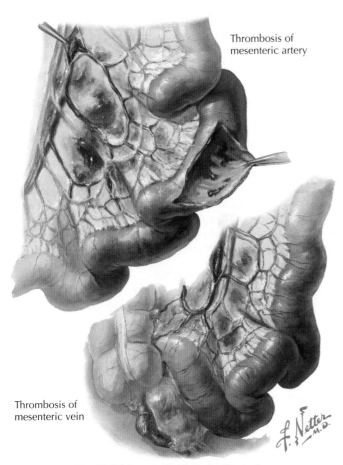

Thrombosis of mesenteric artery

Thrombosis of mesenteric vein

Fig. 46.1 Mesenteric Vascular Occlusion.

Pathophysiology

Ischemic injury to the intestine occurs when it is deprived of oxygen and other nutrients necessary to maintain cellular metabolism and integrity. Reduced blood flow may reflect poor systemic perfusion or may result from local changes in the splanchnic vasculature.

Mesenteric ischemia is a function of the following:

- State of the systemic circulation and extent of collateral blood flow to the intestine.
- Number and caliber of vessels affected, and the ability to supply the needs of the dependent segment of bowel.
- Response of the vascular bed to diminished perfusion, vasoactive substances, local humoral factors, products of cellular metabolism, and the response of the mesenteric vasculature to autonomic stimuli.
- Duration of the insult.
- Metabolic needs of the dependent segment, as dictated by its function and bacterial population.

Acute intestinal ischemia may be classified as occlusive or nonocclusive.

Occlusive mesenteric ischemia most commonly results from an arterial thrombus or an embolus of the celiac or superior mesenteric artery. Although less common, it can also be a consequence of inferior mesenteric artery occlusion or from mesenteric venous occlusion in the same distribution.

1. Arterial embolism accounts for 50% to 60% of cases and is most frequently due to a dislodged left atrial or ventricular mural thrombi, or from a valvular or proximal aortic lesion.
2. Arterial thrombosis accounts for 20% of cases and usually occurs as a superimposed phenomenon in patients with a history of chronic intestinal ischemia from atherosclerotic disease.
3. Mesenteric venous thrombosis accounts for 10% of cases and can be either idiopathic or from hypercoagulable states (e.g. hereditary, malignancy, abdominal surgery).

Nonocclusive mesenteric ischemia is thought to occur as a result of splanchnic hypoperfusion and vasoconstriction. This "low-flow" state is commonly seen in patients after an acute coronary syndrome, cardiogenic or septic shock, and in patients requiring vasopressors. It commonly affects the "watershed" areas of the colon, such as the splenic flexure and rectosigmoid junction.

Clinical Picture

The most common presentation of acute mesenteric ischemia is *severe abdominal pain*, initially colicky and periumbilical, then becoming diffuse and constant. One of the distinctive findings in mesenteric ischemia is that of abdominal pain that is out of proportion to examination, and initially with minimal peritoneal signs. Some patients have surprisingly normal physical findings on abdominal examination despite the severe pain.

Vomiting, anorexia, diarrhea, and constipation also occur frequently but are of little diagnostic help. Examination of the abdomen may also reveal distention; bowel sounds are often normal, even in patients with severe infarction. Gross gastrointestinal bleeding is unusual except in ischemic colitis. Leukocytosis is typical. Later in the disease course, gangrene of the bowel occurs, with diffuse peritonitis, sepsis, and shock.

Diagnosis

Different imaging modalities can be utilized to help in diagnosis. Abdominal plain films in patients with mesenteric ischemia may reveal air-fluid levels and distention. Pneumatosis intestinalis, portal venous gas, and pneumoperitoneum may also be seen with advanced disease.

Although the gold standard for diagnosis is angiography, the most common diagnostic methods of choice are computed tomography (CT) angiography and magnetic resonance (MR) angiography. CT is preferred over MR because of its lower costs, speed, and availability. However, MR angiography may be more sensitive for the diagnosis of mesenteric venous thrombosis and an option for those with an allergy to iodinated contrast.

Treatment and Management

Initial management includes fluid resuscitation, hemodynamic monitoring and support, correction of electrolyte abnormalities, pain control, anticoagulation, and initiation of broad-spectrum antibiotics. Restoration of normal circulation may allow complete recovery if it can be accomplished before irreversible necrosis or gangrene occurs. Unfortunately, infarction and transmural necrosis are frequently found at surgery, necessitating resection. In cases of embolism, the superior mesenteric artery (SMA) is exposed and the arteriotomy is made, and an embolectomy balloon catheter is passed to attempt removal of the embolus. Intravenous fluorescein injection followed by Wood lamp inspection and Doppler ultrasound can assist in assessing the viability of the bowel. More recently, indocyanine green (ICG) fluorescence imaging has also been used to provide intraoperative visual assessment of blood flow to the bowel wall.

In cases of mesenteric thrombosis, revascularization may be performed. A mesenteric bypass can be achieved from the aorta or the iliac artery. The graft material of choice is the saphenous vein. Prosthetic graft should be avoided in patients with nonviable bowel or intra-abdominal contamination.

Patients with nonocclusive ischemia often have extensive necrosis of the intestine resulting from the widespread nature of the ischemic event. The decision to operate is often difficult, given that the typical patient is a poor surgical candidate, with advanced age, sepsis shock, and other serious comorbid conditions. The primary treatment is catheter-directed infusion of vasodilatory agents, with papaverine commonly employed.

In any patient with acute mesenteric ischemia, when bowel viability remains questionable, a second-look operation is commonly performed 24 to 48 hours later.

For patients with chronic mesenteric ischemia, open revascularization with endarterectomy and bypass has been the treatment of choice for many years. In recent decades, endovascular therapy has emerged as a promising modality of intervention. Angiography is performed to visualize areas of mesenteric stenosis or occlusion, pharmacologic agents can be infused, and balloon angioplasty with stent placement can be performed to improve perfusion to the bowel.

Course and Prognosis

Morbidity and mortality from acute mesenteric ischemia remains high, with little improvement despite an aggressive approach. The prognosis in mesenteric venous thrombosis is more favorable than in arterial occlusion, but still serious since further thrombosis and infarction may occur. Medical therapy with antiplatelet and anticoagulation is usually required in these patients to prevent recurrence and progression of the disease.

OTHER VASCULAR LESIONS

Aortic Aneurysm

Aneurysms of the infrarenal aorta are by far the most common arterial aneurysms. Men are affected more than women by a ratio of 4 : 1. Other aneurysms, such as common or internal iliac and femoropopliteal aneurysms, are also frequently present in patients with abdominal aortic aneurysm (AAA).

Etiology

The most common pathologic condition associated with AAA is atherosclerosis. Hypertension and smoking are the most common risk factors. Other less common associated conditions are cystic medial necrosis, syphilis, tuberculosis, bacterial infections, arteritis, and trauma.

Clinical Picture

More than 70% of all infrarenal AAAs are asymptomatic when first discovered, usually as an incidental finding during routine physical examination or radiographic study. Abrupt onset of severe back or abdominal pain is characteristic of aneurysmal expansion or rupture. The incidence of ruptured AAA is 20% to 25% in most series. The typical presentation of such catastrophic disease is midabdominal or diffuse abdominal pain, back pain, pulsatile abdominal mass and hemorrhagic shock.

Treatment and Management

Open surgical repair of AAA has been the gold standard. Due to the complexity of the procedure and the high morbidity and mortality, endovascular aneurysm repair (EVAR) has emerged as the most common modality of repair for the majority AAA today. Diameters greater than 5.5 cm in male and 5.0 cm in women are common indications for repair.

Iliac Artery Aneurysm

Common iliac artery aneurysms frequently occur in continuity or in association with AAAs. Iliac aneurysms occur mainly in the population with atherosclerosis. The natural history of iliac aneurysm is unfavorable, with a high rate of rupture within a few months of diagnosis, possibly because of their large size when diagnosed. Endovascular repair of iliac aneurysms is commonly performed at the same time as endovascular AAA repair with bifurcated and limb extension grafts.

Splanchnic Arterial Aneurysms

Splanchnic arterial aneurysms constitute an uncommon but serious vascular disease. The most common splanchnic vessels involved, in decreasing order of frequency, are the splenic, hepatic, superior mesenteric, celiac, gastroepiploic, jejunal-ileocolic, pancreatic, and gastroduodenal arteries. In general, repair is indicated for splanchnic aneurysms greater than 2 cm or when symptomatic.
- *Splenic arterial aneurysms* account for 60% of all splanchnic arterial aneurysms. Symptoms of left upper quadrant or epigastric pain occur in some patients, and abdominal discomfort has been described in as many as 20%. Repair is indicated in all symptomatic or asymptomatic but greater than 3 cm. Due to very high risk of rupture, women of childbearing age or pregnant should have the aneurysm repaired, regardless of size. Different modalities for repair have been

described. Although open surgical repair with or without splenectomy was the standard of care, most splenic aneurysms today are treated with endovascular embolization and/or stent placement. Laparoscopic aneurysm ligation can also be performed in the hands of skilled minimally invasive surgeons.

- *Hepatic arterial aneurysms* account for 20% of all splanchnic aneurysms, are usually solitary, and are extrahepatic in 80% of patients. Few hepatic aneurysms are symptomatic and manifest as right upper quadrant and epigastric pain.
- *Superior mesenteric artery aneurysms* are the third most common splanchnic aneurysm, accounting for 5.5% of these lesions. In these patients, abdominal discomfort and pain may be present, and is often suggestive of intestinal angina.
- *Celiac arterial aneurysms* account for 4% of all splanchnic aneurysms. Celiac aneurysms can be asymptomatic or can be associated with vague abdominal discomfort.
- *Gastric and gastroepiploic arterial aneurysms* account for 4% of splanchnic aneurysms. Patients usually seek emergency treatment without preceding symptoms.

- *Jejunal, ileal, and colic arterial aneurysms* account for 3% of splanchnic aneurysms. *Pancreatic and gastroduodenal arterial aneurysms* are rare. Many of these aneurysms are undoubtedly asymptomatic and are recognized as incidental findings during arteriography for gastrointestinal bleeding.

ADDITIONAL RESOURCES

Brandt LJ, Boley SJ: Ischemic and vascular lesions of the bowel. In Sleisenger MH, Fordtran JS, editors: *Gastrointestinal disease* (vol 2), Philadelphia, 1993, WB Saunders, pp 1927-1962.

Cameron JL, Cameron AM (2017). *Current surgical therapy.* Philadelphia, PA. Elsevier. ed 12.

Cronenwett Jl, Johnston K (2014). *Rutherford's vascular surgery.* Philadelphia, PA. Saunders; ed 8.

O'Mara CS, Ernst CB: Physiology of the mesenteric circulation. In Zuidema GD, Shackelford RT, editors: *Shackelford's surgery of the alimentary tract,* ed 3, (vol 5), Philadelphia, 1991, Saunders.

Zinner MJ, Ashley SW: *Maingot's abdominal operations,* ed 12, McGraw-Hill Education, 2012.

Alimentary Tract Obstruction and Intestinal Injuries

Mauricio Sarmiento-Cobos, Hira Ahmad, Emanuele Lo Menzo, Raul J. Rosenthal

ALIMENTARY TRACT OBSTRUCTION

Any organic or functional condition that primarily or indirectly impedes the normal propulsion of luminal contents from the esophageal inlet to the anus should be considered an obstruction of the alimentary tract (Fig. 47.1). The spectrum of diseases affecting the alimentary tract and its clinical manifestation is significantly related to the constituent organ(s) involved. Thus, esophageal disorders manifest mainly through their relationship to swallowing. Gastric disorders are dominated by features of nausea and vomiting, and diseases of the small and large intestine manifest primarily through alterations in nutrition and elimination.

Clinical Picture

The most common symptoms resulting from disorders involving the alimentary tract include pain and alterations in bowel habit. Of these symptoms, abdominal pain is the most frequent and variable and may reflect a broad spectrum of problems, from the least threatening to the most urgent.

Abdominal pain of abrupt onset is often encountered in serious illness requiring urgent intervention, whereas a history of chronic discomfort is frequently related to an indolent disorder. Equally important are the changes in pattern, character, progression, location, and its association to meals.

Alterations in bowel habit can result from either disruption of normal intestinal motility or significant structural abnormality. The onset of worsening constipation in an adult with previously regular habits, especially when accompanied by systemic symptoms such as weight loss, suggests an underlying obstructing process, particularly malignancy.

Pathophysiology

In the newborn, various *congenital anomalies*—esophageal or intestinal abnormalities, anal atresias, colonic malrotation, volvulus of the midgut, meconium ileus, and aganglionic megacolon—result in obstruction. Early symptoms that suggest obstruction include increased salivation, feeding intolerance with regurgitation or vomiting, abdominal distention, and failure to pass meconium.

Duodenal obstruction may manifest early in the newborn period or within the first year of life, but sometimes it does not manifest until years into childhood. The common area of blockage is just beyond the ampulla of Vater. On occasion, incarceration occurs in an internal hernia, or a bowel segment may become caught in the ring of a congenital, traumatic, or surgical defect in the diaphragm.

Esophageal diseases such as achalasia can interfere with the normal passage of fluids and solids through the gullet (uppermost row in Fig. 47.1). Fibrotic narrowing has also been observed after anastomotic or plastic procedures at the lower end of the esophagus. A similar picture results from extraluminal pressure on the esophagus by a mass.

Gastric obstruction may be caused by accumulation in the stomach of ingested material, such as trichobezoar and phytobezoar, or development of hypertrophic pyloric stenosis, spastic or cicatricial occlusion related to prepyloric or postpyloric peptic ulcer, or malignant neoplasm.

Small Intestine

Obstruction of the small bowel has four characteristics: abdominal pain, vomiting, abdominal distention, and obstipation. Symptoms are variable, depending on the anatomic level, degree of obstruction, and presence or absence of strangulation.

A foreign body, either ingested by mouth or consisting of a large biliary calculus, may become impacted and result in obstruction. Etiologic mechanisms include postoperative adhesions, congenital peritoneal bands, metastatic tumor implants, bezoars, Meckel diverticulum, and plastic or adhesive peritonitis (tuberculosis, talc granuloma) and occasionally primary neoplasms of the small intestine (carcinoma, lymphosarcoma, Hodgkin granuloma) (fourth row in Fig. 47.1). Iatrogenic intestinal obstruction (anastomotic stenosis, torsion or angulation, anastomosis of incorrect loops) may result from faulty surgical technique.

Large Intestine

Cancer of the large intestine constitutes the most frequent mechanism of obstruction of this viscus. Occasionally, cecal volvulus can be seen if it has a long mesentery or sigmoid volvulus in frail, nursing home patients. A large foreign body inserted rectally (perversion, psychosis) may also obstruct the lumen (sixth row in Fig. 47.1). The most common symptoms of high-grade colonic obstruction are abdominal pain, distention, vomiting, and constipation.

Strictures of the colon may result from cicatricial fibrosis (colitis, diverticulitis) or may occur as postoperative complications (anastomotic stricture). Extraluminal compression, usually caused by primary or metastatic pelvic tumors, may obstruct the lower bowel at the level of the rectosigmoid.

Intestinal Ileus

Nonmechanical impairment of intestinal motor function has been descriptively termed reflex, adynamic, or paralytic ileus. The patient has the syndrome of gastric retention, constipation and failure to pass flatus, abdominal distention, "silent abdomen," and radiographic findings of dilatation of the small and large intestine with gas and accumulated fluid.

- *Reflux ileus* may be encountered in patients with various lesions of the central nervous system. Intestinal atony may follow surgical anesthesia or the trauma of intraabdominal surgical manipulation, extensive rib fractures, or blunt abdominal trauma. Ileus seen in reflex phenomenon includes renal or biliary colic, pneumonia, torsion

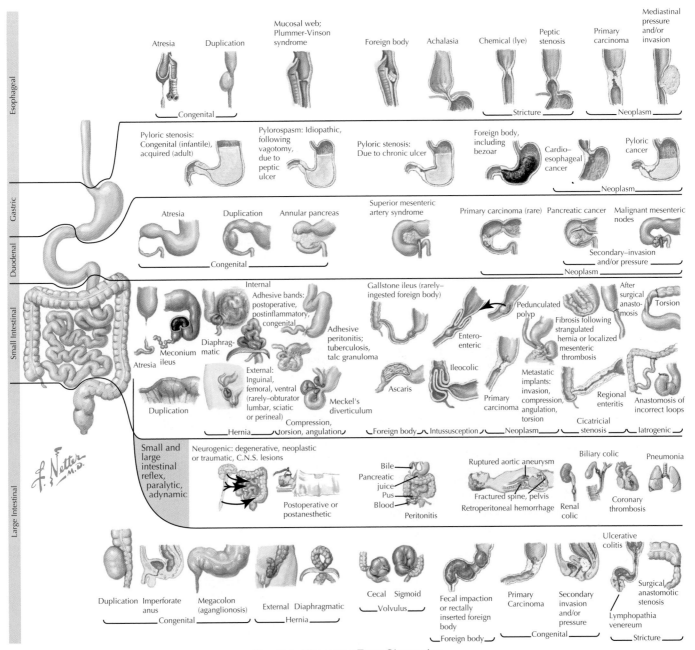

Fig. 47.1 Alimentary Tract Obstruction.

infarction of an ovarian cyst, coronary thrombosis, and retroperitoneal hemorrhage.

- *Paralytic* or *adynamic ileus* occurs most often with purulent peritonitis. Ileus may follow the intraperitoneal extravasation of gastric or duodenal contents, pancreatic juice, bile, and blood.

INJURIES OF THE SMALL INTESTINE

Injuries to the small intestine are common in patients who have experienced penetrating trauma (Fig. 47.2). Diagnosis and management of these types of injuries are relatively simple and direct. Injury to the small bowel secondary to blunt trauma, however, can present a much greater diagnostic dilemma. Associated morbidity is often secondary to the identification and prompt treatment of small-bowel injury.

The small intestine is approximately 6.5 m (21.5 ft) long; the first 40% includes the jejunum, and the remainder is ileum. The ileum is responsible for the absorption of vitamin B_{12} and the reabsorption of bile salts into the enterohepatic circulation. Thus, injuries in ileum pose different long-term challenges than in proximal small bowel. Distal small bowel has a higher anaerobic bacterial load and poses greater risk for postoperative infection.

Clinical Picture

Prompt identification of small bowel injuries depends on a high index of suspicion for injury, particularly in blunt abdominal trauma. In patients with associated head traumas, physical exam is unreliable.

The small intestine is the most frequently injured intraabdominal viscus in patients with penetrating trauma because it occupies most of the abdominal cavity and is highly mobile.

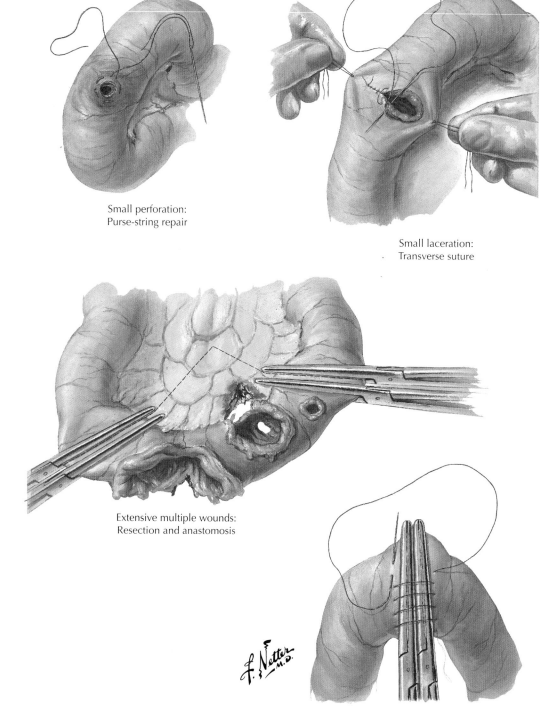

Small perforation:
Purse-string repair

Small laceration:
Transverse suture

Extensive multiple wounds:
Resection and anastomosis

Fig. 47.2 Abdominal Wounds of the Small Intestine.

Diagnosis and Treatment

Traditionally, the diagnosis of penetrating abdominal trauma includes exploratory laparotomy for all penetrating injuries. Evaluation of the entire length of the small bowel begins with the ligament of Treitz and continues to the ileocecal valve. Inspection includes examination of the entire mesentery and identification of hematoma.

Any injuries encountered should be immediately repaired. Small perforations may be repaired primarily in a transverse fashion to the long axis of the bowel to prevent narrowing of the lumen. Resection and primary anastomosis should be performed for multiple injuries in a short segment or for a short segment with massive tissue destruction (see Fig. 47.2). In the presence of mesenteric injuries, management depends on the viability of the corresponding bowel. If a large segment of the bowel is ischemic or if the associated injuries are severe, resection should be limited and should be followed by a planned second-look procedure and delayed anastomosis.

The diagnosis of small-bowel trauma secondary to blunt injury is challenging. The presence of free fluid in the peritoneal cavity in the absence of solid-organ injury is highly suggestive of small-bowel injury. Small intestinal injury may be missed on radiologic studies, particularly if the study is performed in the early postinjury period. Diagnostic laparoscopy has been used for evaluation of peritoneal penetration after stab wounds and diaphragmatic penetration after thoracoabdominal penetrating injuries. Postoperative management of patients with small-bowel injuries is often dictated by the associated injuries. Early enteral nutrition is preferred in the postoperative period, if possible.

INJURIES OF THE COLON

The colon is the second most common abdominal organ injured in penetrating trauma. Even though injury to the colon is rare in blunt trauma, it is associated with a higher risk for complications and increased hospitalization. Furthermore, no diagnostic modality or combination of findings can reliably exclude blunt injury to the colon. Therefore, a surgical approach is recommended early in the evaluation of abdominal trauma suspected to involve the colon (Fig. 47.3).

Treatment and Prognosis

Evolution in the management of colon injury to civilians resulting in significantly reduced deaths is a benefit of lessons learned from warfare. From the Civil War to the Vietnam War, the mortality rate from colonic injury declined from more than 90% to less than 10%. Several factors have contributed to the significant improvement in survival in this patient population, including the use of a diverting colostomy, fluid resuscitation, availability of blood products, and broad-spectrum antibiotics. Infection rates are significantly reduced when prophylactic antibiotics are given before surgery rather than during surgery (7% vs. 33%, respectively).

The *mechanism of injury* is often one of the few factors distinguishing military from civilian injury. Combat lesions frequently result from high-velocity weapons and explosive devices, whereas civilian injuries often result from handguns, stab wounds, and blunt trauma, and thus less severe with better prognosis. The reported mortality rate related to civilian colon injury alone is 1% to 3%. However, the cause of death in victims of colon trauma in the early postoperative period may be associated injuries rather than injury to the colon itself.

The most frequently used scales to classify the severity of colon injury are the Penetrating Abdominal Trauma Index and the Colon Injury Scale (CIS). Patients with CIS grades 1 to 3 are eligible for primary

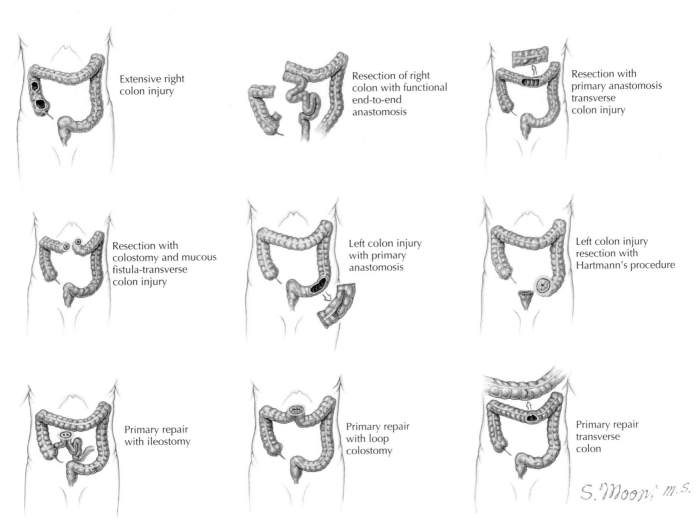

Fig. 47.3 Abdominal Wounds of the Colon.

repair, whereas those with CIS grades 4 and 5 are usually treated with fecal diversion.

The 1979 criteria for mandatory colostomy has since been challenged. In 1996 a prospective, randomized trial showed similar sepsis-related complications of primary repair versus fecal diversion. Moreover, a 2002 Cochrane Review favors primary repair over fecal diversion for the management of penetrating colon wounds. The most recent statement of the Eastern Association for the Surgery of Trauma regarding the management of penetrating intraperitoneal colon injuries recommends primary repair of nondestructive penetrating colon lesions. For destructive colon injuries, resection and anastomosis are recommended for stable patients without major associated trauma. Patients with significant comorbid conditions or severe associated injury have better outcomes when resection and colostomy constitute the treatment of choice (see Fig. 47.3).

Treatment of colon trauma must consider the surgeon's experience, a disciplined approach, the mechanism and extent of injury, the patient's status, and any associated injuries. Additionally, all patients should receive prophylactic antibiotics before surgery.

ADDITIONAL RESOURCES

Al-Salamah SM, Mirza SM, Ahmad SN, Khalid K: Role of ultrasonography, computed tomography and diagnostic peritoneal lavage in abdominal blunt trauma, *Saudi Med J* 23:1350–1355, 2002.

Brohi K: *Injury to the colon and rectum.* http://www.trauma.org/abdo/COLONguidelines.html. (Accessed July 2003).

Bullard Dunn KM, Rothenberger DA, et al: In Charles Brunicardi F, editor: *Schwartz's principles of surgery*, ed 10, New York, NY, 2015, McGraw-Hill.

Cameron JL, Cameron AM: *Current surgical therapy*, ed 12, 2017, Elsevier.

Cayten CG, Fabian TC, Garcia VF, et al: *Patient management guidelines for penetrating intraperitoneal colon injury.* http://www.east.org. (Accessed 1998).

Chappuis CW, Dietzen CD, Panetta TP, et al: Management of penetrating colon injuries: a prospective randomized trial, *Ann Surg* 213:492–497, discussion 498, 1991.

Coleman JJ, Zarzaur BL: *Surgical management of abdominal trauma hollow viscus injury*, vol 97, 2017, Department of Surgery, Indiana University School of Medicine, Indianapolis, IN Surgical Clinics.

Fakhry SM, Brownstein M, Watts DD, et al: Relatively short diagnostic delays (<8 hours) produce morbidity and mortality in blunt small bowel injury: an analysis of time to operative intervention in 198 patients from a multicenter experience, *J Trauma* 48:408–414, 2000.

Filston H: Pediatric surgery. In Sabiston A, editor: *Textbook of surgery*, vol 2, Philadelphia, 1986, Saunders, pp 1253–1298.

Galandiuk S, Smith J, Billeter A, Jorden J: *Shackelford's surgery of the alimentary tract*, ed 7, 2013.

Gonzalez RP, Merlotti GJ, Holevar MR: Colostomy in penetrating colon injury: is it necessary?, *J Trauma* 41:271–275, 1996.

Isselbacber K, Podolsky D: Approach to the patient with gastrointestinal disease. In Fauci AS, editor: *Harrison's principles of internal medicine*, vol 2, ed 14, New York, 1998, McGraw-Hill, pp 1579–1583.

Karulf RE, Fitzharris G: *Colon trauma.* http://www.fascrs.org/coresubjects/2002/karulf.html.

Lannelli A, Fabiani P, Karmdjee BS, et al: Therapeutic laparoscopy for blunt abdominal trauma with bowel injuries, *J Laparoendosc Adv Surg Tech A* 13:189–191, 2003.

McQuay N, Britt LD: Laparoscopy in the evaluation of penetrating thoracoabdominal trauma, *Am Surg* 69:788–791, 2003.

Nelson R, Singer M: Primary repair for penetrating colon injuries, *Cochrane Database Syst Rev* (3):CD002247, 2002.

Pikoulis E, Delis S, Psalides N, et al: Presentation of blunt small intestinal and mesenteric injuries, *Ann R Coll Surg Engl* 82:103–106, 2000.

Rossi P, Mullins D, Thal E: Role of laparoscopy in the evaluation of abdominal trauma, *Am J Surg* 166:707–710, 1993.

Smith LE: Traumatic injuries. In Gordon PH, Nivatvongs S, editors: *Principle and practice for the surgery of the colon, rectum and anus*, ed 2, St Louis, 1999, Quality Medical Publishing, pp 1235–1284.

Stafford RE, McGonigal MD, Weigelt JA, Johnson TJ: Oral contrast solution and computed tomography for blunt abdominal trauma: a randomized study, *Arch Surg* 134:622–626, 1999.

Welch J, Moody FG: Mechanical obstruction of the small and large intestines. In *Surgical treatment of digestive disease*, ed 2, Chicago, 1990, Mosby-Year Book, pp 624–639.

Williams MD, Watts D, Fakhry S: Colon injury after blunt abdominal trauma: results of the EAST multi-institutional hollow viscus injury study, *J Trauma* 55:906–912, 2003.

Abdominal Wall and Abdominal Cavity Hernias

Kandace Kichler, Camila Ortiz Gomez, Emanuele Lo Menzo, Raul J. Rosenthal

The word "hernia" derives from the Greek *hernios,* which means "bud." It indicates a protrusion of organs through an abnormal defect *(opening)* in a natural cavity, being the *opening,* the key part of the definition. In fact, the protrusion may not be recognized in some patients early in the process. The neck of the hernia sac corresponds to the hernial orifice. The dimension of the neck and the volume of the distended sac determine the size of the hernia. The hernia type depends on its location and cause, the mobility of the herniated organ, and the status of the blood supply (Fig. 48.1).

Approximately 20% of males and 0.2% of females acquire hernias during their lifetime. Hernias of the abdominal wall occur only where aponeurosis and fascia are devoid of the protecting support of striated muscle. Some may be acquired through muscular atrophy or surgery. Common sites of herniation are the groin, umbilicus, linea alba, semilunar line of Spiegel, diaphragm, and surgical incisions. Other similar but rare sites of herniation are the peritoneum, superior lumbar triangle of Grynfeltt, inferior lumbar triangle of Petit, and obturator and sciatic foramen of the pelvis.

INGUINAL HERNIAS

Inguinal hernias are by far the most common type of hernia. The highest incidence is during the first year of life, with a second lower peak between ages 16 and 20. The lifetime risk of developing an inguinal hernia is 27% for men and 3% for women. In both men and women, most inguinal hernias are indirect. The hernial *sac* is generally composed of peritoneum and attenuated layers of the abdominal wall. The *ring* is the actual defect and sometimes is the only abnormality palpable on physical examination. The *contents* may vary in different parts of the large and small intestines, bladder, ovaries, and omentum. The proximal part of the sac is the narrowest and is therefore called the *neck,* and the distal part is the *fundus.*

Indirect Inguinal Hernias

Failure of obliteration of the funicular process or processus vaginales during the third trimester of pregnancy leaves a channel open for the formation of an indirect inguinal hernia. However, it does not necessarily imply the development of a hernia; other factors play a role in permitting intraabdominal structures to enter this sac.

On the other hand, the disparity between intraabdominal pressure and resistance of the muscular and fascial structures forming the deep inguinal ring may also explain the origin of the defect. Great examples of this setting are conditions such as pregnancy, ascites, and prolonged coughing in patients with pulmonary emphysema and trauma.

Anatomically, the sac is anterosuperior to the spermatic cord in indirect hernias, and the deep inferior epigastric vessels are displaced medially. In addition, the protrusion of the sac and the widening of the deep ring alter the relationship between the two inguinal rings, which begin to lie perpendicularly.

Direct Inguinal Hernias

Direct inguinal hernias have a different pathophysiologic mechanism than indirect hernias. Although it is considered an acquired condition, with peak prevalence in men age 40 to 50, a congenital developmental abnormality has been identified where the fibers of the lower internal oblique muscle seem to be arranged in a transverse rather than an oblique configuration. Consequently, the conjoint tendon is attached to the rectus muscle at a more superior level, facilitating the formation of a hernia. The protrusion is characteristically medial to the deep epigastric vessels through the posterior wall of the inguinal canal.

Clinical Picture

The spectrum of inguinal hernia symptoms ranges from none to bowel strangulation. In states of rest or recumbency, most hernias are asymptomatic. Physical activity and especially increased intraabdominal pressure elicit symptoms of fullness, pain, or simply a bulge. Occasionally, symptoms may be attributed to the specific organ involved (dysuria in bladder, constipation for sigmoid colon). Predisposing factors to direct hernia include chronic increase in intraabdominal pressure (obesity, ascites, chronic cough, constipation, occupational or recreational weight lifting) and atrophy of the abdominal wall musculature (malnutrition, aging). Usually, symptoms are subtler with direct inguinal hernias.

Diagnosis

History taking and physical examination confirm the diagnosis of hernia. The examination should be conducted with the patient in the supine and upright positions. With the examiner's finger gently invaginating the scrotal skin and covering the superficial ring, the patient is encouraged to abruptly increase abdominal pressure (Valsalva maneuver, cough).

For smaller hernias, especially in women and children, inspection is often more valuable than palpation. Physical examination is more difficult in infants, but a thickened cord at the superficial ring is a reliable sign of hernia, especially if it is unilateral. When a left-sided inguinal hernia develops in a child, there is a 50% chance of bilaterality; however, this does not seem to be true for a right-sided inguinal hernia.

It is important to establish that when the scrotum is swollen ipsilaterally, the clinician must consider the presence of another abnormality such as hydrocele, varicocele, or testicular mass.

Computed tomography (CT) scan of the abdomen can aid the clinician to identify symptomatic inguinal hernias that are otherwise not palpable.

Treatment and Management

Surgery has become the preferred approach for patients of all ages. Surgery for inguinal hernia repair is simpler in infants than in adults.

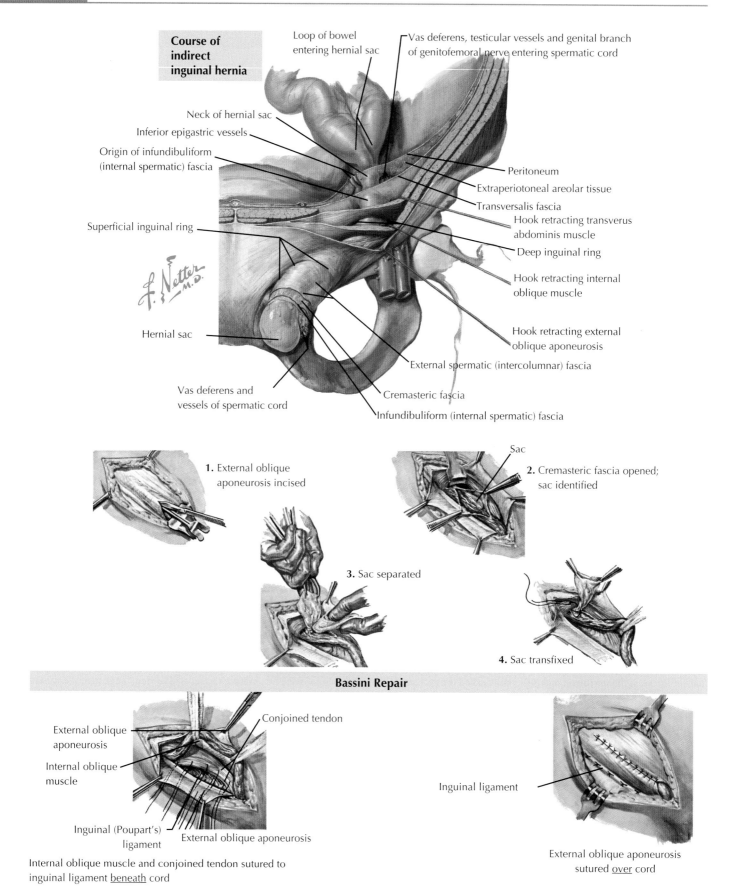

Course of indirect inguinal hernia

Loop of bowel entering hernial sac

Vas deferens, testicular vessels and genital branch of genitofemoral nerve entering spermatic cord

Neck of hernial sac

Inferior epigastric vessels

Origin of infundibuliform (internal spermatic) fascia

Peritoneum

Extraperiotoneal areolar tissue

Transversalis fascia

Hook retracting transverus abdominis muscle

Superficial inguinal ring

Deep inguinal ring

Hook retracting internal oblique muscle

Hernial sac

Hook retracting external oblique aponeurosis

External spermatic (intercolumnar) fascia

Vas deferens and vessels of spermatic cord

Cremasteric fascia

Infundibuliform (internal spermatic) fascia

1. External oblique aponeurosis incised

Sac

2. Cremasteric fascia opened; sac identified

3. Sac separated

4. Sac transfixed

Bassini Repair

External oblique aponeurosis

Conjoined tendon

Internal oblique muscle

Inguinal (Poupart's) ligament

External oblique aponeurosis

Inguinal ligament

Internal oblique muscle and conjoined tendon sutured to inguinal ligament <u>beneath</u> cord

External oblique aponeurosis sutured <u>over</u> cord

Fig. 48.1 Indirect and Direct Inguinal Hernias.

In fact, the proximity of the deep and superficial inguinal rings makes the opening of the aponeurosis of the external oblique muscle unnecessary and dangerous for the cord structures. Isolating the sac is more difficult in female infants because of the smaller size of the sac, in turn making it more difficult to identify anterior to the round ligament.

Numerous surgical techniques have been described. Bassini in Italy and Halsted in the United States established the fundamental principles at the end of the 1800s.

Bassini repair is one of the cornerstones in the evolution of inguinal hernia repair. It involves approximation of the internal oblique, transversalis fascia, and transversus abdominis muscle complex to the inguinal ligament and the ileopubic tract to reinforce the posterior wall of the inguinal canal. *Halsted repair* is almost identical to the Bassini procedure, except for the subcutaneous position of the cord structures and the addition of an extra layer (external oblique aponeurosis) to the repair. This resulted in a high incidence of testicular ischemia and hydrocele, so Halsted modified the original technique, leading to the Halsted II or Ferguson-Andrews procedure.

In 1898 Lotheissen described using the iliopectineal, or Cooper, ligament rather than the inguinal ligament to anchor the triple layer (internal oblique, transversalis fascia, and transversus abdominis muscle) of the Bassini repair. McVay and Anson added, 40 years later, a relaxing incision in the rectus sheath to avert tension. The external oblique was then closed over the cord. This variation has since become more widely used than the Bassini repair, especially for repair of direct hernias.

Treatment of direct hernia is primarily surgical, and multiple techniques have been described. With *lason repair,* the incision is made over the protrusion and is extended to the superficial inguinal ring. The actual repair is accomplished by suturing the conjoint tendon to the inguinal or pectineal ligaments, and the external oblique aponeurosis is imbricated above or below the cord.

Since the introduction of synthetic meshes in the 1950s, interest in the application of *tension-free repair* (e.g., Lichtenstein) in inguinal hernias increased exponentially. Initially used to reinforce conventional repairs, the Marlex mesh was then extended to patients with more challenging hernias, such as large direct or recurrent hernias. The infection rate was reportedly less than 2%, and the recurrence rate was approximately 6%. Later, the primarily repair with a tension-free onlay prosthetic mesh was introduced. Advantages of this technique included decreased postoperative pain, lower recurrence rates, faster return to work and normal activity, and a shorter learning curve than for conventional repairs. Although the possibility of infection was still a concern, subsequent trials failed to show a higher incidence of infection using mesh; they have rather shown a reduced rate of recurrence and likelihood of long-term pain.

Laparoscopic repair was introduced in the early 1990s. Its main advantages were less postoperative pain and more rapid to return to work compared with previous techniques. In addition, laparoscopic hernias present the unique advantage of allowing for bilateral repair during the same operation. The main indications for laparoscopic repair are for bilateral and recurrent hernias. Among the various techniques described, only transabdominal preperitoneal (TAPP) and total extraperitoneal (TEP) repairs remain popular laparoscopic options. The main difference between them is the approach to the preperitoneal space. With the *transabdominal preperitoneal repair,* the transversalis fascia is exposed by way of the intraperitoneal route, whereas with *total extraperitoneal repair,* the dissection is entirely preperitoneal.

Currently there is an additional option for repair available, the robotic-assisted technique. Da Vinci (Intuitive Surgical, Sunnyville, CA) introduced their device into the market in 2000. Since that time, urology and gynecology have mainly used this technology for deep pelvic dissections. The robotic platform has now been used in general surgery and it is used for many abdominal wall hernia repairs, including the inguinal hernia. In a method similar to the TAPP laparoscopic technique, the robot can be docked and the instrument used to reduce the hernia, implant mesh, and close the peritoneal defect. Similar results to the laparoscopic approach are seen in the hands of surgeons trained in and familiar with robotic surgery.

FEMORAL HERNIAS

Femoral hernias are those in which the abdominal viscera protrude through the femoral ring (Fig. 48.2). In most patients a hernia sac is present. These types of hernias are usually unilateral, with a right-sided predominance. Femoral hernias are three times more common in females, although the overall incidence is much lower than for inguinal hernias.

Despite the true etiology of femoral hernia being unknown, two theories have been postulated. The first one states that these hernias are *congenital* and derived from a preformed sac. This is supported by the findings of femoral hernias in fetuses. Conversely, the second theory hypothesizes that the increased intraabdominal pressure plays a key role in *acquiring* this type of defect, explaining the higher incidence of femoral hernias in older, multiparous women and also the embryonic peritoneal protrusion being different from the hernial sac.

Pathophysiologically, the boundaries of the femoral canal are the cribriform fascia and the inguinal ligament anteriorly, the fascia lata over the pectineus muscle and Cooper ligament posteriorly, the femoral vein laterally, and the lacunar (Gimbernat) ligament medially.

The herniating viscus pushes a peritoneal sac and some preperitoneal fat tissue behind the inguinal ligament and through the inguinal ring. It then emerges in the subcutaneous tissue at the level of the fossa ovalis. At this point, the herniated viscus can extend upward to the level of the inguinal hernia. However, the neck is always below the inguinal ligament and lateral to the pubic tubercle. For this reason, a femoral hernia can be mistaken for an inguinal hernia, making reduction difficult if pressure is applied directly upward and toward the superficial ring. The sac may descend anterior to the femoral vessels (prevascular hernia) or behind the vessel (retro vascular hernia). When an aberrant obturator artery is present, the sac may be bisected (bilocular).

Clinical Picture

Femoral hernias are usually small and produce minimal symptoms until they become incarcerated or strangulated. Strangulation is the most common complication of femoral hernias, occurring 10 times more frequently than in inguinal hernias.

Diagnosis

The diagnosis of femoral hernia is made by the presence of a mass at the medial aspect of the thigh, just beneath the inguinal ligament. The mass must be differentiated from an obturator hernia, saphenous vein varix, enlarged lymph node, lipoma, and psoas muscle abscess.

Treatment and Management

The only successful treatment of femoral hernias is surgery. As with other types of hernia, various procedures have been described over the years, indicating the lack of a widely accepted approach. In general, the different approaches can be divided into inguinal and subinguinal, depending on the route chosen to access the hernia. The procedures may also be combined. In general, the *subinguinal* approach requires less dissection and is indicated for patients at high risk. The *inguinal* approach requires more dissection but offers better long-term results.

Most minimally invasive laparoscopic or robotic repairs (TAPP or TEP) address the femoral space, and this hernia can be repaired in this manner. However, incarceration and or strangulation may make this

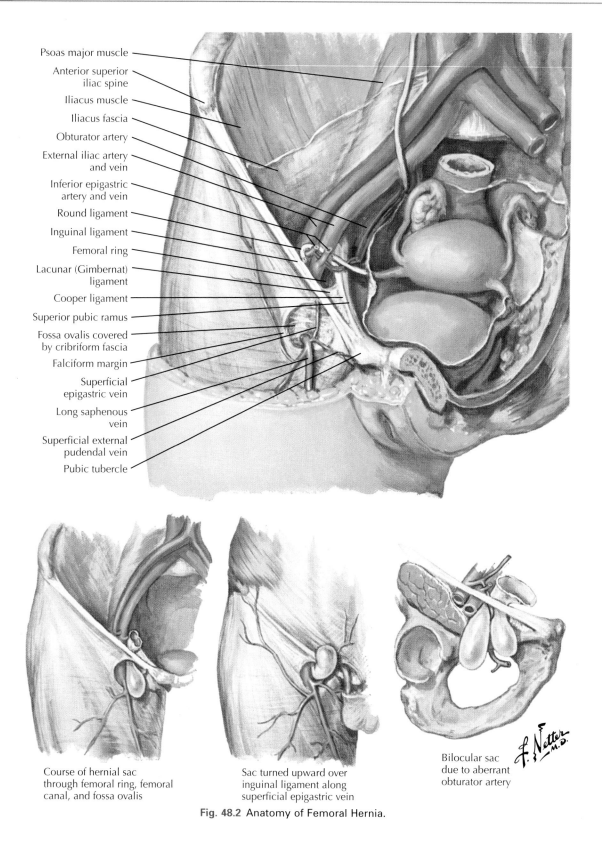

Psoas major muscle

Anterior superior iliac spine

Iliacus muscle

Iliacus fascia

Obturator artery

External iliac artery and vein

Inferior epigastric artery and vein

Round ligament

Inguinal ligament

Femoral ring

Lacunar (Gimbernat) ligament

Cooper ligament

Superior pubic ramus

Fossa ovalis covered by cribriform fascia

Falciform margin

Superficial epigastric vein

Long saphenous vein

Superficial external pudendal vein

Pubic tubercle

Course of hernial sac through femoral ring, femoral canal, and fossa ovalis

Sac turned upward over inguinal ligament along superficial epigastric vein

Bilocular sac due to aberrant obturator artery

Fig. 48.2 Anatomy of Femoral Hernia.

approach more difficult, necessitating a more traditional or open approach, especially if bowel resection is indicated.

VENTRAL HERNIAS

Incisional (ventral) *hernias* result from inadequate healing of a previous surgical incision (Fig. 48.3). Many factors lead to the formation of incisional hernias; obesity being a predominant cause. The bulk associated with a fatty omentum and excessive subcutaneous tissue increases the strain on the surgical wound in the early stages of healing. In addition, many patients with obesity have an associated loss of muscle mass and tone that may result in weakened fascial layers that could not compensate for the strain.

Other factors that can contribute to ventral hernia formation are advanced age, malnutrition, ascites, postoperative hematoma or wound infection, peritoneal dialysis, pregnancy, and conditions that cause increased intraabdominal pressure. Certain medications that blunt the inflammatory response, such as steroids and chemotherapeutic agents, may also contribute to poor wound healing.

Although hernias protruding through very large defects rarely become incarcerated or strangulated, hernias with multiple components may compromise the integrity of their contents. This factor and the high recurrence and complication rates make incisional hernias a complex problem.

Treatment and Management

Primary suture repair of an incisional hernia can occasionally be accomplished for small hernias. However, most ventral hernias are best treated with prosthetic materials. Several materials are available, among which expandable polytetrafluoroethylene (PTFE), polypropylene (Prolene), and polyester are the materials of choice. Timing of surgical repair must be individualized, and, if possible, patients should be in optimal medical condition. Preoperative preparation includes weight loss, smoking cessation, rigid control of diabetes, adequate nutrition, and avoidance of medications that impair wound healing. Previously, in the presence of clean-contaminated conditions, the use of prosthetic materials was absolutely contraindicated; more evidence exists on the safety of these materials in Centers for Disease Control and Prevention (CDC) class 2 conditions. In addition, new biologic and absorbable bioprosthetic materials are now available for these types of situations.

Surgery for ventral hernia repair may be conventional or minimally invasive (laparoscopic or robotic). In general, the advantages of minimally invasive techniques include decreased wound infection, decreased hospital stay, and faster return to work. The limitations of the laparoscopic

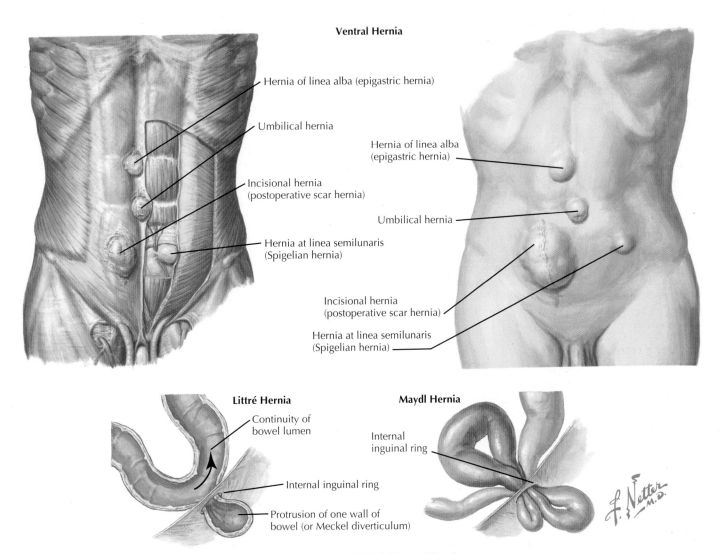

Fig. 48.3 Abdominal Wall: Ventral Hernias.

approach include the simple bridging of the defect with a prosthetic material without closure of it, the higher likelihood of complications related to the adhesiolysis, and the technical difficulty.

Umbilical Hernias

Umbilical hernias are usually present at birth. Patients of African descent are more predisposed to this condition, and, in fact, in the United States, umbilical hernias are eight times more common in African Americans than in Caucasians. Most umbilical hernias close spontaneously, but those that persist in children older than 5 years may need surgical correction.

Umbilical hernias that develop during adulthood are considered *acquired.* Conditions that result in increased intraabdominal pressure, as those previously described, may contribute to umbilical hernias in adults. It is rare for umbilical hernias to be complicated by incarceration or strangulation.

Simple transverse closure of the defect with proper reduction of the sac is generally adequate to treat small (<2.5 cm) umbilical hernias. In larger defects, a mesh is necessary for the repair because it reduces the hernia recurrence rate.

Spigelian Hernias

A Spigelian hernia is an abdominal wall defect located on the outer edge of the *crescent line,* the area between the anterior rectus muscle and the sheaths of the wide muscles of the abdomen in the area, also known as *semilunar or arcuate line.* Spigelian hernias usually occur inferiorly to the semicircular line of Douglas. The lack of posterior rectus fascia below the line of Douglas contributes to inherent weakness in this area. These hernias constitute 0.12% to 2% of all abdominal wall hernias. Classic etiologic factors associated with these defects include obesity, chronic obstructive pulmonary disease, previous surgery, and abdominal trauma.

Spigelian hernias may be found incidentally by ultrasonography and CT; nonetheless, preoperative diagnosis has only a 50% accuracy rate. Spigelian hernias can be successfully repaired during the initial surgery by approximation of the tissues, although prosthetic reinforcement may be used if the defect is large.

Epigastric Hernias

Epigastric hernias are defects of the linea alba above the umbilicus. These are usually small and may be difficult to detect in obese patients. The most common symptom is a painful sensation of "pulling" at the midline on reclining. These hernias are usually repaired by simple closure, with or without mesh. However, the surgeon must keep in mind that more than one defect may exist; therefore proper exposure of the linea alba is mandatory.

Richter Hernia

Any abdominal wall hernia in which the antimesenteric border of the intestine protrudes through the sac may be classified as a Richter hernia. The key characteristic of this type of hernia is that the entire circumference of the intestine is not involved. Symptoms and clinical course vary, depending on the degree of intestinal obstruction. Strangulation can occur as a painful mass, with abdominal distention, nausea, and vomiting.

Although Richter hernia is found predominantly in the femoral canal, the incidence of Richter hernia has increased since the advent of laparoscopy because of unrepaired trocar sites. Proper evaluation of intestinal viability is critical to hernia repair. In patients with compromised viability, intestinal resection is required. The protrusion of more than one loop of intestine (usually two) through the sac is considered a "W" (retrograde) hernia, or Maydl hernia.

Littré Hernia

In Littré hernia, the entire component of the sac must be a Meckel diverticulum. This type of hernia is infrequent and difficult to diagnose. Clinical manifestations of Littré hernia are localized pain over a preexisting hernia with intestinal obstruction, intestinal bleeding, perforation, fistula, and malignancy.

LUMBAR, OBTURATOR, SCIATIC, AND PERINEAL HERNIAS

Lumbar Hernia

Lumbar hernia is an uncommon protrusion in the posterior abdominal wall that occurs in either the inferior (Petit) or the superior (Grynfeltt and Lesshaft) lumbar triangle (Fig. 48.4). Most hernias occur in the superior triangle, which is bordered by the twelfth rib superiorly, the internal oblique muscle anteriorly, and the quadratus abdominis muscle posteriorly. The latissimus dorsi forms the roof, and the transversus abdominis forms the floor. Hernias through the Grynfeltt triangle often develop after flank incisions for kidney surgery. Petit triangle hernias often occur in young, athletic women and usually contain fat, intestine, mesentery, or omentum. Bowel incarceration is the presenting sign in 24% of patients with lumbar hernia. The patient seeks treatment for a "lump in the flank" and reports dull, heavy, localized pain; they tend to become larger and therefore should be repaired when found. Acquired hernias may be caused by direct trauma, penetrating wounds, poor healing of flank incisions, and abscesses. Diagnosis is suspected on identification of a defect in the flank and CT has been advocated as the diagnostic study of choice for suspected lumbar hernia in patients whose condition is stable.

Lumbar hernia should be differentiated from soft tissue tumors, abscesses, hematomas, and renal tumors. Simple suture repair of small hernias is practical, whereas the repair of larger hernias is more demanding. Overlapping and imbricating suture repairs can be performed; however, some large hernias may require mesh reinforcement, pedicle flaps, or free flaps.

Obturator Hernia

The obturator foramen is the largest foramen in the body. Formed by the rami of the ischium and the pubis, it is 2 to 3 cm long and 1 cm wide. A strong quadri lamellar musculoaponeurotic barrier, formed by internal and external obturator membranes and closed by obturator internal and external muscles, contains the obturator nerve, artery, and vein surrounded by fat. Deterioration of the obturator membrane and enlargement of the canal results in the formation of a hernial sac, causing significant intestinal obstruction and incarceration.

An obturator hernia develops in three stages. The first stage is the entry of periperitoneal tissue and fat into the pelvic orifice of the obturator canal. The second stage begins with the development of a dimple in the peritoneum over the internal opening and progresses to the invagination of a peritoneal sac. The third stage begins with the onset of symptoms produced by the entrance of an organ, usually the ileum, into the sac. Three specific signs indicate a strangulated hernia. *Obturator neuralgia* extends from the inguinal crease to the anteromedial aspect of the thigh. The *Howship-Romberg sign* is the classic sign, seen in 25% to 50% of diagnosed strangulated hernias, and is characterized by pain in the medial thigh and occasionally in the hip; flexion of the thigh usually relieves the pain. The *Hannington-Kiff sign* is an absent adductor reflex in the thigh, resulting from obturator nerve compression.

CT is recognized as the standard diagnostic modality, although ultrasonography and magnetic resonance imaging (MRI) can also reliably aid in the diagnosis of obturator hernia. Differential diagnoses

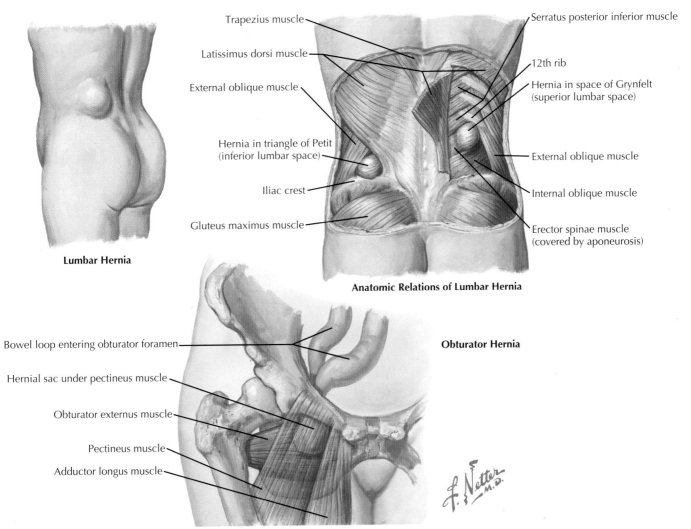

Lumbar Hernia

Anatomic Relations of Lumbar Hernia

Obturator Hernia

Fig. 48.4 Lumbar, Obturator, Sciatic, and Perineal Hernias Image.

include psoas abscess, femoral and perineal hernias, intestinal obstructions, inguinal adenitis, and diseases of the hip joint.

Various approaches to obturator hernia repair have been suggested. The abdominal approach, open or laparoscopic, is preferable when compromised bowel is suspected. The retropubic (preperitoneal) approach is preferred when there are no signs of obstruction. More effective closure of the defect may be obtained by the use of mesh.

Sciatic Hernias

Sciatic hernia is also known as ischiatic hernia, gluteal hernia, hernia incisurae ischiadica, and sacrosciatic hernia. The sciatic notch on the inferior margin of the pelvis is transformed into the greater and lesser sciatic foramina by the sacrospinous and sacrotuberous ligaments. Likewise, the greater sciatic foramen is subdivided by the piriform muscle, forming the suprapiriform and infrapiriform spaces. This anatomic organization leaves, as a result, three possible openings for sciatic hernias.

Clinically, patients have pain patterns that originate mainly in the pelvis but that occasionally radiate to the buttocks and the posterior thigh. Patients rarely exhibit signs such as protrusion, bulge, or saccule because of the small size of the hernial sac. The sac may contain small bowel, ureter, or ovary. Other documented sac contents include Meckel diverticulum, colon, and bladder. Atrophy of the piriform muscle increases the risk for sciatic hernia.

Differential diagnoses include abscess, lipoma, and gluteal aneurysm. Sciatic hernias are usually diagnosed and treated during surgery, with most repairs performed through a transperitoneal or transgluteal approach.

Perineal Hernias

Perineal hernia is another infrequent but well-recognized complication of major pelvic surgery. There are two basic types of perineal hernias: primary and secondary. *Primary,* or anterior, perineal hernias result from acquired weakness of the pelvic floor structures, common in middle-aged women with a history of childbirth. They develop through the urogenital diaphragm with the bulbocavernosus muscle medially, the ischiocavernosus laterally, and the transverse perineal muscle posteriorly. *Secondary,* or posterior, perineal hernias involve a defect between the levator ani and the coccygeus muscle. They are rare, reported in only 1% of patients, and are related to previous surgery, particularly pelvic exenteration, abdominoperineal resection, and perineal prostatectomy. The hernial sac may contain bowel, omentum, or bladder.

Common symptoms of perineal hernias are pain and a reducible bulge, but difficult urination may also be a symptom. Differential diagnoses include soft tissue tumors, cysts, abscesses, and hematomas. Various approaches for surgical repair of perineal hernia have been proposed but not standardized. Although the abdominal or perineal

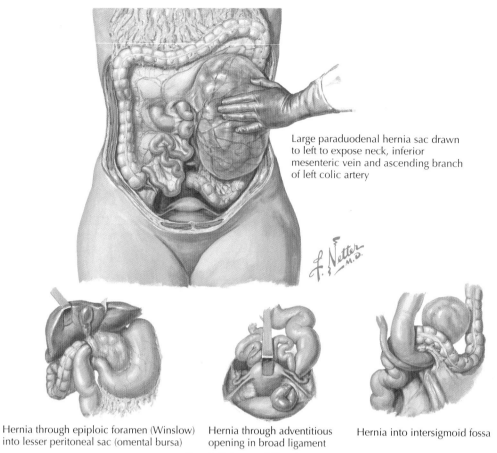

Large paraduodenal hernia sac drawn to left to expose neck, inferior mesenteric vein and ascending branch of left colic artery

Hernia through epiploic foramen (Winslow) into lesser peritoneal sac (omental bursa)

Hernia through adventitious opening in broad ligament

Hernia into intersigmoid fossa

Fig. 48.5 Internal Hernia.

approach can be used, myocutaneous flap or mesh reinforcement is required for repair.

INTERNAL HERNIAS

Congenital Intraperitoneal Hernias

Most intraperitoneal hernias result from anatomic variants that are usually present at birth (Fig. 48.5). Hernias that develop secondarily to alterations in normal intestinal rotation during embryologic development have sacs. These types of hernias are generally *paraduodenal* or *mesocolic*. Hernias that develop through defects in the mesentery or peritoneum do not have sacs. These types of hernia include those through the epiploic foramen, congenital defects in the mesentery of the small and large intestine, and, less commonly, defects in the broad ligaments of the uterus.

Trauma and previous abdominal surgery also cause intraperitoneal hernias. Internal hernias are rarely diagnosed before surgery, regardless of their location. Suspected signs of intestinal obstruction and a palpable mass in the corresponding region may indicate an internal hernia. Preoperative CT scanning may also identify "twisting" or "swirling" of the mesentery, which can indicate the presence of an internal hernia. One of the most remarkable features of internal hernias is that they can be present and remain asymptomatic for the person's lifetime, with diagnosis made only on postmortem study.

The surgical approach should be determined based on the presence of intestinal strangulation or ischemia. The surgeon must be aware that major blood vessels often traverse the neck of the hernial sac; therefore it may be prudent to open the sac beyond the neck to decompress the gut. On the other hand, given the case of an incidentally detected defect, it should be repaired to prevent the development of an internal hernia in the future.

ADDITIONAL RESOURCES

Arregui ME, Nagan RF, editors: *Inguinal hernia: advances or controversies?* New York, 1994, Radcliffe Medical Press, pp 435–436.

Bendavid R: The shouldice method of inguinal herniorrhaphy. In Nyhus LM, Baker RJ, Fischer JE, editors: *Mastery of surgery*, ed 3, Boston, 1987, Little, Brown, pp 1826–1838.

Birgisson G, Park AE, Mastrangelo MJJ, et al: Obesity and laparoscopic repair of ventral hernias, *Surg Endosc* 14:1–5, 2001.

Brian EB, Kimball M: Traumatic lumbar hernia, *South Med J* 93:1067–1069, 2000.

Camps J, Nguyen N, Cornet DA, Fitzgibbons RJ: Laparoscopic transabdominal preperitoneal hernia repair. In Phillips EH, Rosenthal RJ, editors: *Operative strategies in laparoscopic surgery*, Berlin, 1995, Springer, pp 83–87.

Charles EJ, Mehaffey JH, Tache-Leon CA, et al: Inguinal hernia repair: is there a benefit to using the robot? *Surg Endosc* 32(4):2131–2136, 2017.

Cox TC, Huntington CR, Blair LJ, et al: Quality of life and outcomes for femoral hernia repair: does laparoscopy have an advantage? *Hernia* 21(1):79–88, 2017.

Dumanian GA, Denham W: Comparison of repair techniques for major incisional hernias, *Am J Surg* 185:61–65, 2003.

Eubanks S: Hernias. In Townsend CM Jr, Sabiston A, editors: *Textbook of surgery*, ed 16, Philadelphia, 2001, Saunders, pp 783–800.

Fallas MJ, Phillips EH: Laparoscopic near-total preperitoneal hernia repair. In Phillips EH, Rosenthal RJ, editors: *Operative strategies in laparoscopic surgery*, Berlin, 1995, Springer, pp 88–94.

Franklin ME Jr, Abrego D, Parra E: Laparoscopic repair of postoperative perineal hernia, *Hernia* 6:42–44, 2002.

Iraniha A, Peloquin J: Long-term quality of life and outcomes following robotic assisted TAPP inguinal hernia repair, *J Robot Surg*. 1–9, 2017.

John RM, Michael JO, William BS: Sciatic hernia as a cause of chronic pelvic pain in women, *Obstet Gynecol* 91:998–1001, 1998.

Julian EL, Bruce WR, James WJ: Obturator hernia, *J Am Coll Surg* 194: 657–663, 2002.

Julian EL, Kirien TK: Diagnosis and treatment of primary incarcerated lumbar hernia, *Eur J Surg* 168:193–195, 2002.

Katagiri H, Okumura K, Machi J: Internal hernia due to mesenteric defect, *J Surg Case Reports* 2013(5):2013.

Kyzer S, Alis M, Aloni Y, Charuzi I: Laparoscopic repair of postoperative ventral hernia, *Surg Endosc* 13:928–931, 1999.

Lee JS, John A, Gene LC, John ES: Obturator hernia, *Surg Clin North Am* 8:71–84, 2000.

Nyhus L: Recurrent groin hernia, *World J Surg* 13:541–544, 1989.

Öberg S, Andresen K, Rosenberg J: Etiology of inguinal hernias: a comprehensive review, *Front Surg* 4:52, 2017.

Read RC: Inguinofemoral herniation: evolution of repair by the posterior approach to the groin. In Nyhus LM, editor: *Shackelford's surgery of the alimentary tract*, ed 4, Philadelphia, 1996, Saunders, pp 129–137.

Rutledge RH: Cooper ligament repair of groin hernias. In Nyhus LM, Baker RJ, Fischer JE, editors: *Mastery of surgery*, ed 3, Boston, 1987, Little, Brown, pp 1817–1825.

Sanchez Montes I, Deysine M: Spigelian and other uncommon hernia repairs, *Surg Clin North Am* 83:1235–1253, 2003.

Schwartz SI: Abdominal wall hernias. In Schwartz SI, editor: *Principles of surgery*, vol 2, ed 7, New York, 1999, McGraw-Hill, pp 1437–1611.

Stigg KM, Rohr MS, McDonald JC: Abdominal wall, umbilicus, peritoneum mesenteries, omentum and retroperitoneum. In Townsend CM Jr, Sabiston A, editors: *Textbook of surgery*, ed 16, Philadelphia, 2001, Saunders, p 769.

Terranova O, Battocchio F: The bassini operation. In Nyhus LM, Baker RJ, Fischer JE, editors: *Mastery of surgery*, ed 3, Boston, 1987, Little, Brown, pp 1807–1816.

Waite KE, Herman MA, Doyle PJ: Comparison of robotic versus laparoscopic transabdominal preperitoneal (TAPP) inguinal hernia repair, *J Robot Surg*. 10(3):239–244, 2016.

Welsh DRJ: Inguinal hernia repair: a contemporary approach to a common procedure, *Mod Med* 2:49–54, 1974.

49

Abdominal Access

Rene Aleman, Luis F. Zorrilla-Nuñez, Mobola Oyefule,
Emanuele Lo Menzo, Raul J. Rosenthal

ROBOTIC ACCESS

Based on Dr. Halsted's legacy, a surgeon should always protect tissues with exquisite care based on three principles: asepsis, hemostasis, and gentleness. None of the preoperative preparation is as essential as the manner in which details are executed. Gentleness is essential in the performance of any surgical procedure.

However, in recent decades a shift toward the search for less invasive procedures has seen the expansion of laparoscopy. Historically, Kelling was the first to examine the peritoneal cavity with an endoscope in 1901, although it was done in a dog. The first major series of laparoscopies in humans is attributed to Jacobaeus, who in 1911 reported examining both the abdominal and thoracic cavities with a "Lapaothorakoscopie."

Most recently, the technological evolution has brought us computer-assisted remote mechanical devices in the form of robotic surgery. The term *robot* defines a device that has been programmed to perform specific tasks in place of those usually performed by people. In contrast to the use of robotics in industry, the robot does not work autonomously in most surgical applications but rather acts as an interface between the operating surgeon and the patient.

It was largely developed to overcome the limitations of conventional laparoscopy, which include two-dimensional visualization, incomplete articulation of instruments, and limited ergonomics. The robotic platform incorporates high-definition imaging systems, powerful computer processors, and advanced robotic technology surgery with the easier transmission of open surgical skills to laparoscopic surgery. This platform also provides precise and ergonomic control of "wristed" surgical instruments with 7 degrees of freedom in an ergonomically comfortable workstation, and with three-dimensional visualization of surgical anatomy, tremor elimination, and scaling of movement.

The robotic assist surgery (RAS) system is composed of three major hardware components:

1. Surgical (aka patient) cart: contains the mechanical arms (one camera arm, three to four surgical instrumentation arms) that interface with the patient directly at the operating table.
2. Vision cart: usually contains a video monitor (for bedside/assistant visualization), the video processor, a light source, insufflator for CO_2 gas, etc.
3. Surgeon console: contains a "stereoscopic" or binocular visual display that provides high-definition, three-dimensional images with adjustable magnification and fine focus of the operative field and the master controllers.

The most recent iteration of the robotic platform features a second console slave enabling greater assisting and teaching opportunities. An assistant remains at the bedside and changes the instruments as needed, providing retraction as needed to facilitate the procedure.

All patients considered for RAS should undergo preparation for surgery in standard fashion and be carefully evaluated for perioperative risk factors. An emphasis on ample patient education prior to surgery will prepare the patient for a more satisfying surgical experience.

From the physiologic perspective, RAS is similar to standard laparoscopic surgery because the creation of a surgical "working field" will require the development and maintenance of a pneumoperitoneum throughout the procedure.

You must ensure that all three components of the RAS platform are functioning correctly. Once the patient is safely under anesthesia and properly positioned, gaining access to the target surgical anatomy is undertaken in a typical minimally invasive or nonrobotic, laparoscopic fashion. According to individual surgeon preference, a Veress needle, an optical view trocar, or an open, "cut-down" approach is undertaken to gain access to the abdomen and initiate the pneumoperitoneum. Robotic reusable trocars are available from 5- to 13-mm sizes. The robotic endoscopes can be used with standard 12-mm laparoscopic ports or can be used with their respected robotic reusable trocars. The robotic instruments must be used with the robotic reusable trocar cannulas.

Regardless of the initial access technique, upon establishing pneumoperitoneum, the intraabdominal contents are surveyed and carefully assessed for signs of injury due to the initial access maneuver. Once this has been confidently excluded, we can begin placement of additional cannulas under direct visualization. Specific locations and the number/size of the surgical cannulas will be determined by the demands of the surgical procedure and the characteristics of a patient's anatomy. As in laparoscopic surgery, triangulation of the surgical target with respect to the camera and the bilateral working arms is preferred in most situations.

Once all of the cannulas have been placed, the operating table is adjusted into optimal position for the anticipated procedure. In this position, the individual arms of the surgical cart may be prepared for surgical maneuvers in a process called "docking the robot." Visualization is maximized when the center column of the surgical cart is positioned in a straight line behind the target tissue, and the camera is also lined up directly in front of the target tissue. The surgical arms will then be extended over the patient's body and ultimately docked to their designated cannulas.

This results in a final configuration with the camera and all instrument tips pointing directly toward the surgical target with the surgical cart standing directly beyond it. The use of a fourth robotic surgical arm and the placement of additional bedside assistant port(s) are up to the discretion of the operating surgeon. Once docked, the laparoscopic wristed instruments and endoscope can be inserted.

The lack of tactile resistance or feedback must be respected and overcome. The only feedback that the operating surgeon experiences at the surgeon's console is purely visual. Keeping all working instruments in direct and constant visualization is an absolute must for RAS. In addition, careful insertion and removal of surgical instruments by properly trained and knowledgeable assistants is critically important. Furthermore, the surgeon should make a conscious effort to reduce the number of instrument exchanges during the procedure to limit the risk of inadvertent injury and to maximize surgical efficiency.

As with laparoscopic surgery, there has always been an interest in further minimizing the invasiveness of surgery by converting RAS procedures using multiple incisions into a "single-site" operation, using only one small incision.

Single-site laparoscopic surgery required a disoriented "crisscrossing" of surgical instruments, limited surgical views, and poor ergonomics, whereas the RAS platform's capabilities, such as the ability to designate control of individual surgical arms, enhanced surgical visualization, and improved ergonomics, all help to overcome some of the challenges of single-site laparoscopic surgery. Proper patient selection and preoperative planning and optimal equipment setup are the fundamental keys to a successful RAS procedure.

LAPAROSCOPIC ACCESS

Described adeptly as a disruptive innovation, laparoscopy has supplanted laparotomy to become the preferred option for many intraabdominal surgical procedures. Since the early 1990s, general surgeons have used laparoscopy in the treatment of intraabdominal and retroperitoneal pathology. The technique and equipment have greatly improved in the three decades since early adoption, making laparoscopy the most common approach for abdominal operations.

Laparoscopy is superior to laparotomy because it offers measurable advantages such as decreased postoperative pain, decreased incidence of wound complications (hematoma, seroma, fat necrosis, wound dehiscence, evisceration, and hernias), shorter duration of postoperative ileus, and ultimately decreased length of hospital stay. These benefits directly translate to lower cost of surgery, which offsets the initial costs of acquiring laparoscopic instruments. Patient satisfaction is boosted by the ability to largely preserve cosmesis using the smaller incisions afforded by this approach. The principles of laparoscopy are transferable and are now widely used in the fields of robotic and endoluminal surgery.

Indications

Diagnostic laparoscopy, major and minor gastrointestinal (GI) tract resection, non-GI intraabdominal and retroperitoneal tract resection, feeding conduit placement, bariatric surgery, revision surgery, cancer staging.

Contraindications

Inability to tolerate general anesthesia, uncorrected coagulopathy, "frozen" abdomen, hemodynamically unstable patient in extremis.

Morbid obesity and pregnancy, which were conditions thought to be contraindications to laparoscopy, are no longer contraindicated; however, special circumstances will require modification in entry technique and subsequent trocar placement.

Basic Equipment

- Laparoscopic surgery tower typically includes the CO_2 insufflator unit with gas tank, camera processor unit, light source, video camera recorder, electrosurgical unit.
- Video camera with cord
- Veress needle
- Optical trocar
- Hasson cannula
- Gas insufflation tubing
- 0-degree, 30-degree, and 45-degree videoscopes in 3-, 5-, and 10-mm sizes
- Video monitors (minimum of two)
- 3-, 5-, 10-, 12-, and 15-mm trocars with introducing obturators
- S-shaped retractors
- Kocher clamps
- Tonsil clamps
- Laparoscopic instrument set/tray
- Suction irrigator
- Endoscopic removal bag
- Energy devices and corresponding electrosurgical units
- Fog Reduction and Elimination Device (FRED)
- 0-Vicryl suture on a GU-6 needle
- 4-0 Vicryl or 4-0 Monocryl suture on a P-24 needle

Technical Considerations
Gaining Access

Access into the abdominal cavity is gained through open techniques or closed techniques. Although various methods of entry are used by surgeons, multiple studies have concluded that most methods of gaining access when performed by experienced surgeons are noninferior to one another. Each method carried a small but not inconsequential risk of injury to intraabdominal organs; however, the incidence of such occurrences has not been shown to be statistically significant when comparing one method to the next.

Open technique. The open technique is also known eponymously as the Hasson technique (Dr. Hasson, a gynecologist first pioneered this technique in 1989). A 2-cm transverse incision is made in the infraumbilical midline, the subcutaneous tissue is dissected with electrocautery until the anterior fascia is identified at the linea alba. By grabbing on either side of the linea alba with two Kocher clamps, the anterior fascia is tented up and a vertical incision is made through the intervening portion between the Kocher clamps. Once the fascia is entered, an anchoring suture, typically a 0-Vicryl on a GU-6 needle, is placed on either side of the anterior fascia. Blunt dissection is done to expose the peritoneum. Once identified, the peritoneum is tented up in tandem fashion using two tonsil clamps. An incision is made between the tonsil clamps using a curved scissor and the abdominal cavity is entered. A 10-mm Hasson cannula is placed through this opening and advanced until the grooves are snugly in contact with the abdominal wall to provide a secure seal. The cannula is secured to the abdominal wall at its sleeves, using the anchoring stitches placed through the anterior fascia. The obturator is removed, and CO_2 insufflation is begun.

Closed technique using Veress needle. The Veress needle is a particular tool with a spring-activated sheath protecting the sharp bevel. The sharp portion of the needle is designed to penetrate the layers of the abdominal wall without insufflation and, once the resistance of the abdominal wall is surpassed, the spring-activated sheath covers the bevel to protect the intraabdominal organs. After making a stab incision with an 11 blade, the Veress needle is inserted in the midline at the upper border or base of the umbilicus or at Palmer point in the left upper quadrant. Gripped like a pencil, the needle is advanced into the abdominal cavity angled 45 to 90 degrees to the abdominal wall, depending on the adiposity of the patient's abdominal wall, until resistance is met. At the level of the posterior fascia, the operator will feel a "give-in" resistance. The second "give" will occur when the peritoneum is traversed. Once the peritoneum is entered, the blunt protector tip is spring-loaded to prevent injury to intraabdominal organs. After aspirating with a syringe to ascertain that the tip of the needle is not intraluminal to any abdominal structure, 5 mL of saline should be instilled into the hub of the needle, which will flow easily into the abdominal cavity if the tip of the catheter lays freely in the peritoneum. Once access is secured, CO_2 is insufflated into the abdomen at 1 L/min until an intraabdominal pressure of 6 to 7 mm Hg is reached. The rate of insufflation can then be increased to 5 to 6 L/min to obtain the desired goal of 12 to 15 mm Hg.

The Veress needle is removed and replaced with a 5- or 10-mm trocar and corresponding 30-degree videoscope.

Closed technique using optical trocar. The optical trocars have a transparent tip and a hollow obturator to allow the laparoscope to be inserted directly in them. An incision is made in the supraumbilical midline or left subcostal space, depending on the location of intra-abdominal pathology to be addressed. Using a 0-degree scope placed in site of the obturator, the abdominal cavity is entered with direct visualization of major layers. The first layer seen is the subcutaneous adipose layer, followed by the different fascia and muscles layers depending on the location of the incision, the preperitoneal adipose layer, and finally the peritoneum. Once the peritoneum is traversed, the scope can be withdrawn and exchanged for a 30-degree scope. CO_2 insufflation is begun.

Maintaining Pneumoperitoneum

Adequate pneumoperitoneum is achieved and maintained by continuous insufflation of carbon dioxide gas initially at a low rate of 1 L/min until a pressure of 5 to 7 mm Hg is obtained and then at a rate of 3 to 4 L/min until the desired level is reached. Conventionally, we maintain pressures at 12 to 15 mm Hg to gain adequate working space to perform procedures without constraints. Depending on the patient, pressures may need to be reduced for those who do not tolerate high insufflation pressures or increased as in obese patients with more visceral adiposity.

Trocar Placement and Removal

After gaining access into the peritoneal cavity, trocars or working ports are placed under direct visualization. It is important to place trocars in a triangular fashion with respect to the target organ to achieve optimum visualization and to avoid clashing of instruments (Fig. 49.1).

Trocars are also removed under direct visualization to survey for any subdermal bleeding at the port incision sites.

Closing Port Sites

The 5-mm port sites are generally closed in a single layer at the level of the dermis only, because there is a much smaller risk of herniation

Key landmarks of the surface anatomy of the anteriolateral abdominal wall

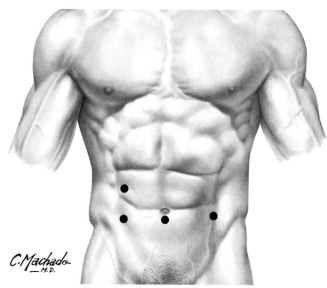

C.Machado
_M.D._

● Standard laparoscopic port placement

Fig. 49.1 Laparoscopic Port Placement.

at these incisions. Using a 4-0 absorbable suture, a simple interrupted stitch is placed in the subcuticular layer, taking care to approximate the skin edges. The knot is concealed as to avoid the potential discomfort for the patient if the knot extrudes through the skin.

Port sites greater than 10 mm are closed in two layers. The fascia is approximated by passing a 0-Vicryl suture laparoscopically with a suture passer device (Carter-Thomason) to create a figure-of-eight stitch. Alternatively, the fascia may be closed by retracting the skin and subcutaneous tissue and placing the 0-Vicryl suture on a GU-6 needle in a figure-of-eight stitch under direct visualization. The skin is then approximated with either interrupted or running subcuticular stitches using a 4-0 absorbable suture. Evidence supports no fascial closure for the 12-mm blunt tip trocars placed off midline, especially above the umbilicus in obese patients, because the risk of herniation is negligible.

OPEN EXPLORATORY LAPAROTOMY APPROACH

Exploration is still the mainstay of treatment for many surgical diseases of the abdominal cavity. Different approaches are meant to provide the best access to the organ or region targeted, minimizing trauma to the patient. A thorough knowledge of the anatomy is paramount. The morbidity of the different incisions varies significantly based on the indication of the exploration, the location of the incision, and the underlying patient's medical history.

At times, no definite diagnosis can be made with the preoperative work-up, and when diagnostic laparoscopy cannot provide a clear understanding of the clinical picture, an exploratory laparotomy remains the ultimate diagnostic tool.

INDICATIONS

There are various reasons to perform an open exploration of the abdominal cavity. Exploratory laparotomy must be performed in a standardized stepwise manner to successfully diagnose and treat the underlying pathology and minimize postoperative complications. Main indications for exploratory laparotomy include the treatment of infectious, traumatic, neoplastic, mechanical, and functional derangements of the abdominal cavity and its contents. In addition, abnormalities of the abdominal wall might require a laparotomy as part of the repair process.

Relevant Anatomy

As described in detail in previous chapters, the layers of the abdominal wall midline include, from superficially to deep, the following structures: skin, Camper superficial fascia, *Scarpa* deep fascia, anterior rectus sheath, *rectus abdominis,* posterior rectus sheath *transversalis* fascia, and peritoneum. Depending on the location within the abdominal wall, these structures might vary. Just below the umbilicus the arcuate line or semicircular line of Douglas marks the limit of the posterior layer of the rectus sheath. In fact, at this level the posterior rectus sheath and *transversalis* fascia move to anterior to the rectus muscle to contribute to the anterior rectus sheath. Another important landmark is the *linea semilunaris* of *Spigelian* line. This is a curvilinear *tendinous* intersection between the lateral aspect of the rectus abdominis muscle and the medial aspect of the external oblique. Within the peritoneal cavity, the transverse mesocolon divides the space into two compartments: the supracolic and the infracolic compartments. The former contains the liver, gallbladder, stomach, spleen, and accompanying neurovasculature. The latter contains the colon, intestines (jejunum and ileum), female reproductive organs, and a retroperitoneal localized bladder, as well as their accompanying neurovasculature. The area posterior to the peritoneum (retroperitoneum) contains the duodenum, pancreas, kidneys, adrenal glands, aorta, and inferior vena cava (IVC).

Technique

Whenever possible the direction of the skin incision should follow that of Langer superficial lines. These are imaginary lines on the skin that correspond to the natural orientation of collagen fibers. Usually these lines are oriented in a parallel fashion to the underlying muscle fibers. The preferred instrument to proceed with the initial incision is the scalpel. However, a systematic review and meta-analysis of 11 trials, comparing the outcomes of abdominal incisions using scalpel or electrosurgery in a total of 3122 patients, concluded that the use of electrocautery resulted in significant lower pain for the first 24 hours after surgery. Moreover, scalpel incisions, if carried out in multiple strokes in different planes, can increase susceptibility for infections.

Upon performing the opening incision, consider a three-step approach for control of superficial bleeding, regardless of abdominal incision selected:

1. Small subcutaneous vessels involved in the opening incision will constrict and blood loss will be under physiologic response control.
2. Cauterize persistent bleeding cautiously and as required.
3. Larger vessels like the inferior epigastric artery should be identified, clamped, and ligated.

Types of Incisions

The type of incision will provide exposure to different anatomic structures and expedite and grant safety to the procedure. Abdominal incisions for laparotomy purposes can be vertical, transverse, or oblique. Vertical incisions are preferred when optimal view of the abdominal cavity is necessary, and it is adequate for exploring supracolic and infracolic compartments. Conversely, transverse and oblique incisions can be performed in any of the abdomen's four quadrants, depending on the site of interest.

Vertical Incisions

The vertical incisions follow a cephalad to caudad direction, as the name implies (Fig. 49.2). They can be in the midline or off the midline.

A midline incision. The midline incision is considered the incision of choice for an exploratory laparotomy because it causes minimal impairment of the abdominal wall by sparing the abdominal wall muscles. It also allows for a satisfactory healing process with minimum postoperative complications. In addition, as the incision follows the linea alba, it allows nerve preservation and minimal bleeding due to the lack of neurovascularity at this site, consequently limiting postoperative pain. The midline incision provides both rapid access and great abdominal cavity exposure.

Of course, anatomic variations of the abdominal wall exist, and bleeding can be encountered in the midline from terminal branches of the thoracoepigastric vein, the superficial inferior epigastric vessels, and the superior epigastric vessels. When necessary, the midline incision has the peculiar advantage of being able to be extended both superiorly toward the xiphoid process and inferiorly toward the pubic tubercle. To avoid possible infections and unwanted scarring, the umbilical scar should not be included in the incision.

Supraumbilical incision (epigastric incision). As the name implies, this incision extends from just above the umbilicus and can reach the xiphoid process of the sternum. This is an ideal incision for organ exposure in the supramesocolic compartment (esophagus, stomach, biliary tree, spleen). When performing a supraumbilical incision, the linea alba is separated along the midline. Typically a substantial layer of preperitoneal fat is then encountered. When the peritoneum is exposed, care should be taken to identify, clamp, divide, and ligate the ligamentum teres of the liver.

Infraumbilical incision (hypogastric incision). The incision carried out below the umbilicus is mostly used to expose the organs in the inframesocolic compartment (small bowel, colon, appendix, female reproductive organs, prostate, urinary system, and retroperitoneal organs). When performing an infraumbilical incision, it is pivotal to remember the lack of a posterior rectus sheath below the line of Douglas, to avoid bowel injuries. When the incision is extended all the way down to the pubis, the identification of the pyramidalis muscles indicates the approaching to the urinary bladder. It is important to proceed with caution because of the risk of injury to the bladder.

Paramedian incision. Paramedian incision provides suboptimal exposure in comparison with a midline incision. It is also laborious, has inferior aesthetic results, and bears a significant risk of dehiscence as compared with a midline incision. Recall that the superficial epigastric vessels run vertically and anteriorly to the rectus abdominis. This entails a surgical site warning for this type of incision, as well as drainage or trocar placement. The need to perform said incision must be valued in terms of benefits-over-risk as to avoid the sectioning of the superficial epigastric vessels. The incision is made 2 to 3 cm lateral to the midline (to the right or to the left), the anterior rectus sheath is incised, the rectus muscle is retracted laterally, the posterior rectus sheath is incised and the peritoneum is exposed. Similar to the midline incision, the paramedian incision obviates nerve endings and transverse sectioning of the rectus muscle. In addition, the paramedian incision can be extended superiorly by curving the incision superiorly alongside the subcostal margin toward the xiphoid process. It is rarely used now.

Vertical muscle-splitting incision. The vertical muscle-splitting incision is made similar to the paramedian incision, with the particularity that the rectus muscle is split. This incision has a distinctive value for rapidness and for reopening previous paramedian incisions. However, the vertical muscle-splitting incision should not extend further than previous paramedian incisions because they may result in significant bleeding and nerve sectioning, consequently compromising the integrity of the abdominal wall.

Transverse and Oblique Incisions

Transverse and oblique incisions have comparatively superior cosmetic results than vertical incisions by following Langer lines of tension. The rectus muscle segmental nerve supply from intercostal nerve is spared during this incision, conveying further benefits related to pain. When properly performed, the transverse and oblique incisions provide good

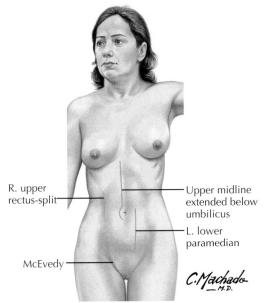

R. upper rectus-split

Upper midline extended below umbilicus

L. lower paramedian

McEvedy

C. Machado
—M.D.

Fig. 49.2 Types of Vertical Incisions.

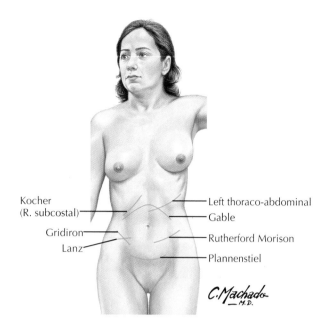

Kocher
(R. subcostal)

Gridiron

Lanz

Left thoraco-abdominal

Gable

Rutherford Morison

Plannenstiel

C.Machado
— M.D.

Fig. 49.3 Transverse and Paramedian Incisions.

exposure of specific organs, yet these incisions limit visibility of upper and lower abdominal viscera. The transverse and oblique incisions are (Fig. 49.3):

- Kocher subcostal incision: right upper quadrant (for hepatobiliary procedures)
- Pfannenstiel infraumbilical incision: hypogastric segment (for gynecologic procedures)
- McBurney and Rockie-Davis incisions: right lower quadrant (for appendectomies and kidney transplantation)
- Subcostal incision: left subcostal incision for left upper quadrant (for splenectomies)
- Rutherford Morrison incision: left lower quadrant (for renal transplant implantation)
- Thoracoabdominal incision: superior exposure of upper abdominal organs (for esophagogastric junction exposure)

Kocher (right subcostal) incision. The right subcostal incision (Kocher incision) exposes the gallbladder and biliary tree, whereas the left subcostal incision exposes the spleen. A bilateral subcostal approach will expose the upper abdomen, for hepatectomies, liver transplantations, gastrectomies, and anterior access of adrenal glands. The incision is done approximately 4 cm below the xiphoid process and extends obliquely parallel to the subcostal margin. This incision has to divide the rectus muscle and corresponding fascia medially and the oblique muscles laterally. Because of the need of muscle division and location underneath the rib cage, this is considered the most painful of the abdominal incisions.

McBurney and Rockie-Davis incisions. Both the McBurney and Rockie-Davis incisions are well suited for appendectomy. The former is oriented obliquely, whereas the latter has a transverse orientation, which conveys better cosmetic results. They are both muscle-sparing incisions and usually have low morbidity. The Rockie-Davis incision can be also used for kidney transplantation.

Pfannenstiel incision. Pfannenstiel incision is mostly suited for gynecologic procedures and access to the retropubic space. More recently this incision, because of its muscle-splitting nature and advantageous cosmetic results, is also used for specimen extraction of laparoscopic-assisted operations (colon in particular). The incision is made in the interspinous crease above the symphysis pubis, affording cosmetic benefits but limiting anatomic exposure.

Rutherford Morrison incision. The Rutherford Morrison incision is placed approximately 2 cm above the left anterior superior iliac spine and extends obliquely toward the midline. This incision renders a place for transplanted kidney in the iliac fossa (when done so extraperitoneally), or exposure of the iliac artery during vascular procedures.

Thoracoabdominal incisions. The thoracoabdominal incisions provide satisfactory exposure of upper abdominal viscera. When the incision is made on the left side, it provides exposure of the left hemidiaphragm, gastro-esophageal (GE) junction, distal pancreas, and spleen, whereas a right-sided incision grants exposure to the right hemidiaphragm, hepatobiliary anatomy, IVC, and proximal pancreas.

ADDITIONAL RESOURCES

Robotic Access

Díaz-Montes TP, Tanner EJ, Fader AN: Instrumentation, platforms, and basic principles of robotics. In Escobar P, Falcone T, editors: *Atlas of single-port, laparoscopic, and robotic surgery*, New York, NY, 2014, Springer.

Hagen ME, Curet MJ: The da vinci surgical® systems. In Watanabe G, editor: *Robotic surgery*, Tokyo, 2014, Springer.

Ohuchida K, Hashizume M: Overview of robotic surgery. In Watanabe G, editor: *Robotic surgery*, Tokyo, 2014, Springer.

Park CW, Portenier DD: Basic setup, principles, and troubleshooting in robotic surgery. In Kroh M, Chalikonda S, editors: *Essentials of robotic surgery*, Cham, 2015, Springer.

Schwartz SI: Chapter 1. A focused history of surgery. In Zinner MJ, Ashley SW, editors: *Maingot's abdominal operations*, ed 12, New York, NY, 2013, Mcgraw-Hill.

Spight DH, Hunter JG, Jobe BA: Minimally invasive surgery, robotics, natural orifice transluminal endoscopic surgery, and single-incision laparoscopic surgery. In Brunicardi F, Andersen DK, Billiar TR, et al, editors: *Schwartz's principles of surgery*, ed 10, New York, NY, 2015, Mcgraw-Hill.

Stetler JL: System control overview and instruments. In Patel A, Oleynikov D, editors: *The SAGES manual of robotic surgery*, Cham, 2018, Springer.

Surgical technique. In Ellison E, Zollinger RM Jr, editors: *Zollinger's atlas of surgical operations*, ed 10, New York, NY, 2016, Mcgraw-Hill.

Laparoscopic Access

Ahmad G, Gent D, Henderson D, et al: Laparoscopic entry techniques, *Cochrane Database Syst Rev* (8):CD006583, 2015.

Baker RJ, Fischer JE: *Mastery of surgery*, Philadelphia, 2001, Lippincott Williams & Wilkins.

Dunne N, Booth MI, Dehn T: Establishing pneumoperitoneum: veress or hasson? The debate continues, *Annals of the Royal College of Surgeons* 93(1):22–24, 2011.

Soper N, et al: *The SAGES manual, Basic Laparoscopy and Endoscopy*, vol 1, ed 3, 2012, Springer Link.

Zollinger RM, Zollinger RM, Zollinger RM: *Zollinger's atlas of surgical operations*, New York, 2003, McGraw-Hill, Medical Pub. Division.

Open Exploratory Laparotomy Approach

Ahmad NZ, Ahmed A: Meta-analysis of the effectiveness of surgical scalpel or diathermy in making abdominal skin incisions, *Ann Surg* 253:8, 2011.

Delcore R, Cheung L: *Acute abdominal pain. ACS surgery: principles and practice 2005*, Chicago, IL, 2005, BC Decker, pp 313–314. ISBN 9780974832746.

Grantcharov TP, Rosenberg J: Vertical compared with transverse incisions in abdominal surgery, *Eur J Surg* 167:260–267, 2001.

Ly J, Mittal A, Windsor J: Systematic review and meta-analysis of cutting diathermy versus scalpel for skin incision, *Br J Surg* 99:613, 2012.

Meeks GR, Trenhaile TR: Management of abdominal incisions, *J Pel Surg* 6:295, 2002.

Seiler CM, Deckert A, Diener MK, et al: Midline versus transverse incision in major abdominal surgery: a randomized, double-blind equivalence trial (POVATI: ISRCTN60734227), *Ann Surg* 249:913–920, 2009.

Small Intestine

Martin H. Floch

50

Anatomy of the Small Intestine

Martin H. Floch

TOPOGRAPHY AND STRUCTURE OF THE SMALL INTESTINE AND TERMINAL ILEUM

The small intestine consists of a retroperitoneal portion, the duodenum, and a mesenteric portion comprising the coils of the jejunum and the ileum (Fig. 50.1). Given that the mesenteric portion of the small intestine is subject to considerable individual and functional variations, its total length varies considerably. The average length for adults is approximately 5 m (15 to 20 feet), 40% of which is accounted for by the upper part, the jejunum, and 60% by the lower part, the ileum.

The *jejunum* begins at the duodenojejunal flexure on the left side of the second lumbar vertebra or, occasionally, somewhat more cranially (see Section II). The *ileum* joins the large intestine in the region of the right iliac fossa. The *duodenojejunal flexure* is situated high up in the inframesocolic zone of the peritoneal cavity and may be partially concealed by the attachment of the transverse mesocolon. Between the duodenojejunal flexure and the ileocolic junction, the parietal line of attachment of the small intestine mesentery runs obliquely from above on the left to below on the right, passing across the lumbar spine, large prevertebral blood vessels (aorta, inferior vena cava), right psoas major, and right ureter.

Because the *mesentery* is only approximately 15 to 20 cm (6 to 8 inches) long at its parietal line of attachment, rather than the several meters (corresponding to length of intestine) along its intestinal attachment, it splays fanlike toward the intestine. Mesentery, consisting of two layers of peritoneum, affords the intestinal coils a wide range of movement. The space between the two layers of peritoneum is filled with connective tissue and fat tissue, the latter varying greatly from one person to another. Embedded in this tissue are blood and lymph vessels running between the intestine and the dorsal wall of the abdomen, along with nerves and mesenteric lymph nodes.

The various portions of the large intestine appear as a horseshoe-shaped arch and form a frame enclosing the convolutions of the small intestine (see Section V). However, this frame may be overlapped ventrally by the coils of the small intestine, particularly on the side of the descending colon. Similarly, depending on their filling and on their relationship to the pelvic organs, the coils of the small intestine may bulge downward into the true pelvis or, if the pelvic organs are greatly distended (e.g., in pregnancy), may be displaced in a cranial direction.

With a greatly variable shape and highly mobile position, the greater omentum hangs like an apron from the greater curvature of the stomach and spreads between the anterior abdominal wall and the coils of the small intestine.

The greater part of the coils of the jejunum lies upward to the left, whereas those forming the ileum are situated lower and to the right side. Because it is attached only to its mesentery, the small intestine is capable of considerable movement. Its coils vary greatly in position even in the same person, depending on the state of intestinal filling and on peristalsis and on the position of the body as observed under x-ray examination after oral introduction of a rubber tube. In accordance with its progressively shortened mesentery, the only position that has a more or less "constant" position is the terminal ileum, which passes from the left across the right psoas major to the site of the ileocolic junction.

GROSS STRUCTURE OF THE SMALL INTESTINE

The freely mobile portion of the small intestine extends from the duodenojejunal flexure to the ileocolic orifice. This portion of the small intestine consists of the jejunum and the ileum, which run imperceptibly into each other; the transition is marked by a gradual change in the diameter of the lumen and by various structural alterations. As with the entire gastrointestinal (GI) tract, the virtually identical walls of the jejunum and ileum consist of five coats: mucosa, submucosa, circular muscularis, longitudinal muscularis, and serosa (Fig. 50.2).

The innermost layer, the mucous membrane, is thickly plicated by macroscopically visible circular or convoluted folds, or *plicae,* known as *circular* or *Kerckring folds* (valves), or valvulae conniventes. These folds vary in height, projecting 3 to 10 mm into the lumen, and run in a transverse direction to the lumen's longitudinal axis. Some plicae extend all the way around the internal circumference, others go only halfway or two-thirds the way around the circumference, and still others spiral around two or even more times. These do not act as a true valve; projecting into the lumen, Kerckring valves will slow down, to a certain extent, the progression of the luminal contents, but their essential function is to increase the absorptive surface area. This principle is all the more obvious because the fold's surface is further equipped with tiny, fingerlike projections, or *villi.*

Below the epithelial surface of the mucosa, but participating in the formation of Kerckring folds and the villi, is the tunica propria, or *lamina propria,* a loose coat of predominantly reticular connective tissue, assuming in some parts a lymphatic character. The lamina propria also contains thin fibers of smooth muscle radiating from the muscularis mucosae and extending upward to the tips of the villi, which have an even surface when these fibers are relaxed but become jagged or indented when the fibers contract. The muscular fibrils act as motors maintaining the pumping function of the villi. Situated in the lamina propria, and especially in the stroma of the villi, are the terminal ramifications of the blood vessels, the central lacteal or lymph vessels of the villi, and nerve fibers. Many solitary lymph nodes are embedded in the lamina propria, which may reach far into the submucosal layer.

The muscularis mucosae separates the mucous membrane from the *submucosal coat* and is composed of two thin, nonstriated muscle layers that keep the movable muscle layer in place. The outer longitudinal

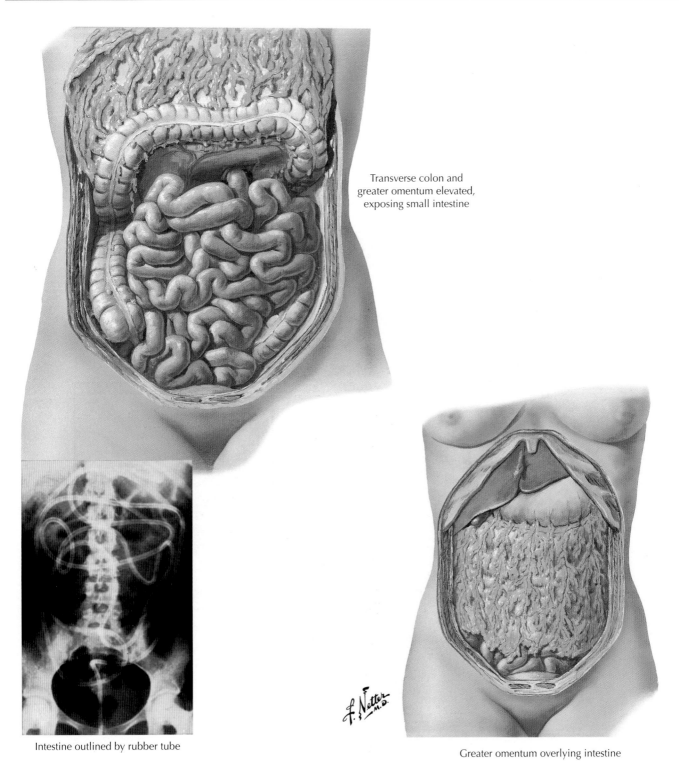

Transverse colon and
greater omentum elevated,
exposing small intestine

Intestine outlined by rubber tube

Greater omentum overlying intestine

Fig. 50.1 Topography and Relations of the Small Intestine.

layer is thinner than the inner circular layer from which the muscle fibers in the core of the villi emanate. Tunica submucosa consists of collagen connective tissue, the fibers of which form a network of meshes. By altering the angles of its meshes, the submucosal network is able to adapt to changes in the diameter and length of the intestinal lumen. The submucosa contains a rich network of capillaries and larger vessels, numerous lymphatics, and the submucous nerve plexus of Meissner. The muscle layer is made of smooth muscle cells.

The thick inner circular layer and the thinner outer longitudinal layer are connected by convoluted transitional fascicles where the layers border on each other. Between the two layers is spread a network of nonmyelinated nerve fibers and ganglion cells, the myenteric plexus of Auerbach.

Serosa is composed of a layer of flat, polygonal epithelia and a subserosa of loose connective tissue. It covers the entire circumference of the intestinal tube, except for a narrow strip at the posterior wall, where

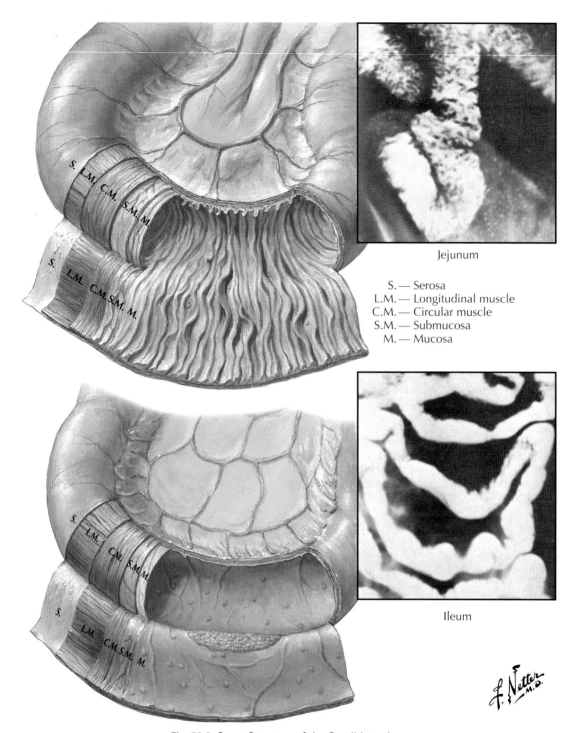

Jejunum

S. — Serosa
L.M. — Longitudinal muscle
C.M. — Circular muscle
S.M. — Submucosa
M. — Mucosa

Ileum

Fig. 50.2 Gross Structure of the Small Intestine.

the visceral peritoneum connects with the two serous layers of the fan-shaped mesentery.

The jejunum and ileum differ in size and appearance. The ileal lumen is narrower and the diameter of the total ileal wall is thinner than in the jejunum. The average diameter of the jejunum is 3 to 3.5 cm, whereas the ileum is 2.5 cm or less. Because of this difference, the intestinal contents show up more clearly through the ileum than through the jejunum. When the abdomen is opened, the jejunum has a whitish red hue, whereas the ileum, during life and after death, takes on a darker appearance. The folds and the villi become smaller and decrease in number as the small intestine continues. In the lower reaches of the ileum, the folds appear only sporadically.

In the jejunum, lymphatic tissue is encountered only in the form of solitary nodules, which appear as pinhead-sized elevations on the surface of the mucosa. They become more numerous and more pronounced as they near the large intestine. In addition, aggregate nodules (Peyer patches) appear, confined to the ileum. Averaging 1 to 1.5 cm wide, Peyer patches are 2 to 10 cm long and vary greatly in number, usually 20 to 30. The ileal mesentery contains more fatty tissue and appears to be thicker than the jejunum.

MICROSCOPIC STRUCTURE OF THE SMALL INTESTINE

The entire mucosal surface of the small intestine is covered with projections 0.5 to 1.5 mm long, the intestinal *villi* (Fig. 50.3). The mass of these villi (estimated at four million for the jejunum and the ileum) accounts for the velvetlike appearance of the intestinal mucosa. In the jejunum, villi are longer and broader than in the ileum. Valleys, or indentations, between the villi result in nonramified pits, each of which harbors one or two tubular structures, the intestinal glands, or *crypts of Lieberkühn.*

The entire inner surface of the small intestine is covered by a single line of epithelial cells, most of which are cylindrical, highly prismatic *columnar cells* with a well-developed cuticular border on the surface. Between these columnar cells are interspersed three other types of cells: goblet cells, Paneth (oxyphilic granular) cells, and enterochromaffin cells. *Goblet cells* secrete an alkaline mucous fluid that coats the entire mucosa. As the small intestine moves closer to the large intestine, healthy anaerobic bacterial organisms tend to live in this mucus and function as probiotics. Most goblet cells are found in the crypts of Lieberkühn or along the lower parts of the villi, but some are located in the upper parts of the villi. The characteristic elements of the floor of the crypts

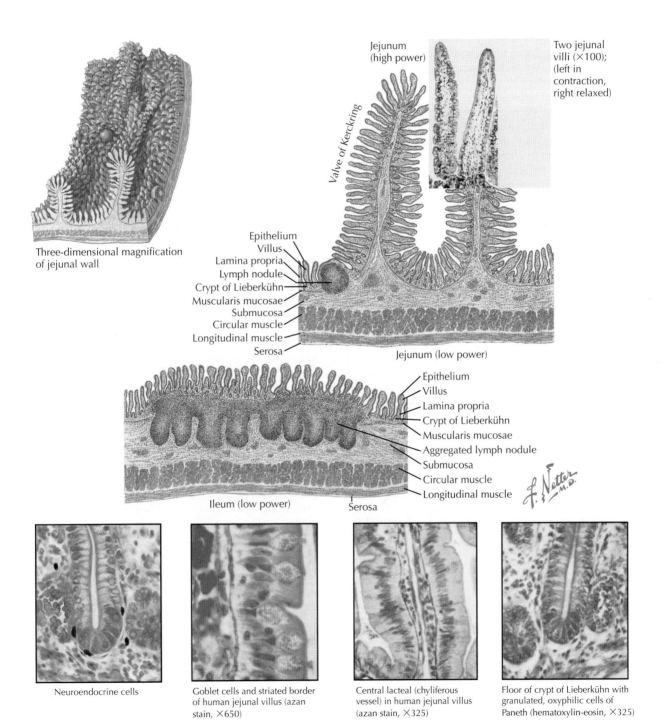

Three-dimensional magnification of jejunal wall

Jejunum (high power)

Valve of Kerckring

Two jejunal villi (×100); (left in contraction, right relaxed)

Epithelium
Villus
Lamina propria
Lymph nodule
Crypt of Lieberkühn
Muscularis mucosae
Submucosa
Circular muscle
Longitudinal muscle
Serosa

Jejunum (low power)

Epithelium
Villus
Lamina propria
Crypt of Lieberkühn
Muscularis mucosae
Aggregated lymph nodule
Submucosa
Circular muscle
Longitudinal muscle
Serosa

Ileum (low power)

Neuroendocrine cells

Goblet cells and striated border of human jejunal villus (azan stain, ×650)

Central lacteal (chyliferous vessel) in human jejunal villus (azan stain, ×325)

Floor of crypt of Lieberkühn with granulated, oxyphilic cells of Paneth (hematoxylin-eosin, ×325)

Fig. 50.3 Microscopic Structure of the Small Intestine.

are *Paneth cells,* also called *oxyphilic granular* cells because of the staining qualities of their granules. They secrete antimicrobial and growth protein substances. The third cell type is *enterochromaffin cells* (argentaffin or argyrophilic), which contain basal staining granules with a high affinity for silver and chromium. Their habitat is the crypts of Lieberkühn, where it is now believed stem cells exist and give rise to all intestinal cells. These cells have a definite neuroendocrine function.

Within the tunica (lamina) propria is a great variety of cells, most of which originate from reticular cells. In addition to the usual connective tissue cells, lymphocytes and plasma cells are present. *Lymphocytes* show a marked tendency to migrate through the epithelium toward the lumen. These cells make up the largest mass of immunoprotective tissue in the body. *Mast cells* are also present in the lamina propria and react to antigens. The *interstitial cells of Cajal* are present in the wall.

The principal task of the GI tract is to serve as an organ of nutrition to satisfy caloric and nutritional requirements. Key steps in digestion occur within the lumen of the small bowel, and then absorption occurs through these epithelial cells. Villi, covered by the epithelial cells, function as the *organelles* of absorption.

The luminal surface of the epithelial cell is covered with fine, projecting rods called *microvilli.* Each epithelial cell contains approximately 1000 microvilli, which increases the cellular surface approximately 24 times. The average length of a microvillus is 1 μm, and the width is 0.07 μm. Covered by a continuation of the cell membrane, microvilli contain, in the core, fine fibrils connected by a network of fibrils called the *terminal web.* Microvilli form a sheet that can be seen under the microscope and that is often lost when the epithelium is damaged, as in celiac disease.

Shortly after the ingestion of a fatty meal, fine lipid droplets are observed in the intermicrovillus spaces, which then are seen in the terminal web; pinocytotic activity subsequently occurs. The droplets seem to proceed and can be found in the main body of the epithelial cell, where they coalesce into large units in vesicles connected to each other by intracellular tubules. The system is referred to as the *endoplasmic reticulum.* Through this reticulum, fat droplets pass toward the lateral cell surfaces, and from the intercellular spaces the droplets traverse the basement membrane to enter the central lacteals of the villi. In the region below the microvilli, the profile of the lateral surface is irregular because of end plates. Toward the base of each cell, the membrane is *plicated,* or underplayed, which means the adjacent cells become interdigitated.

TERMINAL ILEUM

The terminal ileum is the most caudal part of the small intestine and usually lies in the pelvis over the right iliac fossa. It opens sideways from the left into the medial wall of the large intestine (Fig. 50.4). The section of the large intestine caudally or below this junction is a "blind" sac and thus is termed the *cecum.*

In most people, where the ileum joins the large intestine, the peritoneal fold extends from the terminal part of the ileomesentery, across the front of the ileum, to the cecum and lowest part of the ascending colon. This fold is known as the *ileocolic fold,* or *superior ileocecal fold.* It contains the anterior cecal artery and forms the anterior wall of the fossa, correspondingly termed the *ileocolic fossa,* or *superior ileocolic fossa.* The posterior wall of this fossa is made up of the terminal ileum and its mesentery. Its mouth opens downward and somewhat to the left. Another fold, known as the *ileocecal fold,* or *inferior ileocecal fold,* is often encountered in front of the mesoappendix, extending from the lower or right side of the terminal ileum to the cecum. Together with the mesoappendix as the posterior wall, the fold again forms a fossa, the *ileocecal fossa,* or *inferior ileocecal fossa,* of which the fold

represents the interior wall. The ileocecal fold contains no important vessel and therefore has been named the "bloodless" *fold of Treves.* The third peritoneal extension, the mesoappendix, serves as a mesentery of the appendix.

At the ileocecal junction, the terminal ileum is thrust with all its coverings into the wall, invaginates the large intestine, and creates within the lumen of the latter what has been known as the *ileocecal valve.* On exposure of this sphincter at autopsy, the ileal aperture is seen as bounded by two almost horizontal folds, referred to as the upper and lower "lips" of the "valve," in approximately 60% of cases. At both ends of the lips, where they seem to coalesce, two mucosal ridges extend horizontally in the lumen of the large intestine, resembling the crescent-shaped bulbs of the colon. These ridges, known as the *frenulum* of the ileal orifice (ileocecal valve), form the dividing line between the cecum and the ascending colon. In vivo, the ileum may protrude into the large intestine in the form of a rounded *papilla,* the lumen of which assumes a starlike appearance when closed, often compared with the appearance of the cervix protruding into the vagina. When visualized endoscopically, the ileocecal valve may appear closed or open, or at times with motility, it may change shape.

It is thought that the ileocecal valve actually acts as a true sphincter, a sphincter that may be under neural and hormonal control. Dissection of the musculature of the area reveals that some fibers from the mesocolic taenia, ascending from the colon and cecum to the appendix, turn inward and pass into the ileocolic papilla, whereas others turn outward to become continuous with the longitudinal muscle of the ileum. Similarly, the longitudinal muscle of the ileum takes divergent courses, with some fibers passing into the papilla and others joining fibers of the taenia. It is postulated that the circular muscle layer, which is much stronger, closes the sphincter, whereas the longitudinal muscle layer opens it.

Functionally, the ileocecal valve prevents reflux of colonic contents into the small bowel. Motility studies confirm that the terminal ileum and its muscular anatomic structure behave as a valve, allowing ileal contents to empty in a pulsatile manner.

VASCULAR SUPPLY AND DRAINAGE IN THE SMALL INTESTINE

The blood supply to the small and large intestines is extremely variable and, in many cases, uncertain and unpredictable. Variations in the origin, course, anastomoses, and distribution of the intestinal vessels are so common and significant that the conventional textbook descriptions are inadequate and, in many respects, even misleading, similar to descriptions regarding the blood supply of the upper abdominal organs. It is important for surgeons working in this area and for radiologists interpreting angiograms to understand these variations, as detailed in comprehensive anatomy and radiology texts.

Arterial Circulation

The *superior mesenteric artery* arises from the front of the aorta, typically at the level of mid-L1 (first lumbar vertebra), but as far down as the upper third of L2. The distance between the origin of the celiac and superior mesenteric arteries is usually 1 to 6 mm but varies from 1 to 23 mm. Thus contiguous origins of the two vessels are often found, but a common origin from a celiac-mesenteric trunk is rare.

The superior mesenteric artery, passing downward and forward and swinging to the left, particularly in its lower third, gives off a variable number (13 to 21) of intestinal arteries from its convex (left) side, ranging from three to seven (average five) above and 8 to 17 (average 11) below the origin of the ileocolic artery. The first group supplies the jejunum, and the second supplies part of the jejunum and the entire

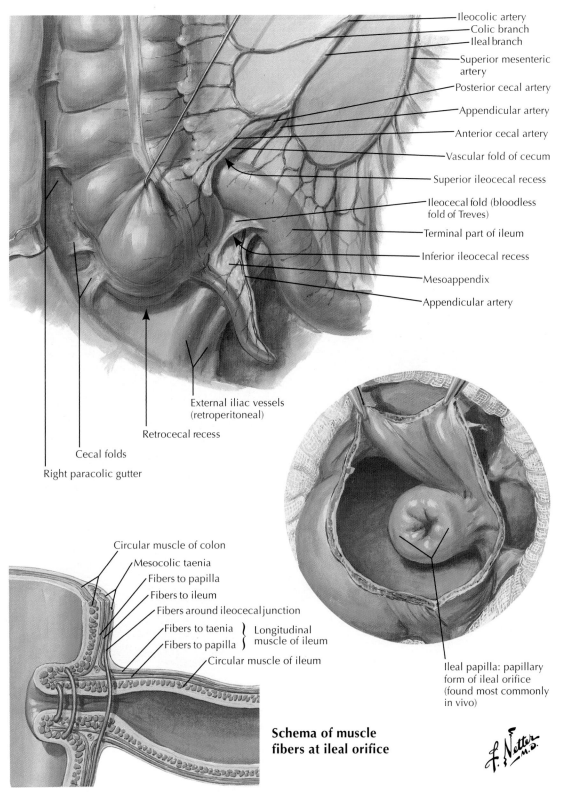

Ileocolic artery
Colic branch
Ileal branch
Superior mesenteric artery
Posterior cecal artery
Appendicular artery
Anterior cecal artery
Vascular fold of cecum
Superior ileocecal recess
Ileocecal fold (bloodless fold of Treves)
Terminal part of ileum
Inferior ileocecal recess
Mesoappendix
Appendicular artery

External iliac vessels (retroperitoneal)

Retrocecal recess

Cecal folds

Right paracolic gutter

Circular muscle of colon
Mesocolic taenia
Fibers to papilla
Fibers to ileum
Fibers around ileocecal junction
Fibers to taenia }
Fibers to papilla } Longitudinal muscle of ileum
Circular muscle of ileum

Ileal papilla: papillary form of ileal orifice (found most commonly in vivo)

Schema of muscle fibers at ileal orifice

Fig. 50.4 Ileocecal Region.

ileum. Intestinal arteries for the jejunum and ileum, running between the layers of the mesentery, follow the pattern shown in Fig. 50.5.

Each vessel courses fairly straight, for a variable distance, before it divides into branches that unite with branches from the adjacent primary stem vessels to form a series of anastomosing arches, the *arterial arcades.*

From these primary arcades arise the secondary and shorter intestinal arteries, which in turn form secondary arcades. Further arcades, although smaller, are formed similarly, essentially by the more distal arteries. In the terminal arcades, small, straight vessels (arteriae rectae) arise. Except for the blood supply of the first part of the duodenum, where the first

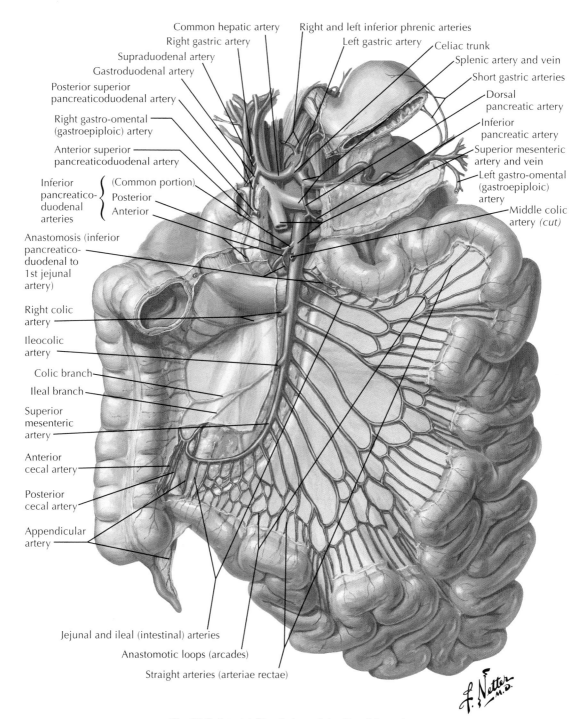

Common hepatic artery

Right gastric artery

Supraduodenal artery

Gastroduodenal artery

Posterior superior pancreaticoduodenal artery

Right gastro-omental (gastroepiploic) artery

Anterior superior pancreaticoduodenal artery

Inferior pancreatico- duodenal arteries { (Common portion) Posterior Anterior

Anastomosis (inferior pancreatico- duodenal to 1st jejunal artery)

Right colic artery

Ileocolic artery

Colic branch

Ileal branch

Superior mesenteric artery

Anterior cecal artery

Posterior cecal artery

Appendicular artery

Right and left inferior phrenic arteries

Left gastric artery

Celiac trunk

Splenic artery and vein

Short gastric arteries

Dorsal pancreatic artery

Inferior pancreatic artery

Superior mesenteric artery and vein

Left gastro-omental (gastroepiploic) artery

Middle colic artery (cut)

Jejunal and ileal (intestinal) arteries

Anastomotic loops (arcades)

Straight arteries (arteriae rectae)

Fig. 50.5 Arterial Circulation of the Small Intestine.

arcade is small with short arteriae rectae, the jejunal arteries are long, have a large caliber, and establish primary and secondary arcades, from which arise multiple long arteriae rectae. Stem arteries for the ileum become progressively shorter, the arcades become smaller, and the arteriae become less elongated.

The vascularization pattern of the jejunum is so characteristically different from the ileum. Through simple inspection of the gut, the examiner can usually distinguish between jejunum and ileum. The jejunum has a thicker wall and a greater digestive surface than the ileum and receives the larger intestinal branches.

The first jejunal branch of the superior mesenteric origin may be large (6 mm in diameter) and may have four large arcades forming branches 6 to 8 cm long and 3 to 4 mm in diameter. However, in many cases the first jejunal branch is small (1 to 2 mm) and is anastomosed with the inferior pancreaticoduodenal artery or shares a common origin. A large primary jejunal artery may be followed by a slender second jejunal artery. The distribution and caliber of the intestinal branches of the superior mesenteric artery vary in the same person; large and small branches alternate without rule or order. Although the first and second jejunal arteries are thought to communicate through an arcade, such an arcade is missing in many patients, in whom the first jejunal artery is found to have no connection with the second.

Anatomic studies show great variation in the arteriae rectae as they pass from the arcades to the walls of the small intestine, entering directly, overlapping, or forming small arcades (see Additional Resources). However, the result is a rich blood supply to the small intestine, where the biologic need for absorption is served.

Venous Drainage

In number, point of origin, and mode of distribution, the veins involved in the drainage of the small intestine follow the same design as the corresponding arteries (Fig. 50.6). Accordingly, the veins have been given the same terminology. An exception is the *superior mesenteric vein,* in that it reaches the right gastroepiploic vein just before entering the portal vein. Other tributaries of the superior mesenteric vein are concordant with the arteries of the same name, which leave the superior mesenteric artery.

In the region where the left colic and upper sigmoid arteries originate from the inferior mesenteric artery, the corresponding vein follows a course of its own, separating from the respective artery. The inferior mesenteric vein takes a straight-upward course, ascending behind the peritoneum, over the psoas muscles, and to the left of the fourth portion

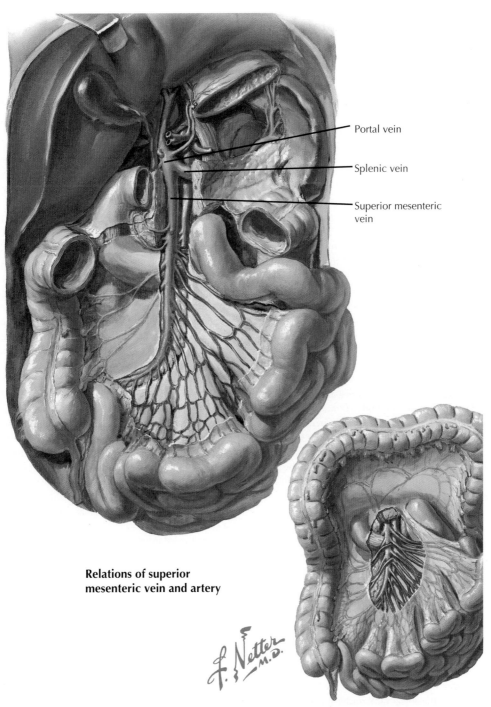

Portal vein

Splenic vein

Superior mesenteric vein

Relations of superior mesenteric vein and artery

Fig. 50.6 Venous Drainage of the Small Intestine.

of the duodenum. The vein continues behind the body of the pancreas to enter most frequently (38% of observed cases) the splenic vein from the latter's union with the superior mesenteric vein (i.e., origin of portal vein). In 29% of persons, the inferior mesenteric vein enters the superior mesenteric vein, and in 32%, it joins the latter and the splenic vein at the junction. In a few persons, a second inferior mesenteric vein has been found. The portal vein, especially variations of its tributaries, is extremely important (see Section IX).

Lymph Drainage

The intramural lymph vessels of the small intestine begin with the central lacteals of the villi. At the base of the villi, the central lacteals join with the lymph capillaries, draining the region of the crypts of Lieberkühn, thus forming a fine network within the tunica propria, in which the first lymphatic valves are already encountered. Many minute branches emerge from this network, penetrating through the muscularis mucosae into the submucosa, where a further network of lymphatic vessels spreads. From this network, in which valves are a conspicuous feature, large lymph vessels receive lymph from the muscle layers and from the serosa and subserosa and pass to the line of attachment of the mesentery, where, together with the arteries and veins, the lymph vessels leave the intestinal wall to enter the mesentery. Lymph vessels of the small intestine have long been referred to as *lacteals* or *chyliferous vessels* because they transport absorbed fat in emulsified form and therefore appear as milky-white threads after the ingestion of fat-containing food.

Lymph vessels of the mesentery drain through masses of *mesenteric lymph nodes,* which number approximately 100 to 200, and constitute the largest aggregate of lymph nodes in the body. They increase in number and size toward the root of the mesentery. In the root of the mesentery, larger lymphatic branches are situated that lead into the superior mesenteric nodes where the superior mesenteric artery arises from the aorta. From the duodenum, the lymph vessels—some of which run through the pancreatic tissue (see Section VII)—pass the lymph nodes lying cranial, caudal, and dorsal to the head of the pancreas. Of these, the upper are known as the *subpyloric* and right *suprapancreatic* nodes, the lower as the *mesenteric root* nodes, and the dorsal as the *retropancreatic* nodes. Lymph flows from these various nodes into the group of celiac lymph nodes.

From the superior mesenteric nodes and the celiac nodes, the lymph passes through the short intestinal or GI lymph trunk, which is sometimes divided, like a river delta, into several smaller, parallel trunks. Lymph then enters the *cisterna chyli,* a saclike expansion of the beginning of the thoracic duct. The intestinal trunk drains not only the entire small intestine but also all organs whose lymph is collected in the celiac and superior mesenteric lymph nodes, especially the stomach, liver, pancreas, and extensive portions of the large intestine.

INNERVATION OF THE SMALL AND LARGE INTESTINES

The nerves supplying the small and large intestines contain sympathetic and parasympathetic efferent and afferent fibers (Figs. 50.7 and 50.8). These nerves have branches of the celiac plexus, the superior and inferior mesenteric plexuses, and the superior and inferior hypogastric plexuses. The *hypothalamus* is a source and terminus of pathways involved in visceral activities, with extensive cortical connections to the premotor areas of the frontal cortex, the cingulate gyrus, and the orbital surfaces of the frontal lobes. Descending fibers important in parasympathetic functioning arise mainly from the anterior region of the hypothalamus and form synapses with cells in the dorsal vagal nuclei and in the second to fourth sacral segments of the spinal cord (S2-S4). Axons of these

cells constitute the *preganglionic* (efferent) fibers in the vagal and pelvic splanchnic nerves, which are distributed to many viscera. Vagus nerves supply those parts derived from the foregut and midgut, and the pelvic splanchnic nerves innervate the parts derived from the hindgut. Intestinal preganglionic fibers carried to the vagal and pelvic splanchnic nerves terminate by relaying around the ganglia cells in the enteric plexuses, and the axons of these ganglionic cells become the *postganglionic* parasympathetic fibers, which, together with the corresponding sympathetic fibers, serve the smooth muscle of the intestinal wall, the intramural vessels, and the intestinal glands.

Fibers descending from the central nervous system (CNS), carrying sympathetic impulses on intestinal activities, relay around lateral cornual cells in the four or five lowest thoracic and the two or three upper lumbar segments of the spinal cord. Axons of these cells, representing the preganglionic sympathetic fibers, emerge from the ventral nerve roots of the corresponding segments and pass in white rami communicates to the adjacent ganglia of the sympathetic trunks. Some fibers relay within these ganglia, whereas others traverse the trunk uninterruptedly, leaving it in medially directed branches as thoracic, lumbar, or sacral splanchnic nerves, which end in the plexuses previously cited to enter synapses with ganglionic cells. Axons of these cells, the postganglionic fibers, accompany the branches of the various arteries supplying the intestine.

The chief segmental sources of the sympathetic fibers innervating different regions of the intestinal tract are indicated in Fig. 50.8, but because of overlap, minor contributions may derive from adjacent segments.

Certain alimentary functions are probably controlled by simple reflex arcs located in the intestinal wall, but other reactions are mediated through more elaborate reflex arcs involving the CNS and consisting of the usual afferent, internuncial, and efferent neurons. Numerous *afferent* fibers of relatively large caliber traverse the enteric plexus without relaying and are carried centripetally through approximately the same sympathetic splanchnic and parasympathetic nerves that transmit the preganglionic, or *efferent,* fibers. Afferent fibers are the peripheral processes of pseudounipolar cells in the inferior vagal ganglia or in the dorsal root ganglia of those spinal ganglia that carry preganglionic intestinal fibers. Central processes enter the brainstem or the spinal cord.

Although insensitive to ordinary tactile, painful, or thermal stimuli, the intestines respond to tension, anoxia, chemicals, and other stimuli. Specialized cutaneous nerve endings in the intestine are absent, except for the Vater-Pacini (pacinian) corpuscles in the adjacent mesentery. As with the efferent fibers, the exact mode of termination of the visceral afferent fibers remains controversial, but *whorl, skein, great, looplike,* and *free* endings have been described in the mucosal, muscular, and serosal coats.

Intrinsic innervation is affected through the enteric plexus in the alimentary tract from the esophagus to the rectum. This plexus consists of small groups of nerve cells interconnected by networks of fibers, and it is subdivided into the *myenteric* (Auerbach) *plexus* and the *submucosal* (Meissner) *plexus*. The Auerbach plexus is relatively coarse, with thicker meshes and larger ganglia at the intersections than the Meissner plexus, which consists of fine meshes with small ganglia. The myenteric plexus lies in the interval between the circular and longitudinal muscular coats and the main (primary) meshes and gives off fascicles of fibers that form finer secondary, and even finer tertiary, plexuses and that ramify within and between the adjacent layers of muscle. Some fibers from the longitudinal intramuscular plexus enter the subserous plexus and constitute a rarified subserous plexus. The submucosal plexus is also subdivided into more superficial and deeper fibers. *Interstitial cells of Cajal* are a network of nonneuronally derived cells from smooth muscles; those in the intramuscular, myenteric plexus and submucosal layers are

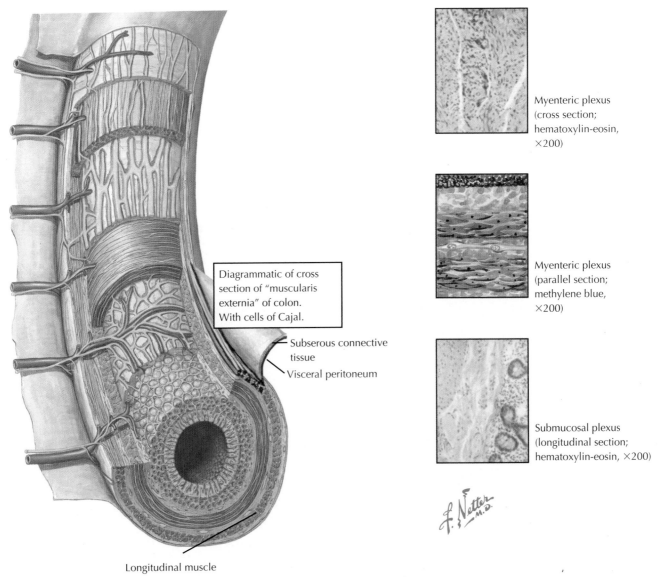

Myenteric plexus (cross section; hematoxylin-eosin, ×200)

Myenteric plexus (parallel section; methylene blue, ×200)

Submucosal plexus (longitudinal section; hematoxylin-eosin, ×200)

Diagrammatic of cross section of "muscularis externia" of colon. With cells of Cajal.

Subserous connective tissue

Visceral peritoneum

Longitudinal muscle

Fig. 50.7 Innervation of the Intestines.

interconnected. Interstitial cells of Cajal are proving important in understanding motility disturbances.

Nerve bundles contain postganglionic sympathetic, preganglionic and postganglionic parasympathetic, and afferent fibers, in addition to elongated dendrites. There is a rich network of dendrites.

The *superior mesenteric plexus* is a continuation of the lowest part of the celiac plexus and surrounds the origin of the superior mesenteric artery. It is interconnected by stout filaments to the celiac and aorticorenal ganglia. The large superior mesenteric ganglia is located usually just above the root of the artery and is incorporated in the commencement of the superior mesenteric plexus. The main plexus divides into subsidiary plexuses corresponding to all the branches of the artery (inferior pancreatic duodenal, jejunal, ileal, ileocolic, right and middle colic), and it innervates those parts of the intestine indicated by their names. Nerves and arteries follow the same route, except for the patterns by which they approach the gut wall. Vessels advance toward the wall and form characteristic arcades, but nerves pass straight outward without arcade formation. This rich network of ganglia and plexuses is distributed throughout the small and large bowel and corresponds to the arteries.

The *superior hypogastric plexus* (presacral nerves), situated in front of the dichotomized aorta and between the divergent common iliac arteries, is a flattened band of intercommunicating nerves extending from the level of the lower border of the third lumbar vertebra (L3) to the upper border of the sacrum, where it ends by dividing into the right and left groups of hypogastric nerves. These nerves are then distributed through the inferior hypogastric plexuses.

Specialized sensory endings exist in the part of the anal canal that develops from the proctodeum and that is supplied by the inferior hemorrhoidal nerve. Sensory endings are absent in the region above the Hilton white line, whereas the afferent fibers end by breaking up to form fibrils or delicate plexuses between the epithelial cells. Thus, below the pectin, this innervation resembles that of the skin, whereas above the pectin, the mucosa is supplied by sympathetic nerves derived from the inferior mesenteric and inferior hypogastric plexuses, following the paths of the hemorrhoidal arteries and the parasympathetic fibers from the pelvic splanchnic nerves. All these nerves convey efferent and afferent fibers to and from the terminal part of the gut. In accord with this difference in nerve supply of the anoderm are the differing sensory responses. The lower part, supplied by somatic nerves, is sensi-

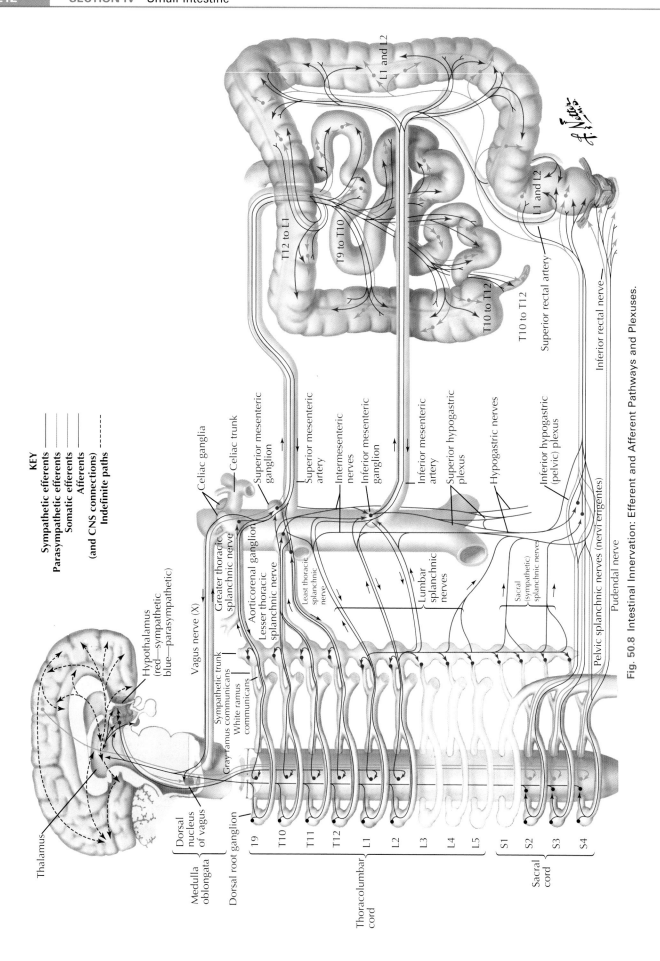

Fig. 50.8 Intestinal Innervation: Efferent and Afferent Pathways and Plexuses.

tive to tactile, painful, and thermal stimuli, whereas the upper part of the anal canal is almost insensitive to such stimuli but responds readily to alternations in tension. From a practical point of view, this neuroanatomic situation explains why an anal fissure is so painful and why, with an injection for hemorrhoids, the puncture is scarcely felt if the needle is inserted through the mucosa.

ADDITIONAL RESOURCES

Bass LM, Wershil B: Anatomy, histology, and developmental anomalies of the small and large intestine. In Feldman M, Friedman LS, Brandt LJ, editors: *Gastrointestinal and liver disease*, ed 10, Philadelphia, 2016, Saunders-Elsevier, pp 1649–1678.

Dinning PG, Costa M, Brooks SJH: Colonic motor and sensory function and dysfunction. In Feldman M, Friedman LS, Brandt LJ, editors: *Gastrointestinal and liver disease*, ed 10, Philadelphia, 2016, Saunders-Elsevier, pp 1696–1712.

Dinning PG, Scott SM: Novel diagnostics and therapy of colonic motor disorders, *Curr Opin Pharmacol* 11:624–629, 2011.

Kornblith PL, Boley SJ, Whitehouse BS: Anatomy of the splanchnic circulation, *Surg Clin North Am* 72:1–30, 1992.

Rosenblum JD, Boytle CM, Schwartz IB: The mesenteric circulation: anatomy and physiology, *Surg Clin North Am* 77:289–306, 1997.

Semrin MG, Russo MA: Anatomy, histology, and developmental anomalies of the stomach and duodenum. In Feldman M, Friedman LS, Brandt LJ, editors: *Gastrointestinal and liver disease*, ed 10, Philadelphia, 2016, Saunders-Elsevier, pp 795–809.

51

Secretory, Digestive, and Absorptive Functions of the Small Intestine

Martin H. Floch

The mucosa of the gut, throughout its entire length, is equipped with secretory cells. The secretory product of the duodenal glands is an alkaline, pale-yellow, viscous fluid consisting essentially of mucus, a primary function of which is to protect the proximal duodenum against the corrosive action of gastric chyme. The glandular apparatus of the jejunum and ileum produces the succus entericus (intestinal juice). The epithelial secretions also contain enzymes, including peptidases, nucleases, nucleosidases, phosphatase, lipase, maltase, sucrase, lactase, and the coenzyme enterokinase, which activates tripsinogen and chymotrypsinogen of pancreatic origin to form active trypsin and chymotrypsin, respectively. The flow of the succus entericus is stimulated by acid secretion in the upper intestine; by local mechanical and chemical stimuli; by the administration of secretin, enterokinin, and pilocarpine; and by sympathectomy.

DIGESTION

In *protein digestion,* the breakdown of food protein begins in the stomach through the action of pepsins, the effectiveness of which depends on the rate of emptying from the stomach and the pH of both the stomach and the duodenum (Fig. 51.1). However, it is apparent from patients who have achlorhydria or who have undergone surgical bypass that gastric proteolysis is not necessary to break down and absorb most proteins. Pancreatic proteolytic enzymes are secreted in the *proenzyme phase.* Through the action of enterokinase, which is secreted in the succus entericus, these enzymes are activated to trypsin, chymotrypsin, elastase, and carboxypeptidases A and B. The final product of the intraluminal enzyme activity yields peptide chains of two to six amino acids, which make up approximately two-thirds of the content, with the other third in the form of simple amino acids. Digestion then occurs further in the *brush border* of the enterocytes as the amino acids and oligopeptides are absorbed. The brush border contains several peptidases, and several within the cytoplasm of the enterocytes complete digestion and some transformation of amino acids for metabolic activity.

Dipeptides are more effectively and actively absorbed than simple amino acids and tripeptides. *Protein absorption* occurs primarily in the duodenum and jejunum and requires a complex transporter system in the brush border with separate sodium-dependent, acid, and basic amino acid systems. Congenital disorders of amino acid transport result in serious growth and developmental disorders and nutritional disease. Epidermal growth factor, neurotensin, cholecystokinin, and secretin enhance transport, whereas somatostatin and vasoactive intestinal polypeptides decrease transport.

The illustrations in Figs. 51.1 and 51.2 are simple. Since that time, there has been a large amount of research and understanding in the mechanisms of absorption. The references in the chapter give the tremendous detail that has arrived at our knowledge base during the past decade. For instance, there is now a relative amount of understanding of protein absorption. Following the lumenal digestion, there is cascade of biochemical events that occur and are described in the references. Interested students should refer to those references if they want to understand the latest knowledge in detail.

The specific method of vitamin B_{12} absorption transport is discussed in Section II.

Digestive and absorptive processes involving the nutrients of *carbohydrates* generally consist of enzymatic cleavage of polysaccharides and oligosaccharides into disaccharides and monosaccharides. The process is relatively simple compared with the digestive and absorptive process that proteins and fats require. *Starches* are the main energy-producing nutrients of all plant foods and consist primarily of amylose and amylopectin. Dietary carbohydrate also includes lactose from milk; fructose, glucose, and sucrose from vegetables and fruits; and sugars as additives in all drinks.

Nonstarch polysaccharides are poorly digested by human enzymes and make up the major component of dietary fiber. Other unavailable carbohydrates that are poorly digested by human enzymes are pectins, gums, lignins, and alginates. These are readily metabolized by the microbiota, and their products can be absorbed through the small and large intestinal mucosa (see Section V).

Starch and sugar digestion occurs with the release of salivary and pancreatic amylases that cleave the α-1,4 link of simple disaccharides and a long-chain starch. The degree of activity of salivary amylase depends on the duration of chewing and the proximity of the enzymes in the chyme, as well as the churning of the stomach. However, the major enzyme breakdown of starch occurs through pancreatic amylase activity in the duodenum, and hydrolysis mainly occurs intraluminally in the proximal small intestine. Monosaccharides and disaccharides are presented to the brush border of the enterocytes, where membrane hydrolysis occurs. Lactase, maltase, sucrase-isomaltase, isomaltase, and trehalase—enzymes in the brush border—are most active in the duodenum and jejunum. These enzymes cleave the disaccharides into glucose, galactose, and fructose, which are transported across the mucosa. Transport is active and passive. Transport mechanisms are controversial, but it is agreed that an active sodium-glucose cotransporter exists and that much of the process is sodium dependent.

The problems of disaccharidase deficiencies result in significant diarrhea and symptomatic syndromes. Disaccharidases are synthesized within the endoplasmic reticulum. The classic deficiency of lactase results in lactose malabsorption. Less common are sucrose- and fructose-absorptive deficiencies, and less common and less well known are the trehalose deficiencies that result from absorption after mushroom ingestion.

During *fat digestion and absorption,* fats are passed into the stomach, where gastric lipase may be active and prefers action at one-ester bonds. The chyme passes the fats into the duodenum, where pancreatic lipase has its greatest activity in both one-ester and three-ester bonds. Approximately 95% of ingested fat is absorbed, undergoing complicated mechanisms to pass into the lymphatics and bloodstream. Intraluminally, the fat is broken down into emulsion droplets, which requires droplets to

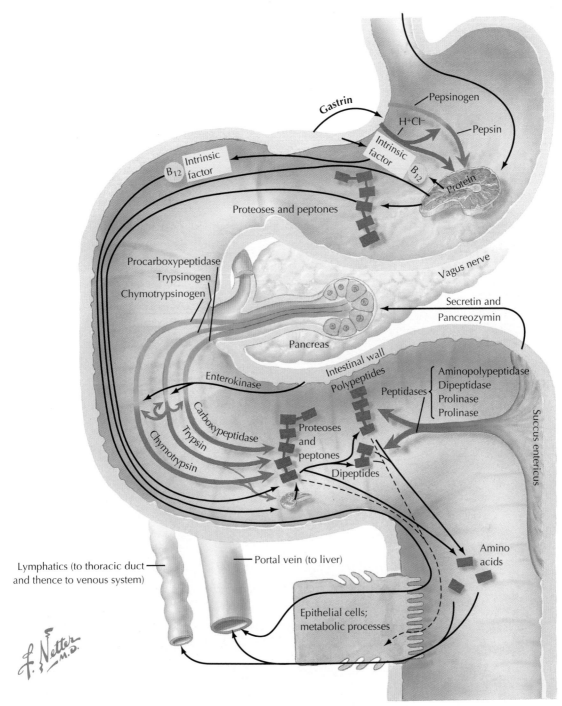

Fig. 51.1 Digestion of Protein.

be coated with a phospholipid. *Lipolysis* begins in the stomach, but pancreatic lipase exerts greater effect. Colipase, lipase, phospholipids, and bile salts are all involved in a complex mechanism of forming *micelles,* and a lipid phase transformed into an aqueous phase permits transport across the brush border. During this process, triglycerides are broken down into diglycerides and monoglycerides, in addition to the monoglycerides and diglycerides present in foods and absorbed. Bile salts are capable of forming micelles because they are ideal emulsifying agents. An unstirred water layer at the surface of the brush border readily permits short-chain or medium-chain fatty acid absorption but limits long-chain fatty acid absorption. Cholesterol, as well as mono-glycerides, diglycerides, and triglycerides, is readily absorbed through

these mechanisms. Once within the enterocytes, triglycerides resynthesize, lipoproteins form, and then chylomicrons form. The material is passed into the lymphatic and portal vein systems to the circulation.

The process of fat digestion and absorption is complex; Fig. 51.1 helps clarify the intraluminal process. The amount of knowledge that has evolved during the past decade is extensive. For instance, the substance called CB36 was first described in 1993, and we now know it is important for the uptake of fatty acids. CB36 is only one part of the complex development of our understanding of fat digestion in the mucosa. The interested reader is referred to the references that describe in detail the cascading of events that occur, along with CB36 and other newly identified enzymes.

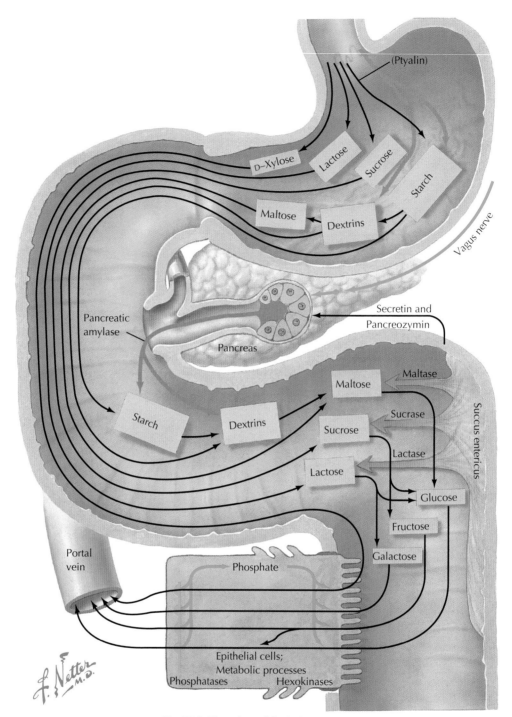

Fig. 51.2 Digestion of Carbohydrates.

It is also now clear that the small intestine has a great ability to adapt to changes through both hypertrophy and development of these transport systems. Again, these are described in detail in the listed references.

ADDITIONAL RESOURCES

Abumrad NA, Davidson NO: Role of the gut in lipid homeostasis, *Physiol Rev* 92:1061–1085, 2012.

Abumrad NA, Nassir F, Marcus A: Digestion and absorption of dietary fat, carbohydrate, and protein. In Feldman M, Friedman LS, Brandt LJ, editors: *Gastrointestinal and liver disease*, ed 10, Philadelphia, 2016, Saunders-Elsevier, pp 1736–1764.

Bishu S, Quigley EMM: Nutrient digestion, absorption and sensing. In Podolsky DK, Camilleri M, Fitz JG, et al, editors: *Yamada's textbook of gastroenterology*, ed 6, West Sussex England, 2016, Wiley-Blackwell, pp 538–555.

Mansbach CM, Siddiqi SA: The biogenesis of chylomicrons, *Annu Rev Physiol* 72:315–333, 2010.

Rao MC, Sarathy J, Sellin JH: Intestinal electrolyte absorption and secretion. In Feldman M, Friedman LS, Brandt LJ, editors: *Gastrointestinal and liver disease*, ed 10, Philadelphia, 2016, Saunders-Elsevier, pp 1713–1735.

Said HM, Trebble TM: Intestinal digestion and absorption of micronutrients. In Feldman M, Friedman LS, Brandt LJ, editors: *Gastrointestinal and liver disease*, ed 10, Philadelphia, 2016, Saunders-Elsevier, pp 1765–1787.

52

Gastrointestinal Hormones and Neurotransmitters

Martin H. Floch

Secretin became the first gastrointestinal (GI) hormone identified in humans in 1902. Since then, a myriad of GI peptides have been identified as hormones. Most have been verified, others have not; regardless, their functions are extremely important. GI hormones act in one of the following four ways:

1. *Endocrine function.* Epithelial cells secrete a substance into the circulation that acts at a distance.
2. *Autocrine function.* The substance secreted by the epithelial cell affects processes in the cell itself.

3. *Paracrine signaling.* The peptide secreted by the cell affects processes in adjacent cells.
4. *Neurocrine function.* Neurons secrete chemical transmitters with peptides into synapses or onto other cell types that signal neurotransmission.

Box 52.1 lists the peptides and hormonal actions identified in the GI tract. Fig. 52.1 demonstrates the diffuse and integrating effects of the peptide hormone substances gastrin, cholecystokinin (CCK), and serotonin.

BOX 52.1 Peptides With Action in the Gastrointestinal Tract

Gut Peptides That Function Mainly as Hormones
- Gastrin
- Ghrelin
- Glucose-dependent insulinotropic peptide (GIP)
- Glucagon and related gene products (GLP-1, GLP-2, glicentin, oxyntomodulin)
- Insulin
- Leptin
- Motilin
- Pancreatic polypeptide
- Peptide tyrosine (PIY)
- Secretin

Gut Peptides That May Function as Hormones, Neuropeptides, or Paracrine Agents
- Cholecystokinin (CCK)
- Corticotropin-releasing factor (CRF)
- Endothelin
- Neurotensin
- Somatostatin

Gut Peptides That Act Mainly as Neuropeptides
- Calcitonin gene-related peptide
- Dynorphin and related gene products
- Enkephalin and related gene products
- Galanin
- Gastrin-releasing peptide (GRP)
- Neuromedin U
- Neuropeptide Y
- Peptide histidine isoleucine or peptide histidine methionine
- Pituitary adenylate cyclase-activating peptide
- Substance P and other tachykinins (neurokinin A, neurokinin B)
- Thyrotropin-releasing hormone (TRP)
- Vasoactive intestinal polypeptide (VIP)

Peptides That Act as Growth Factors
- Epidermal growth factor
- Fibroblast growth factor

- Insulin-like growth factors
- Nerve growth factor
- Platelet-derived growth factor
- Transforming growth factor-β
- Vascular endothelial growth factor

Peptides That Act as Inflammatory Mediators
- Interferons
- Interleukins
- Lymphokines
- Monokines
- Tumor necrosis factor-α

Gut Peptides That Act on Neurons
- CCK
- Gastrin
- Motilin

More Peptide Transmitters Produced in the Gut
- Acetylcholine
- Adenosine triphosphate (ATP)
- Dopamine
- γ-Aminobutyric acid (GABA)
- Histamine
- 5-Hydroxtryptamine (5-HT, serotonin)
- Nitric oxide
- Norepinephrine
- Prostaglandins and other eicosanoids

Other Hormones and Neuropeptides
- Amylin
- Ghrelin
- Guanylin and uroguanylin
- Leptin

Modified from Bohorquez DV, Liddle RA: Gastrointestinal hormones and transmitters. In Feldman M, Friedman LS, Brandt LJ, editors: *Gastrointestinal and liver disease*, ed 10, Philadelphia, 2016, Saunders-Elsevier, pp 36-54.

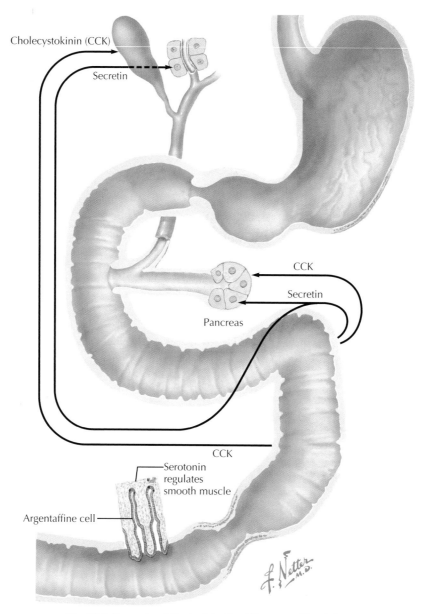

Cholecystokinin (CCK)

Secretin

CCK

Secretin

Pancreas

CCK

Serotonin regulates smooth muscle

Argentaffine cell

Fig. 52.1 Example of Gastrointestinal Hormone Physiology.

Some hormones have reached clinical significance. Produced by specialized G cells, *gastrin* regulates gastric secretion and has two major forms, G_{34} and G_{17}, formed primarily in the gastric antrum and secreted by enterochromaffin cells (see Chapters 38–41). Gastrin secretion into the circulation and production by G cells are stimulated by food, and gastrin acts directly on parietal cells to stimulate acid production. Proteins and high-protein foods have a greater influence than other nutrients on the production of gastrin and on the pH of the stomach. High acid production inhibits gastrin release, and a high gastric pH is a good stimulus for its secretion. Hypergastrinemia occurs in several pathologic states, including Zollinger-Ellison syndrome (see Chapters 19 and 34).

Secretin is a 27-amino acid peptide that stimulates pancreatic fluid and bicarbonate secretion (see Section VII). When the pH is raised in the duodenum, secretin release is inhibited. When gastric acid and chyme pass into the duodenum, secretin secretion is stimulated. Entero-endocrine cells, called *S cells,* produce secretin in the small intestine.

CCK is produced by I cells of the small intestine and is secreted into the blood when food passes into the small bowel. CCK has many actions, including gallbladder stimulation and stimulation of pancreatic secretion, and it helps regulate gastric and intestinal motility. Evidence also indicates that CCK induces satiety, so this hormone has many actions that help regulate feeding. The many forms of CCK include 33-, 58-, and 8-amino acid peptides, with all having biologically similar activities. CCK-A receptors reside primarily in the GI tract. The CCK-B receptor resides in the brain, however, and has been used clinically to stimulate pancreatic secretion in function tests. No disease is known to be associated with CCK.

Vasoactive intestinal polypeptide (VIP; also vasoactive intestinal peptide) has broad activity in the intestine. VIP acts as a vasodilator that increases blood flow, relaxes smooth muscle, and stimulates epithelial cell secretion. It also acts as a chemical messenger that is released from nerve terminals. VIP is chemically related to secretin and glucagons and is an important neurotransmitter. It is not produced by endocrine cells or the GI tract, but rather is produced and released from neurons. VIP has great clinical significance in certain watery diarrhea syndromes (e.g., Verner-Morrison), which demonstrate greatly increased VIP activity.

Glucagon is produced by pancreatic alpha cells and in the ileum and colon by L cells. It has several receptors, and it is known to participate in glucose homeostasis.

Epidermal growth factor (EGF) hormones are numerous throughout the GI tract and help regulate cell growth and activity. EGF hormones are complex, but their action appears to occur primarily through paracrine effects, although some growth factors may have autocrine action. EGF, the first growth factor discovered, is secreted from submaxillary glands and Brunner glands of the duodenum. EGF is believed to act with luminal cells of the GI tract to regulate cell proliferation and thus has an important trophic effect.

Recently recognized GI hormones are amylin, ghrelin, leptin, and guanylin/uroguanylin.

Leptin has 167 amino acid proteins that are secreted from adipocytes. Blood levels usually reflect total body fat stores. Small amounts of leptin are produced by the T-cells of the stomach. They are not thought to be as clinically effective as those produced by the fat cells. Leptin physiology is related to obesity. Obesity physiology is complex and the interested readers are referred to the adjacent references.

Ghrelin is a 28-amino acid peptide produced by the stomach. It is the natural ligand for growth hormone secretagogue receptor. It appears to play a major role in the neurohormonal regulations of food intake and antigen homeostasis. Again, it is complex and the interested reader is referred to the references. Circulating levels decrease after fasting or starvation and increase after feeding.

Motilin is a 22-amino acid peptide produced by endocrine cells of the duodenum. It is not released by the stimulation of food but appears to be secreted into the circulation synchronized with the migrating motor complex. In some clinical situations, it has been correlated with abdominal pain and diarrhea. It is complex and its function is described in the references.

NEUROTRANSMITTERS

Acetylcholine is synthesized in coemergent neurons and is the principle regulator in GI motility and pancreatic secretion. It is stored in nerve terminals and released by depolarization. Once again, its physiology and function in the GI tract is complex and the interested readers are referred to the references.

Understanding the physiology of GI hormones and neurotransmitters is difficult and the interested reader is referred to the appropriate references. Other substances, as well as VIP, are now often associated with significant neural regulation of the GI tract. Particularly, serotonin and somatostatin and their agonists are used clinically.

Somatostatin is found in interneurons and has an inhibitory effect by causing muscle relaxation. *Serotonin* (5-hydroxytryptamine, 5-HT) is found within the myenteric plexus and acts as a transmitter. Recently, 5-HT_4 and 5-HT_3 receptor agonists have been used in the treatment of irritable bowel syndrome (see Chapter 58).

ADDITIONAL RESOURCES

Bohorquez DV, Liddle RA: Gastrointestinal hormones and transmitters. In Feldman M, Friedman LS, Brandt LJ, editors: *Gastrointestinal and liver disease*, ed 10, Philadelphia, 2016, Saunders-Elsevier, pp 36–54.

Cummings DE, Overduin J: Gastrointestinal regulation of food intake, *J Clin Invest* 117:13–23, 2007.

Feng J, Petersen CD, Coy DH, et al: Calcium-sensing receptor is a physiologic multimodal chemosensor regulating gastric G-cell growth and gastrin secretion, *Proc Natl Acad Sci USA* 107:17791–17796, 2010.

Mellitzer G, Beucher A, Lobstein V, et al: Loss of enteroendocrine cells in mice alters lipid absorption and glucose homeostasis and impairs postnatal survival, *J Clin Invest* 120:1708–1721, 2010.

Reimann F, Tolhurst G, Gribble FM: G-protein-coupled receptors in intestinal chemosensation, *Cell Metab* 15:421–431, 2012.

53

Imaging of the Small Intestine

Martin H. Floch

Although the small bowel is long and convoluted, imaging modalities allow its visualization (Figs. 53.1 and 53.2). Barium contrast studies, computed tomography (CT) with enterography, and several forms of endoscopy (direct, wireless capsule, double balloon) are used to visualize select areas.

BARIUM CONTRAST STUDIES

Approximately 16 oz of liquid with very fine, pulverized barium is given to the patient, with serial x-ray films taken before and immediately after the drink, then followed until the terminal ileum is visualized. The test usually is completed in 1 to 2 hours, but some patients have slow transit, and it may take several hours to visualize the terminal ileum. Under fluoroscopy, the radiologist can obtain the many views of the terminal ileal area. The jejunum has characteristic folds, and the ileum is flatter. The jejunum lies primarily in the left side and the ileum in the right side of the abdominal cavity. The terminal ileum has a normal appearance, at times likened to a bird's beak. The jejunum should measure no more than 3 to 3.5 cm in width and the ileum no more than 2.5 to 3 cm in its maximum width. Obstructive lesions, filling defects, irregular mucosa, and the so-called malabsorption pattern (scattered, dilated loops of bowel) can be diagnosed with barium studies. These are described under disease topics in this section.

Enteroclysis, or a small bowel enema, is performed at some centers by inserting a tube into the duodenum and then flooding it with barium contrast solution. This enables the radiologist to better control the timing of images and fluoroscopy so as to identify difficult lesions.

COMPUTED TOMOGRAPHY

CT is used extensively in many institutions. When a contrast dye is given before the procedure, the progress of the dye through the small bowel can be observed on CT scan, similarly discerning lesions seen on contrast barium study. However, CT also allows visualization of the thickness of the bowel wall and any inflammatory response surrounding the wall. Therefore, many radiologists prefer CT to barium contrast study for obtaining initial diagnosis. However, barium contrast can be more helpful if a specific intraluminal lesion must be delineated carefully. CT can also be extremely helpful in diagnosing appendicitis and evaluating the colon and possible inflammatory lesions.

ENDOSCOPY

Endoscopy is used to evaluate the most proximal part of the small bowel and the terminal small bowel through a *colonoscope.* Adding enteroscopes and capsule endoscopy has made visualization possible. The *push enteroscope* is a short scope that can be passed into the proximal or middle jejunum. If it is necessary to visualize the proximal small bowel, this instrument offers direct visualization. The *long enteroscope,* which can pass to the terminal ileum, has been available but has not gained wide use or been successful because it takes an inordinate amount of time to pass the instrument.

Wireless capsule endoscopy (WCE) is now reaching its potential. With this procedure, a small capsule containing a camera captures continuous images in a recorder. The patient swallows the capsule, and the images are recorded. The endoscopist or interpreter must then carefully review all the images. This is time-consuming but allows the identification of small lesions, such as bleeding arteriovenous malformations, as well as strictures and ulcerations. WCE has become the procedure of choice to identify obscure bleeding, early Crohn disease, and small lesions of the bowel. It also complements other imaging studies, often identifying a lesion that is then carefully confirmed by either CT enterography or direct endoscopy (see Fig. 53.2).

Double-balloon endoscopy has not gained wide acceptance because it is a difficult, time-consuming technique. It is done either from above or through the terminal ileum and requires the use of balloons to tease the scope either caudad or aborally. Balloon endoscopy is used to confirm WCE findings or to identify occult gastrointestinal bleeding. Its advantage is that biopsy material can be obtained through the endoscope.

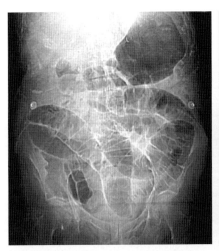

Radiograph demonstrating air-filled loops of distended small bowel.

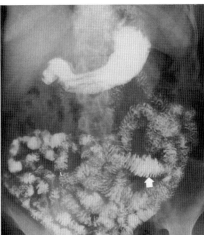

Barium contrast study demonstrating the normal feathery pattern of the jejunum. *Arrow* points to a filled loop with normal valvulae conniventes.

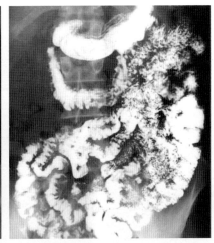

Barium contrast study of a patient with malabsorption syndrome demonstrating the loss of normal folds, clumping of barium, and separation of the meal.

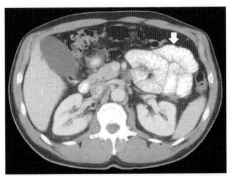

Contrast CT image demonstrating the normal appearance of filled loops of jejunum.

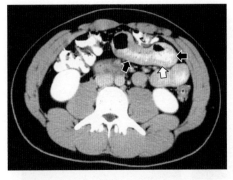

CT image of the abdomen of a patient with Henoch-Schönlein syndrome. The *arrows* point to an abnormal hemorrhagic loop of small bowel.

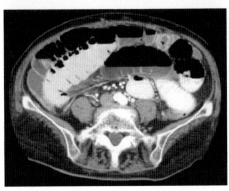

CT image of the abdomen of a patient with small bowel obstruction. Note the large dilated loops of small bowel with fluid levels.

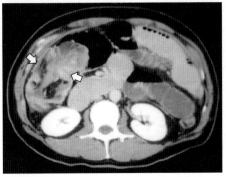

CT image of the abdomen demonstrating small bowel obstruction caused by intussusception *(arrows)*.

Fig. 53.1 Imaging Studies of the Small Intestine. *CT*, Computed tomography.

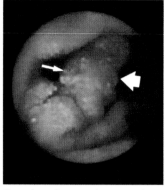

Capsule endoscopy demonstrating polypoid adenocarcinoma of the jejunum (*arrows*).

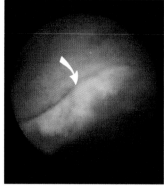

Capsule endoscopy demonstrating large jejunal ulcer *(arrow)*.

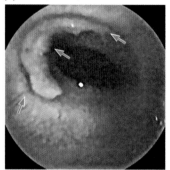

Large Crohn's disease ulcer in ileum.

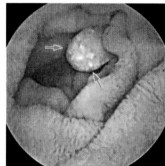

Duodenal polyp.

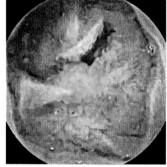

Small bleeding duodenal ulcer.

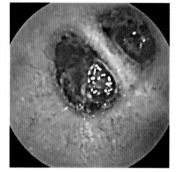

Opening to ileal diverticula.

Fig. 53.2 Wireless Capsule Endoscopy.

ADDITIONAL RESOURCES

de Latour RA, Kilaru SM, Gross SA: Management of small bowel polyps: a literature review, *Best Pract Res Clin Gastroenterol* 31:401–408, 2017.

Feigel DO, Cave D: *Capsule endoscopy*, Philadelphia, 2008, Saunders-Elsevier.

Gore RM, Levine MS: *Textbook of gastrointestinal radiology*, ed 3, Philadelphia, 2008, Saunders-Elsevier.

Gross SA, Stark ME: Initial experience with double-balloon enteroscopy at a U.S. center, *Gastrointest Endosc* 67(6):898–901, 2008.

Gustout CJ: Clinical update: capsule endoscopy, *Gastrointest Endosc* 10:1–4, 2002.

Mata A, Llach J, Castells A, et al: A prospective trial comparing wireless capsule endoscopy and barium contrast series for small-bowel surveillance in hereditary GI polyposis syndromes, *Gastrointest Endosc* 61:721–725, 2005.

Mizell JS, Turnage RH: Intestinal obstruction. In Feldman M, Friedman LS, Brandt LJ, editors: *Gastrointestinal and liver disease*, ed 10, Philadelphia, 2016, Saunders-Elsevier, pp 2159–2170.

Murino A, Despott EJ: Small bowel endoluminal imaging (capsule and enteroscopy), *Frontline Gastroenterol* 8:148–151, 2017.

Savides TJ, Jensen DM: Gastrointestinal bleeding. In Feldman M, Friedman LS, Brandt LJ, editors: *Gastrointestinal and liver disease*, ed 10, Philadelphia, 2016, Saunders-Elsevier, pp 297–335.

Tanaka S, Mitsui K, Tatsuguchi A, et al: Current status of double-balloon endoscopy: indications, insertion route, sedation, complications, technical matters, *Gastrointest Endosc* 66(3 Suppl):S30–S33, 2007.

54

Visceral Reflexes

Martin H. Floch

Visceral reflexes explain a number of clinical signs and symptoms. Afferent impulses from the hypertonic sigmoid initiate reflexes to cranial structures, to the bronchial tree, to the stomach, and to the abdominal skin.

The afferent limb of *viscerosomatic reflexes,* originating from viscera and affecting somatic structures, may be by way of sympathetic or parasympathetic nerves. The efferent limb is usually through somatic nerves or autonomic paths. In *viscerovisceral reflexes,* the afferent and efferent limbs may contain both sympathetic and parasympathetic nerves, but they may be mediated by the intrinsic nerve plexuses only. *Somatovisceral reflexes* involve somatic afferents and sympathetic or parasympathetic efferents to the viscus.

Because they lack a true efferent limb to the arc, *viscerosensory reflexes* are not true reflexes and are believed to result from a shunt or transfer of sensory impulses from autonomic afferents to somatic afferents. Exactly where the shunt or transfer takes place is conjectural. Viscerosensory reflexes explain the phenomena of *referred pain* and *skin hyperalgesia.* In the case of sympathetic reflexes, hyperalgesia occurs in skin areas innervated by the same spinal segment from which the nerve supply of the diseased viscus derives, and in the case of parasympathetic reflexes, it may manifest in more remote areas.

Fig. 54.1 illustrates some of the major visceral reflexes. These are essential in clinical medicine because they explain why somatic or sensory stimuli can cause gastrointestinal symptoms. Pain from muscle or bone may cause vomiting; psychologic or sensory stimuli can cause diarrhea; and abdominal pain can cause headache. The clinician must remember that the symptom may come from a distant stimulus, as listed in Table 54.1.

TABLE 54.1 Origin, Effect, and Clinical Significance of Visceral Reflexes

Reflex	Origin	Effect	Clinical Significance
Viscerosomatic			
Visceromuscular	Diseased abdominal organ	Contraction of voluntary muscles and erectores pili muscles innervated by corresponding spinal segment; also neck and laryngeal muscles	Involuntary guarding suggests underlying visceral irritative process.
Visceroglandular	Diseased abdominal organ	Sweating in area of corresponding dermatomes	Aids in identifying level of visceral involvement.
Viscerovascular	Diseased abdominal organ	Dilatation of blood vessels; dermographia; sense of warmth in corresponding dermatomes	Aids in identifying level of visceral involvement.
Viscerosensory	Diseased abdominal organ	Hyperalgesia in corresponding dermatomes	In absence of distention, explains tenderness and intolerance of tight garments.
Viscerovisceral			
Gastroileocolic and duodenoileocolic	Food entering stomach and duodenum	Stimulation of ileac and colic motility	Accounts for postcoffee defecation reflex; postprandial distress in irritable colon syndrome.
Esophagosalivary and gastrosalivary	Esophagus and stomach	Paroxysmal sialorrhea	Clue to neoplasm of esophagus.
Enterogastric	Distention or irritation of enteric canal	Inhibition of stomach; antral spasm	One of the mechanisms of indigestion; biliousness; nausea.
Cologastric	Distention or irritation of colon	Inhibition of stomach; antral spasm	Instigating epigastric distress in irritable colon syndrome; vomiting in appendicitis.
Urinary tract–gut	Disease of urinary tract	Inhibition and distention of gut	Acute abdominal symptoms may be of genitourinary origin.
Viscerocardiac	Disease of GI organs	Diminution of coronary flow; changes in heart rhythm and rate	Myocardial disturbances (tachycardia, bradycardia, arrhythmia) may occur in GI disorders.
Visceropulmonary	Disease of GI organs	Spasm of bronchioles	Accounts for sense of difficult breathing in irritable colon syndrome.

GI, Gastrointestinal.

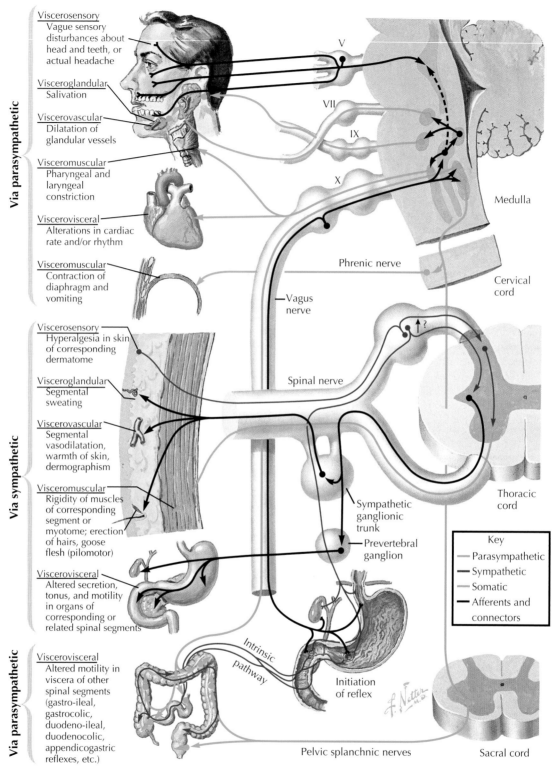

Via parasympathetic

Viscerosensory
Vague sensory disturbances about head and teeth, or actual headache

Visceroglandular
Salivation

Viscerovascular
Dilatation of glandular vessels

Visceromuscular
Pharyngeal and laryngeal constriction

Visceroviseral
Alterations in cardiac rate and/or rhythm

Visceromuscular
Contraction of diaphragm and vomiting

Via sympathetic

Viscerosensory
Hyperalgesia in skin of corresponding dermatome

Visceroglandular
Segmental sweating

Viscerovascular
Segmental vasodilatation, warmth of skin, dermographism

Visceromuscular
Rigidity of muscles of corresponding segment or myotome; erection of hairs, goose flesh (pilomotor)

Visceroviseral
Altered secretion, tonus, and motility in organs of corresponding or related spinal segments

Via parasympathetic

Visceroviseral
Altered motility in viscera of other spinal segments (gastro-ileal, gastrocolic, duodeno-ileal, duodenocolic, appendicogastric reflexes, etc.)

V
VII
IX
X

Medulla

Phrenic nerve

Cervical cord

Vagus nerve

Spinal nerve

Sympathetic ganglionic trunk

Prevertebral ganglion

Thoracic cord

Intrinsic pathway

Initiation of reflex

Pelvic splanchnic nerves

Sacral cord

Key
Parasympathetic
Sympathetic
Somatic
Afferents and connectors

Fig. 54.1 Visceral Reflexes.

ADDITIONAL RESOURCES

Farmer AD, Aziz Q: The brain-gut axis. In Podolsky DK, Camilleri M, Fitz JG, et al, editors: *Yamada's textbook of gastroenterology*, ed 6, Hoboken, New Jersey, 2016, John Wiley and Sons Ltd, pp 227–238.

Millham FH: Acute abdominal pain. In Feldman M, Friedman LS, Brandt LJ, editors: *Gastrointestinal and liver disease*, ed 10, Philadelphia, 2016, Saunders-Elsevier, pp 161–174.

Yarze JC, Friedman LS: Chronic abdominal pain. In Feldman M, Friedman LS, Brandt LJ, editors: *Gastrointestinal and liver disease*, ed 10, Philadelphia, 2016, Saunders-Elsevier, pp 175–184.

55

Congenital Abnormalities of the Small Intestine

Martin H. Floch

Congenital lesions develop in the gastrointestinal (GI) tract and may cause intestinal obstruction (Fig. 55.1). Almost all presentations are in newborns and necessitate immediate surgery. The most common site of complete obstruction or *atresia* (congenital absence or closure) is in the ileum. The duodenum is the second most common site. Obstruction may result from atresia, malrotation of the colon, volvulus, meconium ileus, or imperforate anus.

CLINICAL PICTURE

Vomiting, absence of stool, and abdominal distention are the clinical triad indicating a significant problem in an infant. Certain atresias are evident within the first 24 hours. Malrotation, volvulus, and meconium ileus may manifest immediately. An infant with an imperforate anus produces no stool; diagnosis should be made on initial examination of the newborn.

DIAGNOSIS

Careful examination of the infant and, if necessary, radiographic examination reveal the obvious diagnosis. At times, a barium contrast study (upper or lower) may be necessary to prove the diagnosis.

TREATMENT AND MANAGEMENT

Intestinal obstruction caused by a congenital lesion is life threatening, and surgical intervention is rapidly needed. Atresia requires end-to-end anastomosis to maintain the continuity of the bowel. A malrotation or volvulus requires cutting of the mesentery, and an imperforate anus requires surgery to create an outlet.

Meconium ileus may present differently than the other forms of congenital obstruction in that the mass of meconium can create irregular loops of distended bowel rather than obstruction at the site of the occlusion, such as in atresia. Meconium ileus also may develop in infants born with fibrocystic disease of the pancreas. Less than 10% of infants with cystic fibrosis develop meconium ileus. However, it may occur within the first few months, and the presentation may not be as immediate as with other forms of congenital intestinal obstruction.

PROGNOSIS

If the surgeon is able to perform a corrective procedure, the prognosis is good. However, the problems of infancy and childhood created by a congenital defect may affect growth and development. Early surgery can cause great psychologic stress in the family and can result in long-term psychosocial problems.

Other anomalies of the GI tract, such as abdominal wall defects, intestinal duplication, mesenteric cysts, and omphalomesenteric cysts, are rare. Hirschsprung disease is discussed separately in Section V.

ADDITIONAL RESOURCES

Bass LM, Wershil BK: Anatomy, histology, embryology and developmental anomalies of the small and large intestines. In Feldman M, Friedman LS, Brandt LJ, editors: *Gastrointestinal and liver disease*, ed 10, Philadelphia, 2016, Saunders-Elsevier, pp 1649–1678.

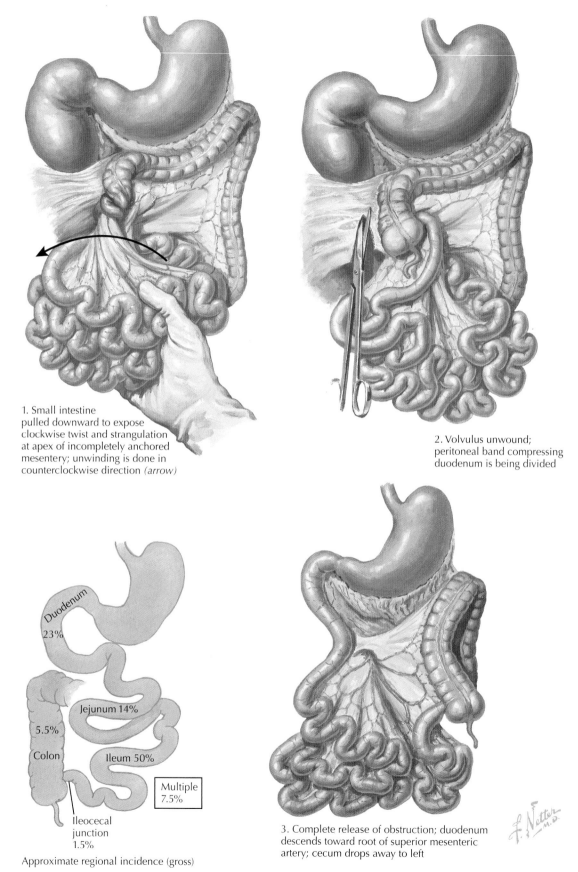

1. Small intestine pulled downward to expose clockwise twist and strangulation at apex of incompletely anchored mesentery; unwinding is done in counterclockwise direction *(arrow)*

2. Volvulus unwound; peritoneal band compressing duodenum is being divided

Duodenum 23%

Jejunum 14%

5.5%

Colon

Ileum 50%

Multiple 7.5%

Ileocecal junction 1.5%

Approximate regional incidence (gross)

3. Complete release of obstruction; duodenum descends toward root of superior mesenteric artery; cecum drops away to left

Fig. 55.1 Congenital Intestinal Abnormalities, Including Malrotation of the Colon With Volvulus of the Midgut.

56

Meckel Diverticulum

Martin H. Floch

The yolk sac is connected to the primitive tubular gut by the *vitelline* (omphalomesenteric) *duct* in early embryonic stages and is normally obliterated about the seventh week of fetal life. Failure of the duct to disappear results in a variety of remnants; the most common presentation is a *sacculation,* or pouch, attached to the ileum and best known as Meckel diverticulum (Fig. 56.1).

Meckel diverticulum is the most frequent congenital anomaly of the gastrointestinal tract and occurs in 1% to 3% of the population. It is located 30 to 90 cm proximal to the ileocecal junction and is always attached to the antimesenteric side of the ileal wall. The diverticulum varies from 1 to 10 cm long and 1 to 3 cm wide. In contrast to the *acquired* intestinal diverticulum, the wall of Meckel diverticulum is composed of all the layers and is thus a true diverticulum. Mucosal lining usually corresponds to that of the ileum, but it may contain ectopic gastric mucosa, or nodules of pancreatic tissue, which can cause serious complications. The rest of the vitelline duct is obliterated in most patients, but it might remain as a fibrous band. The persistence of the entire vitelline duct as a permanent tube leads to an umbilical-intestinal fistula that is usually discovered in infancy.

CLINICAL PICTURE

The clinical picture varies greatly, depending on the complications. Most patients with Meckel diverticulum have no symptoms and no complications. When patients become symptomatic, however, their symptoms vary with the condition. A typical presentation is intestinal bleeding, which is more common in children and often manifests with maroon stools. If the bleeding is slow, melena may be present. Peptic ulceration has been reported when ectopic gastric mucosa is present in the diverticulum. Strangulation, intussusception, torsion, incarceration of Meckel diverticulum into a hernia, and adhesions with obstruction caused by the hernia have all been reported. These findings may present a clinical picture of acute abdomen or chronic pain. Also, neoplasm has been reported to develop in the diverticulum, and all the complications of an intraabdominal neoplasm may be present.

DIAGNOSIS

Diagnosis can be made by technetium-99m pertechnetate imaging. However, if Meckel diverticulum is suspected, computed tomography (CT) is often performed, and the diagnosis is made at scanning. The differential diagnosis includes appendicitis, cholecystitis, diverticulitis, salpingitis, and any other inflammatory condition leading to a colonic or gastroduodenal lesion or pathologic condition of the small bowel. Although the diagnosis is made most frequently through CT, the surgeon is often surprised at laparotomy.

TREATMENT AND MANAGEMENT

The treatment of any symptomatic Meckel diverticulum is surgical resection. It is now possible to reach the lesion easily by laparoscopy, and simple resection is possible. As noted in the reference by Sarasi et al., appendicitis can frequently not be differentiated from Meckel diverticulitis and, therefore, surgery is absolutely necessary.

COURSE AND PROGNOSIS

The prognosis for Meckel diverticulum is excellent for all the abnormalities except neoplasia, which depends on the type of lesion.

ADDITIONAL RESOURCES

Rubin DC, Shaker A: Small intestines: anatomy and structural anomalies. In Podolsky DK, Camilleri M, Fitz JG, et al, editors: *Yamada's textbook of gastroenterology,* ed 6, Hoboken, New Jersey, 2016, John Wiley and Sons Ltd, pp 73–107.

Sanders LE: Laparoscopic treatment for Meckel's diverticulum: obstruction and bleeding is managed with minimal morbidity, *Surg Endosc* 9:724–727, 1995.

Sarosi GA: Appendicitis. In Feldman M, Friedman LS, Brandt LJ, editors: *Gastrointestinal and liver disease,* ed 10, Philadelphia, 2016, Saunders-Elsevier, pp 2112–2122.

St Vil D, Brandy ML, Panic S, et al: Meckel's diverticulum in children: a 20-year review, *J Pediatr Surg* 26:1289–1292, 1991.

Turgeon DK, Barnett JL: Meckel's diverticulum, *Am J Gastroenterol* 85:777–781, 1990.

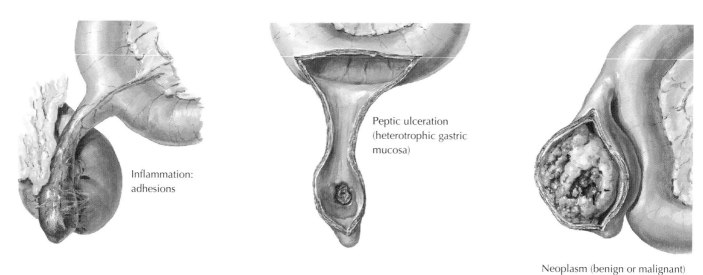

Inflammation: adhesions

Peptic ulceration (heterotrophic gastric mucosa)

Neoplasm (benign or malignant)

Strangulation of bowel loops by knotting of diverticulum

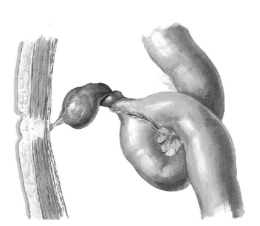

Torsion and strangulation of diverticulum

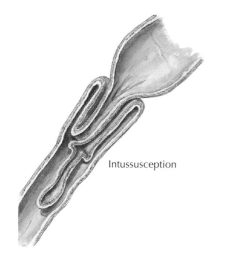

Intussusception

Incarceration in hernia

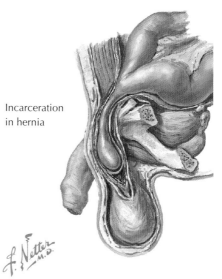

Fig. 56.1 Meckel Diverticulum (Vitelline Duct Remnants).

57

Diverticula of the Small Intestine

Martin H. Floch

A diverticulum of the small bowel is a "blind" outpocket from the hollow viscus that consists of one or more layers (Fig. 57.1). Incidence at autopsy ranges from 0.2% to 0.6%. Diverticula are less common in distal areas of the small bowel. Their etiology is unknown, but most appear to be acquired and to consist of mucosal and submucosal layers only. Colonic diverticulosis is associated with small bowel diverticulosis in 35% to 44% of patients. Complications of inflammation and diverticulitis, obstruction associated with enteroliths, bleeding, perforation, volvulus, bacterial overgrowth, and multiple diverticula have all been reported.

CLINICAL PICTURE

The clinical picture may be an incidental finding and *asymptomatic,* an *acute* complication, or *chronic* symptoms. Symptoms of acute abdomen caused by free perforation, volvulus, or obstruction associated with an enterolith or gastrointestinal (GI) bleeding may cause a patient to seek treatment. Chronic presenting symptoms, including dyspepsia, nausea, occasional vomiting, mild pain, flatulence, and diarrhea, may be caused by bacterial overgrowth or mild inflammation associated with one of the diverticula. Therefore, a broad presenting clinical picture is possible.

Once diagnosed, symptoms should be fully evaluated. Clinicians tend to view diverticula as benign, but they can be a significant finding. Once inflammation occurs in a diverticulum, an acute abdominal infection can result that mimics appendicitis or inflammation, as in Meckel diverticulum. When inflammation develops, erosion of a blood vessel can cause a slow bleed or a massive hemorrhage.

The clinicopathologic correlation of jejunal diverticula is similar to that seen in colonic diverticulosis. The association of jejunal diverticula with steatorrhea and macrocytic anemia has been reported since 1954. There are many cases in the literature of proven bacterial overgrowth and malabsorption. Many patients with jejunal diverticula also have symptoms similar to those of scleroderma, such as esophageal motility disturbances and Raynaud phenomenon.

DIAGNOSIS

The diagnosis is established with small bowel barium contrast study or computed tomography scan with contrast. When chronic anemia or bacterial overgrowth is suspected, studies to evaluate for malabsorption are helpful (see Chapter 62). Anemia and steatorrhea can be demonstrated in patients with bacterial overgrowth.

TREATMENT AND MANAGEMENT

Patients with acute diverticula require surgery, usually by open laparotomy or by laparoscopic surgery when necessary. The treatment for bacterial overgrowth is long-term antibiotic therapy. Ampicillin, tetracycline, or a second- or third-generation drug such as ciprofloxacin can be used daily. It is recommended to alternate antibiotic therapy and "to give the bowel a rest." Some clinicians administer antibiotics every other month to treat this type of bacterial overgrowth. Malabsorption and anemia can be corrected by antibiotic therapy.

COURSE AND PROGNOSIS

Depending on the age of the patient and the acute nature of the clinical situation, the prognosis for diverticulum is similar to that of any condition with a perforated bowel or massive GI hemorrhage. The prognosis for patients with bacterial overgrowth is excellent once therapy is instituted. The mere presence of jejunal or small bowel diverticula without symptoms is benign. However, the clinician should be aware of the risks and should check the patient intermittently for potential insidious complications.

ADDITIONAL RESOURCES

Badnoch J, Bedford PD: Massive diverticula of the upper intestine presenting with steatorrhea and megaloblastic anemia, *Q J Med* 23:462–470, 1954.

DeBree E, Grammatikakis J, Christodoulakis M, Tsiftsis D: The clinical significance of acquired jejunal diverticula, *Am J Gastroenterol* 93: 2523–2528, 1998.

Jexarajah DR, Dunbar KB: Diverticula of the pharynx, esophagus, stomach, and small intestine. In Feldman M, Friedman LS, Brandt LJ, editors: *Gastrointestinal and liver disease,* ed 10, Philadelphia, 2016, Saunders-Elsevier, pp 397–406.

Krishnamurthy S, Kelly MM, Rohrmann CA, Schuffler MD: Jejunal diverticulosis: a heterogeneous disorder caused by a variety of abnormalities of smooth muscle or myenteric plexus, *Gastroenterology* 85:538–547, 1988.

Lobo GN, Braithwaite BD, Fairbrother BJ: Enterolithiasis complicating jejunal diverticulosis, *J Clin Gastroenterol* 29:192–193, 1999.

Rodriguez HE, Ziauddin MF, Quiros ED, et al: Jejunal diverticulosis in gastrointestinal bleeding, *J Clin Gastroenterol* 33:412–414, 2001.

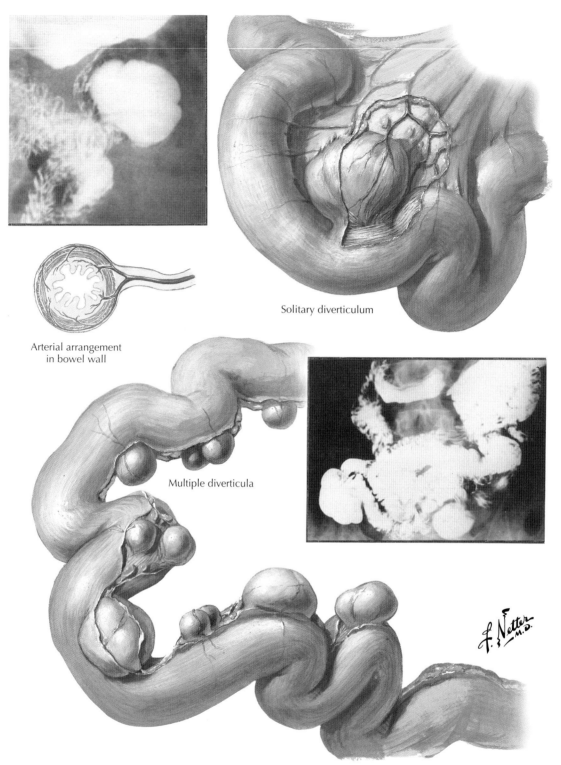

Solitary diverticulum

Arterial arrangement
in bowel wall

Multiple diverticula

Fig. 57.1 Diverticula of the Small Intestine.

58

Motility and Dysmotility of the Small Intestine

Martin H. Floch

Many patients undergo full evaluation for nausea, vomiting, abdominal pain, or dyspepsia, but routine evaluations reveal no abnormalities (see Section II for details of these symptoms and their evaluation). Occasionally, it is readily apparent that a patient may have a true gastric-duodenal motility disturbance (see Chapter 4). Progressive motility from the antrum into the duodenum, then from the duodenum into the small bowel, is important for maintaining normal motor function for absorption and digestion and for cleansing the bowel to prevent bacterial overgrowth (Fig. 58.1).

Any indication of disturbed absorption of nutrients or bacterial overgrowth should lead to further small bowel motility evaluation. True small bowel transit disturbances and dysmotility are rare and difficult to prove. These evaluations are made primarily at selective research centers. However, motility disturbances do exist, and patients can be helped if indications of small bowel dysmotility can be identified.

The small bowel has both a vigorous working longitudinal muscle layer and a circular muscle layer that are governed by an intrinsic nervous system and an extrinsic nervous system modified by the function of the interstitial cells of Cajal. Intrinsic neurons have their cell bodies within the wall and are divided into sensory (afferent) neurons, motor (efferent) neurons, and interneurons, whereas extrinsic neurons are derived from the vagal and spinal pathways of the parasympathetic and sympathetic divisions of the autonomic nervous system.

MEASUREMENTS OF TRANSIT AND MOTILITY

The *lactulose breath test* is used primarily to measure the small intestine's ability to absorb hydrogen or labeled carbon that is freed after the lactulose reaches the distal small intestine; thus, it really is a measure of *orocecal transit time*. These tests are used primarily in research centers and are difficult to interpret in a clinical setting. Some institutions evaluate for scintigraphic orocecal transit time to measure the transit time, but these also are primarily research institution techniques. Barium contrast studies and fluoroscopy have been used, but these are imprecise for determining true transit time and are most effective when there is some obstructive lesion. At times, without any explanation, transit time using barium contrast may be as short as 30 to 45 minutes.

Small bowel *manometry* is used with great skill in research institutions. Gastric and duodenal probes are placed, and metric measurements can be made of antral, pyloric, and duodenal contractions. The normal patterns of motility, a regular and continuous series of contractions (phase 3), occur within the gut during fasting, approximately three cycles per minute in the stomach and 11 cycles per minute in the duodenum. The regular string of contractions lasts several minutes and propagates downward to the bowel from the antrum as a *migrating motor complex* (MMC). Passage of the MMC is followed by a quiescent period (phase 1), and then the contractile pattern becomes irregular (phase 2), which usually occurs during fasting. Immediately upon eating, the fasting pattern of motility is replaced with a fed pattern, both in the stomach and in the small bowel. Contractile activity increases, and there are no migrating bursts of contractions. The increase in contractions in the small intestine mixes intestinal contents and enhances absorption. Although performed mainly at research institutions, these studies are indicated in the diagnosis of subtle intestinal obstruction and in the explanation for small intestinal bacterial overgrowth (Chapter 67), differentiation of intestinal myopathy from neuropathy, gastroparesis refractory to prokinetic agents, and differentiation of visceral pain syndrome from other motility disorders.

Clinicians most often must rely on radiologic transit with barium or computed tomography with contrast to observe small bowel motility. These techniques provide only broad evaluation but can suggest disturbances requiring more sophisticated study and may help guide the clinical treatment course.

DIAGNOSIS

Diseases associated with disordered intestinal motility are nonulcerative dyspepsia (see Chapter 31), irritable bowel syndrome (Chapter 58), chronic intestinal pseudo-obstruction (Chapter 57), partial small bowel obstruction (Chapter 56), gastric resection, acute illness, pregnancy, diabetes, metabolic disturbances, drugs, scleroderma and other connective tissue diseases, neurologic syndromes, rare myopathies, and biliary dyskinesia. Diabetes mellitus often is associated with altered neurotransmission, as can occur with numerous drugs that decrease or alter contractions.

It is important to note that some patients may require evaluation at a research institution that performs the necessary tests. These patients usually have chronic symptoms and have undergone evaluation but now require detailed research studies and analysis.

Colonoscopy offers repeat visualization of the distal ileum. The end of the ileum appears to be wedged into the wall of the colon and at times can be seen to flutter. However, observations on living patients indicate that the ileocecal junction functions as a *true* sphincter, which means it regulates the flow of material from the ileum to the cecum and prevents retrograde passage. However, there is controversy as to whether this is merely a function of the angulation of the anatomy or a true muscular function based on distention of the ileum with a final peristaltic contraction that empties ileal contents into the cecum. At present, no clinical disease entity is known to be related to this physiology.

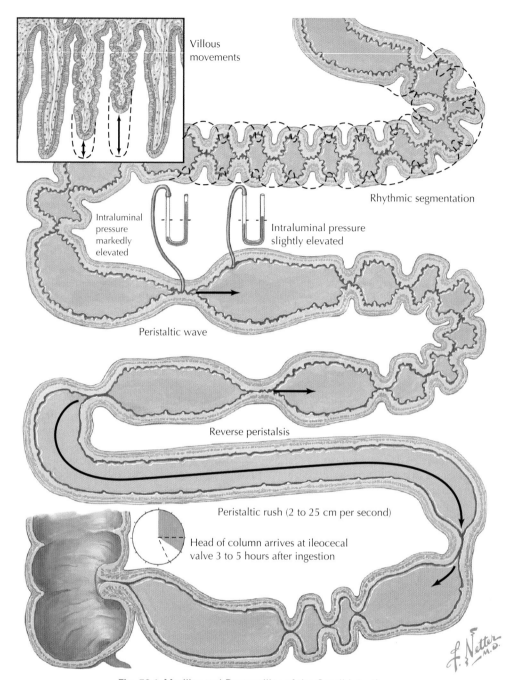

Villous movements

Rhythmic segmentation

Intraluminal pressure markedly elevated

Intraluminal pressure slightly elevated

Peristaltic wave

Reverse peristalsis

Peristaltic rush (2 to 25 cm per second)

Head of column arrives at ileocecal valve 3 to 5 hours after ingestion

Fig. 58.1 Motility and Dysmotility of the Small Intestine.

ADDITIONAL RESOURCES

Andrews JM, Brierly SM, Blackshaw LA: Small intestinal motor and sensory function and dysfunction. In Feldman M, Friedman LS, Brandt LJ, editors: *Gastrointestinal and liver disease*, ed 10, Philadelphia, 2016, Saunders-Elsevier, pp 1679–1695.

Bratton JR, Jones MP: Small intestinal motility, *Curr Opin Gastroenterol* 23:127–133, 2007.

Szarka L: Dysmotility of the small intestine and colon. In Podolsky DK, Camilleri M, Fitz JG, et al, editors: *Yamada's textbook of gastroenterology*, ed 6, Hoboken, New Jersey, 2016, John Wiley and Sons Ltd, pp 1154–1195.

Yamamoto T, Watabe K, Nakahara M, et al: Disturbed gastrointestinal motility and decreased interstitial cells of Cajal in diabetic db/db mice, *J Gastroenterol Hepatol* 23:660–667, 2008.

59

Obstruction and Ileus of the Small Intestine

Martin H. Floch

Intestinal obstruction occurs when the onward passage of intestinal contents is limited by mechanical abnormalities or a functional disturbance (Fig. 59.1). Peristaltic activity may be abolished by reflexes originating from diseased structures within, or remote from, the abdominal cavity. When obstructive lesions occur, some motility may persist. The obstruction may be partial or complete, and when it occurs with vascular compromise, it may indicate simple ischemia or may be attributed to strangulation.

The most common cause of small intestinal obstruction is *adhesions* (>50%). *Herniation* accounts for approximately 25% of obstructions. Adhesions are *extrinsic,* as are hernias, and other causes of extrinsic lesions may be congenital bands, volvulus, or carcinomatosis outside the bowel wall. The remaining 25% of small bowel obstructions are caused by inflammatory lesions, intussusceptions, neoplasms, foreign bodies, or atresias and stenosis. These lesions are primarily *intrinsic* to the bowel.

Ileus occurs when the bowel ceases to pass its contents, becoming *adynamic.* Ileus usually occurs after surgery but also results from inflammatory, metabolic, and neurogenic lesions. It also may be associated with electrolyte imbalances or drug administration. Acute inflammation in the bowel, such as appendicitis, diverticulitis, or peritonitis, can cause loss of motility and ileus. Ileus is also associated with acute pancreatitis, ischemic lesions of the bowel, and, occasionally, chest lesions causing systemic sepsis. Any of the hernias described in Section III can cause intestinal obstruction and manifest acutely.

CLINICAL PICTURE

Depending on the cause, acute obstruction of the bowel may present with abdominal pain, nausea, and vomiting of reflux origin. Abdominal examination reveals increased peristalsis, which gives way to alternating periods of hyperactivity and quiescence until the latter predominates.

In adynamic ileus, peristalsis ceases from the start; therefore the bowel is extremely quiet and emits poor bowel sounds. However, invariably there is increased fluid secretion into the gut and accumulation of gas, with the bowel becoming more and more distended. In patients with *mechanical ileus,* the distention is proximal to the point of obstruction, whereas in patients with *reflex ileus,* the distention is more generalized.

As peristalsis fails, the absorptive functions also fail, permeability is altered, and intestinal bacteria and toxic substances can translocate. Water and electrolytes enter the bowel lumen, aggravating the distention and invariably increasing the vomiting. The overall effect on the patient is dehydration of body tissue and circulatory failure. Patients may become hypotensive and may experience shock and sepsis.

In mild intermittent obstruction, the symptoms are less severe and the only clinical presentation may be recurrent abdominal pain. However, anorexia always correlates with the pain and recurrent bloating of abdominal distention. When obstruction is complete, bowel movements cease. With partial obstruction, the patient may have some bowel movement or even mild diarrhea.

DIAGNOSIS

The clinical picture varies from a mild, partial obstruction to an acute, life-threatening situation. Abdominal radiographs are essential to define the type and degree of obstruction, with films of the patient in the supine and upright positions. Radiographs usually help determine whether the obstruction involves the small intestine, with or without the colon. In patients with ileus, the colon is invariably involved, whereas in patients with mechanical obstruction, the area of the dilated loops of bowel with possible fluid levels can identify the site of the obstruction.

Computed tomography (CT) usually clearly delineates the point of obstruction and invariably makes the diagnosis. CT can define closed-loop obstruction, strangulations, characteristic pictures of volvulus, extrinsic or intrinsic neoplasia, and it can clearly indicate the need for medical or surgical therapy.

When the diagnosis is unclear, contrast studies may be helpful. CT scan is performed with contrast, and the lesions at the point of the obstruction can be identified. However, occasionally, CT findings are unclear, and barium contrast study may be indicated. Barium studies are more feasible in the small intestine than in the large intestine because barium hardens when water is absorbed in the large bowel. Barium should not be used to diagnose a suspected colonic lesion. Absorbable contrast should be used; in the small bowel, lesions can be clearly defined before therapy is indicated.

It is important to confirm the diagnosis of strangulation or impending gangrenous bowel so that the bowel can be saved. This is particularly important in elderly patients, who may have few symptoms before the bowel becomes strangulated and gangrenous.

TREATMENT AND MANAGEMENT

Immediate therapy involves nasogastric suction to treat distention, electrolyte and fluid replacement, and antibiotics to clear infection and prevent sepsis. In adynamic ileus, particularly after surgery, patience and fluid replacement frequently correct the problem.

If the patient is thought to have mechanical obstruction, surgical intervention is indicated for partial and complete obstruction. For complete obstruction, the surgery is performed on an emergency basis to prevent gangrenous bowel.

COURSE AND PROGNOSIS

Ileus may develop after surgery and can last several days. The patient will need reassurance, nasogastric suction, careful electrolyte replacement, and nutritional support. Prognosis is usually good when diagnosis shows

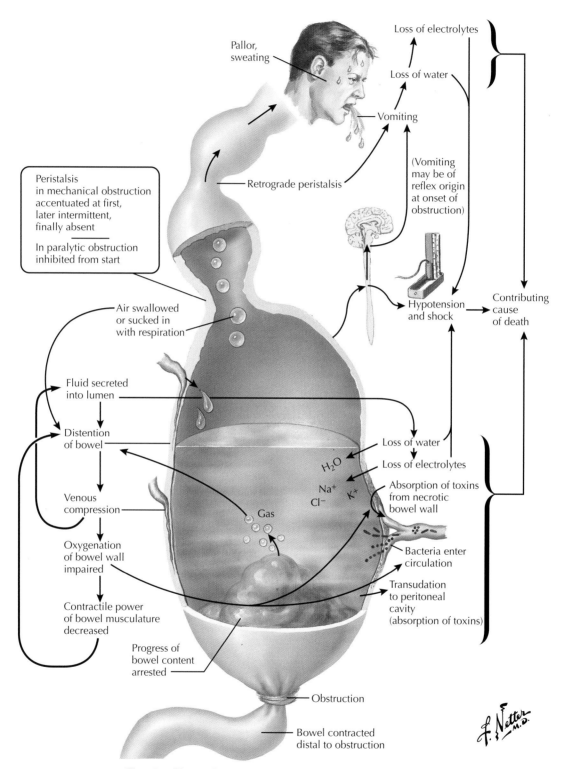

Pallor, sweating

Loss of electrolytes

Loss of water

Vomiting

Retrograde peristalsis

(Vomiting may be of reflex origin at onset of obstruction)

Peristalsis in mechanical obstruction accentuated at first, later intermittent, finally absent

In paralytic obstruction inhibited from start

Hypotension and shock

Contributing cause of death

Air swallowed or sucked in with respiration

Fluid secreted into lumen

Distention of bowel

Venous compression

Oxygenation of bowel wall impaired

Contractile power of bowel musculature decreased

Progress of bowel content arrested

Loss of water

Loss of electrolytes

H_2O

Na^+

Cl^- K^+

Absorption of toxins from necrotic bowel wall

Gas

Bacteria enter circulation

Transudation to peritoneal cavity (absorption of toxins)

Obstruction

Bowel contracted distal to obstruction

Fig. 59.1 Obstruction and Adynamic Ileus of the Small Intestine.

the initial disease to be benign. If the diagnosis indicates malignancy or severe infection and abscess, or conditions such as severe pancreatitis, the prognosis is guarded, and mortality is significant.

If surgery is performed quickly and intervenes in mechanical obstruction, the prognosis is excellent. However, once gangrenous bowel develops, particularly in the elderly patient, the prognosis is guarded. Again, if a malignant lesion causes the obstruction, the prognosis is that for the particular malignancy.

The rapid advent of laparoscopic surgery has facilitated diagnosis, corrected mechanical obstruction, and resulted in shorter postoperative periods. Adynamic ileus rarely requires surgery, but when the bowel remains distended and the patient obtains minimal relief through suction and electrolyte replacement, decompression and drainage may be necessary.

ADDITIONAL RESOURCES

Kelly KA, Sarr MG, Hinder RA: *Mayo clinic gastrointestinal surgery*, Philadelphia, 2004, Saunders.

Margenthaler JE, Longo WE, Virgo KS, et al: Risk factors for adverse outcomes following surgery for small bowel obstruction, *Ann Surg* 243:456–464, 2006.

Mizell JS, Turnage IH: Intestinal obstruction. In Feldman M, Friedman LS, Brandt LJ, editors: *Gastrointestinal and liver disease*, ed 10, Philadelphia, 2016, Saunders-Elsevier, pp 2154–2170.

O'Connor DB, Winter DC: The role of laparoscopy in the management of acute small-bowel obstruction: a review of over 2,000 cases, *Surg Endosc* 26:7–12, 2012.

60

Chronic Intestinal Pseudo-Obstruction

Martin H. Floch

Chronic intestinal pseudo-obstruction (CIPO) is a clinical syndrome that mimics the signs and symptoms of intestinal obstruction (Fig. 60.1). In patients with CIPO, no mechanical obstructive lesion is found on evaluation. CIPO is now thought to be a type of dysmotility and may be related to a functional disturbance in the interstitial cells of Cajal. CIPO may be associated with many disorders of the intestinal or extraintestinal nervous system, including neurologic diseases, small intestinal visceral myopathy, and endocrine and metabolic disorders, and may be precipitated by drugs (Box 60.1). Visceral myopathies and neuropathies are associated with numerous rare congenital abnormalities and are often referred to as *primary* CIPO. Acute colonic pseudo-obstruction (Ogilvie syndrome, false colonic obstruction) is different and presents in critically ill and surgical patients. The list in Box 60.1 is that described in the reference by Camilleri. The reference by Foxx-Orenstein provides a classification slightly differently, yet the same disorders are included in that reference.

CLINICAL PICTURE

CIPO may manifest at any age. Developmental and congenital conditions result in presentation in infancy or early childhood. Associated systemic diseases, such as scleroderma, or paraneoplastic causes may occur later in life. The presenting symptoms are usually obstruction with abdominal distention and pain, vomiting, and inability to have a bowel movement. When the disease is associated with visceral myopathy or neuropathy, pain may become predominant. Rarely, it may be associated with a segmental disease such as megaduodenum or megacolon. An esophageal motility disorder may coexist. Symptoms of those localized lesions, in association with CIPO, may predominate or may obfuscate the diagnosis. In addition, some patients have bacterial overgrowth and can develop malabsorption and diarrhea, with a confusing picture of alternating diarrhea and constipation. Invariably, the physical findings are intestinal obstruction with a distended abdomen, no bowel sounds, and a tympanitic bowel.

DIAGNOSIS

History and physical examination are essential to establish the presence of any neurologic or associated diseases. Often, physical examination reveals weight loss and possibly malnutrition, depending on the degree and chronicity of disease. Radiographs of the abdomen reveal the intestinal obstruction. Patients usually have large, dilated loops of bowel

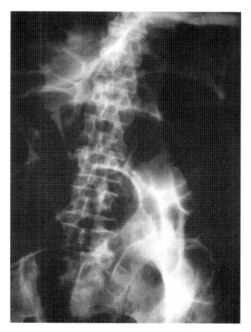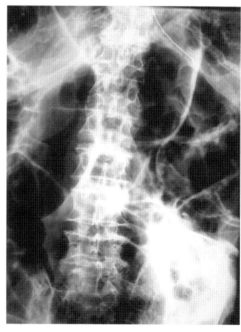

Radiographs of the abdomen demonstrating severe dilatation of overlapping loops of small and large bowel, which is characteristic of CIPO.

Fig. 60.1 Chronic Intestinal Pseudo-Obstruction (CIPO).

BOX 60.1 Clinicopathologic Classification of Chronic Intestinal Pseudo-Obstruction

I. Disorders of the smooth muscle
  A. Primary
    1. Familial visceral myopathies
      a. Type 1 (autosomal dominant)
      b. Type 2 (autosomal recessive, with ptosis and external ophthalmoplegia)
      c. Type 3 (autosomal recessive, with total gastrointestinal tract dilatation)
    2. Sporadic visceral myopathy
    3. Congenital, in infants
  B. Secondary
    1. Progressive systemic sclerosis/polymyositis
    2. Muscular dystrophy syndromes
    3. Systemic lupus erythematosus
    4. Amyloidosis
    5. Radiation injury
    6. Ehlers-Danlos syndrome
    7. Mitochondrial myopathy
  C. Diffuse lymphoid infiltration
  D. Others (muscle cell inclusions; absence of actin)
II. Disorders of the myenteric plexus
  A. Familial visceral neuropathies
    1. Recessive, with intranuclear inclusions (neuronal intranuclear inclusion disease)
    2. Recessive (familial steatorrhea with calcification of the basal ganglia and mental retardation)
    3. Dominant, with neither of the above
    4. POLIP syndrome (*p*olyneuropathy, *o*phthalmoplegia, *l*eukoencephalopathy, *i*ntestinal *p*seudo-obstruction)
    5. Infantile short bowel, malrotation, and pyloric hypertrophy
    6. With progressive neurologic disease at young age
  B. Sporadic visceral neuropathies
    1. Degenerative, noninflammatory (at least two types)
    2. Degenerative, inflammatory (with lymphocytes, plasma cells, or both in myenteric, and sometimes submucosal, plexus)
      a. Paraneoplastic
      b. Infectious (Chagas disease, cytomegalovirus)
      c. Idiopathic
      d. Isolated axonopathy
  C. Developmental abnormalities
    1. Total colonic aganglionosis (sometimes with small intestinal aganglionosis)
    2. Maturational arrest
      a. Isolated to myenteric plexus
      b. With mental retardation
      c. With other neurologic abnormalities
    3. Neuronal intestinal dysplasia
      a. Isolated to intestine
      b. With neurofibromatosis
      c. With multiple endocrine neoplasia, type 2b
  D. Myotonic dystrophy
III. Neurologic disorders
  A. Parkinson disease
  B. Autonomic dysfunction, familial and sporadic
  C. Total autonomic or selective cholinergic dysfunction after Epstein-Barr virus infection
  D. Brainstem tumor
IV. Small intestinal diverticulosis
  A. With muscle resembling visceral myopathy
  B. With muscle resembling progressive systemic sclerosis
  C. With visceral neuropathy and neuronal intranuclear inclusions
  D. Secondary to Fabry disease
V. Endocrine and metabolic disorders
  A. Myxedema
  B. Pheochromocytoma
  C. Hypoparathyroidism
  D. Acute intermittent porphyria
VI. Drugs
  A. Opiates (narcotic bowel syndrome)
  B. Anticholinergics
  C. Phenothiazines
  D. Clonidine
  E. Tricyclic antidepressants
  F. Vinca alkaloids (e.g., vincristine)
  G. Calcium channel blockers
  H. Fetal alcohol syndrome
VII. Miscellaneous
  A. Jejunoileal bypass
  B. Sclerosing mesenteritis
  C. Celiac sprue
  D. Ceroidosis?

From Camilleri M: Acute and chronic pseudo-obstruction. In Feldman M, Friedman LS, Brandt LJ, editors: *Gastrointestinal and Liver Disease*, ed 8, Philadelphia, 2006, Saunders-Elsevier, pp 2679-2702.

with fluid levels. Barium contrast study or computed tomography with contrast media reveals the classic obstructive lesion. Gastric emptying studies or esophageal manometry may further elucidate the associated condition, such as gastroparesis or esophageal symptoms. Complete thyroid evaluation and tests for collagen and vascular diseases should be performed. Finally, it may be necessary to perform a deep biopsy of intestinal muscle; laparoscopy may be helpful.

TREATMENT AND MANAGEMENT

Treatment and management of patients with CIPO depend on whether they have an associated disease. In patients with idiopathic disease and in most with associated disease, standard therapies include prokinetic agents, diet control, and palliative surgery. When obtaining proper nutrition becomes a severe problem, total parenteral nutrition (TPN) on a home basis may be necessary.

Drugs include metoclopramide, 10 to 20 mg three times daily (tid) or four times daily (qid); domperidone, 10 to 20 mg tid or qid (when available); octreotide, 50 to 100 μg daily subcutaneously; and erythromycin, 250 mg tid. These prokinetic agents can be given by mouth or by intravenous injection, depending on the drug and the availability.

Diet therapy varies with the particular condition. During the acute phase, patients are supported intravenously. During the chronic phase, they are usually on low-fat, low-fiber diets with frequent small feedings, gradually progressing to normal feeding as symptoms slowly subside.

Palliative surgery is a drastic procedure that may become necessary to decompress the bowel or to remove or bypass a nonfunctional area.

Colectomy may be used, depending on the degree and type of intestinal involvement. In severely affected patients and those with rare conditions, small intestine transplantation has recently become a treatment consideration, although the procedure is life threatening and offers only limited life expectancy.

COURSE AND PROGNOSIS

When CIPO is associated with another disease, the prognosis of that disease modifies the outcome. Unfortunately, when associated with any significant disease, the finding of CIPO usually heralds the beginning of a fatal prognosis; these patients may die in a few months to a few years. Patients with the idiopathic chronic form may live for many years once a regimen is designed that relieves the obstruction and adequate nutrition can be maintained. Some of these patients receive a combination of prokinetics and nutritional support; life can be maintained, but quality of life decreases. CIPO has a marked effect on the development of children.

ADDITIONAL RESOURCES

Camilleri M: Acute and chronic pseudo-obstruction. In Feldman M, Friedman LS, Brandt LJ, editors: *Gastrointestinal and liver disease*, ed 8, Philadelphia, 2006, Saunders-Elsevier, pp 2679–2702.

Connor FL, DiLorenzo C: Chronic intestinal pseudo-obstruction: assessment and management, *Gastroenterology* 130:S29–S36, 2006.

Foxx-Orenstein AE: Ileus and pseudo-obstruction. In Feldman M, Friedman LS, Brandt LJ, editors: *Gastrointestinal and liver disease*, ed 10, Philadelphia, 2016, Saunders-Elsevier, pp 2171–2195.

Heneyke S, Smith VB, Spitz L, Milla PJ: Chronic intestinal pseudo-obstruction: treatment and long-term follow-up of 44 patients, *Arch Dis Child* 81:21–27, 1999.

Quigley EM: Chronic intestinal pseudo-obstruction, *Curr Treat Options Gastroenterol* 2:239–250, 1999.

Scolapio J, Ukleja A, Bouras E, et al: Nutritional management of chronic intestinal pseudo-obstruction, *J Clin Gastroenterol* 28:306–312, 1999.

Sutton DH, Harrell SP, Wo JM: Diagnosis and management of adult patients with chronic intestinal pseudo-obstruction, *Nutr Clin Pract* 21:16–22, 2006.

61

Irritable Bowel Syndrome and Functional Gastrointestinal Disorders

Martin H. Floch

Irritable bowel syndrome (IBS) is one of a group of functional gastrointestinal (GI) disorders characterized by abdominal discomfort or pain and frequently associated with a change in bowel movements (Fig. 61.1). Worldwide, IBS is the most frequent symptom complex in patients seeking GI consultation. In the United States, it is estimated that more than 3 million office and hospital visits are attributed to this symptom complex.

In disease classification, IBS is thought to be the intestinal or bowel disorder of a group of functional GI disorders that include (1) esophageal disorders such as globus hystericus and functional chest pain; (2) GI disorders such as functional dyspepsia (see Chapter 31), aerophagia, functional vomiting (see Chapter 23), and functional abdominal pain; (3) functional biliary disorders such as sphincter of Oddi dysfunction (see Chapter 139); and (4) anorectal disorders such as anorectal pain and pelvic floor dyssynergia (see Section V).

As understanding of GI physiology broadens, the cause of IBS is thought to be a disturbance in the autonomic and enteric nervous systems of the gut and the gut-brain axis. This disturbance results in abnormal motility and visceral hypersensitivity. Early inflammation of the gut may be a trigger for the onset of the syndrome. The discovery of lactose intolerance has removed many patients from the category of IBS, and, as science evolves, it is certain that other causes may explain the symptoms in select groups of patients. The wide range of food sensitivities and food allergies that exist, as well as slow development of knowledge in this area, may progress and prove helpful in the future.

CLINICAL PICTURE

Three classic symptoms are associated with IBS: abdominal pain, diarrhea, and constipation. Alternating diarrhea and constipation, or diarrhea only, or constipation only, may prevail. In the classic model of the female patient, a woman seeks treatment for recurrent low abdominal pain associated with an inability to have a bowel movement. Constipation is persistent and becomes a lifelong problem. The patient frequently will present with many evaluations that have revealed no significant abnormality. Often, the abdominal pain is relieved by a bowel movement. Patients may or may not notice whether the character of the stool has changed, and often they describe pebblelike stools. However, the pain is persistent and may be nagging or severe, and patients may require pain relief. Characteristic is the history of frequent visits to physician offices, with a work-up that has revealed no disease.

The other common symptom complex is severe diarrhea, noted more often in male patients and consisting of loose or explosive bowel movements that may almost herald incontinence. The diarrhea is associated with severe abdominal cramps, and frequently, patients describe a formed stool on first motion, then liquid stools. Once the diarrhea has stopped, the cramps frequently cease. However, the cramps can be severe and have caused sweating during the bowel movement.

The third pattern is constant, recurrent lower abdominal pain associated with diarrheal bowel movements and, once they have subsided, days of no bowel movements or constipation with a feeling of an inability to evacuate. It is estimated that many patients never report these symptoms to physicians, but, as stated, IBS is one of the major symptom complexes treated by physicians and GI consultants.

DIAGNOSIS

The latest consensus, as expressed in Rome Criteria II and III, is that there should be 12 weeks or more, in the past 12 months, of abdominal discomfort or pain that has two or three features: it must be relieved with defecation, the onset must be associated with a change in frequency of stool, and/or the onset must be associated with a change in the caliber or appearance of the stool. This complex may be associated with increased stool frequency, abnormal forms of stool, marked increased straining or urgency, or a feeling of incomplete evacuation, the appearance of mucus in the stool, or an associated feeling of bloating and abdominal discomfort. The Rome Criteria requires this symptom complex for the diagnosis of IBS.

Some clinicians insist they can make the diagnosis of IBS without a detailed work-up to rule out organic disease. However, most will insist that the diagnosis should not be made without laboratory and imaging evaluation. Certainly, the stool must be free of blood, and a simple microscopic evaluation for leukocytes and overt parasites should be conducted. Screening should be performed to rule out thyroid disease and lactose intolerance. Proponents cite fructose intolerance as a cause in selected patients, and, if suspected, this should be ruled out. Most clinicians will insist that colonoscopy or barium enema evaluation of the colon be performed, depending on the resources available. Furthermore, many will also insist that the small bowel should undergo a screening barium study, or again, depending on the resources, capsule endoscopy or computed tomography of the bowel.

Because the symptoms are recurrent and persistent, conducting a full evaluation is recommended to be able to treat the IBS patient long term. In addition, negative tests reassure the patient that there is no organic disease. Differential diagnosis does include malignancy of the colon, inflammatory bowel disorders, chronic infections, endocrine disorders, and psychiatric disorders.

A theory of bacterial overgrowth or *dysbiosis* has emerged in which some patients have a treatable increase in the small bowel bacterial flora or disturbance in the flora. A lactulose tolerance test is usually positive and is needed to make this diagnosis. Direct bacterial aspiration studies are rarely available, but when performed in research centers, these can prove the small bowel overgrowth. Another theory claims that the normal flora is disturbed, and therefore the addition of probiotic organisms will be helpful. No consensus exists on these theories, but clinicians do treat based on theories, with varied results. There is much experimental

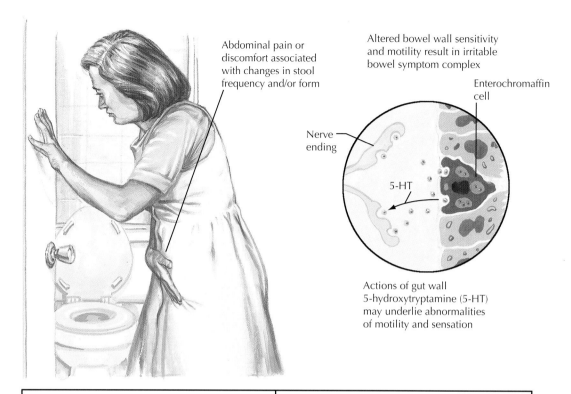

Abdominal pain or discomfort associated with changes in stool frequency and/or form

Altered bowel wall sensitivity and motility result in irritable bowel symptom complex

Enterochromaffin cell

Nerve ending

5-HT

Actions of gut wall 5-hydroxytryptamine (5-HT) may underlie abnormalities of motility and sensation

Rome II diagnostic criteria* for IBS	Symptoms not essential for the diagnosis, but if present increase the confidence in the diagnosis and help to identify subgroups of IBS:
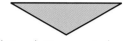	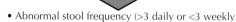
Twelve weeks** or more in the past 12 months of abdominal discomfort or pain that has two out of three features: a. Relieved with defecation b. Onset associated with change in frequency of stool c. Onset associated with change in form (appearance) of stool * In the absence of structural or metabolic abnormalities to explain the symptoms. ** The 12 weeks need not be consecutive.	• Abnormal stool frequency (>3 daily or <3 weekly • Abnormal stool form (lumpy/hard or loose/watery stool) >1/4 of defecations • Abnormal stool passage (straining, urgency, or feeling of incomplete evacuation) >1/4 of defecations • Passage of mucus >1/4 of defecations • Bloating or feeling of abdominal distention >1/4 of days

JOHN A. CRAIG_AD
C. Machado
—M.D.
D. Mascaro

Fig. 61.1 Irritable Bowel Syndrome. *5-HT*, 5-Hydroxytryptamine; *IBS*, irritable bowel syndrome.

evidence that indicates that probiotics, prebiotics, and symbiotics are helpful in treating these patients. An individual clinician must decide either by trial and error or from the literature which they use.

TREATMENT AND MANAGEMENT

There is no single treatment for IBS. Treatment varies with the symptom complex. Because IBS is considered a biopsychologic disorder with abnormal motility and abnormal visceral perceptions, treatments vary. To individualize the treatment, symptoms must be addressed, usually in the categories of constipation, diarrhea, or pain associated with bloating.

The constipated patient is usually first put on a high-fiber diet that requires increased intake of dietary fiber from the usual low amount in Western diets to the normal recommended amounts of 25 to 35 g daily (see Section X). If the constipation is intractable and a work-up reveals no organic cause, laxatives or stimulants must be used (see Chapter 81). The new approach has been to use serotonin (5-HT$_4$) receptor agonists. Tegaserod was a helpful drug but has been removed from the market in the United States.

If diarrhea is the problem, the approach is different. These patients must be carefully evaluated for lactose intolerance, but once that is ruled out, anticholinergics may be tried. If they are not successful, diphenoxylate or loperamide may be used to decrease the number of bowel movements; certain agents are helpful when used before social engagements. Dosage is usually as described with the drug product. Patients may want to take one or two tablets before leaving home.

The 5-HT$_3$ antagonists have now proven to be effective. Alosetron is available and effectively decreases colonic motility. Type 3 alosetron and type 4 tegaserod are first-line serotonin products. We can expect that their future development as antagonists will be helpful in the treatment of IBS.

Clinicians claiming bacterial overgrowth will use rifaximin and other antibiotics in cyclic treatment. This has had varied results, but when correlated with good evidence of overgrowth, it can be helpful.

Proponents of probiotic use have had good results using *Bifidobacterium infantis* in a daily dose, reportedly effective in a double-blind controlled study.

Abdominal pain and bloating can be the predominant factor over the uncontrollable symptom. When treatment of the constipation or diarrhea is unsuccessful and the pain predominates, psychotherapeutic agents may be helpful. Most clinicians use tricyclic antidepressants such as desipramine, 50 mg three times daily, or amitriptyline, 10 to 25 mg twice daily or at bedtime.

COURSE AND PROGNOSIS

IBS can become a lifetime problem. These patients may have abdominal pain with altered bowel movements as children and progress into adulthood with the same symptoms, or they may seek treatment for postinfectious problems that persist for years. Symptoms may resolve with treatment, and then recur years later. However, with understanding, reassurance, and careful treatment, these patients frequently adjust well to their gut abnormality, although their symptoms persist for life. Importantly, many patients with these symptoms never seek medical attention because they learn to control the symptoms. Altered motility and visceral hypersensitivity appear to exist for long periods, even for a lifetime, with exacerbation of severity, but most patients learn to control and live with the symptoms.

ADDITIONAL RESOURCES

Botschuijver S, Roeselers G, Levin E, et al: Intestinal fungal dysbiosis is associated with visceral hypersensitivity in patients with irritable bowel syndrome and rates, *Gastroenterology* 153:1026–1039, 2010.

Chey WD, Lembo AJ, Lavins BJ, et al: Linaclotide for irritable bowel syndrome with constipation: A 26-week, randomized, double-blind, placebo-controlled trial to evaluate efficacy and safety, *Am J Gastroenterol* 107:1702–1712, 2012.

Choi YK, Kraft N, Zimmerman B, et al: Fructose intolerance in IBS and utility of fructose-restricted diet, *J Clin Gastroenterol* 42:233–238, 2008.

Drossman D, Corrazziari E, Delvaux M, et al: *Rome III: the functional gastrointestinal disorders*, 3rd ed, McLean, VA, 2006, Degnon Associates.

Floch MH, Narayan R: Diet and the irritable bowel syndrome, *J Clin Gastroenterol* 35:S45–S54, 2002.

Ford AC, Quigley EM, Lacy BE, et al: Efficacy of prebiotics, probiotics, and synbiotics in irritable bowel syndrome and chronic idiopathic constipation: systemic review and meta-analysis, *Am J Gastroenterol* 109:1547–1561, 2014.

Ford AC, Talley NJ: Irritable bowel syndrome. In Feldman M, Friedman LS, Brandt LJ, editors: *Gastrointestinal and liver disease*, ed 10, Philadelphia, 2016, Saunders-Elsevier, pp 2139–2153.

Halvorson HA, Schlett CD, Riddle MS: Postinfectious irritable bowel syndrome: a meta-analysis, *Am J Gastroenterol* 101:1894–1899, 2006.

Hod K, Ringel Y: Treatment of functional bowel disorders with prebiotics and probiotics. In Floch MH, Ringel Y, Walker WA, editors: *The microbiota in gastrointestinal pathophysiology*, ed 1, New York, NY, 2017, Academic Press-Elsevier, pp 355–364.

Kashyap PC, Macrobal A, Ursell LK, et al: Complex interactions among diet, gastrointestinal transit, and gut microbiota in humanized mice, *Gastroenterology* 144:967–977, 2013.

Koloski NA, Jones M, Kalantar J, et al: The brain-gut pathway in functional gastrointestinal disorders is bidirectional: A 12-year prospective population-based study, *Gut* 61:1284–1290, 2012.

Posserud I, Stotser PQ, Bjornsson ES, et al: Small intestinal bacterial overgrowth in patients with irritable bowel syndrome, *Gut* 56:802–808, 2007.

Staudacher HM, Lomer MCE, Farguharson FM, et al: A diet low in FODMAPs reduces symptoms in patients with irritable bowel syndrome and a probiotic restores bifidobacteriaum species: a randomized controlled trial, *Gastroenterology* 153:936–947, 2017.

Videlock EJ, Chang L: Irritable bowel syndrome. In Podolsky DK, Camilleri M, Fitz JG, et al, editors: *Yamada's textbook of gastroenterology*, ed 6, Hoboken, New Jersey, 2016, John Wiley and Sons Ltd, pp 1495–1521.

Whorwell PJ, Altringer L, Morel J, et al: Efficacy of an encapsulated probiotic *Bifidobacterium infantis* 35624 in woman with irritable bowel syndrome, *Am J Gastroenterol* 102:1581–1590, 2006.

62

Evaluation of the Small Bowel

Martin H. Floch

The rapid development of imaging and histopathologic techniques, in conjunction with an altered pattern of disease and treatments late in the 20th century, has changed the "standard" of testing for small bowel function and anatomy. Testing has now become a sophisticated evaluation performed for outpatients in most clinical practices and in detail at university research centers. Evaluation of the patient thought to have small bowel disease should include the following:

1. Detailed history and physical examination for clues to etiology and physical findings of malabsorption
2. Careful imaging technique
3. Biopsy of the small intestine if needed
4. Biochemical function evaluation
5. Stool analysis for parasitic and infectious etiologies

Key findings in the history and physical examination and analysis are described under each disease. However, small bowel disease must be suspected whenever a patient experiences weight loss, diarrhea, anemia, or any sign or symptom of a selective malabsorption deficiency.

IMAGING TECHNIQUES

In the 20th century, the barium contrast study was used to demonstrate the classic malabsorption pattern, including loss of normal small bowel folds, dilatation of the bowel, and segmentation of the meal. Subtle and dramatic presentations were often recorded. In addition, other defects of the small bowel—including neoplasia, strictures, and diverticula—were frequently demonstrated.

The development of computed tomography (CT) and enterography now allows sophisticated imaging of select areas of the bowel and demonstrates the thickness of the bowel wall and any reaction outside the bowel wall. CT has enhanced the clinician's ability to evaluate for many diseases. At times, however, it is still necessary to do both barium contrast and CT studies.

Endoscopy

The small bowel can be visualized using direct endoscopes, but visualization is usually limited to the duodenum with upper endoscopy, to the proximal jejunum with push enteroscopes, and to the terminal ileum with colonoscopes. Long enteroscopes traversing the entire small bowel are used only in select institutions and have not gained wide acceptance.

Capsule endoscopy is the best procedure for imaging the mucosa (but cannot be used for biopsy) and has proved successful in identifying lesions missed by standard radiographic imaging. It is the preferred technique for occult gastrointestinal (GI) bleeding, to identify such lesions as angiodysplasia, and has found early ulcerations of Crohn's disease, as well as the lesions of nonsteroidal antiinflammatory drug (NSAID) ulcerations. These techniques are discussed in Chapter 36 and relevant disease chapters.

HISTOPATHOLOGY

Small bowel biopsy is essential to confirm the diagnosis of many diseases. Histopathologic evaluation is discussed as it applies to each disease in the corresponding chapter.

BIOCHEMICAL EVALUATION

Sophisticated tests have evolved to define selective malabsorption. However, the clinician in practice can still rely on a battery of simple tests to determine whether bowel function is causing malabsorption. These tests are helpful in differentiating among biliary, pancreatic, and small bowel malabsorption.

A test for carbohydrate malabsorption and small bowel function is the *D-xylose absorption* test (Fig. 62.1). A dose of 5 or 25 g can be given orally; then the urine is collected for 5 hours to determine the amount excreted in the urine. Provided that the patient is well hydrated and has no evidence of bacterial overgrowth, this test reliably assesses small bowel mucosal function. It cannot be used in the patient with renal disease, however, and adequate urinary collections must be ensured. However, if less than 20% of the ingested dose is excreted and a false-positive result is unlikely, D-xylose absorption is a reliable test for determining small bowel malabsorption.

Fat malabsorption is determined best by a *72-hour stool fat collection* while the patient is receiving at least 60 to 80 g of fat. Stool must be collected, and this remains a social problem. Nevertheless, many simple containers are available to help make the collection easier for the patient. The stool should be stored overnight under refrigeration. When this test is conducted carefully, it sets the standard for malabsorption. At least 94% of ingested fat should be absorbed; thus the test is reliable if a 6-g fat excretion in feces is used as the lower limit of normal. From 6 to 8 g should arouse suspicion, and excretion greater than 8 to 10 g indicates malabsorption of fat.

Negative D-xylose and positive stool fat findings usually indicate that the cause is not the small bowel but rather is pancreatic or biliary. Quantitative fecal analysis is the standard; qualitative and semiqualitative tests and breath tests have been too inconsistent to diagnose fat malabsorption. Some clinicians screen for serum β-carotene, but this is merely a screening test. Low β-carotene levels do correlate excellently with malabsorption, and very high levels can be seen in certain thyroid diseases.

The *lactose absorption* test is extremely important in determining whether lactose intolerance or malabsorption exists.

The *breath hydrogen* test is now the standard for lactose testing and is easily done in most laboratories. At baseline, high hydrogen may indicate bacterial overgrowth or a very high intake of dietary fiber substances, but increasing breath hydrogen after the ingestion of a

Schilling Test

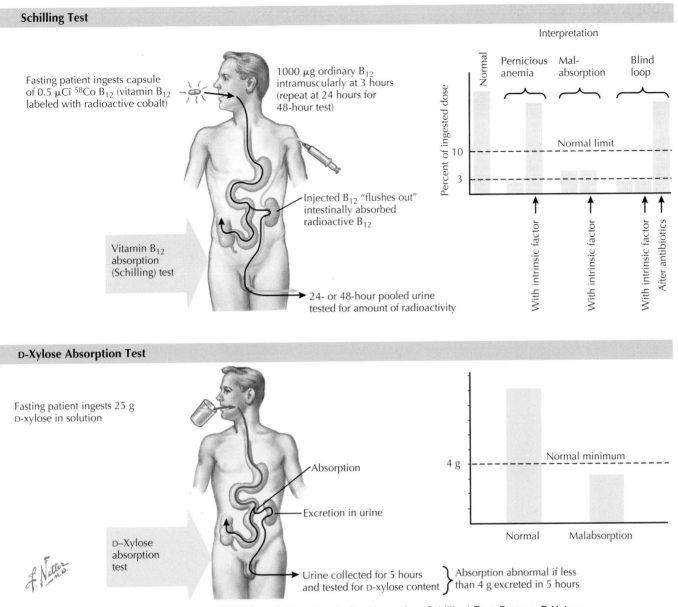

Fasting patient ingests capsule of 0.5 μCi ^{58}Co B$_{12}$ (vitamin B$_{12}$ labeled with radioactive cobalt)

1000 μg ordinary B$_{12}$ intramuscularly at 3 hours (repeat at 24 hours for 48-hour test)

Vitamin B$_{12}$ absorption (Schilling) test

Injected B$_{12}$ "flushes out" intestinally absorbed radioactive B$_{12}$

24- or 48-hour pooled urine tested for amount of radioactivity

Interpretation

Normal

Pernicious anemia

Mal-absorption

Blind loop

Percent of ingested dose

Normal limit

10

3

With intrinsic factor

With intrinsic factor

With intrinsic factor

After antibiotics

D-Xylose Absorption Test

Fasting patient ingests 25 g D-xylose in solution

D–Xylose absorption test

Absorption

Excretion in urine

Urine collected for 5 hours and tested for D-xylose content } Absorption abnormal if less than 4 g excreted in 5 hours

4 g — Normal minimum

Normal   Malabsorption

Fig. 62.1 Evaluation of the Small Bowel: Top, Vitamin B$_{12}$ Absorption (Schilling) Test; Bottom, D-Xylose Absorption Test.

standard dose of lactose is sensitive and specific for lactose intolerance and malabsorption.

Tests for *protein malabsorption* remain difficult to perform. Quantitative *fecal nitrogen* is excellent but is rarely used because it requires stool collection and laboratory analysis. It is actually simple to conduct but is not used by most clinicians. Sophisticated *isotope studies* are used in research laboratories but are rarely used in clinical medicine.

The *Schilling test* is used regularly to determine vitamin B$_{12}$ absorption (see Fig. 62.1). It is based on the observation that small amounts of intestinally absorbed B$_{12}$ are flushed out with the urine when larger quantities administered parenterally are present. Thus B$_{12}$ absorption can be evaluated by measuring radioactivity in a 24-hour urine specimen after the patient has ingested a capsule containing 0.5 μCi of radioactive cobalt with which B$_{12}$ has been labeled. Three hours after administration of the test dose, the patient receives a parenteral injection of 1 mg of ordinary vitamin B$_{12}$. In healthy persons, at least 10%

of the ingested radioactivity appears in the urine within 24 hours. In the absence of *intrinsic factor*, radioactivity excretion is minimal. When intrinsic factor is administered simultaneously with the oral B$_{12}$, radioactivity excretion increases to normal levels. This is the second part of the Schilling test, differentiating pernicious anemia from malabsorption syndrome. A third part is often performed to distinguish bacterial overgrowth, requiring the patient to be treated with antibiotics after the previous parts are done. Excretion improves after the administration of antibiotics, and bacterial overgrowth presumably has caused the malabsorption. Similarly, Schilling results may be abnormal because of pancreatic insufficiency and a lack of freeing R factor. Adding pancreatic enzymes modifies the Schilling test, and results may be normal if the enzymes are added to the oral dose of radioactive vitamin B$_{12}$.

Other breath and permeability tests to evaluate the small intestine are performed at research centers. The *lactulose breath test* is described in Chapter 61.

ADDITIONAL RESOURCES

Benson JA, Culver PJ, Ragland S, et al: The D-xylose test in malabsorption syndromes, *N Engl J Med* 256:335–338, 1957.

Butterworth CE, Perez-Santiago E, Montinez de Jesos J, Santini R: Studies on the oral and parenteral administration of d(+) xylose, *N Engl J Med* 261: 157–162, 1959.

Faigel DO, Cave DR: *Capsule endoscopy*, Philadelphia, 2008, Saunders-Elsevier.

Gore RM, Levine MS: *Textbook of gastrointestinal radiology*, ed 2, Philadelphia, 2000, Saunders.

Hammer HF, Hammer J: Diarrhea caused by carbohydrate malabsorption, *Gastroenterol Clin North Am* 41:611–627, 2012.

Högenauer C, Hammer HF: Maldigestion and malabsorption. In Feldman M, Friedman LS, Brandt LJ, editors: *Gastrointestinal and liver disease*, ed 8, Philadelphia, 2016, Saunders-Elsevier, pp 1788–1823.

Holt PR: Intestinal malabsorption in the elderly, *Dig Dis* 25:144–150, 2007.

Ryan ER, Heaslip IS: Magnetic resonance enteroclysis compared with conventional enteroclysis and computed tomography enteroclysis: A critically appraised topic, *Abdom Imaging* 33:34–37, 2008.

Van de Kamer JH, ten Bokbel Huinik H, Weijens HH: Rapid method for determination of fat in feces, *J Biol Chem* 177:547–552, 1949.

63

Lactose, Fructose, and Sucrose Intolerance

Martin H. Floch

Lactose intolerance occurs when there is a deficiency of lactase in the brush border of the small intestine. When a person with lactase deficiency ingests lactose, the poorly digested lactose is fermented in the small and large intestines, resulting in abdominal bloating, discomfort, or diarrhea (Fig. 63.1).

Lactose, a disaccharide sugar found in milk, is a structural combination of *glucose* and *galactose.* Holzel described defective lactose absorption, which resulted in infant disease in 1959. Later, the clinical picture was also noted in adults.

The incidence of lactose intolerance varies throughout the world. Rates are 85% to 100% in persons of African and Asian descent, 40% to 90% in those of Mediterranean descent, and 5% to 20% in persons of English and Nordic descent. Initially the great ethnic and racial differences were thought to occur because of adaptation, but now genetic differences are believed to be the probable cause.

When lactose is digested, it is normally hydrolyzed in the small intestine. The lactase level appears to fall below 3 U/g tissue for intestinal protein in symptomatic lactase-deficient patients. When the intestinal microflora ferment the lactose, they produce tannic acids, lactic acid, carbon dioxide, and hydrogen. In addition, lactose itself has an osmotic effect in the colon.

CLINICAL PICTURE

The clinical picture varies with the amount of lactose ingested and malabsorbed and the degree of the lactase deficiency. Some patients develop clinical symptoms when they consume very small amounts of lactose, whereas others are less sensitive. Relating this to actual intake of food, some subjects can tolerate a glass of milk, whereas others cannot. The basis for the *lactose tolerance* test is 50 g of lactose, which would be the equivalent of four glasses of milk. Relating this to symptoms, some subjects may never have diarrhea, whereas others will have a violent episode. Those without diarrhea may have mild discomfort, bloating, or cramps after ingesting lactose.

Many persons are lactose intolerant but are unaware of the degree of deficiency. In addition, many are thought to have irritable bowel syndrome (IBS; see Chapter 61). Any patient with postprandial symptoms should undergo lactose tolerance testing.

DIAGNOSIS

Lactose tolerance tests are simple to perform and based on malabsorption resulting in bacterial fermentation in the intestine with hydrogen production. Hydrogen absorption then results in its recovery in expired air. The patient is given a standard dose of 50 g lactose in water. After a baseline hydrogen measurement, expired air is collected every 30 minutes for 3 hours. A 10-ppm increase in hydrogen is classified as a positive finding. There is usually no difficulty in making a positive diagnosis with no false-positive results. At times, patients may be thought to have a high baseline hydrogen level because of a diet very high in fiber or because of bacterial overgrowth in the small intestine. This is taken into consideration during the differential diagnosis.

If the small intestine is damaged because of acute infectious processes, lactose deficiency may be transient and the test result may be positive. However, in an otherwise healthy patient with no acute infectious disease, a positive finding is indicative of lactose intolerance. It is a primary deficiency that occurs in infancy; however, as infants mature into childhood, lactase levels decrease in the small bowel mucosa, and the adult, or acquired, deficiency becomes apparent. If the small bowel is damaged, the enzyme level becomes deficient because of the damage to the small bowel mucosa that occurs in conditions such as celiac disease. Many clinicians believe that the deficiency is increased in inflammatory bowel disease, but this apparently is not true and is merely related to the small patient population. Whenever there is confusion concerning intolerance, a lactose tolerance test should be performed.

Measurement of the breath hydrogen level is the most accurate test. Arriving at the diagnosis by comparing glucose tolerance results with lactose tolerance results (i.e., measuring the blood glucose level after the patient has ingested lactose) was the initial method used. Blood tests are now unnecessary. The breath hydrogen test is readily available and should be used.

TREATMENT AND MANAGEMENT

There are two alternatives for treatment and management. First, removing all lactose-containing foods from the diet may be necessary for extremely sensitive patients. For those who are only mildly sensitive, small amounts of lactose can be ingested without symptoms.

The second alternative is to use lactase substitutes. The enzyme is now readily available worldwide in many over-the-counter products. In addition, in many industrialized countries, milk and milk products are now produced with predigested lactose and are labeled "lactose free."

It is important to review the patient's diet so that the extremely sensitive patient can be fully educated regarding which foods contain lactose. Most are dairy products, and any product containing milk or cheese or made from milk or cheese contains lactose. In modern food production, lactose is frequently used as filler; therefore all labels must be read carefully, and all commercial products must be carefully analyzed to ensure that they do not contain lactose. Also, some pharmaceutical companies add lactose as filler to capsules and pills, which can activate symptoms in patients with extreme sensitivity to lactose. Therefore, for these sensitive patients, the contents of capsules or pills should be checked.

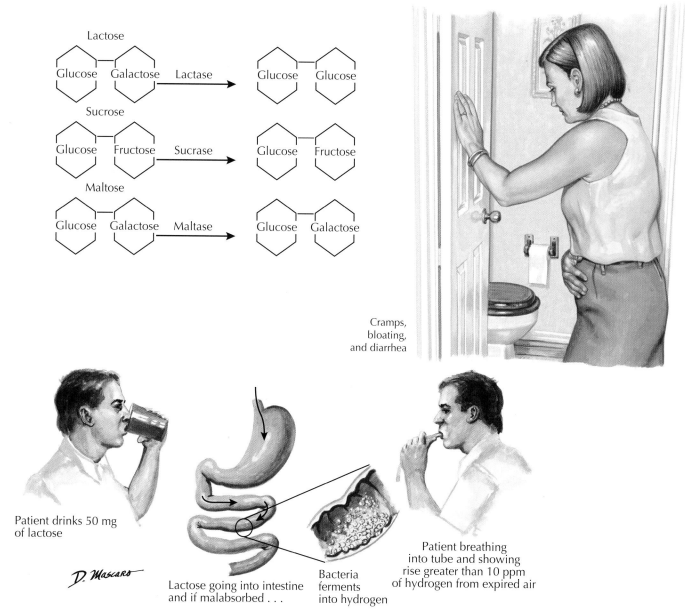

Cramps, bloating, and diarrhea

Patient drinks 50 mg of lactose

Lactose going into intestine and if malabsorbed . . .

Bacteria ferments into hydrogen

Patient breathing into tube and showing rise greater than 10 ppm of hydrogen from expired air

D. Mascaro

Fig. 63.1 Lactose Intolerance.

COURSE AND PROGNOSIS

The removal of lactose from the diet should relieve all symptoms. If not, the diagnosis should be questioned. The availability of lactase substitutes and lactose-free dairy products has been helpful to patients with lactose intolerance. Educating the patient and controlling the diet usually result in relief of symptoms. Prognosis is excellent because this is merely an intolerance that can be corrected.

Patients who remove lactose from their diets should be cautioned about adequate calcium intake, because many have relied on milk and milk products for their calcium supply.

FRUCTOSE INTOLERANCE

Fructose intolerance results from inborn errors of metabolism or is acquired in adulthood. Because of its rarity, fructose intolerance is less understood than lactose intolerance. Some persons definitely have *sucrose*

intolerance, which manifests when disaccharide sucrose is digested to free glucose and fructose. Fructose is present in some fruits and notably present in honey. It is also added to some candies.

Sucrase deficiency in the small bowel, or malabsorption of fructose through the brush border of the enterocytes, results in symptoms. Diarrhea, chronic abdominal pain, and bloating have been reported. Testing for this symptom complex is similar to the lactose breath test except that fructose is used. An increase in hydrogen level indicates malabsorption and usually correlates with the symptoms.

The best treatment is to remove fructose from the diet. In patients with many symptoms, sucrose is also removed. This fructose-intolerant population is more difficult to manage than lactose-intolerant patients.

Physician and patient awareness of possible fructose intolerance has resulted in reports of more cases. As much as 30 g fructose may be present in some sodas and artificially flavored drinks, so it is important to be aware of the possibility of fructose malabsorption and intolerance. A careful study in which patients were advised to reduce sucrose and fructose intake resulted in a significant reduction in symptoms of irritable bowel syndrome. Reducing intake is difficult but can be rewarding.

ADDITIONAL RESOURCES

Gibson PR, Newnham E, Barrett JS, et al: Review article: fructose malabsorption and the bigger picture, *Aliment Pharmacol Ther* 25:349–363, 2007.

Högenauer C, Hammer HF: Maldigestion and malabsorption. In Feldman M, Friedman LS, Brandt LJ, editors: *Gastrointestinal and liver disease*, ed 8, Philadelphia, 2016, Saunders-Elsevier, pp 1788–1823.

Mann NS, Cheung EC: Fructose-induced breath hydrogen in patient with fruit intolerance, *J Clin Gatroenterol* 42:157–159, 2008.

Pasricha PJ: Approach to the patient with abdominal pain. In Podolsky DK, Camilleri M, Fitz JG, et al, editors: *Yamada's textbook of gastroenterology*, ed 6, Hoboken, New Jersey, 2016, John Wiley and Sons Ltd, pp 695–722.

Ryan ER, Heaslip IS: Magnetic resonance enteroclysis compared with conventional enteroclysis and computed tomography enteroclysis: a critically appraised topic, *Abdom Imaging* 33:34–37, 2008.

Sahi T: Genetics and epidemiology of adult-type hypolactasia, *Scand J Gastroenterol* 29(Suppl):7–20, 1994.

Shepherd SJ, Gibson PR: Fructose malabsorption and symptoms of irritable bowel syndrome: guidelines for effective dietary management, *J Am Diet Assoc* 106:1631–1639, 2006.

64

Diarrhea

Martin H. Floch

Since the time of Hippocrates, the term *diarrhea* has been used to designate abnormally frequent passage of loose stools. However, it is a subjective symptom. Patients describe any increased frequency or fluidity to mean diarrhea. It is generally accepted that more than three bowel movements per day represent diarrhea, or a consistency of watery, large-volume liquid, or both. The clinician must obtain an accurate history and ensure that the patient is not reporting incontinence or staining.

The volume of stool in diarrhea is important but is usually difficult to determine. A constipated stool amounts to less than 100 mL/day. In Western societies, with diets of moderate fiber, stool volumes amount to approximately 200 mL daily. When stools are measured in vegetarians or those with a high intake of fiber, the volume may be 400 mL daily. Watery, voluminous stools exceed 500 mL and may reach 1 to 2 L/day in diarrhea.

CLINICAL PICTURE

The presentations of acute and chronic diarrhea are different. The patient with *acute diarrhea* is frequently ill and may have a fever, dehydration, severe abdominal cramps, or uncontrollable passage of watery stools. If the cause is severe gastroenteritis, diarrhea is frequently associated with vomiting.

The patient with *chronic diarrhea* frequently has abdominal cramps or bloating and discomfort associated with an increased number of bowel movements. It is important to ascertain whether movements are nocturnal, because this usually heralds organic disease rather than irritable bowel syndrome (IBS). If the diarrhea has lasted more than 10 to 30 days, it is considered chronic. Chronic diarrhea frequently entails the loss of important nutrients and the beginning of malabsorption syndromes.

In either acute or chronic diarrhea, the patient may appear toxic or dehydrated. When dehydration is a major component, the patient has lost a great amount of water and electrolytes and weight.

DIAGNOSIS

Worldwide, the major cause of diarrhea is infection, which may be acute or chronic. Acute viral or bacterial infections can have a violent onset with severe, watery diarrhea; cholera is a classic form. The chronic diarrheas are caused by (1) lactose and food intolerance, (2) endocrinopathy such as hyperthyroidism, (3) carcinoid-secreting tumors, and (4) IBS. Fig. 64.1 categorizes causes of diarrhea.

With acute infections, gastroenteritis usually is limited, and differential diagnosis is not pursued. However, in epidemics of the common Norwalk virus, rotavirus, or bacterial food contamination or in extensive cholera epidemics, the agent is identified for public health purposes (see Section VI).

There is definite overlap among the inflammatory bowel diseases, such as chronic ulcerative colitis, Crohn disease, and the other colitides (see Section V). It is important to note for the differential diagnosis that these diseases frequently manifest with abdominal cramps; the course may be prolonged; blood may or may not be present in the stool; and testing for an infectious agent in the stool is negative. Although the onset of inflammatory bowel disease may be acute, it usually becomes chronic and then falls into the differential diagnosis of the other metabolic causes listed in Fig. 64.1. IBS associated with diarrhea rather than constipation is common, and with a negative work-up, the final diagnosis becomes apparent.

Whenever the cause of diarrhea is uncertain, it is helpful to determine whether the patient has so-called osmotic or secretory diarrhea. Classic *osmotic* presentations are lactose intolerance and increased intake of magnesium salts or other agents that are poorly absorbed. Classic *secretory* diarrhea is demonstrated by enterotoxins, such as cholera and neuroendocrine tumors, and is seen with surgical and severely damaged bowel. To make this differential, fecal electrolytes and osmolality are determined. The osmolality of colonic fecal water should be approximately that of body fluids; therefore the composite should be no more than 290 mOsm/kg. Osmotic and secretory diarrhea can be differentiated by the "osmotic gap." Secretory diarrhea stool fluid electrolytes reach a level of body fluid electrolytes, whereas the osmolality in the osmotic diarrheas is low and usually caused by ingestion of nonelectrolyte substances. Electrolyte studies of stool are rarely used now because of the difficulty in collection and the confusing analysis attributed to ingested salts, making them impractical. As discussed for malabsorption disorders, chronic diarrhea may be large and muddy and may contain fat, resulting in greasy and foul-smelling stool, which helps in the differential diagnosis (see Chapters 56 and 59).

TREATMENT AND MANAGEMENT

Treatment of acute diarrhea is largely symptomatic and supportive. With extreme diarrhea, or in a patient who has an ileostomy, dehydration may be rapid and may necessitate intravenous fluid and electrolyte replacement. Most patients with gastroenteritis do not require such vigorous therapy. However, fluid replacement is frequently necessary, and in patients with cholera, it is mandatory. Commonly used in Western and Eastern societies, *oral rehydration solutions* are usually based on a high-sodium/potassium electrolyte content associated with simple glucose that enhances absorption in the small intestine. However, other carbohydrates have recently been added to the solutions to enhance short-chain fatty acid absorption from the colon. These solutions aid in the positive absorption of water and electrolytes to treat the excretion caused by diarrheal toxins. Home oral rehydration formulas usually contain 90 to 120 mEq sodium, 25 to 35 mEq potassium, and 25 to 50 g carbohydrate per liter.

Because infectious causes are common, physicians and paramedics often empirically use antibiotic therapy. Using antibiotics without a confirmed infectious cause is not recommended for the short course.

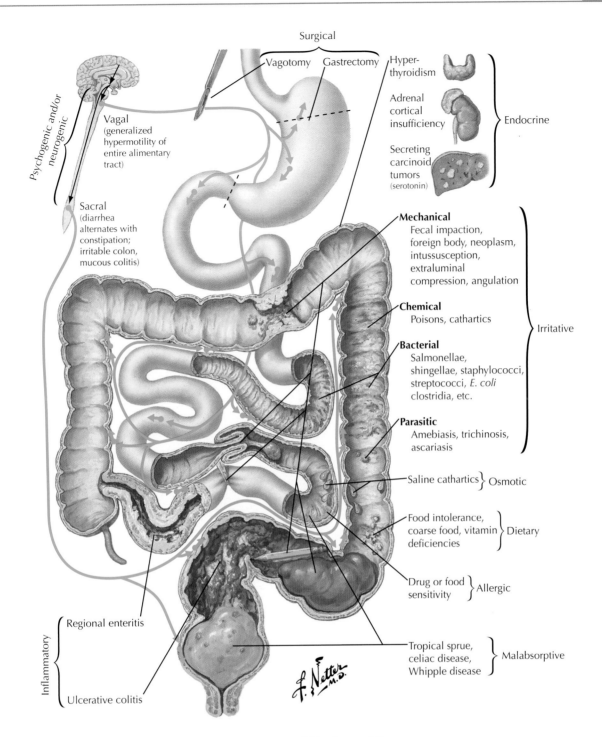

Fig. 64.1 Categories of Diarrhea and Causes.

When the course is prolonged over days into a week, fluoroquinolone is often given and may be effective. As discussed in Section VI, whether to treat salmonellosis is always controversial.

Nonspecific antidiarrheal agents can reduce symptoms. The initial concern about reducing the clearance of pathogens by using such agents has been unsubstantiated. The agents most frequently available are diphenoxylate, 2.5 to 5 mg four times a day (qid); loperamide, 2 to 4 mg qid; codeine, 15 to 60 mg qid; and tincture of opium, 2 to 20 drops qid. Recently, probiotics have been shown to be effective in shortening the course of acute diarrhea. *Lactobacillus* GG and other organisms are recommended.

Treatment of chronic diarrhea and the use of α-adrenergic agonists (e.g., clonidine), octreotide (somatostatin analog), bile salt–binding resins (e.g., cholestyramine), and psyllium seed (to solidify stool) are discussed under particular disease chapters in this section, as well as Sections V and VI.

COURSE AND PROGNOSIS

Although most episodes resolve in a few days, acute infectious diarrhea may result in death in some children and immunocompromised or frail patients. Therefore, although rare, severe dehydration and vascular instability must be treated aggressively. The prognosis for chronic diarrhea is discussed under each particular disease.

ADDITIONAL RESOURCES

Cohen MB: Bacterial, viral, and toxic causes of diarrhea, gastroenteritis, and anorectal infections. In Podolsky DK, Camilleri M, Fitz JG, et al, editors: *Yamada's textbook of gastroenterology*, ed 6, Hoboken, New Jersey, 2016, John Wiley and Sons Ltd, pp 1196–1248.

Dupont HL: Diagnosis and management of Clostridium difficile infection, *Clin Gastroenterol Hepatol* 11:1216–1223, 2013.

Floch MH, Walker WA, Guandalini S, et al: Recommendations for probiotic use—2008, *J Clin Gastroenterol* 42(3 Suppl):S104–S108, 2008.

Hammer HF, Hammer J: Diarrhea caused by carbohydrate malabsorption, *Gastroenterol Clin North Am* 41:611–627, 2012.

Schiller LR, Sellin DH: Diarrhea. In Feldman M, Friedman LS, Brandt LJ, editors: *Gastroenterology and liver disease*, ed 10, Philadelphia, 2016, Saunders-Elsevier, pp 221–241.

Szajewska H, Skorka A, Ruszczynski M, Gieruszczak-Bialek D: Meta-analysis: *Lactobacilllus* GG for treating acute diarrhea in children, *Aliment Pharmacol Ther* 25:871–881, 2007.

Tesjeux HL, Briend A, Butzner JD: Oral rehydration solution in the year 2000: pathophysiology, efficacy, and effectiveness, *Baillieres Clin Gastroenterol* 11:509–515, 1997.

65

Celiac Disease and Malabsorption

Martin H. Floch

Any disease that affects nutrient digestion or small bowel function or that compromises bowel circulation or motility may result in a malabsorption syndrome, which includes systemic vascular, infectious, and neoplastic diseases (Fig. 65.1). This chapter and others in this section discuss common intestinal diseases that cause malabsorption disorders.

Gluten enteropathy, or *celiac disease,* is a malabsorption syndrome that results from gluten-sensitive damage to the intestinal microvilli and villi, producing an abnormal villous architecture and resulting in malabsorption. This disease process exemplifies the classic signs and symptoms of malabsorption disorders. When a person with gluten enteropathy ingests gluten, the epithelium becomes damaged, the cellular maturation of epithelial cells of the villus becomes disturbed, the small bowel mucosa becomes inflamed, and mild villous atrophy to total loss of villi results in atrophic-looking mucosa.

Understanding this classic disease entity leads to an understanding of small bowel function and all its possible diseases. Almost all manifestations of abnormal digestion and absorption and all systemic manifestations, from skin disorders to malignancy, are associated with celiac disease.

Samuel Gee first described celiac disease in 1888 as "celiac affliction," later publicized by Herter in 1908. Finally, in 1950, Dicke and colleagues found that removing wheat from the diet caused the signs and symptoms to disappear. "Celiac disease" should be used only when gluten is demonstrated to be the cause. Some persons have "refractory sprue," in which gluten removal does not reverse the disease. Other names associated with this disorder include "idiopathic steatorrhea" and "celiac sprue."

Celiac disease occurs worldwide, affecting an estimated 1% of the world's population. Ireland has the highest incidence, but recently, a high incidence has been reported in Italy. Gluten enteropathy appears primarily in Europe, North and South America, East Asia, and Australia.

When glutens from wheat, rye, and barley are presented to the intestinal mucosa, they react to form *gliadins,* which can cause the damage. Genetic studies show that a person must have alleles that encode for HLA-DQ2 or HLA-DQ8 proteins. However, many persons have DQ2 or DQ8 human lymphocyte antigen (HLA) gene expression and do not have celiac disease. Patients with celiac disease appear to be able to tolerate oats, which contain some of the biochemical products present in the other grains. Along with oats, patients tolerate rice, corn, sorghum, and millet without intestinal villous damage.

CLINICAL PICTURE

Fig. 65.2 demonstrates all possible presentations and signs/symptoms associated with celiac disease and severe malabsorption. The cardinal presentation of weight loss associated with steatorrhea is seen only occasionally. The clinician should check for celiac disease in the current environment of plentiful food when a patient experiences anemia, osteoporosis, unexplained diarrhea, or any vitamin deficiency, even if weight loss is not apparent. With the availability of numerous serologic tests, latent celiac disease has become more apparent in patients with such conditions as occult anemia, osteoporosis, and some associated malignancies.

DIAGNOSIS

Serum testing has improved the ability to make an early diagnosis of celiac disease and malabsorption syndrome. Immunoglobulin A (IgA) endomysial antibodies and IgA tissue transglutaminase antibodies have reached almost 98% sensitivity and specificity. IgA and IgG antigliadin antibodies are less sensitive and less specific but more helpful.

The standard for diagnosing celiac disease is to demonstrate the histologic lesions on small bowel biopsy. Although initial understanding of this disease resulted from biopsy specimens obtained by suction through tubes or capsules, current biopsy specimens are obtained by punch biopsy at endoscopy. To make the diagnosis, the clinician must be certain that the specimens are obtained from the second or third part of the duodenum, to avoid distortion by glands of the proximal duodenum. Furthermore, adequately sized specimens must be obtained. However, a lesion is not specific for the diagnosis, and significant inflammation or atrophy of villi may be seen in many other disorders, such as tropical sprue and infectious enteropathies. Marked inflammation may also be noted in lymphoproliferative disorders.

Therefore the diagnosis of celiac disease can be elusive, although capsule endoscopy has become an additional tool to help in difficult cases.

Other tests of small bowel absorption, such as the 72-hour stool collection for fecal fat and the D-xylose absorption test (see Chapter 56), are often helpful when there is some confusion about serologic findings. Although imaging was important in the early stages of understanding celiac disease, now it is less helpful; however, it remains useful for ruling out lesions that might be secondary to gluten enteropathy (e.g., malignancy) or for diagnosing other causative disorders (e.g., collagen disease). A diagnosis of gluten enteropathy must be established by serology and histology and demonstration of malabsorption. Finally, many clinicians insist that reversing the primary or secondary findings must be demonstrated on the gluten-free diet.

Dermatitis herpetiformis is a skin disease that produces papulovesicular lesions symmetrically on the extensor surfaces of the extremities, trunk, buttocks, neck, and scalp. It usually manifests in adulthood and is associated with celiac disease in 80% of patients. However, less than 10% of patients with celiac disease have this skin disorder.

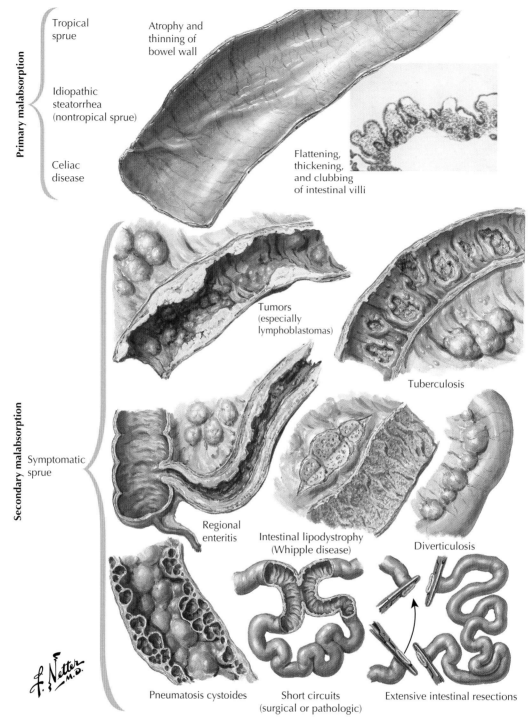

Fig. 65.1 Malabsorption and Celiac Disease: Primary and Secondary Malabsorption.

Other diseases associated with celiac disease include microscopic colitis, although these associations are sporadic and reported without evidence of celiac disease. The most disturbing association is the increased incidence of lymphoma of the bowel and other malignancies. Diligence is required when following up each patient.

Clinical interest has identified two areas which tend to overlap with celiac disease. First is that of tropical malabsorption seen in various countries in Asia and Africa. These patients are identified to have malabsorption.

TREATMENT AND MANAGEMENT

The treatment for celiac disease is a gluten-free diet. There is no other treatment. Removing all gluten from the diet is essential. All diet manuals carry clear recommendations. A celiac society has formed and helps patients to obtain appropriate grains and cereals for cooking and to follow the diet. It has been shown repeatedly that once wheat, barley, or rye is instilled in the small bowel, a lesion develops within hours. Therefore patients may have attacks when they are "fooled" by

Physical findings

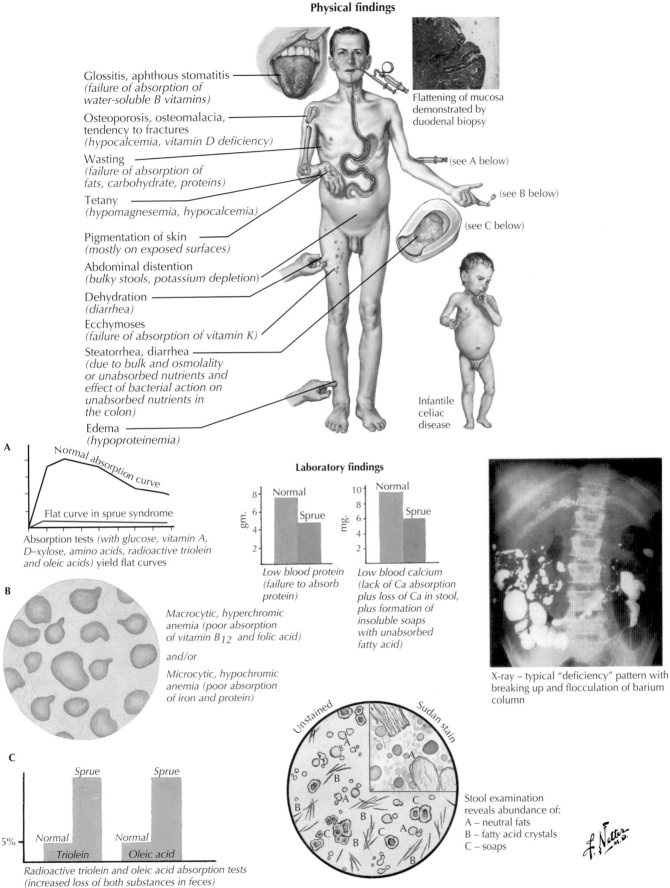

Glossitis, aphthous stomatitis
*(failure of absorption of
water-soluble B vitamins)*

Osteoporosis, osteomalacia,
tendency to fractures
(hypocalcemia, vitamin D deficiency)

Wasting
*(failure of absorption of
fats, carbohydrate, proteins)*

Tetany
(hypomagnesemia, hypocalcemia)

Pigmentation of skin
(mostly on exposed surfaces)

Abdominal distention
(bulky stools, potassium depletion)

Dehydration
(diarrhea)

Ecchymoses
(failure of absorption of vitamin K)

Steatorrhea, diarrhea
*(due to bulk and osmolality
or unabsorbed nutrients and
effect of bacterial action on
unabsorbed nutrients in
the colon)*

Edema
(hypoproteinemia)

Flattening of mucosa
demonstrated by
duodenal biopsy

(see A below)

(see B below)

(see C below)

Infantile
celiac
disease

A

Normal absorption curve

Flat curve in sprue syndrome

Absorption tests *(with glucose, vitamin A,
D–xylose, amino acids, radioactive triolein
and oleic acids)* yield flat curves

Laboratory findings

Normal · Sprue (gm.)

*Low blood protein
(failure to absorb
protein)*

Normal · Sprue (mg.)

*Low blood calcium
(lack of Ca absorption
plus loss of Ca in stool,
plus formation of
insoluble soaps
with unabsorbed
fatty acid)*

B

*Macrocytic, hyperchromic
anemia (poor absorption
of vitamin B$_{12}$ and folic acid)*

and/or

*Microcytic, hypochromic
anemia (poor absorption
of iron and protein)*

X-ray – typical "deficiency" pattern with
breaking up and flocculation of barium
column

C

Sprue · Sprue

Normal · Normal

Triolein · Oleic acid

5%

*Radioactive triolein and oleic acid absorption tests
(increased loss of both substances in feces)*

Unstained · Sudan stain

Stool examination
reveals abundance of:
A – neutral fats
B – fatty acid crystals
C – soaps

F. Netter M.D.

Fig. 65.2 Signs and Symptoms of Malabsorption.

foods that contain any of the incriminating grains. Dietitians are well versed on the disorder and have the adequate educational tools to treat patients.

For patients whose disease is refractory, some clinicians have added glucocorticoids to the therapy.

When a patient is seriously depleted, supplemental therapy is necessary, including vitamin replacement and specific iron or B_{12} (or folic acid) replacement for anemia. Because these deficiencies have been reported in many patients, replacement may be necessary for all nutrients.

COURSE AND PROGNOSIS

Patients who follow a gluten-free diet can have a normal life expectancy. However, the complications of malignancy or the inability to comply with the diet may result in serious morbidity and mortality. Approximately 3% of patients with gluten enteropathy acquire some malignancy, which is an extremely high number. Potential malignancy should be sufficient incentive for patients to comply with a gluten-free diet, but poor compliance is prevalent. Many patients do not comply because they do not have symptoms. However, the high incidence of related malignancy and occult disease indicates that the gluten-free diet is essential to decrease morbidity and mortality in all patients with celiac disease. It is also important to remember that many patients are asymptomatic, and symptoms may not develop until a complication presents.

ADDITIONAL RESOURCES

Benson JA, Culver PJ, Ragland S, et al: The D-xylose test in malabsorption syndromes, *N Engl J Med* 256:335–338, 1957.

Carroccio A, Mansueto P, Iacono G, et al: Non-celiac wheat sensitivity diagnosed by double-blind placebo-controlled challenge: exploring a new clinical entity, *Am J Gastroenterol* 107:1898–1906, 2012.

Collin P, Reunala T, Pukkla E, et al: Celiac disease–associated disorders and survival, *Gut* 35:1215–1220, 1994.

DuBois RN, Lazenby AJ, Yardley JH, et al: Lymphocytic enterocolitis in patients with "refractory sprue," *JAMA* 262:935–938, 1989.

Ghoshal UC, Mehrotra M, Kumar S, et al: Spectrum of malabsorption syndrome among adults & factors differentiating celiac disease and tropical malabsorption, *Indian J Med Res* 36:451–459, 2012.

Green PH, Cellier C: Celiac disease, *N Engl J Med* 357:1731–1743, 2007.

Holmes GK, Stokes PL, Sorahan TM, et al: Celiac disease, gluten-free diet, and malignancy, *Gut* 17:612–618, 1976.

Kelly CP: Celiac diseases. In Feldman M, Friedman LS, Brandt LJ, editors: *Gastrointestinal and liver disease*, ed 10, Philadelphia, 2016, Saunders-Elsevier, pp 1849–1872.

London KE, Scott H, Hansen T, et al: Gliadin-specific HLA-DQ restricted T-cells isolated from the small intestinal mucosa of celiac disease patients, *J Exp Med* 178:187–192, 1993.

Ramakrishna BS: Tropical diarrhea and malabsorption. In Feldman M, Friedman LS, Brandt LJ, editors: *Gastrointestinal and liver disease*, ed 10, Philadelphia, 2016, Saunders-Elsevier, pp 1873–1885.

66

Whipple Disease

Martin H. Floch

Whipple disease is a systemic, infectious disease that primarily affects the small intestine and its lymphatic drainage, although it also has many extraintestinal manifestations, comparable to classic celiac disease (Fig. 66.1). George Whipple first described the clinical syndrome in 1907, but it was not until the bacterium that causes the disease, *Tropheryma whippeli*, was isolated and identified in 1991 and 1992 that full understanding of the entity and its response to therapy became clear. Ribosomal RNA sequences reveal that *T. whippeli* is a novel actinomycete not closely related to other characteristic organisms. The exact sequence of infectivity is not clearly understood, but *T. whippeli* is probably transmitted by the oral route.

CLINICAL PICTURE

Only approximately 700 cases of Whipple disease have been described in the literature, many from the state of Connecticut. However, the syndrome is so classic and the treatment so readily available that it must enter into any differential diagnosis when a male patient has malabsorption syndrome. For unknown reasons, Whipple disease occurs more often in men.

A frequent symptom is the extraintestinal manifestation of *arthritis*. Patients may seek treatment for swollen joints that may be associated with any part of a malabsorption syndrome, usually steatorrhea, but they may also have anemia or weight loss. Early in the disease process, the patient may have arthritis with abdominal bloating or pain. The patient may not be able to describe the steatorrhea clearly but will report diarrhea. Approximately 95% of patients with Whipple disease lose weight, 78% have diarrhea, 65% have arthralgias, and 60% have abdominal pain. Often, the arthralgias predate the other clinical manifestations by several years. Because the organism causes lipodystrophy and lymph nodes are involved, lymph node enlargement is common.

On physical examination, the patient may have abdominal tenderness, hyperpigmentation of the skin, and fever. When the disease is progressive, the patient may have full-blown malnutrition, often because the diagnosis was obscure and attributed to the aging process associated with arthritis. Many reports cite central nervous system involvement with neurologic manifestations, as well as signs of aging, including dementia, ophthalmoplegia, and myoclonus. There have been case reports of cardiac involvement, and fibrinous pericarditis and endocarditis are frequently seen postmortem.

Arthralgias are the primary extraintestinal manifestation and frequently precede full-blown Whipple disease by many years. Arthralgias tend to be migratory and show little evidence of inflammation. However, aspiration of the joints may reveal the organism and lipid-filled macrophages.

DIAGNOSIS

It is important to consider a diagnosis of Whipple disease because it can affect men with arthralgias, which may precede the signs and symptoms of malabsorption. All diseases that may cause malabsorption enter the differential diagnosis once there is evidence of steatorrhea and weight loss. Similarly, all differential diagnoses for arthralgias are present after the intestinal disease develops.

Once the clinician suspects Whipple disease, the diagnosis is confirmed through small bowel biopsy. All test findings that are positive in other malabsorption disorders may be positive in Whipple disease, and the biopsy specimen becomes pathognomonic. Lipid-filled macrophages that stain positively with periodic acid–Schiff (PAS) stain are dramatic and diagnostic. The same lipid deposition occurs in lymph nodes. The bacterium can be demonstrated on electron microscopy. Because it can be fatal if not treated, it is essential that the physician consider Whipple disease.

TREATMENT AND MANAGEMENT

After the discovery that Whipple disease was caused by a bacterium, single-antibiotic therapy proved successful in most patients, but there was a high degree of relapse. *T. whippeli* apparently behaves similarly to mycobacteria and chronic infections. Therefore the current recommendation (and most successful treatment) is a combination of initial treatment and long-term therapy. The current recommendation is penicillin G plus streptomycin, 6 to 24 million U intravenously daily, plus 1 g intramuscularly daily for 10 to 14 days. An alternative for patients sensitive to penicillin is ceftriaxone, 2 g intravenously daily for a similar period. The recommendation for long-term therapy to prevent relapse is maintenance with trimethoprim-sulfamethoxazole, 160 to 800 mg orally two or three times daily for at least 1 year. Tetracycline was initially the drug of choice, but patients often relapsed, and it is no longer a first-line agent. Because of antibiotic allergies and sensitivities, many other regimens are used and described in the literature. The first and second references should be checked carefully if treatment is to be undertaken.

COURSE AND PROGNOSIS

When first described and before antibiotic treatment, Whipple disease was a progressive and unrelenting fatal disease. Antibiotics now make this a curable, treatable disease. Therapy is rewarding, although some neurologic signs, including dementia, may not reverse. The PAS-positive macrophages disappear slowly and may persist up to 1 year (or in

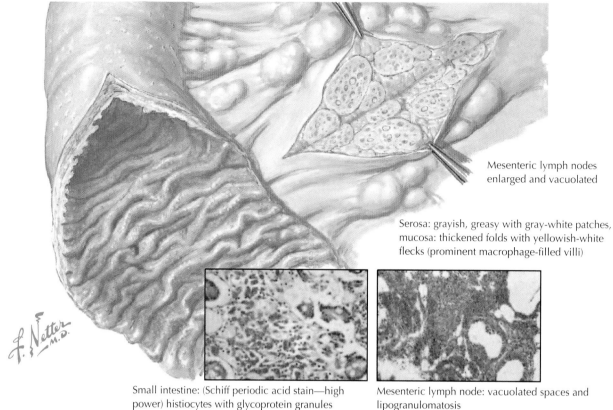

Mesenteric lymph nodes enlarged and vacuolated

Serosa: grayish, greasy with gray-white patches, mucosa: thickened folds with yellowish-white flecks (prominent macrophage-filled villi)

Small intestine: (Schiff periodic acid stain—high power) histiocytes with glycoprotein granules

Mesenteric lymph node: vacuolated spaces and lipogranulomatosis

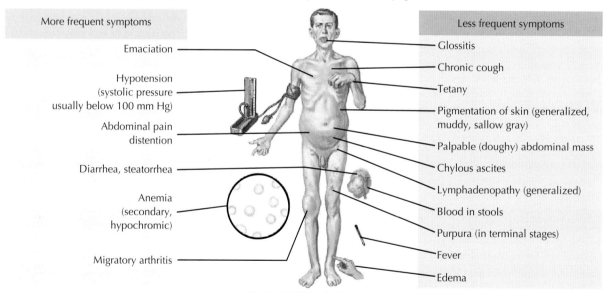

More frequent symptoms

- Emaciation
- Hypotension (systolic pressure usually below 100 mm Hg)
- Abdominal pain distention
- Diarrhea, steatorrhea
- Anemia (secondary, hypochromic)
- Migratory arthritis

Less frequent symptoms

- Glossitis
- Chronic cough
- Tetany
- Pigmentation of skin (generalized, muddy, sallow gray)
- Palpable (doughy) abdominal mass
- Chylous ascites
- Lymphadenopathy (generalized)
- Blood in stools
- Purpura (in terminal stages)
- Fever
- Edema

Fig. 66.1 Whipple Disease.

rare cases, 8 years) before being completely resolved. However, most extraintestinal manifestations and positive signs disappear within 1 year. It is important to remember that long-term antibiotic therapy is usually needed.

ADDITIONAL RESOURCES

Bourke B, Hussey S: Chronic infections of the small intestine. In Podolsky DK, Camilleri M, Fitz JG, et al, editors: *Yamada's textbook of gastroenterology*, ed 6, Hoboken, New Jersey, 2016, John Wiley and Sons Ltd, pp 1249–1263.

Fenollar F, Puechal X, Raoult D: Whipple's disease, *N Engl J Med* 356:55, 2007.

Lagier JC, Lepidi H, Raoult D, et al: Systemic *Tropheryma whipplei:* clinical presentation of 142 patients with infections diagnosed or confirmed in a reference center, *Medicine (Baltimore)* 89:337, 2010.

Maiwald M, von Herbay A, Relman DA: Whipple's disease. In Feldman M, Friedman LS, Brandt LJ, editors: *Gastrointestinal and liver disease*, ed 10, Philadelphia, 2016, Saunders-Elsevier, pp 1886–1895.

67

Small Intestinal Bacterial Overgrowth

Martin H. Floch

The small intestinal bacterial overgrowth (SIBO) syndrome may be caused by a disturbance in gastrointestinal (GI) motility, by an alteration in the anatomy of the intestine, or less likely, by a loss of gastric acid secretion. The disturbance usually causes malnutrition and weight loss from malabsorption. In the healthy small bowel, indigenous bacterial flora growth in the jejunum ranges from 10^2 to 10^5 colony-forming units per milliliter (CFU/mL). Bacteria consist primarily of gram-positive and gram-negative aerobic organisms. Farther down in the small bowel, toward the midileum and into the terminal ileum, the bacterial flora proliferates, and anaerobic organisms increase dramatically, becoming as numerous as the aerobe organisms, and the total counts in the distal ileum can reach 10^8 or 10^9 CFU/mL. Intestinal flora and the increase in anaerobes are discussed in Section VI.

Aerobic and anaerobic organisms proliferate when stasis occurs in the small bowel (Fig. 67.1). *Stasis* results from prolonged strictures or delayed emptying of the small bowel, and organisms are also seen in jejunal diverticula. When the aerobic and anaerobic flora proliferate, they can interfere with absorption, compete for nutrients, and produce substances that cause symptoms. The usual control of the flora is based on gastric acid production and normal motility. Proliferating bacteria can compete for vitamin B_{12}. On the other hand, they can synthesize and produce folic acid. Fat malabsorption caused by interference with enterohepatic bile acid circulation, carbohydrate use by bacteria, and protein malabsorption caused by decreased absorption and use by bacteria all contribute to the malabsorption. Because of bacterial toxic substances, diarrhea might increase.

CLINICAL PICTURE

Clinical features vary with the cause of the SIBO syndrome. For example, if stasis is caused by a stricture with dilatation of the bowel in a patient with Crohn disease, pain and a change in bowel habits would precede the SIBO picture. If the patient has scleroderma, the spectrum of Raynaud phenomenon, esophageal disturbances, and constipation would accompany SIBO. If the patient has small bowel diverticula, the presentation might be malabsorption. In rare cases, the presentation might simply be anemia or malnutrition with no other symptoms before presentation.

The usual causes of SIBO are disturbed anatomy (e.g., blind loops, diverticulosis, strictures), dysmotility (e.g., diabetic enteropathy, scleroderma, pseudointestinal obstruction), and various other conditions in which the small bowel becomes diseased and stasis occurs.

DIAGNOSIS

Diagnosis depends on demonstrating a cause for the bacterial overgrowth and the resulting malnutrition and malabsorption. Radiographic techniques are essential for demonstrating dilated loops of small bowel, diverticula, and strictures. In some patients, bacterial overgrowth can be

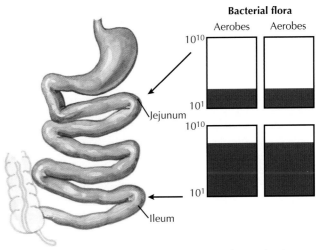

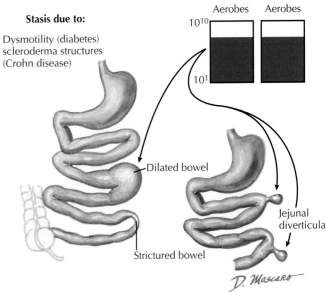

Fig. 67.1 Small Intestinal Bacterial Overgrowth.

documented. Most institutions do not perform colony counts on small bowel aspirates; when available, it is helpful. Currently, however, malabsorption is often documented with breath tests, including the carbon 14 (^{14}C)–bile acid breath test, ^{14}C-xylose breath test, fasting hydrogen breath test, lactulose-hydrogen breath test, and glucose-hydrogen breath test. Use of these tests varies greatly among institutions.

All these tests are relatively simple to perform, but the ^{14}C-xylose breath test appears to be the most sensitive and the most specific. After a 1-g oral dose of ^{14}C-xylose, elevated levels of $^{14}CO_2$ are detected in the breath within 1 hour in more than 85% of patients with SIBO syndrome. Findings on the lactulose-hydrogen breath test and baseline H_2 levels can both be positive, but these measurements appear to be less sensitive than the xylose test. However, they are preferred for pregnant women and children because they do not require significant use of isotopes. In addition, Schilling test findings are classically positive in bacterial overgrowth.

Many clinicians avoid detailed workups. Once they have demonstrated an anatomic reason for bacterial overgrowth, they institute a trial of antibiotic therapy to determine whether the syndrome can be corrected. This is a valid approach when isotope and absorption studies are difficult to conduct.

TREATMENT AND MANAGEMENT

All attempts should be made to correct the cause of the stasis or obstruction. However, this is often difficult surgery that is not feasible or warranted in patients with scleroderma, diabetes, or small bowel dysmotility. Therefore it becomes necessary to use antibiotic therapy for extended periods of time. Most clinicians believe in alternating antibiotic treatment with periods of no treatment. This cyclic therapy has been used in all types of combinations, such as 1 week off and 3 weeks on per month or 1 month on and 1 month off. This type of cyclic therapy has been individualized.

Antibiotics used to treat SIBO include amoxicillin–clavulanic acid, twice daily (bid); cephalexin, 250 mg four times daily (qid), plus metronidazole, 250 mg three times daily; trimethoprim-sulfamethoxazole, bid; or chloramphenicol, 250 mg qid. In addition, ciprofloxacin, norfloxacin, and rifaximin have recently been used successfully in a variety of protocols. Somatostatin and prokinetic agents have also been used to help in dysmotility syndromes. Therapy must be individualized for each patient depending on the disease and disorder causing the bacterial overgrowth.

It is important that the antibiotic selected is well tolerated and can be used cyclically for the individual patient, and that symptoms and malabsorption are relieved by the particular regimen. Some patients are successfully treated for short periods with long intervals between treatment. Each patient should be monitored closely.

Nutritional deficiencies should be corrected. Correcting the bacterial overgrowth will address future deficiencies if therapy is successful. However, any vitamin or mineral deficiencies should be corrected by increased supplements. When bacterial growth decreases, absorption of macronutrients and vitamins corrects any weight loss, as monitored with absorption testing. Outcome evaluation (e.g., use of serum prealbumin) and repeat evaluation for anemia and breath analysis should be performed.

COURSE AND PROGNOSIS

The prognosis for SIBO depends on the disease process causing the overgrowth. If caused by scleroderma, the prognosis is that of scleroderma's natural history. If the cause is Crohn disease or diabetes, all their comorbidities are in effect. Once a regimen is found for the overgrowth, SIBO can be managed, and the morbidity of the primary disease can be decreased with the hope of decreasing mortality risk.

ADDITIONAL RESOURCES

O'Mahoney S, Shanahan F: Enteric bacterial flora and bacterial overgrowth. In Feldman M, Friedman LS, Brandt LJ, editors: *Gastrointestinal and liver disease*, ed 8, Philadelphia, 2006, Saunders-Elsevier, pp 2243–2256.

Quigley EMM: Bacterial overgrowth. In Podolsky DK, Camilleri M, Fitz JG, et al, editors: *Yamada's textbook of gastroenterology*, ed 6, Hoboken, New Jersey, 2016, John Wiley and Sons Ltd, pp 1294–1304.

Quigley E, Quera R: Small intestinal bacterial overgrowth: roles of antibiotics, prebiotics, and probiotics, *Gastroenterology* 130:S78–S90, 2006.

Schiller LR: Evaluation of small bowel overgrowth, *Curr Gastroenterol Rep* 9:373–377, 2007.

68

Short Bowel Syndrome

Martin H. Floch

Short bowel syndrome (SBS) usually occurs when less than 200 cm of small intestine remains after intestinal surgery. Normally the bowel measures 450 to 500 cm (18–20 ft). When an insult occurs to the bowel resulting in surgical removal of major parts, the patient is left with SBS (Fig. 68.1). Although resection of less than 75% of the bowel, leaving larger amounts of the small bowel, may not result in the full SBS, it can still precipitate some aspects of the syndrome. For example, vitamin B_{12} deficiency occurs when there is total ileal resection but an intact jejunum.

Surgery-related causes of SBS that require treatment are vascular compromise, Crohn disease, volvulus, radiation enteritis, trauma to the bowel, and neoplasm. In infants, congenital atresias and stricture are noted, but volvulus with malrotation may be a cause, as well as necrotizing enterocolitis. Fortunately SBS is not common, although the incidence and prevalence of survivors is increasing as therapy improves. At least 40,000 to 50,000 patients with SBS require total parenteral nutrition (TPN) each year, and at least as many are managed without TPN.

CLINICAL PICTURE

The clinical syndrome is usually divided into three phases: acute, adaptation, and maintenance. The acute phase occurs immediately after surgery, when patients require significant amounts of electrolytes and fluids. Features of SBS may include hypovolemia, dehydration, metabolic acidosis, hypoalbuminemia, and deficiencies of potassium, calcium, zinc, magnesium, copper, body acids, fat-soluble vitamins, folic acid, and B_{12}.

The timing, onset, and severity of the clinical manifestations are compounded by numerous variables. One of the major factors is whether other organs are involved. The most significant is whether the colon remains after surgical resection and, if so, how much of the colon is available. Preservation of the ileocecal valve is another major variable.

Phase 1 lasts weeks to months. After that, the patient moves into phase 2, with a variable clinical picture (see Treatment and Management). If major electrolyte and mineral deficiencies develop, clinical evidence may include chronic dehydration. Diarrhea and electrolyte loss may develop when attempts are made to compensate through greatly increased intake. Subtle skin and blood abnormalities may appear because of slowly developing micronutrient and vitamin deficiencies. Weakness, dizziness, unsteady gait, and lack of mental acuity may all be present.

DIAGNOSIS

The diagnosis of SBS clearly can be made at surgery. If SBS is not apparent, the clinician obtains appropriate history and performs simple barium contrast studies to determine bowel length. Less than 200 cm or less than 120 cm of remaining bowel is a clinically arbitrary figure; symptoms and deficiencies are the important factors. Certainly if more than 75% of the bowel remains, SBS is highly unlikely. Nevertheless, selective deficiencies can occur because of ileal resection. Once it is established that less than 200 cm of bowel remains, a correlation must be made with symptoms and deficiencies. To perform these evaluations, a full analysis for anemia, iron and B_{12} absorption, and lactose absorption and tolerance will provide the clinician with a clear therapeutic guideline.

TREATMENT AND MANAGEMENT

During the acute phase, lasting up to 2 months, intravenous electrolyte and nutrient replacement may be essential. It is important to add antisecretory therapy, which includes a proton pump inhibitor, and antimotility therapy, which is usually best administered with the somatostatin analog octreotide. During the acute phase, the patient is evaluated and TPN initiated.

During the adaptation phase, lasting from 2 to 24 months, the bowel begins to adapt by slightly lengthening and increasing individual villous height, thereby increasing the absorptive surface. A major factor in phase 2 is whether the colon is still present and whether the ileocecal valve remains intact. It appears that the jejunum has greater ability to adapt than the ileum.

After the adaptation period, the patient moves into the long-term management (maintenance) period. In phase 3, little changes; determinations are made as to how much can be accomplished by oral feeding and how much TPN will be needed. Some clinicians do use an enteral feeding period during the TPN rest period. Some place a percutaneous gastrostomy or enterostomy tube so that the bowel can be fed slowly during the sleeping hours. However, this creates more discomfort and is socially problematic.

Regulation of oral intake requires trial and error. The goal is to obtain enough energy and protein intake to maintain body homeostasis. Proteins are the key nutrient. An intake of 0.8 to 1.2 mg/kg body weight must be maintained. To metabolize the protein, an adequate amount of energy is essential, usually from a combination of carbohydrates and fats. If the colon is present, medium-chain triglycerides can be absorbed through the colonic mucosa and may be helpful if added to the diet. Otherwise long-chain triglycerides are used. Fat intake may result in more fat excretion in the stool, with the problem of steatorrhea if the colon is present. However, therapy to bind bile salts is usually not warranted, considering how easily the short bowel can become deficient in bile salts. Consequently fat absorption is essential to maintain energy requirements. Carbohydrates in the form of simple and complex polysaccharides are a major energy source. Some patients who cannot

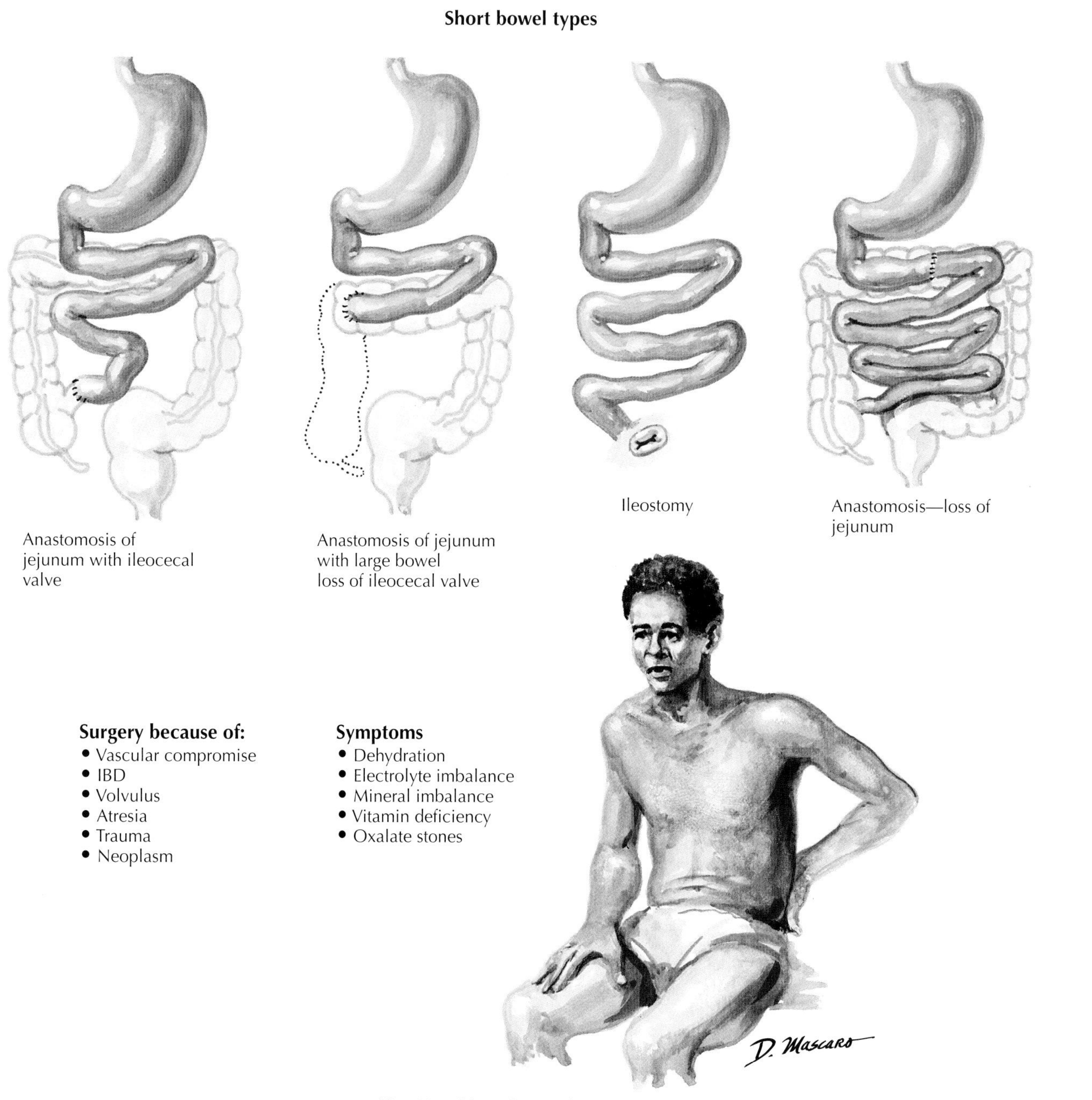

Short bowel types

Anastomosis of
jejunum with ileocecal
valve

Anastomosis of jejunum
with large bowel
loss of ileocecal valve

Ileostomy

Anastomosis—loss of
jejunum

Surgery because of:
• Vascular compromise
• IBD
• Volvulus
• Atresia
• Trauma
• Neoplasm

Symptoms
• Dehydration
• Electrolyte imbalance
• Mineral imbalance
• Vitamin deficiency
• Oxalate stones

Fig. 68.1 Short Bowel Syndrome.

tolerate simple sugars because of bacterial breakdown develop D-lactic acidosis, but this is rare. Most patients can tolerate sugars and complex polysaccharides, which can make up 60% and 70%, respectively, of the energy requirement. Absorption of fat-soluble vitamins may become a problem. However, all vitamins and trace minerals should be replaced in adequate amounts (see Section X).

The degree and amount of nutrient material that can be taken orally varies greatly in patients with SBS. However, after the 2-year period of adaptation, most will require some TPN. For severe cases, the requirement may be total. Most patients may take some of their nutrients orally, and many will have to get at least half their nutritional needs through TPN, thereby requiring a permanent catheter.

When there is an intact colon, increased oxalate absorption can occur because of decreased bile salts, resulting in oxalate nephrolithiasis. Therefore these patients should receive a low-oxalate diet.

Antimotility agents may be helpful during any stage of SBS; they include diphenoxylate, loperamide, codeine, and tincture of opium (see Chapter 64).

Oral hydration solutions might be helpful for select patients. Patients can try 250 mL to 1 L during the adaptive phase and for longer periods if they have selective electrolyte absorption difficulties. However, these are rare situations, and TPN usually corrects these problems.

Whenever bacterial overgrowth is suspected in SBS, as occurs with D-lactic acidosis, intermittent antibiotic therapy may be necessary. Antibiotics used for alternating 2-week or 1-month periods are often tried (see Chapter 67).

It has been suggested that growth hormone increases bowel adaptation, but this is controversial. Nevertheless, some patients may request or attempt this therapy. At present growth hormone is not generally recommended, although it may be tried in low-dose form.

COURSE AND PROGNOSIS

The prognosis in SBS is usually favorable if the duodenum and at least 60 cm of jejunum or ileum remains intact. The presence of an ileocecal valve—by slowing down transit and helping water and electrolyte absorption—greatly enhances the ability of the remaining jejunum or ileum to work effectively. Furthermore, the availability of a colon to absorb electrolytes and some minerals is helpful, and colonic microflora become important. If the colon is present, fermentation of soluble fibers and the usual undigested polysaccharides occurs, producing short-chain fatty acids—primarily butyric, propionic, and acetic. The colon then becomes a digestive organ, and as much as 10% to 20% of caloric requirements can be supplied through the absorption of short-chain fatty acids. Their formation is enhanced by healthy bacterial flora; some clinicians use probiotics to enhance the effectiveness of the microflora in the colon. Consequently the availability of the colon as a digestive organ improves the course and prognosis of SBS.

Comorbidities significantly affect morbidity and mortality. In an elderly patient with another organ illness, the prognosis for long life becomes guarded. Associated diseases or malignancies, severe radiation enteritis, and unrelenting inflammatory bowel disease all increase morbidity. Possible complications of associated chronic liver disease further increases the morbidity and mortality risk.

Finally, the expanding role of transplantation surgery is now offering new insight into the future for patients with SBS. Although still new, small bowel transplantation has been effective in select cases. Its future role remains to be determined, but it is available for patients with intractable disease who cannot be sustained on TPN.

ADDITIONAL RESOURCES

Buchman AL: Short bowel syndrome. In Feldman M, Friedman LS, Brandt LJ, editors: *Gastrointestinal and liver disease*, ed 10, Philadelphia, 2016, Saunders-Elsevier, pp 1832–1848.

Buchman AL, Scolapio J, Fryer J: AGA technical review on short bowel syndrome and intestinal transplantation, *Gastroenterology* 124:1111–1134, 2003.

DiBaise JK, Sudan B: Short bowel syndrome and small bowel transplantation. In Podolsky DK, Camilleri M, Fitz JG, et al, editors: *Yamada's textbook of gastroenterology*, ed 6, Hoboken, New Jersey, 2016, John Wiley and Sons Ltd, pp 1305–1323.

Steiger E: Guidelines for pharmacotherapy in short bowel syndrome, *J Clin Gastroenterol* 40:S73–S106, 2006.

Sundaram A, Koutkia P, Apovin CM: Nutritional management of the short bowel syndrome in adults, *J Clin Gastroenterol* 34:207–220, 2002.

Food Allergy

Martin H. Floch

The terms *food allergy* and food *hypersensitivity* are synonymous. Food "allergy" is distinguished from food "intolerance" in that it includes a true allergic, immunologic response (Fig. 69.1). *Food intolerances* are not immunologic responses. Allergic responses may be acute and may result in anaphylaxis (a rare occurrence) or may be chronic.

Although its incidence is difficult to determine, food hypersensitivity occurs in approximately 2% of the general population and in as many as 6% of young children. However, anecdotal experience indicates a much higher incidence, with many patients not seeking assistance or medical advice because they eliminate foods they identify as causing

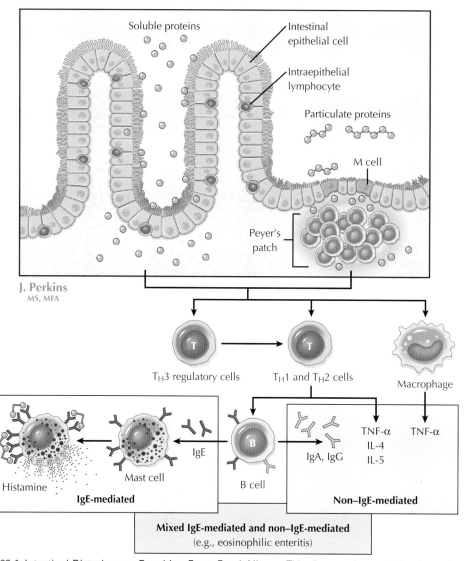

Fig. 69.1 Intestinal Disturbances Resulting From Food Allergy. This diagram demonstrates the entry of proteins through the intestinal epithelium that become attached or react with lymphocytes within Peyer's patches or with macrophages. The reaction is different if it is a T cell or a B cell. The T cells produce non–IgE-mediated reactions through the mechanisms listed in the box on the right. The B cells can stimulate this process or stimulate the IgE-mediated process and activate mast cells. There are also mixed IgE and non–IgE-mediated conditions, such as eosinophilic enteritis.

symptoms. Common foods associated with symptoms are milk, eggs, fish, tree nuts, shellfish, soybeans, fruits, and wheat. Children tend to outgrow the symptoms; in adulthood, the foods most often associated with food hypersensitivity are peanuts, tree nuts, fruits, fish, and shellfish.

The pathophysiology of food allergy is becoming clearer. True hypersensitivity reactions usually are mediated through immunoglobulin E (IgE) and associated with atopy. However, these findings are not essential when an alleged exposure can be demonstrated by an exclusion diet. Although IgG and IgA antibodies are demonstrated in celiac disease, the demonstration of these antibodies in other food allergies has been controversial. Immediate-phase reactions are IgE mediated, with inflammatory mediators released from mast cells. However, some hypersensitivity reactions are non-IgE mediated and involve histamine release from mast cells. Therefore both IgE hypersensitivity and non-IgE hypersensitivity exist. It is also clear that new understandings of the physiology of response are coming forth, particularly, in such areas as calcitonin gene–related peptides (CGRP), where the understanding of nociception is being elaborated.

Non-IgE food allergy is T cell–mediated, but mixed IgE-mediated and non–IgE-mediated conditions appear to involve the gut, including eosinophilic esophagitis, gastritis, or gastroenteritis.

CLINICAL PICTURE

The allergic response may manifest as an emergency anaphylactic reaction (angioneurotic edema, urticaria, asthmatic attacks, allergic rhinitis) or by less dramatic responses (rashes, focal edema. migraine headache). The gastrointestinal tract can certainly react by producing acute symptoms of gastroenteritis or, more chronically, of epigastric distress or diarrhea. The entire spectrum of acute and chronic symptoms may be caused by any of the food allergens. A clear relationship to foods is considered probable in acute, severe, and dramatic reactions; in oral allergy syndromes that produce pruritus; in celiac disease; and in dietary protein-induced enteropathy or enterocolitis in infancy.

Syndromes less dramatic in presentation that require workup include gastroesophageal reflux in infants, eosinophilic esophagitis or gastroenteritis, and enteropathies. Food allergy is often suspected but is extremely difficult to prove or diagnose. The symptoms may be minimal but are persistent and annoying.

DIAGNOSIS

Acute reactions and those temporally associated with symptoms (e.g., pruritus, erythema) are more easily diagnosed. Reactions causing vague symptoms (e.g., migraine, diarrhea) can be difficult. Most allergists and scientists agree that the diagnosis of food allergy can be made from one or more of the following:

1. Clear history and an allergic-like reaction after the ingestion of food
2. Exclusion of any anatomic, functional, metabolic, or infectious cause
3. Finding of certain pathologic features consistent with allergy, such as eosinophilia
4. Confirmation of a relationship between ingestion of a dietary protein and symptoms (e.g., clinical challenges, repeated inadvertent exposures)
5. Evidence of food-specific IgE antibody
6. Failure to respond to conventional therapies and improvement in symptoms with elimination diets

Some clinicians rely on a response to treatment of allergic inflammation with corticosteroids or other drugs. However, the final accepted diagnostic step is elimination of the food to relieve symptoms and a food challenge that recreates the symptomatic picture.

Primary tests for specific IgE antibody or particular foods, the radioallergosorbent test (RAST) and skin-prick test, are frequently used, but their high false-positive rates create confusion. Adjunctive tests such as endoscopic biopsies, absorption studies, and stool analysis for eosinophils are all used but are not pathognomonic. Specific IgE antibody may be used to rule out the potential for severe acute reactions before conducting oral challenges in patients with atopic disease or possible history of severe acute reactions. In patients with chronic symptomatic disorders without atopic disease, food-specific immunoglobulin test results are usually negative. Negative skin-prick tests are the most diagnostic, because the negative predictive value of the skin test is usually greater than 95% and excellent. Unfortunately the positive predictive value of a positive finding is approximately 50%. In vitro tests for a specific IgE with RAST are helpful in evaluating IgE-mediated food allergy. Problems in interpretation are compounded by immunologic cross-reactivity between botanical families and animal species.

Elimination diets are an essential tool in determining whether a food is causing the allergy. There are three types of such diets: (1) elimination of one or several foods suspected of provoking symptoms, (2) elimination of all but a defined group of allowed foods, and (3) use of an amino acid–based formula or the elemental diet. These types of elimination evaluations should be performed by experienced allergists. Failure to have symptoms resolved on the elimination diet would rule out food allergy.

Physician-supervised oral *food challenges* are required for the diagnosis of food allergy. In general, when several foods are under consideration as the cause of symptoms, test results for food-specific IgE are positive, and elimination has resulted in the resolution of symptoms, oral challenge testing for each food eliminated is used to diagnose specific sensitivities and allow expansion of the diet. In the patient with acute anaphylactoid-type reactions but with no evidence of a food-specific IgE suspected of provoking the reaction, a physician-supervised challenge is used to reintroduce the food safely in case of false-negative findings on the skin/RAST test. If suspicion concerning a particular food remains high despite its elimination and without a resolution of symptoms, challenges may be needed for clarification. If tests for specific IgE antibodies are not relevant to the disorder, oral challenges are often the only means of diagnosis. This is the case for most of the gastrointestinal hypersensitivity reactions. Oral challenges are also required to determine when clinical tolerance has developed. However, oral challenges may be optional or contraindicated in some patients, and a physician with experience in the field of food allergy must be consulted.

Research with probiotics indicates that some children have a deficient immune response. Probiotic organisms can stimulate the immune response to correct an allergic response caused by certain foods in infancy and by milk in children.

TREATMENT AND MANAGEMENT

Elimination of the allergic agent is the treatment for food allergy. As discussed, oral challenges may be required to clarify which foods are causing the symptoms. However, judicious use of elimination diets and challenges by experienced physicians can result in adequate control of the problem.

When the responsible foods cannot be identified, some physicians use antihistamines and, in extreme circumstances, corticosteroids to prevent symptoms. Double-blind placebo-controlled food challenges are frequently used and considered by some as the standard by which to diagnose food allergy and thus determine elimination.

Some clinicians use mast cell stabilizers, such as cromolyn sodium and ketotifen fumarate. The key to good management is patient education, with careful instruction on how to eliminate all protein-inciting agents in foods.

Evidence indicates that probiotics may be helpful in the treatment of milk allergy or atopy in children. *Lactobacillus rhamnosus,* also called *Lactobacillus* GG, can be used.

COURSE AND PROGNOSIS

The prognosis is usually excellent in patients who know the food responsible for the allergy and who have eliminated it from the diet. The patient who has experienced an anaphylactoid or severe reaction makes sure that epinephrine injections are available whenever there is potential exposure to an allergen. Patients experiencing chronic conditions may be plagued by the concept of food allergy, especially when specific allergens are not proved. The field is open and prone to questionable diagnostic and therapeutic procedures. However, most credible allergists can set up a program so that their patients can tolerate the diet and receive adequate nutrition despite the elimination of inciting foods. Experience with documented testing indicates that some food allergy reactions can be transient. Therefore patients should be tested after a reasonable time (1 year) to determine whether the allergy persists.

The field of infant allergy reports that most infants requiring hypoallergenic formulas usually become tolerant within 1 to 2 years, and the prognosis is then excellent. These patients are treated by a pediatric allergist.

ADDITIONAL RESOURCES

Atkins D: Food allergy: diagnosis and management, *Prim Care* 35:119–140, 2008.

Bischoff S, Crowe SE: Gastrointestinal food allergy: new insights into pathophysiology and clinical perspectives, *Gastroenterology* 128: 1089–1113, 2005.

Boyce JA, Assa'ad A, Burks AW, et al: Guidelines for the diagnosis and management of food allergy in the United States. Report of the NIAID-sponsored expert panel, *J Allergy Clin Immunol* 126(Suppl 6):S1–S58, 2010.

Brandtzaeg P: Food allergy: separating the science from the mythology, *Nat Rev Gastroenterol Hepatol* 7:380–400, 2010.

Isolauri E, Salminen S: Probiotics: use in allergic disorders, *J Clin Gastroenterol* 42:S91–S96, 2008.

Kirjavainen PV, Salminen SJ, Isolauri E: Probiotic bacteria in the management of atopic diseases: underscoring the importance of viability, *J Pediatr Gastroenterol Nutr* 36:223–227, 2003.

Nowak-Wegrzyn A, Sampson HA: Adverse reactions to foods, *Med Clin North Am* 90:97–127, 2006.

Sicherer SH: Advances in anaphylaxis and hypersensitivity reaction to foods, drugs, and insects, *J Allergy Clin Immunol* 119:1462–1469, 2007.

Spencer NJ, Magnusdottir EI, Jakobsson J, et al: CGRPa within the Trpv1-Cre population contributes to visceral nociception, *Am J Physiol Gastrointest Liver Physiol* 314:G188–G200, 2018. [Epub ahead of print].

Turner JR: Intestinal mucosal barrier function in health and disease, *Nat Rev Immunol* 9:799–809, 2009.

Wang J, Sampson HA: Food allergy, *J Clin Invest* 121:827–835, 2011.

70

Eosinophilic Gastroenteritis

Martin H. Floch

Eosinophilic gastroenteritis is a disease in which tissue eosinophilia occurs in a segment of the gastrointestinal (GI) tract and is associated with GI symptoms (Fig. 70.1). Although first described in 1937, with frequent case reports corroborating the syndrome, the following criteria to establish eosinophilic gastroenteritis were not defined until 1990:

1. The patient must have GI symptoms.
2. Eosinophilic infiltration must be demonstrated on biopsy in one or more areas of the GI tract.
3. The patient should have no eosinophilic involvement of other organs outside the GI tract.
4. The patient should have no parasitic infestation.

Eosinophilic gastroenteritis is a relatively rare disease. The actual incidence is unknown, but most gastroenterologists believe that many cases are unreported. The typical presentation is in the third to fifth decade of life. It may affect any age group, with no apparent gender predilection. The cause of the infiltrate is unknown. It is often associated with a hyperallergic state. Eosinophils may actually damage the GI tract by releasing protein and toxic substances.

Although eosinophils are present in many bowel disorders (e.g., parasitic disease, inflammatory bowel disease), the only evidence in eosinophilic gastroenteritis is the infiltrate in the small bowel. Because it is frequently associated with multiple allergies, the assumption is that patients with eosinophilic gastroenteritis are allergic to some food or substance in the environment. However, this has not been proved. Eosinophilic gastroenteritis is now thought to be a mixture of IgE-mediated and non–IgE-mediated allergic reactions.

Symptoms
- Dyspepsia
- Malnutrition and malabsorption
- Diarrhea
- Weight loss
- Allergy symptoms (asthma)

Biopsy appearance

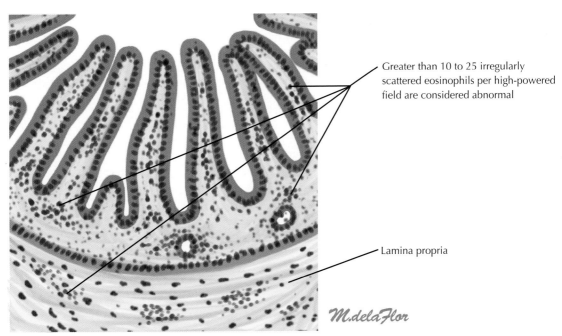

Greater than 10 to 25 irregularly scattered eosinophils per high-powered field are considered abnormal

Lamina propria

Fig. 70.1 Eosinophilic Gastroenteritis.

CLINICAL PICTURE

Most often the stomach and small bowel are involved with the mucosal and submucosal eosinophilic infiltrate. These patients seek treatment for dyspepsia or diarrhea or for mild, intermittent abdominal pain. The syndrome may be intermittent or may be longstanding and accompanied by weight loss and associated malnutrition and malabsorption. Depending on the extent and degree of eosinophil concentration and damage to the stomach and small bowel, erosions and weeping lesions can develop, but these are rarely reported. In young children, an allergy frequently manifests with mild asthma, atopy, severe hay fever, or multiple food intolerances. Almost every part of the GI tract has been involved. Such rare entities as eosinophilic ascites and eosinophilic polyps have been reported.

Eosinophilic esophagitis is usually reported as a separate entity when only the esophagus is involved. It behaves differently from generalized eosinophilic gastroenteritis. Rings form in the esophagus, and symptoms can be chronic. It is treated as a severe reflux disease but also requires topical therapy (see Section I).

DIAGNOSIS

To fulfill the criteria for eosinophilic gastroenteritis, there must be a tissue diagnosis. Once suspicion is raised, upper endoscopy is essential to obtain samples of the esophagus, stomach, and small bowel for biopsy. The clinical picture usually raises the index of suspicion. Peripheral eosinophilia is present in almost 80% of patients, although it may be of low grade and is often overlooked. It is important to rule out parasitic disease. Evaluation for ankylostomiasis, or intestinal parasites, must always be performed. It is also important to rule out other systemic diseases that can cause an eosinophilic infiltrate, such as lymphoma, vasculitis, and Addison disease. Another concomitant finding may be a low serum albumin.

It is important to rule out all other diseases; thus imaging of the upper GI and lower intestinal tracts becomes important. If diarrhea is part of the picture, the usual diarrhea workup for pathogens and colonoscopy are important to obtain biopsy specimens and rule out inflammatory bowel disease.

Biopsy evaluations are critical. Eosinophilic infiltrate may be part of any inflammatory process. Therefore the pathologist must determine whether there is an abnormal increase in eosinophils. Usually more than 10 eosinophils per high-power field (hpf) is considered abnormal, but there are more than 25 eosinophils per hpf in classic eosinophilic gastroenteritis. The infiltrate may be scattered, however, so several areas should undergo biopsy. The appearance of intraepithelial eosinophils is a strong indicator of the syndrome even if the numbers of eosinophils in the lamina propria and submucosa are not high.

Eosinophilic gastroenteritis should not be confused with *hypereosinophilic syndrome* or *diffuse vasculitis,* both of which involve multiple organs.

TREATMENT AND MANAGEMENT

Corticosteroids are the most successful agents once the diagnosis of eosinophilic gastroenteritis is firmly established. Prednisone is begun in relatively high doses and then tapered over 1 to 2 weeks. Most patients respond dramatically, but as many as 15% have relapses and require increasing doses. Many patients are carried with low-dose maintenance prednisone of 5 to 10 mg daily (similar to the treatment of chronic asthma).

Cromolyn sodium has been used with varying success. Because of its safety, cromolyn is often administered before corticosteroids.

If testing reveals a food allergy, it is helpful to eliminate any inciting foods. However, the test for food allergy usually fails in patients with eosinophilic gastroenteritis.

COURSE AND PROGNOSIS

The prognosis for patients with eosinophilic gastroenteritis is excellent. Most patients respond extremely well, and after initial therapy, or within months, they can discontinue prednisone treatment. Relapses occur, but they are usually easily controlled.

ADDITIONAL RESOURCES

Bischoff SC, Mayer J, Nguyen OT, et al: Immunohistochemical assessment of intestinal eosinophil activation in patients with eosinophilic gastroenteritis and inflammatory bowel disease, *Am J Gastroenterol* 94:3521–3529, 1999.

Kalantar SJ, Marks R, Lambert JR, et al: Dyspepsia due to eosinophilic gastroenteritis, *Dig Dis Sci* 42:2327–2332, 1997.

Klein NC, Hargrove R, Sleisinger MH, et al: Eosinophilic gastroenteritis, *Medicine (Baltimore)* 49:299–304, 1970.

Pineton de Chambrum G, Gonzalez F, Canva JY, et al: Natural history of eosinophilic gastroenteritis, *Clin Gastroenterol Hepatol* 9:950–956, 2011.

Rothenberg ME, Habereth Y: Eosinophilic disturbances of the gastrointestinal tract. In Feldman M, Friedman LS, Brandt LJ, editors: *Gastrointestinal and liver disease*, ed 10, Philadelphia, 2016, Saunders-Elsevier, pp 454–463.

Sampson HA: Food allergies. In Feldman M, Friedman LS, Brandt LJ, editors: *Gastrointestinal and liver disease*, ed 10, Philadelphia, 2016, Saunders-Elsevier, pp 148–157.

Talley NJ, Shorter RG, Phillips SF, et al: Eosinophilic gastroenteritis: a clinical pathologic study of patients with disease of the mucosae, musculae, and subserosal tissue, *Gut* 31:54–61, 1990.

Washington MK, Peck RM Jr: Gastritis and gastropathy. In Podolsky DK, Camilleri M, Fitz JG, et al, editors: *Yamada's textbook of gastroenterology*, ed 6, Hoboken, New Jersey, 2016, John Wiley and Sons Ltd, pp 1103–1120.

71

Intussusception of the Small Intestine

Martin H. Floch

Intussusception is the invagination of a portion of the intestine into the contiguous distal segment of the enteric tube (Fig. 71.1). It usually occurs in infants at 4 to 10 months of age and is associated with acute enteritis, allergic reactions, and conditions that cause hypermotility. In older persons, intussusception is associated with a polyp or malignancy, an enlarged Peyer patch or diverticulum (e.g., Meckel), and a large number of rare entities that cause intrusion into the bowel.

Intussusceptions are classified according to the part of the digestive tube that telescopes into the *intussuscipiens,* the receiving part, including ileoileal, jejunoileal, and ileocolic invaginations. The most common is

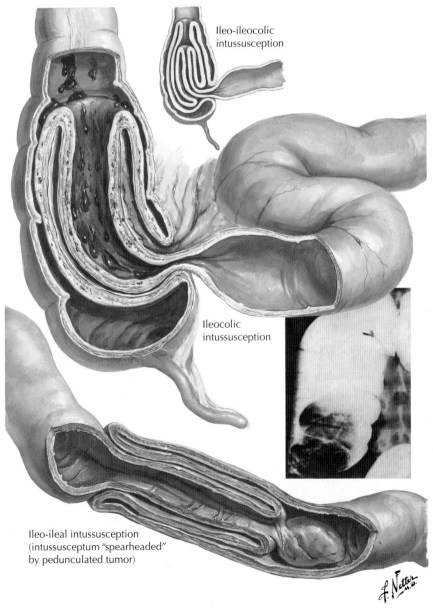

Ileo-ileocolic intussusception

Ileocolic intussusception

Ileo-ileal intussusception (intussusceptum "spearheaded" by pedunculated tumor)

Fig. 71.1 Intussusception of the Small Intestine.

the ileocolic intussusception. A double invagination, or an intussusception within an intussusception, may also occur, called ileoileocolic. How far the *intussusceptum,* the part that becomes ensheathed by the more distal portion, enters the intussuscipiens depends on the length and motility of the mesentery. The intussuscipiens can be compressed, after which edema, peritoneal exudation, vascular strangulation, and, finally, intestinal gangrene can develop.

In children, the most common causes of intussusception are associated infections, and in adults, the most common causes are neoplasms, although these primary causes affect the other group as well. Approximately 30% to 50% of small bowel intussusceptions and 50% to 65% of colonic intussusceptions are associated with malignant neoplasms.

CLINICAL PICTURE

Clinical presentation of intussusception may be alarming, with the sudden development of abdominal pain and cramplike sensations occurring every 10 to 20 minutes. Children may appear to be in shock. In approximately 85% of children, a movable mass may be palpated. If the symptoms progress, blood may be found in the stool. In adults, the presentation may be acute, but often it is intermittent and accompanied by cramplike abdominal pain with nausea and vomiting. With chronic presentation lasting more than 1 week, the patient may lose weight. At times, the chronicity of symptoms can fool the clinician.

DIAGNOSIS

Diagnosis is made and confirmed by radiographic imaging. Ultrasonography is helpful, but barium contrast or computed tomography with contrast media often demonstrates the intussusception. Different radiologic patterns are observed, with classic findings of target lesions, sausage-shaped masses, and associated obstructive phenomena.

TREATMENT AND MANAGEMENT

For most infants and children, intussusception is reduced by pressure from the contrast enema when it is ileocolic. However, the high incidence of neoplasia in adults requires surgical intervention. At times, surgery is performed on an emergency basis to prevent ischemic and gangrenous bowel formation. Once the diagnosis is made, surgical evaluation and intervention are essential. The surgeon may reduce the intussusception when the bowel is entered and then use an end-to-end or end-to-side anastomosis to remove any suspicious lesion. Laparoscopic surgery is now used to perform these resections, although this requires a skilled surgeon.

PROGNOSIS

The immediate prognosis is usually excellent. However, if a neoplasm is identified, the prognosis depends on the type of lesion. A high incidence of polyps in association with intussusception in children and adults may require follow-up monitoring and possibly chemotherapy. When intussusception is associated with hypermotility of viral cause in a child, the prognosis is excellent after the acute infection is controlled.

ADDITIONAL RESOURCES

Maconi G, Radice E, Greco S, et al: Transient small-bowel intussusceptions in adults: significance of ultrasonographic detection, *Clin Radiol* 62:792–797, 2007.

Marinis A, Yaillourou A, Samanides L, et al: Intussception of the bowel: a review, *World J Gastroenterol* 15:407–411, 2009.

Mizell JS, Turnage RH: Intestinal obstruction. In Feldman M, Friedman LS, Brandt LJ, editors: *Gastrointestinal and liver disease*, ed 10, Philadelphia, 2016, Saunders-Elsevier, pp 2154–2170.

Rubin DC, Shaker A: Small intestine: anatomy and structural anomalies. In Podolsky DK, Camilleri M, Fitz JG, et al, editors: *Yamada's textbook of gastroenterology*, ed 6, Hoboken, New Jersey, 2016, John Wiley and Sons Ltd, pp 73–92.

Whitcomb DC, Lowe ME: Hereditary, familial, and genetic disorders of the pancreas and pancreatitic disorders in children. In Feldman M, Friedman LS, Brandt LJ, editors: *Gastrointestinal and liver disease*, ed 10, Philadelphia, 2016, Saunders-Elsevier, pp 944–968.

72

Benign Tumors of the Small Intestine

Martin H. Floch

Benign tumors of the small intestine are rare. In a series of 22,810 autopsies, the incidence was 0.16%. The neoplasms may be located anywhere in the small bowel. *Stromal tumors,* or *leiomyomas,* are more common in the jejunum, and *adenomas* are more common in the ileum. Both are benign but have significant malignant counterparts or potential. Benign tumors may be single or multiple. Adenomas, neurofibromas, and angiomas have a familial occurrence. Leiomyomas and adenomas are most common and, along with lipomas, myomas, some angiomas, and neurogenic tumors, make up more than two-thirds of lesions (Fig. 72.1).

Rarer benign tumors include fibromas, lymphangiomas, myxomas, and osteomas. Tumors may be intraluminal, extraluminal, or intramural. They may vary in size from millimeters to "very large" at 3 cm. Neurogenic tumors tend to appear in multiples, whereas adenomas, lipomas, and leiomyomas tend to appear singly. Neurogenic tumors in the small intestine may be part of a generalized neurofibromatosis (von Recklinghausen disease).

Benign vascular tumors of the small intestine comprise true tumors of blood vessels, or *angiomas,* and congenital vascular malformations, or *hamartomas.* These are difficult to differentiate and may be part of a generalized vascular dysplasia. *Rendu-Osler-Weber syndrome* (hereditary hemorrhagic telangiectasia), a mendelian-dominant disease, includes angiomas of the skin, mucous membranes, and viscera. Another mendelian-dominant inherited syndrome is *Peutz-Jeghers syndrome,* characterized by the association of gastrointestinal (GI) adenomas, polyposis, and a distinct type of mucocutaneous pigmentation (Fig. 72.2). These polyps may be adenomatous or hamartomatous.

Brunner gland hamartomas and nodular lymphoid hyperplasia of the small intestine are benign tumors or polyps. Both are rare and frequently asymptomatic, but they require histologic definition.

CLINICAL PICTURE

In general, many of these benign lesions never cause symptoms, or cause such vague symptoms that a clinical diagnosis cannot be established. Serious clinical symptoms occur usually as a complication, such as intestinal obstruction, necrotic change in the tumor with resultant hemorrhage, infection, rupture, or malignant degeneration (see Fig. 72.2). Intraluminal tumors are likely to cause symptoms earlier than extraluminal tumors. Extraluminal lesions may grow to large dimensions before they become symptomatic. Intraluminal polypoid tumors may lead to obstruction by intussusception. This will manifest with an acute obstructive phenomenon or insidiously, with mild intermittent small bowel obstruction and symptoms of abdominal pain, vomiting, and either diarrhea or constipation. Severity of the symptom depends on the degree of obstruction and the site of the tumor.

Bleeding from the tumor is attributed to necrotic erosion of a vessel. It may be slow and insidious, or it may be massive and result in severe GI bleeding. Extraluminal tumors may rupture into the peritoneal cavity, or they may become necrotic after torsion of a pedicle and thus may lead to intraabdominal hemorrhage or an acute abdomen. In rare cases, fistulae may form through intramural or extraluminal tumors connecting the intestinal lumen with the abdominal cavity, resulting in peritonitis.

Malignant degeneration of benign tumors of the small bowel may occur. Adenomatous lesions are reported to develop into carcinoma in as many as 40% of patients. Similarly, leiomyomas (stromal tumors) are developing into leiomyosarcomas at an increasingly alarming rate.

DIAGNOSIS

Large tumors can be diagnosed easily through barium contrast study or contrast computed tomography. However, small bleeding lesions may often be missed. Small bowel barium studies are often helpful. However, direct-view small bowel endoscopy, double-balloon endoscopy, and capsule endoscopy now make these lesions visible to the endoscopist. Capsule endoscopy has become the procedure of choice to identify lesions early. However, depending on the symptom presentation, a contrast study of the small bowel, enteroscopy, and, if necessary, double-balloon endoscopy and/or capsule endoscopy are indicated. With these tools, a diagnosis should be made.

TREATMENT AND MANAGEMENT

Most benign tumors are asymptomatic and therefore may be incidental findings during work-up. However, once the tumor is identified or symptoms have developed, it is often mandatory to obtain a histologic diagnosis. Laparoscopic surgery has facilitated diagnosis of these lesions, but when small, they may require open laparotomy for identification. If a complication such as intussusception, bleeding, or perforation develops, emergency surgery is essential to remove the lesion.

COURSE AND PROGNOSIS

The prognosis for patients with benign tumors of the small intestine is excellent. However, occasionally a stromal tumor is found to be a leiomyosarcoma, and the prognosis for what appeared to be a benign adenoma becomes one for an adenocarcinoma (see Chapter 73).

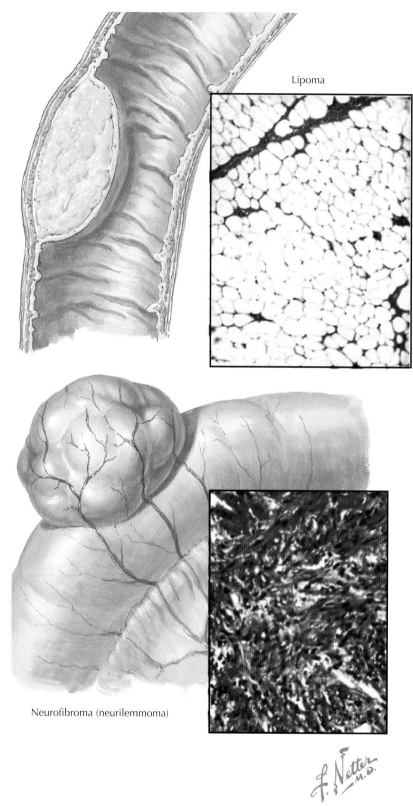

Lipoma

Neurofibroma (neurilemmoma)

Fig. 72.1 Benign Tumors of the Small Intestine.

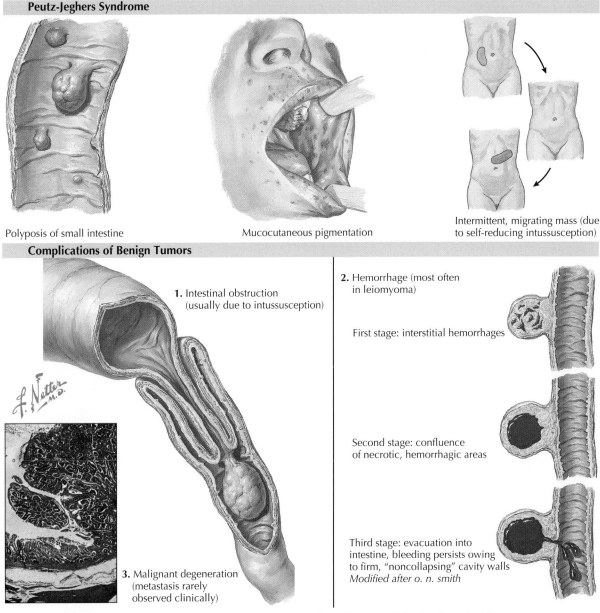

Peutz-Jeghers Syndrome

Polyposis of small intestine

Mucocutaneous pigmentation

Intermittent, migrating mass (due to self-reducing intussusception)

Complications of Benign Tumors

1. Intestinal obstruction (usually due to intussusception)

3. Malignant degeneration (metastasis rarely observed clinically)

2. Hemorrhage (most often in leiomyoma)

First stage: interstitial hemorrhages

Second stage: confluence of necrotic, hemorrhagic areas

Third stage: evacuation into intestine, bleeding persists owing to firm, "noncollapsing" cavity walls
Modified after o. n. smith

Fig. 72.2 *Top,* Peutz-Jeghers Syndrome; *Bottom,* Complications of Benign Intestinal Tumors.

ADDITIONAL RESOURCES

Banck MS, Kanwar R, Kulkarni AA, et al: The genomic landscape of small intestine neuroendocrine tumors, *J Clin Invest* 123:2502–2508, 2013.

Bilimoria KY, Bentrem DJ, Wayne JD, et al: Small bowel cancer in the United States: changes in epidemiology, treatment, and survival over the last 20 years, *Ann Surg* 249:63–71, 2009.

Bresalier RS, Belechaz B: Tumors of the small intestine. In Feldman M, Friedman LS, Brandt LJ, editors: *Gastrointestinal and liver disease*, ed 10, Philadelphia, 2016, Saunders-Elsevier, pp 2196–2212.

Dematteo RP, Ballman KV, Antonescu CR, et al: Adjuvant imatinib mesylate after resection of localised, primary gastrointestinal stromal tumour: a randomized, double-blind, placebo-controlled trial, *Lancet* 373: 1097–1104, 2009.

Feigel DO, Cave DR: *Capsule endoscopy*, Philadelphia, 2008, Saunders-Elsevier.

Gill SS, Heuman DM, Mihs AA: Small intestinal neoplasms, *J Clin Gastroenterol* 33:267–282, 2001.

Kanth P, Grimmett J, Champrine M, et al: Hereditary colorectal polyposis and cancer syndromes: a primer on diagnosis and management, *Am J Gastroenterol* 112:1509–1525, 2017.

Lappas JC, Maglinte DDT, Sandresagaran K: Benign tumors of the small bowel. In Gore RM, Levine MS, editors: *Textbook of gastrointestinal radiology*, ed 3, Philadelphia, 2008, Saunders-Elsevier, pp 845–851.

Maglinte DDT, Lappas JC, Sandresegaran K: Contrast imaging. In Gore RM, Levine MS, editors: *Textbook of gastrointestinal radiology*, ed 3, Philadelphia, 2008, Saunders-Elsevier, pp 755–764.

Mullady DK, Tan BR: A multidisciplinary approach to the diagnosis and treatment of gastrointestinal stromal tumor, *J Clin Gastroenterol* 47: 578–585, 2013.

Tanaka S, Mitsui K, Tatsaguchi A, et al: Current status of double-balloon endoscopy: indications, insertion routes, sedation, complications, technical matters, *Gastrointest Endosc* 66:S30–S33, 2007.

73

Malignant Tumors of the Small Intestine

Martin H. Floch

Malignant tumors of the small intestine are rare. Their frequency in a large autopsy study was lower than 0.1%. Although the small bowel is the largest gastrointestinal organ, less than 5% of malignant tumors arise in the small intestine. The reason for this remains unclear. *Adenocarcinoma* (nonampullary) is the most common malignancy and accounts for 30% to 50% of malignant tumors. Most develop

in the duodenum or the jejunum. Predisposing factors appear to be alcohol intake, Crohn disease, celiac disease, and neurofibromatosis. A predisposing factor appears to be a preexisting adenoma, and more than 40% of patients with familial adenomatous polyposis (FAP) have polyps in the proximal small bowel, and more than 5% develop adenocarcinoma. Fig. 73.1 shows the morphologic

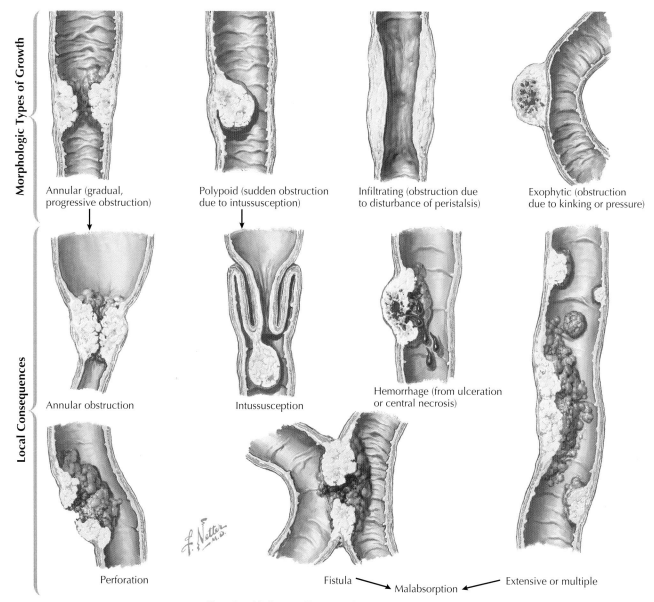

Morphologic Types of Growth

Annular (gradual, progressive obstruction)

Polypoid (sudden obstruction due to intussusception)

Infiltrating (obstruction due to disturbance of peristalsis)

Exophytic (obstruction due to kinking or pressure)

Local Consequences

Annular obstruction

Intussusception

Hemorrhage (from ulceration or central necrosis)

Perforation

Fistula ➔ Malabsorption ⬅ Extensive or multiple

Fig. 73.1 Malignant Tumors of the Small Intestine.

types and local consequences of malignant tumors of the small intestine.

Carcinoma of the ampulla of Vater, together with the other adenocarcinomas, makes up most of the malignancies in the small bowel. Again, these tumors are rare, but they are the most common sites of extracolonic malignancy in FAP. Lymphomas are the third and leiomyosarcomas the fourth most common small intestinal malignancies. Lymphomas make up 15% to 20% of all malignant small bowel tumors, of which non-Hodgkin lymphomas are most common.

Leiomyosarcomas are now classified as *gastrointestinal stromal tumors* (GISTs). It is often difficult for pathologists to define whether these are benign or malignant. Differentiation is usually based on a mitotic index. If there is less than 1 mitosis per 30 high-power fields, metastases are less than 1%. If there are more than 10 mitoses per high-power field, metastases are 100% and 5-year survival rates decrease to 5%, with no 10-year survival reported. A mitotic index between 0 and 10 has grades of 5-year survival and metastases. The GISTs are of great interest (see Chapter 37), and more are being reported. It is not yet clear whether the increase results from better diagnostic studies or whether there is a true increased incidence.

CLINICAL PICTURE

As with benign tumors of the small bowel, the presentation of malignant lesions may be slow and insidious. Patients may have low-grade anemia, slow bleeding, mild abdominal pain, weight loss, and, if there is an infiltrating large lesion, slowly developing malabsorption or intermittent cramps. Patients may have acute symptoms of obstructing intussusception or massive bleed. Patients with malignant lesions usually do not seek emergency treatment but have persistent symptoms over several months.

DIAGNOSIS

As with benign tumors, imaging is paramount for malignant tumors, which are usually easily identified using barium contrast or computed tomography contrast evaluation. Because of their nature, these tumors are usually larger than benign tumors, but enteroscopy, double-balloon enteroscopy, and capsule endoscopy now allow earlier diagnosis if symptoms are also present. Low-grade anemia resulting from slow blood loss from a small lesion may prompt an earlier presentation and permit earlier diagnosis for a better prognosis.

Ampullary lesions may involve bile duct obstruction and jaundice. Because of the position of these lesions, patients may seek treatment early, and the lesions may be resected early. Current endoscopic and endoscopic ultrasound (EUS) techniques may even allow endoscopic resection. EUS now permits determination of tumor depth and is an important technique for evaluation at ampullary sites.

TREATMENT AND MANAGEMENT

It is essential that all tumors be resected. Benign or malignant, the histology must be established; thus resection is imperative. When tumors are very small, attempts to resect by endoscopic techniques may be used. EUS is used in some of these cases.

Once the lesion is resected, histologic analysis will indicate what type of chemotherapy is needed. Chemotherapy is changing rapidly, and the preferred drugs must be determined by the latest oncologic evaluations. This holds true for adenocarcinomas, as well as for lymphomas and leiomyosarcomas.

Therapy for lymphoma is usually more complex. Primary lymphomas should be classified so that management can be determined. Once again, the oncologist provides guidance on the latest therapy.

COURSE AND PROGNOSIS

Findings from a detailed study reveal that the 5-year survival rate for adenocarcinoma of the small bowel is 30% and that the median survival time is less than 20 months. Ampullary adenocarcinoma has a better prognosis, with 5-year survival of 36% and an even better prognosis for patients who undergo early resection.

The overall prognosis for lymphoma varies greatly with the disease stage. In advanced stages, 5-year survival generally ranges from 25% to 30%. However, with radical surgery and rapidly improving drug therapy, 5-year survival has increased, reported as high as 60% to 70%. The prognosis for patients with these tumors is still not good, but advances in chemotherapy may improve prognostic indicators in the future.

ADDITIONAL RESOURCES

Bresalier RS, Belechaz B: Tumors of the small intestine. In Feldman M, Friedman LS, Brandt LJ, editors: *Gastrointestinal and liver disease*, ed 10, Philadelphia, 2016, Saunders-Elsevier, pp 2196–2212.

Cao J, Zuo Y, Chen Z, Li J: Primary small intestinal malignant tumors: survival analysis of 48 postoperative patients, *J Clin Gastroenterol* 42:167–173, 2008.

Howe JR, Karnell LH, Menck HR, et al: The American College of Surgeons Commission on Cancer and the American Cancer Society: adenocarcinoma of the small bowel—review of the National Cancer Data Base, *Cancer* 86:2693–2706, 1999.

Ito K, Fujita N, Noda Y, et al: Preoperative evaluation of ampullary neoplasm with EUS and transpapillary intraductal US: a prospective and histopathologically controlled study, *Gastrointest Endosc* 66:S740–S747, 2007.

Kanth P, Grimmett J, Champrine M, et al: Hereditary colorectal polyposis and cancer syndromes: a primer on diagnosis and management, *Am J Gastroenterol* 112:1509–1525, 2017.

Margalit O, Dubois RN: Neoplasm of the gastrointestinal tract. In Podolsky DK, Camilleri M, Fitz JG, et al, editors: *Yamada's textbook of gastroenterology*, ed 6, Hoboken, New Jersey, 2016, John Wiley and Sons Ltd, pp 587–616.

74

Carcinoid Syndrome and Neuroendocrine Tumors

Martin H. Floch

Eighty percent of gastrointestinal (GI) neuroendocrine tumors are made up of enterochromaffin-like cell carcinoids, duodenal gastrin G-cell tumors, and rectal trabecular L-cell carcinoids. Less common neuroendocrine tumors are gangliocytic paragangliomas, somatostatinomas, lipomas, and schwannomas. Pathologic study has revealed that the term *carcinoid* represents a wide spectrum of neoplasms that originate from different neuroendocrine cells.

Carcinoid tumors of the small intestine that secrete serotonin (5-hydroxytryptamine [5-HT]) are associated with the *carcinoid syndrome.* These neuroendocrine tumors may originate from the foregut, midgut, or hindgut, and the enterochromaffin cells making up the neoplasm may secrete serotonin, gastrin, or adrenocorticotropic hormone. Consequently, they can produce different syndromes. However, the most frequent site for carcinoid tumors is in the GI tract, and the second most common site is the bronchopulmonary system. The most common site within the GI tract is the small bowel, followed by the appendix, with a significant number occurring in the rectum. Neoplasms are usually small and yellowish. Those found in the appendix rarely metastasize, whereas those originating in the small bowel can be more virulent. They can develop anywhere in the GI tract and have been reported in the esophagus, stomach, pancreas, and large bowel.

Carcinoid syndrome occurs when the tumor secretes a large amount of an active substance such as serotonin. Symptoms occur from the carcinoid when the tumors grow larger or when they metastasize. Carcinoid tumors smaller than 1 cm rarely metastasize. Lesions larger than 2 cm should be treated aggressively.

Rectal carcinoids do not result in the carcinoid syndrome, and most are asymptomatic.

CLINICAL PICTURE

Frequently, carcinoids are discovered inadvertently during surgery in the appendix or during a workup. Often, the carcinoids are asymptomatic. In other cases, the carcinoid can cause mild abdominal pain, bleeding, or intussusception, which would then manifest as intermittent abdominal pain or acute obstruction (Fig. 74.1). Rarely, carcinoids manifest as a palpable mass.

When the tumor secretes an active substance, as in approximately 10% of patients, the resulting symptoms are referred to as carcinoid syndrome. The patient typically experiences intermittent abdominal cramps associated with diarrhea, flushing of the face and entire body, and extragastrointestinal symptoms of bronchospasm or even cyanosis.

On physical examination, again rarely or occasionally, a palpable mass heralds the diagnosis. However, most often, there are no findings except when acute intussusception and obstruction occur. In patients with carcinoid syndrome, the physical examination may reveal murmurs of tricuspid valve disease. Carcinoid is associated with fixation of the tricuspid valve leaflets, resulting in typical murmurs. Left-sided heart disease occurs in 10% to 15% of patients. The presentation of the patient with flushing, diarrhea, and tricuspid murmur is classic and almost pathognomonic of the carcinoid syndrome.

DIAGNOSIS

As indicated, often the neuroendocrine tumor is asymptomatic and identified during a work-up for other diseases. However, once symptoms develop, it is essential to perform radiographic contrast studies. These may reveal the site of the tumor. Computed tomography and magnetic resonance imaging are also helpful. Somatostatin-labeled isotope scanning is highly effective for identifying the primary hematostatic sites.

Biochemically, carcinoid syndrome is clearly diagnosed with the finding of more than 10 mg 5-hydroxyindolacetic acid in a 24-hour urine collection.

TREATMENT AND MANAGEMENT

Removing very small lesions is usually curative. Lesions that grow as large as 2 cm have a significant chance to metastasize and require vigorous therapy. The primary lesion must be removed and any metastases treated. Surgical resection of metastatic lesions has resulted in some cures. Chemotherapy has had marginal effect. Chemoembolization and hepatic artery embolization have been effective when performed by experienced practitioners.

Once the carcinoid syndrome evolves, pharmacologic therapy is important, particularly if the lesions cannot be totally removed surgically. Somatostatin receptors are present in more than 80% of carcinoid tumors. The use of *somatostatin* or *octreotide* has proven to be highly effective in relieving the carcinoid syndrome symptoms. Long-acting octreotide injections are now available, making this therapy more feasible and effective. Other inhibitors of serotonin synthesis, such as parachlorophenylalanine and methyldopa, have been used to block the conversion of tryptophan to serotonin. However, the most effective treatment is with somatostatin.

COURSE AND PROGNOSIS

Resecting tumors smaller than 1 cm results in an excellent prognosis. However, if tumors have grown at other sites in the GI tract, metastases occur and the prognosis varies.

The 5-year survival rate for patients with gastric carcinoids is 49% if localized. For pancreatic lesions, which tend to grow large and are discovered late, 5-year survival is 34%. The presentation is variable in the small bowel. When the lesions are larger than 2 cm, metastases have been reported in various series at rates of 33% to 80%. Colon lesions tend to be discovered later, and 5-year survival with these is 42%. Local treatment of rectal carcinoids yields good results; however, if the lesions

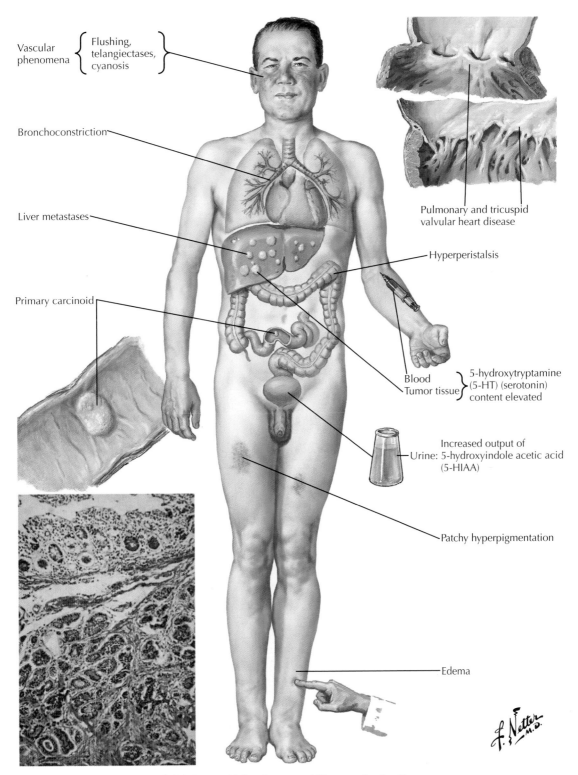

Vascular phenomena { Flushing, telangiectases, cyanosis }

Bronchoconstriction

Liver metastases

Primary carcinoid

Pulmonary and tricuspid valvular heart disease

Hyperperistalsis

Blood Tumor tissue { 5-hydroxytryptamine (5-HT) (serotonin) content elevated }

Increased output of Urine: 5-hydroxyindole acetic acid (5-HIAA)

Patchy hyperpigmentation

Edema

Fig. 74.1 Carcinoid Syndrome and Neuroendocrine Tumors.

are larger than 2 cm, the probability of metastasis is 60% to 80%. When rectal lesions are smaller than 1 cm, the cure rate is 98%.

Overall prognosis for carcinoid tumors varies. Once carcinoids evolve into carcinoid syndrome, the prognosis is guarded.

ADDITIONAL RESOURCES

Falconi M, Bartsch DK, Eriksson B, et al: ENETS consensus guidelines for the management of patients with digestive neuroendocrine neoplasms of the digestive systems: well-differentiated pancreatic non-functioning tumors, *Neuroendocrinology* 95:120–134, 2012.

Jensen RT, Norton JA, Oberg K: Neuroendocrine tumors. In Feldman M, Friedman LS, Brandt LJ, editors: *Gastrointestinal and liver disease*, ed 10, Philadelphia, 2016, Saunders-Elsevier, pp 501–541.

Klimstra DS, Modlin IR, Coppola D, et al: The pathologic classification of neuroendocrine tumors: a review of nonmenclature, grading, and staging systems, *Pancreas* 39:707–712, 2010.

Kulke MH, Meyer RJ: Carcinoid tumors, *N Engl J Med* 340:858–868, 1999.

Modlin IM, Sandor A: An analysis of 8,305 cases of carcinoid tumors, *Cancer* 79:813–829, 1997.

Wang SC, Fidelman N, Nakakura EK: Management of well-differentiated GI neuroendocrine tumors metastatic to the liver, *Semin Oncol* 40:69–74, 2013.

75

Ileostomy, Colostomy, and Gastroenteric Stomas

Martin H. Floch

This chapter discusses ileostomies and colostomies. Gastroenteric anastomoses also are discussed in Chapters 41 to 43 and in Chapter 191. Ileal pouch anal anastomoses are discussed in Chapter 93.

Total or partial *colectomy* with resultant *ileostomy* or *colostomy* is performed primarily to treat inflammatory bowel disease (IBD), familial adenomatous polyposis (FAP), cancer involving pelvic organs, and abdominal trauma. Various types of ileostomies were performed in the past, such as the Kock pouch, but they are no longer popular and rarely used. Temporary colostomies are frequently performed for patients with acute diverticulitis and perforation. These patients often undergo repeat anastomosis and usually have a temporary colostomy for 3 to 6 months. Fig. 75.1 demonstrates the varied function of gastroenteric stomas, depending on the degree of resection.

Since the advent of the Brooke ileostomy, so-called ileostomy malfunction has rarely been seen. The major problem with ileostomy is electrolyte imbalance in the patient with gastroenteritis or food intolerance. After a colostomy has been established and the patient is properly educated to maintain it, colostomy function is compatible with a normal life pattern.

CLINICAL PICTURE

The problems of ileostomy occur when the output may be greatly increased, as occurs in any form of gastroenteritis. The patient can rapidly become dehydrated as the symptoms of abdominal pain and effluence increase but may be corrected when the gastroenteritis is treated.

Colostomy function, once established and regular, rarely represents any problems other than the care of the stoma and peristomal areas. In elderly patients who have undergone colostomy because of incontinence or severe constipation, managing the colostomy is a geriatric care issue. The clinician must always be aware of possible complications, such as intestinal obstruction, from other causes, such as adhesions or recurrent malignancy. When obstruction occurs, it is followed by the classic decrease in output through the ileostomy or colostomy, with resultant distention and all the signs of intestinal obstruction.

DIAGNOSIS

Normal ileostomy output varies from 300 to 800 mL/day. Depending on what the patient eats and drinks, output may increase. However, the ileostomy effluent should be no more than 1 L/day. When it increases dramatically, fluids and electrolytes must be replaced. Ordinarily, sodium chloride and potassium intake are maintained through a regular diet.

Salt loss is a major problem; therefore these patients should be encouraged to increase their salt intake.

When the terminal ileum is resected, vitamin B_{12} malabsorption may occur. Vitamin B_{12} deficiency may be subtle and present as neurologic findings or may be a full-scale megaloblastic anemia. The clinician must be aware of these deficiencies. Vitamin B_{12} should be intramuscularly replaced intermittently in these patients.

TREATMENT AND MANAGEMENT

As mentioned, salt replacement is essential whenever ileostomy effluent increases. Patients with severe output may have to be admitted to an emergency service to receive supplementary intravenous (IV) fluid and electrolyte replacement. After clinical evaluation, most patients can be maintained on adequate oral intake without IV treatment.

The classic World Health Organization liquid formulas that depend on rapid absorption of sodium and glucose can be effective in helping the patient maintain fluid and electrolyte balance. These standard formulas are available in commercial products (e.g., Pedialyte), or they can be made at home (e.g., add salt amount plus table sugar amount to 1 L of fluid, in addition to desired flavoring) (see Chapter 64). Careful monitoring of the patient's blood pressure might be necessary to ensure that vascular compromise has not occurred.

At times, it may be necessary to perform x-ray studies to determine that no obstruction has developed, particularly for patients with a history of adhesions or malignancy. Proper irrigation of the sigmoid colostomy may be necessary to ensure evacuation. This becomes part of the routine colostomy care for patients with low colostomy but not for those with transverse colostomy.

Care of the peristomal skin areas is now routine. All communities have centers from which patients can receive advice for the care of any skin sensitivity or lesions that may occur.

A stoma rarely needs to be revised. However, in certain situations the stoma malfunctions or becomes stenotic, and repair is necessary. This is a surgical decision, and examination is heralded by complaints of pain or symptoms of partial obstruction.

COURSE AND PROGNOSIS

If the ileostomy is performed to manage IBD, trauma, or any benign disease, the prognosis is excellent, and these patients are able to lead a normal life. Similarly, if colostomy is performed for benign disease, patients can live normally. However, if the ostomy is for malignancy or for FAP, monitoring must include checking for recurrence of the neoplasia. Elderly patients often require concomitant geriatric care.

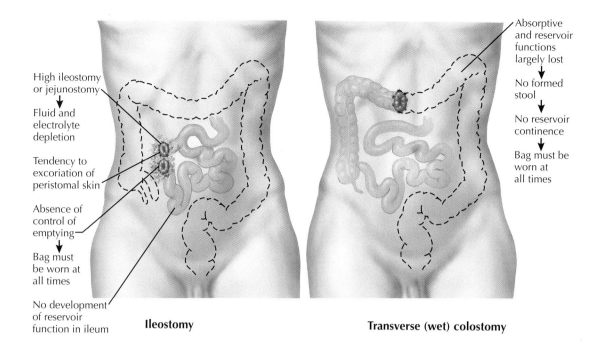

High ileostomy or jejunostomy →
Fluid and electrolyte depletion
Tendency to excoriation of peristomal skin
Absence of control of emptying →
Bag must be worn at all times
No development of reservoir function in ileum

Ileostomy

Absorptive and reservoir functions largely lost →
No formed stool →
No reservoir continence →
Bag must be worn at all times

Transverse (wet) colostomy

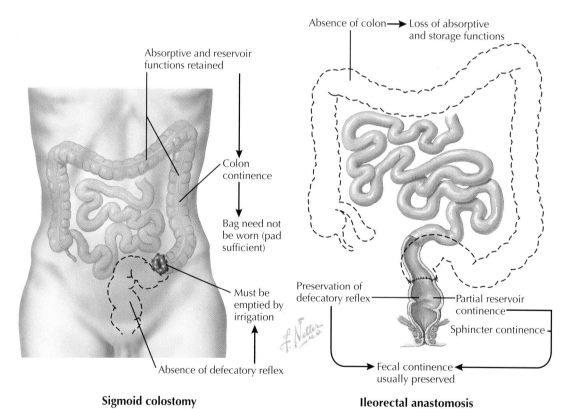

Absorptive and reservoir functions retained →
Colon continence →
Bag need not be worn (pad sufficient)
Must be emptied by irrigation
Absence of defecatory reflex

Sigmoid colostomy

Absence of colon → Loss of absorptive and storage functions

Preservation of defecatory reflex
Partial reservoir continence
Sphincter continence
Fecal continence usually preserved

Ileorectal anastomosis

Fig. 75.1 Physiology of Gastroenteric Stomas.

ADDITIONAL RESOURCES

Araghizadeh F: Ileostomy, colostomy and pouchitis. In Feldman M, Friedman LS, Brandt LJ, editors: *Gastrointestinal and liver disease*, ed 10, Philadelphia, 2016, Saunders-Elsevier, pp 2062–2075.

Brooke BN: Management of ileostomy, including its complications, *Lancet* 2:102–104, 1952.

Kelly KA, Sarr MG, Hinder RA: *Mayo clinic gastrointestinal surgery*, Philadelphia, 2004, Saunders.

Steinhagen E, Colwell J, Cannon LM: Intestinal stomas-postoperative stoma care and peristomal skin complications, *Clin Colon Rectal Surg* 30: 184–192, 2017.

Weise WJ, Serrano EA, Fought J, Gennari FJ: Acute electrolyte and acid-based disorders in patients with ileostomies. A case series, *Am J Kidney Dis* 52: 494–500, 2008.

Colon, Rectum, and Anus

Martin H. Floch

76

Anatomy of the Colon, Rectum, and Anus

Martin H. Floch

THE STRUCTURE AND HISTOLOGY OF THE COLON AND SIGMOID COLON

The large intestine varies in caliber depending on its functional state. Haustra form sacculations that are separated by constricting furrows, so that the lumen bulges and contracts alternately. The caliber is greatest at the commencement of the large intestine (cecum) and narrows toward the rectum. Viewed as a whole, the various parts of the large intestine describe a horseshoe-shaped arc (Fig. 76.1). The total length of the large intestine is approximately 120 to 150 cm (4–5 ft). The four segments of the colon are known as the ascending, transverse, descending, and sigmoid colon. The ascending and descending colon are situated retroperitoneally, and the transverse and sigmoid colon are situated intraperitoneally.

The *ascending colon* averages approximately 15 to 20 cm (6–8 inches) in length and runs in a more or less straight course from the upper lip of the ileocecal valve to the right colic or hepatic flexure, where it passes into the transverse colon. The right colic flexure is usually on the undersurface of the right lobe of the liver. The *transverse colon*, varying from 30 to 60 cm in length, extends from the hepatic flexure to the left colic or splenic flexure, situated slightly more cranially. It lies intraperitoneally and thus is attached to the posterior abdominal wall by a peritoneal fold (mesentery) and the transverse mesocolon, which is very short in the region of the flexures and longest in the middle of the transverse colon. The retroperitoneal *descending colon,* approximately 20 to 25 cm in length, extends downward from the left colic flexure to the iliac crest or beyond it into the left iliac fossa. After running from the angle between the lateral edge of the kidney and the quadratus lumborum muscle and then over the iliac muscle, the colon finally passes in front of the psoas major, crossing the femoral and genitofemoral nerves, and continues with no sharp dividing line into the pelvic colon, or *sigmoid colon,* at which point the colon becomes intraperitoneal again. On its anterior surface, the descending colon is overlapped by the greater omentum and generally by coils of the small intestine.

Corresponding to the structure of the entire intestinal tract, the wall of the colon and cecum consists of a mucosa, a submucosa, a double-layered muscularis, and—depending on its relation to the peritoneum—a serosa and subserosa or an adventitia. The external aspects of the colon, however, differ from those of the small intestine, not only because of its greater caliber but also owing to the appearance of three typical formations: (1) the three taeniae, (2) the haustra, and (3) the appendices epiploicae. The three *taeniae* are longitudinal bands, approximately 8 mm in width, running along the total length of the colon; they exist because the outer muscle layer (i.e., longitudinal muscle) does not constitute a uniform coat. In the region of these three bands, the longitudinal musculature is conspicuous by its thickness, whereas in the spaces between them, it consists merely of a very thin coating. Each taenia is named by reference to its topographic situation in relation to the

transverse colon. The *taenia mesocolica* is situated dorsal to the transverse colon at the line of attachment of the transverse mesocolon and comes to lie dorsomedially on the ascending and descending colon. The *taenia omentalis* is related to the line of attachment of the greater omentum on the ventrocranial surface of the transverse colon and runs along the dorsolateral aspect of the ascending and descending portions. The *taenia libera* is free (not related to any mesenteric or omental attachment) and generally found on the caudal (inferior) surface of the transverse and on the interior aspect of the ascending and descending colon. Where the appendix joins the cecum and where the sigmoid passes into the rectum, the three taeniae merge into one uniform muscle coat, which in the proximal rectum is more strongly developed at its anterior and posterior parts than laterally. Generally the posterior, lateral, and anterior taeniae coalesce into a broad longitudinal band in the region of the middle and lower sigmoid.

The *haustra* are more or less prominent sacculations formed in the spaces between the taeniae. They are separated from each other by constricting circular furrows of varying lengths. The degree of their prominence depends on contraction of the taeniae; the more the taeniae contract, the more marked the haustra intestine becomes, whereas it is almost completely absent when the taeniae are totally relaxed.

The third structural characteristic, the *appendices epiploicae,* consists of grape-shaped subserosal pockets filled with fat and varying in size according to the patient's nutritional state. On the ascending and descending colon, the epiploic appendices are generally distributed in two rows, whereas on the transverse colon, they form only one row along the line of the taenia libera. These fat pads can become extremely large in obese patients.

Corresponding to the furrows between the haustra, visible on the outer surface, the mucous membrane of the large intestine forms crescent-shaped transverse folds known as the *plicae semilunares.* As a rule, the lengths of these semilunar folds correspond to the distance between two taeniae, although they may be longer. Whereas Kerckring folds in the small intestine consist merely of mucosa and submucosa, the plicae semilunares also include the circular muscle layer.

In contrast to the small intestine, the mucosa of the large intestine is not covered with villous projections but contains deep tubular pits that increase in depth toward the rectum and extend as far as the muscularis mucosae. In the submucosa, in addition to the usual structures (blood vessels, lymphatics, Meissner submucosal plexus), numerous solitary lymphatic nodules are present, originating in the reticular tissue with the tunica (lamina) propria and penetrating through the muscularis mucosae into the submucosa. The mucosal epithelium of the large intestine comprises one layer built of tall prismatic cells that, when fixed in a fresh state, display a cuticular border on their surface. Goblet cells are numerous, especially at the base of the pits.

In contrast to the small intestine, the colonic epithelium is relatively simple, but enterochromaffin cells are present, producing serotonin; as

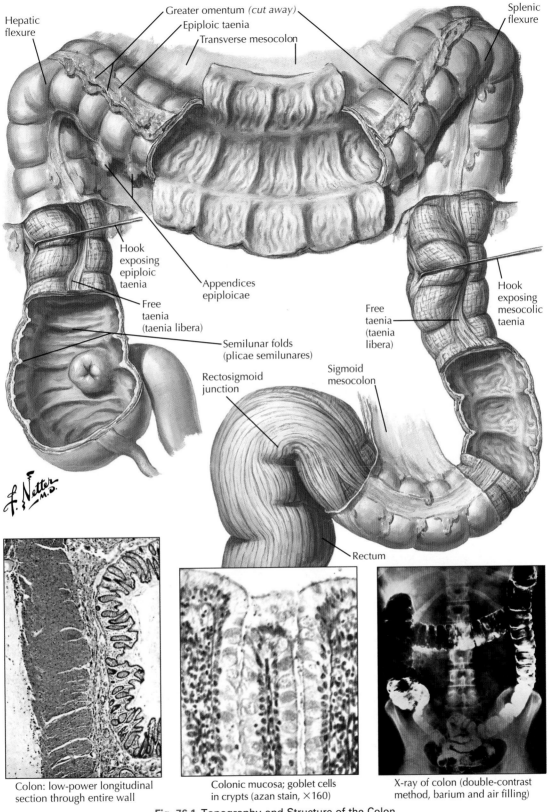

Hepatic flexure

Greater omentum *(cut away)*

Epiploic taenia

Transverse mesocolon

Splenic flexure

Hook exposing epiploic taenia

Free taenia (taenia libera)

Appendices epiploicae

Semilunar folds (plicae semilunares)

Rectosigmoid junction

Sigmoid mesocolon

Free taenia (taenia libera)

Hook exposing mesocolic taenia

Rectum

Colon: low-power longitudinal section through entire wall

Colonic mucosa; goblet cells in crypts (azan stain, ×160)

X-ray of colon (double-contrast method, barium and air filling)

Fig. 76.1 Topography and Structure of the Colon.

are L cells, producing GLI/PYY; and rare D cells, producing somatostatin as well as numerous other substances when studied in detail.

The sigmoid colon is a specialized section of the colon that has a specific motility function, as described in Chapter 83. In populations of the Western world, the sigmoid typically develops diverticula and then the pathology of diverticulitis (see Chapter 90). Colonoscopists are frequently challenged by passage of the instrument through this area because of chronic diverticulosis. Therefore the sigmoid's anatomic structure is of particular importance (Fig. 76.2).

The exact point of commencement of the sigmoid colon—in other words, the transition of descending colon to sigmoid colon—is indefi-

nite. The sigmoid is generally considered to be the part of the large bowel between the descending colon and the rectum that, as a result of its attachment to the mesentery, is freely movable. Because this mesentery is subject to great variations, the extent of the sigmoid also becomes variable. It has been described as beginning at the left iliac crest and the margin of the left psoas muscle or brim of the pelvis minor. Other authorities regard the sigmoid colon as comprising the iliac colon (an iliac portion that has no mesentery) and the pelvic portion (pelvic colon), with a mesentery beginning at the brim of the pelvis minor. The mesenteriolized sigmoid colon generally assumes an omega-shaped flexure arching over the pelvic inlet toward the first or

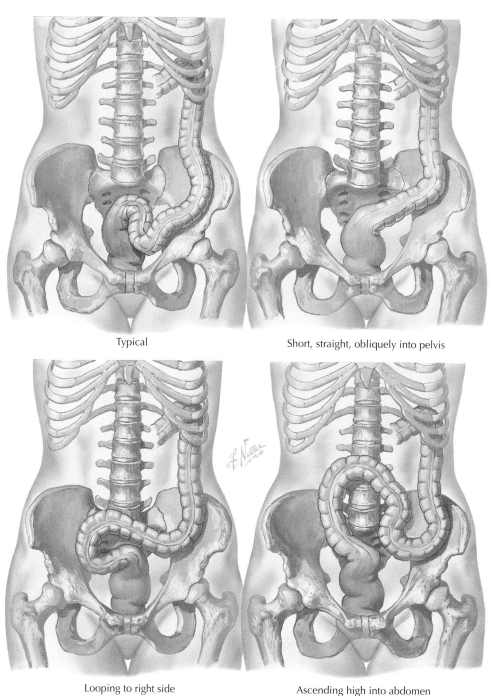

Typical

Short, straight, obliquely into pelvis

Looping to right side

Ascending high into abdomen

Fig. 76.2 Typical Sigmoid Colon and Variations.

second sacral vertebra (S1 or S2) or toward the right side of the pelvis. It finally joins the rectum at an acute angle at about the S3 level. This typical shape of the sigmoid is not a constant finding.

The sigmoid colon may be short, running straight and obliquely into the pelvis, or it may be so long that the loop extends far to the right or, in extreme cases, high into the abdomen. Its average length is approximately 40 cm (16 inches) in adults and 18 cm in children. With the variations mentioned, it may reach 84 cm (and even longer).

The root of the mesentery (i.e., of the mesosigmoid) is variable but, characteristically, starts in the upper left iliac fossa, proceeds downward a few inches, and proceeds mesially and again upward to a point on the psoas muscle, slightly to the left of the fourth lumbar vertebra (L4), where it turns downward into the pelvis. The line of mesenteric attachment takes the shape of an irregular and blunted inverted V. Turning caudally after having reached its highest point, the attachment line of the mesosigmoid courses over the left common iliac artery and vein just above the division of the artery. The length of the mesosigmoid (i.e., distance from root of bowel wall) is extremely variable. A small peritoneal fossa, the *intersigmoid fossa* or recess, is formed by the mesosigmoid while twisting around the vascular pedicle. Rarely, this causes retroperitoneal hernia. Nevertheless, the fossa is a valuable guide to the vascular stalk. The left ureter passes retroperitoneally behind the intersigmoid recess. These relationships are variable but still important when disease occurs in this area.

The looping, arching variations in the sigmoid colon complicate the passage of instruments and make diagnosis difficult when disease occurs in the sigmoid. Diverticulitis can be confused with appendicitis, and diverticulitis with perforation can affect the ureter and pelvic organs.

The mucosa and submucosa of the sigmoid colon are almost identical to the corresponding structures of other parts of the colon. The same holds true for the arrangement of the circular and longitudinal muscle layers except for the most distal parts of the sigmoid colon, where the three flat, longitudinal muscle bands (taeniae), typical of the large intestine, spread out to form the completely encircling longitudinal muscle layer of the rectosigmoid junction. In the same region, the circular layer thickens, in some cases to such an extent that its prominence is alluded to as the "sphincter muscle" of the junction. It is questionable, however, whether this thickening has a true sphincteric function. Throughout the course of the sigmoid colon, the appendices epiploicae of the serous coat diminish gradually in number and size.

The importance of anatomic variations in the sigmoid colon is discussed under colonoscopy (see Chapter 79).

RECTUM AND ANAL CANAL

To understand the numerous diseases and pathologic conditions that occur in the rectal and anal areas, it is essential to understand the details of the anatomy in this area. Functional problems of defecation, vascular disorders of hemorrhoids, and secondary problems of inflammatory bowel disease are all related to this anatomy.

The terminal part of the intestine consists of the rectum and anal canal; the latter extends from the rectosigmoid junction, at the level of the third sacral vertebra (S3), 10 to 15 cm (4–6 inches) downward to the anorectal line (Figs. 76.3 and 76.4). The peritoneal coat continues down from the sigmoid, but only over the anterior and lateral rectal walls, for 1 to 2 cm. A very small mesorectum may occasionally be present, but only close to the rectosigmoid junction. The rectum is thus generally a truly *retroperitoneal* organ.

From the upper anterior rectal surface, the peritoneum is reflected into the interval between the rectum and the bladder in the male or the rectum and uterus in the female, forming the *retrovesical* or *retro-*

uterine recess or pouch, respectively. The depth to which these reflections extend varies an average of 7 cm in males and 4 cm in females. The length and diameter of the rectum vary greatly. The rectum in women is typically much smaller than that in men.

The posterior rectal wall hugs the anterior aspect from the sacrum to the sacrococcygeal articulation, where it comes to lie more or less horizontally over the levator shelf. The anterior wall is comparatively straight and follows, closely aligned, parallel to the posterior cephalic axis of the vagina in the female or the rectogenital septum in the male. The rectal ampullary portion usually has three frequently prominent lateral curvatures, or *flexures.* All three bends correspond to the indentations on the opposite side of the internal rectal wall, which are produced by crescentlike plications of the mucosa and the submucosa, including the circular musculature but not the longitudinal musculature. These more or less marked folds, known as *rectal valves,* encircle approximately one-third to one-half of the rectal circumference. The superior and inferior rectal valves are located on the left side, the superior valves approximately 4 cm below the rectosigmoid junction and the inferior valves approximately 2 to 3 cm above the dentate line. The middle rectal valve usually lies on the right side or slightly above the level of the peritoneal reflection, approximately 6 to 7 cm above the dentate line. Digital examination may reach to the middle valve.

The sphincteric portion of the rectum, often considered to be the upper third of the surgical anal canal, begins at the clinically palpable upper edge of the anorectal muscle ring, usually about 4 cm above the *anal verge,* where the rectum narrows considerably. It extends down to the anatomic *anorectal line* (dentate line), an irregular or undulating demarcation in the rectal mucosa, about 2 to 3 cm above the anal verge. It has been assumed that this line marks the junction of the endodermal primitive gut with the ectodermal proctodeum. However, histologic evidence now shows that this transition of the fetal structures is not abrupt but spreads gradually over several centimeters. Nevertheless the dentate line is visually recognizable, circling the bowel and presenting from 6 to 12 cranial extensions as well as an equal number of intervening caudal sinuosities. The dentate line projects cranially a variable distance, correlative to the rectal columns. These projections may be 1 to 1.5 cm long, and the peninsulas of anoderm they enclose are designated *anal columns.* Interdigitating rectal columns, with their rectal sinuses and anal columns, make a rich network at the junction of the mucosa and the ectodermal tissue. Occasionally the anal columns form papillary projections into the rectal lumen; the name *anal papillae* has been applied to these teatlike processes. In most cases the anal papillae are absent, but when present and exposed to chronic infection, they may hypertrophy and become so prominent as to appear like fibrous polyps, which may even prolapse through the anal canal.

The anatomic anal canal starts at the dentate line and extends to the anal verge, or the margin where the anal tube opens outwardly, or to the circumference. It is difficult to define but is roughly identical to the margin of the anal skin, where hair stops growing.

Within the submucosa of the sphincteric rectal portion, in the submucosal space, lies the internal hemorrhoidal venous plexus. The submucosa is also particularly rich in lymphatics and terminal nerve fibers. Compared with the sigmoid colon, the mucous membrane in the rectum is thicker. It also becomes increasingly red and more vascularized as it reaches the surgical anal canal until its lowermost portion assumes an almost plum color. Its extreme vascularity predisposes it to hemorrhagic disorders.

The cuboidal or columnar epithelium of the rectum extends downward into the upper third of the surgical anal canal, where it changes irregularly above the dentate line into a stratified squamocuboidal type, which directly covers the internal hemorrhoid plexus, the rectal columns, and the sinuses of Morgagni. This epithelial transition zone, which is

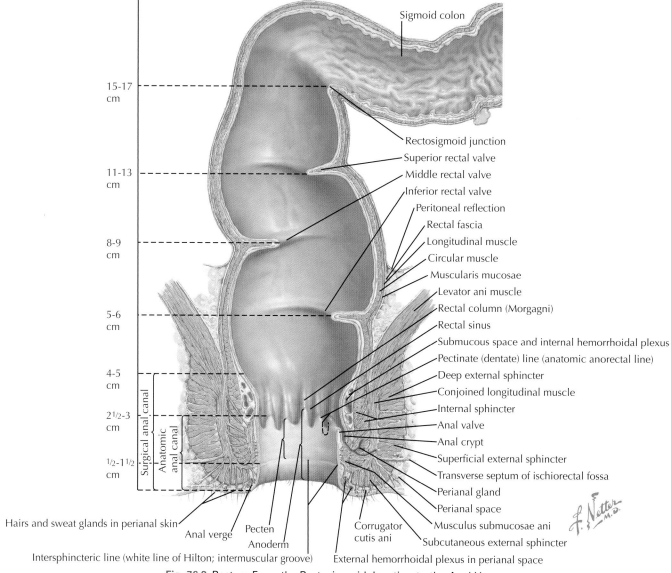

15-17 cm

11-13 cm

8-9 cm

5-6 cm

4-5 cm

2½-3 cm

½-1½ cm

Surgical anal canal

Anatomic anal canal

Sigmoid colon

Rectosigmoid junction
Superior rectal valve
Middle rectal valve
Inferior rectal valve
Peritoneal reflection
Rectal fascia
Longitudinal muscle
Circular muscle
Muscularis mucosae
Levator ani muscle
Rectal column (Morgagni)
Rectal sinus
Submucous space and internal hemorrhoidal plexus
Pectinate (dentate) line (anatomic anorectal line)
Deep external sphincter
Conjoined longitudinal muscle
Internal sphincter
Anal valve
Anal crypt
Superficial external sphincter
Transverse septum of ischiorectal fossa
Perianal gland
Perianal space
Musculus submucosae ani
Subcutaneous external sphincter

Hairs and sweat glands in perianal skin
Anal verge
Pecten
Anoderm
Corrugator cutis ani
External hemorrhoidal plexus in perianal space

Intersphincteric line (white line of Hilton; intermuscular groove)

Fig. 76.3 Rectum From the Rectosigmoid Junction to the Anal Verge.

sometimes referred to as the *anal mucosa,* does not start abruptly and is arranged haphazardly.

In the subepithelial muscular start of the anal canal and the lower rectum, simple tubular and racemose (grapelike) glands may be found, described as perianal glands, intramuscular glands, and anal ducts. Usually the mouths of the ducts open into the bottom of the anal crypts, but the ducts and glands may extend for a variable distance into the adjacent tissues and even into or through the sphincteric muscles ("intramuscular" glands). They are significant as possible sites of anorectal infections and fistulas.

The anorectal musculature is important in understanding many problems with defecation and sphincter control. The significance of the *conjoined longitudinal muscle* for the physiology, pathology, and surgery of the anorectum cannot be overemphasized. Together with the *levator ani muscle,* it exercises its levator and sphincteric action on the anal canal by fibers that take their course through the entire length of the conjoined longitudinal muscle. By its extension at the level of the intermuscular groove and fascial frame in the upper third of the surgical anal canal, the muscle influences the spread of anorectal infec-

tions and the sites of the openings and main tracts of fistulas. Figs. 76.5 and 76.6 help to clarify some of these interrelationships.

The outermost and also most caudad muscular elements of the anal canal belong to the *external anal sphincter,* which is a trilaminar striated muscle. Its three parts—subcutaneous, superficial, and deep—are easily recognized. The *subcutaneous* portion, approximately 3 to 5 mm in diameter, surrounds the anal orifice directly above the anal margin; it is rarely palpable and often discernible as a distinct angular ridge. The male anatomy may show anterior muscular extensions to the median raphe and posterior extensions of the subcutaneous external sphincter may connect with the coccyx. In the female, the subcutaneous portion is more strongly developed, particularly anteriorly, where it forms a prominent angular band that is frequently incised at episiotomy. The subcutaneous portion is functionally integrated with the levator ani muscle through extensions of the conjoined longitudinal muscle, which pass fanlike through it, to terminate as fibers of the corrugator cutis ani. The elliptically shaped *superficial portion,* the next deep layer, is the largest and strongest of the three laminae of the external anal sphincter. It is complex and interdigitating, arises from the tip of the coccyx,

Anal gland and duct opening
into anal crypt

Transition from
squamous to
columnar
epithelium well
above pectinate line

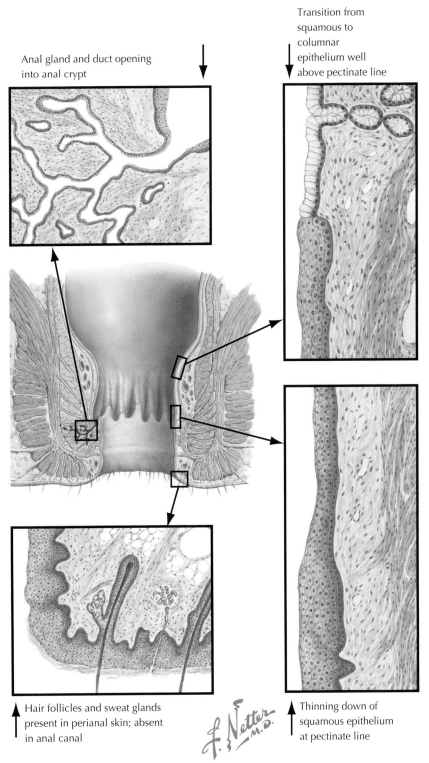

Hair follicles and sweat glands
present in perianal skin; absent
in anal canal

Thinning down of
squamous epithelium
at pectinate line

Fig. 76.4 Histology of the Anal Canal.

and helps form the right and left muscular components of the anococ-cygeal ligament. The *deep portion* of the external anosphincter is mainly an annular muscle bundle usually not attached to the coccyx. It is intimately blended with the puborectalis muscle as the fibers of that muscle pass, sleevelike, around the terminal rectum.

The essential forces that keep the rectoanal canal in position derive from muscles forming the pelvic floor, the levator ani muscle, which

is assumed to be composed of three individual components: pubococ-cygeus, puborectalis, and ileococcygeus muscles. These muscles create a diaphragmatic plane. The action of all these muscles, as demonstrated in Figs. 76.5 and 76.6, are integral for normal defecation. They are also pivotal in retraining when sphincters become incompetent. The levator ani fixes the pelvic floor and acts as a fulcrum, against which increased abdominal pressure—as occurs in lifting, coughing, and defecation—may

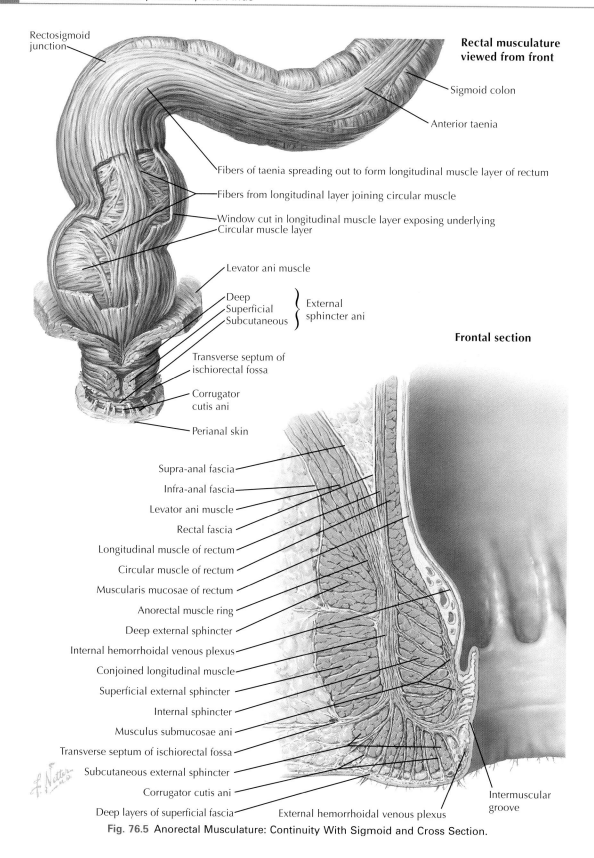

Rectal musculature viewed from front

Rectosigmoid junction

Sigmoid colon

Anterior taenia

Fibers of taenia spreading out to form longitudinal muscle layer of rectum

Fibers from longitudinal layer joining circular muscle

Window cut in longitudinal muscle layer exposing underlying Circular muscle layer

Levator ani muscle

Deep
Superficial
Subcutaneous } External sphincter ani

Transverse septum of ischiorectal fossa

Corrugator cutis ani

Perianal skin

Frontal section

Supra-anal fascia

Infra-anal fascia

Levator ani muscle

Rectal fascia

Longitudinal muscle of rectum

Circular muscle of rectum

Muscularis mucosae of rectum

Anorectal muscle ring

Deep external sphincter

Internal hemorrhoidal venous plexus

Conjoined longitudinal muscle

Superficial external sphincter

Internal sphincter

Musculus submucosae ani

Transverse septum of ischiorectal fossa

Subcutaneous external sphincter

Corrugator cutis ani

Deep layers of superficial fascia

External hemorrhoidal venous plexus

Intermuscular groove

Fig. 76.5 Anorectal Musculature: Continuity With Sigmoid and Cross Section.

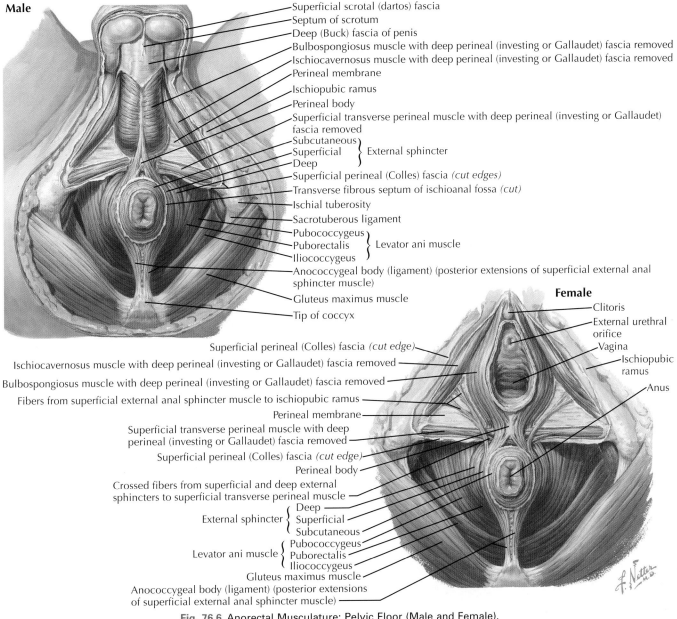

Male

- Superficial scrotal (dartos) fascia
- Septum of scrotum
- Deep (Buck) fascia of penis
- Bulbospongiosus muscle with deep perineal (investing or Gallaudet) fascia removed
- Ischiocavernosus muscle with deep perineal (investing or Gallaudet) fascia removed
- Perineal membrane
- Ischiopubic ramus
- Perineal body
- Superficial transverse perineal muscle with deep perineal (investing or Gallaudet) fascia removed
- Subcutaneous ⎫
- Superficial ⎬ External sphincter
- Deep ⎭
- Superficial perineal (Colles) fascia *(cut edges)*
- Transverse fibrous septum of ischioanal fossa *(cut)*
- Ischial tuberosity
- Sacrotuberous ligament
- Pubococcygeus ⎫
- Puborectalis ⎬ Levator ani muscle
- Iliococcygeus ⎭
- Anococcygeal body (ligament) (posterior extensions of superficial external anal sphincter muscle)
- Gluteus maximus muscle
- Tip of coccyx

Female

- Clitoris
- External urethral orifice
- Vagina
- Ischiopubic ramus
- Anus

- Superficial perineal (Colles) fascia *(cut edge)*
- Ischiocavernosus muscle with deep perineal (investing or Gallaudet) fascia removed
- Bulbospongiosus muscle with deep perineal (investing or Gallaudet) fascia removed
- Fibers from superficial external anal sphincter muscle to ischiopubic ramus
- Perineal membrane
- Superficial transverse perineal muscle with deep perineal (investing or Gallaudet) fascia removed
- Superficial perineal (Colles) fascia *(cut edge)*
- Perineal body
- Crossed fibers from superficial and deep external sphincters to superficial transverse perineal muscle
- External sphincter ⎰ Deep / Superficial / Subcutaneous
- Levator ani muscle ⎰ Pubococcygeus / Puborectalis / Iliococcygeus
- Gluteus maximus muscle
- Anococcygeal body (ligament) (posterior extensions of superficial external anal sphincter muscle)

Fig. 76.6 Anorectal Musculature: Pelvic Floor (Male and Female).

be exerted. Levator ani integration with the other muscles is essential for maintaining the integrity of rectal and urogenital function.

VASCULAR, LYMPHATIC, AND NERVE SUPPLY OF THE LARGE INTESTINE

As in the small intestine and except for the rectum, major arterial vessels that supply the colon are usually paralleled by similar venous vessels, where the venous drainage is rich (Fig. 76.7 and 76.8).

The *middle colic artery,* according to conventional descriptions, arises at the lower border of the pancreas and passes into the right half of the transverse mesocolon, where, at a variable distance from the colonic wall, it typically divides into two branches. One branch courses to the right to anastomose with the ascending branch of the right colic artery and the other branch turns to the left to anastomose with the ascending branch of the left colic artery, derived from the inferior mesenteric artery (see Figs. 76.7 and 76.8). Both divisions of the middle colic

undergo subsequent branchings, forming primary and secondary arcades that direct the arteriae rectae to the transverse colon. This description, however, does not apply to all cases. As a separate branch of the superior mesenteric artery, the middle colic artery, is frequently absent. In such cases the artery is usually replaced by a common right middle colic trunk and occasionally by a branch of the left colic; at times the latter reaches the hepatic flexure. An accessory middle colic artery may be present, generally arising from the aorta above the chief middle colic artery; it usually anastomoses with branches from the left colic artery, forming a secondary arc in the left transverse mesocolon. There may be many variations of these formations.

Conventionally the *right colic artery* is described as rising from the superior mesenteric artery and dividing, halfway between its origin and the ascending colon, into a descending branch that unites with the ileocolic artery and an ascending branch that unites with the left branch of the middle colic artery (see Figs. 76.7 and 76.8). Again, variations are seen in these formations. In as many as 18% of studies, the right

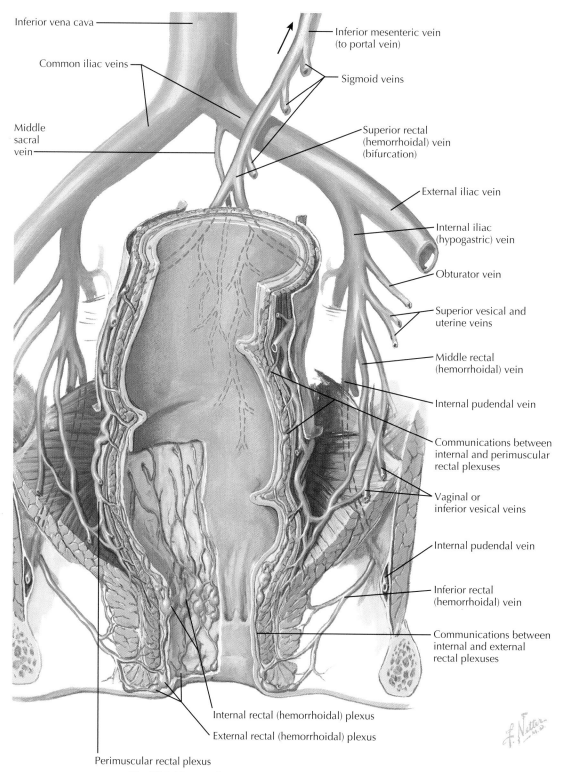

Inferior vena cava

Common iliac veins

Middle sacral vein

Inferior mesenteric vein (to portal vein)

Sigmoid veins

Superior rectal (hemorrhoidal) vein (bifurcation)

External iliac vein

Internal iliac (hypogastric) vein

Obturator vein

Superior vesical and uterine veins

Middle rectal (hemorrhoidal) vein

Internal pudendal vein

Communications between internal and perimuscular rectal plexuses

Vaginal or inferior vesical veins

Internal pudendal vein

Inferior rectal (hemorrhoidal) vein

Communications between internal and external rectal plexuses

Internal rectal (hemorrhoidal) plexus

External rectal (hemorrhoidal) plexus

Perimuscular rectal plexus

Fig. 76.7 Venous Drainage of the Large Intestine and Rectum.

colic artery is entirely absent. There are many variations in the integration of the flow to the right column from the superior mesenteric artery and to the left colon from the inferior mesenteric artery. However, the ileocolic artery, the last branch of the superior mesenteric on its right side, is always present. Therefore, as a rule, there are two chief arterial branches, the ascending colic and the descending ileocolic. Ten different sites of origin and courses are described for the appendicular artery.

The *inferior mesenteric artery* typically arises from the anterior aspect or left side of the aorta, 3 to 5 cm above its bifurcation, which is situated on the level of the lower third of the fourth lumbar vertebra (L4). The inferior mesenteric proceeds down and forks into the last of the sigmoid arteries and the superior rectal artery. This creates a rich blood supply in the rectum (see Figs. 76.7 and 76.8). The sigmoid arteries—in combination with the right pudendal arteries, the rectal arteries, and

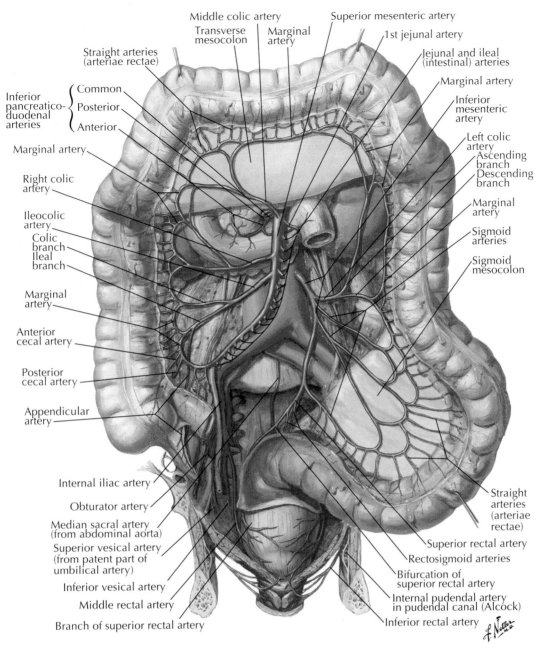

Middle colic artery
Transverse mesocolon
Marginal artery
Superior mesenteric artery
1st jejunal artery
Jejunal and ileal (intestinal) arteries
Straight arteries (arteriae rectae)
Marginal artery
Inferior mesenteric artery
Inferior pancreatico-duodenal arteries { Common / Posterior / Anterior }
Left colic artery
Ascending branch
Descending branch
Marginal artery
Marginal artery
Right colic artery
Ileocolic artery
Colic branch
Ileal branch
Sigmoid arteries
Sigmoid mesocolon
Marginal artery
Anterior cecal artery
Posterior cecal artery
Appendicular artery
Straight arteries (arteriae rectae)
Internal iliac artery
Obturator artery
Median sacral artery (from abdominal aorta)
Superior vesical artery (from patent part of umbilical artery)
Inferior vesical artery
Middle rectal artery
Branch of superior rectal artery
Superior rectal artery
Rectosigmoid arteries
Bifurcation of superior rectal artery
Internal pudendal artery in pudendal canal (Alcock)
Inferior rectal artery

Fig. 76.8 Arterial Circulation of the Large Intestine.

some of the blood vessels that supply the muscles of the pelvis—create a rich arterial blood flow to the rectum and anal area.

The venous drainage of major arteries largely parallels the arterial drainage except for the rectum and anus, where the same veins and arteries are present but rich internal and external *rectal hemorrhoidal plexuses* serve essentially the mucosal, submucosal, and perianal tissue. The plexuses encompass the rectal circumference completely, but the greatest aggregation of small and large veins takes place in the rectal columns. Generally the vessels returning the blood from the plexuses course 10 cm upward in the submucosa. Branches derived from these veins pierce the muscular layer of the rectum and communicate with the perimuscular plexus and directly with the superior rectal vein. Because these piercings of the musculature occur mostly above the level at which the perimuscular plexus connects with the middle rectal veins, it is apparent that the latter assist in draining the internal rectal

plexus. The blood of this plexus returns mostly through the superior rectal vein.

Dilatation of the internal rectal plexus results in internal hemorrhoids (see Chapter 102). Dilatation of the external rectal plexus or thrombosis of its vessels produces external hemorrhoids. The two plexuses (internal and external rectal) are separated by the muscularis submucosa ani and the dense tissue of the rectum, but they communicate with each other through these tissues by slender vessels that increase in size and number with age and that are voluminous in the presence of hemorrhoids. Further, the inferior and middle rectal veins and their collecting vessels, the internal pudendal veins, have valves, whereas the superior rectal veins are devoid of such valves. Increased pressure in the portal vein, as in cirrhosis or other causes of portal hypertension, may reverse the circulation in the superior rectal veins. Portal blood flows through the superior rectal veins, traversing the rectal plexus and then being carried away by the inferior rectal vein and shunted through the internal iliac vein of the cable system.

Lymph Drainage

The lymphatic drainage of the large intestine is complex. The first important regional lymph nodes are the ileocolic, right colic, middle colic, and left colic, pertaining to the respective regions of the large intestine. They start with a chain of nodes, collectively called *pericolic nodes,* which lie along the medial margin of the ascending, transverse, and descending colon; they lie dorsal to these portions of the gut in the retroperitoneal tissue and, to a lesser extent, in the mesosigmoid. Each of these groups of lymph nodes pours its lymph into lymph ducts that run side by side with the respective blood vessels in a median direction toward the large prevertebral vessels. Lymphatics emanating from the rectum and anal canal run in two main directions. In the lower part of the anal canal, they pass over the peritoneum, alongside the scrotum or labia majora and the inner margin of the thigh, to the superior inguinal nodes. The upper part of the anal canal is drained cranially into preaortic and inferior mesenteric nodes.

Innervation

The innervation of the large intestine is similar to that of the small intestine, the central nervous system, and the intrinsic nerves of the colon, as described in Section IV.

ADDITIONAL RESOURCES

Bass LM, Wershil BK: Anatomy, histology, embryology, and developmental anomalies of the small and large intestine. In Feldman M, Friedman LS, Brandt LJ, editors: *Gastrointestinal and liver disease*, ed 10, Philadelphia, 2016, Saunders-Elsevier, pp 1649–1678.

Bharocha AE, Hasler WL: Motility of the small intestine and colon. In Podolsky DK, Camilleri M, Fitz JG, et al, editors: *Yamada's textbook of gastroenterology*, ed 6, Hoboken, New Jersey, 2016, John Wiley and Sons Ltd, pp 367–385.

Mills SE: *Histology for the pathologist*, 4th ed, Philadelphia, 2012, Lippincott, Williams and Wilkins.

Rao SSC: Fecal incontinence. In Feldman M, Friedman LS, Brandt LJ, editors: *Gastrointestinal and liver disease*, ed 10, Philadelphia, 2016, Saunders-Elsevier, pp 251–269.

Vmansky K, Matthews JB: Colon: anatomy and structural anomalies. In Podolsky DK, Camilleri M, Fitz JG, et al, editors: *Yamada's textbook of gastroenterology*, ed 6, Hoboken, New Jersey, 2016, John Wiley and Sons Ltd, pp 93–107.

77

Secretory, Digestive, and Absorptive Functions of the Colon and Colonic Flora

Martin H. Floch

The mucous membrane of the large intestine secretes an opalescent, mucoid, alkaline fluid composed essentially of water, mucus, and electrolytes (Fig. 77.1). Chemical and mechanical irritation enhances the secretion of this fluid. The colonic epithelium also has an excretory function in that it is used as an elimination route for metals (lead, mercury, bismuth; possibly silver and calcium). The mucous gel consists of large mucin glycoproteins, trefoil factors, defensins, secretory immunoglobulins, electrolytes, phospholipids, bacteria, sloughing epithelial cells, and numerous other components still to be identified. This mucoid gel layer serves as a protective coat that is secreted primarily by the goblet cells.

The digestive function of the colon is significant. Varying but usually small amounts of fat and proteins, proteases, peptones, and peptides escape digestion in the jejunum and ileum and may be digested in the colon by the microbiota, which contain the enzymes capable of breaking down these substances. Putrefactive action of bacteria can produce fatty acids. Certain amino acids—primarily tryptophan but also tyrosine, phenylalanine, and histidine—can be digested to form such compounds as skatole, indole, phenol, creosol, and histamine. These products may be absorbed in relatively small amounts by the mucosa and can be transported to the liver, where they are detoxified. They are usually excreted by the kidney in the form of sulfates and glucuronides. The bulk of this material remains in the colonic lumen and leaves the intestine with the feces. Indole, skatole, mercaptan, hydrogen sulfide, and breakdown products of cystine give the feces its unpleasant odor. The color of the feces derives chiefly from stercobilin, the bacterial reduction product of bile pigment.

The greatest activity of fermentation in the colon is the breakdown of starch and nonstarch polysaccharides, such as cellulose. These compounds are not broken down by human enzymes but by enzymes in the microbiota, producing the very important *short-chain fatty acids* (SCFAs). The molecular ratio of *butyric* acid, *acetic* acid, and *propionic* acid is approximately 20:60:20. Diets that include a large proportion of fiber, which contains many nonstarch polysaccharides, nurture the bacterial flora, and more SCFAs are produced. Depending on the amount of soluble or insoluble dietary fiber, the range of intake can be anywhere from 5% to 20% of polysaccharide eaten. This leads to the production of 300 to 800 mmol of SCFA, which makes up as much as 5% to 10% of the host's energy. Most of the bran and insoluble types of fiber are not broken down and remain in the feces to form bulk and hold onto water. Butyric acid is the preferred fuel of colonocytes, and acetic acid and propionic acid are involved in cholesterol synthesis and control when they are absorbed into the hepatic circulation.

The main absorptive function of the colon is to balance the excretion of electrolytes and water by absorbing large amounts of fluid that reach the cecum with sodium. Elaborate mechanisms of epithelial chloride-bicarbonate and sodium-potassium exchange permit homeostatic balancing for the host. A series of sodium-hydrogen exchanges enables sodium absorption. Intercellular cyclic adenosine monophosphate (cAMP) and calcium regulate sodium-hydrogen exchanges. In addition, substances such as nitric oxide, protein kinases, and cytoskeletal proteins all affect sodium-hydrogen exchange. The final effect of water excretion is that the average 1500 to 2000 mL of liquid that reaches the cecum is absorbed and, depending on the amount of dietary fiber and stool bulk from fiber (bacterial or insoluble bran), leaves a stool of 100 to 400 mL. SCFAs are the principal luminal products of the colon; they are heavily involved in this balance of water and electrolyte absorption and enhance sodium absorption. SCFAs appear to be able to diffuse readily across membranes and are absorbed by several mechanisms. Because other water-soluble substances can also be absorbed through these mechanisms, some drugs (e.g., chloral hydrate, anticholinergics, xanthenes, digitalis glycosides) are administered rectally.

The *enteropathic circulation* includes the secretion of bile acids and bile into the upper small intestine, with the major reabsorption occurring in the ileum. It continues to some degree in the ascending colon, where primary and secondary bile acids are reabsorbed.

In summary, a major function of the large intestine is to absorb fluid and balance electrolytes. This occurs primarily in the ascending colon. Colonic flora has a major role in fermenting starch and nonstarch polysaccharides to produce SCFAs. SCFAs are the primary fuel for the colonocyte and are absorbed into the enterohepatic circulation, affecting cholesterol metabolism. Dietary fiber acts to nurture the bacterial flora and to increase the bulk of fecal material so that stool bulk and content are maintained for normal colonic motility and function.

COLONIC MICROFLORA

The gastrointestinal tract and the organisms within its lumen constitute an *ecologic unit*, often referred to as an *intestinal microecology*. The metabolism and function of this ecologic unit affect the host. The four interacting components of the unit are the wall of the gut, the fluid secreted into the lumen, the food that enters the gut, and the intestinal microbiota.

Anaerobic culture and RNA/DNA techniques enable the identification of the most common aerobic and anaerobic organisms in humans. An estimated 500 species reside in the large intestine, and the healthy bowel contains approximately 100 trillion organisms. Although the flora in the distal ileum is rich, it is greatest in the colon. Anaerobes are approximately 100 to 1000 times more abundant than aerobes. New techniques have enabled us to determine that the anaerobic-predominant organisms are made up of the five Bacteroides and Firmicutes. Major anaerobic species are anaerobic cocci, *Bacteroides, Eubacterium, Bifidobacterium, Lactobacillus*, Veillonellae, and *Fusobacterium*. Major aerobic organisms belong to species of *Escherichia, Enterococcus, Streptococcus, Bacillus, Citrobacter*, and *Klebsiella*.

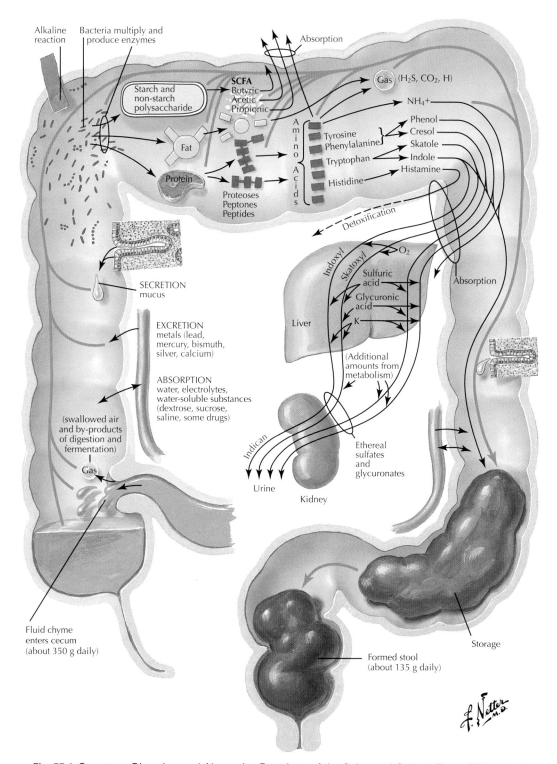

Fig. 77.1 Secretory, Digestive, and Absorptive Functions of the Colon and Colonic Flora. *SCFA,* Short-chain fatty acid.

The major role identified for the bacterial flora is fermenting undigested carbohydrates and converting some fats and proteins into waste products. It is now appreciated, however, that carbohydrate fermentation products are absorbed and can make up as much as 5% to 10% of absorbed energy. Also, a major role for the bacteria is to deconjugate and transfer bile acids to the enterohepatic circulation.

ADDITIONAL RESOURCES

Carroll IM, Ringel-Kulka T, Siddle JP, et al: Alterations in composition and diversity of the intestinal microbiota in patients with diarrhea-predominant irritable bowel syndrome, *Neurogastroenterol Motil* 24:521–530, E248, 2012.

Cummings J: Quantitating short-chain fatty acid production in humans. In Binder HJ, Cummings J, Soergel KH, editors: *Short-chain fatty acids*, London, 1994, Kluwer Academic, pp 11–19.

Floch MH, Gershengoren W, Freedman LR: Methods for the quantitative study of the aerobic and anaerobic intestinal bacterial flora in man, *Yale J Biol Med* 41:50–59, 1968.

Hill C, Shanahan F: The enteric microbiota. In Feldman M, Friedman LS, Brandt LJ, editors: *Gastrointestinal and liver disease*, ed 10, Philadelphia, 2016, Saunders-Elsevier, pp 28–35.

Ho SD, Shekels LL: Mucin and goblet cell function. In Koch TR, editor: *Colonic diseases*, Totowa, NJ, 2003, Humana Press, pp 53–71.

Moote WEC, Holdeman LB: Human fecal flora: the normal flora of 20 Japanese-Hawaiians, *Appl Microbiol* 27:961–979, 1974.

Parkes GC, Rayment NB, Hudspith BN, et al: Distinct microbial populations exist in the mucosa-associated microbiota of sub-groups of irritable bowel syndrome, *Neurogastroenterol Motil* 24:31–39, 2012.

Ramaswamy K, Harig JM, Soergel KH: Short-chain fatty acid transport by human intestinal apical membranes. In Binder HJ, Cummings J, Soergel KH, editors: *Short-chain fatty acids*, London, 1994, Kluwer Academic, pp 93–103.

Sundin J, Rangel I, Fuentes S, et al: Altered faecal and mucosal microbial composition in post-infectious irritable bowel syndrome patients correlates with mucosal lymphocyte phenotypes and psychological distress, *Aliment Pharmacol Ther* 41:342–351, 2015.

Vandeputte D, Falony G, Vieira-Silva S, et al: Stool consistency is strongly associated with gut microbiota richness and composition, enterotypes and bacterial growth rates, *Gut* 65:57–62, 2016.

Wells AL, Sauliner DMA, Gibson GR: Gastrointestinal microflora and interactions with gut mucosa. In Gibson GR, Roberfroid MB, editors: *Handbook of prebiotics*, Boca Raton, Fla, 2008, CRC Press/Taylor & Francis Group, pp 13–38.

78

Probiotics, Prebiotics, and the Microbiota

Martin H. Floch

Probiotics are live microbial food supplements that benefit the individual by improving microbial balance (Fig. 78.1). They are usually strains of lactobacilli or bifidobacteria, but yeasts such as *Saccharomyces* have also been used. Probiotics are typically administered in yogurts, capsules, or powders and have the following properties:

1. Consist of bacteria of human origin
2. Survive passage through the gut
3. Resist stomach secretions, hydrochloric acid, and liver bile acids
4. Produce substances called *adhesins,* which help probiotics adhere to human intestinal cells and help the epithelium prevent invasion by pathogens
5. Have the ability to colonize the human intestinal tract, particularly within the mucous layer
6. Produce antimicrobial substances and antagonize carcinogenic and pathogenic flora
7. Are safe to use in large amounts

The concept of probiotics was first developed by Metchnikoff, who won the Nobel Prize in 1907 for his theory that aging was related to the products of putrefactive bacteria in the intestine. He proposed administering good bacteria to prevent putrefaction and to enhance fermentation. Kiploff promulgated the importance of lactobacilli and, in the last half of the 20th century, Roetger stressed their therapeutic application. Stillwell finally coined the term "probiotic," which was accepted and finally used by Parker. In 1989, Fuller defined probiotics as "microbial supplements that benefit the host animal by improving its intestinal microbial balance." Studies reveal that the benefits of probiotics may derive from local intestinal effects as well as their resultant systemic action.

Numerous organisms are used as probiotics, alone or in combination (Box 78.1). Anecdotal evidence and findings from human and animal experiments propose that all the listed probiotics may be helpful. More studies are becoming available; those usually accepted as clinically important are described here.

Probiotics improve immune status. Their growth clearly increases immunoglobulin A (IgA) production, and they have been used to help treat and prevent childhood infectious diarrhea. They are also reportedly helpful in treating atopy and cow's milk allergy. They are used to prevent and treat antibiotic-associated diarrhea and *Clostridium difficile* colitis, which occurs after antibiotic treatment in a significant percentage of hospital patients. *Lactobacillus* GG and *Saccharomyces* have been used for this purpose.

Genitourinary infections have been prevented and treated successfully with yogurts and *Lactobacillus acidophilus.* Results have been mixed, although studies show excellent findings with vaginal and oral use of different organisms. A combination of eight probiotic organisms, VSL#3 has been used successfully to treat pouchitis (see Chapter 93). Some have treated inflammatory bowel disease with *Escherichia coli* strain Nissle, and others have used *Lactobacillus* in combination with bifido-

bacteria. Probiotics have also been used for irritable bowel syndrome; *Bifidobacterium infantis* is reported as helpful, as are *B. animalis* and *Lactobacillus plantarum* in a yogurt product (Table 78.1).

The gastrointestinal tract is an ecologic unit that is significantly affected by the use of probiotics and foods. Alteration of the bacterial flora can result in disease. The use of prebiotics and probiotics can correct that disease process in select patients. The field of prebiotics has just emerged, and use of prebiotic products to nurture organisms is beginning to prove effective. A combination of a probiotic with a prebiotic is referred to as a *symbiotic.*

The original definition of prebiotics was presented by Gibson and Roberfroid in 1995 and has persisted. "Non-digestible dietary ingredients that beneficially affect the host by selectively stimulating the growth and/or activity of one of a limited number of bacteria in the colon, thus improve host health." This definition includes substances that are natural as well as those produced chemically. This original definition is still accepted. Therefore, many dietary fiber substances are included under it.

Dietary fiber is defined in many places in the literature, but it depends on the chemical analysis employed and the substances that result from

---

BOX 78.1   Probiotic Microorganisms

Lactobacillus Species	*Bifidobacterium* Species
L. acidophilus	B. adolescentis
L. amylovorus	B. animalis
L. casei	B. lactis
L. crispatus	B. bifidum
L. gasseri	B. breve
L. johnsonii	B. infantis
L. paracasei	B. longum
L. plantarum	
L. reuteri	
L. rhamnosus	

Other Lactic Acid Bacteria

Enterococcus faecium
Leuconostoc mesenteroides
Streptococcus thermophilus

Nonlactic Acid Bacteria

Bacillus cereus var. *toyoi*
Escherichia coli strain *Nissle*
Propionibacterium freudenreichii
Saccharomyces cerevisiae
Saccharomyces boulardii

Modified from Floch MH, Hong-Curtiss J: Probiotics in functional foods and gastrointestinal disorders, *Curr Treat Opt Gastroenterol* 5:311-321, 2002.

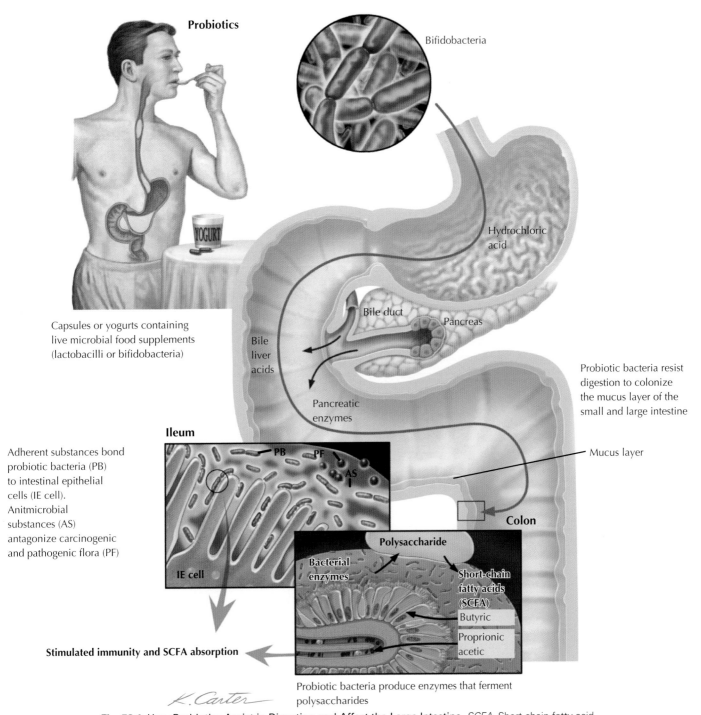

Probiotics

Bifidobacteria

Hydrochloric acid

Bile duct

Pancreas

Capsules or yogurts containing live microbial food supplements (lactobacilli or bifidobacteria)

Bile liver acids

Probiotic bacteria resist digestion to colonize the mucus layer of the small and large intestine

Pancreatic enzymes

Mucus layer

Ileum

Adherent substances bond probiotic bacteria (PB) to intestinal epithelial cells (IE cell). Anitmicrobial substances (AS) antagonize carcinogenic and pathogenic flora (PF)

PB   PF

AS

IE cell

Colon

Polysaccharide

Bacterial enzymes

Short-chain fatty acids (SCFA)

Butyric

Proprionic acetic

Stimulated immunity and SCFA absorption

Probiotic bacteria produce enzymes that ferment polysaccharides

K. Carter

Fig. 78.1 How Probiotics Assist in Digestion and Affect the Large Intestine. *SCFA,* Short-chain fatty acid.

that analysis. The classic definition put forth by Trowell can be summarized as "plant non-starch, polysaccharides that are not digested by human enzymes." This is a simple but good definition and includes cell wall substances such as cellulose, semicelluloses, pectin, lignin, as well as intracellular polysaccharides such as gums and mucilages. The term *resistant starch* is often used but refers again to starch and is not digested by human enzymes that reach the colon.

Probiotics are generally regarded as safe. Others have been approved by the consensus opinion of specialists and recommended for probiotic use. These are listed in Table 78.1.

MICROBIOTA

Reports published by Turnbaugh and colleagues stress the importance of these organisms. There are now publications in the literature that outline the role of these organisms in the gastrointestinal tract, their functions and physiology, and their use. It is clear that the microbiota are pivotal in determining the health, immunologic response, and metabolism of the host. As research evolves, much more information regarding their importance and relation to disease will become known. Research studies have been extensive, and we now know that the

TABLE 78.1 Probiotics With Reported Clinical Relevance

Probiotic	Clinical Relevance
Lactobacillus acidophilus	Prevention of recurrent candidal vaginitis
L. acidophilus LCI	Adherence to human intestinal cells, balancing of intestinal microflora, immune-enhancing
L. acidophilus NCFO1748	Treatment of constipation and decreased food enzymes Prevention of radiotherapy-related diarrhea
L. acidophilus NFCM	Treatment of lactose intolerance, production of bacteriocins, decreased fecal enzyme activity, high lactase activity
L. casei Shirota	Balancing of intestinal bacteria, decreased fecal enzymes, control of superficial bladder cancer
L. rhamnosus GG	Treatment and prevention of rotavirus diarrhea and relapsing *Clostridium difficile* colitis Prevention of acute diarrhea and antibiotic-associated diarrhea Treatment of atopy and milk allergy eczema
Bifidobacterium bifidum	Treatment of rotavirus and viral diarrhea Balancing of intestinal microflora
Lactobacillus reuteri	Colonizing of intestinal tract, shortening duration of rotavirus diarrhea
Saccharomyces boulardi	Prevention and treatment of *Clostridium difficile* colitis and antibiotic-associated diarrhea
Escherichia coli strain Nissle	Used in inflammatory bowel disease to maintain remission
Eight strains VSL 3 (see text and reference)	Decreased recurrence of pouchitis
Lactobacillus plantarum *Bifidobacterium infantis*	Decreased symptoms of irritable bowel syndrome

Modified from Floch MH, Hong-Curtiss J: Probiotics in functional foods and gastrointestinal disorders, *Curr Treat Opt Gastroenterol* 5:311-321, 2002.

microbiota can be used to treat *Clostridium difficile* and liver disease. These are important advances, and the interested reader is referred to the following extensive list of references.

ADDITIONAL RESOURCES

Biblioni R, Fedorak RN, Tannock GW, et al: VSL#3 probiotic-mixture induces remission in patients with active ulcerative colitis, *Am J Gastroenterol* 100:1539–1546, 2005.

Brandt LJ, Aroniadis OC, Mellow M, et al: Long-term follow-up of colonoscopic fecal microbiota transplant for recurrent *Clostridium difficile* infection, *Am J Gastroenterol* 107:1079–1187, 2012.

Donohue D: Safety of probiotic organisms. In Lee YK, Salminen S, editors: *Handbook of probiotics and prebiotics*, ed 2, Hoboken, NJ, 2009, John Wiley & Sons, Inc, pp 75–95.

Eiseman B, Silen W, Bascom GS, et al: Fecal enema as an adjunct in the treatment of pseudomembranous enterocolitis, *Surgery* 44:854–859, 1958.

Floch MH: The role of prebiotics and probiotics in gastrointestinal disease, *Gastroenterol Clin North Am* 47:179–191, 2018.

Floch MH, Binder HJ, Filborn B, Gershengoren W: The effect of bile acids on intestinal microflora, *Am J Clin Nutr* 25:1418–1426, 1972.

Floch MH, Montrose DC: Use of probiotics in humans: an analysis of the literature, *Gastroenterol Clin North Am* 34:547–570, 2005.

Floch MH, Ringel Y, Walker WA: *The microbiota in gastrointestinal pathophysiology; Implications for human health, Prebiotics, Probiotics, and dysbiosis*, Cambridge, MA, 2017, Elsevier Inc.

Floch MH, Walker WA, Guandalini S, et al: Recommendations for probiotic use—2008, *J Clin Gastroenterol* 42:S104–S108, 2008.

Floch MH, Walker WA, Madsen K, et al: Recommendations for probiotic use—2011 update, *J Clin Gastroenterol* 45:S168–S171, 2011.

Floch MH, Walker WA, Sanders ME, et al: Recommendations for probiotic use—2015 update; proceedings and consensus opinion, *J Clin Gastroenterol* 49:S69–S73, 2015.

Gibson CR, Roberfroid MB: Dietary modulation of the human colonic microflora: introducing the concept of prebiotics, *J Nutr* 125:401, 1995.

Gibson GR, Roberfroid MB: *Handbook of prebiotics*, Boca Raton, Fla, 2008, CRC Press/Taylor & Francis Group.

Gionchetti P, Rizzello F, Morselli C, et al: High-dose probiotics for the treatment of active pouchitis, *Dis Colon Rectum* 50:2075–2084, 2007.

Guandalini S: Probiotics for prevention and treatment of diarrhea, *J Clin Gastroenterol* 45:S149–S153, 2011.

Hamilton MJ, Weingarden AR, Sadowsky MJ, et al: Standardized frozen preparation for transplantation of fecal microbiota for recurrent *Clostridium difficile* infection, *Am J Gastroenterol* 107:761–767, 2012.

Lee CH, Steiner T, Petrof EO, et al: Frozen vs. fresh fecal microbiota transplantation and clinical resolution of diarrhea in patients with recurrent *Clostridium difficile* infection: a randomized clinical trial, *JAMA* 315:142–149, 2016.

MacFarlane GT, Cummings JH: Probiotics and prebiotics: can regulating the activities of intestinal bacteria benefit health? *BMJ* 318:999–1003, 1999.

Miele E, Pascarell F, Giannetti E, et al: Effect of a probiotic preparation (VSL#3) on induction and maintenance of remission in children with ulcerative colitis, *Am J Gastroenterol* 104:437–443, 2009.

Miloh T: Probiotics in pediatric liver disease, *J Clin Gastroenterol* 49:S33–S36, 2015.

Reid G: Probiotics, agents to protect the urogenital tract against infection, *Am J Clin Nutr* 73:437S–443S, 2001.

Shukla S, Shukla A, Mehboob S, Guha S: Meta-analysis: the effects of gut flora modulation using prebiotics, probiotics and synbiotics on minimal hepatic encephalopathy, *Aliment Pharmacol Ther* 33:662–671, 2011.

Sood A, Midha V, Makharia GK, et al: The probiotic preparation VSL#3 induces remission in patients with mild to moderately active ulcerative colitis, *Clin Gastroenterol Hepatol* 7:1202–1209, 2009.

Spiller GA: *CRC handbook of dietary fiber in human nutrition*, ed 2, Boca Raton, FL, 1992, CRC Press, pp 15–18.

Surawicz CM, Brandt LJ, Binion DG, et al: Guidelines for diagnosis, treatment, and prevention of *Clostridium difficile* infections, *Am J Gastroenterol* 108:478–498, 2013. quiz 499.

Szajewska H, Guarino A, Hojsak I, et al: Use of probiotics for management of acute gastroenteritis: a position paper by the ESPGHAN working group for probiotics and prebiotics, *J Pediatr Gastroenterol Nutr* 58:531–539, 2014.

Tannock GW: *Probiotics: a critical review*, Wymondham, UK, 1999, Horizon Scientific Press.

Tap J, Derrien M, Tomblom H, et al: Identification of an intestinal microbiota signature associated with severity of irritable bowel syndrome, *Gastroenterology* 152:111–123, 2017.

Thomas DW, Greer FR: American academy of pediatrics committee on nutrition, American academy of pediatrics section on gastroenterology, Hepatology, and nutrition. Probiotics and prebiotics in pediatrics, *Pediatrics* 126:1217–1231, 2010.

Turnbaugh PJ, Ley RE, Hamady M, et al: The human microbiome project, *Nature* 449:804–810, 2007.

Tursi A, Brandimarte G, Papa A, et al: Treatment of relapsing mild to moderately active ulcerative colitis with probiotic VSL#3 as adjunctive to a standard pharmaceutical treatment: a double-blind, randomized, placebo-controlled study, *Am J Gastroenterol* 105:2218–2227, 2010.

Wong VW, Won GL, Chim AM, et al: Treatment of nonalcoholic steatohepatitis with probiotics. A proof-of-concept study, *Ann Hepatol* 12:256–262, 2013.

79

Anoscopy, Sigmoidoscopy, and Colonoscopy

Martin H. Floch

Clinicians can now examine the anal canal, rectum, and colon with ease and with little discomfort to the patient. The indications for each procedure depend on the clinical presentation. For example, red blood on toilet paper or blood dripping into the toilet bowl frequently requires anoscopy and sigmoidoscopy but not colonoscopy. Chronic diarrhea or abdominal pain and signs of intermittent obstruction necessitate colonoscopy (Fig. 79.1).

Use of these techniques for cancer prevention and screening varies throughout the world. Most gastroenterologists agree that colonoscopy is the preferred procedure, whereas occult blood testing and sigmoidoscopy are practiced in many countries as part of colon cancer prevention programs. However, after risk factors (e.g., family history of colon cancer) are identified, colonoscopy is recommended.

ANOSCOPY

Anatomy and abnormalities of the anal canal are examined through anoscopy. The anoscope is a rigid instrument that may be short (proctoscope) or as long as 10 cm (anoscope). Examination requires little preparation, with the patient in the left lateral decubitus position and the buttocks spread by the examiner's left hand. The instrument is gently inserted into the rectum after digital examination. If digital examination is too difficult to perform because of the patient's marked obesity or severe pain, the procedure may have to be limited and deferred to a time when the patient can be sedated and full sigmoidoscopy or colonoscopy performed. After the anoscope or proctoscope is inserted, the anal ring and distal rectum can be carefully inspected. It may be necessary to place the patient in the knee-chest position to spread the buttocks wide. This is especially true with some obese patients, who may feel discomfort in the rectum.

SIGMOIDOSCOPY

Rigid sigmoidoscopes are no longer used. The advent of the flexible sigmoidoscope now permits the prepared patient to be examined in the left lateral decubitus position without sedation, although some clinicians prefer to use mild sedation. After appropriate cleansing, which may include a cathartic or simply a low enema depending on patient cooperation, the instrument is inserted into the rectum after digital examination.

The valves of Houston can be observed and, with appropriate technique, the distal sigmoid loops can be traversed and the flexible instrument can be passed into the descending colon. The instrument is usually passed 60 cm (24 inches) unless there is marked spasm in the sigmoid or an abnormality such as severe diverticular disease prevents passage. Most patients experience some pain as the instrument passes through the sigmoid loop. In approximately 25% of patients, the sigmoid loop is tortuous, creating difficulty for less experienced endoscopists. If it is essential to examine the entire sigmoid in such a patient, sedation and full colonoscopy are indicated. Passage through the difficult sigmoid loops requires training and endoscopic skills in rotating the instrument and the patient (see "Additional Resources").

Aspiration specimens may be obtained for bacteriologic and parasitic study, and mucosal biopsy specimens may be obtained to evaluate for chronic diarrhea, parasitic diseases, and certain systemic diseases.

COLONOSCOPY

Advances in technology and skills now allow examination of the entire colon and the terminal ileum in a single examination. Indications for colonoscopy range from a screening procedure to rule out polyps or early malignancy to evaluation of all symptoms referable to the intestine (Fig. 79.2).

The patient must be well prepared for successful completion of colonoscopy. This includes adequate education and then bowel preparation, in which the entire colon is cleansed. Usually there is a 2-day limitation on intake of fiber-containing foods, with a careful purging of the bowel the day before the examination. Purging agents include magnesium salts, nonabsorbable carbohydrates, and balanced electrolyte solutions in large volume. The type of purge depends on the patient's ability to tolerate substances and the staff's instructional skills.

For routine colonoscopy, sedation is usually required. Rarely, some patients will prefer no sedation, but the average patient requires mild sedation with a narcotic plus a sedative. Some patients are so apprehensive or uncooperative that anesthesia is required.

Bacteremia, which is usually harmless, may develop during the procedure, but for patients who have prosthetic heart valves, previous endocarditis, or recent vascular surgery, antibiotics are used for prophylaxis during and immediately after colonoscopy. Although some controversy exists, antibiotics are not usually recommended for patients with prosthetic joints, pacemakers, or simple mitral valve prolapse. Usual doses are 1 g of ampicillin and 80 mg of gentamicin administered intravenously 10 to 30 minutes before the procedure. Other patients may simply use an oral antibiotic before and several hours after the procedure.

Colonoscopy requires significant training. However, once an endoscopist is skilled, the colon and terminal ileum can be examined and biopsy material obtained for study. Therapeutic colonoscopy is gaining wide acceptance for the removal of polyps, dilatation of certain strictures, reduction of sigmoid volvulus, and intraoperative evaluation to assist in surgery. These procedures are described under the various diseases in Section V.

The endoscopic techniques of passage through a difficult sigmoid or redundant splenic, transverse, or hepatic flexure can be challenging to perform. Most skilled endoscopists are able to evaluate and intubate the terminal ileum, and specimens can be obtained for

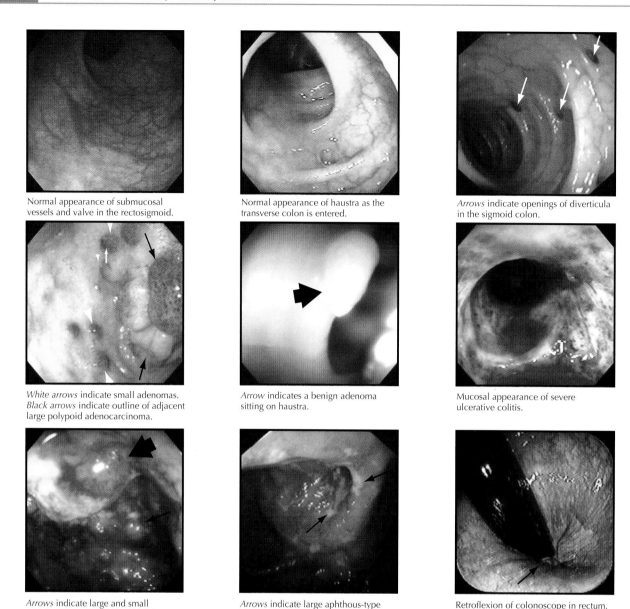

Normal appearance of submucosal vessels and valve in the rectosigmoid.

Normal appearance of haustra as the transverse colon is entered.

Arrows indicate openings of diverticula in the sigmoid colon.

White arrows indicate small adenomas. *Black arrows* indicate outline of adjacent large polypoid adenocarcinoma.

Arrow indicates a benign adenoma sitting on haustra.

Mucosal appearance of severe ulcerative colitis.

Arrows indicate large and small pseudopolyps, as seen in ulcerative colitis.

Arrows indicate large aphthous-type ulcers, as seen in Crohn disease.

Retroflexion of colonoscope in rectum, with mucocutaneous junction visible. *Arrow* indicates small hemorrhoid.

Fig. 79.1 Anoscopic, Sigmoidoscopic, and Colonoscopic Views of Normal Intestinal Structures and Various Lesions.

evaluating diseases in those areas. The complication rate of bleeding or perforation was only 0.35% in a study involving 25,000 diagnostic procedures.

To evaluate the anal ring thoroughly, it is important for the endoscopist to *retroflex* the instrument so that the entire rectal vault can be seen. Because the rectum and anal ring contract as the instrument is pulled through the rectum, small lesions may be missed. These lesions are exposed when the rectal vault is distended and examined from the inside out. It is also easy to obtain biopsy specimens through the retroflexed instrument.

Newer techniques, such as high-resolution endoscopy with chromoscopy and narrow-band imaging, are being used at research and university centers but not widely elsewhere. Capsule endoscopy is rapidly becoming a useful tool.

ADDITIONAL IMAGING METHODS

Radiographic imaging techniques and virtual colonoscopy are helpful but are usually reserved for patients who cannot or choose not to undergo direct endoscopic viewing procedures.

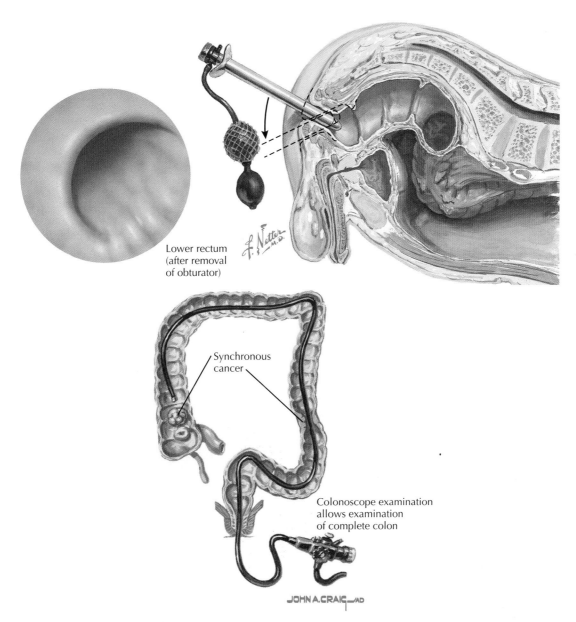

Lower rectum
(after removal
of obturator)

Synchronous
cancer

Colonoscope examination
allows examination
of complete colon

JOHN A.CRAIG—AD

Fig. 79.2 Anoscopy, Sigmoidoscopy, and Colonoscopy.

ADDITIONAL RESOURCES

ASGE Standards of Practice Committee, Banerjee S, Shen B, et al: Antibiotic prophylaxis for GI endoscopy, *Gastrointest Endosc* 67:791–798, 2008.

Barkun A, Chiba N, Enns R, et al: Commonly used preparations for colonoscopy: efficacy, tolerability, and safety—a Canadian association of gastroenterology position paper, *Can J Gastroenterol* 20(11):699–710, 2006.

Bass LM, Wershil BK: Anatomy, histology, embryology, and developmental anomalies of the small and large intestine. In Feldman M, Friedman LS, Brandt LJ, editors: *Gastrointestinal and liver disease*, ed 10, Philadelphia, 2016, Saunders-Elsevier, pp 1649–1678.

Cotton PB: *Advanced digestive endoscopy*, Malden, Mass, 2008, Wiley-Blackwell.

McQuaid KR, Laine L: A systemic review and meta-analysis of randomized, controlled trials of moderate sedation for routine endoscopic procedures, *Gastrointest Endosc* 67:910–923, 2008.

Rex DK: Is virtual endoscopy ready for widespread application?, *Gastroenterology* 125:608–614, 2003.

Rex DK, Lieberman D: ACG colorectal cancer prevention plan: update on CT-colonography, *Am J Gastroenterol* 101:1410–1413, 2006.

Vargo JJ II: Preparation and complications of gastrointestinal endoscopy. In Feldman M, Friedman LS, Brandt LJ, editors: *Gastrointestinal and liver disease*, ed 10, Philadelphia, 2016, Saunders-Elsevier, pp 677–685.

Waye JD, Rex D, Williams CB: *Colonoscopy: principles and practice*, Malden, Mass, 2008, Wiley-Blackwell.

Williams CB: *Practical gastrointestinal endoscopy: the fundamentals*, ed 5, Oxford, England, 2003, Blackwell.

80

Laparoscopy and Laparotomy

Martin H. Floch

Laparoscopy, or peritoneoscopy, is the direct inspection of the peritoneal cavity and its contents by means of an endoscopic instrument introduced through the abdominal wall (Fig. 80.1). The procedure is used in gastroenterology and gynecology to diagnose conditions that cannot be determined with simpler methods. Its major value is that it can frequently obviate the need for exploratory laparotomy.

Modern laparoscopy was preceded by rigid peritoneoscopy. A trocar was placed in the abdominal cavity after it had been insufflated with air and a peritoneoscope was introduced through the trocar to visualize the liver and intraabdominal organs. Today the laparoscope has replaced the peritoneoscope, a flexible instrument that transmits an image from its tip to a monitor. Video-laparoscopy techniques have greatly advanced

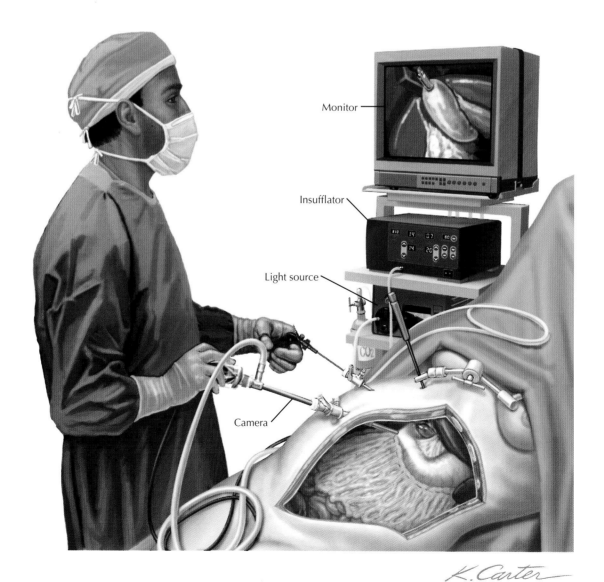

Monitor

Insufflator

Light source

Camera

K. Carter

Fig. 80.1 Laparoscopy (Peritoneoscopy).

and now include laparoscopic therapy and surgery. The broad, ever-expanding indications for diagnostic laparoscopy include assessment of the liver, undiagnosed acute and chronic abdominal pain, and unexplained ascites. Laparoscopy is also used to stage malignancy and obtain guided liver biopsy specimens or specimens of any suspected lesion with the help of radiographic imaging.

Indications for laparoscopy in trauma and therapeutic procedures are also rapidly expanding. Laparoscopic cholecystectomy has been well accepted as the preferred procedure except in complicated cases when the abdomen must be entered. At present technology and skilled laparoscopists also make it possible to explore the common bile duct. The resection of major organs such as the spleen and colon is now common practice and will become even more prevalent as laparoscopists and surgeons develop greater clinical skills. Furthermore, laparoscopic inguinal hernia repair is now standard in many institutions.

With the advent of the need for fundoplication in esophageal reflux disease, laparoscopic fundoplication has become a standard procedure in many institutions. However, this procedure requires implementation by skilled laparoscopic surgeons. Similarly, bariatric surgeons use laparoscopy to do most of their procedures (see Chapters 41 and 191).

Laparoscopy and therapeutic laparoscopy procedures are becoming simpler, and advancing technologic and surgical skills may make them the major standard for most abdominal surgeries.

The main advantage of laparoscopy is that it is less invasive than open surgery. Small lesions measuring 1 mm may be identified and correlated with computed tomography (CT) and magnetic resonance imaging (MRI) findings. Furthermore, direct biopsy is relatively safe and minimizes any possible bleeding. There are some disadvantages stemming from the use of an instrument. In patients who have undergone previous surgery and have multiple adhesions, it is difficult to visualize many of the intraabdominal areas. Organs in the retroperitoneal area and some abdominal areas may not be visualized well. The experience of the laparoscopist and the laparoscopic surgeon is a major factor; the more experience each has, the more can be accomplished.

Although laparoscopy can be performed without anesthesia, a complication is always possible. Therefore the patient must be a candidate for general anesthesia. Local anesthesia with intravenous sedation or inhaled nitrous oxide may be used. Most clinicians prefer using nitrous oxide to create the pneumoperitoneum, but some still prefer carbon dioxide. Laparoscopes with forward viewing range from 2 to 10 mm in diameter, and some have oblique-angled lenses. Other standard instruments used by laparoscopists include scissors, grasping devices, probes, clamps, forceps, retractors, and biopsy forceps.

The patient is invariably in a lithotomy position and a 10- to 15-degree Trendelenburg position when a small skin incision is made for injection. Incisions made to permit entrance of the laparoscope vary depending on the patient's status and any previous surgery.

ADDITIONAL RESOURCES

Katada N, Hinder RA, Raiser F, et al: Laparoscopic Nissen fundoplication, *Gastroenterologist* 3:95–104, 1995.

Kelly NA, Sarr MG, Hinder RA: *Mayo clinic gastrointestinal surgery*, St. Louis, 2003, Elsevier.

O'Conner DB, Winter DC: The role of laparoscopy in the management of acute small-bowel obstructions. A review of over 2000 cases, *Surg Endosc* 26:12–70, 2012.

Parra JL, Reddy KR: Diagnostic laparoscopy, *Endoscopy* 36:289–293, 2004.

Scheidbach H, Schneider C, Huegel O, et al: Laparoscopic sigmoid resection for cancer, *Dis Colon Rect* 45:1641–1647, 2002.

Zorron R, Carvalho G: Laparasocopy and laparotomy. In Podolsky DK, Camilleri M, Fitz JG, et al, editors: *Yamada's textbook of gastroenterology*, ed 6, Hoboken, New Jersey, 2016, John Wiley and Sons Ltd, pp 2693–2702.

81

Stool Examination

Martin H. Floch

Examination of the stool directly and through microscopy and chemical tests can provide much useful information, although patients, physicians, and laboratories tend to avoid stool evaluation (Fig. 81.1).

GROSS AND MICROSCOPIC INSPECTION

An *acholic* stool suggests biliary obstruction; a *tarry* stool indicates gastrointestinal (GI) bleeding; and a *red* stool signifies bleeding from the lower GI tract. The shape of the stool is usually reliably reported by the patient, and the appropriate deductions may be made without the physician observing the stool. Diarrheal stool is loose and watery, but stool associated with malabsorption can be large and greasy, often staining the toilet bowl. The Bristol Stool Scale clearly describes the foam, form, and character of the bowel movement material and has been useful in clinical and research settings (Fig. 81.2). The character of stools is also discussed thoroughly in Chapters 64 (diarrhea) and 85 (constipation).

Microscopic examination of stool can be helpful when inflammatory cells (polymorphonuclear or eosinophilic) are identified. Furthermore, ova and parasites can be identified as eggs or larvae under the microscope.

CHEMICAL ANALYSIS

Chemical analysis of stool is important for assessing *fecal occult blood test* findings. Many different tests are available today, all using a technique similar to the standard *guaiac test*. False-positive results can occur. The patient must not have ingested large amounts of red meat or peroxidase-containing vegetables and fruits (e.g., broccoli, cantaloupe, cauliflower, radishes, turnips). It is also reported that a heavy intake of iron supplements, vitamin C, aspirin, and nonsteroidal antiinflammatory drugs (NSAIDs) gives false-positive results. Guaiac-impregnated slide tests are readily available and used most often. False-negative results can occur from using outdated reagents and old slides.

Stool weight is important in that it is greatly increased in most malabsorption syndromes and in diarrheas of metabolic origin. Stool weight in the person on a low-fiber diet may be as low as 100 g, whereas that in the person on a high-fiber diet can be as high as 300 to 400 g.

Stool electrolyte studies revealing stool osmolality can aid in evaluating various forms of diarrhea. This information is used only to classify diarrhea as secretory. In *secretory diarrhea*, an osmotic gap exists in stool osmolality, approximately 290 mOsm, and is calculated as twice the concentration of sodium plus potassium. Normally the gap is less than 50 mOsm and certainly less than 125 mOsm. Lack of a gap indicates secretory diarrhea.

The chemical analysis of stool can be important for evaluating the malabsorption characteristic of small bowel, pancreatic, or metabolic disease. This requires a 72-hour stool collection. Several kits are available for fat analysis (see Chapter 62). Routine stool staining for fat has been unreliable and is no longer recommended.

BACTERIOLOGIC AND PARASITIC TESTING

Stool culture is important. Stool should be as fresh as possible so that the laboratory can inoculate it on appropriate media. This is the preferred method of identifying bacterial pathogens and is reliable in acute states. *Clostridium difficile* is primarily identified using available toxins. Laboratories should be equipped to identify A and B toxins because the latter can often be missed. Identification of parasites is discussed in Section VI.

ANTIGEN AND GENETIC TESTING

The stool antigen test for *Helicobacter pylori* is as sensitive as other tests to determine the presence of this organism and it can be useful in diagnosing and treating gastric and peptic ulcer disease. The stool antigen test for *Giardia lamblia* is also reliable and helpful in identifying this protozoan, which tends to live in the duodenum and is difficult to identify in stools.

Many laboratories are developing *fecal water tests* to evaluate stool for colon cancer cells and for colon cancer screening. Although these are still too new to be used in clinical practice, they are developing rapidly and should become important soon. Similarly, stool tests are being developed for the genetic analysis of cells, although these are not yet clinically effective tools.

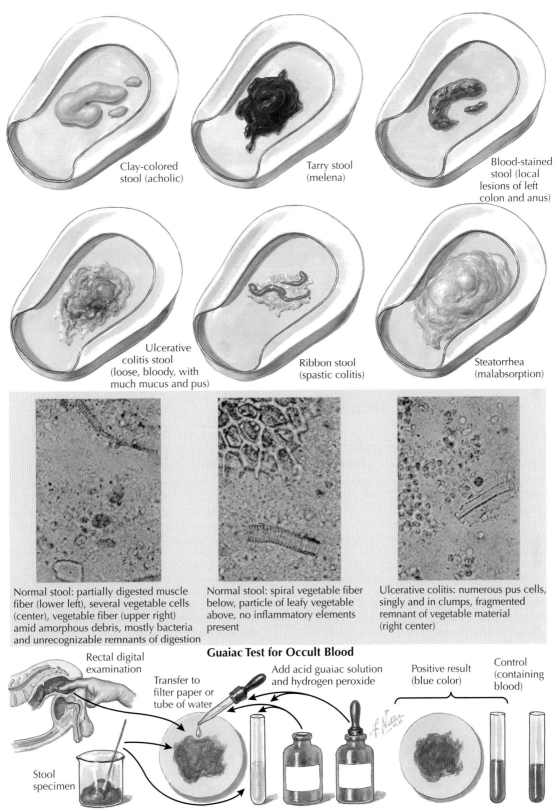

Clay-colored stool (acholic)

Tarry stool (melena)

Blood-stained stool (local lesions of left colon and anus)

Ulcerative colitis stool (loose, bloody, with much mucus and pus)

Ribbon stool (spastic colitis)

Steatorrhea (malabsorption)

Normal stool: partially digested muscle fiber (lower left), several vegetable cells (center), vegetable fiber (upper right) amid amorphous debris, mostly bacteria and unrecognizable remnants of digestion

Normal stool: spiral vegetable fiber below, particle of leafy vegetable above, no inflammatory elements present

Ulcerative colitis: numerous pus cells, singly and in clumps, fragmented remnant of vegetable material (right center)

Guaiac Test for Occult Blood

Rectal digital examination

Add acid guaiac solution and hydrogen peroxide

Transfer to filter paper or tube of water

Positive result (blue color)

Control (containing blood)

Stool specimen

Fig. 81.1 Examination of the Stool.

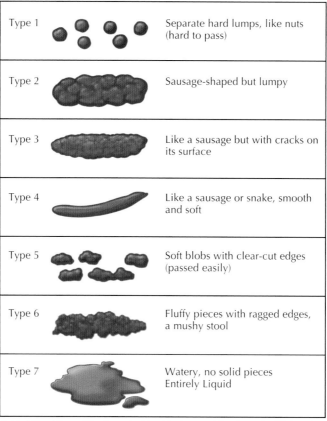

Type 1		Separate hard lumps, like nuts (hard to pass)
Type 2		Sausage-shaped but lumpy
Type 3		Like a sausage but with cracks on its surface
Type 4		Like a sausage or snake, smooth and soft
Type 5		Soft blobs with clear-cut edges (passed easily)
Type 6		Fluffy pieces with ragged edges, a mushy stool
Type 7		Watery, no solid pieces Entirely Liquid

Bristol Stool Form Chart created by Heaton and Lewis at the University of Bristol. Originally published in Scand J Gastroenterol, *32(9):920-924,1997.*

Fig. 81.2 Bristol Stool Form Scale.

ADDITIONAL RESOURCES

Ford CC, Talley NJ: The irritable bowel syndrome. In Feldman M, Friedman LS, Brandt LJ, editors: *Gastrointestinal and liver disease*, ed 10, Philadelphia, 2016, Saunders-Elsevier, pp 2139–2153.

Haine CF, Sears CL: Infectious enteritis and proctocolitis. In Feldman M, Friedman LS, Brandt LJ, editors: *Gastrointestinal and liver disease*, ed 10, Philadelphia, 2016, Saunders-Elsevier, pp 1896–1929.

Hecht GA, Gaspar J, Malaspin M: Approach to the patient with diarrhea. In Podolsky DK, Camilleri M, Fitz JG, et al, editors: *Yamada's textbook of gastroenterology*, ed 6, Hoboken, New Jersey, 2016, John Wiley and Sons Ltd, pp 725–756.

Nair P, Langerholm S, Dutta S, et al: Coprocytobiology: on the nature of cellular elements from stools in the pathophysiology of colonic disease, *J Clin Gastroenterol* 36:S84–S93, 2003.

Rao SSC, Camilleri M: Approach to the patient with constipation. In Podolsky DK, Camilleri M, Fitz JG, et al, editors: *Yamada's textbook of gastroenterology*, ed 6, Hoboken, New Jersey, 2016, John Wiley and Sons Ltd, pp 757–780.

Schiller LR, Sellin JH: Diarrhea. In Feldman M, Friedman LS, Brandt LJ, editors: *Gastrointestinal and liver disease*, ed 10, Philadelphia, 2016, Saunders-Elsevier, pp 221–241.

82

Intestinal Bleeding

Martin H. Floch

Gastrointestinal (GI) bleeding is acute or chronic loss of blood from the upper or lower part GI tract (Fig. 82.1). Acute bleeding may be life threatening, whereas chronic bleeding may be slow or even occult. The GI tract can lose as much as 50 mL of blood daily; it is replaced without anemia but indicates a GI lesion. This chapter discusses lower GI bleeding; Chapter 35 discusses upper GI hemorrhage (see also Section IV).

Lower GI bleeding can be defined as blood loss from below the ligament of Treitz. It accounts for approximately one-fourth to one-third of all bleeding events. The incidence appears to increase with age, with more than a 200-fold increase from the third to the ninth decades of life, and it is more common in men than in women. The mortality rate is less than 5%. Upper GI bleeding has a higher mortality rate than lower GI bleeding.

CLINICAL PICTURE

If a patient has anemia, it is important to examine his or her stool for occult blood. If findings are positive, the GI tract must be ruled out as the probable cause of the anemia. After the upper GI tract is ruled out, the intestine must be investigated. Severe hemorrhages reveal themselves by the appearance of visible blood in the stool. Such blood may be bright red, or it may cause *melena*, a black discoloration, indicating that the blood has been exposed to digestive activity and usually that the bleeding stems from above the ligament of Treitz. Often, however, melena may be from the small bowel or from as far down as the cecum. Red blood in the stool results from severe bleeding. It is important not to be fooled by a black stool caused by the ingestion of iron supplements, bismuth preparations, or foods such as blackberries. Furthermore, red beets, when consumed in large amounts, can produce a red stool.

Patients with occult bleeding usually have few GI symptoms. However, when the symptoms point to the upper GI tract, that workup precedes the lower GI workup. Some patients who are severely anemic may be weak, which usually signifies that occult bleeding has existed for a long time. Acute rectal bleeding that presents as *hematochezia* (blood in feces) and bright-red blood may start with a bout of syncope or as a blood-filled toilet bowl. Patients with acute rectal bleeding must be monitored immediately.

DIAGNOSIS

Once it is established that bleeding is from the intestine, full evaluation of the lower GI tract is indicated. When the patient has anemia or occult bleeding, the diagnostic workup can be done in an orderly fashion. However, if the bleeding is massive, the patient must be immediately stabilized, upper GI bleeding ruled out, and a rapid workup performed. History and physical examination are essential. It is important to note whether abdominal pain or diarrhea is associated with the bleeding and whether the patient has any other GI symptoms. The anal ring must be examined, including anoscopy to rule out severe internal or hemorrhoidal bleeding.

Once the patient has been stabilized, some physicians prefer radio-nucleotide imaging to determine whether the bleeding is from the left or right side of the colon. This usually requires a bleeding rate of more than 1 mL/min. Institutions report varying degrees of success with radionucleotide imaging, and some prefer sigmoidoscopy or colonoscopy. Endoscopy has replaced barium enema examination.

An attempt is made to purge the bowel; then careful colonoscopy is performed. Emergency colonoscopy is reported to make a final diagnosis for colonic lesions in 74% to 90% of patients. If the bleeding is massive and surgery is being contemplated, some clinicians prefer angiography before the colonoscopic examination.

Once the site is identified through angiography, *embolization* can be attempted with polyvinyl alcohol or intraarterial vasopressin. Some studies indicate effectiveness in 79% of patients. Angiographers are now able to place coaxial catheters into the vessel, and microcoils can be used to deliver an embolic agent. This technique appears to lower the risk for bowel ischemia.

The most common cause of intestinal bleeding is *diverticular disease* of the colon. The next most common causes are angiodysplasias, cancer or polyps, and inflammatory bowel disease (IBD). Anorectal, hemorrhoidal, and fissure bleeding are relatively uncommon causes of massive bleeding or anemia, although they are reported in as many as 9% of patients in some series. Other causes are rare and include Meckel diverticulum and intussusception, colitis secondary to ischemia, infections or radiation, and rare entities such as Dieulafoy lesion of the rectum and solitary rectal ulcer. Varices of the colon and rectum are also rarely reported.

Bleeding is usually on the left side but does occur from right-sided lesions; therefore it is important to identify the site if surgery is contemplated.

TREATMENT AND MANAGEMENT

Treatment depends on the lesion. Because diverticular disease is the most common cause of intestinal bleeding, and bleeding stops with minimal transfusion in more than 80% of patients, the prognosis is excellent. However, bleeding may be massive and persistent; therefore—for the surgeon to perform the correct partial colectomy—imaging or angiography must identify whether it stems from the right or the left colon. Angiodysplasias are often embolized or are seen on colonoscopy, and attempts to cauterize or ablate them are possible. Certainly neoplastic lesions can be removed endoscopically. If they are not, surgical resection of the area is required. IBD is treated as described in Chapters 91, 95, and 97. Anorectal disease is treated locally with appropriate therapy (see Chapters 102 and 105).

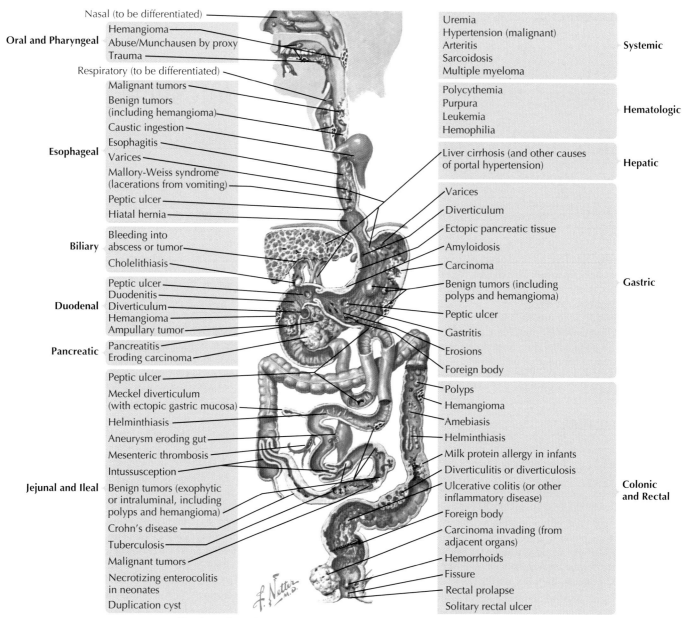

Oral and Pharyngeal
Nasal (to be differentiated)
Hemangioma
Abuse/Munchausen by proxy
Trauma

Esophageal
Respiratory (to be differentiated)
Malignant tumors
Benign tumors (including hemangioma)
Caustic ingestion
Esophagitis
Varices
Mallory-Weiss syndrome (lacerations from vomiting)
Peptic ulcer
Hiatal hernia

Biliary
Bleeding into abscess or tumor
Cholelithiasis

Duodenal
Peptic ulcer
Duodenitis
Diverticulum
Hemangioma
Ampullary tumor

Pancreatic
Pancreatitis
Eroding carcinoma

Jejunal and Ileal
Peptic ulcer
Meckel diverticulum (with ectopic gastric mucosa)
Helminthiasis
Aneurysm eroding gut
Mesenteric thrombosis
Intussusception
Benign tumors (exophytic or intraluminal, including polyps and hemangioma)
Crohn's disease
Tuberculosis
Malignant tumors
Necrotizing enterocolitis in neonates
Duplication cyst

Systemic
Uremia
Hypertension (malignant)
Arteritis
Sarcoidosis
Multiple myeloma

Hematologic
Polycythemia
Purpura
Leukemia
Hemophilia

Hepatic
Liver cirrhosis (and other causes of portal hypertension)

Gastric
Varices
Diverticulum
Ectopic pancreatic tissue
Amyloidosis
Carcinoma
Benign tumors (including polyps and hemangioma)
Peptic ulcer
Gastritis
Erosions
Foreign body

Colonic and Rectal
Polyps
Hemangioma
Amebiasis
Helminthiasis
Milk protein allergy in infants
Diverticulitis or diverticulosis
Ulcerative colitis (or other inflammatory disease)
Foreign body
Carcinoma invading (from adjacent organs)
Hemorrhoids
Fissure
Rectal prolapse
Solitary rectal ulcer

Fig. 82.1 Gastrointestinal Hemorrhage: Causes and Manifestations.

The prognosis in hematochezia is excellent, because 80% stop spontaneously and mortality is well below 5%.

When the colon is not the cause and bleeding comes from the small bowel, it may be caused by neoplasia, which may be identified on radiographic imaging or enteroscopy. The advent of capsule endoscopy has identified ectasias and small lesions caused by Crohn disease that were not seen radiographically. It is now the preferred technique to evaluate occult and sometimes active small bowel bleeding. The closer in time it is done to the bleeding event, the better the diagnostic findings. These tests require treatment of the IBD. If bleeding persists, surgical resection is needed. When a Meckel diverticulum causes bleeding, surgical correction is required, and the prognosis is excellent. If neoplasias of the small bowel are identified, they are usually resected, and the prognosis depends on the nature of the neoplasm (see Section IV).

COURSE AND PROGNOSIS

Depending on the primary disease, the course and prognosis vary for patients with intestinal bleeding. With a benign disorder, the prognosis is excellent. If neoplasia is the cause, the prognosis depends on the type of tumor. A small group of patients with chronic iron-deficiency anemia have recurrent positive stool test results for occult blood and are defined as "occult bleeders." When no lesion is identified, blood replacement and maintenance therapy are performed, and the long-term prognosis is guarded.

ADDITIONAL RESOURCES

Ghassen KA, Jensen DM: Approach to the patient with gastrointestinal bleeding. In Podolsky DK, Camilleri M, Fitz JG, et al, editors: *Yamada's textbook of gastroenterology*, ed 6, Hoboken, New Jersey, 2016, John Wiley and Sons Ltd, pp 797–818.

Jensen DM, Machicado GA, Jutabha R, Kovacs TO: Urgent colonoscopy for the diagnosis and treatment of severe diverticular hemorrhage, *N Engl J Med* 342:78–82, 2000.

Kim ST, Nemcek AA, Vogelzang RL: Angiography and interventional radiology. In Gore RM, Levine MS, editors: *Gastrointestinal radiology*, Philadelphia, 2008, Saunders-Elsevier, pp 117–140.

Savides TJ, Jensen DM: Gastrointestinal bleeding. In Feldman M, Friedman LS, Brandt LJ, editors: *Gastrointestinal and liver disease*, ed 10, Philadelphia, 2016, Saunders-Elsevier, pp 297–335.

Strate LL, Ayanian JZ, Kotler G, Syngal S: Risk factors for mortality in lower intestinal bleeding, *Clin Gastroenterol Hepatol* 6:1004–1010, 2008.

Wald A: Other diseases of the colon and rectum. In Feldman M, Friedman LS, Brandt LJ, editors: *Gastrointestinal and liver disease*, ed 10, Philadelphia, 2016, Saunders-Elsevier, pp 2298–2315.

83

Motility and Dysmotility of the Large Intestine

Martin H. Floch

Normal colonic motility involves the integrated function of many components: the central nervous system (CNS); the colonic nervous system; the circular and longitudinal involuntary muscle of the colon, sigmoid, and rectum; and the voluntary muscle of the pelvis and rectum. This complex system of neuromuscular activity is further integrated with impulses arising in the upper gastrointestinal (GI) and small bowel tracts and is influenced by GI hormone activity (see Chapter 58).

Various types of colonic movements can be differentiated (Fig. 83.1). There appears to be a receptive relaxation of the cecal musculature as the terminal ileum evacuates its contents and permits the accommodation of adequate quantities of intestinal chyme before the activation of stretch receptors. Adaptive relaxation in other parts of the colon provides similar accommodation of the fecal contents without distress and without premature propulsion, which does occur in the rectum when the rectum becomes filled. Such a *reservoir of continence* function is a property particularly of the descending colon, and it is this feature that renders colostomy a fairly tolerable and practical condition.

Contraction of the longitudinal muscular bands (taeniae) shortens the bowel and forms pleats or sacculations (haustra), in which the residues of the chyme are retained to allow time for the absorption of water and a number of digestive products. This function is abetted by contractions of the circular muscle, which may create small indentations within the haustra. These contractions of the longitudinal and circular musculature must be considered analogous to the rhythmic segments of the small bowel. There are *nonpropulsive* movements of segmental contractions and *propulsive* movements that arise in proximal segments and pass in a caudad direction, obliterating some haustra. *Mass peristalsis,* analogous to the peristaltic rush of the jejunum or ileum, occurs only two or three times in a 24-hour period and is initiated by (or related to) the gastrocolic reflex and propels colonic contents toward the rectosigmoid colon.

The innervation of the colon is similar to that of the small bowel (see Chapter 53). Extrinsic nerves exert an effect on the intrinsic nerve network, which appears to function autonomously and is capable of coordinating movements of adjacent segments necessary for peristaltic progression. These effects may be altered in many pathologic conditions. The broad concept that the parasympathetic nerves generally augment, and the sympathetic nerves inhibit, muscular contraction is acceptable as a working hypothesis, but it becomes more complex when the intrinsic nervous system of the colon is considered.

Understanding the *interstitial cells of Cajal* has helped clarify colonic physiology. They serve two important functions as smooth muscle pacemakers: controlling myogenic activity and mediating or amplifying the effects of the enteric neurons. The cells of Cajal are spread throughout the muscle and are nonneuronal, being derived from smooth muscle.

Dietary factors affect regional transit; a solid-food diet hinders transit through the cecum and ascending colon, whereas a mixed diet, particularly liquids, is stored in the ascending and the transverse colon. The volume and consistency of the contents affect the rate of emptying and correlate with stool frequency and weight. Chemical substances and distention can stimulate propulsive activity. *Antiperistaltic waves* assist in retaining contents within the colon.

Transit of material through the colon is normally slow, and contents move from the cecum to the rectum over 24 to 48 hours. In general, transit appears to be faster in men than in women and faster in younger women than in middle-aged or older women. *Propulsion* varies tremendously among persons. The material does tend to dwell in the rectosigmoid colon, indicating storage in this area. In some patients, radiographic observations reveal a marked delay in the ascending or the transverse colon. As the volume increases in the ascending colon, retroperistaltic patterns decrease and give way to aboral propulsive contractions.

The functions of the rectum, anus, and pelvic floor are discussed in Chapter 84.

Manometry of the colon is largely restricted to research centers and has not proved to be adaptable or helpful in clinical situations. These centers can demonstrate abnormalities in the interdigestive migratory motor complex and relate them to functional abnormalities. Using motility-measuring material and an electronic barostat is helpful in understanding the physiology but is not readily adaptable to clinical situations.

DISORDERS OF COLONIC MOTILITY

Three major areas of colonic motility disorders concern clinicians: constipation, diarrhea, and irritable bowel syndrome, as discussed in Chapters 61, 64, and 85. Disturbances in anorectal motility are discussed in Chapter 84.

Colonic motility disturbances can be secondary to nonmotor disorders, such as occur with endocrinopathy and neurologic disease. Furthermore, once the intestine is diseased, motility is also easily disturbed, and either digestion or absorption becomes altered. This occurs when inflammation in the intestinal tract caused by acute or chronic disease alters the balance of the neuromuscular activity and severely alters the motility of the colon.

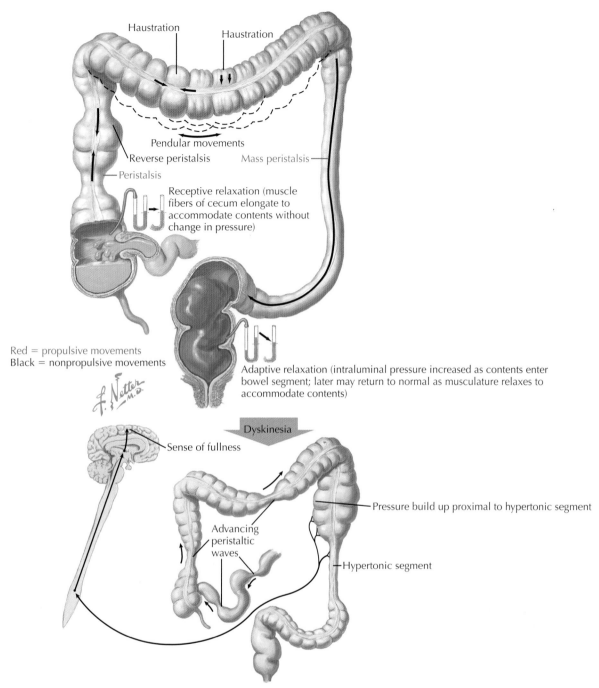

Haustration Haustration

Pendular movements
Reverse peristalsis Mass peristalsis
Peristalsis

Receptive relaxation (muscle fibers of cecum elongate to accommodate contents without change in pressure)

Red = propulsive movements
Black = nonpropulsive movements

Adaptive relaxation (intraluminal pressure increased as contents enter bowel segment; later may return to normal as musculature relaxes to accommodate contents)

Dyskinesia

Sense of fullness

Advancing peristaltic waves

Pressure build up proximal to hypertonic segment

Hypertonic segment

Fig. 83.1 Motility and Dysmotility of the Large Intestine.

ADDITIONAL RESOURCES

Bharucha AE, Hasler WL: Motility of the small intestine and colon. In Podolsky DK, Camilleri M, Fitz JG, et al, editors: *Yamada's textbook of gastroenterology*, ed 6, Hoboken, New Jersey, 2016, John Wiley and Sons Ltd, pp 367–389.

Dinning PG, Costa M, Brookes SJH: Colonic motor and sensory function. In Feldman M, Friedman LS, Brandt LJ, editors: *Gastrointestinal and liver disease*, ed 10, Philadelphia, 2016, Saunders-Elsevier, pp 1696–1712.

Rao SSC, Parkman HP, McCallum RW: *Handbook of gastrointestinal motility and functional disorders*, New York, 2015, Slack Inc.

Szarka L: Dysmotility of the small intestine and colon. In Podolsky DK, Camilleri M, Fitz JG, et al, editors: *Yamada's textbook of gastroenterology*, ed 6, Hoboken, New Jersey, 2016, John Wiley and Sons Ltd, pp 1154–1195.

84

Normal Defecation and Pathophysiology of Fecal Incontinence

Martin H. Floch

NORMAL DEFECATION

A peristaltic wave moving the contents of the left colon into the rectum is usually considered the initial phenomenon in the sequence of events in defecation (Fig. 84.1).

The urge to defecate, when residue accumulates in the rectum, normally occurs at intervals varying from several times daily to every fourth or fifth day. When the rectum fills with approximately 400 mL in a healthy person with intact nerves and reflexes, the urge to defecate is usually uncontrollable. Most people feel an urge daily, usually in the morning after breakfast, after waking from sleep, assuming the erect position, and moving about. Ingesting food and liquids favors the initiation of *mass peristalsis* (gastrocolic reflex). Increased intrarectal pressure brings about a reciprocal relaxation of the anal sphincters, which may be counteracted by voluntary contraction of the external sphincter,

permitting the delay of defecation. Prolonged delay may result in a temporary reduction in the intensity of the urge. The entire act of defecation comprises a series of contractions and relaxations of muscles in the rectum and the pelvis.

When the urge to defecate occurs, the person usually assumes a squatting position, which facilitates a reflex contraction of the hamstrings. The squatting position supports an increase in intraabdominal pressure, which is accomplished by contraction and fixation of the diaphragm, closure of the glottis, and contraction of the muscles of the abdominal wall. Voluntary control of contraction of the external sphincter is released, and the fecal mass is expelled by the increasing rectal contraction, which leads to an intrarectal pressure of 100 to 200 mm Hg. Simultaneously, the muscles of the pelvic floor contract and contribute to the forces that increase the intraabdominal pressure. The contents of the left colon, or part of it, may be emptied in

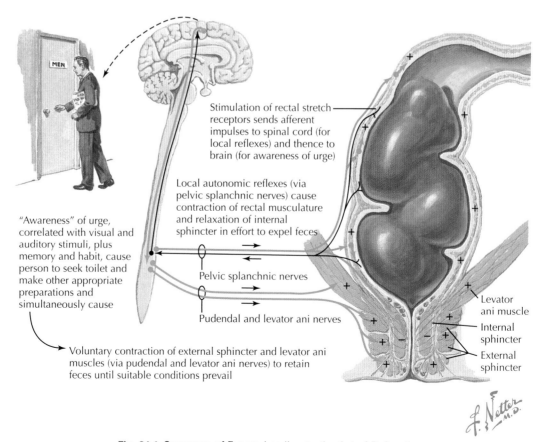

Stimulation of rectal stretch receptors sends afferent impulses to spinal cord (for local reflexes) and thence to brain (for awareness of urge)

Local autonomic reflexes (via pelvic splanchnic nerves) cause contraction of rectal musculature and relaxation of internal sphincter in effort to expel feces

Pelvic splanchnic nerves

Pudendal and levator ani nerves

"Awareness" of urge, correlated with visual and auditory stimuli, plus memory and habit, cause person to seek toilet and make other appropriate preparations and simultaneously cause

Voluntary contraction of external sphincter and levator ani muscles (via pudendal and levator ani nerves) to retain feces until suitable conditions prevail

Levator ani muscle
Internal sphincter
External sphincter

Fig. 84.1 Sequence of Events Leading to the Act of Defecation.

a single continuous peristaltic progression, or the anorectal structures may return to the resting state after the first bolus has been evacuated until another contraction of the colon delivers more fecal material into the rectum.

This integrated function involves neurons of the motor cortex, sympathetic and parasympathetic pathways, and numerous reflex mechanisms (Fig. 84.2). Electromyographic studies indicate that musculature of the pelvic floor behaves as a single muscle during defecation and that the anorectal angle created by the puborectalis muscle produces a functional obstruction to prevent accidental loss of stool.

Disease and malfunction of the anal sphincter and rectum and anal manometry are discussed in Chapter 104.

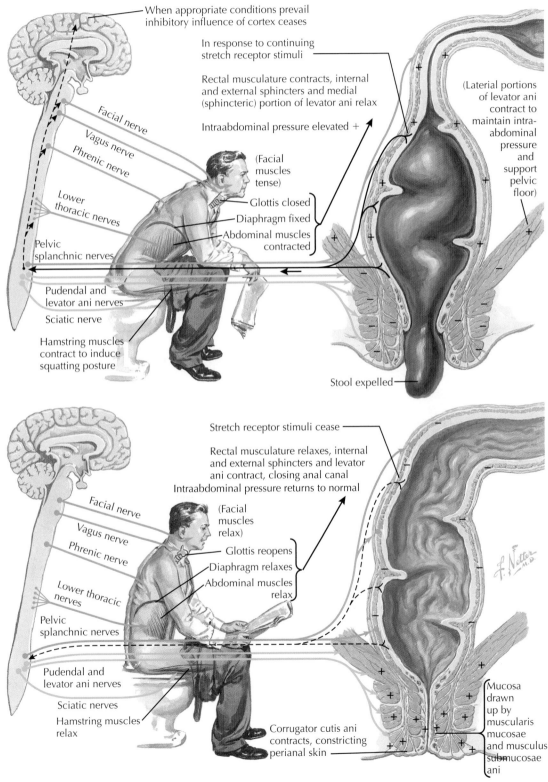

Fig. 84.2 Neuronal Functions and Anatomic Correlations in Defecation.

FECAL INCONTINENCE

After transection of the spinal cord above the origin of the lumbar sympathetic nerves—during the period of spinal shock, which supervenes immediately and lasts for some weeks—the rectum and sphincters are completely paralyzed and the patient is incontinent (Fig. 84.3). Thereafter, the tonus of the sphincters returns and defecation occurs reflexively by way of the lumbosacral center. Because voluntary contraction of the external sphincter is no longer possible and distention of the rectum no longer perceived, the patient has no control over the

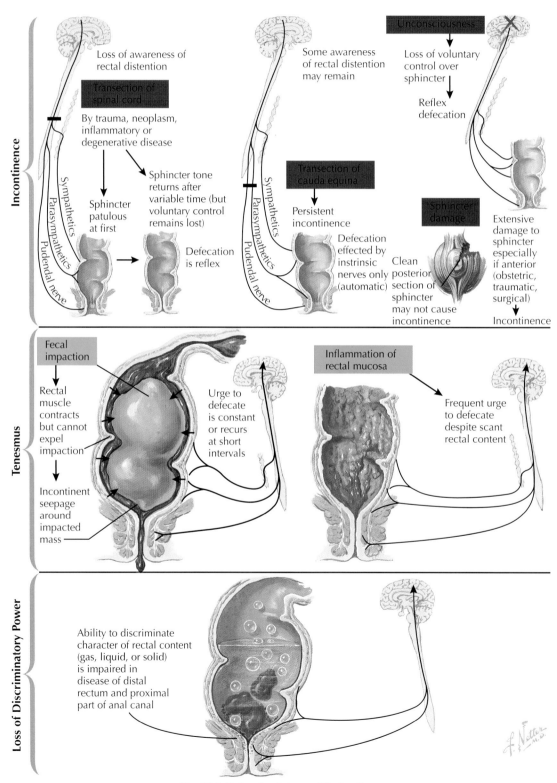

Fig. 84.3 Pathophysiology of Defecation.

act of defecation. This poses a difficult problem in paraplegic patients that is usually managed by the regular use of enemas and digital evacuation of the rectum.

When the cord lesion involves the cauda equina, with destruction of the sacral innervation, the reflexes are abolished and defecation becomes automatic or dependent entirely on intrinsic nervous mechanisms. In these patients, the rectum still responds to distention, although with limited force, and the reciprocal relaxation of the already patulous sphincters enables feces to be extruded. Some awareness of rectal distention may be present if the transection is below the lumbar sympathetic outflow, and the persistence of sympathetic connections in the absence of a sacral outflow may contribute to the sluggishness of rectal contractions.

The presence of excretory material in the rectum is not in itself sufficient to excite the urge to defecate. The content must be sufficiently large to exceed the threshold of the distention stimulus characteristic of the person. In many patients with regular bowel movements, digital examination reveals a considerable mass of varying consistency in the rectum. However, the accumulation of a large mass in a greatly dilated rectum, especially in older persons, suggests loss of tonicity of the rectal musculature, which could be attributed to the long-standing habit of ignoring or suppressing the urge to defecate or to the degeneration of nerve and muscle pathways involved in defecation reflexes. Painful lesions of the anal canal (e.g., ulcers, fissures, thrombosed hemorrhoidal veins) impede defecation by exciting a spasm of the sphincters and by voluntary suppression to avoid the resultant pain.

Dietary factors greatly affect defecation. Persons who eat diets high in fiber (30–50 g daily) will have loose stools and easy defecation, whereas subjects eating low-fiber diets will have small, hard, infrequent stools. The type of fiber also affects the character of the stool and defecation. Diets high in insoluble fiber, such as the African maize diet, will produce soft and watery stools, whereas diets high in soluble fiber will produce increased gases because of fermentation, with a softer, more gellike stool.

Distention of the rectum often provokes a repeated, almost continuous urge to defecate (tenesmus), but the rocklike character of the feces prevents molding for passage through the sphincters. If the condition cannot be dealt with by rectal infusions of oil or by surface-acting agents such as dioctyl sodium sulfosuccinate (docusate sodium), digital evacuation is often necessary.

The constant urge to defecate in the absence of appreciable content in the rectum may be caused by external compression of the rectum, intrinsic neoplasms, and particularly inflammation of the rectal mucosa.

Fecal incontinence occurs when voluntary control of the external sphincter fails because of a large bolus of feces (see Chapter 107). This occurs most often when there is a rapid, sudden transit. Rapid transit occurs in infectious diarrheas and in irritable bowel syndrome. Incontinence may also be caused by damage of the anal sphincter or the pelvic musculature (see Chapters 104 and 105). Fecal incontinence, the involuntary passage of stool to the anus, is estimated to occur in approximately 7% of the general population in the form of soiling but in less than 1% in the form of gross incontinence, although the incidence in nursing homes is as high as 50%. Soiling usually results from some abnormality in the anal sphincter, but large amounts of feces are a result of damage to the anal sphincter or severe neuropathy.

A detailed workup includes physical examination of the anal ring. If the gross pathology is not defined, pelvic magnetic resonance imaging (MRI), barium defecography, anal sonography, and anal manometry may be helpful; if surgery is needed, electromyography or pudendal nerve terminal motor latency testing may be used. These tests may not be readily available in clinical offices and are used primarily in university or research centers (see "Additional Resources").

The treatment of incontinence depends on the associated cause. If there is anal disease, the treatments discussed in the appropriate chapters on anal disorders are used. If caused by other conditions, treatment is provided as discussed under the specific condition, but typically a general pattern develops in which a trial of either diphenoxylate or loperamide is indicated. Patients may rely on rectal colon plugs or may use diapers, depending on the degree of incontinence. Studies have shown diapers, often used in nursing homes, to be helpful in decreasing the incidence of incontinence in those patients where no definite cause can be established.

Attempts at using biofeedback training to control incontinence have shown varied success. However, it can be extremely helpful when the pelvic musculature needs to be strengthened.

Finally, there are surgical alternatives for strengthening the musculature or bypassing the rectum with an ostomy.

ADDITIONAL RESOURCES

Bharucha AE, Hasler WL: Motility of the small intestine and colon. In Podolsky DK, Camilleri M, Fitz JG, et al, editors: *Yamada's textbook of gastroenterology*, ed 6, Hoboken, New Jersey, 2016, John Wiley and Sons Ltd, pp 367–389.

Bharucha AE, Wald A: Anorectal disease. In Podolsky DK, Camilleri M, Fitz JG, et al, editors: *Yamada's textbook of gastroenterology*, ed 6, Hoboken, New Jersey, 2016, John Wiley and Sons Ltd, pp 1629–1652.

Dinning PG, Costa M, Brookes SJH: Colonic motor and sensory function. In Feldman M, Friedman LS, Brandt LJ, editors: *Gastrointestinal and liver disease*, ed 10, Philadelphia, 2016, Saunders-Elsevier, pp 1696–1712.

Rao SSC, American College of Gastroenterology Practice Parameters Committee: Diagnosis and management of fecal incontinence, *Am J Gastroenterol* 99:1585–1604, 2004.

Wald A: Clinical practice. Fecal incontinence in adults, *New Engl J Med* 356:1648–1655, 2007.

85

Constipation

Martin H. Floch

Constipation can generally be defined as fewer than three bowel movements per week. However, if it is included as a "functional disorder" in accordance with the Rome II criteria, the definition would state that the diagnosis of constipation requires at least 12 weeks of symptoms during the preceding 12 months and that two of the following criteria should be present: straining, lumpy or hard stool, sensation of incomplete evacuation, sensation of anorectal obstruction, and fewer than three bowel movements per week.

Constipation is a symptom. Therefore interpretation is subjective regarding sensations of bowel movement and stool size.

In the United States, studies indicate that there are approximately 2.5 million patient visits to physicians' offices per year for constipation. Most people living in industrialized countries have one bowel movement per day, and it varies in weight from 120 to 130 g. However, there is great individual variation. In general, stool weight is related to the transit time, and colonic transit is usually delayed in most patients with constipation.

Etiologies or pathophysiologic mechanisms that cause constipation can be classified into six groups: (1) inadequate intake of dietary fiber, (2) drug-induced constipation, (3) metabolic and endocrine problems, (4) neurologic problems, (5) local or systemic disease involving the intestine, and (6) functional disorder or irritable bowel syndrome (IBS) (Fig. 85.1).

CLINICAL PICTURE

Because constipation is a subjective interpretation, patient reports vary greatly. However, as defined, the stool must be small or infrequent. The symptom must be correlated with the cause. If the patient is otherwise healthy, the constipation is usually part of a functional gastrointestinal disorder and the patient has many symptoms, but none of organic cause. If the constipation has an organic cause, the symptoms will be associated with metabolic, neurologic, or local disease. For example, if the patient has Parkinson disease, the associated tremors will accompany constipation. If it is associated with severe rectal pain, the problems of anal ring disease will be evident. If the constipation is associated with severe hypothyroidism, the patient would also report weakness and other symptoms of the endocrine disorder.

DIAGNOSIS

Diagnosis depends on the initial history and physical findings. If evident on physical examination, an associated disease usually explains the constipation. If no disease is evident, the workup includes history, colonoscopy or barium study of intestine, and transit time using opaque markers or colonic scintigraphy. Thorough evaluation of anorectal function requires inspection of the area and, if necessary, anorectal manometry and defecography.

The importance of *transit time* to evaluate the function versus the symptom is essential in making the diagnosis of any organic obstructive disease versus a functional disorder. The transit time is simple to measure and requires swallowing Sitz markers, which are then traced by simple abdominal x-ray films for 5 days. The clinician can determine whether there is slow, even transit or whether an obstruction exists and should be evaluated.

TREATMENT AND MANAGEMENT

If the constipation has an organic cause, that disease must be treated to treat the constipation. It is often difficult to withdraw drugs that the patient might need; thus the constipation may require treatment even if the patient is taking a narcotic and pain-relieving therapy. The treatment of constipation is dietary, behavioral, pharmacologic, or surgical. Drugs used to treat constipation are described in Chapter 86 (see Box 86.1).

When constipation is caused by fiber deficiency, results of *dietary treatment* are often successful. Dietary fiber intake should be increased to 20 to 25 g, if tolerated by the patient without abdominal discomfort. Fiber increase should be gradual. Foods that include fiber substances are listed in Chapter 188, but often it is important to recommend a high-fiber cereal in the morning, depending on the patient's work and eating habits. Dietary recommendations then can be made to increase the intake of fruits, vegetables, and grains. A high-fiber breakfast cereal plus four to five portions of fruits or vegetables can easily reach the 25-g average of daily dietary fiber needed to maintain normal colon function.

When fiber does not solve the problem, *pharmacologic therapy* may or must be instituted. Pharmacologic agents available are listed in all drug formularies and derive from seven categories: bulk formers, emollients, lubricants, saline products, stimulants, hyperosmolar agents, and prokinetic agents (see Chapter 86). It is a challenge for a physician to select the correct combination of therapies. Most recently, work with 5-HT$_4$ antagonists has shown some promise, although tegaserod (Zelnorm), the latest drug in this category, was taken off the US market although it did help some patients. A chloride channel absorption–blocking agent, lubiprostone (Amitiza), has proved helpful to some patients.

In children with constipation, *behavioral change and retraining* may be helpful in as many as 50% to 75% of patients. Enemas and laxation are used to empty the bowel frequently and are gradually withdrawn as the child learns the behavior of regular defecation.

In patients with functional disorders and certain psychiatric disorders, successful treatment can be accomplished if the individual's psychologic state is treated.

Indications for *surgical treatment* are relatively few, but it may be successful in some patients. Certainly for organic causes such as

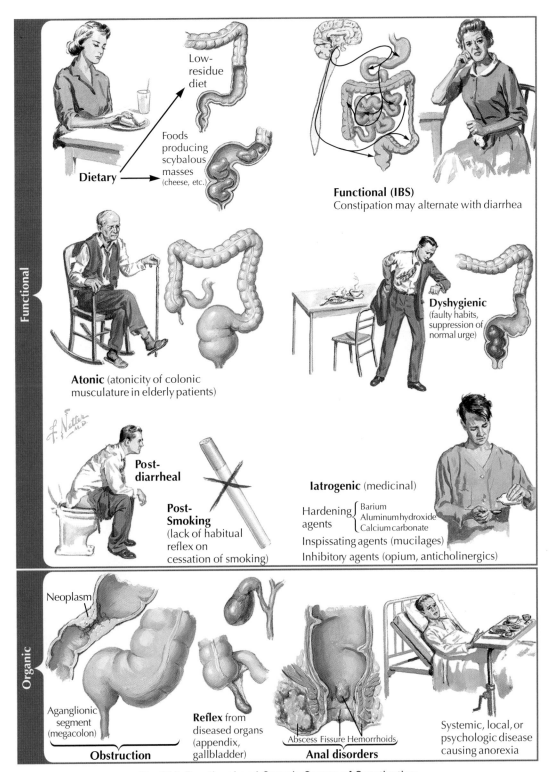

Fig. 85.1 Functional and Organic Causes of Constipation.

Hirschsprung disease, surgery is needed. Some patients with severe colonic inertia are refractory to all therapies, and in rare, severely intractable cases, ileorectal anastomosis or cecostomy is used.

Treating constipation in a patient with a functional disorder or one taking drugs is often challenging. Some patients require simple laxation, whereas others require different combinations of laxation. The clinician should start simply with one of the agents described in the seven cat-egories and then add a wetting or osmotic agent. If that is unsuccessful, stimulants can be added. An example would be to begin with magnesium hydroxide (Milk of Magnesia) or polyethylene glycol (MiraLax) on a daily or an every-other-day basis. If this fails, a wetting agent or an osmotic agent, such as lactulose, can be tried. If that does not succeed, a stimulant such as senna extract or a trial of a new agent such as lubiprostone could be attempted.

COURSE AND PROGNOSIS

Most cases of simple constipation can be treated by dietary means with increased soluble fibers, insoluble fibers, or both. When this approach fails and a cause cannot be determined, therapy that incorporates behavioral approaches or pharmacologic agents is necessary. Surgery is rarely indicated.

ADDITIONAL RESOURCES

Bharucha AE, Pemberton JH, Locke GR 3rd.: American gastroenterological association technical review on constipation, *Gastroenterol* 144:218–238, 2013.

Lembo AJ: Constipation. In Feldman M, Friedman LS, Brandt LJ, editors: *Gastrointestinal and liver disease*, ed 10, Philadelphia, 2016, Saunders-Elsevier, pp 270–296.

Lembo AJ, Schneier HA, Shiff SJ, et al: Two randomized trials of linaclotide for chronic constipation, *New Engl J Med* 365:527–536, 2011.

Rao S, Lembo AJ, Schiff SJ, et al: A 12-week, randomized, controlled trial with a 4-week randomized withdrawal period to evaluate the efficacy and safety of linaclotide in irritable bowel syndrome with constipation, *Am J Gastroenterol* 107:1714–1724, 2012.

Rao SSC, Camilleri M: Approach to the patient with constipation. In Podolsky DK, Camilleri M, Fitz JG, et al, editors: *Yamada's textbook of gastroenterology*, ed 6, Hoboken, New Jersey, 2016, John Wiley and Sons Ltd, pp 757–780.

Singh S, Heady S, Coss-Adame E, Rao SS: Clinical utility of colonic manometry in slow transit constipation, *Neurogastroenterol Motil* 25:487–495, 2013.

Szarka L: Dysmotility of the small intestine and colon. In Podolsky DK, Camilleri M, Fitz JG, et al, editors: *Yamada's textbook of gastroenterology*, ed 6, Hoboken, New Jersey, 2016, John Wiley and Sons Ltd, pp 1154–1195.

86

Effects of Drugs on the Colon

Martin H. Floch

Folklore and society have maintained the philosophy that regular bowel movements are essential to health. Consequently people have attempted to maintain bowel regularity and to experience a "good" bowel movement by using laxatives and drugs that affect the gastrointestinal (GI) tract, particularly the colon (Fig. 86.1 and Box 86.1).

Drugs may cause colonic injury. Enemas can actually damage the mucosa of the colon, especially when substances are added to the enema that can be injurious, such as hydrogen peroxide or caustic soaps. Routine laxatives such as those containing senna may color the bowel and cause melanosis coli. Oral contraceptives, vasopressin, ergotamine, cocaine,

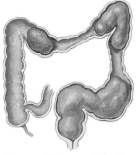

Bulk agents (bran, psyllium, methylcellulose) provide increased size, promote peristalsis by distention

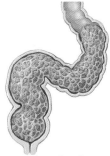

Wetting agents (dioctyl sodium sulfosuccinate) soften stool by coating and dispersion of component particles

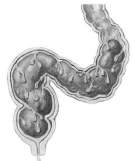

Mineral oil lubricates and mixes with stool to soften it

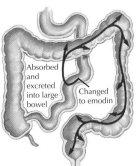

Emodins (cascara, senna, aloes) stimulate large bowel peristalsis and secretion by irritation

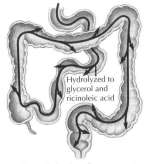

Castor oil and derivatives stimulate activity of small and large bowel by irritation

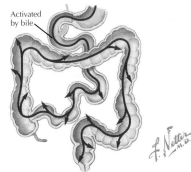

Phenolphthalein stimulates peristalsis and secretion by irritation; site of major action undetermined, probably widespread

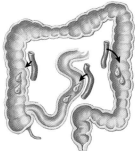

Salines (magnesium sulfate, citrate, and hydroxide; sodium phosphate) draw and hold fluid in lumen osmotically, also have some irritant action

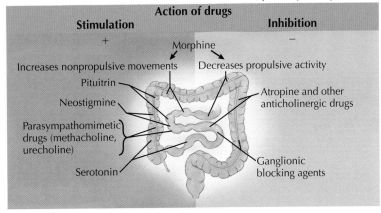

Fig. 86.1 Effects of Drugs on the Large Intestine.

BOX 86.1 Cathartic/Stimulant/Laxative Drug Categories

Bulk Agents
Bran (wheat fiber): retains water
Psyllium (ispaghula): nurtures and increases size of microflora
Guarana
Sterculia
Methylcellulose (inert chemical)

Nonabsorbed Sugars
Lactulose (osmotic; nurtures flora)
Lactitol (osmotic)

Salts (Extract Water)
Magnesium citrate
Magnesium hydroxide (Mg[OH]$_2$)
Sulfate (SO$_4$)
Sodium sulfate (NaSO$_4$)

Polyethylene Glycol (Retains Water)
Cleansing: 1 L
Daily: 250 mL

Anthranoid Compounds
Aloe
Cascara
Senna
Castor oil

Polyphenolic Compounds
Phenolphthalein
Bisacodyl
Sodium picosulfate

Detergents
Docusate sodium

Liquid Paraffin (Lubricant)
Mineral oil

Prokinetic Agents (Stimulate Motility)
Tegaserod (Zelnorm)[a] (5-HT$_4$ agonist)

Chloride Channel Blocker
Lubiprostone (Amitiza)

[a]Pulled from US market.

dextroamphetamine, digitalis, neuroleptics, and alosetron have all been shown to cause an ischemic condition and ischemic colitis. Nonsteroidal antiinflammatory drugs (NSAIDs), cyclooxygenase (COX-2) inhibitors, certain antibiotics, and chemotherapy can cause a single or numerous ulcerations in the bowel. So-called cathartic colon may result from frequent and abusive use of laxatives. The colon can become shortened or dilated from laxative abuse.

Drugs may affect the motor and secretory activities in the intestine directly or indirectly. The classic parasympathomimetic drug *metha-choline* and the agents that inhibit hydrolysis of acetylcholine by blocking cholinesterase action (*physostigmine* and *neostigmine*) stimulate intestinal contractions. *Atropine* and a legion of synthetic anticholinergic drugs block the transmission of parasympathetic stimuli to the effector organs and thus inhibit intestinal contractions. Drugs that stimulate or inhibit the effects of sympathetic nerves are less active in the GI tract than other systems. Therefore sympathomimetic drugs would have to be used in very large doses to affect intestinal motility. *Ganglionic blocking agents*, interfering with the transmission of nerve impulses at the sympathetic and the parasympathetic ganglionic synapses, inhibit intestinal contractions.

Morphine and all related opiates, used for centuries as antidiarrheal agents, generally decrease the propulsive motility and increase tonus, particularly of the large intestine, sometimes to the point of spasms, which may explain the abdominal discomfort associated with opiates.

The endless number of drugs and preparations that promote defecation are called *cathartics* and are frequently listed as "laxatives" or "purgatives." Classification according to different mechanisms or actions is usually the basis for their selection in a given clinical situation (see Box 86.1 and Chapters 83–85).

ADDITIONAL RESOURCES

Drossman DA, Morris CB, Edwards H, et al: Diagnosis, characterization, and 3-month outcome after detoxification of 39 patients with narcotic bowel syndrome, *Am J Gastroenterol* 107:1426–1440, 2012.

Lembo AJ: Constipation. In Feldman M, Friedman LS, Brandt LJ, editors: *Gastrointestinal and liver disease*, ed 10, Philadelphia, 2016, Saunders-Elsevier, pp 270–296.

Schiller LR, Sellin JH: Diarrhea. In Feldman M, Friedman LS, Brandt LJ, editors: *Gastrointestinal and liver disease*, ed 10, Philadelphia, 2016, Saunders-Elsevier, pp 221–241.

87

Megacolon and Hirschsprung Disease

Martin H. Floch

Megacolon is divided into the congenital and acquired types. The congenital form is Hirschsprung disease and includes classic, short-segment, and ultrashort-segment types as well as total colonic aganglionosis (Fig. 87.1).

Acquired megacolon includes many disorders. However, *idiopathic* acquired megacolon has no cause and is often associated with an acute form of Ogilvie syndrome (see Chapter 60). Acquired forms are also associated with a variety of neurologic diseases, intestinal smooth muscle disease, and metabolic disorders (see Chapter 59).

Congenital megacolon usually presents during infancy (although it is now well documented in adolescents and adults). It is more common in males than in females and classically has an *aganglionic* segment in the rectum or sigmoid with a dilated segment above. Findings from anal manometry are classically abnormal. The pathophysiology is attributed to a loss of ganglionic cells in the segment of bowel. It is reported as being linked with both dominant and recessive inheritance. In addition, patients have classic cases of the idiopathic form.

CLINICAL PICTURE

Constipation is the symptom that drives the parent or patient to seek medical advice. Functional constipation brings more children to medical attention than does aganglionic megacolon, but the differential diagnosis includes these two conditions. Great variations in clinical signs and symptoms are expected, but typical situations are readily characterized. The child with chronic functional constipation is a healthy-looking youngster of normal body appearance, whereas a child with aganglionic megacolon appears to be chronically ill, has a protuberant abdomen, and bears the stigma of malnutrition in growth and development. However, well-documented cases of normal growth and development show the disease progressing into adolescence, with rare reports in adults, up to age 40.

Typically, the child or adolescent has never had a normal bowel movement and requires laxatives and enemas to evacuate. Occasionally the presentation is diarrhea, characterized by liquid stool moving around an impaction. On rectal examination, the sphincter may be normal or relaxed, and stool or a dilated rectum is palpated; fecal impaction is often severe, and the rectal sphincter may be extremely tight.

DIAGNOSIS

The diagnosis is usually straightforward in the classic infant presentation. In early childhood or adolescence or in adulthood, however, making the diagnosis becomes more difficult. Barium enema shows the classic presentation of a narrowed segment with dilated bowel above. It is now known that in the atypical presentations, the aganglionic or narrowed segment may be extremely short and may involve only the internal anal sphincter.

Proctosigmoidoscopy and colonoscopy reveal a dilated sigmoid. At times, if the dilatation is of long standing, it may be difficult to examine the entire bowel endoscopically. However, no obstructive lesions are demonstrated. If the fecal impaction is chronic, traumatic ulceration of the mucosa may be noted. Barium contrast enema may reveal the narrow segment and confirm the suspected diagnosis, but further evaluation is needed before surgery can be performed.

In the classic presentation, physiologic testing reveals that the anal sphincter fails to relax after distention of the rectum. This may be helpful when the narrowed segment is not easily demonstrated. However, manometry has not been universally reproducible.

The diagnosis of Hirschsprung disease is definitively made by examining biopsy specimens that reveal *aganglionosis*, or a patchy area, in the segment. Often suction or punch biopsy is attempted first, but deeper biopsy is required to confirm the diagnosis. However, the observation of ganglion cells on colon biopsy tends to rule out the diagnosis of Hirschsprung disease.

Acquired megacolon is often confused with congenital megacolon (Hirschsprung disease). Certainly when the rectum is greatly dilated and short-segment Hirschsprung disease is suspected, the diagnosis depends on biopsy and histologic interpretation. When the two conditions are difficult to distinguish, full-thickness biopsy is essential.

TREATMENT AND MANAGEMENT

Classic megacolon requires surgical correction, the treatment of choice. The goal of surgery is to establish regular defecation. Therefore the aganglionic segment must be removed.

COURSE AND PROGNOSIS

When the presentation and findings are not classic and are seen in early childhood or adolescence, the patient will have had numerous trials of laxatives. The adult patient will have undergone repeated laxative and probably enema therapy. Some patients can be managed by laxative and enema evacuation to provide comfort and to ensure that the bowel is not dilated and causing obstruction to normal digestion and absorption.

Because of the great variation in presentations and laxative programs used, course and prognosis vary. In the classic case of Hirschsprung disease, the prognosis is good after successful surgery. Long-term follow-up studies reveal an approximately a 90% cure rate, with residual fecal soiling in some cases. Even though course and prognosis can vary greatly, especially in older age groups, the prognosis is good if the aganglionic segment can be removed.

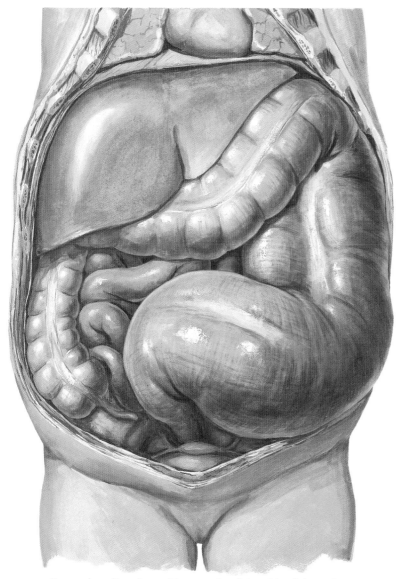

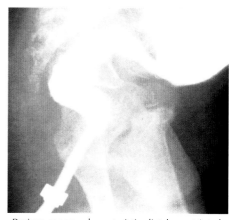

Barium enema; characteristic distal constricted segment

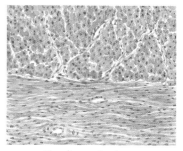

Ganglion cells absent

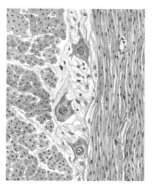

Ganglion cells present between longitudinal and circular muscle layers

Tremendous distention and hypertrophy of sigmoid and descending colon; moderate involvement of transverse colon; distal constricted segment

Fig. 87.1 Megacolon (Hirschsprung Disease).

ADDITIONAL RESOURCES

Barnes PRH, Lennard-Jones JE, Howley PR, Todd IP: Hirschsprung's disease and idiopathic megacolon in adults and adolescents, *Gut* 27:534–541, 1996.

Bass LM, Wershil BK: Anatomy, histology, embryology, and developmental anomalies of the small and large intestine. In Feldman M, Friedman LS, Brandt LJ, editors: *Gastrointestinal and liver disease*, ed 10, Philadelphia, 2016, Saunders-Elsevier, pp 1649–1678.

Foxx-Orenstein AE: Ileus and pseudo-obstruction. In Feldman M, Friedman LS, Brandt LJ, editors: *Gastrointestinal and liver disease*, ed 10, Philadelphia, 2016, Saunders-Elsevier, pp 2171–2195.

Kim HJ, Kim AY, Lee CW, et al: Hirschsprung disease and hypoganglionosis in adults: radiologic findings and differentiation, *Radiology* 247:428–434, 2008.

88

Volvulus, Sigmoid, and Cecum

Martin H. Floch

Intestinal volvulus is the rotation of a segment of bowel around its mesentery (Fig. 88.1). This usually causes a closed-loop obstruction and may cause vascular compromise. Primary volvulus of the colon usually occurs in the sigmoid colon and in the cecum; the other parts of the large bowel are well fixed in the posterior abdominal wall.

SIGMOID VOLVULUS

Sigmoid volvulus is a comparatively rare form of intestinal obstruction in the Western world, occurring more frequently in middle-aged and elderly patients. It is more common in eastern Europe and Asia, presumably reflecting different dietary habits. Cultures with diets high in bulky vegetables have a higher incidence of sigmoid volvulus. The high-fiber bulk causes a larger fecal residue and results in a more distended and elongated bowel that is prone to rotation.

In the United States, patients with sigmoid volvulus are usually constipated and frequently use laxatives. Sigmoid volvulus develops more frequently in patients with neurologic or psychiatric disorders such as Alzheimer or Parkinson disease. Chronic symptoms may be difficult to differentiate from the patient's usual constipation. However, onset of symptoms is usually sudden, with lower abdominal pain, obstipation, and abdominal distention. When vascular compromise occurs, ischemia and peritoneal signs may evolve rapidly. Possible ischemia and perforation, as well as acute volvulus, mandate rapid evaluation.

Once abdominal distention raises the index of suspicion, immediate radiographic evaluation of the abdomen is necessary (see radiograph in Fig. 88.2). The classic dilated sigmoid loop may be seen on a simple obstructive series. Usually no feces are present in the rectum, but there may be dilatation of other loops in the colon. Plain x-ray films of the abdomen confirm the diagnosis in more than 60% of patients. If there is any doubt, an absorbable-dye enema can assist in the diagnosis. *Barium should not be used* because it may result in perforation. Computed tomography can also make the diagnosis promptly.

Management of sigmoid volvulus consists of attempted enemas, use of a rectal tube, and flexible sigmoidoscopes or colonoscopy to decompress and detorse the sigmoid bowel. The success rate using a flexible sigmoidoscope is 95% to 98%, depending on the endoscopist's experience. The colonoscope is usually not necessary unless the shorter sigmoidoscope cannot reach the suspected area. If bowel is ischemic, immediate surgery should be seriously considered to relieve any compromise in the vasculature.

In rare cases the symptoms may be mild and recurrent, and a thorough evaluation is necessary. A long loop of sigmoid may twist, necessitating surgical correction. Twisting of this loop may be discovered only by chance.

The recurrence rate for sigmoid volvulus is approximately 40% and is high even after endoscopic decompression. Therefore if symptoms recur, elective resection is recommended. It is important to consider whether the patient is ambulatory or institutionalized. If the patient experiences vascular compromise and gangrene has set in, mortality is very high (>50%). Surgical evaluation and the timing of surgery are extremely important in predicting the course and progress for each patient.

VOLVULUS OF THE CECUM

Volvulus of the cecum is an abnormal rotation of the cecum from an apparent anomalous attachment to the mesentery, resulting in increased mobility (see Fig. 88.2). It occurs infrequently in Western countries, where it accounts for approximately 1% of cases of intestinal obstruction. As with volvulus of the sigmoid, volvulus of the cecum appears to be more common in populations that have a diet high in vegetables and fibrous foods. Persistent loading of the bowel with a large fecal mass may play a role in the etiology.

The predisposing factor is inadequate fixation of the cecum and the ascending colon to the posterior abdominal wall, a result of an incomplete embryologic third stage of intestinal rotation. Twisting of the mesentery may be loose and intermittent without becoming complete. When it is complete, however, the vessels may strangulate and the bowel may become gangrenous.

A variant of cecal volvulus called *cecal bascule* can occur when the ascending colon fills up without twisting. It accounts for approximately 10% of cases of cecal volvulus. Although this type is not a true volvulus, cecal bascule can present with the same symptoms.

Patients with volvulus of the cecum are usually younger than those with sigmoid volvulus; most are 20 to 40 years of age. Onset with severe central abdominal pain is usually sudden, and vomiting soon follows. The pain is constant but intermittently severe. Symptoms are rarely sporadic. If the pain ceases it is presumed that the volvulus has resolved, but it may then recur spontaneously. On examination, the abdomen is usually distended. In most patients the distended cecum may be distinguished as a palpable tympanic swelling in the midabdomen.

The best way to diagnose volvulus of the cecum is by viewing plain x-ray films of the abdomen, which reveal a greatly distended central coil, possibly with a fluid level. Loops of ileum behind it may be obstructed. Plain abdominal radiographs and clinical status confirm the diagnosis in 50% of patients. In some patients, a diatrizoate (Gastrografin) barium enema or computed tomography is necessary to delineate the site of obstruction. Use of all the studies still yields a

Pathogenesis of sigmoid volvulus

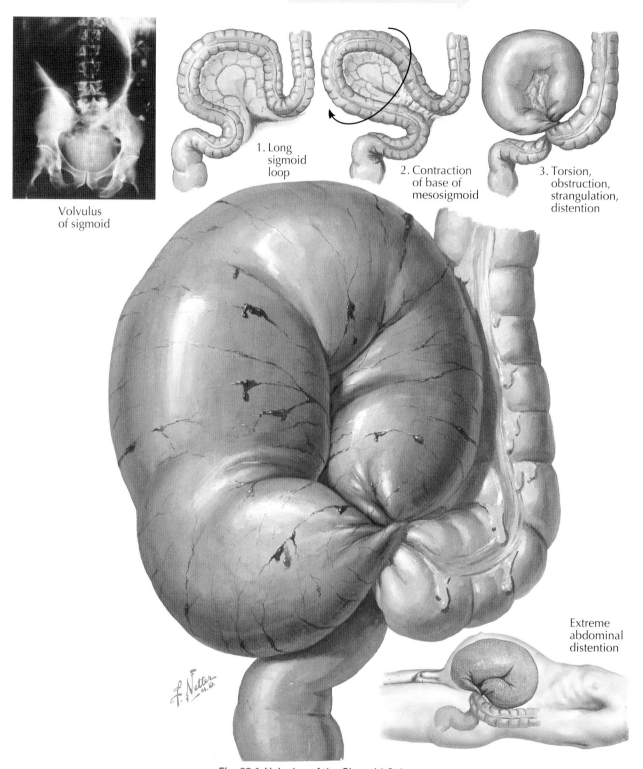

Volvulus
of sigmoid

1. Long
sigmoid
loop

2. Contraction
of base of
mesosigmoid

3. Torsion,
obstruction,
strangulation,
distention

Extreme
abdominal
distention

Fig. 88.1 Volvulus of the Sigmoid Colon.

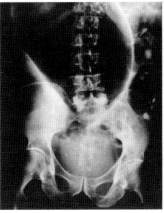
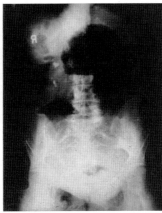

Volvulus of sigmoid   Volvulus of cecum

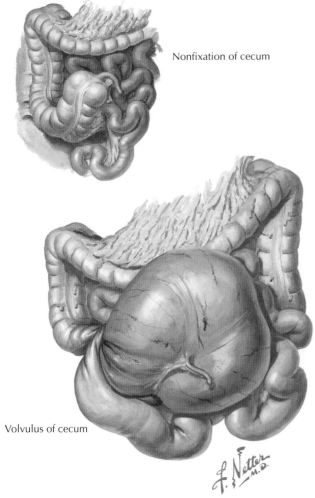

Nonfixation of cecum

Volvulus of cecum

Fig. 88.2 Volvulus of the Cecum.

diagnosis in only 60% to 90% of patients. However, with the picture of abdominal pain, abdominal distention, vomiting, constipation, and the dilated loop, there is enough suspicion to warrant immediate laparotomy. One study reported that as many as 25% of patients have gangrenous bowel at laparotomy. Therefore there should be no delay when the suspicion is significant.

After the diagnosis is made, especially if gangrene is suspected, laparotomy and resection are urgent. When there is no suspicion of peritonitis or gangrene, attempts at reducing the volvulus with colonoscopy are indicated. However, this is less successful than in sigmoid volvulus. Consequently most surgeons believe that surgery is indicated without delay when cecal volvulus is suspected. Surgical detorsion is performed, followed by cecal fixation to prevent recurrence. Depending on the patient and the condition, right hemicolectomy with cecal resection may be indicated to eliminate possible recurrence.

The mortality rate may be as high as 10%, and if gangrene develops, it may approach 40%. These statistics emphasize the need for early surgery to treat volvulus of the cecum.

ADDITIONAL RESOURCES

Delabrousse E, Sarlieve P, Sailley N, et al: Cecal volvulus, CT findings and correlation with pathophysiology, *Emerg Radiol* 14:411–415, 2007.

Mizell JS, Turnage RH: Intestinal obstruction. In Feldman M, Friedman LS, Brandt LJ, editors: *Gastrointestinal and liver disease*, ed 10, Philadelphia, 2016, Saunders-Elsevier, pp 2154–2170.

Umansky K, Mathews JB: Colon: anatomy and structural anomalies. In Podolsky DK, Camilleri M, Fitz JG, et al, editors: *Yamada's textbook of gastroenterology*, ed 6, Hoboken, New Jersey, 2016, John Wiley and Sons Ltd, pp 93–107.

89

Diseases of the Appendix: Inflammation, Mucocele, and Tumors

Martin H. Floch

Inflammatory changes of the vermiform appendix are the most frequent cause of laparotomy in western countries, where the incidence of appendicitis is approximately 10 times that in eastern countries.

The *appendix* is part of the cecum, and its abdominal marking usually lies in the transition of the outer to the middle third of an imaginary line drawn from the anterosuperior iliac spine to the umbilicus (the McBurney point). However, because of embryologic development and the mobility of the cecum, the appendix may lie anywhere in the abdominal cavity (Fig. 89.1). Furthermore, it is a rudimentary organ, narrow and thin, and may be positioned retrocecally or may fall into the pelvis. The layers of the appendix are the same as those in other parts of the intestinal tract, but it is not enwrapped by visceral peritoneum, and the longitudinal muscle envelops the entire circumference.

It is proposed that obstruction of the lumen of the appendix followed by infection is the cause of acute appendicitis. In the initial stage, acute appendicitis is confined to the mucous membranes, which become edematous and hyperemic, and are invaded by white blood cells (WBCs). If the inflammatory process subsides, which rarely occurs, but involves other coats of the appendix in an acute suppurative process, the whole organ becomes enlarged, and a fibrinous or fibropurulent exudate covers the appendix. *Abscesses* may form in the appendiceal wall and lead to gangrenous appendicitis. Necrosis and putrefaction of the entire appendiceal tissues may lead to perforation. Once infected material spills into the abdominal cavity, peritonitis may form a periappendiceal abscess or diffuse peritonitis. Depending on the position of the appendix, it may spill into the pelvis or any location in the abdominal cavity.

Rarely, the suppurative process may heal without medical attention. The resultant fibrosis of the wall can lead to the formation of a future cyst or *mucocele* when mucus is secreted into the fibrosed area. This type of cystic tumor may be benign but must be differentiated from adenocarcinoma. Malignant tumors can spill into the entire abdominal cavity, causing pseudomyxoma peritonei.

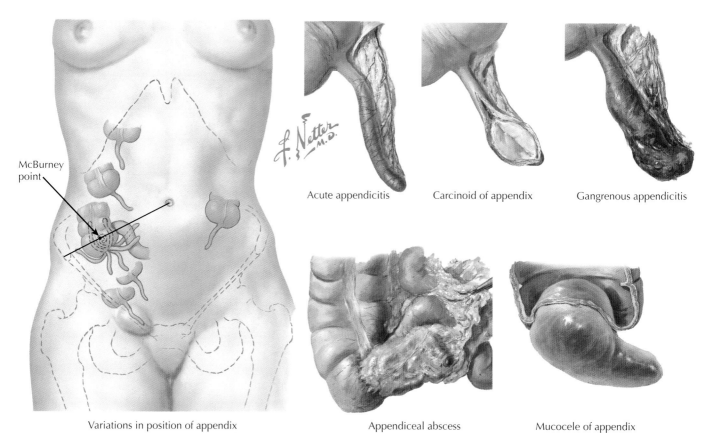

McBurney point

Variations in position of appendix

Acute appendicitis   Carcinoid of appendix   Gangrenous appendicitis

Appendiceal abscess   Mucocele of appendix

Fig. 89.1 Variations in Position and Diseases of the Appendix.

CLINICAL PICTURE

The classic clinical picture of appendicitis is periumbilical pain that radiates to the right lower quadrant and may be associated with nausea or vomiting. The picture usually evolves over 24 hours and may be associated with fever, but the pain is usually persistent, grows in intensity, and is associated with significant nausea or vomiting. Unfortunately most cases are not typical, and symptoms are often vague. In elderly persons, the picture may be masked, and the acute signs may not be present until massive perforation appears. Also, the appendix may be positioned in different parts of the abdominal cavity, and symptoms may be atypical, such as left-lower-quadrant pain, right-upper-quadrant pain, or even left-upper-quadrant pain (see Fig. 89.1).

All diagnosticians should consider appendicitis in any presentation of acute abdominal pain or mild nausea and vomiting. Appendicitis does not cause violent vomiting or extensive diarrhea and thus should not be confused with severe acute gastroenteritis.

DIAGNOSIS

When clinical findings point to appendicitis, surgical intervention is indicated. Studies show that a higher index of complexity in diagnosis leads to more perforations. Atypical presentations, as previously described, occur in approximately 20% of patients. Good clinical practice indicates that simple laparotomy or laparoscopy should be performed rather than waiting for perforation.

The differential diagnosis includes Meckel diverticulitis, cecal diverticulitis, mesenteric lymphadenitis, and ileitis. Other causes—such as renal, sigmoid, and gynecologic disease—can be diagnosed by careful examination and imaging techniques.

Computed tomography (CT), especially with helical imaging, has become the most accurate diagnostic test for appendicitis, proving positive in greater than 90%, and can be extremely helpful when the diagnosis is uncertain. Ultrasound examination may also yield high accuracy, but the procedure is operator-dependent and varies from institution to institution. However, when appendicitis is suspected during pregnancy and x-ray imaging should be avoided, ultrasound is used. Helical CT will make the diagnosis and help rule out any complications, such as perforation or abscess, or any renal or gynecologic disease.

It is also useful to conduct a simple WBC count. The WBC count is elevated in approximately 80% of patients with appendicitis. A normal WBC count usually alerts the diagnostician to look for other causes of the pain.

TREATMENT AND MANAGEMENT

Treatment is surgical removal of the appendix. Unfortunately, if perforation has occurred, local drainage of the abscess may be required. In rare, fascinating cases, obstruction of the appendix occurs because of parasites, such as pinworms. The parasitic infestation should be treated along with the appendicitis (see Section VI).

Simple excision of the appendix can be accomplished with a small incision. Also, surgeons adept in laparoscopic surgery now perform appendectomies with ease. The choice depends on the patient and the surgeon. Both procedures produce equally excellent results provided that no complications arise.

COURSE AND PROGNOSIS

Once the correct diagnosis has been made and there is no perforation, patients usually leave the hospital within 24 to 48 hours and can return to full activity in 2 weeks. However, if perforation occurs, mortality rates increase and can become significant in elderly patients. Complication rates may be as high as 12% to 20%. Mortality as high as 30% has been reported in the elderly population. Therefore, physicians need to make an early diagnosis and intervene to prevent complications.

Tumors of the appendix other than mucocele and cystadenocarcinoma do occur at significant rates (see Chapter 99). Carcinoid of the appendix is the most common appendiceal tumor (see Chapter 74).

ADDITIONAL RESOURCES

Kelly K, Sarr M, Hinder R: *Mayo Clinic gastrointestinal surgery*, Philadelphia, 2004, Elsevier.

Sarosi GA Jr: Appendicitis. In Feldman M, Friedman LS, Brandt LJ, editors: *Gastrointestinal and liver disease*, ed 10, Philadelphia, 2016, Saunders-Elsevier, pp 2112–2122.

Sherman CB, McQuaid K: Approach to the patient with acute abdomen. In Podolsky DK, Camilleri M, Fitz JG, et al, editors: *Yamada's textbook of gastroenterology*, ed 6, Hoboken, New Jersey, 2016, John Wiley and Sons Ltd, pp 781–796.

Silen W, editor: *Cope's early diagnosis of the acute abdomen*, ed 22, New York, 2010, Oxford University Press.

Squires R, Poster R: Acute abdomen. In Townsend CM, Beauchamp RD, Evers BM, Mattox KL, editors: *Sabiston textbook of surgery: the biological basis of modern surgical practice*, ed 19, Philadelphia, 2012, Elsevier.

90

Diverticulosis

Martin H. Floch

DIVERTICULAR DISEASE OF THE COLON

Diverticulosis of the colon is an acquired condition that results from herniation of the mucosa through defects in the muscle coats (Fig. 90.1). Defects are usually located where the blood vessels pierce the muscular wall to gain access to the submucosal plane. These vessels enter at a constant position, just on the mesenteric side of the two lateral taeniae coli, so diverticula typically occur in two parallel rows along the bowel. Appendices epiploicae (omentales) are also situated in this part of the circumference.

Diverticula probably arise from pulsion as a result of increased intraluminal pressure from uncoordinated peristalsis or inadequate luminal contents, possibly resulting from a low-fiber diet. Diverticula do not occur in the rectum but may be found throughout the entire colon. They are more common in the left side and usually affect the sigmoid colon. Diverticula are relatively rare in persons younger than 40 years of age but are common (60%) in persons older than 60 living in Western countries. The incidence is dramatically higher in Western countries, where the diet is much lower in fiber; this decreased fiber intake results in decreased colonic luminal content, and pressure from wall contraction is transmitted to the wall rather than to the luminal content. Therefore the formation of diverticula is related to fiber deficiency. The fact that contractions and their force are greatest in the sigmoid supports the theory that diverticula are more prominent in the sigmoid than in the rest of the bowel. Associated with chronic diverticula formation is the gradually increased deposition of connective tissue by *elastin*, resulting in thickening of the sigmoid, with some bowel rigidity where large amounts of elastin are deposited.

Although diverticula may form in the second or third decade of life, they are usually asymptomatic at that time.

Clinical Picture

If discovered during a barium enema examination, computed tomography (CT) scan, or colonoscopy performed for other clinical reasons (e.g., gastrointestinal [GI] bleeding, irritable bowel syndrome [IBS]), diverticula are assumed to be asymptomatic. Approximately 60% of the Western population older than 80 years of age have significant but asymptomatic diverticula formation. Furthermore, the high percentage of patients with IBS often includes those who have some diverticula formation, but not diverticulitis (see Chapter 90).

Many physicians assume that the diverticula are not causing symptoms when in reality they may cause mild symptoms. In addition, many patients with diverticula have symptoms but do not develop acute or chronic diverticulitis. Some may report a low-grade, dull ache in the left lower quadrant or a change in bowel habit. Some thought to have IBS may have diarrhea or constipation. However, diverticula are rarely thought to cause such symptoms unless temperature and white blood cell (WBC) count are elevated or imaging findings demonstrate spasm in the area of the diverticula.

On the basis of its natural history, diverticular disease is now classified into *asymptomatic, symptomatic uncomplicated,* and *complicated* types.

Diagnosis

The diagnosis of diverticula formation is made through barium enema examination, CT, or colonoscopy. When diverticula are discovered incidentally, no further diagnostic evaluation is needed. However, if the diverticula are accompanied by symptoms and the discovery was made during a barium enema or CT study, colonoscopy may be necessary. It may also be necessary to perform a WBC count and to monitor the patient carefully to identify any associated inflammation.

Treatment and Management

Most clinicians do not treat diverticula when they are discovered incidentally. Diverticula can result from a low-fiber diet, so all patients with diverticula should be advised to increase their fiber intake to 25 to 35 g daily (see Chapter 188). There is no evidence that increased fiber intake will reverse the formation of diverticula, but increased intake should prevent further progression and increased fiber in the bowel should decrease the pressure on the bowel wall.

Course and Prognosis

In western societies there is a concomitant increase in diverticula with age, and 60% of the population has diverticula by age 85. Studies also reveal that 5% to 20% of patients develop true inflammation associated with the diverticula. Asymptomatic diverticula are benign and have an excellent course and prognosis.

In patients who do have complications, the course and prognosis vary.

DIVERTICULITIS AND ITS COMPLICATIONS AND DIVERTICULAR BLEEDING

Diverticulitis

The formation of diverticula may be considered to represent the first stage of the disease process. *Diverticular disease* represents the entire spectrum of, first, diverticula formation and then diverticulitis with its complications (Fig. 90.2). For unclear reasons, inflammation in and around the diverticula occurs in only a small percentage of patients. Obstruction at the mouth of the diverticulum was thought to result in diverticulitis, similar to appendicitis, but this is no longer the accepted theory, and some believe that chronic inflammation precedes clinical diverticulitis.

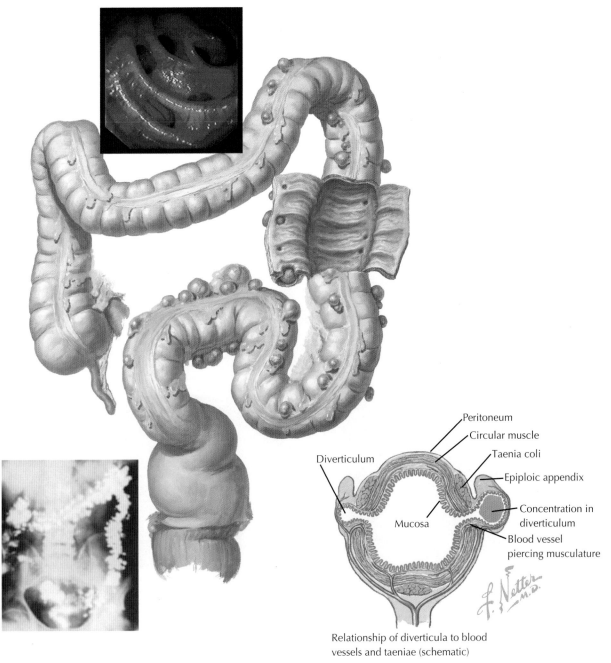

Peritoneum
Circular muscle
Taenia coli
Epiploic appendix
Diverticulum
Concentration in diverticulum
Mucosa
Blood vessel piercing musculature

Relationship of diverticula to blood vessels and taeniae (schematic)

Fig. 90.1 Colonoscopic View of Diverticula.

Once diverticulitis develops, it may manifest as symptomatic disease or may progress to cause complications, with pericolitis (microabscess), pericolic phlegmon, pericolic abscess, pelvic or intraabdominal abscess, and free perforation leading to bowel obstruction, fistulization, or bacteremia and septicemia. Any of these complications may occur after inflammation begins in the diverticula.

Clinical Picture

The clinical presentation depends largely on the degree and extent of the inflammation. The most common presentation is left-lower-quadrant pain associated with low-grade fever, mild leukocytosis, and obstipation. Symptoms vary, however, depending on the severity of the inflammation.

If the pathologic process is localized in the left lower quadrant, the pain will present as left lower quadrant pain. The pain may be mild or severe and is usually associated with a decreased number of bowel movements or intestinal obstruction. Occasionally patients have mild diarrhea. If the obstructive symptoms persist, nausea or vomiting may occur. Depending on the site of the diverticula, the pain may be distributed across the midabdomen or to the suprapubic and right side of the colon. Any fever is usually low grade, but a temperature greater than 102°F (38.8°C) indicates that the process is extensive or that bacteremia or septicemia may be present.

The classic picture is tenderness in the left lower quadrant with or without a palpable mass. However, if *rebound* occurs and if the mass is very tender, an abscess may have formed. Diffuse rebound can indicate

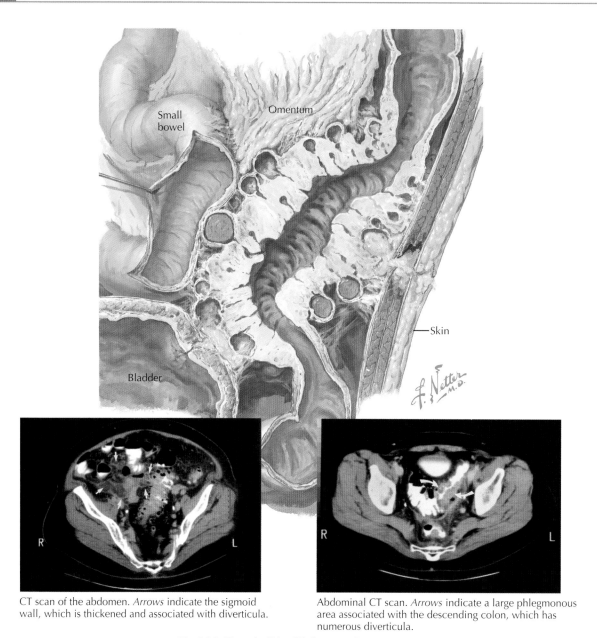

CT scan of the abdomen. *Arrows* indicate the sigmoid wall, which is thickened and associated with diverticula.

Abdominal CT scan. *Arrows* indicate a large phlegmonous area associated with the descending colon, which has numerous diverticula.

Fig. 90.2 Diverticulitis. *CT,* Computed tomography.

peritonitis and perforation. Examination of the rectum usually reveals no significant findings.

Diagnosis

Laboratory results often reveal an elevated WBC count with a predominance of polymorphonuclear leukocytes. In elderly or immunocompromised patients, leukocytosis may not be present. Depending on the symptoms (obstructive more than inflammatory), the differential diagnosis includes carcinoma of the colon, pelvic mass of gynecologic origin, or atypical appendicitis. At this point, radiologic evaluation is critical. Barium enema examination is not indicated and may even be contraindicated because of potential perforation and leakage from the pressure. CT currently is the best technique; it reveals the location of any abscess formation, any sign of perforation, and any thickening of the bowel associated with diverticula. Furthermore, CT clearly reveals the extent of the disease by demonstrating the gray areas in the mesentery adjacent to the diverticula. Colorectal examination findings are often negative, and pelvic examination may be necessary to rule out gynecologic disease; again, CT can help in defining the disease.

In rare cases it is impossible to differentiate between diverticulitis and Crohn disease or carcinoma. The diagnosis of the so-called overlap syndrome, in which both diverticula and Crohn disease are present in the sigmoid, can be made only by a pathologist. Because perforation may result from colonoscopy, as from barium enema, medical treatment is pursued until diagnostic colonoscopy can be performed. At times, especially when toxicity or perforation is suspected, the clinical situation indicates surgical intervention; then a definitive diagnosis is made at laparoscopy.

Diverticulitis is unusual in younger people, especially those under age 40. When it does occur in this age group, it may have a virulent course, with as many as two-thirds of these patients requiring surgical intervention in the past. However, recent studies indicate that the course is becoming less severe in younger patients and that a conservative approach may be followed.

Treatment and Management

Uncomplicated symptomatic diverticulitis is usually treated with bowel rest, antibiotic therapy, and slow progression from clear liquids to a low-fiber diet and then to a high-fiber diet. Once complications are present, however, vigorous treatment is indicated. The patient may require hospital admission, with intravenous antibiotics the preferred therapy and broad enough to cover the spectrum of aerobic and anaerobic microflora; this is essential. At present, most institutions use gentamicin plus another broad-spectrum antibiotic.

If an abscess has formed, percutaneous drainage should be considered. When drainage is unsuccessful or is used only as a temporizing measure, surgical intervention is necessary. Indications for surgery include uncontrollable sepsis, perforation, obstruction, fistula, and uncontrolled hemorrhage as well as persistent symptoms of diverticulitis in the patient receiving antibiotic therapy. Two-stage procedures are most common at present. A colostomy is created, and after an extended period (usually months), the continuity of the bowel is recreated. However, one-stage resections are used when the segment is small, with minimal inflammation, or when the patient has symptoms without signs of abscess inflammation.

Course and Prognosis

There are some caveats with therapy. Diverticulitis in the immunocompromised patient may manifest with few signs and symptoms; therefore treatment may be delayed, and morbidity and mortality may increase dramatically. Also, the index of suspicion should be high when the patient has abdominal pain, fever, or obstipation.

The risk for recurrent symptoms of diverticulitis or attacks ranges from 7% to 45%. It is thought that a high-fiber diet will reduce the risk, with a 70% chance of response to medical therapy after a first attack but only a 6% chance after the third attack. Thus some recommend resection of the sigmoid after two attacks of uncomplicated diverticulitis. However, treatment of recurrent attacks is changing, and some now believe that these cases, if uncomplicated, can be followed medically. Based on early reports, some are using mesalamine (5-aminosalicylic acid) to decrease attacks, although this recommendation is still under research. Mortality rates range from 3% to 35%, depending on the patient population. Early diagnosis, appropriate therapy, and surgical intervention (when indicated) are essential.

Diverticular Hemorrhage

Diverticula are the most common cause of massive colonic bleeding in Western societies. An estimated 3% to 5% of patients with diverticular disease will have severe blood loss. In most patients, bleeding occurs from a single diverticulum. Surprisingly, the diverticula that bleed are often on the right side but are not inflamed. The most persistent finding is thinning of the wall of the diverticulum, with erosion of a vessel. Patients typically have massive lower GI bleeding.

There are standard therapeutic protocols for GI hemorrhage, as well as a standard workup, but the clinician should determine whether the bleeding is from the right or the left side of the colon, because surgical intervention may be necessary. Therefore radionucleotide imaging, arteriography, and colonoscopy should all be used to determine the location of the bleeding. Barium contrast has no place in this evaluation.

Therapeutically, arteriography can be used to inject sclerosing agents to occlude the bleeding vessel. If this is not successful and the bleeding is not controlled, surgical intervention is necessary. Usually angiography identifies the site, and vasopressin infusions or embolization of a vessel can be used to stop the bleeding. If these measures do not succeed, surgical intervention will be required. If the segment can be identified, rebleeding will be relatively rare. Segmental resection, when possible, is associated with lower morbidity than hemicolectomy. Unfortunately surgical mortality is 9% to 11% and depends on comorbid conditions and the patient's age. When the site of bleeding cannot be identified, morbidity and mortality rates increase to approximately 35%, and a total colectomy must be considered. Fortunately most cases of diverticular hemorrhage resolve spontaneously, and massive bleeding is relatively rare.

ADDITIONAL RESOURCES

Alny TP, Howell DA: Diverticular disease of the colon, *N Engl J Med* 302:324–329, 1980.

Bhukel TP, Stollman NH: Diverticular disease of the colon. In Feldman M, Friedman LS, Brandt LJ, editors: *Gastrointestinal and liver disease*, ed 10, Philadelphia, 2016, Saunders-Elsevier, pp 2123–2138.

Everhart JE, Ruhl CE: Burden of digestive diseases in the United States part II: lower gastrointestinal diseases, *Gastroenterology* 136:741–764, 2009.

Floch CL: Diagnosis and management of acute diverticulitis, *J Clin Gastroentol* 40:S136–S144, 2006.

Floch MH, White JA: Management of diverticular disease is changing, *World J Gastroenterol* 12:3225–3228, 2006.

Hughes LE: Postmortem survey of diverticular disease of the colon, *Gut* 10:326–335, 1969.

Painter NS, Burkett BP: Diverticular disease of the colon: a 20th century problem, *Clin Gastroenterol* 4:3–21, 1975.

Sheth AA, Longo W, Floch MH: Diverticular disease and diverticulitis, *Am J Gastroenterol* 103(6):1550–1556, 2008.

Strate LL: Diverticulosis and dietary fiber: rethinking the relationship, *Gastroenterology* 142:205–207, 2012.

Strate LL: Lifestyle factors and the course of diverticular disease, *Dig Dis* 30:35–45, 2012.

Strate LL, Modi R, Cohen E, Spiegel BM: Diverticular disease as a chronic illness: evolving epidemiologic and clinical insights, *Am J Gastroenterol* 107:1486–1493, 2012.

Tursi A: New physiopathological and therapeutic approaches to diverticular disease of the colon, *Expert Opin Pharmacother* 8:299–307, 2007.

91

Ulcerative Colitis

Martin H. Floch

Ulcerative colitis (UC) is a disease of unknown etiology characterized by diffuse mucosal inflammation of the large bowel (Fig. 91.1). The disease is variable in extent, severity, and clinical course, and knowledge of many aspects remains incomplete. The incidence and prevalence of UC vary with geography and race. Most studies have been performed in North America and England; incidence varies from 0 to 10 per 100,000, with prevalence as high as 200 per 100,000 population.

Environmental and genetic factors undoubtedly create an altered immune response that results in inflammation of the mucosa of the bowel. Although infectious etiologies have been suspect and do cause an acute colitis, no organism has been identified as the cause of the chronic idiopathic form. It is also clear that genetic factors have a greater influence in Crohn disease than in UC. Nevertheless, alterations in the T-cell and cytokine responses unquestionably occur in UC patients. The lesion may be limited to the rectum *(proctitis)* or may extend from the rectum into the left side and then into the transverse colon *(universal colitis* or *pancolitis).*

CLINICAL PICTURE

The cardinal sign of UC is usually *diarrhea,* often associated with bleeding. Onset may be sudden, or bowel habits may change gradually. Sudden onset is often confused with disease of infectious etiology. In reality, many of the early descriptions of chronic UC followed infections with dysentery, but after the infectious organisms were clear, a chronic disease evolved. Gradual onset or progression of disease may be associated with elevated temperature, pain and cramps in the lower abdomen, and gradual weight loss. If the bleeding is severe, the patient will have anemia. If the symptoms are persistent and severe, anorexia, nausea, and occasional vomiting may follow, leading to weight loss and possible malnutrition, depending on when the patient seeks treatment. Rarely, the diseased bowel may distend and present as toxic megacolon.

Atypical presentations of UC can involve the skin, joints, eyes, or liver and may precede full-blown colonic involvement. In children, the presentation may simply be growth failure.

DIAGNOSIS

The clinical presentation of diarrhea and blood loss should result in a thorough evaluation of diarrhea, including stool cultures, stool for ova and parasites, and blood workup for anemia and infectious agents. Once this initial screening is accomplished, endoscopy is essential. The appropriate endoscopic and biopsy evaluations in UC can be obtained through sigmoidoscopy, but many gastroenterologists perform the examination with a colonoscope and obtain a full evaluation of the entire colon. However, this may not be necessary to make the diagnosis of UC, in which the lesion begins in the rectum and progresses into the left side of the colon.

Biopsy material reveals the classic lesions of nonspecific UC and can differentiate among infectious, ischemic, and possibly Crohn colitis. The latter may be difficult to differentiate on mucosal biopsy. The advent of serologic markers as part of the clinical diagnostic armamentarium has been helpful. Finding an elevation of perinuclear antineutrophil cytoplasmic antibody (pANCA) is helpful diagnostically. Classic patterns have been described; the finding of anti–*Saccharomyces cerevisiae* antibody (ASCA) is helpful, and the combination of positive pANCA and negative ASCA findings has a positive predictive value for UC of 88% to 92%. New markers are being evaluated, but interpretations continue to be controversial.

Radiographic imaging can be helpful, but often does not make the diagnosis of UC. Computed tomography reveals thickening of the bowel, and barium enema examination reveals classic spicules of the mucosa, strictures, or loss of haustral markings. Histologic diagnosis, however, is still necessary. Therefore, most clinicians choose colonoscopy over barium enema, although the latter is helpful in select cases. Barium enema and colonoscopy may be traumatic for patients with acute or toxic UC, so caution is warranted, and initial evaluation should be performed with gentle sigmoidoscopy.

TREATMENT AND MANAGEMENT

Numerous drugs are available to treat UC. Initial treatment usually starts with a variety of antiinflammatory agents, such as sulfasalazine (the former top choice) or mesalamine. When control is not obtained in a reasonable time, clinicians turn to corticosteroids or budesonide and then immunosuppressive agents, which include 6-mercaptopurine or azathioprine, methotrexate, and cyclophosphamide. Several centers have used probiotics with some success. Most recently, antitissue necrosis factor agents and biological agents have been added to treatment. These are usually used in research centers, but many clinicians have tried them after initial failure with the other agents. The biologics include infliximab (Remicade, Janssen), adalimumab (Humira, AbbVie), certolizumab pegol (Cimzia, UCB), golimumab (Simponi, Janssen), natalizumab (Tysabri, Biogen), vedolizumab (Entyvio, Takeda), and most recently ustekinumab. All of these are truly experimental but are being used in research.

If all medical treatment fails, or the course is fulminant and unrelenting (e.g., severe bleeding, toxic megacolon), surgery is appropriate. Numerous subtleties associated with UC, including its varied complications, occurrence during pregnancy, and malignant potential, are discussed elsewhere.

COURSE AND PROGNOSIS

The usual course of UC is benign in most patients, who are treated on an ambulatory basis with antiinflammatory or immunosuppressive agents. Research and university centers may use sophisticated indices

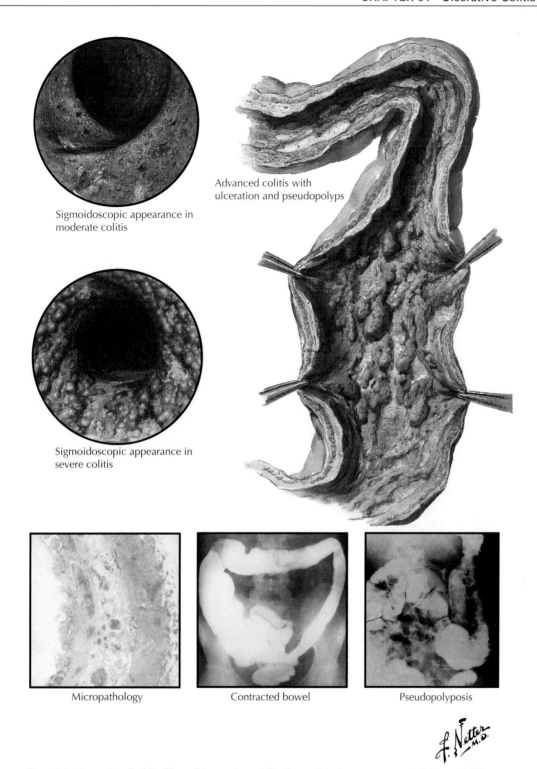

Sigmoidoscopic appearance in
moderate colitis

Advanced colitis with
ulceration and pseudopolyps

Sigmoidoscopic appearance in
severe colitis

Micropathology   Contracted bowel   Pseudopolyposis

Fig. 91.1 Ulcerative Colitis: Sigmoidoscopic and Radiographic Appearance and Advanced Disease.

to evaluate the course and endpoints of treatments. Most clinicians do not use these indices in daily practice. However, if a patient must be admitted for hospital care during the first year of the disease, the probability of further admissions and surgery increases. An estimated 30% of UC patients undergo surgery. Their lifetime incidence of colorectal cancer approaches 6%, and the cancer-related mortality rate is approximately 3%. Considering the incidence and prevalence of UC, these percentages are significant, and patients should be aware of all the possibilities in this chronic disease.

Histologic diagnosis of UC or inflammatory bowel disease (IBD) is imprecise and often difficult to make (Fig. 91.2). In addition, the factors that differentiate UC from Crohn disease are often not evident through simple mucosal biopsy. However, when accepted criteria are present, a diagnosis can be made. The following factors define UC:

- *Distorted mucosal architecture,* as evidenced by crypt distortion with or without crypt atrophy. In severe cases, mucosal erosions and ulcerations can be seen.

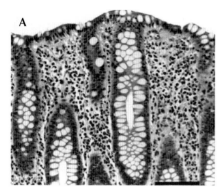

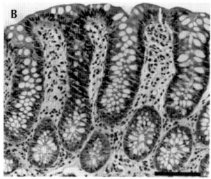

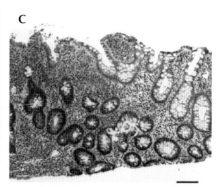

Mononuclear cell infiltration in the lamina propria. (A) Upper limit of "mild" mononuclear cell infiltration.

(B) Upper limit of "minimal" mononuclear cell infiltration.

(C) Borderline figure narrowly judged as "focal" mononuclear cell infiltration. (Hematoxylin and eosin; bar = 100 μm.)

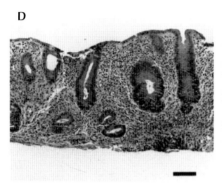

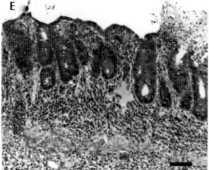

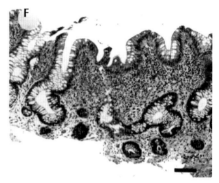

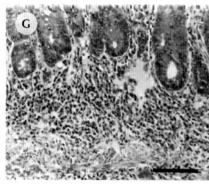

Crypt architectural abnormalities and basal plasmacytosis (D and E). Typical figures judged as "presence" of crypt atrophy, which was recognized by generally increased distance of more than one crypt diameter between crypts (D), or a general increase in the distance between crypts and the muscularis mucosae (E). (F) Typical figure judged as "presence" of crypt distortion, which was recognized by branched crypts with nonparallelism. (G) Typical basal plasmacytosis. (Hematoxylin and eosin; bar = 100 μm.)

Fig. 91.2 Ulcerative Colitis: Histologic Diagnosis and Dysplasia. (Schematic modified from Itzkowitz S: Colon carcinogenesis in inflammatory bowel disease: applying molecular genetics to clinical practice, *J Clin Gastroenterol* 36:S70-S74, 2003; histologic images from Tanaka M, Riddell RH, Salto H, et al: Morphologic criteria applicable to biopsy specimens for effective distinction of inflammatory bowel disease from other forms of colitis and of Crohn's disease from ulcerative colitis, *Scand J Gastroenterol* 34:55-67, 1999.)

- *Inflammatory cell infiltrate in the lamina propria,* which is usually lymphoplasmacytic in what is described as the "chronic" form and neutrophilic or eosinophilic in the "acute" form. So-called crypt abscesses are usually described in the acute form and contain neutrophils (see Fig. 91.2). The intensity of the white blood cell (WBC) infiltrate ranges from mild to severe. An often-described, ambiguous feature is an excess of intraepithelial neutrophils or lymphocytes, in which the infiltrate in the lamina propria is not severe. *Basal plasmocytosis,* when at least three plasma cells are found below the crypt area, may be a significant finding.
- *Mucin depletion, distal Paneth cell metaplasia,* and areas of *intense eosinophilia* have been described in UC. Detailed analysis of clinical status with histologic findings has revealed that crypt atrophy, crypt distortion, basal plasmocytosis, and severe mononuclear cell infiltra-

tion, with Paneth cell metaplasia distal to the hepatic flexure, were significant findings in UC, with sensitivity greater than 99% and specificity greater than 97%. In addition, the presence of epithelioid granulomas revealed a sensitivity of 86% to 94% and specificity of 97% to 100% for Crohn disease.

Other colitides that can be diagnosed by mucosal biopsy may confuse the differential diagnosis of UC, but usually these are distinguished by unique characteristics. *Infectious colitis* causes an acute inflammatory response, but rarely are crypt areas distorted. *Chronic ischemic colitis* can cause ulceration similar to UC, but also usually shows lamina propria fibrosis, and the classic inflammatory response is minimal or absent. *Chronic radiation disease* and *chronic graft-versus-host disease* may elicit similar responses. However, the history in these patients is significant. Nonsteroidal antiinflammatory drugs (NSAIDs) have been associated with acute or chronic colitis, along with microscopic, lymphocytic, and collagenous colitis, but rarely with crypt architectural disturbance.

Numerous eosinophils in the clinical and endoscopic findings of UC may further confuse the diagnosis. *Eosinophilic gastroenteritis* may be included in the differential diagnosis (see Chapter 70). In many UC patients, the biopsy material shows many eosinophils; degree and distribution may be confusing. Classically, eosinophils represent a response to allergic or parasitic disease. However, their presence in UC is of uncertain significance, and no clinical distinguishing features exist to necessitate different treatment.

DYSPLASIA

The presence of dysplasia in mucosal biopsy material from patients with UC is classified as high, low, or indeterminate. Studies reveal that pathologists' interpretations vary greatly, as do reports among institutions. Although it is difficult to differentiate the three categories, certain criteria can establish a category. The clinician must emphasize the importance of a correct diagnosis to the pathologist interpreting the specimens.

Low-grade dysplasia can be defined as "nuclear crowding," with some stratification of nuclear pleomorphism and hyperchromasia. The glandular architecture is minimally abnormal. *High-grade dysplasia* has more marked nuclear pleomorphism, hypochromasia, and stratification, and there may or may not be architectural abnormalities such as villi-formed surfaces. As seen in Fig. 91.2, it may be difficult and completely arbitrary when uncertainty exists in defining low-grade and high-grade dysplasia. Whenever there is marked inflammation and apparently significant reparatory changes, it may be difficult or impossible to distinguish reactive changes from true dysplasia. In these patients, a diagnosis of *indefinite dysplasia* is made.

Dysplasia often resembles adenoma; it may be impossible to distinguish them. So-called sporadic adenomas may develop in areas of UC and thus may enter into the clinical decision process. If a sporadic adenoma develops in an area distant from active UC, such as in the right colon, and if the colitis is present only in the left colon, the sporadic adenoma can be considered as truly benign. Patients with dysplastic lesions appear to have UC longer (>10 years) and are more likely to have active disease.

Dysplasia and Monitoring in Inflammatory Bowel Disease

It is now apparent that there are molecular factors for colitis-associated colon cancer (see Fig. 91.2). The bowel with no dysplasia presumably goes through a formation process of indefinite dysplasia, low-grade dysplasia, high-grade dysplasia, and then carcinoma. *Aneuploidy* (altered DNA content) and microsatellite instability develop, and tumor-suppressor genes such as *APC* and *p*53 become altered. Other changes in genetic regulation, such as induction of the K-*ras* oncogene, and loss of other functioning tumor-suppressor genes, in addition to the *p*53 gene function, appear to permit adenoma to progress to carcinoma.

Therefore, the question is whether careful surveillance can prevent cancer in IBD patients. Most pathologists and clinical gastroenterologists conclude that the increased incidence of colorectal cancer in UC patients warrants careful monitoring and surveillance. If no dysplasia or adenoma formation is seen on first colonoscopy, it is safe to monitor the patient every 2 years. Most accept that because the incidence of carcinoma increases after UC is present for 10 years, surveillance should be considered annually. Although no random clinical trials have been conducted, several cohort and case series indicate that monitoring does have a role in preventing cancer. Surveillance colonoscopy includes

thorough evaluation of the colon, with specimens for mucosal biopsy taken every 5 to 10 cm. Physicians disagree on the number of biopsy specimens needed, but most agree at least 10 areas should be sampled. Controversy surrounds whether low-grade dysplasia is an indication for surgery, but most agree that the presence of high-grade dysplasia, or adenoma within active disease, warrants total colectomy.

EXTRAINTESTINAL MANIFESTATIONS

Extraintestinal manifestations of UC are numerous and the complications can be severe, with significant morbidity and mortality (Fig. 91.3). This chapter lists all the complications, but detailed discussions of each may be found throughout this text and in the literature.

An epidemiologic study of more than 1000 patients with UC reveals that the overall prevalence of extraintestinal manifestations is 21%, and that incidence increases with increased severity of illness. More than one extracolonic manifestation occurred in approximately 25% of patients. The cause of the extracolonic manifestations is unknown; Box 91.1 lists the sites most often involved. However, the literature includes reports of scattered cases in the bronchopulmonary, renal and genito-urinary, cardiac, endocrine, and neurologic organs.

The clinical presentation of each of these extracolonic manifestations is typical of the disease without UC. Manifestation may occur without active disease, but it occurs more frequently when disease activity is increased. Therefore, it is imperative that the disease be controlled and treated to ameliorate the extraintestinal manifestations.

BOX 91.1   Extraintestinal Sites of Ulcerative Colitis Involvement

Joints (7%)[a]
- Arthritis
- Sacroiliitis
- Ankylosing spondylitis
- Hypertrophic osteoarthropathy
- Osteoporosis/osteomalacia
- Granulomatous synovitis
- Rheumatoid arthritis
- Osteonecrosis
- Steroid-induced myopathy

Skin (2.6%)
- Erythema nodosum
- Pyoderma gangrenosum
- Psoriasis

Eyes (1.6%)
- Uveitis/iritis
- Episcleritis
- Chorioretinitis
- Retinal vascular disease

Hepatobiliary (11%)
- Primary sclerosing cholangitis
- Steatosis
- Cholelithiasis
- Cholangiocarcinoma
- Autoimmune hepatitis
- Pericholangitis

[a]Percentage of UC patients affected.

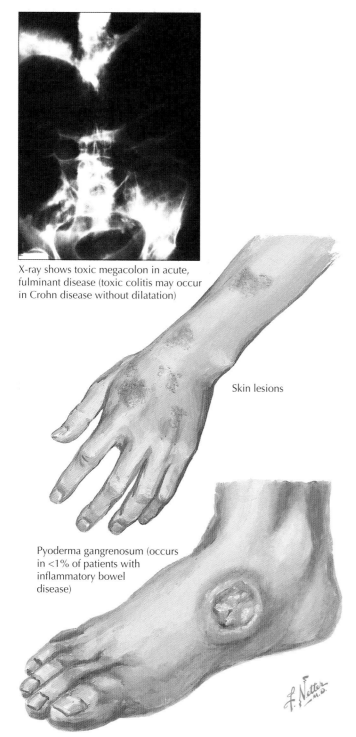

X-ray shows toxic megacolon in acute, fulminant disease (toxic colitis may occur in Crohn disease without dilatation)

Skin lesions

Pyoderma gangrenosum (occurs in <1% of patients with inflammatory bowel disease)

Fig. 91.3 Ulcerative Colitis: Extraintestinal Manifestations and Complications.

Pyoderma gangrenosum is a classic manifestation for which intensive therapy may be necessary. Treatment of the pyoderma may require corticosteroids, which would not be used for the disease itself. Once again, each manifestation must be treated individually, in accordance with the experience readily available in the literature. Biological therapy is now being used more frequently in an attempt to control the symptoms rapidly when steroids are not immediately effective.

Importantly, disease manifestation may change. The best example is *sclerosing cholangitis*, which may occur before UC develops. It is hypothesized that this is part of an autoimmune process relating to the disturbance of the immunologic response in UC patients. Sclerosing cholangitis may progress to liver failure and liver complications, resulting in liver transplantation. Patients with UC are able to tolerate liver transplantation. UC appears to come under control with the combined treatments and therapies involved during transplantation, and patients may do well with their IBD and are able to sustain transplantation and recover. Reports indicate that as many as 4% of IBD patients develop sclerosing cholangitis.

An increased incidence of *osteoporosis* is also reported in IBD patients. Treatment with steroids and some immunosuppressive drugs aggravates osteoporosis. Therefore, patients must be diligently placed on calcium and vitamin D intake and any necessary bone-stimulatory drugs.

Major Complications

Major complications of chronic UC are massive bleeding, perforation with or without dilatation, carcinoma, and perianal disease. Fortunately, *massive hemorrhaging* from the bowel is not as frequent as once believed. However, when a massive hemorrhage does occur and bleeding does not stop with standard intravenous therapy, colectomy may be necessary. Slow bleeding with its attendant anemia is more prevalent. Iron-deficiency anemia is most common and is treated with iron replacement. Deficiencies of other vitamins or of folic acid that occur with sulfasalazine therapy are treated with replacement of those vitamins.

Free perforation usually complicates toxic megacolon; therefore, toxic dilated bowel requires immediate surgical intervention when medical therapy fails. A colonic diameter greater than 6 to 7 cm may indicate toxic colon. When the patient is febrile, has abdominal distention, and has a high pulse rate or a greatly elevated WBC count, emergency surgery may be required. Actually, the patient's condition should be stabilized and medical treatment attempted, but careful observation is necessary to ensure that perforation does not occur, because mortality rates can be as high as 40% to 50% with perforation. Surprisingly, toxic megacolon, which was thought to result from drug therapy (e.g., opiates, anticholinergics), seems to occur most often in first episodes of colitis. Free perforation may result from small lesions, which require good surgical support with appropriate surgical intervention as each case indicates. Again, morbidity and mortality are high.

Strictures occur in chronic UC, and most are short (<2–5 cm). Once a stricture is identified, the clinician should investigate whether a lesion is local (e.g., from scarring) or is caused by malignant infiltration. Because stent placement may be attempted, obtaining a specimen through biopsy or resection of the area is recommended, so as not to overlook a malignancy.

Perianal disease occurs frequently in UC patients. The main problem related to UC is irritation of the anal ring with resultant cryptitis, fissures, and perianal irritation. It is essential to control the diarrhea to control the irritation of the anal ring. After the disease is controlled, perianal disease usually subsides. Treatment of perianal disease is discussed in Chapters 102, 104, and 105.

Numerous extraintestinal manifestations and disease complications affect the quality of life of patients with UC. Although many are not life threatening, the burden is great on these patients. Reassurance and frequently psychotherapy are needed for them to cope with the recurrent manifestations of the disease. When the quality of life is seriously affected, colectomy should be considered. However, complications or extraintestinal manifestations such as sclerosing cholangitis can occur even after total colectomy. Fortunately, the rate of extraintestinal manifestations and complications is less than 50%, and those unaffected can lead normal lives.

Abscesses and fistulae are much more common in Crohn disease (20%–40%) than in nonspecific UC (see Chapters 95 and 96).

Fecal microbial transplant has been attempted and reported as successful in remission of UC, but it is early in the use of this therapy.

SURGICAL TREATMENT

The American College of Gastroenterology Practice Guidelines on treatment of UC states, "Absolute indications for surgery are exsanguinating hemorrhage, perforation, and documented or strongly suspected carcinoma. Other indications for surgery are (1) severe colitis with or without toxic megacolon, unresponsive to conventional maximal medical therapy, and (2) the patient with less severe, but medically intractable symptoms or intolerable steroid side effects."

Although indications seem clear in clinical practice, one unclear area is the *suspicion of cancer*. Some clinicians believe that low-grade dysplasia is an indication for colectomy, and most believe that high-grade dysplasia is a clear indication for total colectomy in UC patients.

Clinical Picture

Eventually, the patient who is undergoing extensive medical therapy for UC and who requires large doses of steroids or medication, whether continuous or intermittent, must consider surgery. The choice is frequently up to the patient. Some patients do not want to deal with the lifestyle-limiting effects of a chronic disorder and choose surgery, whereas others fear surgery. However, surgery can relieve the symptoms of UC and cure the disease.

Diagnosis

The clinician must be certain of the diagnosis when referring a patient with UC for surgery. The extent of the disease is clearly evaluated on colonoscopy, and histologic and biopsy specimens can make a definitive diagnosis. Unfortunately, as many as 20% to 50% of patients have indeterminate diagnoses. The surgeon cannot be sure whether these patients have Crohn colitis or UC; the type of surgery to perform then becomes debatable. Serologic examination may be 97% to 100% specific for Crohn colitis and 80% to 90% specific for UC. Therefore, serologic findings that demonstrate high ASCA level raise the index of suspicion that the patient has Crohn colitis. The small bowel should be evaluated if time permits. If the patient has acute hemorrhage or acute perforation, a two-stage procedure should be performed to give the patient an ileostomy, with an ileal pouch inserted later. All physicians involved in patient evaluation should determine whether they are dealing with nonspecific UC or Crohn colitis.

Treatment and Management

It is estimated that approximately 30% of UC patients will require surgery. During the past decade, ileal pouch anastomosis has become the treatment of choice. However, some patients do not have the appropriate body build for a pouch, or they may have a relative contraindication. For these patients, total colectomy with ileostomy is the treatment of choice (see Chapters 92 and 93). With either procedure, the patient will be free of UC unless it is a variant form or is indeterminate, or unless Crohn ileitis develops after surgery. Ileostomy is a safe procedure, and long-term analysis now reveals that ileoanal pouches are safe, although some patients do experience pouchitis. Surgery may be performed even in patients with sclerosing cholangitis.

Fig. 91.4 demonstrates the ileostomy site and the removal of the rectum with closure of the perianal area. This is usually a two-stage procedure. After the ileostomy is created, the patient is given several months to recover, and then the rectum is removed and the perineum closed. This procedure is associated with less sexual dysfunction than other procedures and does not hinder female reproduction. Details of ileal pouch anal anastomosis are described in Chapter 93.

ADDITIONAL RESOURCES

Abaghizadeh F: Ileostomy, colostomy and pouches. In Feldman M, Friedman LS, Brandt LJ, editors: *Gastrointestinal and liver disease*, ed 10, Philadelphia, 2016, Saunders-Elsevier, pp 2062–2075.

Bohl JL, Sobba K: Indications and options for surgery in ulcerative colitis, *Surg Clin North Am* 95:1211–1232, 2015.

Collins PD, Mpofu C, Watson AJ, Rhodes JM: Strategies for detecting colon cancer or dysplasia in patients with inflammatory bowel disease, *Cochrane Database Syst Rev* (19):CD000279, 2006.

Costello SP, Soo W, Bryant RV, et al: Systemic review with meta-analysis: faecal microbiota transplantation for the induction of remission for active ulcerative colitis, *Aliment Pharmacol Ther* 46:213–224, 2017.

Derwa Y, Gracie DJ, Hamlin PJ, Ford AC: Systemic review with meta-analysis: the efficacy of probiotics in inflammatory bowel disease, *Aliment Pharmacol Ther* 46:389–400, 2017.

Ferrante M, Declerck S, De Hertogh G, et al: Outcome after proctocolectomy with ileal pouch–anal anastomosis for ulcerative colitis, *Inflamm Bowel Dis* 14:20–28, 2008.

Fichera A, Finlayson E, Magglori L, Michelassi F: Surgical treatment of inflammatory bowel disease. In Podolsky DK, Camilleri M, Fitz JG, et al, editors: *Yamada's textbook of gastroenterology*, ed 6, Hoboken, New Jersey, 2016, John Wiley and Sons Ltd, pp 1450–1478.

Hanauer SB: Combination therapy for inflammatory bowel disease, *Gastroenterol Hepatol* 13:296–298, 2017.

Hanauer SB, Podolsky DK: Ulcerative colitis. In Podolsky DK, Camilleri M, Fitz JG, et al, editors: *Yamada's textbook of gastroenterology*, ed 6, Hoboken, New Jersey, 2016, John Wiley and Sons Ltd, pp 1378–1417.

Olsson R, Danielsson A, Jarnerot G, et al: Prevalence of primary sclerosing cholangitis in patients with ulcerative colitis, *Gastroenterology* 100:1319–1323, 1991.

Osterman MT, Lichtenstein GR: Ulcerative colitis. In Feldman M, Friedman LS, Brandt LJ, editors: *Gastrointestinal and liver disease*, ed 10, Philadelphia, 2016, Saunders-Elsevier, pp 2023–2061.

Tanaka M, Riddell RH, Saito H, et al: Morphologic criteria applicable to biopsy specimens for effective distinction of inflammatory bowel disease from other forms of colitis, and of Crohn's disease from ulcerative colitis, *Scand J Gastroenterol* 34:55–67, 1999.

Vleggaar FP, Lutgens MW, Claessen MM: The relevance of surveillance endoscopy in long-lasting inflammatory bowel disease (review), *Aliment Pharmacol Ther* 26(Suppl 2):47–52, 2007.

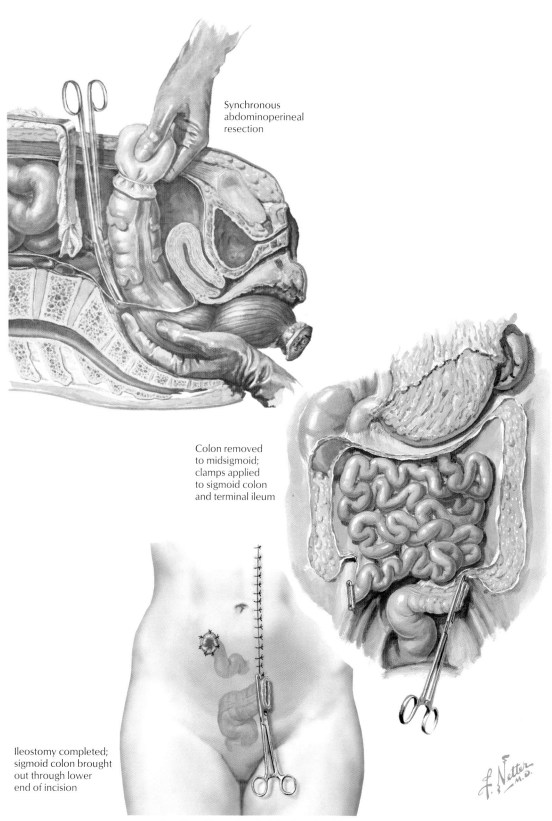

Synchronous abdominoperineal resection

Colon removed to midsigmoid; clamps applied to sigmoid colon and terminal ileum

Ileostomy completed; sigmoid colon brought out through lower end of incision

Fig. 91.4 Ulcerative Colitis: Surgical Treatment.

92

Ileostomy and Colostomy

Martin H. Floch

Colostomies are performed for numerous reasons, including obstructive lesions caused by cancer, severe diverticulitis, severe intractable constipation, and trauma. Ileostomies are performed for the same reasons, but permanent ileostomy is reserved almost exclusively for patients with ulcerative colitis and diffuse polyposis of the colon. Although ileal pouch anal anastomosis (IPAA) is now the preferred procedure (see Chapter 93), some patients may not be surgical candidates for IPAA or may not be able to tolerate the pouch and must be converted to an ileostomy. Both ileostomies and colostomies may be permanent or temporary, depending on the clinical indication.

Because it involves the removal of the colon, *ileostomy* often results in more complications than colostomy. Colostomy excreta usually have a free or an intermittent flow that may be facilitated by simple irrigation. Ileostomy effluent has a free flow that should range from 800 to 1000 mL/day, depending on the diet. Ileostomy effluent may be dramatically increased in patients with gastroenteritis. Complications of ileostomies include malfunctioning, prestomal ileitis, irritation of the peristomal skin, and obstruction.

CLINICAL PICTURE

The carefully placed ileostomy is usually situated in the right lower quadrant. Most patients become well versed in taking care of the site. Fig. 92.1 demonstrates the method of placing an appliance over the fistula. Most patients become comfortable with it and empty the appliance several times daily.

DIAGNOSIS

The diagnosis of an obstructive lesion is the same as for any intestinal obstruction. After ileostomy, however, a patient may have an early obstruction, and the ileal discharge first may increase because of bowel dilatation and increased intestinal secretions. Examination of the stoma with a small finger or an endoscope can reveal the dilated ileum, and radiographic studies can confirm the findings. Surgery is indicated to remove any obstruction.

Prestomal ileitis fortunately occurs rarely, but patients with this condition may also exhibit features of mechanical obstruction. They may become dehydrated or at times anemic. Ileal mucosa may demonstrate ulcerations. It is thought that prestomal ileitis is often a recurrence of Crohn disease. However, it may be difficult to determine whether there is an obstruction at the stoma site or whether Crohn disease has recurred.

TREATMENT AND MANAGEMENT

When an obstruction or prestomal ileitis is suspected, endoscopy and medicosurgical intervention are indicated, depending on the cause. If the condition appears to be inflammatory, medical treatment should help resolve the problem. However, if it is mechanical, surgical intervention is necessary, and resection of the stoma must be considered.

Care of the peristomal area is a routine part of postoperative nursing. Most institutions have a specialized nurse to educate patients. Emollient salves and skin care are administered for lesions.

Most people who undergo ileostomy can lead normal lives. Occasionally, it is necessary to revise a stoma. Most surveys indicate that approximately 90% of patients are satisfied after ileostomy, but some require a revision to the procedure. Patients learn to change their diets and to limit their intake of foods not digested by human enzymes, such as high-fiber foods of insoluble fiber, including fruits and grains. Most patients learn to chew their food thoroughly so that it does not obstruct the stoma. However, every clinician has occasionally treated a patient who has swallowed unchewed nuts that caused obstruction. Patients learn what to do and what not to do.

COURSE AND PROGNOSIS

The major disease for which the ileostomy or colostomy is performed dictates the prognosis. If the disease is malignant, it may result in a poor outcome. If the disease is benign or is caused by trauma, the patient can lead a normal life. Colostomy presents less risk for dehydration if gastroenteritis occurs. Ileostomy patients must be monitored carefully. If severe enteritis occurs and the ileostomy effluent is not controlled by simple medication, patients frequently need intravenous replacement of fluid and electrolytes.

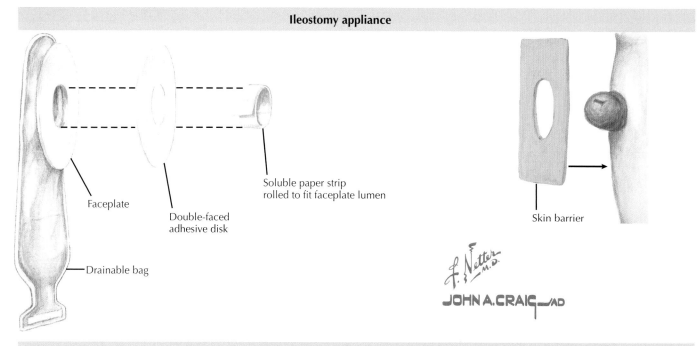

Ileostomy appliance

Faceplate

Double-faced
adhesive disk

Soluble paper strip
rolled to fit faceplate lumen

Drainable bag

Skin barrier

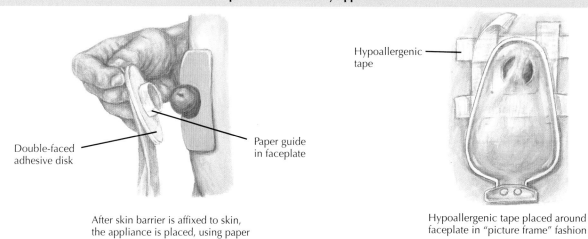

Components of ileostomy appliance

Double-faced
adhesive disk

Paper guide
in faceplate

Hypoallergenic
tape

After skin barrier is affixed to skin,
the appliance is placed, using paper
strip guide to align faceplate lumen
over stoma

Hypoallergenic tape placed around
faceplate in "picture frame" fashion

Fig. 92.1 Ileostomy and Colostomy.

ADDITIONAL RESOURCES

Abaghizadeh F: Ileostomy, colostomy and pouches. In Feldman M, Friedman LS, Brandt LJ, editors: *Gastrointestinal and liver disease*, ed 10, Philadelphia, 2016, Saunders-Elsevier, pp 2062–2075.

Evans JP, Brown MH, Wilkes GH, et al: Revising the troublesome stoma: combined abdominal wall recontouring and revision of stomas, *Dis Col Rect* 46:122–126, 2003.

Fulham J: Providing dietary advice for the individual with a stoma, *Br J Nurs* 17:S22–S27, 2008.

Gordon P, Nivatvonas S: *Principles and practices of surgery: colon, rectum and anus*, New York, 2007, Informa Healthcare.

Steinhagen E, Colwell J, Cannon LM: Intestinal stomas-postoperative stoma care and peristomal skin complications, *Clin Colon Rectal Surg* 30:184–192, 2017.

93

Ileal Pouch Anal Anastomosis and Pouchitis

Martin H. Floch

The surgical treatment of choice for patients requiring colectomy for ulcerative colitis or familial adenomatous polyposis (FAP) is *restorative proctocolectomy* with ileal pouch anal anastomosis (IPAA). The "pouch" is an ileal reservoir that acts as a neorectum to store fecal material and to avoid constant output from the ileostomy. Anastomosis of the ileal-to-rectal mucosa is controversial, but most surgeons prefer *mucosectomy*, bringing the ileal mucosa to the anal skin line. This is best accomplished with suturing, but some prefer stapling.

There are three types of pouches—J, S, and W—but the J pouch has become the most popular (Fig. 93.1). Unfortunately, as many as 40% of patients who undergo this procedure develop at least one episode of *pouchitis*, and 60% of these patients may have recurrent disease. Only 15% of patients with pouchitis have chronic disease that requires maintenance therapy.

Patients with IPAA to manage FAP rarely experience pouchitis. Furthermore, pouchitis appears to occur more frequently in patients with extraintestinal manifestations of colitis. Patients with primary *sclerosing cholangitis* have the highest prevalence of pouchitis.

CLINICAL PICTURE

Pouchitis causes diarrhea, lower abdominal pain, and bloody discharge. Patients may have fever, associated malaise, and nausea. Some lose weight or have night sweats or extraintestinal arthritis. When patients are routinely observed through sigmoidoscopy, some are found to have active pouchitis but few or no symptoms.

DIAGNOSIS

Because pouchitis consists of a triad of variable clinical (history), endoscopic, and histologic criteria, many clinicians use a *pouchitis disease activity index* consisting of a series of points assigned to the criteria (Box 93.1). Scores higher than seven points indicate pouchitis. Clinicians also use this index to monitor the progress of therapy.

Positive histologic findings are necessary for a diagnosis of pouchitis, but this is controversial among pathologists, and most patients with pouches have low-grade inflammation. Therefore, the pouchitis activity index is helpful. Severe cases, determined by histologic findings, involve acute inflammatory infiltrates with crypt abscesses and ulceration. Most clinicians consider a diagnosis of pouchitis unwarranted if the inflammation and ulceration are found only through routine sigmoidoscopy, or if the patient does not have clinical symptoms or an increased number of stools or rectal bleeding. Therefore, the history (clinical) component is important for making the diagnosis. The Cleveland Clinic group defines *irritable pouch syndrome* as disease activity index less than 7 and little evidence of pouchitis other than its symptoms.

TREATMENT AND MANAGEMENT

Again, 60% of patients with pouchitis have recurrent attacks, and as many as 15% have significant long-term problems.

The primary treatment for pouchitis has been *metronidazole.* Initial studies demonstrated a change in the bacterial flora, with an increase in aerobic organisms and a decrease in anaerobes, as well as a decrease in the normal probiotic organisms. Metronidazole was excellent in inducing remissions, but symptoms recurred. Many clinicians used broad-spectrum coverage of ciprofloxacin and ampicillin if unable to use metronidazole, or if its use might have caused complications. Some clinicians have used other antiinflammatory agents, such as mesalamine, and some have had to use steroid enemas or steroids systemically to control symptoms.

The use of *probiotic agents* has been promising; one study reported almost 100% induction of remission and maintenance of the asymptomatic state. However, therapy requires large doses of VSL#3 daily, consisting of eight probiotic organisms. Studies over several years have

BOX 93.1 Pouchitis Disease Activity Index[a]	
Criterion	**No. of Points**
History (Clinical)	
One or two more stools than usual	1
More than three stools	2
Daily bleeding	1
Occasional fecal urgency or cramps	1
Usual fecal urgency or cramps	2
Fever	1
Endoscopy	
Edema	1
Granularity	1
Friability	1
Loss of vascularity	1
Mucus	1
Ulceration	1
Histology	
Mild PMN infiltrate	1
Moderate PMN infiltrate and crypt abscesses	2
Severe PMN infiltrate and crypt abscesses	3
Less than 25% ulceration/low-power field	1
25% to <50%/low-power field	2
More than 50% ulceration/low-power field	3

[a]Score greater than 7 points indicates pouchitis.
PMN, Polymorphonuclear leukocyte.

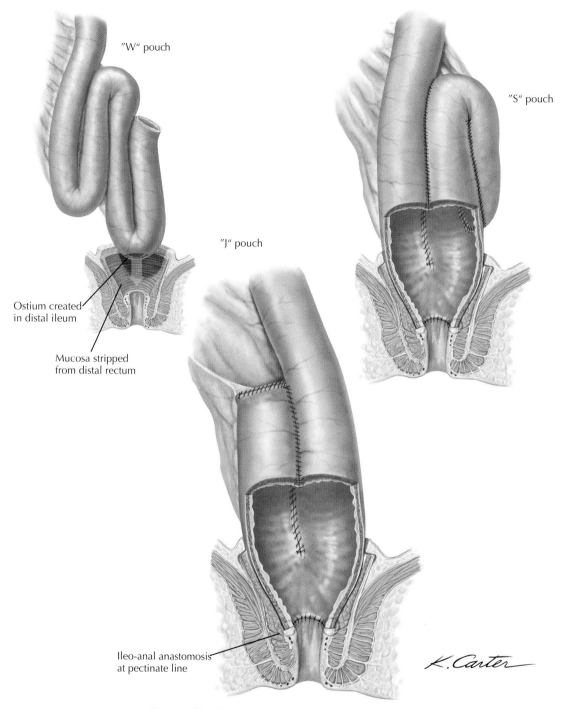

"W" pouch

"S" pouch

"J" pouch

Ostium created
in distal ileum

Mucosa stripped
from distal rectum

Ileo-anal anastomosis
at pectinate line

K. Carter

Fig. 93.1 Ileal Pouch Anal Anastomosis and Pouchitis.

proved the effectiveness of this therapy, but long-term evaluations are still necessary.

Previous data analysis showed that metronidazole was effective therapy for active pouchitis, but that VSL#3 was effective for maintaining remission in chronic pouchitis. With judicious use of antibiotics and probiotics, pouchitis symptoms can be controlled.

It is important to monitor the pouch because dysplasia may develop. The incidence of dysplasia is unknown because IPAA has been broadly used for less than 10 years. Nevertheless, possible dysplasia in some patients indicates that pouches must be serially monitored.

Removal of the pouch and ileostomy rarely becomes necessary. Some studies report revision in as many as 2% to 3% of patients.

COURSE AND PROGNOSIS

Prognosis after IPAA is excellent. The Mayo Clinic reports that 94% of patients have successful outcomes. Nocturnal incontinence occurs in approximately 10% of patients, at least one episode of pouchitis occurs in 48% of patients, and cumulative pouch failure at 1 and 10 years occurs at rates of 2% and 9%, respectively. The most common early postoperative problems are bowel obstruction, urinary tract infection, and wound sepsis.

Postoperative impotence and retrograde ejaculation are noted in up to 3% of men with pouches. Pregnancy and delivery are well tolerated by women with pouches.

ADDITIONAL RESOURCES

Abaghizadeh F: Ileostomy, colostomy and pouches. In Feldman M, Friedman LS, Brandt LJ, editors: *Gastrointestinal and liver disease*, ed 10, Philadelphia, 2016, Saunders-Elsevier, pp 2062–2075.

Fichera A, Finlayson E, Magglori L, Michelassi F: Surgical treatment of inflammatory bowel disease. In Podolsky DK, Camilleri M, Fitz JG, et al, editors: *Yamada's textbook of gastroenterology*, ed 6, Hoboken, New Jersey, 2016, John Wiley and Sons Ltd, pp 1450–1478.

Floch MH: Probiotics, irritable bowel syndrome, and inflammatory bowel disease, *Curr Treat Opt Gastroenterol* 6:283–288, 2003.

Gionchetti P, Rizzello F, Venturi A, et al: Oral bacterial therapy as maintenance treatment in patients with chronic pouchitis: a double-blind, procedure-controlled trial, *Gastroenterology* 119:305–309, 2000.

Osterman MT, Lichtenstein GR: Ulcerative colitis. In Feldman M, Friedman LS, Brandt LJ, editors: *Gastrointestinal and liver disease*, ed 10, Philadelphia, 2016, Saunders-Elsevier, pp 2023–2061.

Sandborn WJ, McLeod R, Jewel DP: Medical therapy for induction and maintenance of remission in pouchitis: a systemic review, *Inflamm Bowel Dis* 5:33–39, 1999.

Sandborn WJ, Tremaine WJ, Batts KP, et al: Pouchitis after ileal pouch anastomosis: a pouchitis disease activity index, *Mayo Clin Proc* 69:409–413, 1994.

94

Differentiating Features of Ulcerative Colitis and Crohn Disease

Martin H. Floch

A classification of *inflammatory bowel disease* (IBD) based on scientific data has not gained acceptance. An early attempt was made to classify IBD according to two categories: (1) ulcerative colitis (UC) and Crohn disease; and (2) collagenous colitis, eosinophilic enteritis, Behçet disease, transient colitis, microscopic colitis, prestomal ileitis, pouchitis, and solitary rectal ulcer. None of these entities had a definitive etiology, resulting in overlap and confusion.

Most authorities group these IBD entities into *UC, Crohn disease,* and *indeterminate colitis.* However, IBD study still has no classification, with difficult clinical situations in which patients seem to have overlapping diseases, such as diverticulitis and Crohn disease. Nevertheless, because the etiology of each is unknown and because the most common disease entities are UC and Crohn disease, this chapter discusses the differentiating factors because these are important for clinical management and determining the course and prognosis of each. Many of the same therapeutic regimens are used for UC and Crohn disease, with subtle variations, and the clinician should understand the differences (Fig. 94.1).

The differential diagnosis of UC and Crohn disease greatly overlaps, and for indeterminate colitis, a differentiation cannot be made. Furthermore, the IBD pattern appears to be changing with the changing environment and more information. The following differentiating features and comparisons, however, have held over the past few decades.

PRESENTING SYMPTOMS

Patients with UC often have diarrhea that contains mucus or blood. At times, the patient may appear to have infectious gastroenteritis. However, the diarrhea persists even after therapeutic trials. Rarely, an extraintestinal manifestation, such as migratory joint pain, pyoderma gangrenosum, or acute toxic megacolon, may be the presenting symptom.

Patients with Crohn disease usually have abdominal pain and a change in bowel habits. They may have diarrhea. The presentation of Crohn colitis may be similar to that of UC. However, the diffuseness of Crohn disease may result in extracolonic symptoms in many patients. If Crohn disease has developed in the small bowel, symptoms of pain, fever, mass, or anemia may be present. If extracolonic symptoms include joint pain or liver disease, these may be the presenting symptoms.

GENETICS AND HEREDITY

UC and Crohn disease are complex genetic disorders with multiple contributing genes. Linkage studies implicated some unique genomic regions containing IBD susceptibility genes, with some unique to Crohn disease, some unique to UC, and some unique to both diseases. IBD II, on chromosome 12q, is observed more in UC. IBD I, on chromosome 16q, contains the Crohn disease-susceptible gene *NOD2/CARD15.* Patients of European descent show three major coding-region polymorphisms within *NOD2/CARD15.* One copy of the risk allele means the patient has a twofold to fourfold risk for Crohn disease, but with a double-dose carriage, the risk increases to 20-fold to 40-fold. Patients with ileal disease, earlier age of onset, and stricturing carry the *NOD2/CARD15* allele. The genetic evaluation of these two diseases is constantly being studied and more detailed discussions are available in the references below.

Ethnic, racial, family, and twin studies reveal a leveling off in incidence and prevalence of UC and an increasing rate of Crohn disease. In addition, nonwhite persons appear to have a consistently lower rate of Crohn disease. The prevalence of Crohn disease per 100,000 population is 43.6 among white persons, 29.8 among black persons, 4.1 among Hispanic persons, and 5.6 among Asian persons. Furthermore, Jewish persons in the United States seem to be at greatest risk for twofold to fourfold higher incidence and twofold to ninefold higher prevalence. Family studies show IBD clusters within families, suggesting that genetics plays a major role. First-degree relatives have about a 10-fold to 15-fold increased risk. The risk overlaps; one family member may acquire Crohn disease and another, UC. In addition, asymptomatic family members appear to have an increased rate of positive serologic findings. Monozygotic twin concordance for Crohn disease is reported to be as high as 42% to 58%, a key factor supporting a major genetic influence.

GROSS AND MICROSCOPIC PATHOLOGY

UC is a diffuse mucosal inflammatory disease limited to the colon. UC almost always affects the rectum and appears to spread from the rectum aborally. There are rarely "skipped" areas, and the disease is contiguous. Studies of large numbers of UC patients reveal that approximately 45% have gross rectal and sigmoid involvement, and 37% have involvement of the entire colon (17% on left side only). UC is mucosal, so biopsy of the mucosa reveals the classic histology. Although some cases are confusing, the most typical findings can usually distinguish acute infectious-limiting disease. Patients with UC have distorted crypt architecture, atrophy of crypts, mixed-lymphocytic plasma cells, and neutrophilic infiltrates with varying degrees of eosinophilia. Although often present, crypt abscesses are not pathognomonic of UC.

Gross findings in Crohn disease, when involving only the colon, may be similar to those of UC, but often manifest with aphthous-type ulcerations. Ulcerations are deeper in Crohn disease than in UC. The disease is *transmural* in that inflammation penetrates the entire wall of the colon. Classic histologic findings reveal granulomas and a variety of histologic changes, including some similar to those in UC. However, the defining feature is that Crohn disease is transmural. This may not be appreciated on simple mucosal biopsy, but it certainly is present on larger specimens. Furthermore, because of Crohn transmural nature, gross findings include fibrosis, stricturing, and classic "skipped" areas. The rectum may or may not be involved. Defining gross features also

Ulcerative colitis

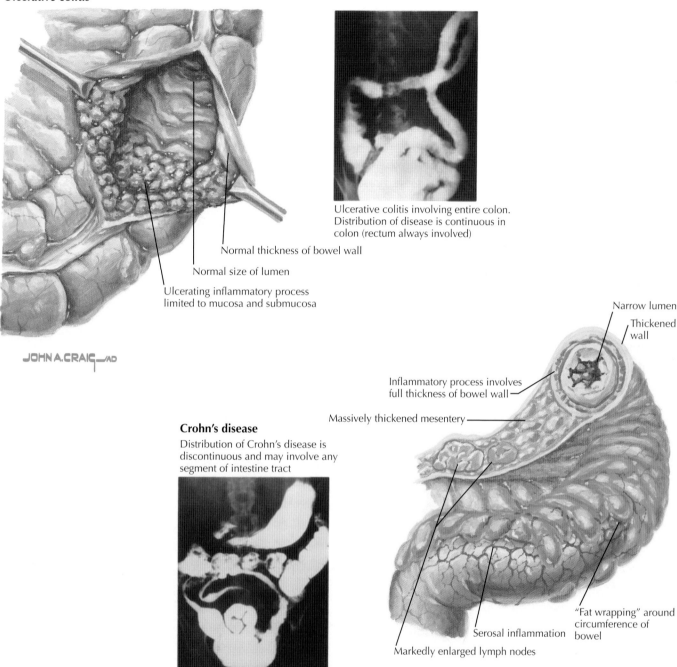

Normal thickness of bowel wall

Normal size of lumen

Ulcerating inflammatory process limited to mucosa and submucosa

Ulcerative colitis involving entire colon. Distribution of disease is continuous in colon (rectum always involved)

JOHN A. CRAIG—AD

Crohn's disease

Distribution of Crohn's disease is discontinuous and may involve any segment of intestine tract

Narrow lumen

Thickened wall

Inflammatory process involves full thickness of bowel wall

Massively thickened mesentery

"Fat wrapping" around circumference of bowel

Serosal inflammation

Markedly enlarged lymph nodes

Fig. 94.1 Differentiating Features of Ulcerative Colitis and Crohn Disease.

includes lesions with deeper ulceration than in UC. Once the small bowel is involved, the patient unquestionably has Crohn disease.

In biopsy material, changes in the M-cell population in the epithelium overlying Peyer patches, prominent lymphoid aggregates, and dilated submucosal lymphatics and granulomas are pathognomonic of Crohn colitis and are not seen in UC.

ENDOSCOPIC FINDINGS

The classic endoscopic finding in UC is a friable, finely ulcerated mucosa that may be limited to the rectum *(proctitis)* or that may extend aborally to any point in the large bowel.

In Crohn disease, the endoscopic finding may be similar to that of UC. Often in Crohn disease, however, ulcerations are deeper, there are skipped areas of normal and abnormal bowel in the colon, and the rectum appears normal. Also, areas of erythema and ulceration are scattered around the colon.

SEROLOGIC FINDINGS

Although serologic findings are not always positive, the serologic pattern can be helpful. Approximately 80% of patients with UC and as many as 45% of patients with Crohn disease have perinuclear antineutrophil cytoplasmic antibody (pANCA). Anti–*Saccharomyces cerevisiae* antibody

(ASCA) occurs in 60% to 70% of patients with Crohn disease and is specific in that it rarely occurs in UC patients.

Positive ASCA and negative pANCA help determine that the disease is Crohn colitis if simple mucosal biopsy does not elucidate the diagnosis and the classic skipped areas are absent. Strong positive pANCA and negative ASCA help determine that the disease is UC. This combination might have a predictive value in 95% to 96% of patients. Newer antibody tests are being developed and may become helpful in some cases.

Although the clinician cannot easily observe the serologic differences, UC is more of an antibody-mediated hypersensitivity, whereas Crohn disease shows an ongoing T-helper cell type 1 response with excessive interleukin-12, interferon-γ, and tissue necrosis factor-α.

INDETERMINATE COLITIS

Even with clear identification of clinical and histologic factors distinguishing UC from Crohn colitis, some patients develop Crohn disease in the remaining small bowel after ileal pouch anal anastomosis (IPAA) for UC. These patients are then categorized as having indeterminate colitis. The clinician cannot determine which form of colitis is present,

and variations of both Crohn disease and UC may be observed in the same patient over the course of the disease.

Another indeterminate area is the overlap of *diverticular disease* with colitis. When these diseases cannot be differentiated pathologically and seem to occur together, they are cured when the area is resected. Therefore, the pathology may be confusing, but the course indicates the disease is neither the classic ulcerative type nor Crohn type of colitis (see Chapter 90).

ADDITIONAL RESOURCES

Ferrante M, Henckaerts L, Joossens M, et al: New serological markers in inflammatory bowel disease are associated with complicated disease behavior, *Gut* 56:1394–1403, 2007.

Osterman MT, Lichtenstein GR: Ulcerative colitis. In Feldman M, Friedman LS, Brandt LJ, editors: *Gastrointestinal and liver disease*, ed 10, Philadelphia, 2016, Saunders-Elsevier, pp 2023–2061.

Sands BE, Siegel CA: Crohn's disease. In Feldman M, Friedman LS, Brandt LJ, editors: *Gastrointestinal and liver disease*, ed 10, Philadelphia, 2016, Saunders-Elsevier, pp 1990–2022.

Sartor RB: Mechanisms of disease: pathogenesis of Crohn's disease and ulcerative colitis, *Nat Clin Pract Gastroenterol Hepatol* 3:390–407, 2006.

95

Crohn Disease, Complications and Surgical Therapy

Martin H. Floch

Crohn disease is a transmural inflammation of the gastrointestinal (GI) tract characterized by granulomas. It involves primarily the colon and the ileum *(regional enteritis)* but may involve any part of the GI tract (Fig. 95.1). Approximately 40% of patients have a pattern that involves the small and large intestines, 30% have only small bowel involvement, and 25% have large bowel involvement.

The incidence of Crohn disease appears to be slightly higher in females. In Western countries, the incidence now ranges from 6 to 10 per 100,000 population, with a prevalence rate of 130 per 100,000, and reports indicate the incidence is rising. However, the incidence is much lower in Japan, South America, and Africa.

The cause of Crohn disease is unknown. However, most authorities believe an infectious, environmental, or at times drug (nonsteroidal antiinflammatory drug [NSAID]) trigger results in an altered immune inflammatory response in the correct genetic setting. Most cases are diagnosed in patients younger than age 40. Often, however, the disease goes undiagnosed or is mild until a complication develops later in life.

Because Crohn disease involves transmural inflammation, it appears to "skip" areas in the GI tract. A healthy area of small or large bowel can be adjacent to a diseased area (see Fig. 95.1). Transmural inflammation may lead to internal or external fistulization. Genetic susceptibility is apparent; as many as 25% of patients have a positive family history of Crohn disease. The *NOD2/CARD15* gene of chromosome 16, found in monocytes involved in the immune response to pathogenic organisms, appears responsible for the increased susceptibility.

CLINICAL PICTURE

The major presenting symptoms in Crohn disease are abdominal pain, diarrhea or change in bowel habits, and weight loss. Symptoms vary greatly. In ulcerative colitis (UC), diarrhea is the overriding factor. The bowel pattern varies with the area of the intestine involved. When the terminal ileum is involved, the major presenting symptom is usually right lower quadrant pain, which can be confused with appendicitis. At times, the abdominal pain may be diffuse, but it varies with the area of the bowel involved.

Because of the chronicity of the symptoms, most patients lose weight. Depending on the extent of Crohn disease, the symptoms can be accompanied by obstruction, and thus obstipation and abdominal distention; by perianal rectal drainage resulting from fistulization; or in rare cases, by anemia from blood loss and malabsorption. Symptoms vary depending on the site of GI disease.

Physical examination may reveal no findings or a mass in the right lower quadrant. The patient with Crohn disease may have diffuse tenderness or obstruction or may be anemic, pale, and febrile. Once again, physical findings depend on the extent of disease. Atypical presentations from extraintestinal manifestations may be seen.

DIAGNOSIS

Initial laboratory evaluation may reveal anemia, elevated erythrocyte sedimentation rate and C-reactive protein, leukocytosis, and thrombocytosis, again depending on the extent of disease. If the patient is losing weight and has diarrhea, hypoalbuminemia may be present.

The next step in the diagnosis involves examining the GI tract. Symptoms will determine whether to begin with endoscopy. If the patient has diarrhea, colonoscopy will likely reveal the classic aphthous ulcerations of the bowel and "skipped" areas. Histologic examination may confirm the diagnosis. Most colonoscopists can examine the terminal ileum. Biopsy can be performed on that area to confirm or rule out a diagnosis of terminal ileitis.

Barium contrast studies or computed tomography (CT) can be used to image the GI tract. Either technique may make the diagnosis of Crohn disease, or either may be needed to complement the other's findings. Barium studies may reveal a classic stricture or an inflamed loop of bowel. Most often, Crohn disease is in the terminal ileum, but skipped areas may be present. Barium studies may also reveal strictures and enteroenteric fistulae. Because of the symptoms, or possibly a masked presentation, the clinician may prefer CT or may need CT to complement findings of the barium study. CT classically reveals evidence of the increasing fat pad deposition noted in most pathology specimens and the "smudgy" area outside the bowel. The bowel wall shows areas of thickness, depending on the site of involvement.

If the patient has perianal or anal disease, anoscopy should be performed in addition to colonoscopy to determine the sites of fistulization and fissures.

Serologic markers are now available and have been helpful in confirming, and at times making, the diagnosis. About 60% to 70% of patients with Crohn disease have elevated anti–*Saccharomyces cerevisiae* antibody (ASCA) levels. However, ASCA has specificity greater than 95%. If the perinuclear antineutrophil cytoplasmic antibody (pANCA) is negative, the patient almost certainly has Crohn disease.

Capsule endoscopy is gaining wide acceptance and can demonstrate ulceration and stricture of the small bowel. Because some are subtle, small bowel changes can be missed on barium contrast studies or CT scans. Push enteroscopy, with scopes of distance, often do not cover the entire small bowel. Double-balloon enteroscopy may be helpful in uncertain cases, and biopsy material can be obtained. Positive findings on capsule endoscopy in conjunction with positive serologic markers strongly suggest that the patient has Crohn disease.

Extraintestinal manifestations develop in approximately 25% of the patients. These may complicate Crohn disease, may occur at any time during the disease, or may be a presenting finding, to which the clinician must be alert. Areas involved are the skin, eyes, liver, and musculoskeletal system. In addition, other areas of the gut are reportedly involved,

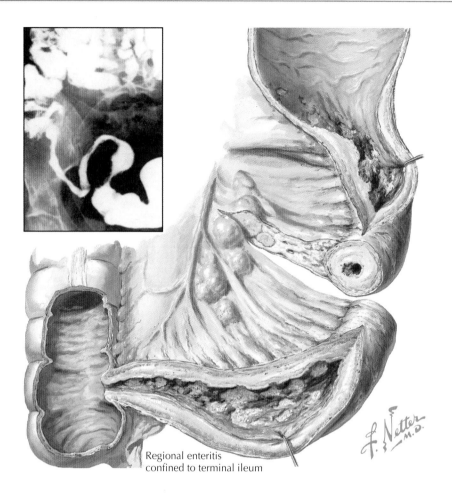

Regional enteritis
confined to terminal ileum

Regional variations

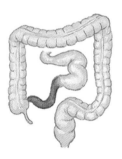

Terminal ileum

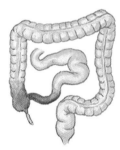

Involving cecum

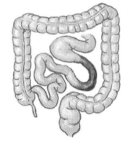

Upper ileum
or jejunum

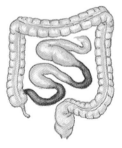

"Skip" lesions

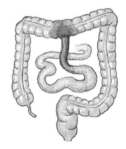

At ileocolostomy

Fig. 95.1 Crohn Disease (Regional Enteritis).

including the mouth, esophagus, stomach, and duodenum. The most dramatic extraintestinal manifestations are pyoderma gangrenosum and perianal tags (skin), uveitis, iritis, and conjunctivitis (eye), and peripheral arthritides, sacroiliitis, and osteoporosis (bones). Primary sclerosing cholangitis may be the presenting symptom if Crohn disease develops later in life.

Diseases that can mimic Crohn disease include bowel lymphomas, other malignancies, tuberculosis of the bowel, and at times, a chronic *Yersinia* infection. However, laboratory test results and endoscopy can differentiate these diseases readily.

TREATMENT AND MANAGEMENT

Pharmacologic treatment for Crohn disease includes a host of immunosuppressive agents (see Chapter 97). Nutritional management is discussed in Section X.

Nutritional management for patients with Crohn disease is different than that for patients with UC. In Crohn disease, patients may achieve remission on elemental diets; UC patients do not. Although it is slow and medical therapy is faster, nutritional management is effective. The decision to stay with medical therapy when the disease is insidious and causes changes in the activities of daily living is difficult. Surgery can be effective and can cause remission of symptoms, but surgical intervention has limits.

COURSE AND PROGNOSIS REQUIRING SURGERY

Crohn disease results in high morbidity and diminished quality of life, but it does not greatly shorten a patient's life span. It is estimated that 70% of patients will require some type of surgical procedure during their lifetime. However, most patients can achieve remission with one of the therapeutic medical regimens. When surgery is necessary, patients frequently achieve remission. When repeated surgeries and resections are necessary, short bowel syndrome may develop.

Failure to thrive in children, malnutrition, and anemia are problems associated with Crohn disease. Diligent medical and nutritional therapy can maintain good quality of life in most patients.

The most common complications of Crohn disease are abscesses and fistulae, obstruction, and perianal disease (Fig. 95.2). Abscesses develop in 15% to 20% of patients and arise from an infected area. Fistulae are more common and develop in 20% to 40% of patients, and most are enteroenteric or enterocutaneous.

Antibiotic and medical treatment may be helpful and in some studies have proved effective, but surgical therapy is often necessary. Obstruction is a common complication, and although stents and dilatation are attempted, surgical intervention is necessary to relieve progressive obstruction, which is most common in the small bowel. Perianal disease is probably the most difficult complication to treat. Antibiotics, bowel rest, and intensive medical therapy, including antitissue necrosis factor, vary in their ability to heal fistulae. Hemorrhage and free perforation are rare but do occur. At times, bleeding may be occult and may require treatment.

An estimated 60% of patients with Crohn disease will require some form of surgery within 10 years of diagnosis. These data are several decades old, however, and new, more dramatic medical therapies may be able to avert the need for surgery in some patients. Nevertheless, the list of indications for surgery is long, and its necessity becomes apparent in individual patients (Box 95.1).

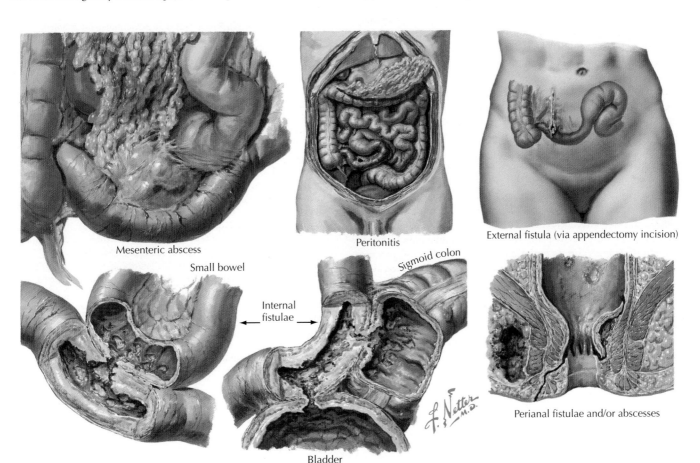

Mesenteric abscess

Small bowel

Internal fistulae

Sigmoid colon

Bladder

External fistula (via appendectomy incision)

Peritonitis

Perianal fistulae and/or abscesses

Fig. 95.2 Crohn Disease: Complications.

BOX 95.1   Indications for Surgery for Crohn Disease

Medical management failure
Intestinal obstruction
    Partial or complete
Intestinal fistulae
    Symptomatic enteroenteric fistula
    Enterocutaneous fistula
    Enterovesical fistula
    Enterovaginal fistula
Intraabdominal abscess
Inflammatory mass
Hemorrhage
Perforation
Perineal disease
    Perianal abscess
    Superficial fistula-in-ano unresponsive to medical therapy
    Complex fistula-in-ano unresponsive to medical therapy

From Hurst RB: Surgical management of inflammatory bowel disease. In Cohen RV, editor. *Inflammatory Bowel Disease,* Totowa, NJ, 2003, Humana Press, pp 157-200.

CLINICAL PICTURE OF COMPLICATIONS

The clinical presentation varies with each complication. Symptoms and physical findings of pain, elevated temperature, abdominal mass, and rectal abnormality combined with CT findings confirm the diagnostic impressions and indicate which medical or surgical therapy is needed.

When bowel resection is needed to remove obstruction, there should always be an attempt to limit the amount of bowel resected. At times, however, there are "skipped" areas, and several segments have to be resected. Severe recurrent obstruction leads to significant resection and short bowel syndrome (see Chapter 68).

Enteroenteric fistulae and internal fistulae are not an indication for surgery unless symptomatic. Fistulization of the skin, bladder, or vagina may require a more aggressive or a surgical approach because other organ systems are involved.

If an abscess forms intraabdominally, medical management may still be effective. However, if the abscess can no longer be controlled, surgical drainage and resection are necessary.

Treatment of perianal disease is discussed in Chapter 96.

Finally, it must be emphasized that patients with Crohn disease are at increased risk for adenocarcinoma of the colon and the small bowel. If screening demonstrates dysplasia, careful consideration must be given to resection. This is easier to perform in colon disease, but suspicious lesions in the small bowel must be investigated. Resection is indicated if the lesions may be neoplastic.

COURSE AND PROGNOSIS AFTER SURGERY

Surgery for Crohn disease is not curative. Endoscopic evidence for recurrence ranges from 28% to 73% at 1 year and 77% to 85% at 3 years after ileal resection. Studies from various institutions give different rates, but most clinicians believe that Crohn disease will recur within 5 years. Unfortunately, if repeat surgery is necessary, short bowel syndrome and malabsorption may develop. Recurrences are most likely to occur close to the area of resection. However, long-term studies have not been conducted to evaluate the effectiveness of the newer biological therapies postoperatively to prevent recurrent resection.

Surgical treatment for Crohn colitis includes segmental resection, subtotal colectomy with ileoproctostomy, or if performed because of an uncertain primary diagnosis, ileorectal anal anastomosis and total colectomy with ileostomy. Older studies report recurrence in approximately 75% of patients at 10 years; again, long-term studies of the newer therapies are needed to determine whether repeat surgical treatment is necessary. Nevertheless, total colectomy with ileoanal anastomosis is not recommended for patients with Crohn colitis because of the high recurrence rate in the area of the new pouch. Unfortunately, some patients with indeterminate colitis inadvertently undergo total colectomy with an ileoanal procedure only to experience a recurrence of ileitis. Laparoscopic surgery can be performed for Crohn disease and ileocolic resection. Early studies reveal that laparoscopic surgery results in lower incidence of minor complications and shorter periods of postoperative recovery. Indications for the use of laparoscopic surgery do not differ from those for open surgery.

ADDITIONAL RESOURCES

Borelli O, Cordischi L, Cirulli M, et al: Polymeric diet alone versus corticosteroids in the treatment of active pediatric Crohn's disease: a randomized controlled open-label trial, *Clin Gastroenterol Hepatol* 4:744–753, 2006.

Colombel JF, Sanborn WJ, Rutgeerts P, et al: Adalimumab for maintenance of clinical response and remission in patients with Crohn's disease: the CHARM trial, *Gastroenterology* 132:52–65, 2007.

Fichera A, Finlayson E, Magglori L, Michelassi F: Surgical treatment of inflammatory bowel disease. In Podolsky DK, Camilleri M, Fitz JG, et al, editors: *Yamada's textbook of gastroenterology*, ed 6, Hoboken, New Jersey, 2016, John Wiley and Sons Ltd, pp 1450–1478.

Froehlich F, Juillerat P, Pittet V, et al: Maintenance of surgically induced remission of Crohn's disease, *Digestion* 76:130–135, 2007.

Johnson T, Macdonald S, Hill SM, et al: Treatment of active Crohn's disease in children using partial enteral nutrition with liquid formula: a randomized controlled trial, *Gut* 55:356–361, 2006.

Melmed GY, Targan SR: Crohn's disease: clinical manifestations and management. In Podolsky DK, Camilleri M, Fitz JG, et al, editors: *Yamada's textbook of gastroenterology*, ed 6, Hoboken, New Jersey, 2016, John Wiley and Sons Ltd, pp 1418–1449.

Murphy SJ, Ullman TA, Abreu MD: Gut microbes in Crohn's disease: getting to know you better?, *Am J Gastroenterol* 102:397–398, 2008.

Sanborn WJ, Rutgeerts P, Enns R, et al: Adalimumab induction therapy for Crohn disease previously treated with infliximab: a randomized trial, *Ann Intern Med* 146:829–838, 2007.

Sands BE, Siegel CA: Crohn's disease. In Feldman M, Friedman LS, Brandt LJ, editors: *Gastrointestinal and liver disease*, ed 10, Philadelphia, 2016, Saunders-Elsevier, pp 1990–2022.

Siebold F: ASCA: genetic marker, predictor of disease, or marker of a response to an environmental agent?, *Gut* 54:1212–1213, 2005.

96

Perianal Disease in Crohn Disease

Martin H. Floch

Anorectal Crohn disease may consist of fissures, ulcers, abscesses, fistulae, strictures, edematous skin tags, and benign skin tags (Fig. 96.1). The overall prevalence is 36%, but it is 46% when the colon is involved and only 25% when the small bowel is involved. Often, one of these lesions may appear before there is evidence of intestinal disease.

CLINICAL PICTURE

The patient may have only mild diarrhea or may have severe rectal pain or bulging abscesses. A simple skin tag may be enlarged and painless but can be rectally disfiguring ("elephant ears"). Such pain is severe and necessitates emergency treatment.

Physical examination on the exterior can reveal the lesion. It is important to test for local tenderness and look for discharge from a fistula. At times, it may be too difficult to perform a rectal examination, but the anal ring can be teased, and often a small fissure can be demonstrated without entering the anal ring. Bulging of a large abscess is obvious.

DIAGNOSIS

To diagnose a fissure, the fissure must be seen, but its presence can be suspected when there is great tenderness on digital examination. Anoscopy may have to be delayed or performed only with sedation. It is important to rule out any malignant lesion during early presentation in a patient who has not undergone endoscopic examination of the anal ring, and anesthesia may be necessary to evaluate the rectum.

TREATMENT AND MANAGEMENT

Therapy for fissures, edematous skin tags, and associated hemorrhoidal problems is local, as described in Chapters 102 to 107. Topical treatment may be successful, but if it does not result in improvement, surgical intervention may be necessary. Ischiorectal abscesses require prompt incision and drainage. Most heal, but as many as 35% develop a fistula-in-ano. Although many Crohn lesions do not heal, most do resolve.

The goal of therapy in perianal disease is relief of local pain and preservation of the sphincter. Although abscesses must be drained, the presence of a fistula does not necessarily require more surgery. Aggressive medical therapy helps healing. Local cleansing, Sitz baths, suppositories, and cleansing ointments to the area all are important.

Fissures and fistulae have healed with antibiotic therapy. Metronidazole has been effective in as many as 75% of patients, but several months of therapy are required, and disease does tend to recur. Lesions also heal with adequate disease control; therefore, vigorous immunosuppression or biological therapy is indicated.

If medical therapy fails, surgical drainage and placement of setons and mushroom catheters may be necessary. This therapy usually requires months, but healing occurs slowly. Occasionally, more aggressive surgery is necessary and includes fistulotomy. If perianal disease is severe and incontinence develops, proctectomy is necessary. Removal of the fecal flow eventually leads to healing.

ADDITIONAL RESOURCES

Abdelnaby A, Downs JH: Diseases of the anorectum. In Feldman M, Friedman LS, Brandt LJ, editors: *Gastrointestinal and liver disease*, ed 10, Philadelphia, 2016, Saunders-Elsevier, pp 2316–2336.

Beck DE, Roberts PL, Saclarides TJ, et al, editors: *The ASCRS textbook of colon and rectal surgery*, 2nd ed, New York, 2011, Springer.

Ingle SB, Loftus EV Jr: The natural history of perianal Crohn's disease, *Dig Liver Dis* 39:963–969, 2007.

Keighley MRB, Williams NS: *Surgery of the anus, Rectum and colon*, 3rd ed, Philadelphia, 2007, Saunders Ltd.

Sands BE, Siegel CA: Crohn's disease. In Feldman M, Friedman LS, Brandt LJ, editors: *Gastrointestinal and liver disease*, ed 10, Philadelphia, 2016, Saunders-Elsevier, pp 1990–2022.

Steele SR: Operative management of Crohn's disease of the colon including anorectal disease, *Surg Clin North Am* 87:611–631, 2007.

Vermeire S, Van Assche G, Rutgeerts P: Perianal Crohn's disease: classification and clinical evaluation, *Dig Liver Dis* 39:959–962, 2007.

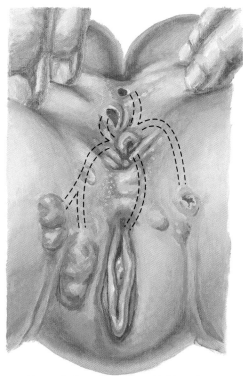

Unusually located (often multiple) anal fistulae, abscesses, ulcers, and edematous hemorrhoidal skin tags

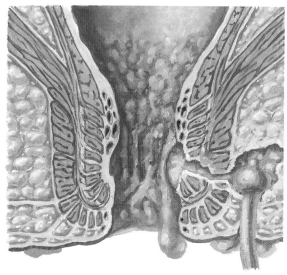

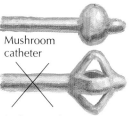

Mushroom catheter

Malecot catheter (allows ingrowth of fibrous tissue, making removal difficult)

Abscess drained by placing small mushroom catheter as close to anus as possible to avoid subsequent long fistula tract

JOHN A.CRAIG—AD

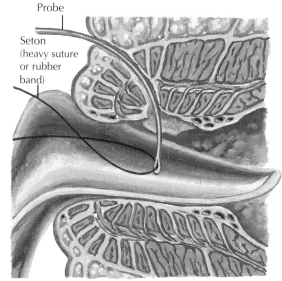

Probe

Seton (heavy suture or rubber band)

Sepsis of fistula tract controlled by placing seton (avoids fistulotomy wounds, which heal poorly)

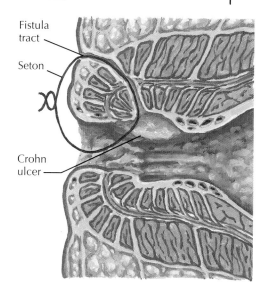

Fistula tract

Seton

Crohn ulcer

Seton left in place between internal and external openings to prevent abscess formation and further destruction of sphincter mechanism

Fig. 96.1 Crohn Disease: Perianal Disease.

97

Drug Therapy for Inflammatory Bowel Disease

Martin H. Floch

Pharmacologic agents used for the treatment of inflammatory bowel disease (IBD) are similar for both ulcerative colitis (UC) and Crohn disease, with two major differences. Rectally instilled topical agents are effective in UC, but usually not in Crohn disease, and certainly not in Crohn ileitis. Nutritional therapy, such as the use of elemental and polymeric diets for the induction of remission, has been effective in Crohn disease, but not in UC. With these differences in mind, most drugs can be used for patients with UC or Crohn disease. The clinician's experience in the use of medications facilitates successful management. Importantly, US Food and Drug Administration (FDA) approval may apply only to some uses of these drugs, but most practitioners use the drugs based on the literature.

Management of UC tends to vary with the severity and extent of illness; active disease is treated more vigorously than inactive disease (Box 97.1). Inactive clinical symptomatic disease may reflect *complete remission,* with no evidence of a pathologic condition or with a low-grade, chronic condition. In either case, maintenance therapy is recommended.

Depending on patient tolerance and physician preference, topical therapy in the form of enemas or suppositories is often effective for acute and maintenance therapy. Some patients cannot tolerate topical therapy, and oral medications are necessary. When severe or fulminant disease progresses, intravenous (IV) therapy is necessary. Nutrition therapy has no role in patients with UC other than to maintain adequate energy and nutrient intakes.

The same medications in UC therapy are used for patients with Crohn disease, with some variations (Box 97.2). The increased incidence of perianal disease requires different approaches, and the effectiveness of infliximab has been more dramatic and is used earlier in Crohn disease. In addition, complete bowel rest and elemental or polymeric liquid diets have been effective in inducing remission when patients or clinicians do not want to use corticosteroid therapy. Although nutritional therapy is slower, significant studies have shown that it works.

Table 97.1 outlines proven drug therapies for IBD.

DRUG THERAPIES

Aminosalicylates

The broad group of medications known as aminosalicylates relies on *5-aminosalicylic acid* (5-ASA) as its active compound. In the past, *sulfasalazine* was the preferred choice and dependent on the bacterial release of 5-ASA from sulfapyridine. Because the intolerance rate was 10% to 15%, the need to remove sulfa from the compound led to the development of other forms of 5-ASA therapy.

Therefore, conjugated, unconjugated, and rectal forms are now available, as well as a formulation that can be given once daily. It appears that delayed-release (DR) *mesalamine* in several compounds can be used in the small bowel, whereas all the others, plus the DR form, are

effective in colon disease. Otherwise, the effectiveness of these medications is comparable, and remission and maintenance rates of 35% to 95% have been reported.

It is important to remember that the 5-ASA compounds are associated with complications. They may cause diarrhea, and some clinicians prefer not to use them in patients with severe, acute UC. Many reports cite impaired renal function from 5-ASA use; therefore, renal function should be monitored in patients receiving long-term therapy.

BOX 97.1 Pharmacologic Treatment of Active Ulcerative Colitis to Control Symptoms or Induce Clinical Remission

Mild to Moderate Disease
- *Distal Colitis*
  - Sulfasalazine or 5-ASA (oral or topical)
  - Topical corticosteroid (or in combination with oral therapy)
- *Pancolitis*
  - Sulfasalazine or oral 5-ASA

Moderate to Severe Disease
- *Distal Colitis*
  - Topical or oral 5-ASA
  - Topical corticosteroid (or in combination with oral therapy)
  - Prednisone
- *Pancolitis*
  - Prednisone
  - Azathioprine or 6-MP

Severe to Fulminant Disease
- *Distal Colitis or Pancolitis*
  - Infliximab or other biological[a]
  - Intravenous corticosteroids
  - Intravenous cyclosporine

Maintenance Therapy
- *Distal Colitis*
  - Sulfasalazine or 5-ASA (oral or topical)
  - Azathioprine or 6-MP
- *Pancolitis*
  - Sulfasalazine or oral 5-ASA
  - Azathioprine or 6-MP

[a]*Adalimumab, certolizumab, or natalizumab.*
5-ASA, 5-Aminosalicylic acid; *6-MP,* 6-mercaptopurine.
Modified from Stein RB, Hanauer SB: Medical therapy for inflammatory bowel disease. *Gastroenterol Clin North Am* 28:297, 1999.

BOX 97.2 Pharmacologic Treatment of Active Crohn Disease to Induce Clinical Remission or Control Symptoms

Mild to Moderate Disease
- Sulfasalazine or 5-ASA
- Metronidazole
- Prednisone
- Azathioprine or 6-MP
- Infliximab or other biological[a]

Severe Disease
- Prednisone
- Intravenous corticosteroids
- TPN or elemental diet
- Infliximab or other biological[a]
- Intravenous cyclosporine

Perianal or Fistulizing Disease
- Metronidazole or alternative antibiotic
- Azathioprine or 6-MP
- Infliximab or other biological[a]
- TPN on temporary basis

Maintenance Therapy
- Sulfasalazine or 5-ASA
- Metronidazole or ciprofloxacin
- Azathioprine or 6-MP
- Infliximab or other biological[a]

[a]*Adalimumab, certolizumab, or natalizumab.*
5-ASA, 5-Aminosalicylic acid; *6-MP*, 6-mercaptopurine; *TPN*, total parenteral nutrition.
Modified from Stein RB, Hanauer SB: Medical therapy for inflammatory bowel disease. *Gastroenterol Clin North Am* 28:297, 1999.

Corticosteroids

Corticosteroids are the most effective drugs to induce remission of IBD, but they are not preferred for maintenance therapy. Many patients with chronic or severe disease require long-term corticosteroid therapy and may develop the associated complications. Great effort should be made to use an immunomodulator to replace corticosteroids if patients become dependent on their use.

There are increasing reports that a single course of IV corticosteroid therapy will induce remissions as effectively as other maintenance therapies. More research is needed on this form of therapy. Corticosteroids are also rapidly effective in topical form, when disease is limited to the rectum or the distal colon. Topical corticosteroid or mesalamine is the drug of choice for proctitis.

Immunomodulators

Azathioprine and *6-mercaptopurine* (6-MP, actively produced from metabolized azathioprine) are effectively used for maintenance therapy in UC and Crohn disease. Doses are variable, and patients must be checked carefully for any hematologic complications. However, long-term therapy with these drugs has proved to be relatively safe. *Cyclosporine* has been used for severe disease when patients are hospitalized and are not responsive to IV corticosteroids. Cyclosporine can induce a remission of symptoms, and patients may be placed on oral cyclosporine or other immunosuppressive agents. However, this is drastic therapy, and these patients are close to undergoing total colectomy or surgery.

Methotrexate has been used less frequently; studies show mixed benefit. Large doses are necessary to induce remission of symptoms. Some clinicians use methotrexate when other therapies are failing.

Biologicals

Infliximab (antitumor necrosis factor–a antibody) has been shown to be effective in the treatment of Crohn disease and UC. It must be administered intravenously. Usually, the patient receives three treatments of 5 or 10 mg/kg body weight at 2-week intervals; then it is decided whether to administer long-term maintenance therapy, with doses every 8 weeks. Because allergic and possible hematologic adverse effects may develop, infliximab must be used with caution. However, its wide use in rheumatoid arthritis has given gastroenterologists confidence about its safety. Infliximab has been effective for many patients who could not tolerate other maintenance or corticosteroid therapy and is now accepted as corticosteroid-sparing therapy.

Natalizumab, an α_4-integrin, was shown in early trials to be effective in inducing remission and improving quality of life. It was taken off the market because of cases of progressive multifocal leukoencephalopathy (PML). Natalizumab has now been placed back on the market and joins infliximab, *adalimumab*, and *certolizumab* as other biological therapy choices. Extensive research is now being done to decide the best biological drugs and select clinical situations in which biologicals may be effective against IBD.

An increased incidence of lymphoma has been suspected with the use of infliximab, but recent evaluations indicate the immunomodulator may be incriminated. Intensive evaluation is forthcoming.

Placebo

All the acute and chronic trials with biologicals have been matched against placebo. Placebos have worked in 5% to 50% of the trials. Therefore, all the previously mentioned drugs have statistical significance, but patients with IBDs have been shown to enter remission, which is maintained without therapy, through placebo medication.

NONDRUG THERAPIES

Forms of therapy other than pharmaceutical agents have included *probiotics, fish oils,* and *nutrient supplements* and *antioxidants.* These are mentioned in the chapters on the particular diseases for which they are used. It must be stressed, however, that these therapies are not *pharmacologic* agents and have not been exposed to the rigorous controls applied to the pharmaceutical industry.

PREGNANCY AND FERTILITY

Because IBD is a disease of the young, the concern of an effect on pregnancy or fertility is always present.

Most drugs are categorized into pregnancy classes A, B, C, and D. The actual disease process is associated with only a slight increase in spontaneous abortion. Statistical data reveal that sulfasalazine, mesalamine, and corticosteroids appear safe during pregnancy. Furthermore, a recent study reports statistically significant safety with the use of 6-MP. Sulfasalazine has been shown to affect sperm and thus is contraindicated in men who hope to father children. Other information on drugs in spermiogenesis is minimal. The long-term effect of biologicals is not yet known.

Classifications change with the most recent information available; therefore, the pregnancy class of a drug should be checked with the physician prescribing and the pharmacy delivering the drug to a pregnant patient.

TABLE 97.1   Oral Drug Therapy of Proven Value in Inflammatory Bowel Disease

Drug	Site	Ulcerative Colitis	Crohn Disease
Aminosalicylates			
Topical (Enemas and Suppositories)			
Mesalamine	Rectum to distal colon	+ +	
Azo-Bond Compounds			
Sulfasalazine (sulfapyridine + 5-ASA)	Colon	+ +	+ +
Olsalazine (5-ASA dimer)	Colon	+ +	+ +
Balsalazide (5-ASA + 4-ABBA)	Colon	+ +	+ +
Mesalamine			
Delayed release (Asacol)	Ileum, colon	+ +	+ +
Multi Matrix delivery system (Lialda)	Ileum, colon	+ +	+ +
Sustained release (Pentasa)	Stomach to colon	+ +	+ +
Steroids			
Topical			
Hydrocortisone suppositories	Rectum, distal colon	+ +	+ +
Hydrocortisone, prednisone, and betamethasone enemas	Rectum, distal colon		
Systemic (PO or IV)			
Prednisone, methylprednisolone, hydrocortisone	Stomach to colon	+ +	+ +
Immunomodulators			
Azathioprine	Stomach to colon	+ +	+ +
6-MP	Stomach to colon	+ +	+ +
Cyclosporine	Stomach to colon	+	+
Methotrexate	Stomach to colon	+	+
Antibiotics			
Metronidazole	Stomach to colon	+	+ +
Ciprofloxacin	Stomach to colon	+	+ +
Biologicals			
Infliximab (IV) (anti-TNF-α)	Stomach to colon	+ +	+ +
Natalizumab (α_4-integrin)	Stomach to colon	+ + ?	+ +
Adalimumab	Stomach to colon	+ + ?	
Certolizumab	Stomach to colon	+ + ?	

ABBA, 4-Aminobenzoyl-beta-alanine; *5-ASA*, 5-Aminosalicylic acid; *6-MP*, 6-mercaptopurine; *IV*, intravenous; *PO*, oral; *TNF*, tumor necrosis factor. +, *Effective*; + +, *very effective.*

ADDITIONAL RESOURCES

Behm BW, Bickston SJ: Tumor necrosis factor-alpha antibody for the maintenance of remission in Crohn's disease, *Cochrane Database Syst Rev* (1):CD006893, 2008.

Francella A, Dyan A, Bodian C, et al: The safety of 6-mercaptopurine for childbearing patients with inflammatory bowel disease: a retrospective cohort study, *Gastroenterology* 124:9–17, 2003.

Hanauer SB, Podolsky DK: Ulcerative colitis. In Podolsky DK, Camilleri M, Fitz JG, et al, editors: *Yamada's textbook of gastroenterology*, ed 6, Hoboken, New Jersey, 2016, John Wiley and Sons Ltd, pp 1378–1417.

Ho GT, Smith L, Aitken S, et al: The use of adalimumab in the management of refractory Crohn's disease, *Aliment Pharmacol Ther* 27:308–315, 2008.

Melmed GY, Targan SR: Crohn's disease: clinical manifestations and management. In Podolsky DK, Camilleri M, Fitz JG, et al, editors:

Yamada's textbook of gastroenterology, ed 6, Hoboken, New Jersey, 2016, John Wiley and Sons Ltd, pp 1418–1449.

Osterman MT, Lichtenstein GR: Ulcerative colitis. In Feldman M, Friedman LS, Brandt LJ, editors: *Gastrointestinal and liver disease*, ed 10, Philadelphia, 2016, Saunders-Elsevier, pp 2023–2061.

O'Sullivan NA, O'Morain CA: Nutritional therapy in Crohn's disease, *Inflamm Bowel Dis* 4:45–53, 1998.

Sands BE, Siegel CA: Crohn's disease. In Feldman M, Friedman LS, Brandt LJ, editors: *Gastrointestinal and liver disease*, ed 10, Philadelphia, 2016, Saunders-Elsevier, pp 1990–2022.

Targan SR, Feagan BG, Fedorak RN, et al: Natalizumab for the treatment of active Crohn's disease: results of the ENCORE trial, *Gastroenterology* 132:1672–1683, 2007.

98

Microscopic Colitis (Lymphocytic or Collagenous Colitis)

Martin H. Floch

Microscopic colitis is a syndrome in which patients have (1) chronic diarrhea, (2) normal findings on colonoscopy and a normal-appearing mucosa, (3) histologic evidence of increased cellular infiltrate in the lamina propria, and (4) either (a) full-blown *lymphocytic colitis* with intraepithelial lymphocytes and increased infiltrate in the lamina propria or (b) *collagenous colitis* with a collagen band below the epithelium larger than 10 mm (Fig. 98.1).

Microscopic colitis has been difficult to define, but numerous reports have clarified the syndrome. Initially described as "collagenous" colitis, with watery diarrhea and deposition of collagen, it was later noted that many patients with chronic watery diarrhea have a lymphocytic infiltrate and a definite intraepithelial lymphocytic infiltrate. During the past decade, many patients have been described with watery diarrhea responsive to therapy and with increased infiltrate only in the lamina propria. It is important to note that watery diarrhea and absence of gross findings on colonoscopy are components of the syndrome. Histologic examination of the biopsy specimen shows no distortion of the crypts, as seen in ulcerative colitis.

One study found microscopic colitis in 9.5% of patients with watery diarrhea. Incidence is reported as 4.2 per 100,000 population, with the lymphocytic type three times more common than the collagenous form. The cause and etiology remain unknown, but it is thought that microscopic colitis is associated with toxins, drugs, or latent autoimmune enteropathy, as well as various diseases (e.g., celiac). Almost 30% of patients with celiac disease have been reported to have some form of microscopic colitis; thus, a similar cause is suspected.

CLINICAL PICTURE

The cardinal feature of microscopic colitis is watery diarrhea, generally manifesting during the sixth decade of life. Less than 50% of patients have abdominal pain along with diarrhea, and less than 33% experience weight loss. Reports indicate an association with lansoprazole and cholestyramine, omeprazole, nonsteroidal antiinflammatory drugs (NSAIDs), and celiac disease.

The effects of watery diarrhea can be severe, and many patients become hypokalemic. Systemic inflammation is rare. Microscopic colitis appears to be twice as prevalent in women as in men.

DIAGNOSIS

The diagnosis is made through histopathology. Often, a patient with low-grade watery diarrhea receives a diagnosis of irritable bowel syndrome on the basis of normal gross colonoscopy findings, but no biopsy specimen was taken because the mucosa looked normal. Mucosal biopsy of the colon must be performed to determine whether a patient with watery diarrhea has microscopic colitis. More detailed research will allow a determination of the incidence and prevalence of the disease.

The histopathology of microscopic colitis has been controversial. An initial criterion was "increased collagen deposition," and then the "presence of intraepithelial lymphocytes" was added as a criterion. It is now accepted that increased levels of lymphocytes and plasma cells, with the possibility of eosinophils in the lamina propria, correlating with the clinical picture and resolving with treatment, make the diagnosis. The pathologist must determine whether crypt distortion has occurred. If so, the diagnosis would be nonspecific ulcerative colitis.

TREATMENT AND MANAGEMENT

Eliminating any agent thought to cause microscopic colitis is paramount. The medications most often used are *mesalamine* and *budesonide,* with the latter favored in a recent study. Trials have been conducted using bismuth subsalicylate, antibiotics, and other agents, but 5-aminosalicylic acid (5-ASA) compounds can induce remission. Some experts prefer a 4- to 8-week trial of bismuth subsalicylate before administering mesalamine. It may be necessary to use prednisone to induce remission if bismuth subsalicylate and mesalamine fail to do so. Some reports show that calcium channel blockers can be helpful.

It is important to document microscopically that the patient's condition has returned to normal with therapy or with withdrawal of a suspected etiologic agent.

COURSE AND PROGNOSIS

Recent large studies indicate the difficulty of determining the relevance of histopathologic findings to the clinical course. All microscopic colitides seem to behave similarly. The course of microscopic colitis is benign, and most patients respond to mesalamine, budesonide, bismuth subsalicylate, and if needed, corticosteroids or an experimental therapeutic agent.

More than 70% of patients experience long-term cessation of diarrhea. Other patients, however, experience relapse and require repeat therapy after being in remission. In either case, the prognosis is excellent.

Lymphocytic colitis

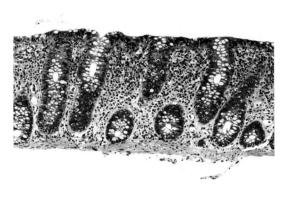

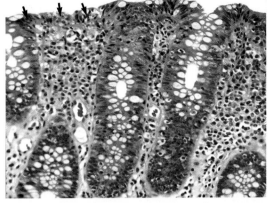

Low-power microphotograph of lymphocytic colitis that shows increased lymphocytic and round cell infiltration in the lamina propria. The crypts appear normal.

High-power microphotograph of lymphocytic colitis (same patient and biopsy as in figure at left). *Arrows* indicate the classic infiltrate of lymphocytes in the epithelium.

Collagenous colitis

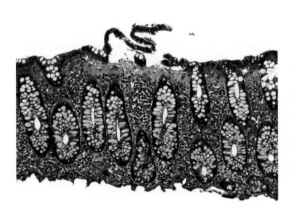

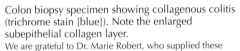

Colon biopsy specimen showing collagenous colitis (trichrome stain [blue]). Note the enlarged subepithelial collagen layer.
We are grateful to Dr. Marie Robert, who supplied these photomicrographs.

High-power microphotograph of collagenous colitis that shows an enlarged (pink) collagen layer and an increased lymphocytic infiltrate in the lamina propria. The *arrow* indicates a cellular element (fibroblast nucleus) entrapped in the enlarged collagen layer.

Fig. 98.1 Microscopic Colitis: Lymphocytic and Collagenous.

ADDITIONAL RESOURCES

Lindstrom CG: Collagenous colitis with watery diarrhea: a new entity, *Pathol Urol* 11:87–91, 1976.

Pardi DS, Loftus EV Jr, Smyrk TC, et al: The epidemiology of microscopic colitis: a population-based study in Olmstead County, Minnesota, *Gut* 56:504–508, 2007.

Stewart MJ, Seow CH, Storr MA: Prednisolone and budesonide for short- and long-term treatment of microscopic colitis: systematic review and meta-analysis, *Clin Gastroenterol Hepatol* 9:881–890, 2011.

Stroehlein JR: Microscopic colitis, *Curr Treat Options Gastroenterol* 3:231–236, 2007.

Wald A: Other diseases of the colon and rectum. In Feldman M, Friedman LS, Brandt LJ, editors: *Gastrointestinal and liver disease*, ed 10, Philadelphia, 2016, Saunders-Elsevier, pp 2297–2315.

Yen EF, Pardi DS: Microscopic colitis and other miscellaneous inflammatory and structural disorders of the colon. In Podolsky DK, Camilleri M, Fitz JG, et al, editors: *Yamada's textbook of gastroenterology*, ed 6, Hoboken, New Jersey, 2016, John Wiley and Sons Ltd, pp 1479–1494.

99

Neoplasms of the Large Bowel: Colon Polyps and Colon Cancer

Martin H. Floch

COLON POLYPS

A colon *polyp* is any elevation of the colon mucosal surface (Fig. 99.1). It may be of any size, sessile or pedunculated, and benign or malignant. *Benign polyps* are categorized as neoplastic, nonneoplastic, and submucosal. *Neoplastic polyps* are usually considered premalignant, and most are adenomas. *Adenomas* may be classified histologically as tubular, tubulovillous, or villous. The polyp may demonstrate low-grade or high-grade dysplasia. High-grade dysplasia in a polyp is often referred to as "intermucosal carcinoma (malignant)," or *carcinoma in situ.*

Nonneoplastic polyps include mucosal, hyperplastic, and inflammatory (pseudopolyps) types, hamartomas, and other rare types. *Submucosal polyps* are lipomas, lymphoid collections, leiomyomas, hemangiomas, fibromas, and rare presentations of endometriosis, pneumatosis cystoides intestinalis, colitis cystica profunda, or metastatic lesions.

The prevalence of colorectal neoplasia varies worldwide: 30 to 40 per 100,000 population in the United States; 15 to 30 per 100,000 in Europe; and less than 5 to 10 in South America and Asia. The prevalence varies with the population being studied.

Hereditary polyposis syndromes show that colorectal neoplasia has a *genetic* component (see Chapter 100). The progression of normal mucosa to neoplasia is associated with a loss of the *APC* gene in the cell, and the progression to carcinoma is associated with K-*ras, DCC,* and *p53* activity. The genetic component is complex; the interested reader is referred to the Additional Resources. It is estimated that up to 20% of neoplastic polyps result from genetic effects. Strong epidemiologic evidence shows that *dietary* factors play a major role in polyp formation through the microflora and intestinal microbiologic relationships. Diets with high levels of fat and red meat and low levels of fiber are associated with a higher incidence of neoplastic polyp formation. Australian patients who combined a low-fat diet with increased bran intake had a lower incidence of recurrent polyps; increased bran or low-fat diet alone did not result in a decrease. Not all studies are in agreement, but the very low incidence of neoplastic polyps in societies whose diets are high in fiber and low in saturated fats is incriminating for these nutrient factors. Dietary carcinogens and micronutrient deficiencies are also thought to play a role, but no proof of a cause-and-effect sequence is yet available.

Polyps usually develop in the rectum and the sigmoid and descending colon. Incidence seems to be greater on the right side of the colon. Most polyps can progress from an adenoma to a carcinoma, *flat adenomas* have a potential for malignancy, and the amount of severely dysplastic tissue in a polyp is related to its size. Flat polyps are of great interest to endoscopists because of their malignant potential and because they are more challenging to identify and remove completely. Polyps shown on histologic examination to contain villous elements are associated with a higher incidence of malignancy. Therefore, patients with flat adenomas and polyps with significant villous elements are at higher risk for malignancy.

Patients with hyperplastic or inflammatory polyps are also at risk for carcinoma. *Serrated polyps,* a combination of hyperplastic and adenomatous elements, are being found with increasing frequency and have malignant tendencies. Most submucosal polyps are benign. Many patients with carcinoids, metastatic lesions, melanomas, lymphomas, and Kaposi sarcoma have malignant polypoid formation in the colon. Except for its association with some malabsorption syndromes, lymphoid hyperplasia has no malignant significance.

Clinical Picture

Polypoid lesions are often accompanied by occult or gross bleeding. Depending on their position, they may cause intussusception or obstruction of the bowel; therefore, they rarely cause pain. Usually, polyps are detected during colonoscopic or barium enema screening for other symptoms. If the polyp is large, which is now unusual, the patient experiences a change in bowel habits and obstruction. Large lesions are rarely benign. Unlike benign polyps, malignant formation is life threatening.

Three findings with a polyp are important in risk for malignancy: size (>2 cm), histologic type (villous formation), and degree of dysplasia (severe).

Screening

The diagnosis of colon polyps can be made through sigmoidoscopy, colonoscopy, barium enema, or virtual colonoscopy (Fig. 99.2). The diagnosis is made when symptoms indicate the need for a polyp search or a screening procedure to prevent colon cancer. Screening allows small lesions to be detected and removed before they can advance to carcinoma.

Screening procedures include fecal occult blood testing, digital rectal examination, sigmoidoscopy, colonoscopy, and virtual colonoscopy. All may detect a lesion, but *colonoscopy* results in the greatest yield and enables biopsy and possible removal and identification of the polyp. Therefore, colonoscopy is the screening procedure of choice for most gastroenterologists. Statistical evidence shows that a combination of fecal occult blood testing and sigmoidoscopy can be as effective as colonoscopy or double-contrast barium enema in preventing mortality from colon cancer, if cost is an issue and colonoscopy is unavailable. Endoscopy and stool screening procedures are described in Chapters 79 and 81. However, there is now a 10-year study involving the Veterans Administration to evaluate effectiveness of colonoscopy as compared to fecal immunochemical tests in reducing the mortality from colon cancer. The study just began and will be finished in 10 years (see references). We hope that this study will answer the question which is better and how often it is done.

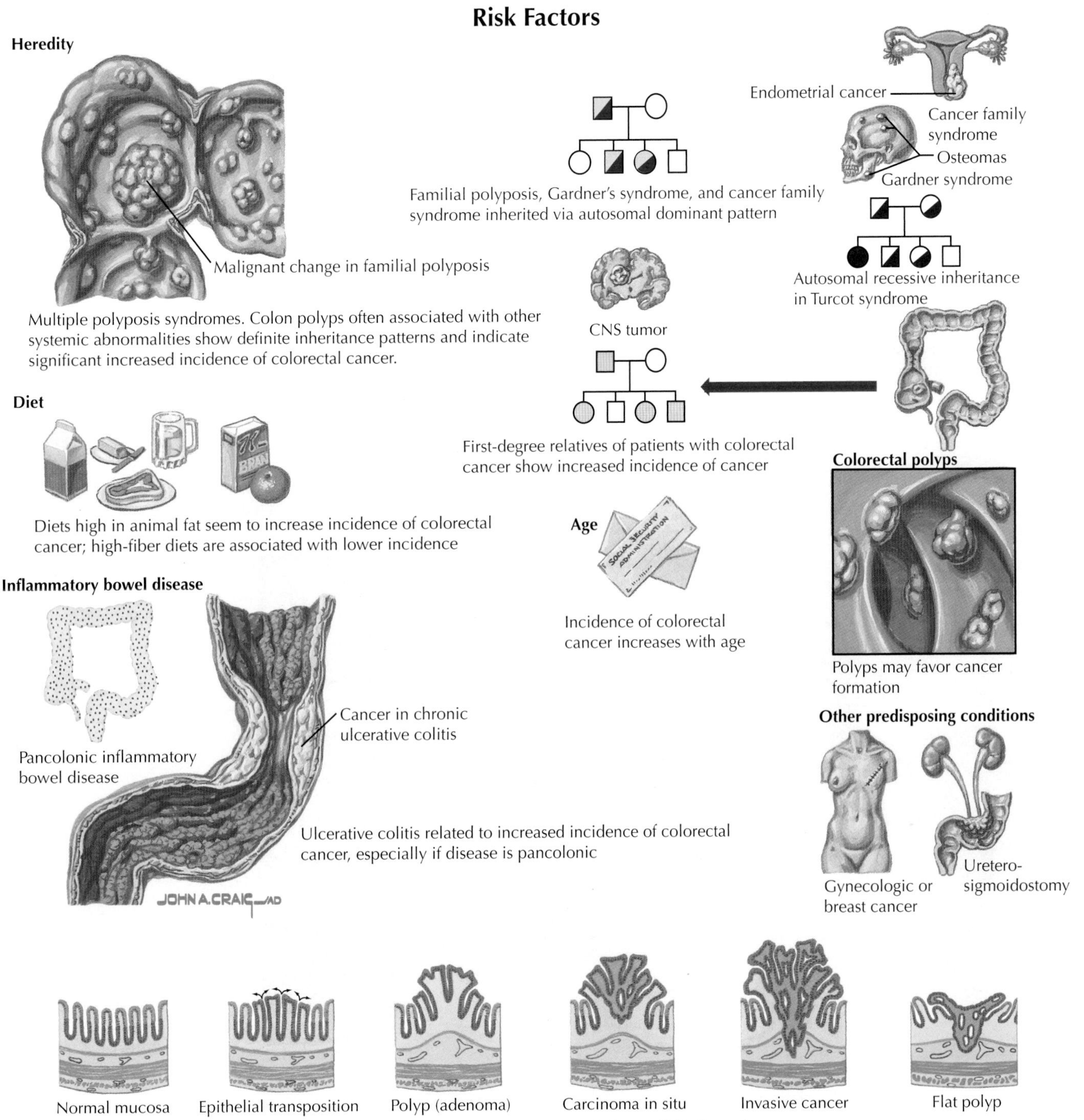

Risk Factors

Heredity

Malignant change in familial polyposis

Multiple polyposis syndromes. Colon polyps often associated with other systemic abnormalities show definite inheritance patterns and indicate significant increased incidence of colorectal cancer.

Familial polyposis, Gardner's syndrome, and cancer family syndrome inherited via autosomal dominant pattern

Endometrial cancer

Cancer family syndrome

Osteomas

Gardner syndrome

Autosomal recessive inheritance in Turcot syndrome

CNS tumor

First-degree relatives of patients with colorectal cancer show increased incidence of cancer

Colorectal polyps

Polyps may favor cancer formation

Diet

Diets high in animal fat seem to increase incidence of colorectal cancer; high-fiber diets are associated with lower incidence

Age

Incidence of colorectal cancer increases with age

Other predisposing conditions

Gynecologic or breast cancer

Uretero-sigmoidostomy

Inflammatory bowel disease

Pancolonic inflammatory bowel disease

Cancer in chronic ulcerative colitis

Ulcerative colitis related to increased incidence of colorectal cancer, especially if disease is pancolonic

JOHN A. CRAIG—AD

Normal mucosa | Epithelial transposition | Polyp (adenoma) | Carcinoma in situ | Invasive cancer | Flat polyp

Fig. 99.1 Neoplasms of the Large Bowel: Colon Polyps. *CNS,* Central nervous system.

Treatment and Management

Once identified, a polypoid lesion should be removed. Most lesions smaller than 3 cm can be removed during endoscopy. Biopsy, *snaring,* elevating the polyp with water injection and removing it piecemeal, and cauterization are all used effectively to ablate polyps. It is hoped that the entire polyp has been removed; the removed tissue is evaluated histopathologically for possible carcinoma in situ. The histopathology is important to ensure that all neoplastic tissue and highly dysplastic or serrated lesions are removed with no possibility of spread. The histology and correlation with genetic and growth factors (e.g., microsatellite

instability, hereditary nonpolyposis colorectal cancer [HNPCC]) are important (see "Additional Resources"). Complication rates of screening procedures are low.

After a polyp is removed, the question is how often colonoscopy should be repeated. If there is any question about total removal, or if the colonoscopy was difficult, a repeat procedure is performed within 1 year. However, if there is only a single polyp, the question is whether repeat colonoscopy should be performed in 3 to 5 years. Recent studies reveal that small tumors can grow rapidly. A physician or patient may want a repeat examination in 3 years, but if examination findings are excellent, screening can be delayed until 5 years, with fecal occult blood

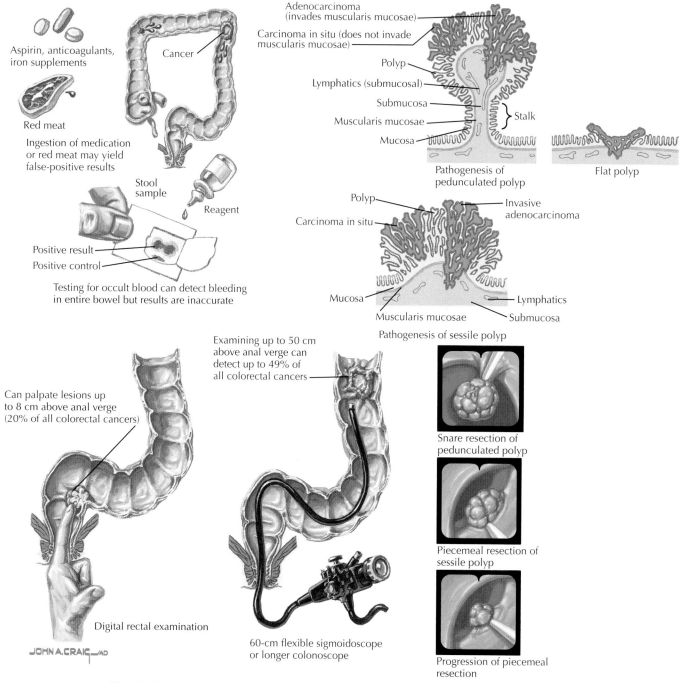

Aspirin, anticoagulants, iron supplements

Red meat

Ingestion of medication or red meat may yield false-positive results

Cancer

Stool sample

Reagent

Positive result

Positive control

Testing for occult blood can detect bleeding in entire bowel but results are inaccurate

Adenocarcinoma (invades muscularis mucosae)

Carcinoma in situ (does not invade muscularis mucosae)

Polyp

Lymphatics (submucosal)

Submucosa

Muscularis mucosae

Mucosa

Stalk

Pathogenesis of pedunculated polyp

Flat polyp

Polyp

Carcinoma in situ

Invasive adenocarcinoma

Mucosa

Muscularis mucosae

Lymphatics

Submucosa

Pathogenesis of sessile polyp

Can palpate lesions up to 8 cm above anal verge (20% of all colorectal cancers)

Examining up to 50 cm above anal verge can detect up to 49% of all colorectal cancers

Snare resection of pedunculated polyp

Piecemeal resection of sessile polyp

Digital rectal examination

JOHN A.CRAIG—AD

60-cm flexible sigmoidoscope or longer colonoscope

Progression of piecemeal resection

Fig. 99.2 Neoplasms of the Large Bowel: Screening Techniques and Treatment of Colon Polyps.

testing in the "off" years. The guidelines are clear, but variations occur depending on each patient's health and circumstances.

The patient identified with polyps should be treated for risk prevention and possible polyp chemoprevention. The patient should also be advised to maintain adequate weight, decrease the intake of foods high in polyunsaturated fat, and increase the intake of foods high in dietary fiber. An 81-mg dose of aspirin daily seems effective in decreasing the risk for cancer. Other chemopreventive agents, such as nonsteroidal antiinflammatory drugs (NSAIDs [e.g., sulindac, COX-2 inhibitors]), and increased calcium intake show some statistical effectiveness, but low-dose aspirin is the most widely accepted chemopreventive regimen.

Course and Prognosis

In the United States, vigorous screening programs in conjunction with colonoscopic removal of polyps and small lesions, combined with chemopreventive agents, can decrease the incidence of colon cancer and related deaths. In other countries, incidence and mortality appear to be stabilizing, but vary with environmental and economic conditions.

The chemopreventive agents include aspirin, celecoxib, and now statins. These drugs can be associated with cardiovascular complications and gastrointestinal bleeding, and their use and selection depend on the physician's recommendations for the individual patient.

COLON CANCER

Cancer of the colon is a major cause of morbidity and mortality in Western countries with similar dietary and lifestyle habits. Colon cancer is believed to be an acquired genetic disease caused by exposure to environmental carcinogens. A genetic instability occurs, followed by mutational changes that produce neoplastic clones. Free from homeostatic growth controls, the cancer increases with time and total carcinogenic exposure. The clinical result is that cancer incidence rises as an exponential function of age. Deaths from colorectal cancer typically begin to increase slowly in the fifth decade of life, rising steeply with advancing age. In the United States, 56,700 persons died of colorectal cancer in 2001; the incidence varies greatly with the population, from 30% to 35% per 100,000.

The prevalence in whites is highest in the ascending colon and cecum (22% in men, 27% in women) and in the sigmoid colon (25% in men, 23% in women). The incidence is approximately 3 to 4 per 100,000 population in undeveloped countries of Asia and 35 per 100,000 in some areas in the United States. The epidemiologic association of high-fat, high-meat, low-fiber diets correlates with worldwide incidence discrepancies. Nutrients such as calcium, selenium, and antioxidant vitamins may decrease this incidence, but chemoprevention programs based on these substances have not yet been effective.

Colorectal cancer develops throughout the large bowel. Approximately 45% of cases are observed in the rectum and sigmoid, but the distribution seems to be increasing on the right side, with as many as 25% in the cecum and ascending colon. Alterations in K-*ras, APC, DCC,* and *p*53 genes have all been demonstrated in association with malignant transformation. Other significant genetic findings are unfolding. Syndromes such as *HNPCC,* or Lynch syndrome, are being discovered and understood. Families with this syndrome must be followed closely. Patients at particular risk for colorectal cancer are those who have polyposis syndromes.

Clinical Picture

Family history of cancer of the colon, polyps, or inflammatory bowel disease (IBD) raises the index of suspicion for colorectal cancer in patient with classic signs, such as rectal bleeding, change in bowel habits, signs of obstruction, or anemia in the presence of occult blood (Fig. 99.3).

Diagnosis

Any patient with clinical suspicion of colon cancer must undergo colonoscopic evaluation. Findings from the physical examination, which must include digital rectal examination, may indicate the need for endoscopic evaluation. If the patient has an anorectal lesion (see Chapter 101), diagnosis can be made through proctoscopy or sigmoidoscopy. Even if the patient has a low lesion, however, full colonoscopic examination should be performed because synchronous lesions develop in as many as 30% of patients; treatment depends on understanding the distribution of a polyp or a malignant lesion anywhere in the colon. If full examination is not possible, contrast air enemas can be used with absorbable media or with barium if there is no chance of obstruction. Large biopsy specimens should be obtained for diagnosis. Evaluation should be followed by computed tomography (CT) of the abdomen and by chest evaluation to stage the cancer for the appropriate treatment. Endoscopic ultrasound can be helpful, particularly in the rectum, in staging the disease to determine whether it has extended through the wall and whether nodes are present.

Many lesions can mimic those of colon cancer, including benign tumors, areas of diverticulitis, IBD, masses caused by parasites, and other tumors of the colon, such as lymphoma, carcinoid, Kaposi sarcoma, and extrinsic lesions involving the peritoneum. When direct biopsy material cannot be obtained, biopsy through laparoscopy or laparotomy is necessary to determine appropriate treatment.

Full serum chemistry profiles are needed to determine whether the patient has anemia. Carcinoembryonic antigen (CEA) level may be elevated, and CEA level does have some relationship to outcome.

Colorectal cancer is a major clinical problem, but preventive and control measures can be effective. Recent data indicate that its incidence is stabilizing, probably associated with intensive screening programs in the United States. Any patient with a suspicious lesion or with a high-risk background should undergo colonoscopic screening. Fecal occult blood testing, sigmoidoscopic examination, and barium contrast enemas have been shown to be effective in large screening programs. However, most gastroenterologists prefer colonoscopy. If it is unavailable, fecal occult blood testing and sigmoidoscopy can be used for screening, and barium air contrast can be used for diagnostic evaluation. Contrast studies are more effective at detecting larger cancerous lesions than small, benign polyps. In fact, before the advent of colonoscopy, the barium air contrast procedure was used for preoperative evaluation.

Staging

To determine the correct treatment for a patient with colon cancer, the disease must be staged. The malignancy may be limited to an area within a polyp, often referred to as *carcinoma in situ.* Lesions may be limited to the muscularis mucosae, or they may extend into the muscularis propria or into the subserosa. Lesions also may invade and perforate the peritoneum and other organs. Lymph nodes may or may not be involved. The classification commonly used is the tumor-node-metastasis (TNM) classification (Box 99.1). However, the Dukes stages are still popular and categorize lesions as limited to the bowel wall (Dukes A), extending through the wall (B), extending to nodal or regional metastases (C), and extending to distant metastases (D).

Approximately 20% of colon cancer tumors are poorly differentiated or undifferentiated, and 10% to 20% may have a strong mucinous cellular element. Each factor usually indicates poor outcome.

Treatment

Surgical resection is the primary therapy for any neoplastic lesion of the colon. Fig. 99.4 demonstrates the segmental and hemicolectomy resections usually performed.

Before surgery, blood screening, CT, and colonoscopic or barium contrast study should be performed. CEA is not used for diagnostic purposes, but is helpful in monitoring postoperative care. Anemia must be treated. Any evidence of another tumor in the colon will govern the surgical decision on how much of the colon to resect.

Adjuvant therapy is not used for carcinoma in situ or for stage I disease. Some clinicians do not want or advise adjuvant therapy in stage II, but most do recommend it when the mucosa is invaded. Numerous therapeutic regimens are available, but levamisole plus 5-fluorouracil (5-FU) is effective in increasing survival for patients with Dukes stages B and C tumors. Five-year survival rates according to Dukes classification are 99% for stage A, 85% for stage B, 67% for stage C, and 14% for stage D. Of all patients with colon cancer, approximately 70% have resectable disease that can be cured, but 45% of these surgical patients experience recurrent disease. In patients with stage C tumors, adjuvant therapy has improved recurrence rates from 63% to 47% and has reduced mortality in approximately 33% of treated patients compared with controls. The addition of leucovorin to the available drugs has resulted in continued success in treatment. A 5-FU/leucovorin combination for 6 months for all patients with stage III is now suggested (see Bresalier in "Additional Resources").

Again, CEA is useful only as a preoperative staging and a postoperative follow-up tool. It is not useful for screening, but a sharp increase

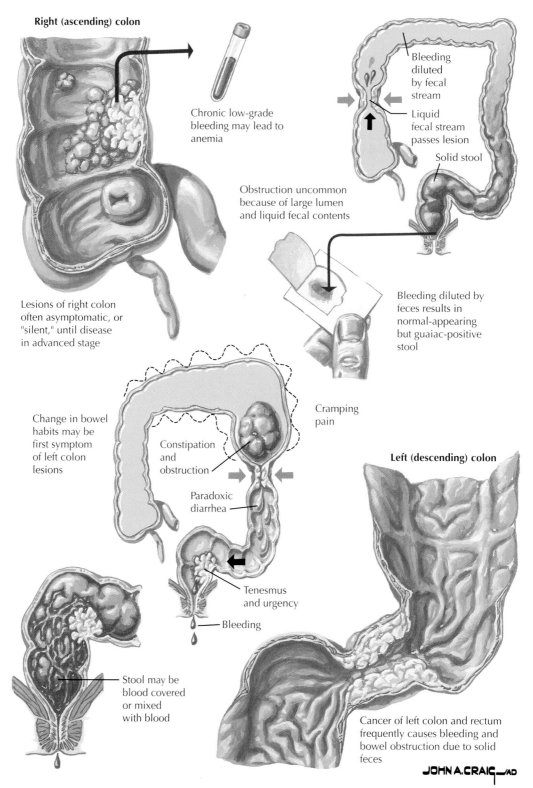

Right (ascending) colon

Chronic low-grade bleeding may lead to anemia

Bleeding diluted by fecal stream

Liquid fecal stream passes lesion

Solid stool

Obstruction uncommon because of large lumen and liquid fecal contents

Lesions of right colon often asymptomatic, or "silent," until disease in advanced stage

Bleeding diluted by feces results in normal-appearing but guaiac-positive stool

Cramping pain

Change in bowel habits may be first symptom of left colon lesions

Constipation and obstruction

Paradoxic diarrhea

Left (descending) colon

Tenesmus and urgency

Bleeding

Stool may be blood covered or mixed with blood

Cancer of left colon and rectum frequently causes bleeding and bowel obstruction due to solid feces

JOHN A. CRAIG—AD

Fig. 99.3 Clinical Manifestations of Colorectal Cancer.

BOX 99.1 Colorectal Cancer Staging (American Joint Committee on Cancer Tumor-Node-Metastasis Classification)

Stage 0
Carcinoma in situ, intraepithelial, or invasion of lamina propria[a] (Tis N0 M0).

Stage I
Tumor invades submucosa (T1 N0 M0); Dukes A.
Tumor invades muscularis propria (T2 N0 M0).

Stage II
Tumor invades muscularis propria into submucosa or into nonperitonealized pericolic or perirectal tissues (T3 N0 M0); Dukes B.[b]
Tumor perforates the visceral peritoneum or directly invades other organs or structures and/or perforates visceral peritoneum.[c]

Stage III
Any degree of bowel wall perforation with regional lymph node metastasis.
N1 metastasis in one to three regional lymph nodes.
N2 metastasis in four or more regional lymph nodes.
Any T N1 M0; Dukes C.[b]
Any T N2 M0.

Stage IV
Any invasion of the bowel wall with or without lymph node metastasis, but with evidence of distant metastasis.
Any T, any N M1; Dukes D.

[a]Tis includes cancer cells confined within the glandular basement membrane (intraepithelial) or lamina propria (intraepithelial) with no extension through the muscularis mucosae into the submucosa.
[b]Dukes stage B (corresponds to stage II) is a composite of better (T0 N0 M0) and worse (T4 N0 M0) prognosis groups, as is Dukes stage C (corresponds to stage III) (any T N1 M0 and any T N2 M0).
[c]Direct invasion in T4 includes invasion of other segments of the colorectum by way of the serosa, such as invasion of the sigmoid colon by carcinoma of the cecum.
M0, No distant metastasis; *M1,* distant metastasis; *MX,* distant metastasis cannot be assessed; *N0,* no regional lymph node metastasis; *NX,* regional lymph nodes cannot be assessed; *TNM,* tumor-node-metastasis.
Modified from Feldman M, Friedman LS, Brandt LJ, editors: *Gastrointestinal and liver disease,* ed 8, Philadelphia, 2006, Saunders-Elsevier, p 2784.

---

in CEA level after surgery or a decrease as a result of treatment does have statistical clinical significance.

Radiation treatment appears to have little role in colon cancer, but it has a definite role in rectal cancer, as discussed in Chapter 101.

Course and Prognosis

Postsurgical follow-up should include CT, colonoscopy, and CEA determinations. The incidence of metachronous colorectal cancer ranges from 1% to 5%. Therefore, colonoscopy is essential for patient follow-up. The first follow-up should occur 1 year after surgery, and then, depending on the patient's status, serial follow-up should occur at 1, 2, or 3 years. The incidence of recurrent cancer is high whenever the tumor has penetrated the wall and the nodes have become involved (stage III or above). Therefore, follow-up is essential to rule out metastasis and to determine whether further surgery or chemotherapy is necessary.

Metastatic disease holds a poor prognosis. The major site of metastasis is the liver; more than 80% of patients who die of metastatic colorectal cancer have liver involvement. Aggressive approaches to resect a single metastasis and even multiple metastases have resulted in some success. Patients with untreated hepatic metastases have a median survival of approximately 10 to 11 months. Mortality from surgery for resection of liver metastases is less than 5%, increasing the 5-year survival rate for patients to 25% to 35%, depending on the series evaluated.

Unfortunately, chemotherapy has not proved successful for these patients; with a wide range of reported responses, the maximum improvement rate is 20%. New chemotherapeutic agents have been developed and others are emerging, and although therapy now includes aggressive surgery, results are still uncertain.

Initial dietary studies reveal an increased rate of recurrence in patients who continue to eat a Western diet. This work is preliminary but should encourage patients with stage III colon cancer to eat a high-fiber, non-Western type of diet.

ADDITIONAL RESOURCES

Alberts DS, Ritenbaugh C, Story JA, et al: Randomized, double-blinded, placebo-controlled study of wheat bran fiber and calcium on fecal bile acids in patients with resected adenomatous colon polyps, *J Natl Cancer Inst* 88:81–92, 1996.

Burt RW, Jasperson KW: Polyposis syndromes. In Podolsky DK, Camilleri M, Fitz JG, et al, editors: *Yamada's textbook of gastroenterology,* ed 6, Hoboken, New Jersey, 2016, John Wiley and Sons Ltd, pp 1583–1607.

East JE, Saunders BP, Jass JR: Sporadic and syndromic hyperplastic polyps and serrated adenomas of the colon: classification, molecular genetics, natural history, and clinical management, *Gastroenterol Clin North Am* 37:25–46, 2008.

Garber III JJ, Chung DC: Polyps of the colon and rectum. In Podolsky DK, Camilleri M, Fitz JG, et al, editors: *Yamada's textbook of gastroenterology,* ed 6, Hoboken, New Jersey, 2016, John Wiley and Sons Ltd, pp 1537–1553.

Itzkowitz SH, Potack J: Colonic polyp and polyposis syndrome. In Feldman M, Friedman LS, Brandt LJ, editors: *Gastrointestinal and liver disease,* ed 10, Philadelphia, 2016, Saunders-Elsevier, pp 2213–2247.

Jacobs ET, Thompson PA, Martinez ME: Diet, gender, and colorectal neoplasia, *J Clin Gastroenterol* 41:731–746, 2007.

Koushik A, Hunter DJ, Spiegelman D, et al: Fruits, vegetables and colon cancer risk in a pooled analysis of 14 cohort studies, *J Natl Cancer Inst* 99:1471–1483, 2007.

Luther J, Chan AT: Malignant tumors of the colon. In Podolsky DK, Camilleri M, Fitz JG, et al, editors: *Yamada's textbook of gastroenterology,* ed 6, Hoboken, New Jersey, 2016, John Wiley and Sons Ltd, pp 1554–1582.

Makinen MJ: Colorectal serrated adenocarcinoma, *Histopathology* 50:131–150, 2007.

McGarr SE, Ridlon JM, Hylemon PB: Diet, anaerobic bacterial metabolism and colon cancer: a review of the literature, *J Clin Gastroenterol* 39:98–109, 2005.

Pasche B: Familial colorectal cancer: a genetics treasure trove for medical discovery, *JAMA* 299:2564–2565, 2008.

Surgical resection of colon cancer

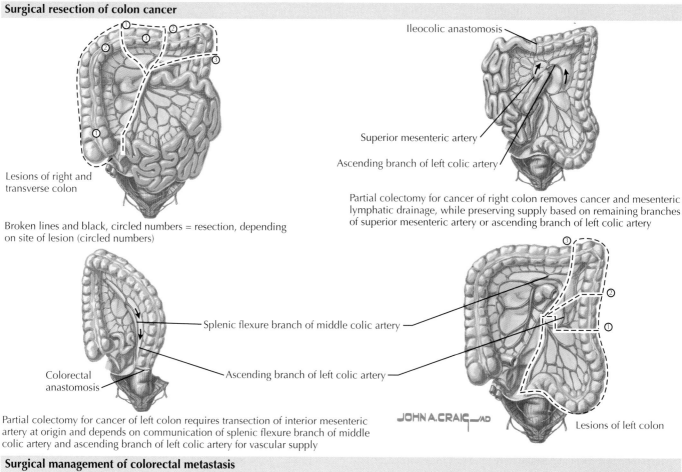

Lesions of right and transverse colon

Broken lines and black, circled numbers = resection, depending on site of lesion (circled numbers)

Ileocolic anastomosis

Superior mesenteric artery

Ascending branch of left colic artery

Partial colectomy for cancer of right colon removes cancer and mesenteric lymphatic drainage, while preserving supply based on remaining branches of superior mesenteric artery or ascending branch of left colic artery

Splenic flexure branch of middle colic artery

Colorectal anastomosis

Ascending branch of left colic artery

Partial colectomy for cancer of left colon requires transection of interior mesenteric artery at origin and depends on communication of splenic flexure branch of middle colic artery and ascending branch of left colic artery for vascular supply

JOHN A.CRAIG—AD

Lesions of left colon

Surgical management of colorectal metastasis

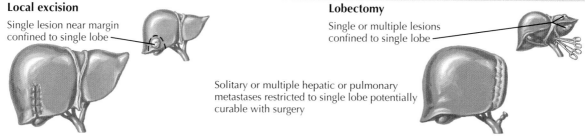

Local excision

Single lesion near margin confined to single lobe

Lobectomy

Single or multiple lesions confined to single lobe

Solitary or multiple hepatic or pulmonary metastases restricted to single lobe potentially curable with surgery

Fig. 99.4 Typical Surgical Resections for Colon Cancer and Management of Colorectal Metastasis.

Potter JD: Fiber and colorectal cancer: where to now?, *N Engl J Med* 340: 223–224, 1999.

Poynter MPH, Gruber SB, Higgins PDR, et al: Statins and the risk of colorectal cancer, *N Engl J Med* 352:2184–2192, 2005.

Riegert-Johnson DL, Johnson RA, Rabe KG, et al: The value of MUTYH testing in patients with early-onset microsatellite stable colorectal cancer referred for hereditary nonpolyposis colon cancer syndrome testing, *Genet Test* 11:361–365, 2007.

Rostom A, Dube C, Lewin G, et al: Nonsteroidal and anti-inflammatory drugs and cyclooxygenase-2 inhibitors for primary prevention of colorectal cancer: a systematic review prepared for the U.S. Prevention services task force, *Ann Intern Med* 146:376–389, 2007.

Soetikno RM, Kaltenbach T, Rouse RV, et al: Prevalence of nonpolypoid (flat and depressed) colorectal neoplasms in asymptomatic and symptomatic adults, *JAMA* 299:1027–1035, 2008.

Spring KJ, Zhao ZZ, Karamatic R, et al: High prevalence of sessile serrated adenomas with *BRAF* mutations: a prospective study of patients undergoing colonoscopy, *Gastroenterology* 131:1400–1407, 2006.

Vasen HF: The lynch syndrome (hereditary nonpolyposis colorectal cancer) (review), *Aliment Pharmacol Ther* 26(Suppl 2):113–126, 2007.

100

Familial Adenomatous Polyposis and Polyposis Syndromes

Martin H. Floch

Gastrointestinal (GI) polyposis is the presence of multiple polypoid lesions in the GI tract (Fig. 100.1). Numerous syndromes have now been classified (Box 100.1).

Familial adenomatous polyposis (FAP) is the most common and best known of the polyposis syndromes. It has an autosomal dominant inheritance pattern, and it occurs from germline mutations of the *APC* gene (see "Additional Resources" for details on the genetics of these disorders). The prevalence is approximately 3 cases per 100,000 population. There appears to be no geographic or significant ethnic variation.

Recently, a germline *MYH* mutation has been described with a syndrome similar to that in patients who do not have the *APC* mutation. These patients were identified in the United Kingdom with a clinical syndrome similar to FAP. The significance of this genetic finding requires further evaluation.

BOX 100.1 Gastrointestinal Polyposis Syndromes

Inherited Polyposis Syndromes
- *Adenomatous Polyposis Syndromes*
  - Familial adenomatous polyposis (FAP)
  - Variants of FAP
  - Gardner syndrome
  - Turcot syndrome
  - Attenuated adenomatous polyposis coli
- *Hamartomatous Polyposis Syndromes*
  - Peutz-Jeghers syndrome
  - Juvenile polyposis
  - Syndromes related to juvenile polyposis
  - Cowden disease
  - Bannayan-Ruvalcaba-Riley syndrome
  - Rare hamartomatous polyposis syndromes
  - Hereditary mixed polyposis syndrome
  - Intestinal ganglioneuromatosis and neurofibromatosis
  - Devon family syndrome
  - Basal cell nevus syndrome

Noninherited Polyposis Syndromes
- Cronkhite-Canada syndrome
- Hyperplastic polyposis syndrome
- Lymphomatous polyposis
- Nodular lymphoid hyperplasia

Modified from Feldman M, Friedman LS, Brandt LJ, editors: *Gastrointestinal and Liver Disease*, ed 10, Philadelphia, 2016, Saunders-Elsevier, p 2214.

CLINICAL PICTURE

Patients with GI polyposis often have a family history of the syndrome or rectal bleeding, diarrhea, or abdominal pain. Most patients seek treatment in the fourth decade of life if the family history is unknown. If a patient has a variant syndrome, disease manifestation may be that of the syndrome, such as a bone lesion in Gardner syndrome, a neurologic lesion in Turcot syndrome, or an intussusception in Peutz-Jeghers syndrome. The details of the syndromes listed in Box 100.1 are not described in this chapter; they are unique to those particular syndromes, particularly when associated polyps and lesions develop outside the colon.

DIAGNOSIS

Multiple polyps in the colon can be identified during endoscopy. Colonoscopy is essential for evaluating the degree and extent of the polyps and for ruling out malignant transformation. Polyposis may be detected through barium air contrast study, but colonoscopy is still essential to rule out malignant changes in any of the polyps. Once polyposis syndrome is identified, upper endoscopy and upper barium contrast studies should be performed to rule out gastric and duodenal polyps. Polyps can occur in any location. The rate of occurrence in the duodenal area is 3% to 5% in FAP. Up to 2% of patients may have pancreatic or thyroid carcinoma. Hepatoblastoma has similarly been reported in up to 1.6% of patients.

Genetic testing has become available worldwide, but methods change rapidly. Laboratories can be identified through the Internet (www.gtest.org). Although testing is sophisticated and is not performed regularly in most clinical settings, it is recommended when the clinical diagnosis is uncertain, when polyposis syndrome appears certain but the patient has no family history, and when relatives are tested in a family with FAP.

TREATMENT AND MANAGEMENT

Once polyposis syndrome is diagnosed, treatment depends on the particular syndrome. In FAP, the patient may have few polyps that gradually increase in number. It is essential that the patient undergo colon screening if genetic testing indicates the potential for FAP or if a first-degree relative has FAP. Screening should occur early, by age 10 to 12 years. If polyps are not found, screening can be performed at longer intervals. If polyps are found, the timing of colectomy varies. Clinicians prefer to wait until adulthood, but given the high risk for colon cancer in these patients, ileal pouch anal anastomosis (IPAA) is now recommended early and in place of colostomy, particularly because there is a lower incidence of pouchitis in these patients than in those who undergo the procedure for ulcerative colitis. Some clinicians still

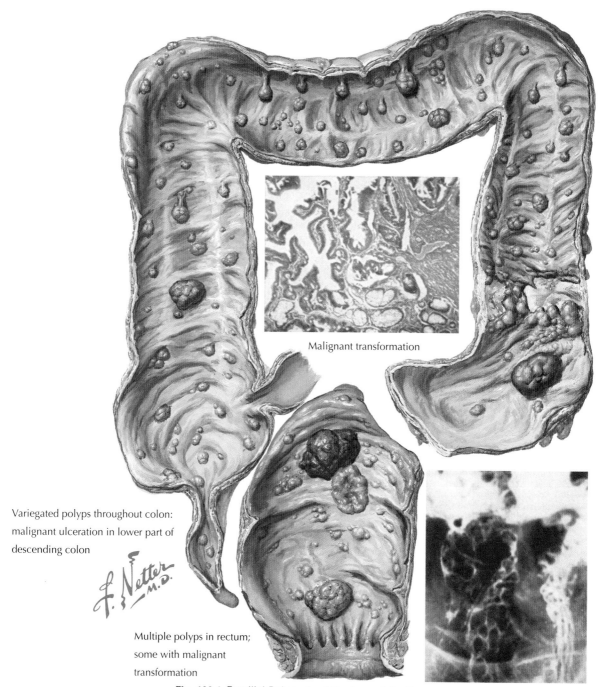

Malignant transformation

Variegated polyps throughout colon:
malignant ulceration in lower part of
descending colon

Multiple polyps in rectum;
some with malignant
transformation

Fig. 100.1 Familial Polyposis of the Large Intestine.

prefer total colectomy with ileorectal anastomosis. However, the risk for rectal carcinoma is always present, thus the IPAA recommendation (see Chapter 93).

In all other polyposis syndromes, colon screening is recommended at different intervals. Given the high rates of duodenal lesions and duodenal adenocarcinoma in patients with FAP, however, upper endoscopy evaluation should be performed regularly.

improves dramatically if the patient undergoes total colectomy. Duodenal cancer and desmoid tumors are the major complications and mortality risks after colectomy. Other cancers are reported, but the rate of carcinomatosis does not increase in these patients. Rectal cancer occurs in a high percentage of patients with polyposis syndrome, so they must be placed under careful surveillance or, even better, should undergo IPAA after colectomy.

COURSE AND PROGNOSIS

With early screening and surgical correction, the prognosis for patients with polyposis syndromes should improve. Life expectancy for a person with untreated FAP is not much longer than 40 years, but it

ADDITIONAL RESOURCES

Abaghizadeh F: Ileostomy, colostomy and pouches. In Feldman M, Friedman LS, Brandt LJ, editors: *Gastrointestinal and liver disease*, ed 10, Philadelphia, 2016, Saunders-Elsevier, pp 2062–2075.

Bulow S, Bulow C, Vasen H, et al: Colectomy and ileorectal anastomosis is still an option for selected patients with familial adenomatous polyposis, *Dis Colon Rectum* 51:1318–1323, 2008.

Burt RW, Jasperson KW: Polyposis syndromes. In Podolsky DK, Camilleri M, Fitz JG, et al, editors: *Yamada's textbook of gastroenterology*, ed 6, Hoboken, New Jersey, 2016, John Wiley and Sons Ltd, pp 1583–1607.

Desai TK, Barkel D: Syndromic colon cancer: lynch syndrome and familial adenomatous polyposis, *Gastroenterol Clin North Am* 37:47–72, 2008.

Itzkowitz SH, Potack J: Colonic polyp and polyposis syndrome. In Feldman M, Friedman LS, Brandt LJ, editors: *Gastrointestinal and liver disease*, ed 10, Philadelphia, 2016, Saunders-Elsevier, pp 2213–2247.

Levin B, Lieberman DA, McFarland B, et al: Screening and surveillance for early detection of colorectal cancer and adenomatous polyps, 2008: a joint guideline from the American cancer society, the US multi-society task force on colorectal cancer, and the American college of radiology, *Gastroenterology* 134:1570–1595, 2008.

Vassen HF, Moslein G, Alonso A, et al: Guidelines for the clinical management of familial adenomatous polyposis (FAP), *Gut* 57:704–713, 2008.

101

Rectal Cancer

Martin H. Floch

Rectal cancer appears to be a different disease than colon cancer. Mortality from rectal cancer in the United States is slowly decreasing, even though the incidence is slowly increasing. This indicates that early detection and treatment of rectal polyps may be preventing the formation of malignant lesions. Furthermore, there appears to be an epidemiologic difference between rectal and colon cancer, because the incidence of rectal cancer is similar for Japan and the United States but different for colon cancer. Treatment and response to treatment differ in the rectum and the colon.

CLINICAL PICTURE

Patients with rectal cancer seek treatment for bleeding or difficulty with defecation. Rectal examination usually reveals a lesion. The lesion may be soft or polypoid and therefore may be missed on rectal examination, but it is clearly seen on proctoscopy (Fig. 101.1). Once rectal cancer has developed, it is invariably symptomatic. Rectal polyps can be asymptomatic but, fortunately, are noted during cancer screening and are removed through sigmoidoscopy or colonoscopy. Again, this may be a reason for the declining incidence of rectal cancer.

DIAGNOSIS

The diagnosis of rectal cancer is made through visualization of the lesion by sigmoidoscopy or colonoscopy and biopsy of the lesion. Colonoscopy is recommended to rule out other colon lesions before initiating therapy. Synchronous lesions are present at significant rates. Ultrasound is now recommended to evaluate the extent of the lesion, stage the lesion, and determine whether nodes are present. Once the lesion is identified, a full workup should be performed to evaluate for metastasis, including computed tomography (CT) of the abdomen and pelvis.

TREATMENT AND MANAGEMENT

It is generally well accepted that surgery is still the best therapy for rectal cancer. Smaller lesions that show no evidence of metastasis can be excised, but most authorities believe that any lesion larger than Dukes stage A (stage I) requires wide excision. Also, preoperative combined-modality therapy is now preferred and accepted as beneficial. Past studies revealed that patients undergoing resection for cure had 2- and 5-year survival rates of 56% and 43%, respectively, if they underwent preoperative radiation therapy. Recent studies have confirmed the importance of preoperative chemoradiation for patients with advanced disease. Chemoradiation is effective in downstaging most lesions and permits a better cure rate. Downstaging after chemoradiation can be accomplished in 60% to 90% of patients, with a complete resectability rate of approximately 60% and a pathologic response rate of 10% to 20%.

COURSE AND PROGNOSIS

The course and prognosis of rectal cancer depend completely on the stage at which the disease is recognized. Again, early removal of simple rectal polyps seems to have decreased the incidence of rectal carcinoma. Dukes stage A lesions can be resected locally if there is no evidence of metastasis. Patients with lesions categorized as Dukes stage B (stage II) and greater should undergo preoperative chemoradiation to downstage the disease. Cure depends largely on the extent of the lesion and whether metastasis has occurred. Prognosis is poor if there is preoperative nodal involvement. Prognosis is better if downstaging results in no evidence of local metastases.

Diagnosis of rectal cancer

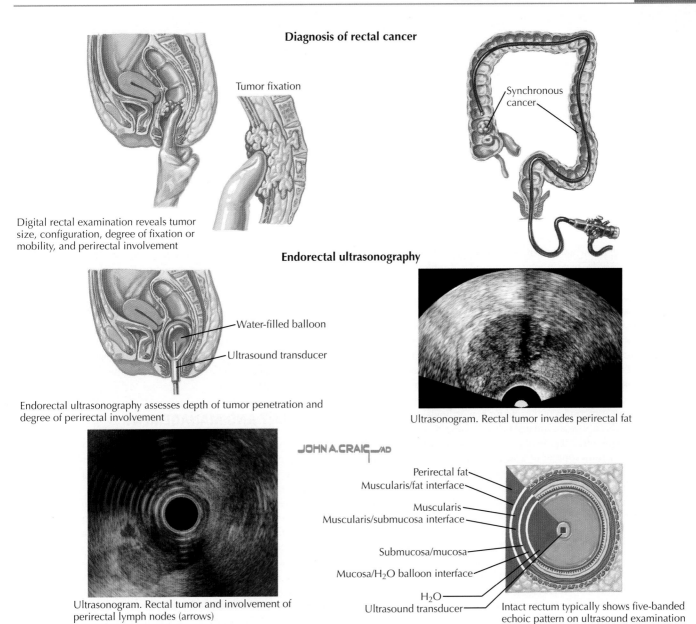

Tumor fixation

Digital rectal examination reveals tumor size, configuration, degree of fixation or mobility, and perirectal involvement

Synchronous cancer

Endorectal ultrasonography

Water-filled balloon

Ultrasound transducer

Endorectal ultrasonography assesses depth of tumor penetration and degree of perirectal involvement

Ultrasonogram. Rectal tumor invades perirectal fat

JOHN A. CRAIG—AD

Ultrasonogram. Rectal tumor and involvement of perirectal lymph nodes (arrows)

Perirectal fat
Muscularis/fat interface
Muscularis
Muscularis/submucosa interface
Submucosa/mucosa
Mucosa/H_2O balloon interface
H_2O
Ultrasound transducer

Intact rectum typically shows five-banded echoic pattern on ultrasound examination

Fig. 101.1 Rectal Cancer.

ADDITIONAL RESOURCES

Bresalier RS: Colorectal cancer. In Feldman M, Friedman LS, Brandt LJ, editors: *Gastrointestinal and liver disease*, ed 10, Philadelphia, 2016, Saunders-Elsevier, pp 2248–2296.

Daniels IR, Fisher SE, Heald RJ, Moran BJ: Accurate staging, selective preoperative therapy and optimal surgery improves outcome in rectal cancer: a review of the recent evidence, *Colorectal Dis* 9:290–301, 2007.

Levine MS, Rubesin SE: Plain and contract radiology. In Podolsky DK, Camilleri M, Fitz JG, et al, editors: *Yamada's textbook of gastroenterology*, ed 6, Hoboken, New Jersey, 2016, John Wiley and Sons Ltd, pp 2721–2742.

Luther J, Chan AT: Malignant tumors of the colon. In Podolsky DK, Camilleri M, Fitz JG, et al, editors: *Yamada's textbook of gastroenterology*, ed 6, Hoboken, New Jersey, 2016, John Wiley and Sons Ltd, pp 1554–1582.

102

Hemorrhoids

Martin H. Floch

Hemorrhoids are varicose dilatations of the radicals of the superior or inferior plexus of the hemorrhoidal veins. Varicosities are accompanied, in varying degrees, by hypertrophy and round cell infiltration of the perivascular connective tissue. Approximately 50% of the population is affected. Hemorrhoids usually develop in persons between 25 and 55 years of age, and they seldom develop in children.

Factors in hemorrhoid formation include (1) genetic predisposition, (2) absence of valves in the portal venous system attributed to the erect human posture, and (3) conditions that cause transient or constant increased pressure or stasis within the rectal venous plexuses, such as straining from constipation, frequency of bowel movements from diarrhea, rectal tumors or strictures, pregnancy, and pelvic tumors that increase pressure. Varicosities of the inferior hemorrhoidal plexus cause *external hemorrhoids* that are situated below the pectinate line and are covered by the modified skin of the anus. Formation of a thrombus within a vein, or from rupture of a vein with extravasation of blood into the cellular tissue, causes a thrombotic external hemorrhoid, which is an acute variety of the external type. This usually results from straining and appears as a sudden, painful lump that can be seen as a round, bluish, tender swelling (Fig. 102.1). When these resolve, they remain as skin tags.

Internal hemorrhoids are enlargements of the veins of the superior hemorrhoidal plexus. In early stages, they do not protrude through the anal ring, and they are seen only on endoscopic evaluation. In later stages, they may protrude through the anal canal, and if they protrude through the anal ring and persist, they can become ulcerated.

CLINICAL PICTURE

The clinical picture of a thrombosed external hemorrhoid is one of a painful, tender mass. Its onset is usually sudden. However, most hemorrhoids manifest as simple rectal bleeding, with blood seen on the toilet tissue or in the toilet bowl. At times, the bleeding might be brisk enough to result in bright-red blood in the toilet bowl. It is rarely severe enough to cause anemia. Internal hemorrhoids are usually reducible, but when they cannot be reduced, they may become strangulated, and vessels may become thrombosed, resulting in a very tender, painful presentation.

DIAGNOSIS

Simple external thrombosed hemorrhoids can be readily observed on inspection. Often, the anal ring is too tender to permit full rectal examination, but when full examination is possible, no lesions are felt inside the anal ring. Inspection and digital examination are essential in all evaluations of external hemorrhoids. If anemia or significant bleeding develops, endoscopic examination is essential. Proctologic or sigmoidoscopic examination is required when internal hemorrhoids are suspected: these are visualized in the rectal vault.

Hemorrhoids are graded from 1 to 4 depending on severity. When hemorrhoids are recurrent and prolonged, a full diagnostic evaluation is warranted. Complete blood count should be performed to check for anemia, with full colonic examination to rule out any associated malignancy. Computed tomography of the pelvis may also be important if an associated tumor may be causing intraabdominal pressure and formation of the hemorrhoid.

TREATMENT AND MANAGEMENT

Depending on the symptoms, initial treatment is invariably medical for grades 1 and 2 hemorrhoids. A tender, severe, thrombosed hemorrhoid that is not reduced within 24 to 48 hours might require lancing for relief of the pain. Medical therapy usually includes stool softeners, increased dietary fiber to soften stools, sitz baths with or without salts in warm water, astringents such as witch hazel, and topical analgesics. If patients cannot change their diet, supplements such as psyllium seed are encouraged.

Many clinicians add hydrocortisone suppositories or creams or mesalamine suppositories to reduce the inflammatory reaction surrounding the internal or external hemorrhoids. These are effective but need to be used for at least 1 to 2 weeks. Temporary relief of pain from external hemorrhoids can be obtained by using sprays (e.g., benzocaine 20%) or ointments (e.g., dibucaine 1%).

When conservative medical therapy fails, surgery is usually necessary. Surgical procedures include rubber band ligation, injection sclerotherapy, cryosurgery, electrocoagulation, photocoagulation, and hemorrhoidectomy. Meta-analysis of controlled, randomized trials reveals that rubber band ligation is superior to sclerotherapy, and that patients undergoing ligation are unlikely to require therapy later. Furthermore, although it results in better responses than rubber band ligation, hemorrhoidectomy also causes more pain and complications. Most clinicians and proctologists recommend rubber band ligation as first-line surgical treatment.

COURSE AND PROGNOSIS

Most hemorrhoids resolve with medical therapy, but many patients require surgery. After surgery, the acute situation is under control, but some patients may have mild, recurrent bleeding that is usually controlled by medical therapy. Occasionally, repeat surgery is needed.

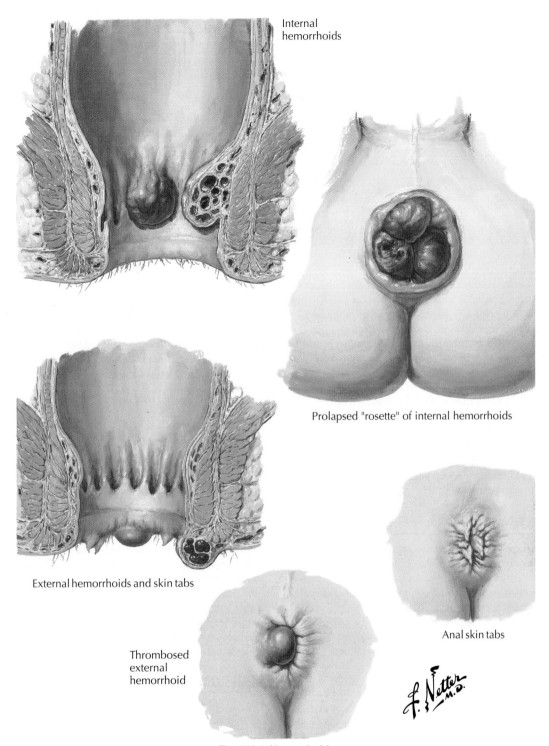

Internal hemorrhoids

Prolapsed "rosette" of internal hemorrhoids

External hemorrhoids and skin tabs

Thrombosed external hemorrhoid

Anal skin tabs

Fig. 102.1 Hemorrhoids.

ADDITIONAL RESOURCES

Abdelnaby A, Downs MJ: Diseases of the anorectum. In Feldman M, Friedman LS, Brandt LJ, editors: *Gastrointestinal and liver disease*, ed 10, Philadelphia, 2016, Saunders-Elsevier, pp 2316–2336.

Beck DE, Roberts PL, Saclarides TJ, et al, editors: *The ASCRS textbook of colon and rectal surgery*, 2nd ed, New York, 2011, Springer.

Chand M, Nash GF, Dabbas N: The management of haemorrhoids, *Br J Hosp Med* 69:35–40, 2008.

Rivadeneira DE, Chalasani S, Rafferty JL, et al: Practice parameters for the management of hemorrhoids (revised 2010), *Dis Colon Rectum* 54:1059–1064, 2011.

103

Rectal Prolapse and Procidentia

Martin H. Floch

Prolapse of the rectum is a condition in which one or more layers of the rectum or anal canal protrudes through the anal orifice (Fig. 103.1). It can be partial or complete. *Partial prolapse* involves only the mucosa, which usually extends no more than $\frac{1}{2}$ to 1 inch (2.5 cm) outside the anal canal. *Procidentia* is total prolapse, involving all the layers of the rectum. The mass is larger and bulbous, and it may eventually contain a hernial sac of peritoneum with a segment of bowel in the interior. Rectal prolapse is uncommon in children, but it may occur during infancy. Although usually idiopathic, it may be associated with congenital defects. Prolapse occurs with defecation, usually reduces spontaneously with conservative treatment, and is self-limited.

Rectal prolapse in adults occurs more often in women than in men. It is associated with poor pelvic musculature tone, chronic straining, fecal incontinence, and often neurologic or traumatic damage associated with the pelvis. Its etiology remains unknown, but a defect in the supporting structures may permit increased intraabdominal pressure to produce the prolapse. In elderly or debilitated persons, prolapse is usually caused by a loss of sphincteric tone.

CLINICAL PICTURE

Patients usually seek treatment for rectal staining or incontinence. Careful history reveals they can feel there is prolapse of tissue with defecation. Degree of prolapse varies by patient. When it is significant, it is troublesome. Prolapse is often associated with straining and with a sensation of incomplete evacuation and of the mass.

Complete rectal prolapse (procidentia) is large, and patients seek treatment fearing that the mass they can sense is malignant. The mass can cause pain and bleeding.

DIAGNOSIS

Examination with the patient in the left lateral position and straining slightly often reveals the prolapse and a weak anal sphincter. At times, the diagnosis cannot be made in this position, and the patient must be placed in the upright position, or sitting, so that straining will produce the prolapse. A detailed workup is needed to rule out malignancy and should include colonoscopic examination and computed tomography of the pelvis to ensure that no perirectal lesion increases intraabdominal pressure on the rectum.

Procidentia necessitates digital rectal examination, and an attempt should be made to reduce the mass. It may be tender, and the patient may need sedation to undergo the examination. For these patients, a colorectal surgeon should be involved in evaluating the procidentia.

TREATMENT AND MANAGEMENT

Very small prolapses can be handled medically by making sure that straining is reduced to a minimum. If the prolapse is significant and recurrent, it must be removed surgically.

Numerous surgical procedures are available for rectal prolapse. Some are simple and others are complex, involving a combined procedure in which the rectum is fixed to the sacral hollow and the redundant sigmoid colon is removed. The type of procedure and the outcome vary and depend on the degree of the prolapse and the experience of the colorectal surgeon.

In very elderly patients, simple extraabdominal approaches through perineal rectosigmoidectomy are possible. Some studies of these approaches in this select patient group have shown great success.

COURSE AND PROGNOSIS

Many persons live with a small degree of prolapse and are able to control their bowel movements. When incontinence becomes a problem, or when the prolapse is complete, various surgical interventions are possible. Studies report 80% good to excellent results with no mortality. A 90% success rate is reported in very elderly patients who require an extraabdominal approach. If the patient has uncontrolled prolapse and colostomy is necessary, prognosis depends on the debilitating disease, but colostomy is usually successful.

ADDITIONAL RESOURCES

Bharucha AE, Wald A: Anorectal diseases. In Podolsky DK, Camilleri M, Fitz JG, et al, editors: *Yamada's textbook of gastroenterology*, ed 6, Hoboken, New Jersey, 2016, John Wiley and Sons Ltd, pp 1629–1652.

Gourgiotis S: Baratsis s: rectal prolapse, *Int J Colorectal Dis* 22:231–243, 2007.

Lembo AJ: Constipation. In Feldman M, Friedman LS, Brandt LJ, editors: *Gastrointestinal and liver disease*, ed 10, Philadelphia, 2016, Saunders-Elsevier, pp 270–296.

Madiba TE, Baig MK, Wexner SD: Surgical management of rectal prolapse, *Arch Surg* 140:63–73, 2005.

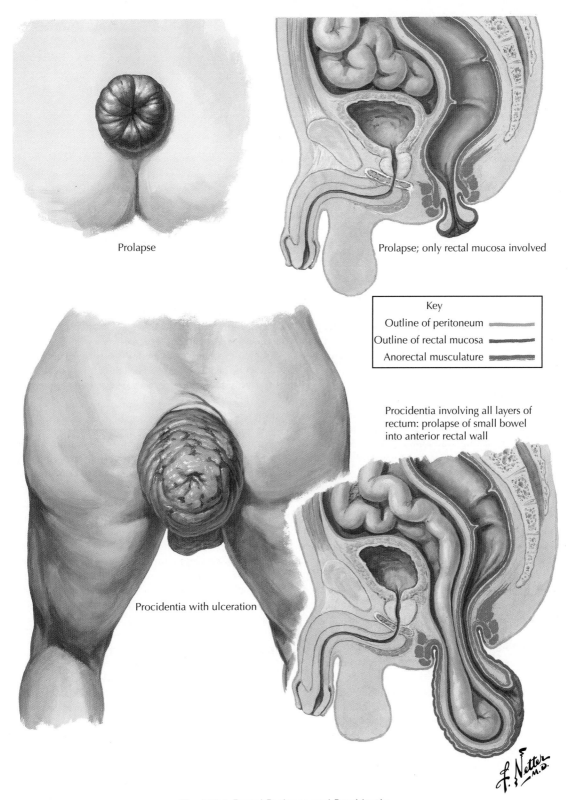

Prolapse

Prolapse; only rectal mucosa involved

Key		
Outline of peritoneum		
Outline of rectal mucosa		
Anorectal musculature		

Procidentia involving all layers of rectum: prolapse of small bowel into anterior rectal wall

Procidentia with ulceration

Fig. 103.1 Rectal Prolapse and Procidentia.

104

Anal Fissure, Pruritus Ani, Papillitis, and Cryptitis

Martin H. Floch

ANAL FISSURE

Anal fissure is a tear of the skin in the distal anal canal, usually in the posterior midline (Fig. 104.1). Occasionally, it is in the anterior midline. When not in the midline, anal fissure is often associated with an abnormality such as Crohn disease, human immunodeficiency virus (HIV) infection, tuberculosis, syphilis, or anal malignancy. Fissures usually are acute but may become chronic. The cause of an anal fissure typically is unknown, but it is clearly associated with increased resting anal pressure. Identifying this physiology has led to some of the most recent treatments. The exact incidence is not known, but anal fissure is relatively common.

Clinical Picture

The classic presentation of anal fissure is acute, severe pain on defecation that may persist for hours after passage of the fecal bolus. Bleeding may be associated with the fissure, with blood on the toilet paper or in the bowl. However, the pain is significant and is the hallmark of the clinical presentation.

Diagnosis

The diagnosis of anal fissure is best made by spreading apart the patient's buttocks with gloved fingers. Digital rectal examination is extremely painful and should be avoided. If the fissure is seen and is in the midline, it is not secondary to other diseases, and treatment can be used as a therapeutic trial. At times, a sentinel skin tag lies distal to the fissure. Endoscopy should be deferred until the patient is asymptomatic. If there is any uncertainty about the diagnosis, sedation and anesthesia may be necessary to enable appropriate examination of the patient.

Treatment and Management

Many options exist for treating anal fissure. The therapy chosen often depends on the experience of local physicians. Medical therapy should be tried first, including a course of sitz baths, psyllium fiber supplements to soften the stool, or emollient suppositories. Treatment may be successful in 27% to 44% of patients. Some clinicians have used sitz baths plus bran supplementation, at least 15 g daily, which has also been successful. Use of 2% lidocaine ointment plus 2% hydrocortisone cream has proved to be successful in approximately 60% of patients.

When simple medical therapy does not succeed, other options include topical therapy. Topical nitrates (0.2% glyceryl trinitrate) and calcium channel blockers have proved effective, with more data on the nitrates. Healing has been reported in as many as 77% of patients with the use of four suppositories for 8 weeks. These agents significantly lower anal sphincter pressure.

Botulin toxin (Botox) has yielded excellent results and healing rates of 82% and 79% at 3 and 6 months, respectively. Other studies have resulted in slightly lower percentages, and recurrence has been reported with botulin toxin.

If medical therapy for anal fissure does not succeed, surgery is warranted. Most patients heal after lateral internal sphincterotomy. Some may experience incontinence, although the rate of this surgical complication is extremely low.

Course and Prognosis

As indicated, outcomes are excellent for most patients with anal fissure, and cure rates range from 50% to 70% after medical therapy and 70% to 90% after surgical therapy. Some fecal incontinence may occur after surgical treatment, but recurrence is low.

Simple posterior or anterior fissure is benign, but clinicians should always be on guard that perianal disease may be the first manifestation of Crohn disease or a venereal disease (see Chapter 106).

PRURITUS ANI

Pruritus ani is a symptom that may accompany any anorectal disease, but frequently no evidence of primary disease is found. Perianal itching without any apparent cause is thought to be neurodermatitis. When a cause is identified, it should be treated. Causes of pruritus ani include parasitic infections, local irritants (e.g., food allergies), and dermatologic conditions (e.g., psoriasis, atopic dermatitis, moisture collecting in obese person).

Treatment for pruritus ani is whichever therapy is necessary for the primary disease and symptoms. For troublesome pruritus, the patient should discontinue irritating soap and use hypoallergenic soap instead, apply a hydrocortisone cream regularly, keep the anal area clean, and use a protective ointment such as zinc oxide. Severe chronic pruritus can be treated.

PAPILLITIS AND CRYPTITIS

Inflammatory processes of the papillae usually start in one of the crypts and cause pain disproportionate to the size and severity of the lesion. In acute *papillitis*, the area is swollen, edematous, and congested. In the chronic stage of papillitis, the area becomes fibrosed and hypertrophied. Gradually, the hypertrophic papillae may develop a stalk and then change to a so-called fibrous polyp, which may produce the sensation of a foreign body in the anal canal.

Cryptitis may remain restricted to circumscribed reactions in and around the crypts, or it may spread to the surrounding tissues, including the formation of abscesses and fistulae (see Chapter 105). Symptoms of cryptitis occasionally resemble those of a fissure and often include itching and radiation of pain, which is aggravated by defecation. Visualization of the cryptitis and any purulent discharge or granulation of tissue, or of the hypertrophied papillae, is necessary. Treatment is usually successful with medical regimens to decrease local irritation by using hydrocortisone or mesalamine suppositories, softening the stool through psyllium or bran intake, and using relaxing agents, if necessary.

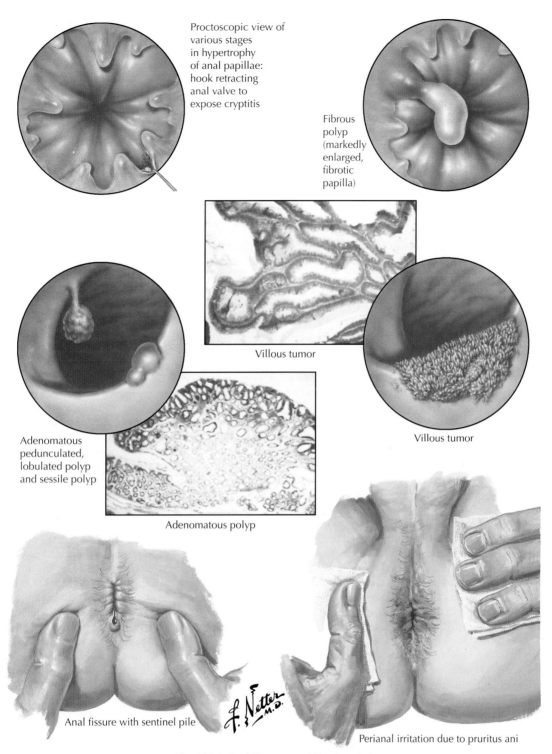

Proctoscopic view of various stages in hypertrophy of anal papillae: hook retracting anal valve to expose cryptitis

Fibrous polyp (markedly enlarged, fibrotic papilla)

Villous tumor

Villous tumor

Adenomatous pedunculated, lobulated polyp and sessile polyp

Adenomatous polyp

Anal fissure with sentinel pile

Perianal irritation due to pruritus ani

Fig. 104.1 Anal Fissure and Pruritus Ani.

ADDITIONAL RESOURCES

Abdelnaby A, Downs MJ: Diseases of the anorectum. In Feldman M, Friedman LS, Brandt LJ, editors: *Gastrointestinal and liver disease*, ed 10, Philadelphia, 2016, Saunders-Elsevier, pp 2316–2336.

Bharucha AE, Wald A: Anorectal diseases. In Podolsky DK, Camilleri M, Fitz JG, et al, editors: *Yamada's textbook of gastroenterology*, ed 6, Hoboken, New Jersey, 2016, John Wiley and Sons Ltd, pp 1629–1652.

Brisinda G, Cadeddu F, Brandara F, et al: Randomized clinical trial comparing botulinum toxin injections with 0.2% nitroglycerin ointment for chronic anal fissure, *Br J Surg* 94:162–167, 2007.

Freuhauf H, Fried M, Wegmueller B, et al: Efficacy and safety of botulinum toxin A injection compared with topical nitroglycerine ointment for the treatment of chronic anal fissure: a prospective randomized study, *Am J Gastroenterol* 101:2107–2112, 2005.

Savides TJ, Jensen DM: Gastrointestinal bleeding. In Feldman M, Friedman LS, Brandt LJ, editors: *Gastrointestinal and liver disease*, ed 10, Philadelphia, 2016, Saunders-Elsevier, pp 297–348.

105

Anorectal Abscess and Fistula

Martin H. Floch

Localized infection with a collection of pus in the anorectal area is designated an *anorectal abscess.* Usually, it results from the invasion of the normal rectal flora into the perirectal or perianal tissues. The pathologic process seems to start with inflammation of one or more of the crypts (see Chapter 104), spreads to the anal ducts and anal glands, and then spreads submucosally, subcutaneously, or transsphincterally to the surrounding tissue. This sequence of events closes with the spontaneous rupture of the abscess, either into the anorectal canal or through the perianal skin, if the abscess has not been drained surgically. After the abscess has perforated, the cavity and its outlet shrink, leaving a tubelike structure, an *anorectal fistula,* which invariably is the result of the abscess. Therefore, the abscess is the acute phase, and the fistula is the chronic phase.

The *levator ani plane,* demarcating the various perineal pelvic spaces, is used to classify anorectal abscesses according to localization. Retrorectal, pelvirectal, and submucosal abscesses belong to the *supralevator* abscesses and have a somatic sensory nerve supply; therefore, these cause a sensation of discomfort from pressure rather than from pain in the anorectal region. *Infralevator* abscesses may produce signs of toxemia and prostration. *Retrorectal* and *pelvirectal* abscesses originate from infectious processes in other pelvic organs and thus are not anorectal lesions in the strict sense, although they usually rupture into the rectum or the anal canal. Infralevator abscesses are also divided according to site into subcutaneous, intramuscular, fistulorectal, and cutaneous abscesses. The fistula is called *complete* when both openings, the primary and the secondary, can be detected and are accessible. Such a complete variety usually connects the rectal lumen with the anal or perianal skin. If there is only one opening, it is called a *blind* fistula or a sinus.

Fig. 105.1 depicts the various types of fistulas (or fistulae) and the *Goodsall-Salmon law,* in which an imaginary transverse line across the center of the anus can be used to predict the location of the tract and the primary opening.

Anorectal abscess and fistula are associated with specific diseases, such as Crohn disease, malignancy, radiation proctitis, leukemia, lymphoma, tuberculosis, actinomycosis, and lymphogranuloma venereum. Other diseases may cause a similar picture, such as diverticulitis and Bartholin abscesses.

CLINICAL PICTURE

Swelling in the perianal area accompanied by acute pain are the most common symptoms. The patient reports that a change in sitting position, moving, or a bowel movement makes the pain worse. Onset is usually slower than in fistula formation, and the patient may experience fever and fatigue. Discharge from the abscess may occur. Chronic purulent discharge is a major problem. Depending on the site and the amount of drainage, the abscess may be minor or large, and the perianal area may be excoriated.

DIAGNOSIS

Endosonography and magnetic resonance imaging (MRI) can be extremely helpful in delineating the extent of the abscess and the fistulous tracts.

TREATMENT

Healthy persons with small, superficial abscesses can undergo outpatient drainage under local anesthesia. Past treatments used setons, but this form of therapy alone is now used less often and is combined with other therapy, such as infliximab. For large abscesses or those in patients with underlying disease, surgery is necessary. Standard surgical treatment is usually performed on an emergency basis. Mortality is as high as 50% if surgery is delayed and a necrotizing anorectal infection develops.

Although antibiotics may not be necessary for small lesions, most clinicians believe antibiotics are important, especially if the patient has an underlying associated disease. Antibiotic therapy must treat the aerobic and the anaerobic flora and therefore is usually a combination of drugs.

Postoperative management consists of routine surgical management and may include warm baths, prevention of any constipation, and appropriate nutrition. Novel therapies have been developed to close fistulae. Fibrin glue has been reported to be successful in up to 69% of patients. This therapy has worked after initial failures with other therapies.

Finally, special consideration must be given to patients with Crohn disease. The primary disease must be treated, which may include 5-acetylsalicylic acid (5-ASA) products, immunosuppressive agents, or biologicals and antibiotic therapy. Infliximab (antitumor necrosis factor-α) has been used successfully. Attempts at healing fistulae in patients with Crohn disease through bowel rest or enteral feedings have shown some success, but the fistulae tend to return when regular foods are added. Newer studies indicate a relationship between genetic variants of *NOD2/CARD15* and antibiotic response.

COURSE AND PROGNOSIS

Surprisingly, MRI has been shown to predict clinical outcome based on the initial severity of the fistulous tracts. As indicated, if there is delay in treatment, mortality may increase to as much as 50%. If treatment is introduced early in a relatively healthy patient, the prognosis is good. However, if there is associated significant morbidity, such as severe diabetes or autoimmune disease, the fistula and the abscess can constitute significant comorbidity, leading to death. Therefore aggressive therapy is indicated in these patients.

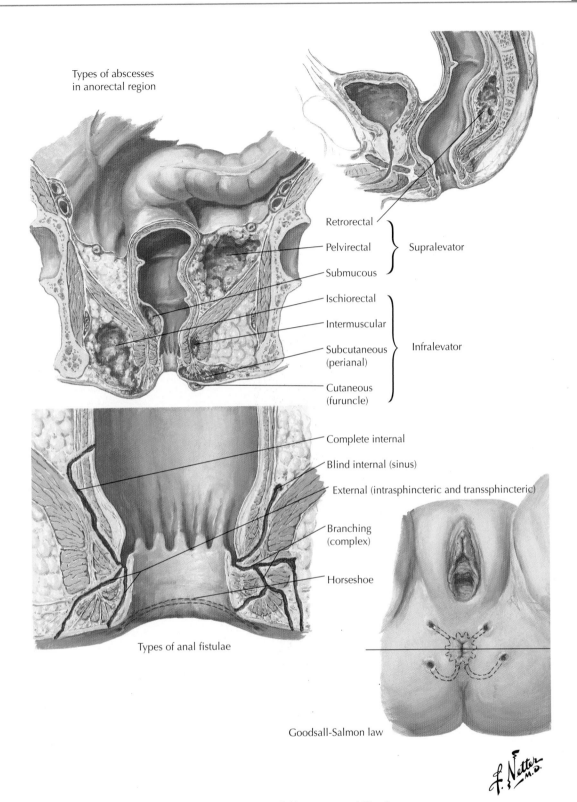

Types of abscesses
in anorectal region

Retrorectal ⎫
Pelvirectal ⎬ Supralevator
Submucous ⎭

Ischiorectal ⎫
Intermuscular │
Subcutaneous ⎬ Infralevator
(perianal) │
Cutaneous ⎭
(furuncle)

Complete internal

Blind internal (sinus)

External (intrasphincteric and transsphincteric)

Branching
(complex)

Horseshoe

Types of anal fistulae

Goodsall-Salmon law

Fig. 105.1 Anorectal Abscesses and Fistulae.

ADDITIONAL RESOURCES

Abdelnaby A, Downs MJ: Diseases of the anorectum. In Feldman M, Friedman LS, Brandt LJ, editors: *Gastrointestinal and liver disease*, ed 10, Philadelphia, 2016, Saunders-Elsevier, pp 2316–2336.

Angelberger S, Reinisch W, Dejaco C, et al: *NOD2/CARD15* gene variants are linked to failure of antibiotic treatment in perianal fistulating Crohn's disease, *Am J Gastroenterol* 103:1197–1202, 2008.

Bharucha AE, Wald A: Anorectal diseases. In Podolsky DK, Camilleri M, Fitz JG, et al, editors: *Yamada's textbook of gastroenterology*, ed 6, Hoboken, New Jersey, 2016, John Wiley and Sons Ltd, pp 1629–1652.

Hyder SA, Travis SP, Jewell DP, et al: Fistulizing anal Crohn's disease: results of combined surgical and infliximab treatment, *Dis Colon Rectum* 49:1837–1841, 2006.

Sandborn WT, Fazio VW, Feagan BG, Hanauer SB: AGA technical review on perianal Crohn's disease, *Gastroenterology* 125:1508–1530, 2003.

Schwartz DA, Herdman CR: The medical treatment of Crohn's perianal fistulas (review), *Aliment Pharmacol Ther* 19:953–967, 2004.

Schwartz DA, White CM, Wise PE, Herline AJ: Use of endoscopic ultrasound to guide combination medical and surgical therapy for patients with Crohn's perianal fistulas, *Inflamm Bowel Dis* 11:727–732, 2005.

106

Lymphogranuloma Venereum and Sexually Transmitted Proctitis

Martin H. Floch

Lymphogranuloma venereum (LGV) and sexually transmitted proctitis are relatively uncommon in the general population, occurring more often in male homosexuals and promiscuous heterosexuals. Certain infections are typically seen when proctitis is identified in a patient with a history of promiscuous sexual activity (Table 106.1). LGV is rare but leads to a pathologic condition that can be confused with other granulomatous diseases (Fig. 106.1). Because of social reasons, there has been a great variation in the incidence of LGV. While incidences decreased for a while, it has now recurred (see "Additional Resources").

LYMPHOGRANULOMA VENEREUM

The organism that causes LGV is *Chlamydia trachomatis*. Worldwide, *C. trachomatis* accounts for approximately 50 million new infections of LGV each year. It is the leading bacterial cause of sexually transmitted disease (STD) in the United States. *C. trachomatis* is divided into three biovars based partly on host susceptibility and DNA homology. The trichoma biovar and the LGV biovar cause human infections, whereas the third biovar does not. The trichoma biovar multiplies in columnar epithelial cells, and the LGV strains also are capable of multiplying in macrophages. The biovars have been subdivided into 15 serovars, which appear to cause specific infections. Anorectal LGV infections occur in homosexual men and heterosexual women engaging in anal intercourse. Infection also may be spread by infected vaginal secretions in women or through lymphatic spread from genital infection.

Clinical Picture

The clinical picture for patients with LGV can vary greatly, from absence of symptoms to severe granulomatous disease (see Fig. 106.1). Variation occurs with the different serovars. If LGV leads to proctocolitis,

TABLE 106.1 Common Organisms Causing Sexually Transmitted Proctitis[a]

Organism	Common Symptoms and Signs	Investigations	Recommended First Line Treatment
Gonorrhoea	Commonly asymptomatic. Pruritus ani, constipation, mucopurulent anal discharge with or without bleeding, rectal pain, and tenesmus.	Culture (gold standard) NAAT (not validated, always confirm with culture)	Cefixime 400 mg stat or ceftriaxone 250 IM or spectinomycin 2 g IM
Chlamydia (non-LGV serovars)	Commonly asymptomatic. Pruritus ani, mucoid discharge, perianal pain.	NAAT (not validated)	Azithromycin 1 g stat or doxycycline 100 mg bd for 1 week
LGV	Systemic symptoms (fever and malaise). Purulent, often bloodstained anal discharge. Severe pain, tenesmus, constipation. Symptoms and signs may be mistaken for those of inflammatory bowel disease.	NAAT as for chlamydia—refer to reference lab if positive for typing	Doxycycline 100 mg bd for 3 weeks
Syphilis	Primary syphilis—anorectal chancres commonly asymptomatic, may be associated with pain or discomfort, itching, bleeding, discharge, and tenesmus. Secondary syphilis—snail track ulcers and mucous patches. Perianal condylomata lata. Generalized rash, fever, and lymphadenopathy may be present.	Dark ground microcopy if ulcer present. Serological tests: RPR/VDRL > 70% sensitive in primary syphilis, 100% sensitive in secondary syphilis EIA/TPPA/TPHA > 70% sensitive in primary syphilis, 100% in secondary syphilis. Stay positive after treatment and in latent infection	Procaine penicillin IM 750 mg daily for 10 days or benzathine penicillin 2.4 g IM stat or doxycycline 100 mg bd for 14 days. Advice should be sought if the patient is HIV infected as treatment regimens may vary.
Herpes simplex virus	Vesicular lesions, severe pain, difficulty in passing a bowel motion, tenesmus, discharge, viraemic symptoms such as fever and lymphadenopathy.	Viral culture or PCR	Acyclovir 200 mg 5 × daily for 5 days

[a]It should be noted that more than one infection may be present.
bd, Twice daily; *EIA*, enzyme immunoassay; *HSV*, herpes simplex virus; *IM*, intramuscular; *LGV*, lymphogranuloma venereum; *NAAT*, nucleic acid amplification testing; *PCR*, polymerase chain reaction; *RPR*, rapid plasma reagin test; *STI*, sexually transmitted infections; *TPPA*, *Treponema pallidum* particle agglutination; *TPHA*, *Treponema pallidum* haemagglutination assay; *VDRL*, Venereal Disease Research Laboratories.
Hamlyn E, Taylor C. Sexually transmitted proctitis. *Postgraduate Medical Journal*. 2006;82(973):733-736.

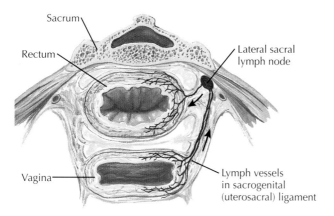

Pathway of spread of lymphogranuloma
(lymphopathia) venereum from upper vagina
and/or cervix uteri to rectum via lymph vessels

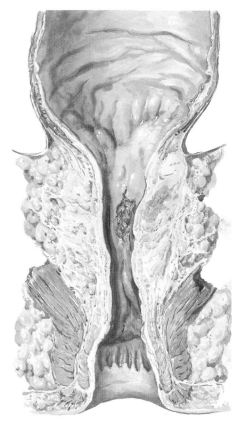

Long tubular stricture of rectum

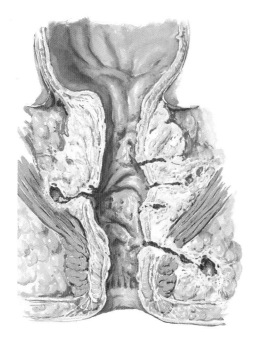

Stricture of rectum
with multiple
blind sinuses

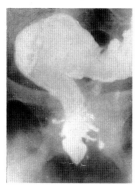

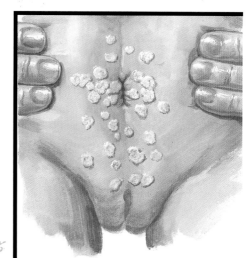

Condylomata lata (2° syphilis)

Fig. 106.1 Lymphogranuloma Venereum.

patients may have severe itching, discharge, diarrhea or constipation, rectal bleeding, fever, lymphadenopathy, and lower abdominal pain. If left untreated, LGV may progress to perirectal abscess with fibrosis stricture, stenosis, and Crohn disease presentation. At times, obstruction of the lymphatic system can cause marked hemorrhoids or perianal condylomata.

Diagnosis

In any patient with suspected sexually transmitted proctitis, the differential diagnosis should include all possible conditions. Certainly, in any patient with Crohn disease with an appropriate history, LGV should be suspected. Diagnosis is made by culture of the rectal exudate and identification of infected cells with a fluorescein-labeled monoclonal antibody to chlamydial antigens.

A fourfold increase in the titer in acute and convalescent sera has been used as supportive evidence of infection. However, positive serology alone does not make the diagnosis of LGV because a high percentage of adults have antibodies to *C. trachomatis*. Therefore, a single serum sample is usually of little diagnostic value.

Treatment and Management

Treatment is effective with tetracycline, doxycycline, and erythromycin. Resistant *C. trachomatis* strains have been reported. However, current treatment of non-LGV biovars is 100 mg of doxycycline twice daily for 7 to 10 days. A single 1-g dose of azithromycin appears to be as effective as a 7-day course of doxycycline for genital infections and uncomplicated rectal infections. Some recommend a 21-day course of doxycycline. If a patient has full-blown rectal disease with strictures, long-term antibiotic therapy plus surgery may be necessary.

SEXUALLY TRANSMITTED PROCTITIS

Table 106.1 describes the organisms that can cause sexually transmitted proctitis. Furthermore, in the patient with human immunodeficiency virus (HIV), a wide range of organisms may be involved in producing the same symptoms. The diagnosis must be made by identifying the causative organism. Treatment is then specific for the organism (see Section VI). Although antibiotics may cause acute and fulminating colitis, most cases are usually self-limiting. *C. trachomatis* infection can be confused with Crohn granulomatous disease, and treatment and prognosis vary with each. Also, antibiosis can mimic fulminant colitis, and the other infections can cause persistent and recurrent proctitis.

ADDITIONAL RESOURCES

Cohen MB: Bacterial, viral, and toxic causes of diarrhea, gastroenteritis, and anorectal infections. In Podolsky DK, Camilleri M, Fitz JG, et al, editors: *Yamada's textbook of gastroenterology*, ed 6, Hoboken, New Jersey, 2016, John Wiley and Sons Ltd, pp 1196–1248.

Collins L, White JA: Lymphogranuloma venereum, *BMJ* 332:66, 2006.

Dal Conte L, Mistrangelo M, Cariti C, et al: Lymphogranuloma venereum: an old, forgotten re-emerging systemic disease, *Panminerva Med* 56:73–83, 2014.

Isaksson J, Carlsson O, Airell A, et al: Lymphogranuloma venereum rates increased and chlamydia trachomatis genotypes changed among men who have sex with men in Sweden 2004-2016, *J Med Microbiol* 66:1684–1687, 2017.

Montgomery EA, Kalloo AN: Endoscopic mucosal biopsy—histopathological interpretation. In Podolsky DK, Camilleri M, Fitz JG, et al, editors: *Yamada's textbook of gastroenterology*, ed 6, Hoboken, New Jersey, 2016, John Wiley and Sons Ltd, pp 2980–3051.

Parra-Sanchez M, Garcia-Rey S, Pueyo Rodriguez I, et al: Clinical and epidemiological characterisation of lymphogranuloma venereum in southwest Spain, 2013-2015, *Sex Transm Infect* 92: 629–631, 2016.

Stamm WE, Jones RB, Batteiger BE: *Chlamydia trachomatis* (trachoma, perinatal infections, lymphogranuloma venereum, and other genital infections). In Mandel GL, Bennett JE, Dolin R, editors: *Mandel, Douglas, and Bennett's principles and practice of infectious diseases*, ed 6, Philadelphia, 2005, Churchill Livingstone–Elsevier, pp 2239–2256.

van Hal SJ, Hillman R, Stark DJ, et al: Lymphogranuloma venereum: an emerging anorectal disease in Australia, *Med J Aust* 187:309–310, 2007.

107

Fecal Incontinence

Martin H. Floch

Fecal incontinence is the involuntary passage of fecal material. It may be a single occurrence, but when recurrent, incontinence can be devastating. Several surveys indicate that fecal incontinence may occur in 7% to 15% of the population. It is more frequent in women than in men. In acutely ill hospital patients, the rate of fecal incontinence is as high as 33% to 43%. It is the leading cause of admission of patients to nursing homes, where episodes of incontinence occur in approximately 20% of residents. Box 107.1 lists some of the many causes of fecal incontinence.

Incontinence associated with infectious diarrhea or a bout of irritable bowel syndrome is different from incontinence that results from traumatic injury of the anal sphincter or from neurologic disease in a nursing home patient. Normal continence depends on normal function of the internal anal sphincter and the external sphincter and puborectalis muscle, as well as normal neurologic innervation for rectal sensation and distention (see Chapter 84). When any of these functions is significantly disturbed, incontinence can occur.

CLINICAL PICTURE

The patient with fecal incontinence may seek treatment after having a large, uncontrolled, loose bowel movement or after regular fecal staining or recurrent episodes of significant incontinence, or the patient may be brought in by a family member and may be unaware of any rectal staining. It is important to be certain that the patient has fecal incontinence and not merely anal discharge of mucus or blood. Certainly, the latter infers an abnormality other than a true loss of stool.

DIAGNOSIS

The patient's history is essential to determine whether trauma to the rectum has occurred or whether the patient has a neurologic disorder. In addition, inspection and examination of the rectum are essential. The voluntary squeeze response on digital rectal examination can help to localize the problem to the internal or external sphincter. Voluntary contraction suggests an internal sphincter problem, with a disturbance in the autonomic nervous system or with smooth muscle function, as occurs in patients with diabetes or scleroderma. Striated muscle may be affected because of neuropathy or longstanding damage.

If the diagnosis is not obvious, as in traumatic injury, a combination of anal ultrasound and anal manometry can be helpful (see algorithm in Fig. 107.1). Both procedures are usually performed in special centers, but these are limited in number. Magnetic resonance imaging (MRI) is the best way to determine whether the integrity of the internal anal sphincter has been compromised. Although endosonography appears to be more accurate and costs less, MRI is available in many areas and may be the only modality that clearly defines the anatomy. Defecography may be used to evaluate the rectoanal angle but adds little to the treatment algorithm.

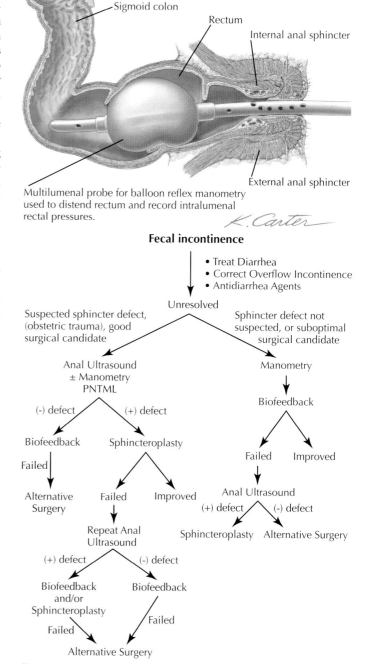

Multilumenal probe for balloon reflex manometry used to distend rectum and record intralumenal rectal pressures.

Fig. 107.1 Fecal Incontinence. *PNTML,* Pudental nerve terminal motor latency. (Algorithm from Soffer E: Practical approach to fecal incontinence, *Am J Gastroenterol* 95:1879, 2000.)

BOX 107.1 Causes of Fecal Incontinence

Normal Sphincters and Pelvic Floor
- Diarrhea
- Infection
- Inflammatory bowel disease
- Intestinal resection

Anatomic Derangements and Rectal Disease
- Congenital abnormalities of anorectum
- Fistula
- Rectal prolapse
- Anorectal trauma
- Injury
- Childbirth injury
- Surgery (including hemorrhoidectomy)
- Sequelae of anorectal infections, Crohn disease

Neurologic Diseases
Central Nervous System Disease
- Dementia, sedation, mental disease
- Stroke, brain tumors
- Spinal cord lesions
- Multiple sclerosis
- Tabes dorsalis

Peripheral Nervous System Disease
- Cauda equina lesions
- Polyneuropathies

- Diabetes mellitus
- Shy-Drager syndrome
- Toxic neuropathy
- Traumatic neuropathy
- Idiopathic incontinence
- Perineal descent
- Postpartum
- Altered rectal sensation (site of lesion unknown)
- Fecal impaction
- Delayed-sensation syndrome

Skeletal Muscle Diseases
- Myasthenia gravis
- Myopathies, muscular dystrophy

Smooth Muscle Dysfunction
Abnormal Rectal Compliance
- Proctitis caused by inflammatory bowel disease
- Radiation proctitis
- Rectal ischemia
- Fecal impaction

Internal Anal Sphincter Weakness
- Radiation proctitis
- Diabetes mellitus
- Childhood encopresis

Modified from Feldman M, Friedman LS, Schlesinger MH, editors: *Gastrointestinal and Liver Disease*, ed 7, Philadelphia, 2002, Saunders.

Anal manometry is important for both diagnosis and treatment and is very provider dependent (see Fig. 107.1). After documenting weakness or incompetence of the sphincters, biofeedback therapy can be used effectively to correct many causes of incontinence.

TREATMENT AND MANAGEMENT

Medical therapy includes appropriate bowel management. Uncontrollable diarrhea, overflow incontinence from impaction, and other obvious causes should be treated medically. Biofeedback should be tried if the situation indicates that it can help the patient's condition (see algorithm).

If the sphincter has been significantly damaged, surgical therapy and repair are indicated. Many techniques are available, and successful repair depends on the surgeon's skill and experience. Colostomy is a last resort but may be necessary when other therapies fail and it is determined that this would be best for the patient.

COURSE AND PROGNOSIS

As indicated by its cause, if incontinence occurs in an elderly patient or in a young patient with a neurologic disorder, outcome is poor, and appropriate hygiene is necessary. If incontinence is caused by sphincter damage, biofeedback mechanisms and surgical repair may correct the situation. However, biofeedback is labor intensive with variable success and requires skilled therapists or physicians.

ADDITIONAL RESOURCES

Bellicini N, Malloy PJ, Caushaj P, Koslowski P: Fecal incontinence: a review, *Dig Dis Sci* 53:41–46, 2008.

Bharucha AE, Seide BM, Zinsmeister AR, Melton LJ III: Relation of bowel habits to fecal incontinence in women, *Am J Gastroenterol* 103:1470–1475, 2008.

Bharucha AE, Wald A: Anorectal diseases. In Podolsky DK, Camilleri M, Fitz JG, et al, editors: *Yamada's textbook of gastroenterology*, ed 6, Hoboken, New Jersey, 2016, John Wiley and Sons Ltd, pp 1629–1652.

Brown SR, Wadhawan H, Nelson RL: Surgery for faecal incontinence in adults, *Cochrane Database Syst Rev* (7):CD001757, 2013. doi:10.1002/14651858.CD001757.

Hannaway CD, Hull TL: Fecal incontinence, *Obstet Gynecol Clin North Am* 35:249–269, 2008.

Heymen S, Scarlett Y, Jones K, et al: Randomized, controlled trial shows biofeedback to be superior to alternative treatments for patients with pelvic floor dyssynergia-type constipation, *Dis Colon Rect* 50:428–441, 2007.

Rao SS: Advances in diagnostic assessment of fecal incontinence and dyssynergic defecation, *Clin Gastroenterol Hepatol* 8:910–919, 2010.

Rao SSC: Fecal incontinence. In Feldman M, Friedman LS, Brandt LJ, editors: *Gastrointestinal and liver disease*, ed 10, Philadelphia, 2016, Saunders-Elsevier, pp 251–269.

Scott SM, Gladman MA: Manometric, sensorimotor, and neurophysiologic evaluation of anorectal function, *Gastroenterol Clin North Am* 37:511–538, 2008.

Wald A: Fecal incontinence in adults, *N Engl J Med* 356:1648–1655, 2007.

Infectious and Parasitic Diseases of the Alimentary Tract

C. S. Pitchumoni

108

Human Immunodeficiency Virus and Gastrointestinal Tract

C. S. Pitchumoni

Acquired immunodeficiency syndrome (AIDS) has been a devastating pandemic since the late 20th century, caused by the human immuno-deficiency virus (HIV). HIV-1 is the most prevalent type worldwide. HIV-2 is less prevalent and less pathogenic, found principally in western Africa. Globally, HIV continues to be a major public health problem. The availability of highly active antiretroviral therapy has reduced the number of complications and their severity, while prolonging life expectancy, but it is not yet a cure. Because of the prolongation of life, many chronic complications of the disease, such as coinfection with hepatitis B/C, are increased.

The mode of infection is variable depending on the geographic area. Blood, breast milk, semen, and vaginal secretions can transmit the disease. In the United States as well as other developed nations, the most frequent mode of transmission is having unprotected anal or vaginal sex with an infected individual. According to the Centers for Disease Control and Prevention (CDC), about 67% of people diagnosed with HIV in 2014 in the United States were gay and bisexual men. Globally speaking, other more common risks include sharing contaminated needles, blood transfusions, and medical procedures involving unsterile cutting or piercing and organ transplantation in unsafe environments.

The three stages of HIV infection are as follows. The first stage, Acute HIV, develops within 2 to 4 weeks of acquiring infection. The symptoms include fever, headache, rash, fatigue, swollen lymph nodes, malaise, and ulceration in the mouth, esophagus, or genitals. In the chronic stage (asymptomatic HIV), the virus continues to multiply at low levels, but the patient is infective. Without highly active retroviral therapy (HAART), chronic HIV infection progresses to AIDS in 10 or more years. With the evolution of the disease, HIV infection reduces the number of CD4 cells in the body (normal 500 to 1600 cell/mm³). When the number falls below 200 cells/mm³, the HIV infection has progressed to AIDS.

With the availability of HAART since 1996, the clinical spectrum has changed. HAART is composed of a combination of three to four drugs. The individual components of HAART are reverse transcriptase inhibitors, protease inhibitors, and fusion inhibitors. The components of HAART attack the viral life cycle at different points. However, the prohibitive cost of HAART has excluded a large number of patients in developing nations from the benefits. These patients still develop the classic complications of HIV disease of the pre-HAART era.

IHAART produces a logarithmic fall in the circulating HIV load with appreciable increases in CD4 lymphocyte counts. A notable reduction of many complications is associated with identification of a few new complications often related to HAART. Currently the life-span of an HIV patient is about the same as someone who does not have HIV disease. A clinician practicing in a major metropolitan city in the United States with a large number of immigrants is still likely to observe the spectrum of HIV manifestations of both the pre-HAART as well as the post-HAART era.

The terms HIV and AIDS are interchangeably used in the following discussion.

GASTROINTESTINAL MANIFESTATIONS OF HIV/AIDS

The symptoms of gastrointestinal involvement signify the progression of HIV infection to acquired immunodeficiency syndrome. The entire GI tract, including the liver, gallbladder, biliary tree, and the pancreas, are variably involved. Infectious esophagitis is discussed separately in the next chapter.

Table 108.1 summarizes the clinical manifestations of the organs involved and their etiological associations.

Stomach

The symptoms of gastric involvement are nonspecific. Nausea, vomiting, early satiety, and anorexia are predominant. The prevalence of *Helicobacter pylori* is probably lower. As a result of chronic gastritis, the secretion of gastric acid and intrinsic factor is reduced. Achlorhydria may

TABLE 108.1 Gastrointestinal Complications of HIV		
Location	**Pathology**	**Etiology**
Esophagus	Dysphagia Odynophagia (esophagitis)	Candida CMV Herpes simplex Varicella-Zoster Mycobacteria Histoplasma *Pneumocystis jirovecii* Idiopathic ulcerations
Stomach	Achlorhydria (gastritis)	*H. pylori* CMV Kaposi sarcoma
Liver	Hepatitis (acute/chronic)	Coinfections with hepatitis C Drug induced Peliosis hepatis
Biliary tree	Cholangiopathy	Acalculous cholecystitis (CMV, cryptosporidium, microsporidia) Cholangitis
Pancreas	Pancreatitis	Drug induced (didanosine, pentamidine)
Small intestine/ Large intestine	Acute and chronic diarrheal syndromes	*C. difficile* CMV Cryptosporidium Mycobacterium avium complex HIV enteropathy

contribute to malabsorption of iron, B12, and certain medications (e.g., the absorption of ketoconazole is markedly limited in achlorhydria). CMV gastritis and Kaposi sarcoma are other manifestations. The incidence of AIDS-related lymphoma has decreased with HAART.

Small and Large Bowel

Chronic diarrhea is a major manifestation of HIV disease. HIV associated diarrhea may be due to the involvement of the small bowel, large bowel, or both. A pure small bowel diarrhea is characterized by large volume, watery stool and quite debilitating. Profound malnutrition and malabsorption may occur. Diarrhea due to the involvement of the large intestine is associated with frequent small volume stools not enough to cause dehydration. Colonic causes of diarrhea may be associated with hematochezia. Tenesmus is a feature if the rectum is involved. Although steatorrhea is an underdiagnosed entity encountered with HIV disease, it can be detected with fecal fat estimation testing. The incidence of enterocolitis has decreased considerably with the advent of HAART.

Chronic diarrhea may be caused by an infection from a bacterial, viral, or protozoal pathogen. The frequently encountered bacterial pathogens are *Salmonella* spp, *shigella*, *Campylobacter jejuni*, *Escherichia coli*, and *Listeria monocytogenes*. *Clostridium difficile* is another cause of bacterial diarrhea. Other causes of enterocolitis are *Aeromonas*, *Plesiomonas*, *Yersinia*, and *Vibrio*. *Mycobacterium avium complex* and *Mycobacterium tuberculosis* have been noted to be the cause of diarrhea in advanced stages of HIV. Other opportunistic pathogens of importance are *Cryptosporidium*, *microsporidia* spp. (such as *Enterocytozoon bieneusi* and *Encephalitozoon intestinalis*), *Cystoisospora*, *Cyclospora*, *Entamoeba histolytica*, and *Giardia lamblia*. Giardiasis is not more common or severe in HIV disease. *Cryptosporidium* causes a chronic large volume watery diarrhea. The diagnosis is made by modified acid-fast stains, immunofluorescence assays, and enzyme immunoassays of the stool. *Isospora* and *Cyclospora* cause small bowel diarrhea, which may be severe and chronic in advanced disease. Both infections are diagnosed by the modified acid-fast stain of the stool or by duodenal biopsy. *Entamoeba histolytica* infection is rare, but the nonpathogenic *Entamoeba dispar* is often seen in 20% of patients. Cytomegalovirus is the most frequent cause of viral diarrhea in HIV. However, it is much less common with HAART. CMV involvement of the intestine has a variable presentation. It may be subclinical, cause chronic diarrhea, or result in fulminant colitis. Toxic megacolon, massive hemorrhage, or perforation can occur in severe colitis. CMV colitis occurs with a low CD4 count of <100. The diagnosis is established by colonoscopy, mucosal biopsy for viral culture, and histopathology. CMV colitis is localized to the area proximal to the splenic flexure. The culture of blood, stool, and urine are not useful.

Once an infectious cause for diarrhea is excluded, AIDS enteropathy is diagnosed. AIDS enteropathy has no identifiable cause and is pathogen negative. AIDS enteropathy may be associated with prominent villous atrophy, crypt architectural distortion and a decrease in crypt/villous ratio.

Liver

Because of their overlapping modes of infection and prolonged survival with HAART, there is an increasing number of patients diagnosed with HIV and hepatitis B or C coinfection. These diseases share common modes of infection, such as IV drug abuse, homosexuality, and exposure to paid commercial sex partners. In the United States, although estimates vary, nearly 25% of the 1.2 million HIV infected population is coinfected with HCV. HCV viral load is noted to be higher in coinfection with HIV as compared with HCV infection alone. Interestingly, after HAART, end-stage liver disease has become a significant problem because of prolonged survival. The progress of liver fibrosis with coinfection is rapid. Approximately 5% to 10% of the HIV patients have active HBV infection.

The timing of treatment of coinfection is controversial. The current recommendation is that HAART be started first. Anti-HCV therapy should be initiated after a full response from HAART with an increase in CD4 count. With the recent availability of HCV direct-acting antivirals (DAAs), treatment of hepatitis C has become simpler with a much better response. The efficacy and adverse event rates among those with HIV/HCV coinfection are similar to those observed with HCV monoinfection. The treatment of hepatitis B virus is unsatisfactory.

As would be expected, the incidence of drug-induced liver disease is high, but the majority of cases are mild asymptomatic enzyme elevations. Peliosis hepatis, a rare condition characterized by cystic, blood-filled spaces in hepatic parenchyma, occurs rarely in advanced AIDS. Patients with HIV are more likely to develop metabolic syndrome and hence nonalcoholic steatohepatitis.

Biliary Tree and the Gallbladder

The common AIDS-associated biliary disorders are acalculous cholecystitis and cholangiopathy, considered together as AIDS cholangiopathy (AC). With the advent of the HAART, the incidence of AIDS cholangiopathy is very low. The diagnosis of AC is dependent on a combination of clinical, biochemical, and radiologic evidence of bile duct abnormalities. AIDS cholangiopathy occurs in patients with a CD4 count < 50 cells/mm^3. The etiology of AIDS cholangiopathy is unknown, but often it is an enteric infection that leads to portal bacteremia. Cholangitis is known to be associated with opportunistic infections like CMV, cryptosporidium, and microsporidia. Patients present with fever, right upper quadrant pain, and tenderness, and an elevated serum alkaline phosphatase level. Ultrasound scan reveals a thickened or edematous gallbladder with obliteration of the lumen without gallstones. Imaging studies like MRI/ERCP may show papillary stenosis with or without sclerosing cholangitis, and a long extra hepatic stricture. Endoscopic retrograde cholangiopancreatography may be needed for therapeutic purposes.

Although rare, the use of Atazanavir in HAART may cause symptomatic cholelithiasis.

Pancreas

Acute pancreatitis a complication of HIV is more frequent with antiretroviral therapy. The drugs related to HIV therapy that cause acute pancreatitis are nucleoside reverse transcriptase inhibitors (NRTIs) (didanosine, stavudine) and rarely with protein inhibitors via induction of hypertriglyceridemia. The risk of acute pancreatitis increases in patients with a low CD4 counts and high viral loads.

ADDITIONAL RESOURCES

Andrade HB, Shinotsuka CR, da Silva IRF, et al: Highly active antiretroviral therapy for critically ill HIV patients: A systematic review and meta-analysis, *PLoS ONE* 12(10):e0186968, 2017.

Center for Disease Control and Prevention: *Today's HIV/AIDS epidemic.* https://www.cdc.gov/nchhstp/newsroom/docs/factsheets/todaysepidemic-508.pdf. August 2016.

Lackner AA, Mohan M, Veazey RS: The gastrointestinal tract and AIDS pathogenesis, *Gastroenterology* 136(6):1965–1978, 2009.

Shmagel KV, Saidakova EV, Shmagel NG, et al: Systemic inflammation and liver damage in HIV/hepatitis C virus coinfection, *HIV Med* 17(8):581–589, 2016.

Wilcox CM, Saag MS: Gastrointestinal complications of HIV infection: changing priorities in the HAART era, *Gut* 57:861–870, 2008.

World Health Organisation: *Media center, HIV/AIDS.* http://www.who.int/mediacentre/factsheets/fs360/en/. Updated November 2017.

Infectious Esophagitis

C. S. Pitchumoni

Infectious esophagitis may be caused by fungal, bacterial, or viral agents. The three most common causes are *Candia albicans,* herpes simplex virus (HSV 1 and HSV 2), and cytomegalovirus (CMV). The most common predisposing factor for infective esophagitis caused by any one or more of the previously mentioned agents is acquired immunodeficiency syndrome (AIDS). With the advent of highly active antiretroviral therapy (HAART), the incidence of opportunistic infections has become rare. Other causes of immunodeficiency such as uncontrolled diabetes mellitus, chronic renal failure, and solid organ transplantation can be associated with infectious esophagitis.

CANDIDA ESOPHAGITIS

Candida is a part of the normal flora in the human gastrointestinal tract. *Candida* spp., primarily *C. albicans,* are the most common agents in causing esophagitis. In addition to human immunodeficiency virus (HIV) disease, other factors that predispose to Candida esophagitis include advanced age, frequent antibiotic use, inhaled or ingested corticosteroids, poorly controlled diabetes mellitus, adrenal dysfunction, alcoholism, head and neck radiotherapy, hematologic malignancies, and motility disorders such as achalasia and scleroderma. Routine prophylactic antifungal therapy has reduced the incidence of Candida esophagitis in patients undergoing solid organ/bone marrow transplantation. Odynophagia (painful swallowing) with or without dysphagia is the classic symptom. Although oral thrush may be seen in many patients, absence of it does not exclude the infection. Esophagogastroscopy is diagnostic and is needed in all patients with alarm symptoms (dysphagia, weight loss, and bleeding) and those who do not respond to empiric therapy. Esophagoscopy shows white mucosal plaquelike lesions. Confirmatory biopsy shows the presence of yeast and pseudohyphae with invasion of mucosal cells. Empiric therapy is appropriate in AIDS patients on the basis of patient's history. However, nearly 50% of the patients may not respond because of the high incidence of coinfection with CMV and HSV in particular when the CD4 count is less than 200 cell/mm^3. The treatment of oropharyngeal candidiasis without AIDS is with antifungal lozenges or solutions of nystatin 600,000 U four times daily or clotrimazole 10 mg five times daily. Fluconazole 200 to 400 mg a day for 2 to 3 weeks is recommended in immunosuppressed patients, as well as those not responding to the previously mentioned empiric therapy. Posaconazole 400 mg twice daily followed by 400 mg once daily is an option in patients who have refractory disease.

CYTOMEGALOVIRUS-INDUCED ESOPHAGITIS

The predisposing factors for CMV esophagitis are almost the same as for candida esophagitis. In particular, patients who have undergone organ transplantation (bone marrow transplantation), those undergoing long-term dialysis, and those on prolonged steroid therapy. CMV esophagitis presents with odynophagia, but fever and substernal chest pain may be associated features. Esophagoscopy shows large solitary, deep ulcers usually in the distal esophagus. Histopathology shows intranuclear cytoplasmic inclusion bodies. The treatment is with intravenous gancyclovir 5 mg/kg or foscarnet 90 mg/kg. Therapy with oral valgancyclovir is an option in patients with a relapse.

HERPES SIMPLEX ESOPHAGITIS

HSV esophagitis (HSE) occurs frequently in patients who have undergone solid organ or bone marrow transplantation. The presenting symptoms are odynophagia and/or dysphagia, fever, and retrosternal chest pain (50% of the patients). The diagnosis is established by endoscopic demonstration of esophageal ulcers. These ulcers are usually punctate but may coalesce and have a volcano-like appearance. The treatment of HSE is with oral acyclovir 200 mg five times a day or 400 mg three times a day for 1 to 2 weeks. In the immunocompetent, HSE may be self-limiting and resolves within 2 weeks.

ADDITIONAL RESOURCES

Center for Disease Control and Prevention: Candida *infections of the mouth, throat, and esophagus,* Last updated: August 4, 2017. https://www.cdc.gov/fungal/diseases/candidiasis/thrush/index.html.

Patel NC, Caicedo RA: Esophageal infections: an update, *Curr Opin Pediatr* 27(5):642–648, 2015.

Wilcox CM: Overview of infectious esophagitis, *Gastroenterol Hepatol (N Y)* 9(8):517–519, 2013.

Typhoid Fever (Paratyphoid Fever, Enteric Fever)

C. S. Pitchumoni

Salmonella typhi (S. typhi) causes classic typhoid fever, and serotypes paratyphi A, B, or C cause the less severe, paratyphoid fever. Transmission of the organism occurs from human feces or urine, but flies or shellfish such as oysters and clams can transmit the organism (Fig. 110.1). Fecal contaminations of water supply or street-vended foods are major causes of epidemics in the developing nations.

An estimated 21 million cases of typhoid occur worldwide every year, with approximately 200,000 deaths. Although infrequent in the United States, 5700 cases occur annually, mostly in international travelers. After an acute episode, chronic carrier state occurs in 5% of cases. The disease elucidates many pathophysiologic phenomena of infectious diseases in the small bowel.

CLINICAL PICTURE

The disease is insidious in onset and presents with fever, headache, constipation, malaise, chills, and myalgia. Diarrhea and vomiting are infrequent and mild in character (Fig. 110.2). The pulse rate is usually slow, inconsistent with the high temperatures. The characteristic temperature pattern shows an increase each day and drops by the subsequent morning. The peaks and troughs rise progressively over time.

Depending on where the intestinal Peyer patches are swollen and ulcerated, the abdominal pain may be periumbilical, in the right lower quadrant, or diffuse. Characteristically, the spleen is enlarged, swollen, and easily palpable. Faint salmon colored macules (Rose spots) may develop on the chest and abdomen.

In the second week of the disease, the temperature plateaus to 103 to 104°F and the patient looks debilitated. As the fever persists into the third week, patients may become delirious and possibly dehydrated. The patient is severely anorexic and discharges diarrheic or classic "pea soup" stool, and has a distended, tender abdomen. Untreated patients who survive start to improve gradually in the fourth week as temperatures decline. The natural history of the untreated severe disease is 4 weeks to 1 month.

A chronic carrier state has been reported in patients with gallstones. Salmonella spp. creates a biofilm that is responsible. A classic historical example is that of Marry Mallon, or typhoid Mary, a cook in New York city who infected at least 54 people.

DIAGNOSIS

Typhoid fever should be high up in the differential diagnosis of fever in any patient who travels from an endemic area. Diagnosis is usually made by isolating *S. typhi* or *S. paratyphi* from blood cultures, stool, or urine. Blood cultures are positive in 50% to 70% of patients. Although bone marrow culture yields a 90% positivity, it is extremely painful and not very popular. Stool culture is positive in approximately 85% to 90% of patients within the first week of onset. Organisms can be obtained from punch biopsies of the rose spots. Widal is a serological antigen specific test and is not very helpful in patients from endemic areas. A seropositivity may indicate a previous infection. Accurate diagnosis of typhoid fever remains problematic. A highly specific polymerase chain reaction (PCR) assay with 100% specificity is not easily available. Newer tests are being developed using immunodiagnostic assays.

TREATMENT AND MANAGEMENT

Mortality in untreated classic enteric typhoid fever may be as high as 30% of patients, but with prompt and appropriate treatment, it has been reduced to 1% to 4%. Treatment of choice was *chloramphenicol*, ampicillin, amoxicillin, and trimethoprim sulfamethoxazole. However, the current drug of choice is fluoroquinolones. They are less expensive, have good tissue penetration, achieve high concentration in the gall bladder (where the organism is in a carrier state), and offer rapid therapeutic response. However, there is an increase in the multidrug resistant (MDR) strain in the Indian subcontinent. Third-generation cephalosporin and azithromycin are options. Chloramphenicol, although known to cause agranulocytosis in 1 in 10,000 patients, is widely used because of its low cost.

Chronic carrier state occurs in 1% to 5% of typhoid fever patients and more in females above the age of 50 years. Therapeutic options include amoxicillin or ampicillin plus probenecid. Patients with gallstones require cholecystectomy.

Because some organisms have developed resistance to chloramphenicol, ciprofloxacin and amoxicillin are alternative therapies. Oral quinolone and parenteral third-generation cephalosporins have also been substituted to treat resistant organisms.

Two types of vaccines are available for typhoid in oral (Ty21a, a live vaccine) and parenteral (Vi capsular polysaccharide) forms. WHO recommends vaccination for international travelers and for children in endemic areas.

COURSE AND PROGNOSIS

Most complications occur in the third or fourth week of infection. Intestinal perforation may occur at the site of ulceration from infected lymphoid tissue. Rare complications have included GI bleeding, acalculous cholecystitis, endocarditis, pericarditis, liver and splenic abscesses, and spontaneous rupture of the spleen. The leukocytosis that may occur in children resolves, as do the leukopenia and anemia in adults.

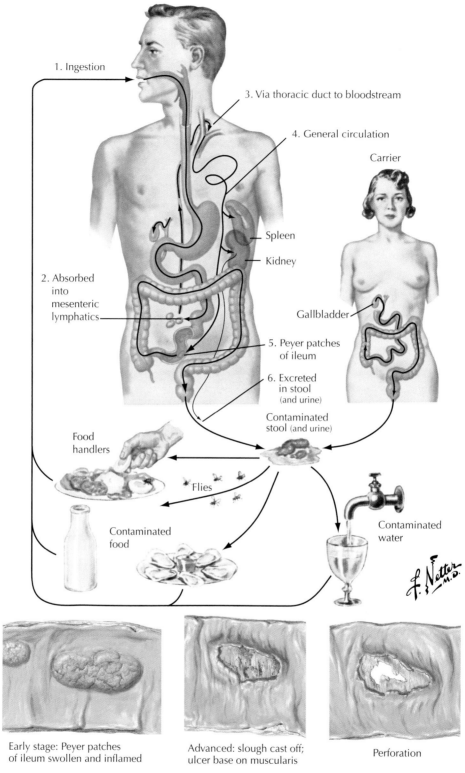

1. Ingestion

3. Via thoracic duct to bloodstream

4. General circulation

Carrier

Spleen

Kidney

2. Absorbed into mesenteric lymphatics

Gallbladder

5. Peyer patches of ileum

6. Excreted in stool (and urine)

Contaminated stool (and urine)

Food handlers

Flies

Contaminated food

Contaminated water

Early stage: Peyer patches of ileum swollen and inflamed

Advanced: slough cast off; ulcer base on muscularis

Perforation

Fig. 110.1 Typhoid Fever: Transmission and Pathologic Lesions.

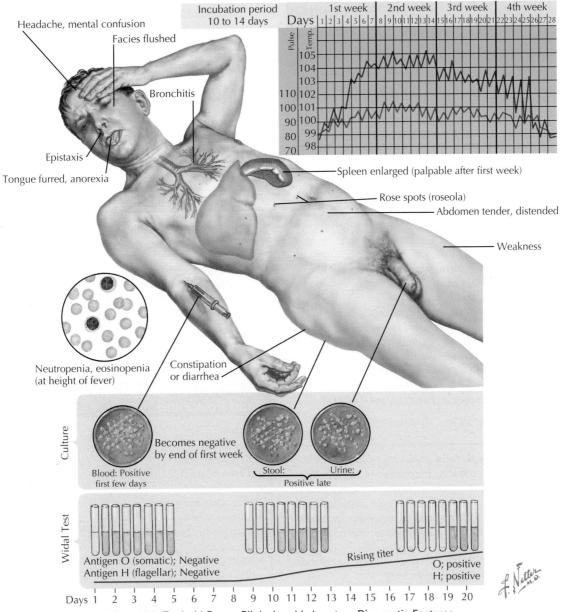

Fig. 110.2 Typhoid Fever: Clinical and Laboratory Diagnostic Features.

ADDITIONAL RESOURCES

Buckle GC, Walker CL, Black RE: Typhoid fever and paratyphoid fever: Systematic review to estimate global morbidity and mortality for 2010, *J Glob Health* 2(1):010401, 2012.

Centers for Disease Control and Prevention—National Center for Health Statistics: *Typhoid fever.* https://www.cdc.gov/typhoid-fever/sources.html. (Accessed 25 April, 2014).

Galán JE: Typhoid toxin provides a window into typhoid fever and the biology of salmonella typhi, *Proc Natl Acad Sci USA* 113(23):6338–6344, 2016.

Gonzalez-Escobedo G, Marshall JM, Gunn JS: Chronic and acute infection of the gall bladder by salmonella typhi: understanding the carrier state, *Nat Rev Microbiol* 9(1):9–14, 2011.

Harris JB, Ryan ET: Enteric fever and other causes of fever and abdominal symptoms. In Mandell GL, Bennett JE, Dolin R, editors: *Mandell, Douglas and Bennett's principles and practice of infectious diseases*, ed 8, Philadelphia, 2015, Elsevier–Churchill Livingstone, pp 1270–1282.

111

Food Poisoning and Enteric Pathogens

C. S. Pitchumoni

Food poisoning is characterized chiefly by acute gastroenteritis developing within hours or days of ingesting contaminated food. The food may contain either live organisms that grow within the host and can be designated *infectious,* or more often, preformed *toxins* produced by organisms growing in the food. In addition, foods such as mushrooms, fish, and mussels may contain poisonous components.

An estimated 38 to 78 million food poisonings occur annually in the United States, resulting in approximately 325,000 hospitalizations and 2000 to 5000 deaths, influenced by comorbidities. This chapter emphasizes gastroenteritis, but other foodborne illnesses affecting other organ systems exist. Depending on the area and the outbreak, about 50% of foodborne poisonings can be attributed to bacteria and 50% to viral agents (importantly norovirus; Box 111.1 and Table 111.1).

CLINICAL PICTURE

The causative organisms may be toxin producing or invasive to the mucosa. The common toxin-producing organisms are *Staphylococcus aureus, Bacillus cereus, Clostridium perfringens,* enterotoxigenic strains of *Escherichia coli* and *Vibrio cholerae, Campylobacter jejuni,* and *Salmonella* and *Shigella* spp. The invasive bacterial organisms are usually *Salmonella* or *Shigella* and sometimes *Campylobacter, Vibrio,* invasive *E. coli,* or *Yersinia enterocolitica.*

Figs. 111.1 and 111.2 depict the clinical symptoms and presentation in the infection and toxin types of food poisoning.

Symptoms vary depending on patient's age, comorbidities, and the toxin. The severity of diarrhea or vomiting may vary; for example, *B. cereus* toxin can produce primarily a diarrhea-type or a vomiting-type food poisoning. If onset of disease is short after consuming the suspected food, the organism is toxin producing; if onset is delayed, the organism is infectious.

DIAGNOSIS AND TREATMENT

Diagnosis largely depends on obtaining culture of stool and, in select patients, other bodily secretions. Because these infections are relatively short-lived, serology is of little value, except that it may be helpful for studying epidemics (see Table 111.1).

Cholera

Cholera is usually caused by *V. cholerae,* a curved gram-negative rod capable of causing death within hours. Once these bacteria invade the intestine, their virulent toxin increases adenylate cyclase activity, which prevents water absorption and increases fluid and electrolyte secretion, rapidly dehydrating the patient. Daily fecal output can be as much as 20 L. Without fluid replacement, the patient can die. Other strains of *Vibrio* are rampant on the Indian subcontinent. Occasionally cases are reported in the southern United States. There also have been epidemics in South America.

A majority of patients can be treated successfully with prompt administration of oral rehydration solution, as prescribed by WHO/UNICEF. The standard ORS powder sachet is dissolved in 1 L of water, and up to 6 L/day may be needed to treat dehydration. A typical oral rehydration solution for adults contains 124 mmol/L of sodium, 16 mmol/L potassium, 90 mmol/L chloride, and 48 mmol/L bicarbonate, resulting in

---

BOX 111.1 Organisms That Cause Food Poisoning

Bacteria
- *Brucella* spp.
- *Campylobacter* spp.
- *Escherichia coli,* O157:H7
- *E. coli,* non-O157:H7
- Listeria monocytogenes
- *Salmonella typhi*
- Nontyphoidal *Salmonella* spp.
- *Shigella* spp.
- *Vibrio cholerae*
- Noncholera *Vibrio* spp.
- *Vibrio vulnificus*
- *Yersinia enterocolitica*

Bacterial Toxins Produced by:
- *Bacillus cereus*
- *Clostridium botulinum*
- *Clostridium perfringens*
- *Staphylococcus aureus*
- *Streptococcus* spp.

Parasites
- *Cryptosporidium parvum*
- *Cyclospora cayetanensis*
- *Giardia lamblia*
- *Toxoplasma gondii*
- *Trichinella spiralis*

Viruses
- Norwalklike virus
- Rotavirus
- Astrovirus
- Hepatitis A virus

TABLE 111.1   **Foodborne Illness-Causing Organisms in the United States**[a]

Organism	Common Name of Illness	Onset Time After Ingesting	Signs and Symptoms	Duration	Food Sources
Bacillus cereus	*B. cereus* food poisoning	10–16 h	Abdominal cramps, watery diarrhea, nausea	24–48 h	Meats, stews, gravies, vanilla sauce
Campylobacter jejuni	Campylobacteriosis	2–5 days	Diarrhea, cramps, fever, and vomiting; diarrhea may be bloody	2–10 days	Raw and undercooked poultry, unpasteurized milk, contaminated water
Clostridium botulinum	Botulism	12–72 h	Vomiting, diarrhea, blurred vision, double vision, difficulty in swallowing, muscle weakness. Can result in respiratory failure and death	Variable	Improperly canned foods, especially home-canned vegetables, fermented fish, baked potatoes in aluminum foil
Clostridium perfringens	Perfringens food poisoning	8–16 h	Intense abdominal cramps, watery diarrhea	Usually 24 h	Meats, poultry, gravy, dried or precooked foods, time and/or temperature-abused foods
Cryptosporidium	Intestinal cryptosporidiosis	2–10 days	Diarrhea (usually watery), stomach cramps, upset stomach, slight fever	May be remitting and relapsing over weeks to months	Uncooked food or food contaminated by an ill food handler after cooking, contaminated drinking water
Cyclospora cayetanensis	Cyclosporiasis	1–14 days, usually at least 1 week	Diarrhea (usually watery), loss of appetite, substantial loss of weight, stomach cramps, nausea, vomiting, fatigue	May be remitting and relapsing over weeks to months	Various types of fresh produce (imported berries, lettuce, basil)
Escherichia coli producing toxin	*E. coli* infection (common cause of "travelers' diarrhea")	1–3 days	Watery diarrhea, abdominal cramps, some vomiting	3–7 or more days	Water or food contaminated with human feces
E. coli O157:H7	Hemorrhagic colitis or *E. coli* O157:H7 infection	1–8 days	Severe (often bloody) diarrhea, abdominal pain and vomiting. Usually, little or no fever is present. More common in children 4 years or younger. Can lead to kidney failure	5–10 days	Undercooked beef (especially hamburger), unpasteurized milk and juice, raw fruits and vegetables (e.g., sprouts), and contaminated water
Hepatitis A	Hepatitis	28 days average (15–50 days)	Diarrhea, dark urine, jaundice, and flulike symptoms (i.e., fever, headache, nausea, and abdominal pain)	Variable, 2 weeks–3 months	Raw produce, contaminated drinking water, uncooked foods and cooked foods that are not reheated after contact with an infected food handler; shellfish from contaminated waters
Listeria monocytogenes	Listeriosis	9–48 h for gastrointestinal symptoms, 2–6 weeks for invasive disease	Fever, muscle aches, and nausea or diarrhea. Pregnant women may have mild flulike illness, and infection can lead to premature delivery or stillbirth. The elderly or immunocompromised patients may develop bacteremia or meningitis.	Variable	Unpasteurized milk, soft cheeses made with unpasteurized milk, ready-to-eat deli meats
Noroviruses	Variously called viral gastroenteritis, winter diarrhea, acute nonbacterial gastroenteritis, food poisoning, and food infection	12–48 h	Nausea, vomiting, abdominal cramping, diarrhea, fever, headache. Diarrhea is more prevalent in adults; vomiting more common in children.	12–60 h	Raw produce, contaminated drinking water, uncooked foods and cooked foods that are not reheated after contact with an infected food handler; shellfish from contaminated waters

Continued

TABLE 111.1   **Foodborne Illness-Causing Organisms in the United States[a]—cont'd**

Organism	Common Name of Illness	Onset Time After Ingesting	Signs and Symptoms	Duration	Food Sources
Salmonella	Salmonellosis	6–48 h	Diarrhea, fever, abdominal cramps, vomiting	4–7 days	Eggs, poultry, meat, unpasteurized milk or juice, cheese, contaminated raw fruits and vegetables
Shigella	Shigellosis or Bacillary dysentery	4–7 days	Abdominal cramps, fever, and diarrhea. Stools may contain blood and mucus.	24–48 h	Raw produce, contaminated drinking water, uncooked foods and cooked foods that are not reheated after contact with an infected food handler
Staphylococcus aureus	Staphylococcal food poisoning	1–6 h	Sudden onset of severe nausea and vomiting. Abdominal cramps. Diarrhea and fever may be present.	24–48 h	Unrefrigerated or improperly refrigerated meats, potato and egg salads, cream pastries
Vibrio parahaemolyticus	V. parahaemolyticus	4–96 h	Watery (occasionally bloody) diarrhea, abdominal cramps, nausea, vomiting, fever	2–5 days	Undercooked or raw seafood, such as shellfish
Vibrio vulnificus	*V. vulnificus* infection	1–7 days	Vomiting, diarrhea, abdominal pain, bloodborne infection. Fever, bleeding within the skin, ulcers requiring surgical removal. Can be fatal to persons with liver disease or weakened immune systems.	2–8 days	Undercooked or raw seafood, such as shellfish (especially oysters)

[a]While the American food supply is among the safest in the world, the federal government estimates that there are about 48 million cases of foodborne illness annually—the equivalent of 1 in 6 Americans each year. And each year these illnesses result in an estimated 128,000 hospitalizations and 3000 deaths. The chart includes foodborne disease-causing organisms that frequently cause illness in the United States. As the chart shows, the threats are numerous and varied, with symptoms ranging from relatively mild discomfort to very serious, life-threatening illness. While the very young, the elderly, and persons with weakened immune systems are at greatest risk of serious consequences from most foodborne illnesses, some of the organisms shown pose grave threats to all persons.
From U.S. Food and Drug Administration. https://www.fda.gov/downloads/Food/FoodborneIllnessContaminants/UCM187482.pdf (Accessed April 2018).

passive absorption of the electrolytes and fluid and preventing massive dehydration. Patients with severe cholera require intravenous therapy and should be given when ORS is not possible. Often the need for fluid replacement is underestimated. Administration of 200 mL/kg of isotonic fluid, oral or intravenous, in the first 24 hours is recommended. Antibiotics (tetracycline, ciprofloxacin, and doxycycline) are adjunctive therapy in moderate to severely ill patients and after adequate hydration. Zinc supplementation reduces the duration of diarrhea and the volume of stool in children. The currently available oral cholera vaccine plays an important role in preventing epidemics.

Before the advent of fluid replacement, cholera vaccine, and antibiotics, cholera mortality was as high as 50% to 75%, but is now less than 1% with proper therapy.

Salmonellosis

Nontyphoidal salmonellosis is a common cause of foodborne enteric infections in the industrialized world, accounting for 93.8 million foodborne illnesses and 155,000 deaths per year. It is caused by *Salmonella enteritidis, Salmonella typhimurium,* and other serologic types. The food sources of infection are cheese, contaminated raw produce, eggs, meat, poultry, unpasteurized milk, or juice.

Based on clinical patterns in salmonellosis, *Salmonella* infection can be grouped into typhoidal *Salmonella* and nontyphoidal *Salmonella.* Gastroenteritis is the most common manifestation of *Salmonella*

infection worldwide, followed by bacteremia and enteric fever (discussed elsewhere).

The salmonellae do not seem to grow extensively in the intestine, but rather invade the lymph and phagocytic tissue. The clinical picture is composed of nonbloody diarrhea, vomiting, nausea, headache, abdominal cramps, and myalgia. Rarely the disease may be complicated by cholecystitis, acute pancreatitis, perforation of terminal ileum, and appendicitis. Any diarrhea is usually self-limiting, lasting 3 to 7 days, and the symptoms are largely resolved within 72 hours; however, organisms may exist in stool for 1 month.

Antibiotics are usually not recommended for routine *Salmonella* infection because of the increased risk for bacterial resistance, and the disease is self-limiting. However, it may be necessary to treat severely ill patients with comorbidities. If the patient has bacteremia, antibiotic therapy is indicated for 7 to 14 days, often with two antibiotics; choices include ampicillin, amoxicillin, trimethoprim-sulfamethoxazole, cefotaxime or ceftriaxone, chloramphenicol, and fluoroquinolones. If a patient has an intravascular infection, a 6-week course of antibiotics is indicated.

Other Bacterial Pathogens

The enteropathogenic, enteroinvasive, and enterohemorrhagic forms of *E. coli* produce different types of syndromes (see Additional Resources). *Shigella* produces a classic, bacillary form of dysentery.

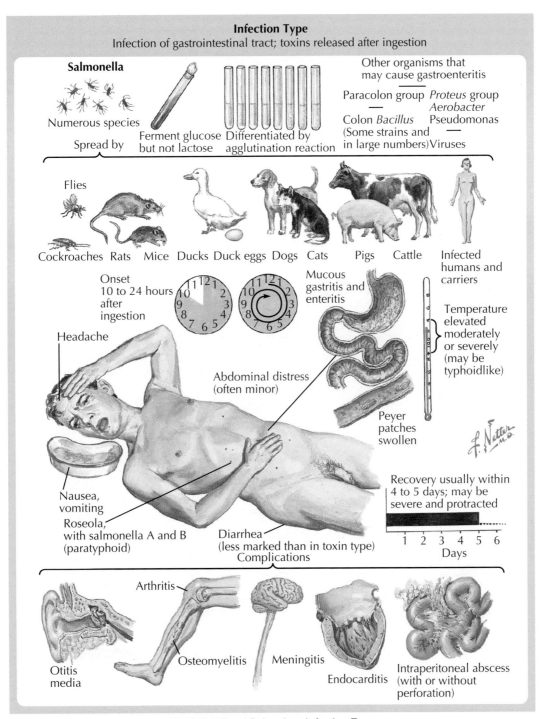

Infection Type
Infection of gastrointestinal tract; toxins released after ingestion

Salmonella

Numerous species

Spread by

Ferment glucose but not lactose

Differentiated by agglutination reaction

Other organisms that may cause gastroenteritis

Paracolon group *Proteus* group
— *Aerobacter*
Colon *Bacillus* Pseudomonas
(Some strains and —
in large numbers)Viruses

Flies

Cockroaches Rats Mice Ducks Duck eggs Dogs Cats Pigs Cattle Infected humans and carriers

Onset 10 to 24 hours after ingestion

Headache

Mucous gastritis and enteritis

Temperature elevated moderately or severely (may be typhoidlike)

Abdominal distress (often minor)

Peyer patches swollen

Nausea, vomiting

Roseola, with salmonella A and B (paratyphoid)

Diarrhea (less marked than in toxin type)

Recovery usually within 4 to 5 days; may be severe and protracted

1 2 3 4 5 6
Days

Complications

Otitis media

Arthritis

Osteomyelitis

Meningitis

Endocarditis

Intraperitoneal abscess (with or without perforation)

Fig. 111.1 Food Poisoning: Infection Type.

The interested reader is referred to the appropriate resources for *C. perfringens*, *Campylobacter*, *Listeria*, *Yersinia*, and *B. cereus* infections. As a caveat in modern society, *B. cereus* can come from fried rice that is not fresh or that is kept at low-grade refrigeration for 24 to 48 hours.

Viral Pathogens

Viral pathogens causing food poisoning are as common as bacterial pathogens and include five groups: rotaviruses, caliciviruses (Norwalk viruses), enteric adenoviruses, astroviruses, and toroviruses (enveloped single-stranded RNA that causes 3% of diarrhea in children). Symptoms and syndromes are similar for all these viruses, with some different epidemiologic findings. Norwalk viruses are more common in adults, whereas rotaviruses, adenoviruses, astroviruses, and toroviruses are more common in infants and children. Adenoviruses also are associated with upper respiratory infection and may cause vomiting, diarrhea, and severe dehydration over 5 to 7 days.

Laboratory diagnosis is primarily made using immunoassay or electron microscopy. Successful growth of these viruses routinely in the laboratory has not been accomplished.

Treatment of viral food poisoning is largely supportive. When diarrhea is severe, replacing electrolytes and fluids is essential. Most cases

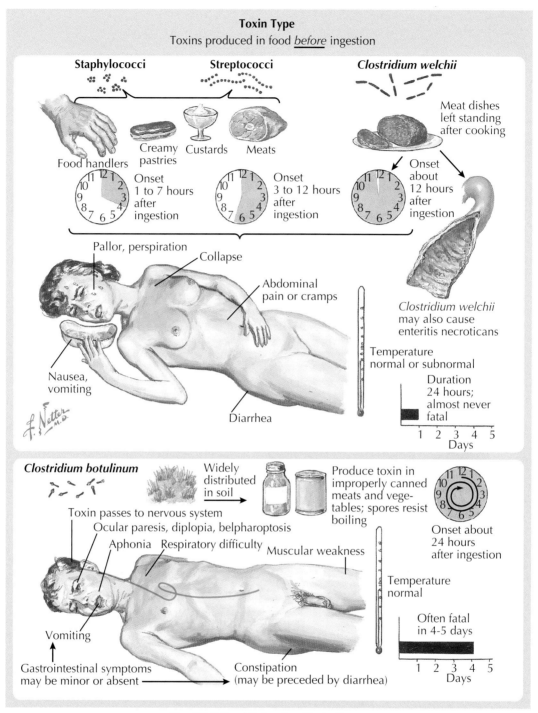

Fig. 111.2 Food Poisoning: Toxin Type.

resolve spontaneously. However, for patients with comorbidities and infants, the dehydration may be life threatening, especially when fluid replacement is not possible.

TRAVELER'S DIARRHEA

With millions of people traveling to and from developing nations, traveler's diarrhea (TD) is a frequently encountered clinical entity. Typically TD symptoms are self-limiting and last for less than 3 days. Traveler's diarrhea is defined as the passage of three or more unformed stools with one or more associated gastrointestinal symptoms (abdominal pain, cramping, and distention) in an individual with a history of recent travel usually to a developing nation with poor sanitation. The incidence of TD is higher in individuals from developed nations (who lack immunity), in the age group 15 to 30 years, those on proton pump inhibitor therapy (low gastric acidity), and within the first 2 weeks of travel. TD is mostly a fecally-orally transmitted disease caused by bacterial (enterotoxigenic *E. coli* [ETEC], enteroaggregative *E. coli* [EAEC], *Campylobacter* spp., *Shigella* spp. and *Salmonella* spp.), viral (Norovirus, Rotavirus), or parasitic (*Giardia duodenalis, Cryptosporidium parvum, Entamoeba histolytica, Cyclospora cayetanensis*) pathogens. The stool culture often shows multiple pathogens. A large proportion of traveler's diarrhea is due to *E. coli*, which produces a heat labile (LT) and heat stable (ST) toxin. The ST type of *E. coli* poisoning is frequent in Guatemala, Mexico, and India. Importantly, campylobacter, an important cause of TD, is ciprofloxacin resistant in Asia.

Although not routinely used, a multiplex quantitative PCR test is available to detect common pathogens.

The management of TD is prevention by appropriate food hygiene. Bismuth subsalicylate provides protection against TD. Antibiotic chemoprophylaxis with fluoroquinolone (resistance in India) or rifaximin helps. Adequate hydration with oral fluid intake is important in preventing and treating dehydration associated with TD.

COURSE AND PROGNOSIS

Because transmission is through the oral and fecal routes, prevention is the best cure. When a pandemic or epidemic of food poisoning seems to be evolving, exposure to contaminated persons must be avoided. Oral rehydration solutions are effective and, if the diarrhea causes dehydration, should be used before intravenous therapy becomes necessary.

ADDITIONAL RESOURCES

Giddings SL, Stevens AM, Leung DT: Traveler's diarrhea, *Med Clin North Am* 100(2):317–330, 2016.

Harris JB, LaRocque RC, Qadri F, et al: Cholera, *Lancet* 379(9835):2466–2476, 2012.

Hohmann EL: Nontyphoidal salmonellosis, *Clin Infect Dis* 15(32):263–269, 2001.

Jiang ZD, DuPont HL: Etiology of travelers' diarrhea, *J Travel Med* 24(suppl_1):S13–S16, 2017.

Mody RK, Griffin PM: Foodborne disease. In Mandell GL, Bennett JE, Dolin R, editors: *Mandell, Douglas and Bennett's principles and practice of infectious diseases*, ed 8, Philadelphia, 2015, Elsevier–Churchill Livingstone, pp 1283–1296.

Switaj TL, Winter KJ, Christensen SR: Diagnosis and management of foodborne illness, *Am Fam Physician* 92(5):358–365, 2015.

112

Clostridium difficile and Other Antibiotic-Associated Diarrhea

C. S. Pitchumoni

The use of antibiotics causes diarrhea by three mechanisms. Mild diarrhea is a side effect of many antibiotics, more often seen with broad-spectrum antibiotics and when multiple antibiotics are used simultaneously. Antibiotic-associated hemorrhagic colitis may rarely occur following the use of penicillins. A good example is the hemorrhagic colitis associated with ampicillin-clavulanic acid use caused by the bacteria *Klebsiella oxytoca*. However, *Clostridium difficile*–associated disease (CDAD) is one of the important causes of antibiotic-associated diarrheal disorders of tremendous public health importance.

In the United States, *C. difficile* is one of the leading causes of nosocomially acquired diarrheal syndromes. CDAD is increasing in its incidence and severity. Some recent observations on the epidemics are of concern. Once, CDAD was predominantly a hospital-acquired disease. Currently, community-acquired CDAD is increasing, one-quarter of the cases being nursing home acquired. The recurrence rate has increased, as well as the severity of the disease along with the indications for colectomy for toxic megacolon or intestinal perforations.

C. difficile is a spore-forming, gram-positive, anaerobic, toxin-producing bacteria. *C. difficile* colonizes the intestinal tract in up to 15% of healthy adults (Fig. 112.1).

PATHOGENICITY

The transmission of the disease is by fecal-oral contamination through the ingestion of spores. The spores survive gastric acidity, and they germinate into vegetative cells in the intestine of susceptible hosts. The organisms then infiltrate the mucus layer and adhere to the epithelial cells. *C. difficile* produces two cytotoxins, toxin A (TedA) and toxin B (TedB). The toxins cause diminished transepithelial resistance, fluid accumulation, and destruction of the intestinal epithelium. A new hypervirulent strain (Quebec strain, *C. difficile* BI/NAPI 027) produces a third toxin, a binary toxin (CDT) that causes a severe form of the disease.

RISK FACTORS

The leading cause of CDAD is antibiotic exposure. Antibiotic therapy causes dysbiosis of the healthy gut microbiota and predisposes to CDAD. Dysbiosis causes a loss of resistance associated with alterations of endogenous bacteria. The most frequently implicated antibiotics are fluoroquinolones, ampicillin-amoxicillin, and clindamycin. Almost all antibiotics including administration of intravenous (IV) vancomycin are reported to predispose to CDAD.

Other risk factors are advanced age, hospitalization, exposure to long-term care facility, recent gastrointestinal surgery, tube feedings, therapy with proton pump inhibitors (PPIs) and antimotility drugs, inflammatory bowel diseases (IBDs), malignancies as well as chemotherapy and immune suppression, and mechanical ventilation.

CLINICAL FEATURES

The spectrum of *C. difficile* disease is wide. Most of the cases are mild in nature, the diarrhea disappearing without any treatment and escaping a diagnosis. In typical cases, the diarrhea is characterized by foul-smelling watery stools with mucus. Bloody diarrhea is rare. Associated symptoms are nausea, vomiting, and dehydration. Mild leukocytosis is frequent, and a leukemoid reaction is rare. CDAD is not always mild. Toxic megacolon associated with fulminant colitis, intestinal perforation, and multiple organ failures are seen in severe cases. Despite appropriate treatment, one recurrence occurs in 15% to 20% of cases, and secondary relapses occur in 45% after the first relapse. Multiple recurrences occur in nearly 5% of the patients who had an episode of CDAD. The mortality rate in CDAD has been increasing.

The severity of the disease is influenced by the age of the patient, nutritional status, low serum albumin, comorbidity, and bacterial genotype (BI/NAPI 027 strain).

DIAGNOSIS

Current opinion on the diagnosis of CDAD is as follows. Only stools from patients with diarrhea should be tested for *C. difficile*. The exception is a patient suspected to have the disease with paralytic ileus when rectal swabs can be tested. An algorithm recommended by experts is provided. Stool antigen testing, once popular, has lost its utility because of its inability to separate the commensal organism from the pathogenic organisms. Much better tests are currently available. Stool toxin assay is fast and superior. The stool culture is performed in epidemics.

See Table 112.1 for a critical evaluation of available tests for the diagnosis of *C. difficile* colitis.

TREATMENT

The following is a summary of current guidelines from the American College of Gastroenterology recommendations.

A large majority of patients have only a mild and self-limiting disease that does not need any treatment. In those with symptoms of colitis, the diagnosis of *C. difficile* colitis must be established before implementation of antimicrobial therapy. Empiric therapy for CDAD is acceptable only if the pretest probability is very high.

If the patient is currently on antibiotic therapy, it should be discontinued. The use of antiperistaltic agents should be strictly avoided. Supportive care includes adequate hydration, electrolyte replacement, and venous thromboembolism prophylaxis.

Patients with mild to moderate disease should be treated with metronidazole 500 mg orally three times a day for 10 days. Those with severe CDAD should be treated with vancomycin 125 mg orally four times a day for 10 days. Failure to respond to metronidazole therapy

A. Currently popular algorithm

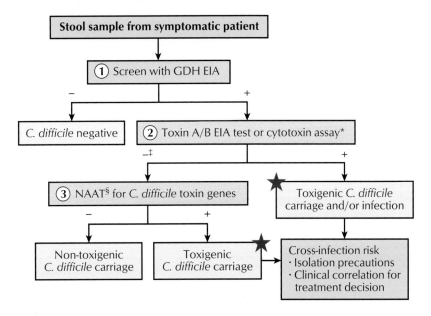

B. Newer algorithm already popular in many U.S. centers

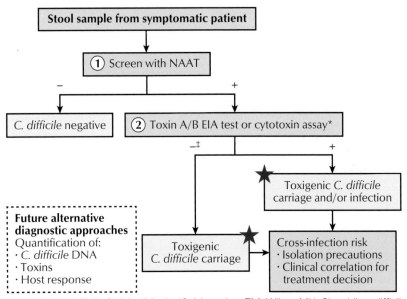

Fig. 112.1 *Clostridium difficile* Colitis. (Martin JS, Monaghan TM, Wilcox MH: Clostridium difficile infection: epidemiology, diagnosis and understanding transmission. *Nat Rev Gastroenterol Hepatol* 13(4):206-216, 2016.)

within 5 to 7 days prompts a change of antibiotic to vancomycin. A surgical specialist should evaluate patients with a suspected toxic megacolon.

In IBD patients with suspected CDAD, empiric therapy for CDAD along with therapy for the flare of IBD should be initiated.

The first recurrence of CDAD should be treated with the same regimen that was used in the treatment of the initial episode. In severe cases, as well as for a second recurrence, vancomycin therapy is needed. A pulse regime of vancomycin prescribed for recurrences consists of standard therapy at a dose of 125 mg four times daily for 10 days followed by 125 mg daily pulsed every 3 days for 10 doses.

In case of the third recurrence, the patient should be evaluated for fecal microbiota transplant (FMT) that has become popular. FMT uses a healthy stool to restore the colonic microbiome to a state resistant to CDAD. The success rates for FMT after a single infusion are high.

Therapy with probiotics is always an adjunct to the standard antibiotic regimen. The use of *Saccharomyces boulardii* reduces the number of recurrences. A trial of *Lactobacillus plantarum* has also demonstrated an appreciable clinical benefit. There is no role for IV immunoglobulin in the treatment of CDAD.

Surgery is indicated in the management of complications such as toxic megacolon or perforation.

TABLE 112.1 **Evaluation of Available Tests for *Clostridium difficile* Colitis**

Test	Methodology	Advantage	Disadvantage
Stool antigen (glutamate dehydrogenase assay)	Latex agglutination or immunochromatographic	Preliminary test Rapid test < 1 hr	Alone is nonspecific Needs to be done in combination with toxin detection tests
Toxin testing	1. Tissue culture 2. Enzyme immunoassay toxin A or B or both (A–, B+ strains exist)	Detects toxin B only Rapid Relatively inexpensive	Costly and requires 48 hr and possibility of recovering nontoxigenic strains. Relative insensitivity (less than tissue culture and PCR)
Molecular tests	FDA-approved real-time PCR assay	Fast test Highly sensitive and specific for toxin B producing *Clostridium difficile* colitis Positive predictive value 94%, negative predictive value of 99%	Expensive
Stool culture	Culture (needed only in cases of relapse or ineffective drug therapy)	Most sensitive Used in outbreaks	Too many false-positives

FDA, US Food and Drug Administration; *PCR*, polymerase chain reaction.

The treatment of patients with CDAD includes infection control practices to prevent the spread of the disease. Patients continue to shed organisms for some days even after diarrhea disappears. Hospital-based infection control program, antibiotic stewardship, and contact precautions for all patients with should be enforced. Proper hand hygiene cannot be overemphasized. Alcohol-based hand lotions are not enough to kill the spores. Thorough hand washing between examination of patients with soap and water is the most effective procedure.

ADDITIONAL RESOURCES

Hryckowian AJ, Pruss KM, Sonnenburg JL: The emerging metabolic view of clostridium difficile pathogenesis, *Curr Opin Microbiol* 35:42–47, 2017.

Martin JS, Monaghan TM, Wilcox MH: Clostridium difficile infection: epidemiology, diagnosis and understanding transmission, *Nat Rev Gastroenterol Hepatol* 13(4):206–216, 2016.

Martínez-Meléndez A, Camacho-Ortiz A, Morfin-Otero R, et al: Current knowledge on the laboratory diagnosis of clostridium difficile infection, *World J Gastroenterol* 23(9):1552–1567, 2017.

Napolitano LM, Edmiston CE Jr: Clostridium difficile disease: diagnosis, pathogenesis, and treatment update, *Surgery* 162(2):325–348, 2017.

Surawicz CM, Brandt LJ, Binion DG, et al: Guidelines for diagnosis, treatment, and prevention of clostridium difficile infections, *Am J Gastroenterol* 108(4):478–498, 2013.

113

Gastrointestinal Tuberculosis

C. S. Pitchumoni

Tuberculosis (TB) is caused by *Mycobacterium tuberculosis* and historically is one of the oldest known human afflictions. According to the World Health Organization (2013), globally the annual incidence of TB was 8.6 million, and 1.3 million died in 2012. TB is the ninth leading cause of death worldwide, ranking above HIV/AIDS. In 2016 there were an estimated 1.3 million deaths from TB among HIV negative persons, and an additional 374,000 among HIV positive people. The countries with the highest incidence are India, Indonesia, China, and Philippines.

There are two forms of the mycobacterium complex, *M. tuberculosis* (the causative agent predominantly for TB in the human beings) and *M. bovis* (mostly found in cattle but a rare pathogen in the human). Pasteurization of cow's milk has resulted in the marked decline of *M. bovis* infection in most parts of the world. HIV infection may be complicated by tuberculosis, with a 20 times greater risk. In Africa, TB occurs in 20% to 26% of the HIV-infected population.

Although predominantly a pulmonary disease, TB also involves the central nervous system (tuberculous meningitis), lymphatic system, genitourinary system, bones and joints (Pott disease of the spine), and the gastrointestinal tract. The gastrointestinal tract, including the liver and pancreas, may be affected by tuberculosis. Extrapulmonary TB is noted in 15% of the cases worldwide. In the Unites States, one-fifth of the cases of TB are extra pulmonary, of which 5% are peritoneal.

Abdominal TB usually occurs in four forms: (1) tuberculous lymphadenopathy, (2) peritoneal, (3) gastrointestinal (GI), and (4) visceral (involving the genitourinary system, liver, spleen, and pancreas). Often a combination of two or more of the above occurs in a single patient. In tuberculous lymphadenopathy, the most frequently involved lymph nodes are mesenteric, omental, porta hepatis, celiac, and peripancreatic. Peritoneal TB may present in three forms: (1) the wet ascitic type is the most common, associated with large amounts of high-density free or loculated fluid with high protein content due to its inflammatory nature; (2) the fixed fibrotic type involving the omentum and mesentery shows matted bowel loops on imaging; (3) the dry plastic type has fibrous peritoneal reaction and adhesions.

The three modes of involvement of the gastrointestinal tract are (1) through ingestion of infected food material or sputum, (2) hematogenous spread from a tuberculous foci, and (3) direct spread to the peritoneum from an adjacent foci.

The ingested tuberculous bacteria in a susceptible individual invade the intestinal tract (Fig. 113.1). The mucosal layer of the GI tract once infected with bacilli results in the formation of epithelioid tubercles. After 2 to 4 weeks, the tubercles undergo caseous necrosis and cause ulcerations. Invasion of the gut occurs primarily in lymphoid tissue. Therefore Peyer patches are susceptible. Terminal ileum, rich in lymphoid tissue, is most susceptible to intestinal TB. Morphologically, the intestinal tuberculosis may be either ulcerated or hypertrophic. In the *ulcerated* type, after invasion of the lymphoid follicles of Peyer patches, ulceration slowly develops. A necrotic base forms in the ulcer, which may perforate, or spread into the peritoneum. The less common *hypertrophic* type leads to extensive granuloma formation and fibrosis. In the colon, it can form a "napkin ring" lesion mimicking carcinoma.

TB peritonitis may occur from dissemination or direct extension. Caseating granulomas are characteristic of the disease. TB involvement of the appendix has been reported.

CLINICAL PICTURE

The most common symptoms of intestinal TB are abdominal pain, fever, anorexia, diarrhea, weight loss, constipation, bloating, and infrequently gastrointestinal hemorrhage. When TB is located in the stomach or duodenum, symptoms referable to these organs may predominate. The intestinal type being the most common, abdominal pain is the predominant symptom. Colorectal TB maybe characterized by linear fissured transverse or circumferential ulcers covered with dull white or yellow exudates.

Esophageal TB is rare and presents as solid food dysphagia. Hepatic TB is also rare and affects approximately 1% of all TB cases, but more in HIV patients. It presents with nonspecific symptoms of fever, hepatomegaly, abdominal pain, and weight loss. The biochemical features are an elevated alkaline phosphatase and gamma-glutamyltransferase.

DIAGNOSIS

A high index of suspicion is needed to consider abdominal TB in the evaluation of a patient with vague gastrointestinal symptoms. Demographic data like country of origin, immunity status, diabetes, treatment with biologics, steroid therapy, malnutrition, smoking, alcoholism, HIV disease, and a family history of tuberculosis suggest a high risk. Incarcerated and institutionalized individuals are also at a high risk for the development of TB.

Tests that are available include histopathology, culture, T-SPOT TB test, and enzyme linked immunosorbent assay (ELISA). Culture, although specific for TB, has a low yield and is time-consuming. It may take up to 6 weeks for culture. T-SPOT or QuantiFERON testing detects the in vitro production of interferon-gamma by peripheral blood mononuclear cells in response to *M. tuberculosis*-specific antigens. It has a sensitivity of 70% to 90%.

Useful radiological studies are barium imaging of the gastrointestinal (GI) tract, computed tomography (CT) scan, CT enteroscopy, colonoscopy with ileal intubation, and biopsy. A definitive diagnosis is demonstration of tuberculous granuloma. If granuloma is noncaseating, it is difficult to differentiate intestinal TB from Crohn disease.

Ultrasound facilitates the diagnosis of abdominal and hepatic TB by identifying enlarged lymph nodes and ascites that can be sampled for further analysis. The ascitic fluid is exudative (>3 g%), with a

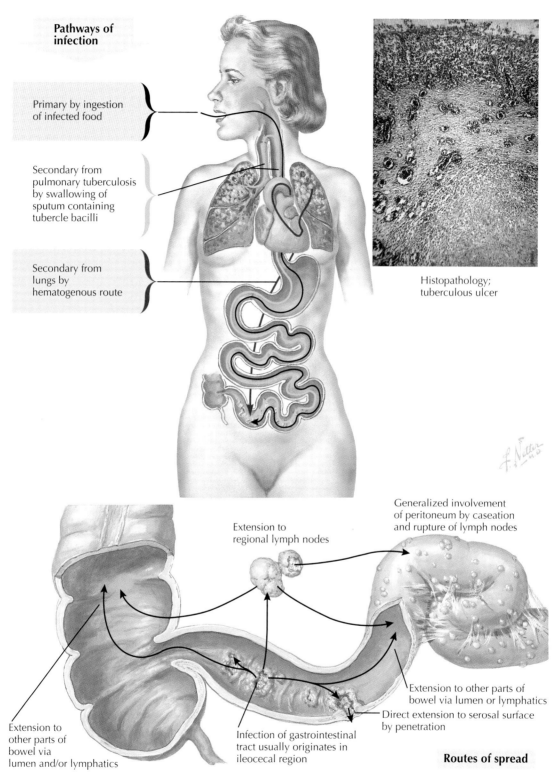

Pathways of infection

Primary by ingestion of infected food

Secondary from pulmonary tuberculosis by swallowing of sputum containing tubercle bacilli

Secondary from lungs by hematogenous route

Histopathology; tuberculous ulcer

Generalized involvement of peritoneum by caseation and rupture of lymph nodes

Extension to regional lymph nodes

Extension to other parts of bowel via lumen or lymphatics

Direct extension to serosal surface by penetration

Extension to other parts of bowel via lumen and/or lymphatics

Infection of gastrointestinal tract usually originates in ileocecal region

Routes of spread

Fig. 113.1 Gastrointestinal Tuberculosis: Pathways of Infection and Routes of Spread.

serum-ascites album gradient of <1.1 g%. Adenosine deaminase activity evaluated in the ascitic fluid is a specific marker for TB.

Laparoscopic examination of the peritoneum allows direct visualization and biopsy of the characteristic granulomas. It can establish the diagnosis in 80% to 90% of patients.

The purified protein derivative (PPD) skin testing (Mantoux test) gives supportive evidence for abdominal TB in 55% to 70%; if positive, however, a negative tuberculin test is observed in one third of the patients. At times, the differential diagnosis can be difficult. It may include Crohn disease, lymphoma, carcinoma, diverticular disease, appendicitis, and other infections of the GI tract. One of the following criteria is necessary to make a firm diagnosis:

- Growth of the organism from infected tissue
- Histologic demonstration of *M. tuberculosis* in tissue
- Histologic demonstration of granulomas with caseating necrosis
- Typical gross pathologic findings in the bowel
- Histologic findings of granulomas with caseation necrosis in associated lymph nodes.

TREATMENT AND MANAGEMENT

Medical management of abdominal TB involves 6 months of antitubercular therapy, with 2 months of isoniazid, rifampicin, pyrazinamide, and ethambutol, followed by 4 months of isoniazid and rifampicin.

In case of development of multidrug-resistant TB, the first-line oral agents like pyrazinamide, rifabutin, and ethambutol are used. Treatment is usually continued for at least 6 months. Other drugs are now becoming available, including amikacin, levofloxacin, cycloserine, ethionamide, kanamycin, capreomycin, and *p*-aminosalicylic acid.

Laparoscopic surgery may be needed in patients with peritoneal obstructive tuberculosis.

COURSE AND PROGNOSIS

Prognosis depends on the TB patient's comorbidities and basic immune status. Therapy with multiple antibiotics is usually successful when started early in the disease course. In severely affected HIV patients, TB may be fatal. If TB is suspected early, treatment should be started, pending histologic and microbiologic confirmation, because early treatment is critical for immunocompromised patients. Even with resistance to antibiotics, treatment can be successful because numerous drugs are effective.

ADDITIONAL RESOURCES

Chugh SN, Jain V: Abdominal tuberculosis—current concepts in diagnosis and management. In Singal RK, editor: *Medicine update (volume 17, 2007)*, 2007, Jaypee Brothers Pvt Ltd, pp 600–608.

Debi U, Ravisankar V, Prasad KK, et al: Abdominal tuberculosis of the gastrointestinal tract: revisited, *World J Gastroenterol* 20(40):14831–14840, 2014.

Evans RP, Mourad MM, Dvorkin L, Bramhall SR: Hepatic and intra-abdominal tuberculosis: 2016 update, *Curr Infect Dis Rep* 18(12):45, 2016.

Global tuberculosis report 2017: World Health Organization.

114

Abdominal Actinomycosis

C. S. Pitchumoni

Actinomycosis of the abdomen is most often caused by a gram-positive anaerobic bacterium, *Actinomyces israelii.* However, many other species can cause the same syndrome. *Actinomyces* as commensals colonize the oral cavity, upper gastrointestinal tract, and female urogenital tract. Abdominal and genital actinomycosis is increasing in incidence with the use of intrauterine device (IUD). There are three major types of clinical infection syndromes in humans: cervicofacial (15%–60%), thoracic (15%–30%), and abdominal (20% including liver abscess). Rarely, the central nervous system may be involved. The intraabdominal actinomycosis presents with a vague symptomatology mimicking abdominopelvic neoplasia, clinically as well as radiologically. The intraabdominal form often occurs without any detectable cause but rarely may occur after gastrointestinal surgical procedures, endoscopic procedures, or trauma. Actinomycosis is an indolent, slowly progressive disease, and hence the diagnosis may be delayed by months to years.

The most common site in the gastrointestinal tract is in the ileocecal valve area, but any part may be involved. Mucosal involvements being rare, endoscopic procedures are not helpful in the diagnosis, and lymph nodes are seldom involved. It is assumed that once the disease is present in the abdominal cavity, drainage into the liver is the cause of liver abscess. Fortunately, when the disease manifests, it usually is in only one organ and is not disseminated. When infection occurs, other organs may be involved in the abscess formation.

Actinomyces is a part of the indigenous flora. Infections develop when the patient is in a susceptible state, such as during surgery, trauma, debilitating disease (e.g., malignancy, diabetes mellitus), or chronic corticosteroid therapy.

CLINICAL PICTURE

Most patients have pain, weight loss, and fever, and they may have anorexia and chills if there is visceral involvement. Hepatic *Actinomyces* is nonspecific and varied, and thus must be considered in any patient with hepatic abscess, or it may accompany chronic fistula or manifest as an indurated mass or abscess.

DIAGNOSIS

Usually the clinical picture is confusing, and the diagnosis is difficult and is only made after surgical exploration or drainage of an abscess.

Because abdominal *Actinomyces* has a predilection for the right lower quadrant, it must be considered in any confusing presentation of Crohn disease, tuberculosis of the ileum, or appendicitis. Classic symptoms include indurated mass, sinus tract and fistula, and abscesses (Fig. 114.1). Abdominal *Actinomyces* can mask carcinoma of the cecum or appendix.

Routine hematological and biochemical studies are not helpful, but mild leukocytosis, anemia, and elevated erythrocyte sedimentation rate may be present. An elevated alkaline phosphatase indicates a hepatic abscess. Cultures are positive in only 25% to 50% of patients. Gram staining reveals beaded, branched, or gram-positive filamentous rods. The organisms also may be recovered from the blood. Suspected diagnosis is confirmed by fine needle aspiration or core biopsy, demonstrating the characteristic disease and sulfa granules. Sulfa granules are actually microcolonies of the organism, and classic eosinophilic material at the edges of the granules represents the host response.

Gallium-67 citrate scintigraphy exhibits an increased uptake and radioactivity in the infected foci. Other radiologic findings can be misleading, as they mimic abdominopelvic neoplasia.

TREATMENT AND MANAGEMENT

Once the diagnosis of actinomycosis is established, long-term antibiotic therapy is instituted. Standard treatment is intravenous penicillin G over 2 to 6 weeks, followed by oral penicillin V (2–4 g/day) for 6 to 12 months. In pregnant women, erythromycin is given. Patients allergic to penicillin can be given doxycycline, minocycline, or clindamycin. Additional surgical treatment may be warranted in cases of necrosis or abscess.

COURSE AND PROGNOSIS

Because the disease course is indolent, abdominal actinomycosis requires long-term therapy. Monitoring with computed tomography may be essential to follow therapeutic progress. If abdominal *Actinomyces* is associated with a malignancy, the course of the malignancy predicts the prognosis. However, if associated with chronic disease (e.g., diabetes mellitus), actinomycosis may be cured. Recurrence of the disease may occur with duration of therapy of less than 3 months.

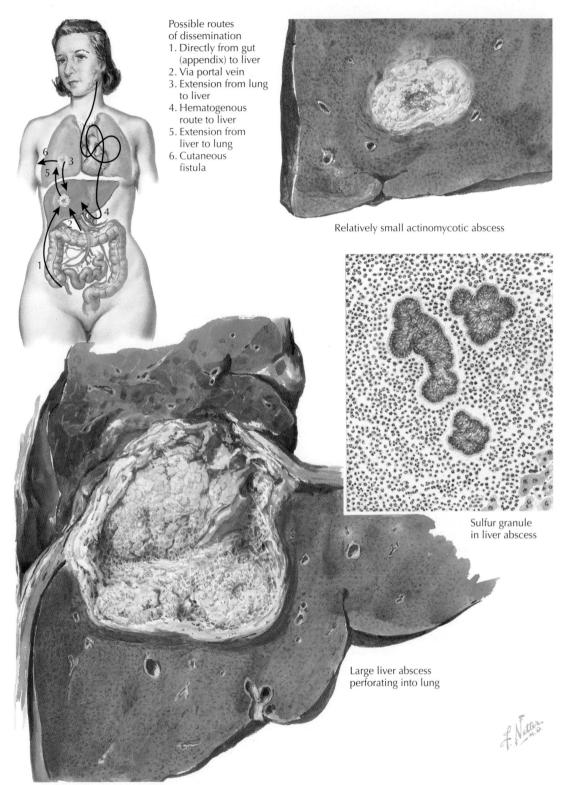

Possible routes
of dissemination
1. Directly from gut
   (appendix) to liver
2. Via portal vein
3. Extension from lung
   to liver
4. Hematogenous
   route to liver
5. Extension from
   liver to lung
6. Cutaneous
   fistula

Relatively small actinomycotic abscess

Sulfur granule
in liver abscess

Large liver abscess
perforating into lung

Fig. 114.1 Abdominal Actinomycosis.

ADDITIONAL RESOURCES

Könönen E, Wade WG: Actinomyces and related organisms in human infections, *Clin Microbiol Rev* 28(2):419–442, 2015.

Montori G, Allegri A, Merigo G, et al: Intra-abdominal actinomycosis, the great mime: case report and literature review, *Emerg Med Health Care* 3:2, 2015.

Russo TA: Agents of actinomycosis. In Mandell GL, Bennett JE, Dolin R, editors: *Mandell, Douglas and Bennett's principles and practice of infectious diseases*, ed 8, Philadelphia, 2015, Elsevier–Churchill Livingstone, pp 2864–2873.

Sung HY, Lee IS, Kim SI, et al: Clinical features of abdominal actinomycosis: a 15-year experience of a single institute, *J Korean Med Sci* 26(7):932–937, 2011.

Wong VK, Turmezei TD, Weston VC: Actinomycosis, *BMJ* 343:2011.

115

Amebiasis

C. S. Pitchumoni

Worldwide, amebiasis is caused by *Entamoeba histolytica* (*E. histolytica*) and is the third most common parasitic disease, affecting 50 million people and causing 100,000 deaths per year. It is highly prevalent in Central America, South America, Africa, and Asia. In the United States, *E. histolytica* represents the third most frequently identified protozoan infection from human specimens (1.2 cases per 100,000 persons), following *Giardia lamblia* and *Cryptosporidium parvum.* Although *Blastocystis hominis* is more common than the above three, the pathogenicity is controversial (Fig. 115.1). Amebiasis is spread through the fecal-oral route by contaminated food and water (see Fig. 115.1). Populations in countries with poor sanitation have the highest infection rates. An estimated 50,000 cysts are produced annually in a patient with invasive *E. histolytica.* The cysts are highly infective.

Entamoeba dispar is a noninvasive type of amoeba and is limited to the intestine. Its infection rate is estimated to be 7- to 10-fold higher than that of *E. histolytica.*

The *E. histolytica* trophozoites are liberated from the ingested cysts, and they become invasive. They may spread through the colonic mucosa, causing colitis, and enter the portal circulation to spread to the liver and form liver abscess, or disseminate to other sites. Hepato-pulmonary amebiasis (empyema, broncho-hepatic fistula, or extension of pleuropulmonary abscess and acute pericarditis), followed by cerebral and cutaneous amebiasis, is the most common type of extraabdominal amebiasis.

CLINICAL PICTURE

Most patients with intestinal amebiasis present with diarrhea that may be mild or may be full-blown colitis with bloody bowel movements, tenesmus, and cramps. In rare cases, it may become fulminant, and toxic colitis may develop. Only 10% of patients harboring *E. histolytica* have symptoms, others become chronic carriers. Abdominal pain and tenderness are common, but fever occurs in only 40% of patients. Incidental diagnosis of amebic colitis has been reported after surgical exploration in patients with toxic megacolon. The incidence of perforation is high when a colitis patient is treated with steroids with a presumptive diagnosis of ulcerative colitis. Colonic amebiasis mimics other causes of infectious diarrhea, inflammatory bowel disease, ischemic colitis, diverticulitis, and AV malformation. Ameboma is a mass of granulation tissue with peripheral fibrosis, located often in the ileocecal region. Ameboma may present with a colonic obstruction that mimics a carcinoma, Crohn disease, ileocecal tuberculosis, lymphoma, and Kaposi sarcoma.

DIAGNOSIS

Early diagnosis is based on clear identification of the organisms in the patient's stool. Patients with active colitis have erythrophagocytic form of trophozoites. Chronic carriers pass the cystic form in stool. When extraintestinal disease occurs, E. histolytica may or may not be present in feces, and stool examination is not helpful. Routine laboratory tests cannot distinguish between the nonpathogenic *E. dispar* and *E. histolytica.* Leukocytosis may or may not be present. Eosinophilia is not present.

A fecal antigen detection test (*E. histolytica* II ELISA) has a superior sensitivity as compared with stool microscopy. The test can also distinguish between *E. histolytica* and *E. dispar.* The PCR is superior in sensitivity but is complex and expensive. Serological tests are less sensitive in intestinal amebiasis as compared with hepatic abscess. Endoscopic diagnosis of amebic colitis can be difficult because its appearance may mimic other forms of colonic disease. Histologically, invasion by the organism through the mucosa and submucosa produces the characteristic flask shaped ulcer with a broad base composed of fibrin and cellular debris.

The differential diagnosis for any patient with colitis should include an evaluation for *E. histolytica,* especially in areas of the world where the infection is prevalent and in select areas of developed countries with poor sanitation and immigrant populations.

During the workup of the patient with an extraintestinal manifestation, such as a liver abscess, aspirated material becomes important for the diagnosis. Nearly 60% of the patients with amebic liver abscess do not have a concomitant amebic colitis, and hence stool examination for cyst/vegetative forms and/or endoscopy have little value. The liver abscess is initially identified through abdominal ultrasound, computed tomography, and magnetic resonance imaging. A diagnostic/therapeutic aspiration of the abscess has limited utility. However, aspiration may be needed when rupture of the abscess is thought to be imminent, differentiation between amebic and pyogenic abscess is critical, or there is a lack of response to antiprotozoal therapy. Sigmoidoscopy or stool examination may be negative in hepatic amebiasis and not useful.

TREATMENT AND MANAGEMENT

Treatment varies with the type of amebiasis. Asymptomatic cyst passers can be treated with luminal agents such as iodoquinol, 650 mg three times daily for 20 days; paromomycin, 500 mg three times daily for 7 days; or diloxanide furoate, 500 mg three times a day for 10 days (drug not currently available for use in the United States). If a patient has acute colitis, metronidazole (750 mg) plus one of the luminal agents is recommended for 7 to 10 days.[a]

For amebic liver abscess, metronidazole, 750 mg three times daily intravenously or orally, plus one of the luminal agents, is recommended for 7 to 10 days. Tinidazole, 800 mg three times orally daily for 5 days, is an alternative and is used frequently in other parts of the world.[a] Paramomycin is a nonabsorbable aminoglycoside and is a drug of choice in pregnant women.

---

[a]Pediatric doses are given according to weight (kg).

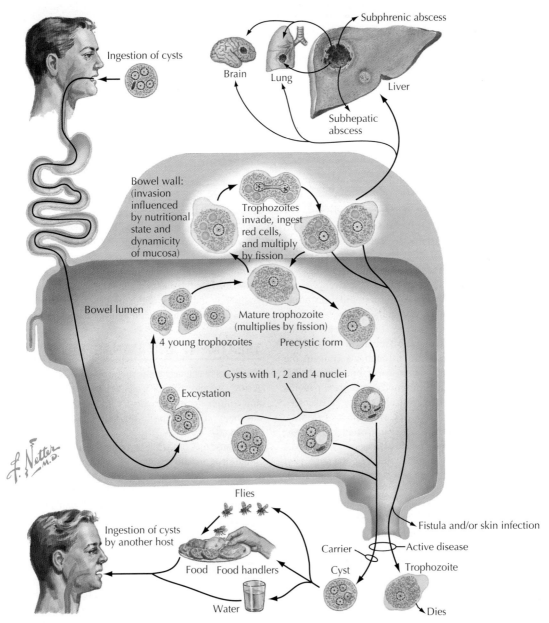

Fig. 115.1 Amebiasis: Fecal-Oral Spread of Disease.

With adequate treatment and early, diligent therapy, the mortality rate from liver abscess falls to less than 1%. The response is usually dramatic, within 3 days. Percutaneous drainage may be necessary, especially if an abscess might have ruptured. Emetine, a medication once popular in the treatment of amebiasis, is associated with potential cardiac toxicity. Dehydroemetine is effective in tissue infections like liver abscess, but not in luminal disease, and is preferred to emetine due to its lower toxicity. Dehydroemetine is available in the United States only from the Centers for Disease Control and Prevention.

PROGNOSIS

The prognosis is guarded for patients with amebiasis and HIV infection or autoimmune disease, but it is good for patients with amebiasis and minimal comorbidity.

ADDITIONAL RESOURCES

Haque R, Huston CD, Hughes M, et al: Amebiasis, *N Engl J Med* 348(16): 1565–1573, 2003.

Haque R, Mollah NU, Ali IK, et al: Diagnosis of amebic liver abscess and intestinal infection with the techlab entamoeba histolytica II antigen detection and antibody tests, *J Clin Microbiol* 38(9):3235–3239, 2000.

Hechenbleikner EM, McQuade JA: Parasitic colitis, *Clin Colon Rectal Surg* 28(2):79–86, 2015.

Gonzales ML, Dans LF, Martinez EG: Antiamoebic drugs for treating amoebic colitis, *Cochrane Database Syst Rev* (2):CD006085, 2009.

Mohapatra S, Singh DP, Alcid D, et al: Beyond O&P times three, *Am J Gastroenterol* 113:805–818, 2018.

Stanley SL Jr: Amoebiasis, *Lancet* 361(9362):1025–1034, 2003.

116

Giardia lamblia and Other Protozoan Infections

C. S. Pitchumoni

Giardia lamblia, also called *Giardia intestinalis* (or *G. duodenalis*), is a flagellated intestinal protozoan (Fig. 116.1). In the United States an estimated 1.2 million individuals are reported to develop gastrointestinal symptoms annually because of giardial infection. *G. lamblia* is the most frequently identified intestinal parasite in the United States.

The life cycle of *G. lamblia* includes a trophozoite (active) phase in the intestine, which encysts to a cystic phase. The cysts are transmitted easily in water or through contamination from numerous hosts, including domestic and wild animals as, for example, the beaver has gained attention as a potential source of Giardia contamination of lakes, reservoirs, and streams. The infection occurs through ingestion of the cysts via waterborne, foodborne, and person-to-person transmission. Infants, children, elderly persons, and immunocompromised patients are at high risk for infection. Other risk factors include day-care centers, immunodeficiency disorders, and men having sex with men (MSM). Hikers, backpackers, and campers who drink untreated water from lakes, streams, or wells also have a high chance of developing the infection. As few as 10 cysts may result in infection. Once the cysts pass through the stomach, acid stimulates them to form trophozoites, which enter the duodenum and attach to the mucosa. Some persons in areas with high infection rates develop immunity. *Giardia* attaches to the intestinal cells by virtue of its ventral disc. Once attached, it can cause a pathologic response, resulting in the clinical disease spectrum. Trophozoites multiply by binary fission, and when exposed to a hostile environment in the intestine, they can encyst. A heavily infected host may pass thousands of cysts into the environment.

CLINICAL PICTURE

Once *G. lamblia* trophozoites are formed in the duodenum, they cause symptoms. The incubation period lasts 7 to 14 days, but cysts do not appear in the stool until 1 week after symptoms develop. Hosts may be asymptomatic carriers, or they may acquire acute, self-limiting diarrhea or chronic diarrhea with complications. The short-lived diarrhea may go unnoticed or is ignored. Chronic diarrhea occurs in 25% to 30% of the patients, and a modest weight loss of 10 lbs can occur in 50% of the patients. The most severe presentations have been in children younger than 2 years and in persons with immunodeficiency or immunoglobulin A (IgA) deficiency. There is an association between secretory IgA deficiency and giardiasis and nodular lymphoid hyperplasia. Lactose intolerance occurs in 40% of patients that may persist for months. In school-age children, the infection may cause zinc deficiency.

DIAGNOSIS

Whenever a patient has prolonged diarrhea and has visited (or lives in) an endemic area for giardiasis or when an epidemic of giardial diarrhea exists in the community, the diagnosis of *G. lamblia* infection should be pursued. Cysts or trophozoites can be identified in the stool or duodenal aspirates, but the yield is usually very low, and identification varies in laboratories from 25% to 75%, depending on the technician's skill. The most reliable test now used is the stool antigen for *Giardia.* Currently, examination of duodenal aspirate or mucosal biopsy specimen is seldom performed for the diagnosis of giardia. When malabsorption develops, endoscopy and biopsy of the duodenum are indicated to rule out other diseases in the differential diagnosis of malabsorption.

TREATMENT AND MANAGEMENT

The drugs of choice include metronidazole, tinidazole, and nitazoxanide. A single 2-g dose of tinidazole is proven to have superior clinical efficacy and compliance as compared with metronidazole. Metronidazole can also be used at 250 mg (5 mg/kg for children) three times daily (tid) for 7 days.

Because metronidazole is contraindicated in pregnancy, paromomycin is the drug of choice, even though it is less effective than the other antibiotics. Some patients may require several courses of therapy because of resistant infection and should be evaluated for common variable immunodeficiency. Lactose intolerance should be ruled out when diarrhea persists. B_{12} deficiency noted in patients with heavy giardial infection usually corrects itself after the eradication of the parasite.

OTHER INTESTINAL PROTOZOANS

Dientamoeba fragilis is a flagellated protozoan that does not appear to form cysts. It is transmitted from person to person. Although rare, it can cause diarrhea with abdominal pain, anorexia, fatigue, and fever. Its exact incidence and pathologic significance remain evasive. Once identified, *D. fragilis* should be treated with iodoquinol, 650 mg orally (PO) tid for 20 days, or paramomycin (25–35 mg/kg/day orally in three divided doses for 7 days) or metronidazole, 500 to 750 mg tid for 10 days.

Balantidium coli is a ciliated protozoan (see Fig. 116.1), and infections have been reported after transmission from pigs. It is uncommon cause of diarrhea, but on occasion the bacterium has been reported to be invasive. If *B. coli* is found in the stool in a symptomatic patient, treatment is indicated. Tetracycline, 500 mg PO four times a day for 10 days, is the drug of choice. Alternatives are metronidazole and iodoquinol.

Blastocystis hominis is a parasite frequently found in stools; whether it can be pathogenic is controversial. Some clinicians think that after *B. hominis* is identified and treated, another organism is identified as the actual cause of the symptoms, and that cure results from treating the unknown organism. Regardless, when *B. hominis* is associated with diarrhea, it must be treated. The drug of choice is usually metronidazole (750 mg PO tid for 10 days) or iodoquinol (650 mg PO tid for 20 days). Trimethoprim-sulfamethoxazole and nitazoxanide are alternatives.

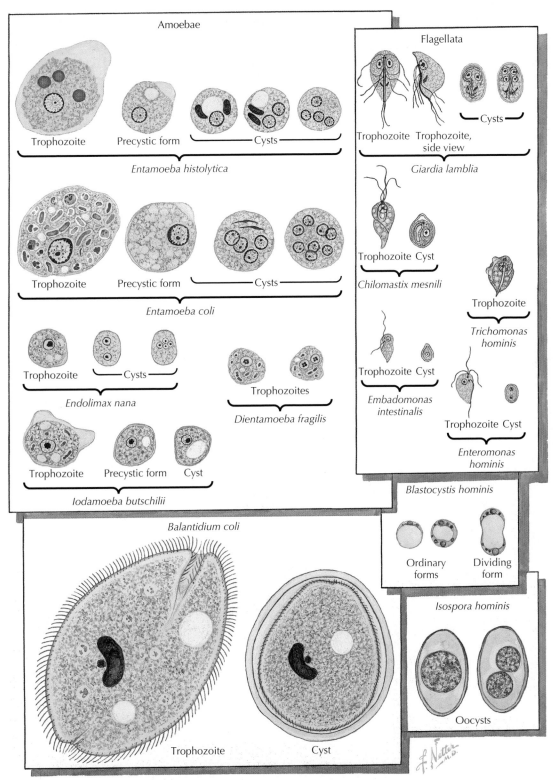

Fig. 116.1 *Giardia lamblia* and Other Protozoans.

INTRACELLULAR PROTOZOAN PARASITES

They are more prominent in elderly persons and immunocompromised patients. *Cryptosporidium parvum*, *Cyclospora cayetanensis*, and two species of microsporidia, *Enterocytozoon bieneusi* and *Encephalitozoon intestinalis*, are invasive organisms that can cause full-blown diarrhea along with fever, abdominal pain, and weight loss.

The cryptosporidiosis infection in the immunocompetent patients accounts for 2.2% of the cases of diarrhea in developed countries and 6.1% in developing countries. The infection spreads through the fecal-oral route. Many outbreaks of cryptosporidiosis have been associated with contaminated drinking water in the United States. In immunocompetent patients, the diarrhea is self-limiting, but in patients with CD4 count less than 50 cells/μL a fulminant infection occurs. The diarrhea is usually watery and associated with abdominal pain, nausea, vomiting, and fever. The diagnosis is made by identifying the organisms in the stool examination. However, immunofluorescent and enzyme immunoassay tests are superior in sensitivity and specificity and now commonly used in diagnostic laboratories. Treatment options depend on immune status. Treatment with nitazoxanide 500 mg BD PO for 3 days in immunocompetent patients is effective. In HIV patients a combination of antiparasitic therapy (nitazoxanide or paramomycin combined with azithromycin) with antiretroviral therapy is beneficial.

Isospora belli is related to *Cryptosporidium* and *Sarcocystis* and may cause protracted diarrhea, particularly in immunocompromised patients. Occasionally, *I. belli* has been identified in traveler's diarrhea. This obligate intracellular coccidian protozoan is found worldwide, but its infection rate is low and its epidemiology poorly understood. Its presentation may be similar to that of cryptosporidiosis or giardiasis, and the diagnosis of *I. belli* infection is made from examining stool samples or, when invasive, biopsy specimens of the small bowel.

Sarcocystosis, caused by protozoa of the *Sarcocystis* genus, is a rare infection in humans and is reported primarily in developing countries. It can cause necrotizing enteritis and, as with other protozoans, is diagnosed by the discovery of oocysts in the stool or the parasite in biopsy specimens.

ADDITIONAL RESOURCES

Cabada MM, White AC Jr: Treatment of cryptosporidiosis: do we know what we think we know?, *Curr Opin Infect Dis* 23(5):494–499, 2010.

Fletcher SM, Stark D, Harkness J, et al: Enteric protozoa in the developed world: a public health perspective, *Clin Microbiol Rev* 25(3):420–449, 2012.

Hill DR, Nash TE: Giardia lamblia. In Mandell GL, Bennett JE, Dolin R, editors: *Mandell, Douglas and Bennett's principles and practice of infectious diseases*, ed 8, Philadelphia, 2015, Elsevier–Churchill Livingstone, pp 3154–3160.

Minetti C, Chalmers RM, Beeching NJ, et al: Giardiasis, *BMJ* 355:i5369, 2016.

Mohapatra S, Singh DP, Alcid D, Pitchumoni CS: Beyond O&P times three, *Am J Gastroenterol* 113:805–818, 2018.

Soares R, Tasca T: Giardiasis: an update review on sensitivity and specificity of methods for laboratorial diagnosis, *J Microbiol Methods* 129:98–102, 2016.

117

Intestinal Helminths: Trichuriasis

C. S. Pitchumoni

Intestinal helminths are common worldwide, but the most important and common soil transmitted helminthic infections are by *Ascaris lumbricoides, Trichuris trichiura,* and the two hookworm species *Ancylostoma duodenale* and *Necator americanus.*

Trichuris trichiura is commonly known as the "whipworm" because of its morphology. Its life cycle is simpler than that of the other helminths (Fig. 117.1). *Trichuris* eggs are ingested in contaminated food and water (see Fig. 123.1). They mature in the distal small bowel and then pass into the colon. Adult worms migrate to the cecum and the appendix, where they live, copulate, and deposit eggs. The eggs pass through the feces to complete the life cycle.

Trichuriasis currently affects an estimated 1 billion persons worldwide, with most infections concentrated in the tropics or the semitropics. *Trichuris trichiura* most often infects humans, who are the only host of the species. It is identified in approximately 1% of stool specimens in the United States, most often in young children. Most humans harbor only a few worms, but the infection can be extremely heavy in some patients. The life span of the worm can range from 1 to 8 years, and each female may produce as many as 3000 to 20,000 eggs. The eggs may penetrate or attach to the mucosa and cause a significant pathologic response.

CLINICAL PICTURE

Mild *Trichuris* infections are asymptomatic. However, when the worm burden reaches more than 50 to 100, it may cause lower abdominal pain, diarrhea, distention, anorexia, and weight loss within a year. In children, it may cause dysentery. In developing countries, chronic infection can impair growth, and anemia may be severe and prolonged if trichuriasis is untreated.

Children with heavy infection can experience frequent, painful passage of stool that contains a mixture of mucus, water, and blood. Rectal prolapse is a known complication.

A beneficial role has been hypothesized for *Trichuris* (and perhaps other parasites) infection in childhood in regulating the gut immunology and reducing the burden of Crohn disease. *Trichuris suis* ova in treating Crohn disease and ulcerative colitis, bronchial asthma, and other allergic disorders is an interesting observation that needs to be further studied for clinical application.

DIAGNOSIS

Diagnosis of trichuriasis is usually made easily by the characteristic presence of eggs in stool specimens. The eggs are easy to identify because of their large number. It is surprising for an endoscopist to see the worms on sigmoidoscopy or colonoscopy, but they often can be seen hanging into the intestinal lumen. The accompanying anemia is iron deficient and microcytic, and is usually associated with low-grade eosinophilia.

TREATMENT AND MANAGEMENT

The present drugs of choice for trichuriasis are mebendazole, 100 mg orally twice daily for 3 days or 500 mg for one dose, and albendazole, 400 mg orally for 3 days. Cure rates with these drugs are approximately 40%. The worm burden is decreased with single-dose therapy, but decreasing the worm burden is often difficult, and 3-day therapy is required for any attempt at a cure. Repeat stool analysis should be performed.

PROGNOSIS

The prognosis is excellent. However, clinicians must remember that clearing the worm burden can be difficult and that repeat therapy may be necessary.

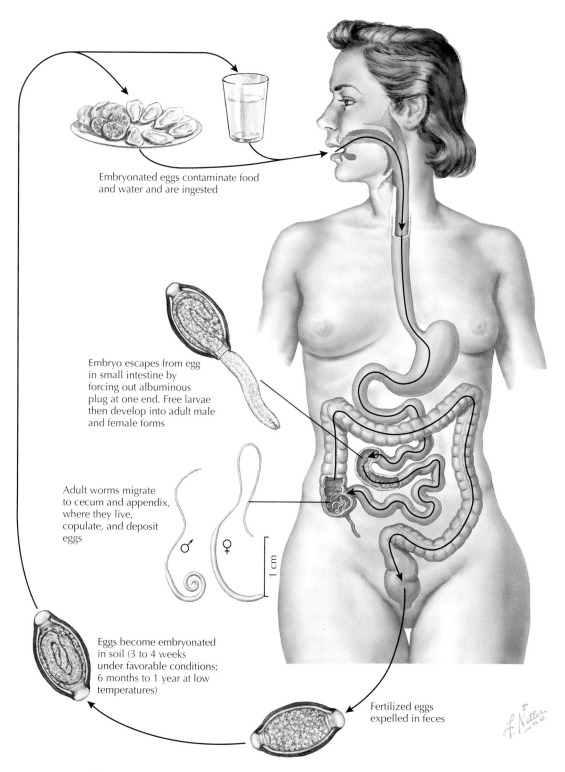

Embryonated eggs contaminate food and water and are ingested

Embryo escapes from egg in small intestine by forcing out albuminous plug at one end. Free larvae then develop into adult male and female forms

Adult worms migrate to cecum and appendix, where they live, copulate, and deposit eggs

♂ ♀

1 cm

Eggs become embryonated in soil (3 to 4 weeks under favorable conditions; 6 months to 1 year at low temperatures)

Fertilized eggs expelled in feces

Fig. 117.1 Trichuriasis: Life Cycle of Trichuris Nematode Helminth (Whipworm).

ADDITIONAL RESOURCES

Centers for Disease Control and Prevention: *Parasites—Trichuriasis (also known as whipworm infection)*. Last updated January 10, 2013. https://www.cdc.gov/parasites/whipworm/.

Maguire JH: Intestinal nematodes (Roundworms). In Mandell GL, Bennett JE, Dolin R, editors: *Mandell, Douglas and Bennett's principles and practice of infectious diseases*, ed 8, Philadelphia, 2015, Elsevier–Churchill Livingstone, pp 3199–3207.

Mohapatra S, Singh DP, Alcid D, Pitchumoni CS: Beyond O&P times three, *Am J Gastroenterol* 113:805–818, 2018.

118

Enterobiasis

C. S. Pitchumoni

Enterobiasis is caused by the pinworm *Enterobius vermicularis.* This nematode is probably the most common parasite to host on humans because it flourishes in temperate and tropical climates.

The small, spindle-shaped, white round adult worms inhabit the cecum and appendix, and adjacent parts of the large and small intestines; their heads attach to the intestinal mucosa. A male worm measures 2 to 5 mm in length, and the female 9 to 11 mm. The female produces eggs in its ovary and releases them into a reservoir, or uterus, where fecundation takes place. When the reservoir is filled, the worm detaches itself from the bowel wall and migrates down the colon to the rectum. Some parasites are expelled with feces, but others migrate through the anal canal and, while crawling, deposit eggs in the perianal and the genito-crural folds. On average, one female deposits 11,000 eggs. Within hours of passage, the eggs enter an infective stage, and they may be passed to humans by hand contact, from sheets and pillowcases, or directly onto food and water (Fig. 118.1; see also Fig. 123.1). Once the eggs are ingested, the larvae escape from the eggs into the stomach and the duodenum, molt twice, and pass into the large intestine to complete the life cycle.

CLINICAL PICTURE

Most pinworm infections are asymptomatic. School-age children are commonly affected, and it is a leading cause of malnutrition and growth retardation in children in developing nations. Severe anal itching in children is a common manifestation. However, adults also may be infected and may seek treatment for the same symptom. Perianal reactions by large burdens of worms can be intense. When they migrate from the perianal area, the worms can cause vaginitis, appendicitis, and rarely affect the peritoneum and ovary.

DIAGNOSIS

Demonstrating the *E. vermicularis* ova in feces or on a perianal specimen (using a strip of transparent tape) establishes the diagnosis. The test should be performed on three consecutive mornings right after the infected person wakes up and before he/she does any washing. The Centers for Disease Control and Prevention (CDC) does not recommend stool examination for O and P, since the yield is low.

TREATMENT AND MANAGEMENT

The drug of choice for treating enterobiasis is albendazole (400 mg), mebendazole (100 mg), Ivermectin (200 µg/kg), or pyrantel pamoate (11 mg/kg, maximum up to 1 g). The worms live from 7 to 13 weeks, and treatment is usually successful if the patient is not reinfected. A second dose is given in 2 weeks. However, reinfection is a major problem. Sheets and pillowcases must be cleaned thoroughly, and all infected family members must be treated to prevent reinfection. At times, the entire household, including curtains and floors, must be cleaned to eradicate the eggs.

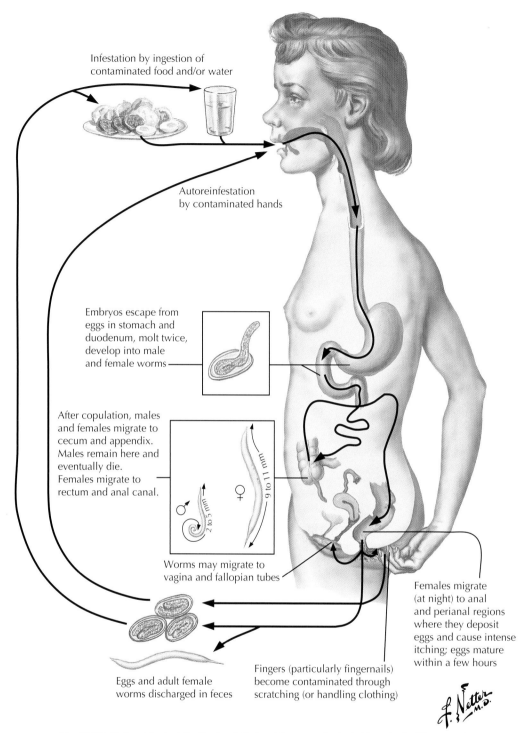

Infestation by ingestion of contaminated food and/or water

Autoreinfestation by contaminated hands

Embryos escape from eggs in stomach and duodenum, molt twice, develop into male and female worms

After copulation, males and females migrate to cecum and appendix. Males remain here and eventually die. Females migrate to rectum and anal canal.

Worms may migrate to vagina and fallopian tubes

Females migrate (at night) to anal and perianal regions where they deposit eggs and cause intense itching; eggs mature within a few hours

Eggs and adult female worms discharged in feces

Fingers (particularly fingernails) become contaminated through scratching (or handling clothing)

Fig. 118.1 Enterobiasis: Life Cycle of *Enterobius vermicularis* Nematode (Pinworm).

ADDITIONAL RESOURCES

Centers for Disease Control and Prevention: *Parasites—Enterobiasis (also known as pinworm infection).* https://www.cdc.gov/parasites/pinworm/diagnosis.html. Last updated January 10, 2013.

Maguire JH: Intestinal nematodes (Roundworms). In Mandell GL, Bennett JE, Dolin R, editors: *Mandell, Douglas and Bennett's principles and practice of infectious diseases*, ed 8, Philadelphia, 2015, Elsevier–Churchill Livingstone, pp 3199–3207.

Mohapatra S, Singh DP, Alcid D, Pitchumoni CS: Beyond O&P times three, *Am J Gastroenterol* 113:805–818, 2018.

119

Ascariasis

C. S. Pitchumoni

An estimated 807 to 1221 million people in the world are infected with *Ascaris lumbricoides*, the largest helminth to infect humans. The adult male measures 15 to 25 cm and is smaller than the female, which may be as large as 35 cm. These helminths may live for 10 to 18 months and usually copulate in the lumen of the small intestine; the mature female may produce up to 200,000 eggs daily.

The infection occurs when eggs are ingested from contaminated food or water. The eggs pass into the duodenum, where they liberate a larva that penetrates the small intestine and may reach the lungs (Fig. 119.1; see also Fig. 123.1).

A patient may have hypersensitivity reaction in the lung, causing the clinical manifestation of *Löffler syndrome,* which is usually self-limiting. Löffler syndrome manifests as an eosinophilic accumulation in the lung as a response to a parasitic infection. The larvae pass into the bronchi and are swallowed. They mature in the small intestine, where they copulate, and their eggs are passed into feces to complete the life cycle.

CLINICAL PICTURE

Once the worms reach the lower intestine, the symptoms of ascariasis develop depending on the worm load and the location of the parasite. Most of the patients with ascaris infection are asymptomatic or have mild abdominal discomfort, nausea, dyspepsia, or loss of appetite. A heavy worm load may cause weight loss or malnutrition. Complications of chronic ascariasis include intestinal obstruction, obstruction of bile and pancreatic ducts, appendicitis, intestinal perforation, intussusception, and bowel necrosis requiring emergent surgical intervention. The worms can also migrate to the pancreatic and biliary systems, resulting in duct obstruction with jaundice, cholecystitis, cholangitis, and/or pancreatitis, referred to as *hepatobiliary ascariasis.* Intestinal obstruction is common in children. Live worms have been noted in sputum and vomitus.

DIAGNOSIS

The diagnosis of ascariasis is made by demonstration of the larvae, ova, or worms on stool microscopy, combined with peripheral eosinophilia (in tissue migration phase). In the pulmonary phase, eosinophils and Charcot-Leyden crystals may be found in sputum, and larvae also have been recovered from sputum. Lung involvement precedes any intestinal phase by 8 to 10 weeks, but eggs do not appear in the feces in the early stage.

The large adult worms and the characteristic eggs are easy to identify on stool examination.

TREATMENT AND MANAGEMENT

The pulmonary phase of ascariasis, although self-limited, may require treatment to control all symptoms, sometimes necessitating the use of steroids. Anthelmintic treatment is ineffective for pneumonia. The most important intervention to reduce the burden of intestinal ascariasis is to prevent infection, in areas of the world that have poor sanitation. Mass chemotherapy in epidemic areas has been tried, but there is no substitute for improved sanitation. The drug of choice for treatment of the intestinal phase is albendazole, 400 mg orally (PO) once; mebendazole, 100 mg PO twice daily for 3 days or 500 mg once; or ivermectin, 200 μg/kg PO once. Safety in children or pregnant women remains to be established.

PROGNOSIS

The prognosis of early diagnosed ascariasis is excellent.

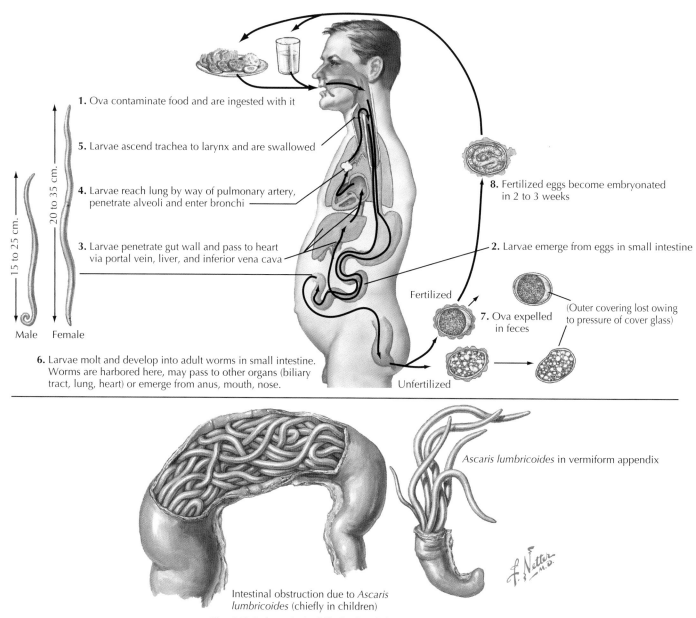

1. Ova contaminate food and are ingested with it

5. Larvae ascend trachea to larynx and are swallowed

4. Larvae reach lung by way of pulmonary artery, penetrate alveoli and enter bronchi

3. Larvae penetrate gut wall and pass to heart via portal vein, liver, and inferior vena cava

8. Fertilized eggs become embryonated in 2 to 3 weeks

2. Larvae emerge from eggs in small intestine

Fertilized

7. Ova expelled in feces

(Outer covering lost owing to pressure of cover glass)

Unfertilized

15 to 25 cm.

20 to 35 cm.

Male   Female

6. Larvae molt and develop into adult worms in small intestine. Worms are harbored here, may pass to other organs (biliary tract, lung, heart) or emerge from anus, mouth, nose.

Intestinal obstruction due to *Ascaris lumbricoides* (chiefly in children)

Ascaris lumbricoides in vermiform appendix

Fig. 119.1 Ascariasis: Life Cycle of *Ascaris lumbricoides.*

ADDITIONAL RESOURCES

Centers for Disease Control and Prevention. *National center for Health Statistics. Parasites—Ascariasis.* https://www.cdc.gov/parasites/ascariasis/index.html. Last updated May 24, 2016.

Khuroo MS, Rather AA, Khuroo NS, Khuroo MS: Hepatobiliary and pancreatic ascariasis, *World J Gastroenterol* 22(33):7507–7517, 2016.

MacGuire JH: Intestinal nematodes (Roundworms). In Mandell GL, Bennett JE, Dolin R, editors: *Mandell, Douglas and Bennett's principles and practice of infectious diseases,* ed 8, Philadelphia, 2015, Elsevier–Churchill Livingstone, pp 3199–3207.

120

Strongyloidiasis

C. S. Pitchumoni

Strongyloidiasis, caused by the nematode *Strongyloides stercoralis* (*S. stercoralis,* threadworm), is prevalent in Asia, Africa, Oceania, South America, Southern Europe, and southeastern states of the United States (Kentucky, Virginia, Tennessee, and North Carolina). In the United States, the predisposing factors for the infection include immigrants and military veterans who have lived in endemic areas, and patients with malnutrition, chronic obstructive pulmonary disease (COPD), chronic renal failure, alcoholism, or underlying malignancies. The mode of infection is by contact with contaminated soil with free living larvae that penetrate the skin and migrate throughout the body prior to the lungs and finally to the small intestine. The larvae from the lungs are coughed up and swallowed, and reach the small intestine. Here they mature into the adult female worm, which can produce rhabditiform larvae by means of parthenogenesis. Larvae are also found in the heart, liver, gallbladder, brain, genitourinary organs, and nervous system (Fig. 120.1). The larvae are then swallowed and enter the duodenum, where the adults attach to or penetrate the wall. The female worm is tiny—no more than 2 mm in length. It enters the small bowel mucosa, where it can extrude eggs (see Fig. 123.1). A sexual cycle of development then occurs in which the rhabditiform larvae develop into males and females, and pass eggs into the soil, which then form filariform larvae that can restart the cycle.

However, a short life cycle can occur in which the rhabditiform larvae mature and penetrate the skin in the perianal area and autoinfect the host. Parasitologists debate these varieties in the life cycle. Autoinfection is well documented, and rhabditiform larvae do develop adult sexual forms in soil.

Hyperinfection can occur if large numbers of organisms enter the host, usually in an immunocompromised patient or when one is treated with corticosteroids. The worms are able to regulate their own populations, but when a host is treated with corticosteroids, the eggs produce increased amounts of ecdysteroid substances (a steroid structurally similar to androgens) in host tissue, which allow proliferation of adult female worms and eggs and a massive number of larvae. Hyperinfection has been associated with millions of adult worms or filarial larvae in the mucosa of the small and large intestines.

CLINICAL PICTURE

Most patients with strongyloidiasis are asymptomatic, and larvae may be fortuitously encountered in the stool. However, if the infestation persists, symptoms may affect many organs. The patient may have a characteristic cutaneous lesion at the site in the perianal area by autoinfection or on the feet if the infection occurred through the soil. When the immune status is compromised, strongyloidiasis causes hyperinfection syndrome and disseminated disease, which can be life threatening. Hyperinfection may be precipitated in those on steroid therapy, human T-cell leukemia-lymphoma virus, hematologic malignancies, and transplant patients. Patients with hyperinfection may have gastroenteritis with severe diarrhea, abdominal pain, and malabsorption. The symptoms may mimic ulcerative colitis. Peripheral eosinophilia, a feature of classic strongyloidiasis, is absent in hyperinfection syndrome. The multisystem involvement includes maculopapular or urticarial rash, pulmonary symptoms such as pneumonitis, and CNS symptoms such as meningitis and brain abscesses. Since the clinical picture is varied, the astute clinician must be alert to suspect the infection.

DIAGNOSIS

Eosinophilia is invariably present. If there is clinical suspicion of strongyloidiasis in a patient with eosinophilia, the stool should be screened carefully for larvae, although the sensitivity of the test is low. Many techniques are used to identify the larvae, and the yield depends on the parasitology laboratory. Currently an enzyme linked immunoassay with 90% sensitivity, although with a lower specificity, is recommended by the CDC. An assay that uses luciferase immunoprecipitation system to identify IgG antibodies to a recombinant *Strongyloides* antigen and *S. stercoralis* immunoreactive antigen and has a 100% sensitivity and specificity.

TREATMENT AND MANAGEMENT

The drug of choice for strongyloidiasis is *ivermectin,* 200 µg/kg/day orally for 2 days. Safety in children less than 15 kg (33 lb) in weight or in pregnant women remains to be determined. Ivermectin is well tolerated compared with the previously used thiabendazole, which is no longer available in many countries. An alternative drug, albendazole, 400 mg twice daily for 7 days, is reported to be less effective.

Treatment of hyperinfection syndrome requires ivermectin for at least 7 days after the stool, sputum, and urine samples become negative.

ADDITIONAL RESOURCES

Centers for Disease Control and Prevention—National Center for Health Statistics. *Parasites—Strongyloides* 2015; https://www.cdc.gov/parasites/strongyloides/. (Accessed 13 April 2015).

Kassalik M, Mönkemüller K: Strongyloides stercoralis hyperinfection syndrome and disseminated disease, *Gastroenterol Hepatol (N Y)* 7(11):766–768, 2011.

MacGuire JH: Intestinal nematodes (Roundworms). In Mandell GL, Bennett JE, Dolin R, editors: *Mandell, Douglas and Bennett's principles and practice of infectious diseases,* ed 8, Philadelphia, 2015, Elsevier–Churchill Livingstone, pp 3199–3207.

Marathe A, Date V: *Strongyloides stercoralis* hyperinfection in an immunocompetent patient with extreme eosinophilia, *J Parasitol* 94:759–760, 2008.

Mendes T, Minori K, Ueta M, et al: Strongyloidiasis current status with emphasis in diagnosis and drug research, *J Parasitol Res* 2017:5056314, 2017.

Mohapatra S, Singh DP, Alcid D, et al: Beyond O&P times three, *Am J Gastroenterol* 113:805–818, 2018.

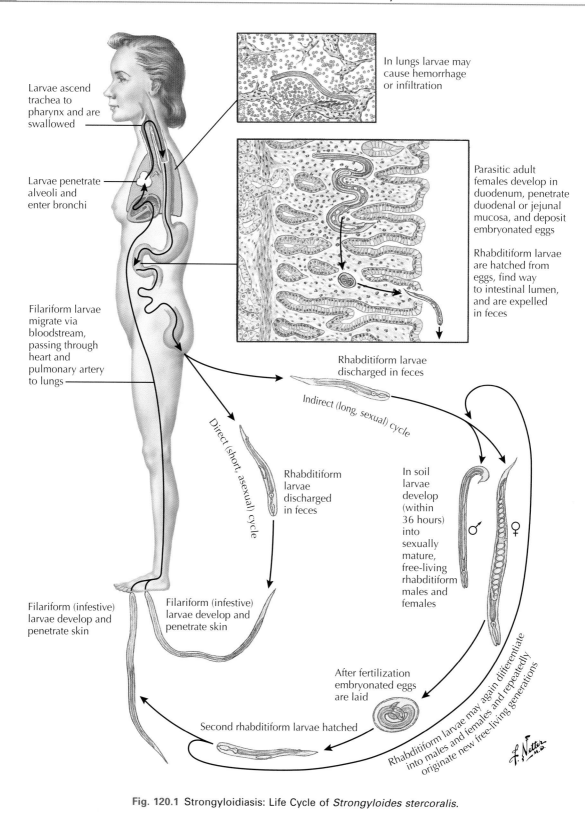

Larvae ascend trachea to pharynx and are swallowed

Larvae penetrate alveoli and enter bronchi

Filariform larvae migrate via bloodstream, passing through heart and pulmonary artery to lungs

Filariform (infestive) larvae develop and penetrate skin

In lungs larvae may cause hemorrhage or infiltration

Parasitic adult females develop in duodenum, penetrate duodenal or jejunal mucosa, and deposit embryonated eggs

Rhabditiform larvae are hatched from eggs, find way to intestinal lumen, and are expelled in feces

Rhabditiform larvae discharged in feces

Indirect (long, sexual) cycle

Direct (short, asexual) cycle

Rhabditiform larvae discharged in feces

In soil larvae develop (within 36 hours) into sexually mature, free-living rhabditiform males and females

Filariform (infestive) larvae develop and penetrate skin

After fertilization embryonated eggs are laid

Second rhabditiform larvae hatched

Rhabditiform larvae may again differentiate into males and females and repeatedly originate new free-living generations

Fig. 120.1 Strongyloidiasis: Life Cycle of *Strongyloides stercoralis.*

121

Hookworm Disease (Necatoriasis and Ancylostomiasis)

C. S. Pitchumoni

Hookworm disease is caused by either of two nematodes, *Necator americanus* (New World hookworm) or *Ancylostoma duodenale* (Old World hookworm). *N. americanus* is found in the Western Hemisphere in tropical and subtropical areas and also in Africa and Asia. *A. duodenale* is found in the Mediterranean region and in parts of Europe and Asia; it is rarely, if ever, seen in the Western Hemisphere. The worms measure 7 to 9 mm, but *Ancylostoma* may be much larger than *Necator* and is more prolific, producing 10,000 to 30,000 eggs.

The life cycles of *A. duodenale* and *N. americanus* are essentially the same (Fig. 121.1), and the infection is acquired by skin penetration when walking barefoot in soil contaminated with hookworms. The worms attach to the small intestine, where they feed on the blood and lymph of the host, and the fertilized female lays eggs. Large numbers of eggs are passed in the feces. Rhabditiform larvae develop in warm moist soil, and the larvae penetrate human skin, pass through the circulation to the lungs, and are then swallowed to complete the life cycle in the duodenum (see Fig. 123.1). The worms may live for years in the host.

An estimated 1 billion persons harbor hookworms, which surprisingly were not identified as human parasites until the mid-19th century. They heavily infect children but can be unusually virulent and cause chronic infections and anemia in elderly persons. They probably are a major cause of iron deficiency anemia worldwide. Each worm can cause 0.03 to 0.26 mL of blood loss per day. *Ancylostoma* is larger and more aggressive in its drainage. Hookworms develop in tropical and subtropical areas, where larvae can grow in the soil.

CLINICAL PICTURE

Anemia is the distinguishing characteristic of hookworm infestation. The anemia relates to the burden of the infestation. Young children in underdeveloped countries may experience the impaired growth and development resulting from anemia, whereas elderly persons may experience the debilitating effects of anemia.

The filariform larvae penetrate the skin, and a local inflammatory reaction may develop (ground itch). As the larvae migrate through the lungs, they may cause hypersensitivity pneumonia and Löffler eosinophilic syndrome characterized by dry cough and asthmatic wheezing. When the worms inhabit the duodenum, they may cause abdominal pain, nausea, vomiting, and diarrhea. Eosinophilia is usually, but not always, present. When the worm burden exceeds the host's intake of iron and protein, iron deficiency anemia and protein malnutrition develop. In children, hookworm infection may cause growth retardation and intellectual and cognitive impairment.

The migratory phase of the larvae may encompass creeping eruption or cutaneous larva migrans, typically caused by canine or feline hookworm larvae (*Ancylostoma braziliense*). In some parts of the world, such as Australia, the dog hookworm (*Ancylostoma caninum*) has been reported to cause eosinophilic gastroenteritis.

Most patients have only mild infection; thus the infestation may go unnoticed or the patient might have only mild anemia. Large infestations can cause severe symptoms.

DIAGNOSIS

The diagnosis of hookworm disease is made on finding the characteristic eggs in the stools, combined with peripheral eosinophilia on complete blood count. Classic concentration techniques are used to find the eggs, and they are easily identified in most parasitology laboratories. Hookworm eggs of all types are similar, and the species is distinguished by identifying the larvae or the actual worm.

TREATMENT AND MANAGEMENT

Many drugs are available to rid the host of hookworms, but results may be variable. Mebendazole, 100 mg twice daily for 3 consecutive days or 500 mg once, and albendazole, 400 mg in a single dose, are highly effective. However, these drugs are associated with rare toxicity and thus are discouraged in patients with blood dyscrasia, leukopenia, or liver disease. Therefore pyrantel pamoate, 11 mg/kg (maximum 1 g), can be given daily for 3 days.

It may be necessary to institute iron replacement therapy if a patient has experienced continuous blood loss, and anemia should be monitored in any patient with chronic infestation. Children with impaired growth should be followed closely to ensure that hookworm was the cause and that it is corrected by iron and blood replacement.

COURSE AND PROGNOSIS

The prognosis is excellent once the host is rid of the hookworm burden. It is important that prevention be part of the therapy because reinfection can occur. Unfortunately, in parts of the world where sanitation and social conditions do not permit improvement to the environment, reinfection occurs. At present, there is no vaccine to prevent hookworm infection.

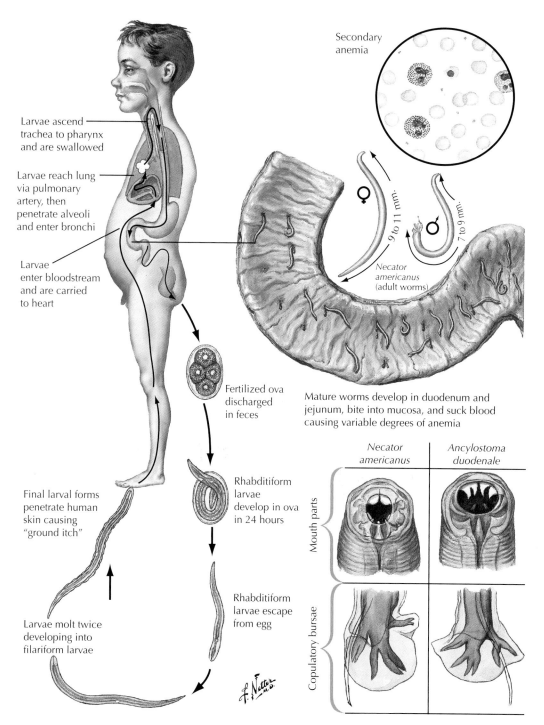

Larvae ascend trachea to pharynx and are swallowed

Larvae reach lung via pulmonary artery, then penetrate alveoli and enter bronchi

Larvae enter bloodstream and are carried to heart

Final larval forms penetrate human skin causing "ground itch"

Larvae molt twice developing into filariform larvae

Fertilized ova discharged in feces

Rhabditiform larvae develop in ova in 24 hours

Rhabditiform larvae escape from egg

Secondary anemia

Necator americanus (adult worms)

9 to 11 mm.

7 to 9 mm.

Mature worms develop in duodenum and jejunum, bite into mucosa, and suck blood causing variable degrees of anemia

	Necator americanus	*Ancylostoma duodenale*
Mouth parts		
Copulatory bursae		

Fig. 121.1 Hookworm Disease: Life Cycle of *Necator americanus* (Necatoriasis) and *Ancylostoma duodenale* (Ancylostomiasis).

ADDITIONAL RESOURCES

Centers for Disease Control and Prevention. *Treatment Guidelines from The Medical Letter,* Vol. 11 (Suppl), 2013.

Drugs for parasitic infections, New Rochelle, NY, 2007, Medical Letter.

Elliott DE: Intestinal worms. In Feldman M, Friedman LS, Brandt LJ, editors: *Gastrointestinal and liver disease,* ed 8, Philadelphia, 2006, Saunders-Elsevier, pp 2435–2457.

Keiser J, Utzinger J: Efficacy of current drugs against soil-transmitted helminth infections: systematic review and meta-analysis, *JAMA* 299:1937–1948, 2008.

MacGuire JH: Intestinal nematodes (Roundworms). In Mandell GL, Bennett JE, Dolin R, editors: *Mandell, Douglas and Bennett's principles and practice of infectious diseases,* ed 8, Philadelphia, 2015, Elsevier–Churchill Livingstone, pp 3199–3207.

Mohapatra S, Singh DP, Acid D, Pitchumoni CS: Beyond O&P times three, *Am J Gastroenterol* 113:805–818, 2018.

122

Tapeworms (Cestodes)

C. S. Pitchumoni

The four clinically important cestodes, or flatworms, are *Taenia saginata* (beef tapeworm), *Taenia solium* (pork tapeworm), *Diphyllobothrium latum* (fish tapeworm), and *Hymenolepis nana* (dwarf tapeworm). The tapeworms live in the intestine of vertebrates (the primary or definitive host) but spend a part of their lifecycle in animals (intermediate hosts). The term proglottid refers to one of the segments of a tapeworm formed by a process of strobilation (a form of asexual reproduction) in the neck region of the worm which contains both male and female reproductive organs. The scolex is the worm's head that attaches to the intestine of the primary host. The scolex is covered with hooks or suckers that characterize the worm.

Table 122.1 summarizes the data on the mode of infection, clinical features, diagnostic methods, and management of the four clinically important tapeworms.

TAENIA INFECTIONS

Taenia solium

T. solium, or pork tapeworm, causes clinical manifestations both by the adult and larval stages. Eating infected undercooked pork is the source of infection. The muscle contains cysticercus stage (when the scolex is inverted in the sac) of the organism and as the meat is digested; cysticercus breaks down, releasing a scolex that attaches to the upper jejunum (Fig. 122.1). The adult form develops in 10 to 12 weeks. As a hermaphrodite, it reproduces by self or cross fertilization. The mature proglottids and eggs are released in the feces which are then consumed by the pig. In the pig, eggs hatch into oncospheres and can migrate to the striated muscle where they form the cysticerci.

TABLE 122.1 Clinical Data, Diagnosis, and Management of Cestode Infections

Parasite	Mode of Infection (Consumption of Infected)	Clinical Features	Diagnosis (Stool Examination)	Management
Taenia saginata (beef tapeworm) Europe, Asia, Australia, Canada	Undercooked meat (beef)	• Asymptomatic • Abdominal pain, diarrhea	Eggs and proglottid	Praziquantel[a] Alternatively Niclosamide[b]
Taenia solium (pork tapeworm) Latin America, eastern Europe, sub-Saharan Africa, India, and Far East	Raw/undercooked pork	• Disseminated infection (cystecercosis) • Skeletal muscle, brain, subcutaneous tissue, myocardium may be infected	Eggs and proglottid (Coproantigen ELISA test as an early indicator for treatment failure)	Albendazole 400 mg orally thrice daily for 3 days Praziquantel[a]
Diphyllobothrium latum (fish tapeworm) Scandinavia, Baltic countries, Japan, and Swiss lakes region	Undercooked freshwater fish	• Asymptomatic • Abdominal discomfort • Vomiting • Weight loss • Intestinal obstruction • Gallbladder disease • Megaloblastic anemia (B_{12} deficiency)	Eggs and proglottid (characteristic central uterus)	Single dose of Niclosamide[b] or Praziquantel[a]
Hymenolepis nana (dwarf tapeworm) Asia, southern and eastern Europe, southern America, and Africa. In the US institutionalized, immunocompromised, and malnourished patients	Contaminated food Only tapeworm that is transmitted from human to human	• Asymptomatic • Children with heavy infection have abdominal cramps, anorexia, dizziness, and diarrhea	Eggs (characteristic double membrane)	Praziquantel[a] or Niclosamide[b]

[a]Praziquantel 5 to 10 mg/kg single dose orally.
[b]Niclosamide 2 g single dose orally.
ELISA, Enzyme-linked immunosorbent assay.
From Bustos JA, Rodriguez S, Jimenez JA, et al: Detection of *Taenia solium* taeniasis coproantigen is an early indicator of treatment failure for taeniasis. *Clin Vaccine Immunol* 19(4):570-573, 2012.

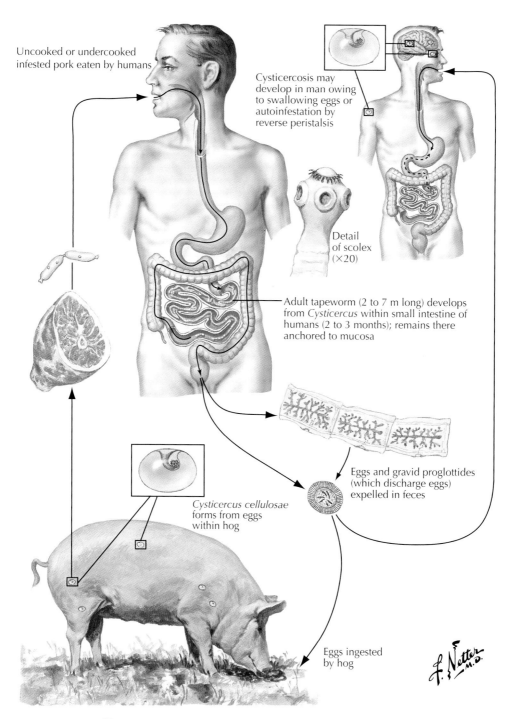

Uncooked or undercooked
infested pork eaten by humans

Cysticercosis may
develop in man owing
to swallowing eggs or
autoinfestation by
reverse peristalsis

Detail
of scolex
(×20)

Adult tapeworm (2 to 7 m long) develops
from *Cysticercus* within small intestine of
humans (2 to 3 months); remains there
anchored to mucosa

Eggs and gravid proglottides
(which discharge eggs)
expelled in feces

Cysticercus cellulosae
forms from eggs
within hog

Eggs ingested
by hog

Fig. 122.1 Pork Tapeworm Infection: Life Cycle of *Taenia solium.*

T. solium can also cause autoinfection, when the person acquires infection when in contaminated feces. This is the cause of dissemination of cysts and neurocysticercosis.

The gastrointestinal symptoms are nonspecific, and most of the patients remain asymptomatic. Abdominal pain, nausea, and vomiting are the chief complaints, which are relieved by eating small amounts of food. Weight loss, caused by loss of appetite, is more noticeable in children than in adults. Neurocysticercosis can cause neurologic abnormalities which presents as hemiparesis, seizures, and sensory disturbances.

Taenia saginata

T. saginata is also known as beef tapeworm, and the infection occurs upon ingestion of infected larval cysts found in the meat of cattle. The life cycle of *T. saginata* is almost similar to that of *T. solium,* but there is no autoinfectivity (Fig. 122.2). The infection is mostly asymptomatic, but a small number have reported abdominal cramps or malaise. The proglottids of *T. saginata* are motile and can be found in the perineum, clothing, or after passing feces. These events are often psychologically disturbing and can have anxiety-associated symptoms.

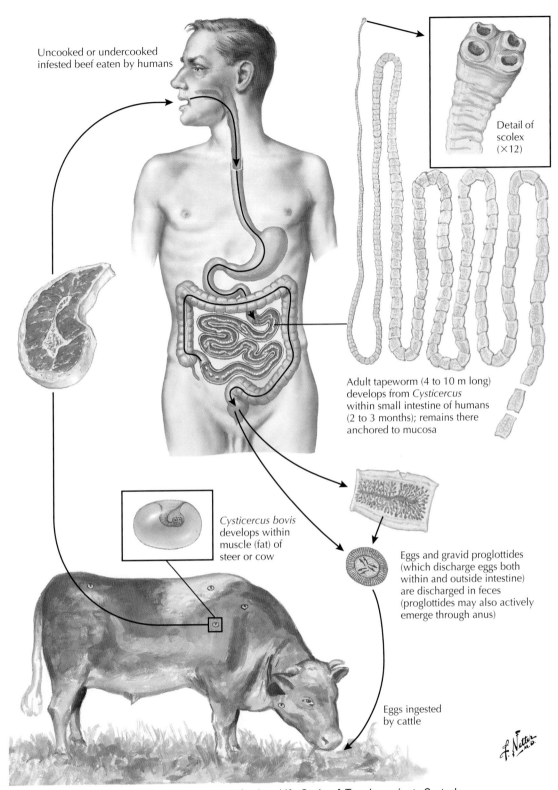

Uncooked or undercooked infested beef eaten by humans

Detail of scolex (×12)

Adult tapeworm (4 to 10 m long) develops from *Cysticercus* within small intestine of humans (2 to 3 months); remains there anchored to mucosa

Cysticercus bovis develops within muscle (fat) of steer or cow

Eggs and gravid proglottides (which discharge eggs both within and outside intestine) are discharged in feces (proglottides may also actively emerge through anus)

Eggs ingested by cattle

Fig. 122.2 Beef Tapeworm Infection: Life Cycle of *Taenia saginata* Cestode.

Diphyllobothrium latum

D. latum (broad tapeworm/fish tapeworm) is the most important of the many *Diphyllobothrim* worm that infect human beings. Areas endemic for *D. latum* include Siberia, Scandinavia, Japan, and Chile. Although there is a decrease in the incidence of diphyllobothriasis in several countries, there is a reemergence in Russia, South Korea, Japan, and South America. Human *D. latum* worms are large, reaching nearly 40 feet (12 m) in length.

The parasite eggs that reach the fresh water, embryonate and release the free-swimming larvae (coracidia). Coracidia are ingested by the water fleas (Cyclops) and develop into plerocercoid larvae (Fig. 122.3).

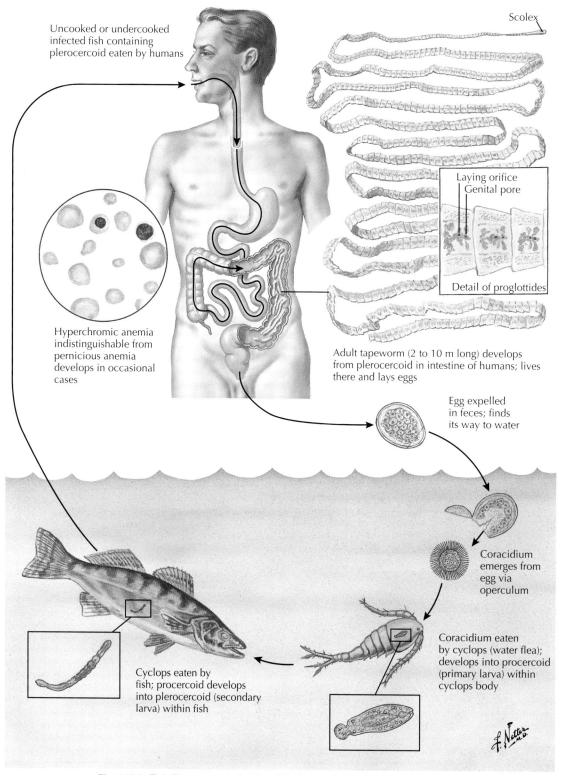

Fig. 122.3 Fish Tapeworm Infection: Life Cycle of *Diphyllobothrium latum.*

These are consumed by the freshwater fish, and the parasite turns into an infective plerocercoid form. The plerocercoid larvae are embedded in fish. The infection is acquired by eating uncooked freshwater fish. Consumption of dry or smoked fish and "raw bar" foods such as ceviche, sushi, and sashimi has caused small epidemics in developed nations. The symptoms of the infestation are nonspecific and include weakness, dizziness, salt craving, and abdominal discomfort. The parasite dissoci-ates the B_{12}-intrinsic factor complex in the gut lumen, making B_{12} unabsorbable, and uses B_{12}. Folate deficiency may also occur.

Hymenolepis nana

H. nana (Fig. 122.4) is the smallest but the most common tapeworm to colonize people. It has a worldwide distribution, with highest preva-lence in hot and arid regions. Transmission occurs by direct infection

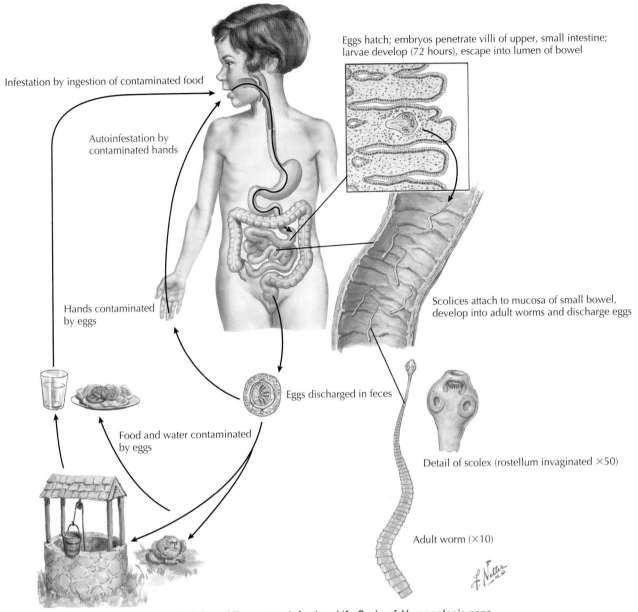

Infestation by ingestion of contaminated food

Eggs hatch; embryos penetrate villi of upper, small intestine; larvae develop (72 hours), escape into lumen of bowel

Autoinfestation by contaminated hands

Hands contaminated by eggs

Scolices attach to mucosa of small bowel, develop into adult worms and discharge eggs

Eggs discharged in feces

Food and water contaminated by eggs

Detail of scolex (rostellum invaginated ×50)

Adult worm (×10)

Fig. 122.4 Dwarf Tapeworm Infection: Life Cycle of *Hymenolepis nana*.

from person to person and self-inoculation. The self-inoculation or the autoinfection allows for colonization to persist for years. There is no intermediatory host, and thus it is found in the institutionalized persons in the United States. Ingestion of infested fleas, beetles, mealworms, and cockroaches allows for transmission, although this is a rare occurrence.

Most people infested with *H. nana* are asymptomatic but heavy worm load can cause anorexia, abdominal pain, and diarrhea.

ADDITIONAL RESOURCES

King CH, Fairley JK: Tapeworms (Cestodes). In Mandell GL, Bennett JE, Dolin R, editors: *Mandell, Douglas and Bennett's principles and practice of infectious diseases*, ed 8, Philadelphia, 2015, Elsevier–Churchill Livingstone, pp 3227–3236.

123

Other Helminth Infections:
Trichinella spiralis and Flukes

C. S. Pitchumoni

TRICHINOSIS

The most common *Trichinella* species in the United States is *Trichinella spiralis,* which is almost worldwide in its distribution. However, other *Trichinella* species infect humans in Africa and in the arctic regions. Humans become infected by eating undercooked pork meat. The main reservoir is the pig.

The life cycle of *Trichinella* has an intestinal phase and a muscular phase. When the uncooked meat is eaten, larvae are released in the small intestine, where they go through four phases of development to adulthood. After approximately 1 week, the adult female worms produce larvae which cross the intestinal wall, spread via blood vessels, and settle in the striated muscle. A single worm may produce as many as 1500 larvae. The second-generation larvae can survive in the host for many years. In the United States the number of trichinosis cases reported each year is usually less than 50.

Clinical Picture

During the initial stage of trichinosis, a patient may have mild gastroenteritis with nausea, vomiting, or abdominal pain, and diarrhea. This phase may last up to 1 week. When the larvae enter the muscle, myalgia, fever, periorbital edema, and systemic signs of allergic response develop. The more larvae present, the more severe will be the disease. Generalized edema may develop, and proteinuria can follow. Central nervous system signs and symptoms, cardiomyopathy, and extraocular muscle involvement occur in patients with moderate to severe infection.

Muscle tenderness can be readily detected, along with an unusually high white blood cell count, increased level of immunoglobulin E, muscle enzymes (creatinine kinase and lactate dehydrogenase) and significant eosinophilia. In pregnant women, *Trichinella* infection can cause abortion or premature delivery.

Diagnosis

The diagnosis of trichinosis is made by obtaining muscle tissue and demonstrating the parasitic complexes. The diagnosis can also be made by detecting *Trichinella*-specific DNA using polymerase chain reaction. After approximately 2 weeks, enzyme-linked immunosorbent assay can detect the antibodies in some patients.

Treatment and Management

Albendazole (400 mg twice daily for 8–14 days) or mebendazole (200–400 mg three times a day for 3 days, followed by 400–500 mg three times a day or 10 days) are recommended as the first-line treatment. If symptoms are severe, corticosteroids may be helpful in decreasing inflammation.

Prevention and Control

Prevention is still the best method for avoiding trichinosis. All meat should be cooked thoroughly at 58.5°C for 10 minutes. Freezing also kills the worms, but the meat must be frozen at −20°C for at least 3 days. One species, *Trichinella nativa,* is resistant to freezing. Hunters and humans who eat wildlife should be cautious because they are particularly susceptible to *Trichinella* infestation if they eat meat that is not cooked properly.

FLUKE INFECTIONS

Flukes are trematodes with complex life cycles. The most common are the schistosomes (blood flukes), affecting the liver. Rarer fluke infections involve liver flukes and other intestinal flukes.

Liver Flukes

The clinically important human liver flukes are *Clonorchis sinensis, Opisthorchis viverrini,* and *Fasciola hepatica.* An important intestinal fluke is *Fasciolopsis buski.* Humans become infected because they eat raw freshwater fish. Liver flukes live in the biliary tract, and eggs pass into stool. There are two intermediate hosts: snails, then freshwater fish. It is estimated that as many as 7 million people are infected in some parts of Asia. Fluke infection of the liver is associated with cholangitis, cholecystitis, cholelithiasis, hepatocellular carcinoma, and cholangiocarcinoma.

F. hepatica can infect humans who eat watercress contaminated with excysted metacercariae. Snails are the intermediate host, and herbivorous mammals are easily infected. Larvae in the small intestine can penetrate the gut, migrate through the peritoneal cavity, and enter the liver. They then migrate through the liver and enter the bile ducts, where they spend the rest of their lives. Patients may have acute infections that can appear as acute hepatitis. Diagnosis is usually confirmed by finding the ova in the bile or the stool. Fig. 123.1 shows ova of *C. sinensis* and *F. hepatica,* as well as those of intestinal helminths described in previous chapters.

Intestinal Fluke

F. buski is the intestinal fluke. It is seen throughout Asia and infects humans, pigs, and dogs. Snails are the intermediate host, and the cercariae subsist on water plants. Ingestion of the plants results in the encystment of larvae and the formation of mucosal abscesses in the small intestine. Diagnosis is made by finding the eggs in the stool, and the treatment of choice is praziquantel.

Clinical Picture

Flukes may live in the bile ducts for as long as 10 to 30 years. They may cause liver enlargement and every type of biliary condition, including adenomas, fibrosis, and stricture of the bile ducts.

Diagnosis and Treatment

The diagnosis of fluke infection is made by identifying ova in the stool or in bile obtained by endoscopic retrograde cholangiopancreatography. The treatment of choice is praziquantel.

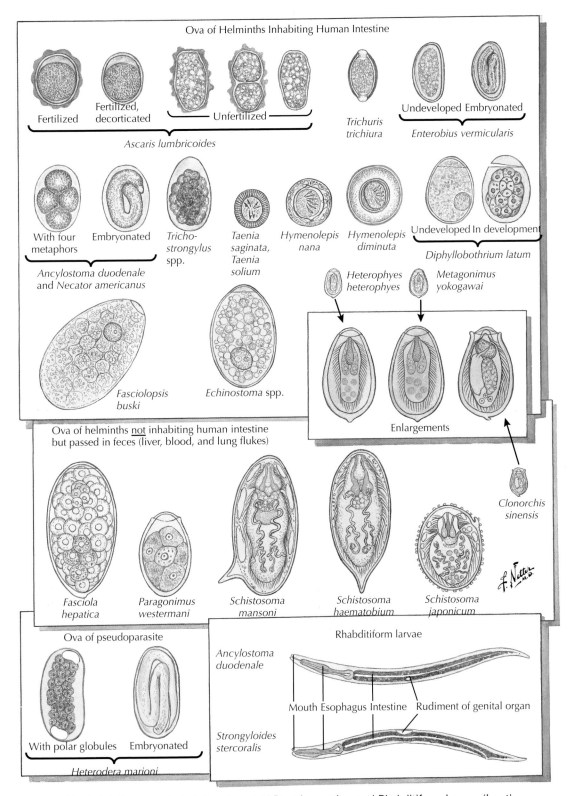

Fig. 123.1 Ova of Helminth Parasites and Pseudoparasites and Rhabditiform Larvae *(Inset).*

ADDITIONAL RESOURCES

Fürst T, Keiser J, Utzinger J: Global burden of human food-borne trematodiasis: a systematic review and meta-analysis, *Lancet Infect Dis* 12(3):210–221, 2012.

Kazura JW: Tissue nematodes (trichinellosis, dracunculiasis, filariasis, loiasis, and onchocerciasis). In Mandell GL, Bennett JE, Dolin R, editors: *Mandell, Douglas and Bennett's principles and practice of infectious diseases,* ed 8, Philadelphia, 2015, Elsevier–Churchill Livingstone, pp 3208–3215.

Xia J, Jiang SC, Peng HJ: Association between liver fluke infection and hepatobiliary pathological changes: a systematic review and meta-analysis, *PLoS ONE* 10(7):e0132673, 2015.

Pancreas

C. S. Pitchumoni

124

Development and Anatomy of the Pancreas

C. S. Pitchumoni

One of the earliest references to the pancreas as a distinct organ occurs in the Talmud, which refers to the organ as "the finger of the liver." Aristotle (384–322 BCE) believed the organ had the sole function of protecting the neighboring vessels. Herophilus of Chaldikon, in the third century BCE, made some initial anatomic descriptions. Almost 200 years later, Rufus of Ephesus used the term "pancreas" (pan, all; kreas, flesh). George Wirsung described the structure of the major pancreatic duct in humans in 1642 CE. Approximately 100 years later, Giovanni Santorini described the accessory pancreatic duct. Paul Langerhans discovered the endocrine pancreas in 1869 CE. In 1889 Oskar Minkowski and Joseph von Mering observed that pancreatectomized dogs developed diabetes and died soon afterward. In 1921 Frederick Banting and Charles Best discovered insulin at the University of Toronto.

The pancreas arises from two diverticula of the foregut, in a region that later becomes the duodenum (Fig. 124.1). Early in the fifth week of gestation, a larger dorsal bud develops proximally just above the level of the hepatic diverticulum. The ventral outpouch appears soon afterward. Growing fairly rapidly and extending into the dorsal mesentery of the duodenum near the developing omental bursa, the dorsal pancreatic bud passes in front of the developing portal vein. Because of the more rapid growth of the duodenum, the ventral bud, together with the developing *common bile duct* (CBD), rotates backward behind the duodenum. When the rotation is completed, the original ventral bud comes to lie close to, below, and somewhat behind the dorsal pancreas, and eventually its tip lies behind the superior mesenteric vein and the root of the portal vein.

From the larger dorsal bud originates the cephalad part of the head, as well as the neck, body, and tail of the pancreas, whereas the caudate part of the head and the uncinate process derive from the smaller ventral bud. Ducts develop in both buds but anastomose. During the seventh week, the dorsal and ventral buds fuse, enclosing the vena cava. The secretions of the neck, body, and tail are subsequently shunted into the duct of the smaller ventral pancreas, which becomes the principal pancreatic *duct of Wirsung*. Only the upper portion of the head is finally drained by the original duct of the dorsal pancreas, the accessory *duct of Santorini*.

The pancreas in the adult is 14 to 18 cm long, 2 to 9 cm wide, and 2 to 3 cm thick and extends transversely across the abdomen from the concavity of the duodenum to the spleen. It has four parts: head, neck, body, and tail (Fig. 124.2). Located deep in the epigastrium and the left hypochondrium behind the lesser omental sac, approximately on the level of the first and second lumbar vertebrae (L1-L2), the gland escapes physical examination. The head is globular and has an inferior extension, and the *lingula* (uncinate process) projects hooklike to the left and is crossed anteriorly by the superior mesenteric vessels. Covered anteriorly by the pylorus and transverse colon, the head fits snugly into the loop of the duodenum, so that the CBD passes either through a groove or through the substance of the gland. The posterior surface of the head touches the inferior vena cava, left renal vein, and aorta. The splenic artery and vein extend along its upper border. Its anterior surface, covered by serosa, is separated by the omental bursa from the posterior wall of the stomach. The inferior surface, below the attachment of the transverse mesocolon, is related to the duodenojejunal junction and to the splenic flexure of the colon. The posterior surface is in contact with the aorta, splenic vein, and left kidney, where the body tapers off into a short tail.

The lymphatics of the pancreas arise as fine periacinar and perilobular capillary networks extending along the blood vessels to the surface of the gland. Direct lymphatic connections exist wherever the pancreas is attached to other organs.

The arterial blood supply to the head of the pancreas, together with the duodenum, is by an anterior and posterior pancreaticoduodenal arcade formed by the union of anterior and posterior branches of the superior and inferior pancreaticoduodenal arteries. Inferior and superior pancreatic arteries supply the neck and the body. The splenic artery supplies the tail and body of the pancreas through several branches.

The pancreas has a rich nerve supply. The sympathetic nerves reach the pancreas through the greater and lesser splanchnic trunks arising from the fifth to the ninth thoracic ganglion through the greater splanchnic nerve. The parasympathetic fibers reach the pancreas through the vagi. Pancreatic nerves influence hormonal secretions playing a role in glucose metabolism. They also control exocrine pancreatic secretions and digestion and absorption of food.

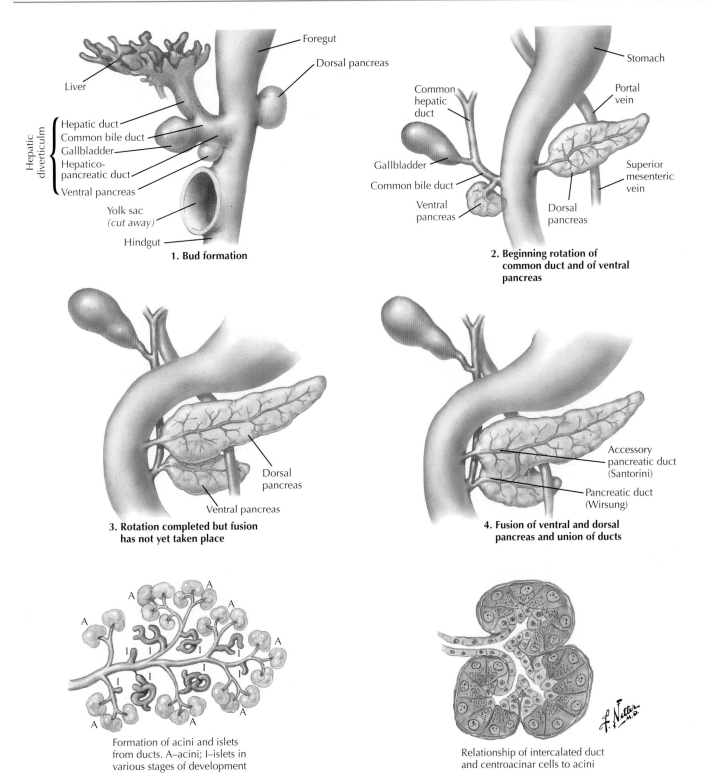

1. Bud formation

2. Beginning rotation of common duct and of ventral pancreas

3. Rotation completed but fusion has not yet taken place

4. Fusion of ventral and dorsal pancreas and union of ducts

Formation of acini and islets from ducts. A–acini; I–islets in various stages of development

Relationship of intercalated duct and centroacinar cells to acini

Fig. 124.1 Development and Anatomy of the Pancreas.

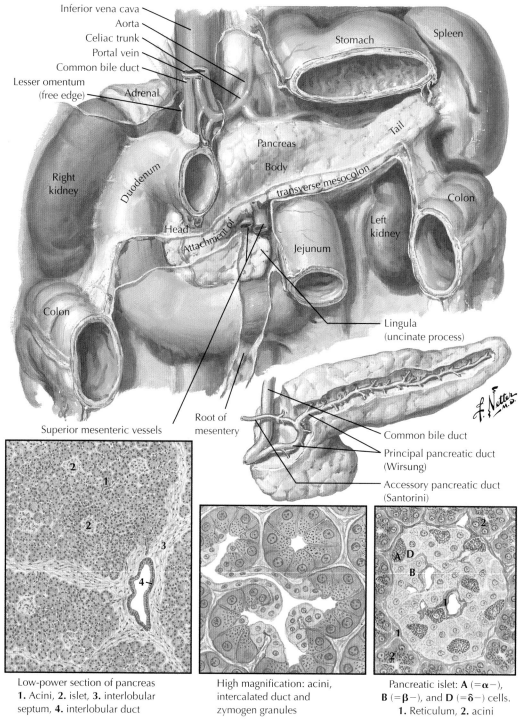

Inferior vena cava
Aorta
Celiac trunk
Portal vein
Common bile duct
Lesser omentum
(free edge)
Adrenal

Stomach
Spleen

Pancreas

Body
Tail

Right
kidney

Duodenum

transverse mesocolon

Colon

Head
Attachment of

Jejunum

Left
kidney

Lingula
(uncinate process)

Colon

Superior mesenteric vessels

Root of
mesentery

Common bile duct

Principal pancreatic duct
(Wirsung)

Accessory pancreatic duct
(Santorini)

Low-power section of pancreas
1. Acini, **2.** islet, **3.** interlobular
septum, **4.** interlobular duct

High magnification: acini,
intercalated duct and
zymogen granules

Pancreatic islet: **A** (=**α**−),
B (=**β**−), and **D** (=**δ**−) cells.
1. Reticulum, **2.** acini

Fig. 124.2 Anatomy of the Pancreas.

ADDITIONAL RESOURCES

Bockman DE: Anatomy of the pancreas. In Go VLW, editor: *The pancreas: biology, pathobiology, and disease,* New York, 1993, Raven Press, pp 1–8.

Bockman DE: Nerves in the pancreas: what are they for? *Am J Surg* 194(4): S61–S64, 2007.

Dudeja V, Christein JD, Jensen EH, Vickers SM: Exocrine pancreas. In Townsend CM, Beuachamp RD, Evers BM, Mattox KL, editors: *Sabiston textbook of surgery,* ed 20, Philadelphia, 2017, Saunders–Elsevier, pp 1520–1555.

Longnecker D: Anatomy and histology of the pancreas. *Pancreapedia: Exocrine Pancreas Knowledge Base,* 2014. *Version 1.*

125

Pancreatic Ducts and Exocrine and Endocrine Organs

C. S. Pitchumoni

The pancreas is an integrated organ with endocrine and exocrine functions. The acinar cells make up almost 90% of the gland's mass, ductal tissue approximately 5%, and 10^5 to 10^6 islets of Langerhans occupy approximately 2% of the pancreas. The arrangement of the pancreatic ducts within the gland varies considerably and even more so in relationship with the terminal common bile duct (CBD) (Fig. 125.1). Occasionally, the relative size of the two ducts (Santorini and Wirsung) is reversed so that the duct of Santorini remains the main duct. The accessory duct ordinarily inserts into the duodenum proximally, on a separate papilla (minor), but may enter through the papilla of Vater. The main pancreatic duct enters the duodenum either through a separate orifice or through a common channel, the ampulla of Vater.

The main pancreatic duct begins in the tail. Centrally located, it courses to the right through the body and neck and is joined by tributaries that usually enter at right angles, alternating from opposite sides. In the head, the main duct usually turns caudally and dorsally and comes close to or joins the CBD while coursing through the substance of the pancreas. The main duct usually drains the tail, neck, and body and the caudal and dorsal portions of the head. Magnetic resonance cholangiopancreatography (MRCP) is the most common noninvasive imaging test. Measurements based on MRCP studies are important with regards to ductal diameters. Diameters of 3.5 mm at the head, 2.5 mm in the body, and 1.5 mm in the tail and a length of 14 to 18 cm should be considered normal. As age advances, the size of the head, body, and tail of the pancreas shrinks. Pancreatic anteroposterior (AP) diameter significantly decreases with aging which is as a result of pancreatic fibrosis. Pancreatic ductal ectasia in relation to aging is not a uniform observation.

The *sphincter of Oddi* is formed by smooth muscles surrounding three sites: the lower end of the CBD, the major pancreatic duct, and the ampulla.

Pancreas divisum is a congenital variant of the ductal morphology in which the dorsal and ventral pancreatic ducts do not fuse. This abnormality is reported in up to 14% of autopsy studies and in 2% to 7% of patients undergoing endoscopic retrograde cholangio pancreatography (ERCP). In pancreas divisum, the bulk of the enzyme flow occurs through the accessory papilla, which is narrower than the main duct. If the orifice is too small or is stenotic, the intraductal pressure is increased and may give rise to pancreatitis.

Annular pancreas is a rare malformation in which a band of pancreatic tissue surrounds the descending portion of the duodenum, with smooth continuation to the head of the pancreas. Partial obstruction of the duodenum may be a clinical presentation in childhood or later. *Heterotopia* of the pancreas is healthy pancreatic tissue developing in an abnormal location with no vascular, neuronal, or anatomic continuity with the main pancreas.

The *exocrine pancreas* is a compound acinar gland, similar in structure to the salivary gland, which lacks islets of Langerhans. The functional units consist of an acinus and its draining duct, and the units are separated by fine, connective tissue septa that have blood vessels, lymphatics, nerves, and secretory ducts. The nucleus of the acinar cell is located near the broad base. The cytoplasm is basophilic and contains numerous acidophilic, highly refractile zymogen granules, which contain the proenzymes. The *acinar cells* of the pancreas are among the richest cells of the body in RNA content and have the highest protein turnover. The most enigmatic *centroacinar cells* of the pancreas are smaller than acinar cells. They are located at the junction of acini and ducts. These ductal cells are devoid of zymogen granules. Carbonic anhydrase is associated with bicarbonate production and is present in the centroacinar cells and in the ductal epithelium. Intercalated ducts, which partially penetrate and drain the acini, are lined by centroacinar and clear cells. Intralobular ducts are also lined by cells with clear cytoplasm. Centroacinar cells play an important role in regulating the contents of distal ductal lumen.

Pancreatic stellate cells (PSCs) located within the periacinar spaces contribute to all pancreatic cells under physiologic conditions. The stellate cells are rich in vitamin A and are necessary to maintain normal pancreatic architecture. PSC activation occurs in pancreatic injury by alcohol, smoking, and other factors. PSC stimulation results in an active state of the cells (myofibroblastic) which play a role in the pathogenesis of pancreatic injury, repair, and pancreatic cancer.

The *pancreatic islets (islets of Langerhans)*, scattered over the gland but especially in the body and tail, consist of cells structurally and functionally different from those of the exocrine parenchyma. Adult human islets consist of 10% alpha (α) cells, 70% beta (β) cells, 15% pancreatic polypeptide (PP) cells, and 5% delta (δ) cells. The α cells secrete glucagon; the β cells, insulin; the PP cells, PP; and the β cells, somatostatin.

ADDITIONAL RESOURCES

Andren-Sandberg A, Hardt PD: Second giessen international workshop on interactions of exocrine and endocrine pancreatic diseases. Castle of rauischholzhausen of the justus-liebig-university, Giessen (Rauischholzhausen), Germany. March 7-8, 2008, *JOP* 9(4):541–575, 2008.

Apte MV, Pirola RC, Wilson JS: Pancreatic stellate cells: a starring role in normal and diseased pancreas, *Front Physiol* 3:344, 2012.

Ballian N, Hu M, Liu S, Brunicardi C: Proliferation, hyperplasia, neogenesis and neoplasia in the islets of Langerhans: a review, *Pancreas* 35:199–206, 2007.

Beer RL, Parsons MJ, Rovira M: Centroacinar cells: at the center of pancreas regeneration, *Dev Biol* 413(1):8–15, 2016.

Johnson LR: Pancreatic secretion. In Johnson LR, editor: *Gastrointestinal physiology*, ed 7, Philadelphia, 2007, Mosby-Elsevier, pp 85–95.

Özcan S: microRNAs in pancreatic β-cell physiology, *Adv Exp Med Biol* 887:101–117, 2015.

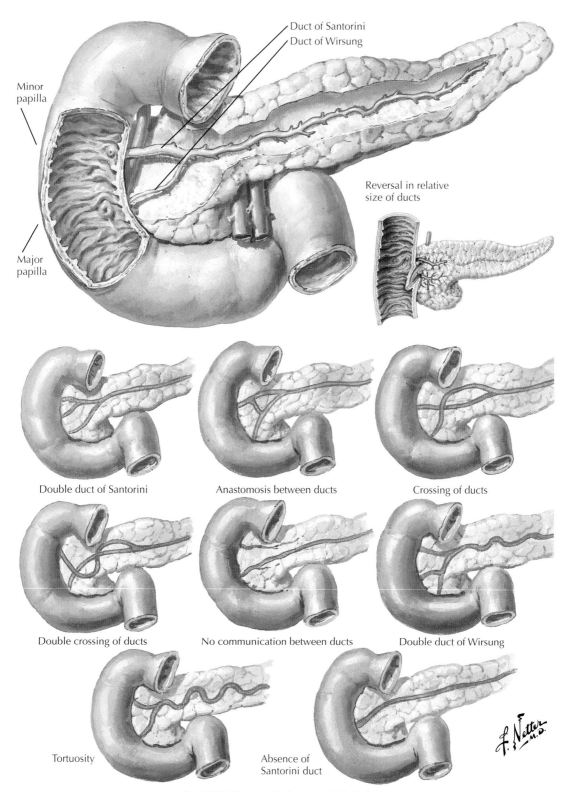

Duct of Santorini

Duct of Wirsung

Minor papilla

Major papilla

Reversal in relative size of ducts

Double duct of Santorini

Anastomosis between ducts

Crossing of ducts

Double crossing of ducts

No communication between ducts

Double duct of Wirsung

Tortuosity

Absence of Santorini duct

Fig. 125.1 Pancreatic Ducts and Variations.

126

Pancreatic Physiology

C. S. Pitchumoni

The pancreas is an integrated organ with three components, which are the endocrine, exocrine, and exocrine ductal part. Acinar cell secretion is regulated by the islets through paracrine and endocrine secretions. In addition to the islets and acinar cells, the role played by centroacinar cells (CACs) is being increasingly recognized. The CACs are located within the center of acinii at the ductular terminus. The CACs play a major role in regulating the contents of the distal ductal lumen.

Each day, 1 to 2.5 L of colorless, bicarbonate-rich fluid is secreted by the exocrine pancreas. The pancreatic secretion is regulated in three phases: cephalic, gastric, and intestinal. The intestinal phase is the most important in regard to ductal secretion. The pancreas secretes approximately 0.2 to 0.3 mL of juice each minute in the interdigestive phase, which can increase to 3.15 mL/min in response to hormonal stimulation and a meal (Fig. 126.1). Digestive enzymes are secreted by the acinar cells, and a large volume of bicarbonate-rich solution is produced by the centroacinar and ductal cells. Intracellular Ca^{2+} modulates acinar cell function. Pancreatic enzymes are packed in zymogen granules in the apical pole. The role of the pancreatic secretion is to digest fat, proteins, and starch. Together with bile, it is responsible for fat absorption.

The basal bicarbonate concentration at low secretory rates is approximately 30 to 60 mmol/L, increasing to as high as 135 mmol/L after stimulation by gastric acid entering the duodenum. The bicarbonate secretion helps to neutralize the gastric acid entering the duodenum, thus providing an ideal pH for the digestive enzymatic action. It also prevents the inactivation of bile acids by gastric acid. The bicarbonate concentration of the ductal secretion is more than five times of the serum value. The gene *cystic fibrosis transmembrane conductance regulator (CFTR)* is a critical player in HCO_3^- secretion.

The pancreatic secretion is rich in proteins and has a concentration of 7 mg/mL after stimulation of cholecystokinin (CCK). The acinar cells secrete 17 different proteins. Only amylase and lipase are secreted in the active form; all the proteolytic enzymes are secreted as inactive proenzymes.

Pancreatic amylase hydrolyzes dietary starch, glycogen, and other carbohydrates (except cellulose) to produce disaccharides and a few trisaccharides. Digestion of starch by pancreatic amylase is a continuation of the process initiated by salivary amylase.

Pancreatic lipase hydrolyzes neutral fat into fatty acids and monoglycerides. Lipase has a molecular weight of 48,000 daltons and isoelectric point of 6.5, a major difference from salivary or gastric lipase, which is stable at acid pH. Pancreatic lipase activity decreases from a maximal value at pH 7.5 to total inhibition at pH 4.5. *Colipase* is secreted as a proenzyme and activated by tryptic digestion, and it enhances lipase activity in the presence of bile salts. Pancreatic colipase is believed to be helpful in anchoring the pancreatic lipase to the lipid droplets and micelles. The breakdown products of fat digestion have low solubility in water, but the solubility is substantially enhanced after micelle formation by primary bile acids. Cholesterol esterase of pancreatic secretion hydrolyzes the ester bonds to yield free cholesterol. Phospholipases split lecithin to lysolecithins and free fatty acid.

Proteolytic enzymes (trypsinogen, chymotrypsinogen, carboxypeptidase, and several elastases) secreted as zymogens degrade dietary proteins into amino acids and oligopeptides composed of up to six amino acid residues. *Trypsinogen* is converted to trypsin by the intestinal brush border enzyme enterokinase. Active trypsin then converts other zymogens into their active forms. Three forms of trypsinogen have been identified in human pancreatic juice—cationic, anionic, and intermediate—representing more than 20% of the total proteins of pancreatic juice. Proteolytic enzymes secreted as zymogens degrade dietary proteins into amino acids and oligopeptides composed of up to six amino acid residues. To protect the pancreas from autodigestion, the acinar cells also produce trypsin inhibitors. Proteases also play a part in clearing the complex dietary B_{12} with R-binding protein so that intrinsic factor can bind with vitamin B_{12} for further absorption in the terminal ileum.

Pancreatic secretion is regulated by interdependent hormonal and neuronal mechanisms. Two intestinal hormones, *secretin* and CCK, stimulate the ductular secretion and the acinar cells, respectively. Neuronal influence occurs through not only hormonal release but also by direct cholinergic control of the exocrine pancreas. There is also a paracrine influence in the acinar cells. Pancreatic secretion has three phases: cephalic, gastric, and intestinal. In the gastric phase, vagovagal reflex effects are seen from the stomach to the pancreas. A *pyloropancreatic reflex* mechanism for pancreatic protein secretion is also reported. Food in the antrum of the stomach is a strong stimulant of pancreatic enzymes, in addition to its role in stimulating gastrin production. The most important phase of pancreatic secretion is the intestinal phase.

Secretin, the first peptide hormone identified, in 1902, is released in response to acid chyme and, to a lesser extent, by sodium oleate and bile acids, entering the duodenum with pH less than 4.5 to 5. Secretin-producing cells (S cells) are located in the duodenal and jejunal mucosa. Secretin stimulates the water and bicarbonate (145 mEq/L concentration) secretion in the duodenum, pancreatic and biliary ducts. Secretin also inhibits food stimulated gastrin release and lower esophageal sphincter pressure.

CCK is produced by intestinal I cells located in the duodenum and jejunum. The secretion of CCK is stimulated predominantly by products of partial protein digestion, proteases, and peptones and, to a small extent, by long-chain fatty acids and hydrochloric acid. There is a negative feedback inhibition of CCK release by pancreatic proteases in the duodenum.

CCK primarily stimulates the acinar cells by acting on neuronal pathways. Acetylcholine is a major stimulant. Vagotomy or administration of atropine greatly reduces the pancreatic enzyme response to food in the intestine. CCK suppresses appetite and food intake.

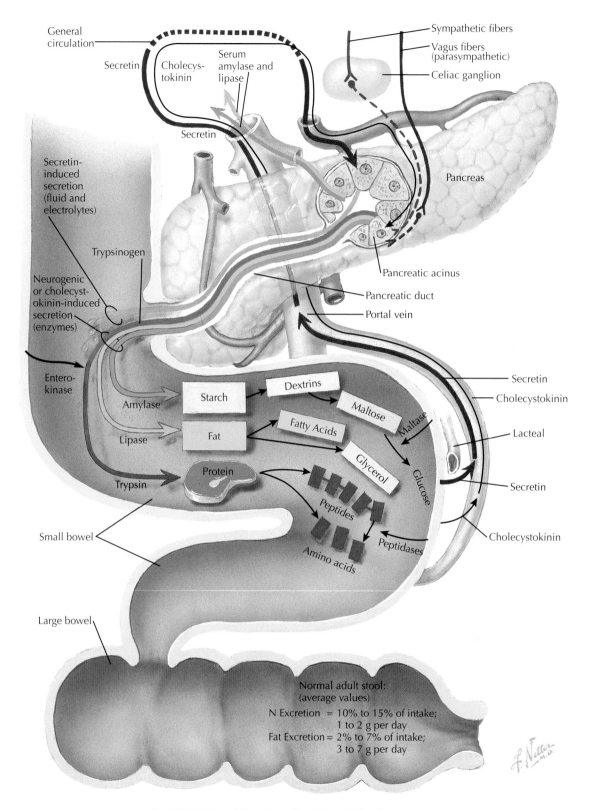

Fig. 126.1 Normal Secretory Functions of the Pancreas.

TABLE 126.1 Pancreatic Hormones

Hormones	Producing Cells	Primary Target Cells	Hormonal Effects	Regulation
Glucagon	α cells	Liver, adipose tissue	1. Promotes glucose synthesis, glycogen breakdown, and increases blood glucose 2. Mobilizes lipid reserves	1. Stimulated in response to low blood glucose concentrations. 2. Inhibited by somatostatin.
Insulin	β cells	Most cells	1. Promotes uptake of glucose by most cells 2. Promotes storage of lipid and glycogen (anabolic and lipogenic effect)	1. Stimulated by high blood glucose concentration, parasympathetic stimulation and high levels of amino acids. 2. Inhibited by somatostatin and sympathetic stimulation.
Somatostatin	δ cells of pyloric antrum, duodenum and pancreatic islets	Islet cells, digestive epithelium	1. Inhibits insulin and glucagon 2. Slows the rate of absorption and enzyme secretion	Stimulated by protein rich meal.
Pancreatic polypeptide (PP)	F cells in the head of the pancreas.	Digestive organs	1. Inhibits gallbladder contraction 2. Regulates production of pancreatic enzymes 3. Influences rate of nutrient absorption	Autonomic control (parasympathetic stimulation) and released following feeding/hypoglycemia.

The islet hormones of importance are insulin, glucagon, somatostatin, neurotensin, PP fold family of peptides (pancreatic polypeptide [PP], neuropeptide Y, and peptide YY).

Somatostatin is produced by the delta cells of the pancreas and is a potent inhibitor of (1) pancreatic bicarbonate and enzyme secretion and (2) other gastrointestinal hormones (gastrin, CCK, secretin, motilin, and vasoactive intestinal polypeptide). Another inhibitory agent is *calcitonin gene–related peptide,* localized in endocrine or paracrine cells and nerve fibers of the pancreas. PP produced by the F cells of the islets inhibits pancreatic secretion, as does *peptide YY,* released from the ileum or colonic mucosa. Peptide YY release is in response to free fatty acids and carbohydrates in the ileum. Vasoactive intestinal peptide (VIP) localized in pancreatic nerve fibers functions as a vagal neurotransmitter. An important function of VIP is to increase blood flow by vasodilatation and influence pancreatic secretion.

The functions of pancreatic hormones are summarized in Table 126.1. Glucagon-like peptide 1 (GLP-1) is peptide hormone produced in the intestinal epithelial endocrine L cells. GLP-1 is released in response to meal intake. GLP-1 stimulates insulin secretion (an incretin hormone) and inhibits glucagon secretion, limiting postprandial glucose excursions. GLP-1 also appears to be a physiological regulator of appetite and food intake.

The pancreatic stellate cells (PSCs) are spatial cells that play a critical role in pancreatic fibrosis, chronic pancreatitis, and pancreatic cancer. In health, PSCs preserve the normal architecture of that pancreatic tissue by regulating the synthesis and degradation of extracellular matrix proteins.

The endocrine functions of pancreatic hormones, insulin, and glucagon related to maintenance of blood glucose and diabetes are not discussed here.

Evidence indicates that *insulin* and *glucagon* influence pancreatic enzyme synthesis and release. Distinct insulin receptors are identified in the acinar cells. Glucagon exerts an inhibitory effect on pancreatic secretion.

ADDITIONAL RESOURCES

Afroze S, Meng F, Jensen K, et al: The physiological roles of secretin and its receptor, *Ann Transl Med* 1(3):29, 2013.

Apte M, Pirola RC, Wilson JS: Pancreatic stellate cell: physiologic role, role in fibrosis and cancer, *Curr Opin Gastroenterol* 31(5):416–423, 2015.

Asakawa A, Inui A, Yuzuriha H, et al: Characterization of the effects of pancreatic polypeptide in the regulation of energy balance, *Gastroenterology* 124:1325–1329, 2003.

Beer RL, Parsons MJ, Rovira M: Centroacinar cells: at the center of pancreas regeneration, *Dev Biol* 413(1):8–15, 2016.

Brownlee IA, Forster DJ, Wilcox MD, et al: Physiological parameters governing the action of pancreatic lipase, *Nutr Res Rev* 23(1):146–154, 2010.

Pallagi P, Hegyi P, Rakonczay Z Jr: The physiology and pathophysiology of pancreatic ductal secretion: the background for clinicians, *Pancreas* 44(8):1211–1233, 2015.

Pandol SJ: Neurohumoral control of exocrine pancreatic secretion, *Curr Opin Gastroenterol* 20:435–436, 2004.

127

Cystic Fibrosis

C. S. Pitchumoni

Cystic fibrosis (CF) is a progressive genetic disease transmitted by an autosomal recessive mechanism. Among Caucasians, the frequency is 1 in 2000 to 3000 live births but much less in African Americans (1:15,000) and Asian Americans (1:30,000). The carrier rate in Caucasians is 1 in 25. Individuals with one copy of the nonfunctioning CF gene are asymptomatic carriers but do not suffer from the disease. Early diagnosis and management of CF have improved the quality of life and life expectancy to 40 years.

The classic form of CF is characterized clinically by sinopulmonary disease, *exocrine pancreatic insufficiency,* and male infertility and biochemically by abnormal sweat electrolytes (Fig. 127.1). Depending on the degree of genetic mutation, the disease may have the classic picture or features involving only the pancreas. Approximately 5% of individuals with CF are diagnosed after age 16 years because they lack classic symptoms.

Mutations are found in the *CFTR* (cystic fibrosis transmembrane conductance regulator) gene, located on the long arm of chromosome 7. The abnormality in genetic mutation can be either reduced quantity or reduced function of the CFTR protein. The resulting abnormalities in epithelial ion and water transport are associated with derangements in airway mucociliary clearance and other cellular functions related to normal cell biology. The genetic defect causes increased sodium chloride content in sweat and increased electrical potential difference across the respiratory epithelium. The secretions become viscid, sticky, and dry and obstruct the ducts, leading to dysfunction at the organ level. In the pancreas, the secretions precipitate within the ducts, causing blockage and duct dilatation. Epithelial cells lacking *CFTR* fail to produce the normal level of the ubiquitous regulator nitric oxide, contributing to increased sodium reabsorption, enhanced inflammatory response, and inefficient destruction of bacteria.

CLINICAL PICTURE

In classic CF the clinical features are (1) persistent pulmonary infection, (2) chronic pancreatic insufficiency, and (3) elevated sweat chloride. In a small number of patients (<2%) with atypical CF, only one organ system (infertility or chronic pancreatitis) may be affected. During infancy, CF manifests as *meconium ileus* (obstruction of distal ileum or proximal colon with thickened viscid meconium), meconium peritonitis or prolonged jaundice caused by steatosis, and biliary obstruction caused by thick mucus. After infancy, failure to thrive associated with respiratory insufficiency and frequent, bulky, foul-smelling oily stools should alert to the possibility of CF secondary to exocrine pancreatic insufficiency. Deficiencies of fat-soluble vitamins A, D, E, and K and prolonged prothrombin time occur.

CF-related diabetes, a common comorbidity, occurs in approximately 20% of adolescents and 40% to 50% of adults due to insulinopenia. However, CF-related diabetes is a distinct clinical entity sharing the features of type 1 and type 2 diabetes.

Recurrent bronchopulmonary infections in infancy and early childhood and colonization of the lungs with *Haemophilus influenzae, Staphylococcus aureus, Pseudomonas aeruginosa,* and *Burkholderia cepacia* are important features. Severe bronchiectasis, massive hemoptysis, and spontaneous pneumothorax are complications. A high incidence of nasal polyps is a classic association.

In adulthood, gastrointestinal symptoms become prominent. Intestinal obstruction near the ileocecal junction (distal intestinal obstruction syndrome) from accumulation of solid stool and intussusception may occur. Rectal prolapse is common. In children and adults, recurrent small bowel obstruction termed *meconium ileus equivalent* occurs. Other gastrointestinal problems include elevation of serum liver enzymes, cirrhosis with portal hypertension, and increased risk for cholelithiasis. Computed tomography may show "fatty replacement" of the pancreas.

Mutation of the *CFTR* gene is a risk factor for chronic pancreatitis, often considered "idiopathic." Although all CF patients are at risk for pancreatitis, the majority of patients with classic CF, the "pancreas insufficient" (PI) group, develop pancreatitis in utero, leading to pancreatic destruction by early childhood, and they are at low risk for subsequent attacks of acute pancreatitis. However, the "pancreas sufficient" (PS) group is particularly vulnerable to attacks of acute and chronic pancreatitis (appears to be idiopathic) later in life, explaining the frequent incidence of pancreatitis in adult CF patients.

Hepatic steatosis and gallstones, focal biliary stricture, and common bile duct (CBD) obstructions are the hepatobiliary manifestations. Portal hypertension, splenomegaly, esophageal varices and bleeding, and hepatic encephalopathy develop in advanced disease.

DIAGNOSIS

A clinical picture consistent with CF with laboratory evidence of *CFTR* dysfunction confirms the diagnosis. In many Western countries, newborns are screened for CF by measuring immunoreactive trypsinogen levels in blood, which are elevated in infants with CF but normal in adult PS patients with CF.

The sweat electrolyte test, for the diagnosis of CF, should be performed only in a specialized laboratory by experienced personnel. An electrolyte concentration greater than 60 mEq/L is confirmatory.

Although there are hundreds of mutations of the *CFTR* gene, most US laboratories screen for 20 to 30 of the common mutations.

TREATMENT AND MANAGEMENT

A multidisciplinary approach is needed to offer intensive symptomatic management. Nutritional support, treatment of exocrine insufficiency, and appropriate therapy for bronchopulmonary infections and other complications are important. Proper planning for adulthood, education, and occupation are other important considerations.

Clinical Features of Cystic Fibrosis

Infancy:	Meconium ileus Meconium peritonitis Jaundice
Beyond infancy:	Failure to thrive
Childhood:	Recurrent bronchopulmonary infections
Adult:	(40% of CF patients currently)
GI Manifestations: **Hepatobiliary manifestations:**	Fatty liver (30%–50%) Cirrhosis (5%–15%) Portal hypertension (1%–8%) Cholelithiasis/sludge (12%–24%) Sclerosing cholangitis/ductal calculi Microgallbladder (30%)
Pancreatic manifestations:	Exocrine insufficiency (85%–90%) Recurrent acute pancreatitis Diabetes mellitus (30%–50%) Calculi (7%)
Others:	GERD, peptic ulcer Distal intestinal obstruction syndrome Pneumatosis intestinalis Rectal mucosal prolapse

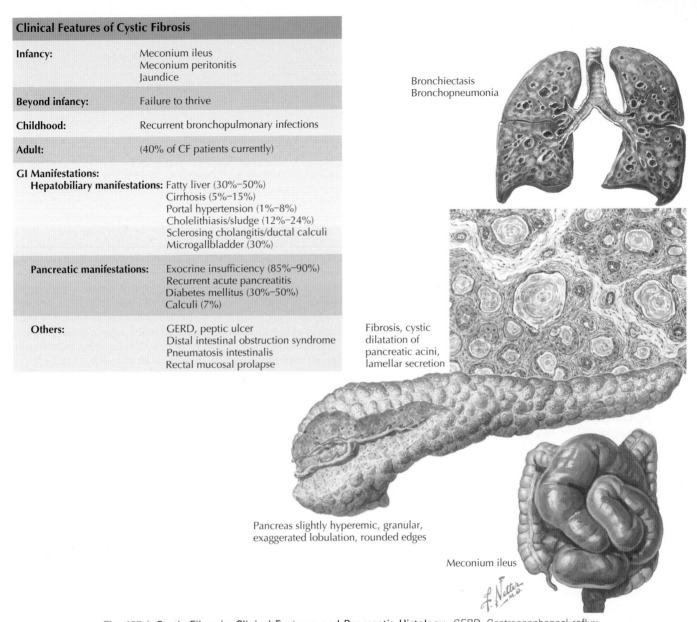

Bronchiectasis
Bronchopneumonia

Fibrosis, cystic dilatation of pancreatic acini, lamellar secretion

Pancreas slightly hyperemic, granular, exaggerated lobulation, rounded edges

Meconium ileus

Fig. 127.1 Cystic Fibrosis: Clinical Features and Pancreatic Histology. *GERD,* Gastroesophageal reflux disease; *GI,* gastrointestinal.

Along with a high-calorie, balanced diet, supplementary oral pancreatic enzyme therapy in adequate dose is important to manage steatorrhea. To correct deficiencies of fat-soluble vitamins, a double-dose multivitamin preparation should be administered, along with vitamins E and K in water-soluble form. Medium-chain triglyceride supplementation is particularly needed in infants. The use of pancreatic preparations with a high concentration of proteolytic enzymes is reported to cause colonic stricture in children.

Aggressive management of bronchopulmonary problems is important. Lung or heart-lung transplantation is an option for a few patients. Ursodeoxycholic acid therapy improves bile flow and ameliorates liver function abnormalities.

Personalized genotype-directed therapies (e.g., ivacaftor) are currently being evaluated.

COURSE AND PROGNOSIS

Overall, with early diagnosis and aggressive management, the prognosis for CF has greatly improved, and many patients survive until the third

or even fourth decade of life. All patients with at least one severe mutation of the *CFTR* gene should be longitudinally assessed for progressive pancreatic dysfunction.

Other congenital diseases of the pancreas of clinical importance include pancreas divisum (Chapter 125) and hereditary pancreatitis (Chapter 129).

ADDITIONAL RESOURCES

Boyle MP: Adult cystic fibrosis, *JAMA* 298:1787–1793, 2007.

De Boeck K, Vermeulen F, Dupont L: The diagnosis of cystic fibrosis, *Presse Med* 46(6 Pt 2):e97–e108, 2017.

Krysa J, Steger A: Pancreas and cystic fibrosis: the implications of increased survival in cystic fibrosis, *Pancreatology* 7:447–450, 2007.

Ong T, Ramsey BW: New therapeutic approaches to modulate and correct CFTR, *Pediatr Clin North Am* 63(4):751–764, 2016.

128

Acute Pancreatitis

C. S. Pitchumoni

ETIOLOGY AND CLINICAL PICTURE

Acute pancreatitis (AP), an inflammatory disorder of the pancreas characterized clinically by abdominal pain and biochemically by elevated levels of serum amylase and lipase, may present as a mild, self-remitting disorder or as a fulminant disease with many local and systemic complications. The revised Atlanta classification of 2012 addresses a number of issues of the disease in adults (Table 128.1). The new classification defines the severity, complications, and management and clarifies terminologies.

The diagnosis of AP requires two out of the three following features: (1) epigastric pain radiating to the back (pancreatic pain), (2) increase in levels of serum amylase and or lipase at least three times greater than the normal values, and (3) imaging findings by contrast enhanced computed tomography (CT) of abdomen or magnetic resonance imaging (MRI) or abdominal ultrasound.

AP may be interstitial edematous or necrotizing based on imaging findings.

Hemorrhage is only a complication of severe AP; thus the term "hemorrhagic pancreatitis" is no longer used.

ETIOLOGY

Alcoholism and gallstone disease account for almost 80% of cases of AP (Box 128.1). Gallstone pancreatitis is caused by migration of stones, biliary sludge, or microlithiasis from the gallbladder through the common bile duct (CBD) to the ampulla of Vater and transient ductal obstruction. The sequelae of ductal obstruction are refluxed biliary-pancreatic secretions, and premature activation of intracellular trypsinogen to trypsin and release of active trypsin into the gland triggering an attack of AP. The pathogenesis of alcoholic pancreatitis is unclear and may involve direct toxic effects on the acinar cells and/or alterations in the composition of pancreatic secretion causing protein plugs and intraductular obstruction. The natural history of alcoholic pancreatitis demonstrates a long history (more than 5 years) of heavy alcohol consumption (more than four to five drinks daily, approximately greater than 80 g/day). Cigarette smoking is an added factor in the pathogenesis of pancreatitis. Hypertriglyceridemia with triglyceride levels usually greater than 1000 mg/dL is a rare cause of AP (see Box 128.1).

There are many other causes for AP, and a few of them are discussed here. Endoscopic retrograde cholangiopancreatography (ERCP)-induced pancreatitis is the most common and feared complication of the procedure, occurring in 2% to 8% of patients. Risk factors include female gender, younger age, history of previous post-ERCP pancreatitis, normal serum bilirubin, sphincter of Oddi dysfunction, multiple pancreatic duct contrast injections, difficulty in cannulation, and precut sphincterotomy (in particular, minor papilla sphincterotomy); these can be additive. The

TABLE 128.1 Severity of Acute Pancreatitis Atlanta Classification 2013

Severity	Organ Involvement
Mild	Absence of organ failure Absence of local complications
Moderate	Local complications and/or Transient organ failure < 48 h
Severe	Persistent organ failure > 48 h

Local complications: Absence of peripancreatic fluid collection, pancreatic pseudocyst, acute necrotic collection, pleural effusion.

Organ failure: failure of three or more major organs, respiratory, cardiac, renal and other organ systems (hepatic, hematologic, and neurologic)

Banks PA, Bollen TL, Dervenis C, et al: Classification of acute pancreatitis—2012: revision of the Atlanta classification and definitions by international consensus. *Gut* 62:102-111, 2013.

BOX 128.1 Etiologic Associations for Acute Pancreatitis

Chronic alcoholism
Gallstones
Drug-induced causes
Infectious agents (viral, bacterial, parasitic)
Trauma
Hypertriglyceridemia
Hypercalcemia
Post-ERCP[a]
Autoimmune
Genetic
Pancreatic divisum
Idiopathic causes
Pancreatic cancer
Rare causes
Postsurgical
Toxic injury: exposure to organophosphorus
Anatomic abnormality: pancreas divisum
Vascular diseases
Scorpion bite *(Tityus trinnitatis)* in Trinidad
Eating disorders: bulimia, anorexia nervosa, refeeding pancreatitis
Diabetic ketoacidosis (DKA)
Chronic renal failure
Hypothermia

[a]Endoscopic retrograde cholangiopancreatography.

mechanism of drug-induced pancreatitis is not clear. Many drugs, including azathioprine, sulfonamides, sulindac, tetracycline, didanosine, pentamidine, estrogens, furosemide, acetylsalicylic acid (ASA) compounds, valproic acid, and glucagon-like peptide-1 receptor agonists (GLP-1) drugs (sitagliptin and exenatide), cause AP. Hypercalcemia, diabetic ketoacidosis, and chronic renal failure are other etiologic factors. *Pancreas divisum* is an infrequent cause. Ampullary tumors and pancreatic cancer may present as AP in the older adult. At least one-third of the cases of idiopathic pancreatitis are secondary to microcrystals. Genetic mutations associated with genes encoding cationic trypsinogen (PRSS 1), serine protease inhibitor Kazal type 1 (SPINK1), and cystic fibrosis transmembrane conductance regulator (CFTR) are involved as primary or associated factors in the pathogenesis of acute as well as chronic pancreatitis. Traumatic AP may develop after penetrating or blunt injury to the abdomen or after abdominal surgery.

CLINICAL PICTURE

The cardinal manifestation of AP is sudden onset of epigastric abdominal pain that is moderate to severe and that lasts for many hours to days. The characteristic radiation of the pain straight to the back is moderately relieved by sitting forward or lying down on one side with knees flexed. Nausea, vomiting, low-grade fever, and tachycardia are associated features. Based on the severity of AP, the disease may be classified into three types: (1) Mild AP is self-limiting and requires only a brief hospitalization. There is no organ failure. (2) Moderately severe AP is associated with transient organ failure lasting less than 48 hours or local (peripancreatic fluid collection) or systemic complications. (3) Severe AP, seen in 15% to 25% patients, is characterized by organ failure greater than 48 hours. Physical examination of the abdomen in early stages may show mild to moderate tenderness on palpation with hypoactive or even absent bowel sounds, depending on the severity of illness. Abdominal rigidity is not a feature of AP. Examination of the chest may reveal findings of pleural effusion, more often on the left side but occasionally on both sides. Other findings may include atelectasis, pneumonia, or congestive heart failure. Scleral icterus; subcutaneous fat necrosis over the buttocks, trunk, and extremities; lipemia retinalis; and eruptive xanthomas (indicative of preexisting hyperlipidemias) are rare. Ecchymotic discoloring of the flanks (Grey Turner sign) or periumbilical region (Cullen sign) are rare and nonspecific.

Additional physical findings depend on the etiologic factor (e.g., alcoholic vs. biliary or hyperlipidemic), degree of severity, stage of illness (at onset vs. 2 weeks later), and complications (cholangitis, pancreatic necrosis).

DIAGNOSIS

Uncomplicated cholecystitis, perforated peptic ulcer disease, splenic infarction, and intestinal ischemia may mimic AP. Serum *amylase* or *lipase* levels at least three times greater than normal values on initial evaluation of a patient with recent onset of abdominal pain is almost diagnostic of AP and is unlikely to be secondary to other causes. Box 128.2 lists other causes of hyperamylasemia. As a single test, serum lipase estimation is superior to estimating amylase.

It is important to note that in hypertriglyceridemic pancreatitis, serum amylase levels may be normal or only modestly elevated. Nonspecific hyperamylasemia and hyperlipasemia also occur in nonpancreatic disorders. Although high levels are often considered specific, falsely elevated lipase levels are as common as falsely elevated amylase levels. In macroamylasemia, the molecular weight of serum amylase is greater than 150,000 daltons (normal range, 50,000–55,000). Renal clearance is affected, and serum amylase level is disproportionately elevated above

---

BOX 128.2 Selected Causes of Elevated Serum Amylase Levels (Hyperamylasemia)

Pancreatitis
Diabetic ketoacidosis (DKA)
Mumps
Perforated bowel
Intestinal obstruction
Cholecystitis
Appendicitis
Peritonitis
Inflammatory bowel disease
Renal failure
Ruptured ectopic pregnancy
Ovarian tumor, cyst
Salpingitis
Post-ERCP[a]
Pancreatic cancer

[a]Endoscopic retrograde cholangiopancreatography.

---

the near-normal or below-normal urinary amylase level. The initial evaluation includes hemoglobin/hematocrit (Hb/Hct) levels, leukocyte count, and aspartate transaminase, alanine transaminase, alkaline phosphatase serum bilirubin, blood urea nitrogen (BUN), creatitine, serum calcium, and albumin. It is appropriate to repeat Hb/Hct and leukocyte count, as well as blood urea nitrogen, creatinine, calcium, and albumin levels in 24 hours to help determine the adequacy of initial therapy (in particular the intravenous [IV] hydration) and prognosis. Once a diagnosis of AP is made, there is very little value in repeating serum amylase or lipase serially.

IMAGING PROCEDURES

It is important to perform initial chest x-ray. Chest x-ray film may show elevation of the diaphragm, pleural effusion (occasionally bilateral), and atelectasis. Evidence of pericardial effusion, congestive heart failure, or acute respiratory distress syndrome may be seen later in the disease course. Abdominal radiography is needed in excluding only other causes of abdominal pain. Its value is in excluding other causes of acute abdominal pain associated with or without elevated serum amylase levels.

Abdominal ultrasound is a valuable initial diagnostic procedure in all patients with AP. Gallbladder stones, choledocholithiasis, dilated CBD, and sometimes enlargement of the pancreas can be identified. When the diagnosis of AP is clear and appears to be uncomplicated and mild, no indication exists for CT within the first 72 hours of admission. However, the indications for an early CT are (1) when the history of abdominal pain is not clear (e.g., disoriented patient), (2) when the history is atypical and other causes of abdominal pain exist, and (3) when the patient is reporting to the hospital a few days after the onset of abdominal pain. The CT scan helps in diagnosis and to exclude other causes of acute abdominal pain, to grade the severity of AP, and to evaluate pancreatic and extrapancreatic intraabdominal complications (Fig. 128.1). Rapid-sequence, contrast-enhanced CT with 5-mm slicing is highly recommended as the best imaging study to visualize the inflammatory changes associated with AP. MRI and magnetic resonance cholangiopancreatography provide good evaluation of the biliary system to assess duct size and to rule out a stone in the CBD. The diagnosis of sterile or infected pancreatic necrosis (IPN) is differentiated using CT, especially with fine-needle aspiration of the necrotic area. A contrast-enhanced CT is needed if symptoms do not resolve in a few days to evaluate pancreatic necrosis and other local complications.

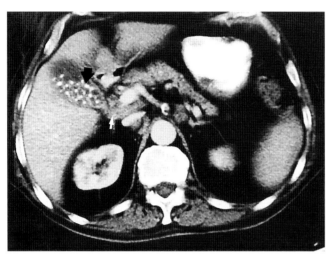

Mild biliary pancreatitis. Note stones in gallbladder *(black arrow)* and swollen pancreas *(white arrow)*.

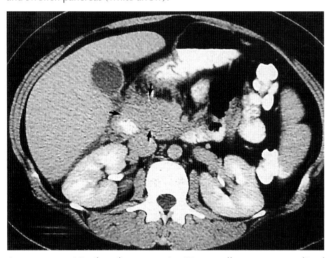

Acute pancreatitis of moderate severity. Note swollen pancreas outlined by *arrows.*

Fig. 128.1 Acute Pancreatitis: Computed Tomography Images of Mild and Moderately Severe Disease.

TREATMENT AND MANAGEMENT

If early evaluation of prognostic markers suggests the possibility of moderately severe or severe AP, the patient has to be treated in an intensive care. Single markers of prognosis or multiple scoring systems are available. Once popular, Ranson criteria are not routinely used currently in clinical practice. Older age, associated comorbid conditions, obesity, pleural effusion, spontaneous ecchymosis, admission dehydration (hematocrit > 44 mg/dL, BUN > 20 mg/dL, creatinine > 1.8 mg/dL) suggest the potential for severe AP. Clinically useful scoring systems are those in the revised Atlanta criteria, American College of Gastroenterology practice guidelines, Acute Physiology and Chronic Health Evaluation (APACHE) II score, or the simple bedside index for severity of AP (Boxes 128.3 and 128.4).

A C-reactive protein rise of greater than 90 mg/dL from admission or an absolute value of greater than 190 mg/dL at 48 hours predicts severe disease with the greatest accuracy. However, this is not useful in early evaluation of severity.

Principles of therapy include managing pain, correcting fluid and electrolytes imbalances, and providing nutritional support.

BOX 128.3 Scoring System for Bedside Index of Severity in Acute Pancreatitis

Score one point for each of the following criteria:
- Blood urea nitrogen level > 8.9 mmol/L
- Impaired mental status
- Systemic inflammatory response syndrome is present (see Box 128.4)
- Age > 60 years
- Pleural effusion on radiography
  A score of more than three indicates an increased risk of death.

Reused with permission from Park JI, Jeon TJ, Ha TH, et al: Bedside index for severity in acute pancreatitis: comparison with other scoring systems in predicting severity and organ failure. *Hepatobiliary Pancreat Dis Int* 12(6):645-650, 2013. Table 1.

BOX 128.4 How to Determine if Systemic Inflammatory Response Syndrome Is Present

Systemic inflammatory response syndrome is present if two or more of the following criteria are met:
- Heart rate > 90 beats/min
- Respiration rate > 20 breaths/min or partial pressure of carbon dioxide is <32 mm Hg
- Body temperature < 36°C or > 38°C
- Leukocyte count < 4 or > 12 ↔ 109/L, or >10% immature neutrophils (bands)

Reused with permission from Singh VK, Wu BU, Bollen TL, et al: Early systemic inflammatory response syndrome is associated with severe acute pancreatitis. *Clin Gastroenterol Hepatol* 7:1247-1251, 2009. Table 1.

Management of pain: Morphine (10 mg/4 h subcutaneously) is generally advocated over mepridine because of its shorter half-life and absence of neuromuscular side effects. There is no evidence for its presumed adverse effect on the sphincter of Oddi. Hydromorphine or fentanyl may be used. Patient controlled analgesia is an option when the pain is severe. Abdominal pain is relieved by meperidine, 25 to 50 mg intramuscularly every 4 to 6 hours as needed. Repeated doses of meperidine rarely cause seizures, and many physicians prefer hydromorphone 0.2 to 0.6 mg (based on a 70-kg patient) every 2 to 3 hours. Patients with prior opiate exposure may tolerate higher doses.

Only patients with protracted vomiting or severe AP need a nasogastric tube placement to keep their stomach empty to prevent aspiration. It is advisable to place patients on no oral feeding (NPO) initially, usually for a brief period of 1 or 2 days. When pain relief occurs and the patient feels hungry, oral feeding maybe started. Early oral feeding is superior to prolonged NPO status. Nutritional support, preferably enteral, should be provided only to patients with severe pancreatitis and is not needed in patients with mild or moderate disease. Nasogastric feeding is safer and better tolerated as compared with nasojejunal feeding. Incidences of multiple organ dysfunction syndrome, systemic inflammatory response syndrome (SIRS), and pancreatic infection, as well as the length of stay in the intensive care unit (ICU), are significantly lower with early enteral feedings.

Adequate and early fluid replacement is critical in the management of AP. IV Ringer lactate is somewhat superior to normal saline. Hydration at 5 to 10 mL/kg per hour is advisable. The aim of early hydration is to prevent hemoconcentration and elevated BUN and creatinine and reduce pancreatic necrosis.

There is no role for prophylactic antibiotic therapy in patients with AP and in sterile necrosis. Antibiotic therapy is needed for those with evidence of ascending cholangitis.

Patients with uncomplicated gallstone pancreatitis should undergo elective cholecystectomy in the same hospitalization soon after resolution of the acute episode of pancreatitis. Patients with severe biliary pancreatitis should be managed in the intensive care unit from the beginning. Cholecystectomy may be electively performed later.

Urgent ERCP with papillotomy and stone extraction is indicated in those with demonstrated dilated CBD with evidence of an impacted stone and impending ascending cholangitis.

COMPLICATIONS

Severe AP is associated with multiple systemic complications and local complications in and around the pancreas intraabdominally. A severe AP is predicted by prognostic markers and criteria discussed earlier.

Systemic Complications

Systemic complications in AP occur in two peaks in the course of the disease. The systemic manifestations are attributed to a variety of proinflammatory and antiinflammatory mediators released from the pancreas and other sources. The first peak during the first 7 to 8 days occurs from the disease onset, connected with early dysfunction of organs is not related to morphologic severity seen in imaging studies. It is purely a functional one. The development of organ failure is related to presence of SIRS. SIRS is characterized by a temperature less than 36°C (96.8°F) or greater than 38°C (100.4°F), heart rate greater than 90 beats per minute, respiratory rate greater than 20/min, and white blood cell (WBC) count less than 4000/mm³ or greater than 12,000/mm³. The second peak of severity occurs from the second week of the disease closely related to necrosis and sepsis (Box 128.5).

Hypoxemia is frequently seen in AP. Pleural effusion is a marker of severity. Usually, pleural effusion resolves without any specific treatment. Pulmonary infiltrates, left lower lobe consolidation, and atelectasis are frequent radiologic findings. The pathogenesis of *acute respiratory distress*

syndrome is multifactorial, and patients often require ICU support. The pathogenetic factors of cardiac manifestations include hypovolemia and metabolic disturbances (e.g., hyperkalemia, hypomagnesemia, and hypophosphatemia).

Hypocalcemia, with calcium levels less than 8 mg/dL, correlates strongly with poor prognosis. The pathogenesis of hypocalcemia is multifactorial.

The systemic complications are tabulated (see Box 128.5).

Intraabdominal Complications

Pancreatic and other intraabdominal complications occur 7 to 21 days after the onset of AP, while treatment for the acute attack is in progress (see Box 128.5). The terminologies described later are based on the revised Atlanta classification.

The fluid collections can be either acute or chronic and sterile or infected.

Acute pancreatic fluid collections (APFCs) located in the peripancreatic area occur in edematous pancreatitis during the first 4 weeks. In APFC, there is only fluid with no necrotic material. APFCs do not need any specific management, and most of them resolve. If APFC has not resolved, it develops a well-marked capsule and becomes a pseudocyst.

Pancreatic pseudocyst is an encapsulated collection of fluid with a well-defined inflammatory wall usually outside the pancreas with no necrosis. It can complicate the course of both acute and chronic pancreatitis. Pseudocysts develop in less than 10% of the cases following edematous pancreatitis. Approximately 60% of the pseudocysts resolve spontaneously (Fig. 128.2). Symptomatic pseudocysts, cysts that grow during observation, and cysts compressing adjacent viscera or infected pseudocyst should undergo surgical, endoscopic, or percutaneous drainage. Complications of a pseudocyst include enlargement and pressure on adjacent organs, rupture, pancreatic ascites, pleural effusions, and aneurysm formation in blood vessels and hemorrhage. Communication with the pancreatic ductal system occurs in approximately 25% of pseudocysts. Endoscopic transmural drainage with endoscopic ultrasound guidance is a major advancement.

Abdominal CT and fine-needle aspiration of the suspected area establishes the diagnosis. Surgical drainage is required. Percutaneous drainage of pus may be helpful. With appropriate therapy, the prognosis is better than for IPN.

The fluid collections in necrotizing pancreatitis maybe either acute necrotic collections (ANCs) or walled-off necrosis (WON, previous terms "necroma" and organized pancreatic necrosis).

ANCs occur in the first 4 weeks and are heterogenous and nonencapsulated and contain nonliquefied material. ANC is defined as diffuse or focal areas of nonviable pancreatic parenchyma of more than 3 cm in size or 30% of the pancreas. Patients both sterile and infected may be characterized clinically by fever, leukocytosis, and persistent abdominal pain (see Fig. 128.2). Most patients with sterile necrosis improve with conservative treatment. The use of prophylactic antibiotics to prevent infection in sterile pancreatitis is not recommended.

IPN: in approximately a third of patients, pancreatic necrosis becomes infected. The diagnosis is by clinical features, or by fine-needle aspiration and/or CT scan appearance. The CT-guided fine-needle aspiration is a safe, effective, and accurate method in distinguishing infected and sterile necrosis. IPN is associated with a mortality rate of approximately 30% and is virtually always an indication for treatment. Without intervention, mortality approaches 100%. Early surgical necrosectomy is not indicated and is associated with a high mortality. Intravenous antibiotics (imipenem or ertapenem) with endoscopic or percutaneous drainage is an acceptable and preferable initial therapeutic strategy for patients with IPN.

BOX 128.5 Complications of Acute Pancreatitis

Systemic
- Pulmonary: hypoxemia, pleural effusion, acute respiratory distress syndrome
- Cardiac: shock, pericardial effusion, electrocardiograph changes, arrhythmias
- Hematologic: disseminated intravascular coagulation, thrombotic thrombocytopenic purpura
- Renal: azotemia, oliguria, myoglobinuria
- Metabolic: hypocalcemia, hyperglycemia, acidosis, hypoalbuminemia
- Central nervous system: psychosis, Purtscher retinopathy
- Peripheral: rhabdomyolysis, fat necrosis, bone necrosis, arthritis

Intraabdominal
- Pancreatic
  - Necrosis: (sterile vs. infected; nonviable parenchyma)
  - Fluid collections: peripancreatic or pseudocyst (infection, rupture, hemorrhage, abscess)
- Local Nonpancreatic
  - Pancreatic ascites: high-protein, high-amylase ascites
  - Contiguous involvement: gastrointestinal bleeding, thrombosis of splenic vein, colonic infarction, lower gastrointestinal (GI) bleeding
  - Obstructive jaundice
  - Abdominal compartment syndrome

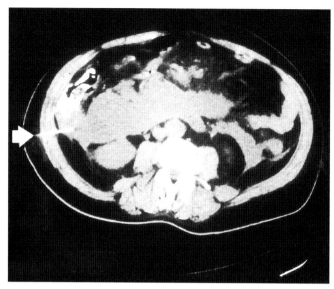

Needle *(arrow)* to aspirate necrotic pancreas.

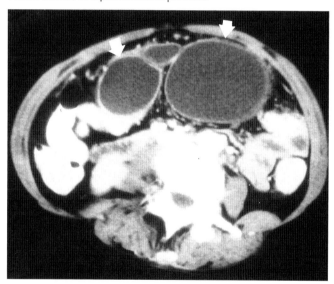

Large pseudocysts (see *arrows*).

Fig. 128.2 Complications of Acute Pancreatitis: Computed Tomography Images of Necrosis and Pseudocysts.

WON is a mature, encapsulated collection of pancreatic and/or peripancreatic necrosis that has developed a well-defined inflammatory wall that develops after 4 weeks. In contrast to pseudocyst, WON has a part of the pancreatic parenchyma and presents with thick contents (pancreatic necrotic debris). Management is same as for pancreatic necrosis.

Other rare intraabdominal complications are pancreatic ascites and abdominal compartment syndrome. The pathogenesis of abdominal compartment syndrome is attributable to visceral edema caused by over hydration, pancreatic ascites, and paralytic ileus.

ADDITIONAL RESOURCES

Afghani E, Pandol SJ, Shimosegawa T, et al: Acute pancreatitis—progress and challenges: a report on an international symposium, *Pancreas* 44(8): 1195–1210, 2015.

Banks PA, Bollen TL, Dervenis C, et al; Acute Pancreatitis Classification Working Group: Classification of acute pancreatitis—2012: revision of the Atlanta classification and definitions by international consensus, *Gut* 62(1):102–111, 2013.

Forsmark CE, Vege SS, Wilcox CM: Acute pancreatitis, *N Engl J Med* 375(20): 1972–1981, 2016.

Foster BR, Jensen KK, Bakis G, et al: Revised atlanta classification for acute pancreatitis: a pictorial essay, *Radiographics* 36(3):675–687, 2016.

Lankisch PG, Weber-Dany B, Maisonneuve P, et al: Frequency and severity of acute pancreatitis in chronic dialysis patients, *Nephrol Dial Transplant* 23(4):1401–1405, 2008.

Piorkowski RJ, Qayyum A, Yarmish GM: ACR Appropriateness Criteria® acute pancreatitis, *Ultrasound Q* 30(4):267–273, 2014.

Rau BM, Bothe A, Kron M, et al: Role of early multisystem organ failure as major risk factor for pancreatic infections and death in severe acute pancreatitis, *Clin Gastroenterol Hepatol* 4:1053–1061, 2006.

Schorn S, Ceyhan GO, Tieftrunk E, et al: Pain management in acute pancreatitis. *Pancreapedia: Exocrine Pancreas Knowledge Base*, 2015.

Tenner S, Baillie J, DeWitt J, et al; American College of Gastroenterology: American College of Gastroenterology guideline: management of acute pancreatitis, *Am J Gastroenterol* 108(9):1400–1415, 1416, 2013.

van Dijk SM, Hallensleben NDL, van Santvoort HC, et al: Acute pancreatitis: recent advances through randomised trials, *Gut* 66(11):2024–2032, 2017.

Whitcomb D: Acute pancreatitis, *N Engl J Med* 354:2142–2150, 2006.

Working Group IAP/APA Acute Pancreatitis Guidelines: IAP/APA evidence-based guidelines for the management of acute pancreatitis, *Pancreatology* 13(4 Suppl 2):e1–e15, 2013.

Wu BU: Prognosis in acute pancreatitis, *CMAJ* 183(6):673–677, 2011.

Wu BU, Johannes RS, Sun X, et al: The early prediction of mortality in acute pancreatitis: a large population-based study, *Gut* 57(12):1698–1703, 2008.

129

Chronic Pancreatitis

C. S. Pitchumoni

DISEASE FORMS AND CLINICAL PICTURE

The cardinal manifestations of chronic pancreatitis (CP) are recurrent or persistent abdominal pain that lasts for months to years, accompanied by diabetes, steatorrhea, and pancreatic calculi. Morphologically, the disease is characterized by destruction and loss of exocrine parenchyma that may be focal, segmental, or diffuse, as well as by fibrosis of the pancreas (Fig. 129.1). These changes may be associated with strictures and dilatation of segments of the pancreatic duct and with intraductal protein plugs or calculi.

The epidemiology of CP parallels the prevalence of alcohol abuse in the community. In the United States, almost 75% of cases of CP are associated with chronic alcoholism, which is thus the most important etiologic factor.

Although the pathogenesis of pancreatic injury is still speculative, current data indicate that acinar cells are injured first, with subsequent development of secretory changes and morphologic alterations such as fibrosis, ductular abnormalities, and stone formation.

Pancreatic stellate cells (PSCs) play a critical role in pancreatic fibrosis, a consistent histologic feature of CP. PSCs are located within the periacinar spaces of the pancreas. PSCs maintain normal tissue architecture via regulation of the synthesis and degradation of extracellular matrix (ECM) proteins in normal physiology. Toxic metabolites, unopposed free-radical injury, and genetic mutations that promote premature activation of trypsinogen to trypsin within the acinar cell are associated with the pathogenesis of CP. Three genes are currently believed to play a major role: cationic trypsinogen gene (*PRSS1*; 7q35), *CFTR*, and *SPINK1*.

Forms of Disease

In *chronic alcoholism,* onset of CP usually occurs after 15 or more years of 80 to 150 g of daily alcohol consumption. Individual susceptibility varies, and only approximately 10% of alcoholics who drink heavily develop clinical pancreatitis, but a larger number may have histologic changes in the pancreas. The susceptibility for pancreatic injury is increased with cigarette smoking and genetic abnormalities.

Tropical calculous pancreatitis (TCP) is a nonalcoholic form of CP that occurs mostly in children and young adults of many developing nations. The pathogenesis of TCP is unknown. Genetic factors (mainly *SPINK1* mutations) in association with many other environmental factors are suspected.

Hereditary pancreatitis (HP) is one of the most common causes of recurrent pancreatitis in children. Episodes of abdominal pain typically occur within the first two decades of life, but the onset may occur later in life. Relatives of patients often have pancreatic calculi, steatorrhea, or diabetes. A major milestone in the history of HP is the recent discovery of an abnormal gene and the feasibility of identifying the genetic abnormality. HP is generally caused by gain-of-function mutations in the cationic trypsinogen gene (PRSS1), although rare kindreds have

been identified with other known or unknown etiologies. The most dreaded complication of HP is a 50- to 70-fold increased risk for pancreatic cancer.

Autoimmune pancreatitis (AIP) (lymphoplasmacytic sclerosing pancreatitis [LPSP], idiopathic duct centric chronic pancreatitis [IDCP], tumefactive CP) is a rare form of steroid responsive fibroinflammatory type of CP. AIP includes two variants, type 1 characterized predominantly by LPSP and types two by IDCP. Clinicopathologic features of the two types overlap to some extent. An autoimmune etiology is suggested because of its response to steroid therapy, the presence of various auto antibodies, and association with other autoimmune diseases.

Type 1 AIP is a systemic disease, more frequent than type 2. The clinical presentation may be as acute or chronic obstructive jaundice. The onset of the disease is after the sixth decade of life. The multisystem involvement includes pancreas, bile ducts, kidneys, retroperitoneum, lymph nodes, and salivary glands. The serum immunoglobulin G4 (IgG4) level is increased to twice the upper limit of normal.

Radiologic features are diffuse enlargement, hypoechogenicity of the pancreas (sausage-shaped pancreas), and a thickened bile duct. Magnetic resonance cholangiopancreatography (MRCP) or endoscopic retrograde cholangiopancreatography (ERCP) shows narrowing of the pancreatic and biliary duct systems mimicking sclerosing cholangitis. Histopathologically AIP is characterized by periductular lymphoplasmacytic infiltrate, predominant IgG4 cells, storiform fibrosis, and obliterative phlebitis. The HISORT (pneumonic) criteria stands for histology, imaging, serology, other organ involvement, and finally a response to steroid therapy. A major differential diagnosis is from pancreatic cancer.

Type 2 is a pancreas-specific disease seen equally in both sexes. In younger individuals the disease presents with obstructive jaundice and pancreatitis. Elevated IgG4 is not a constant feature. The diagnosis is mainly by histology.

AIP responds to steroid therapy dramatically; the dose and duration of therapy are determined by clinical response.

Idiopathic pancreatitis has two subsets. The *juvenile* form is characterized by male preponderance, age of onset before 25 years, and a long history of recurrent attacks of abdominal pain. Hallmarks of CP, such as calculi formation, pancreatic insufficiency, and diabetes, develop 25 to 28 years after onset. The prognosis is poor because of the absence of a removable cause. *Late-onset* (usually after age 60) idiopathic CP *(senile pancreatitis)* may be painless, diagnosed by incidental discovery of calculi during routine abdominal radiography or during work-up of a patient with steatorrhea of uncertain etiology.

Other rare causes of CP include obstruction, hyperlipidemia, pancreas divisum, hyperparathyroidism, gastrectomy, and celiac disease.

Clinical Picture
Recurrent Abdominal Pain

Postprandial pain is the dominant symptom in approximately 85% of patients with CP and the most common reason they seek medical

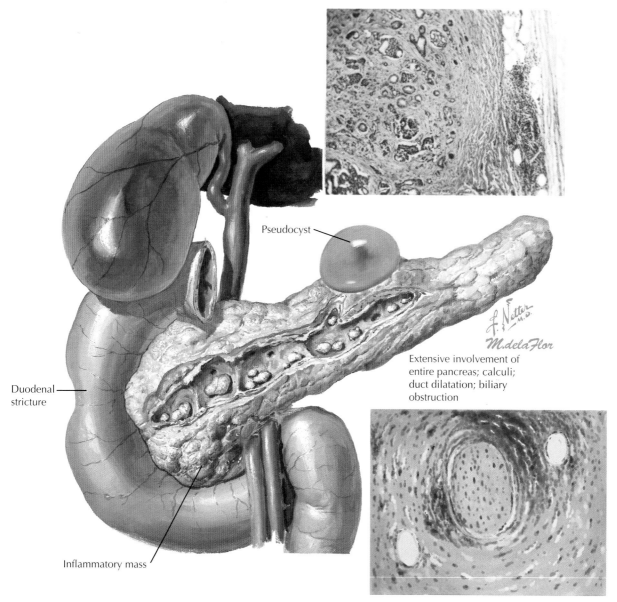

Pseudocyst

Duodenal stricture

Extensive involvement of entire pancreas; calculi; duct dilatation; biliary obstruction

Inflammatory mass

Neuronal inflammation

Fig. 129.1 Chronic Pancreatitis.

attention. Pain can be debilitating and intractable, often leading to functional incapacity, drug and alcohol addiction, poor quality of life, and even suicidal tendencies. Steady, boring, and agonizing pain in the epigastrium or sometimes in the left upper quadrant with radiation directly to the back, between the twelfth thoracic (T12) and second lumbar (L2) vertebrae, or to left shoulder is the typical presentation. Patients sit up and lean forward to the so-called pancreatic position or lie in the knee-chest position on the side to obtain a partial relief of pain. The severity and frequency of painful attacks vary. The duration of pain-free intervals is unpredictable, from weeks to many months. Pain may decrease or disappear, become stable, or worsen with advancing disease.

Pancreatic pain appears to be multifactorial in pathogenesis, accounting for the difficulty encountered in pain management. Intraductal or interstitial hypertension, neuronal hypertrophy, perineural inflammation, and ongoing pancreatic injury are proposed mechanisms. Treatable complications such as pseudocyst and common bile duct (CBD) obstruction may contribute to the pain.

Malabsorption

Steatorrhea does not occur until enzyme secretion is reduced to less than 10% of normal. Lipolytic activity decreases more quickly than does tryptic activity, and it explains why steatorrhea occurs sooner and is more severe than protein malabsorption. In addition to reduced secretion of pancreatic enzymes, patients with severe CP have decreased bicarbonate secretion. The stools may be bulky and formed, in contrast to the frank, watery diarrhea seen in malabsorptive disorders secondary to small intestinal causes. Oil droplets in the stool are often reported in CP. B_{12} deficiency in CP patients occurs and is related to pancreatic protease deficiency.

Diabetes

Diabetes develops in almost 30% of patients with alcoholic pancreatitis 10 years after onset of disease. Diabetes in CP is an example of acquired β and α-cell insufficiency associated with insulin resistance. Ketosis is rare, but other complications (e.g., nephropathy, retinopathy) are as common as in type 2 diabetes, and neuropathy may be more common in view of the addictive effect of alcoholism.

DIAGNOSIS

The diagnosis of CP in its early stage remains a clinical challenge. CP should be considered in all patients with unexplained upper abdominal pain. Only a few patients will have the classic triad of pancreatic calculi, diabetes mellitus, and steatorrhea initially. In most patients, the diagnosis is made based on a typical history of pancreatic type of abdominal pain with a longstanding history of alcoholism. Physical examination findings in alcoholic pancreatitis are nonspecific.

Elevations of serum amylase or lipase levels are often not seen except in acute exacerbations and in early stages of CP. The secretin stimulation test, which involves placement of a tube into the duodenum, although considered the "gold standard," is performed by very few centers.

The imaging tests available are plain radiography, ultrasound or computed tomography (CT) of the abdomen, endoscopic ultrasound (EUS), MRCP, and ERCP. All imaging modalities have limited sensitivity or specificity. Plain film of the abdomen, including a chest film, is the initial radiologic study in all patients to detect pancreatic calculi and to exclude other intraabdominal causes of pain. Pancreatic calculi, although rare in early stages, are highly specific for the diagnosis of CP and make other tests unnecessary. CT abdomen has a sensitivity from 74% to 90% and a specificity of 80% to 90%. CT findings include pancreatic ductal dilatation, parenchymal atrophy, and intraductal stones (often called pancreatic calcification). Because it is noninvasive and widely available, abdominal CT is often performed to exclude other intraabdominal disorders and to identify complications such as pseudocyst, splenic artery aneurysms, enlarged CBD, intrahepatic ducts, and neoplastic masses. Small calculi missed on plain radiographs are identified on CT. Patchy atrophy of the pancreas, fatty replacement, and pancreatic ductal dilatation are visible in advanced cases. Helical CT using a pancreas-optimized protocol is recommended.

ERCP is not and early diagnostic test because of its invasive nature, need for sedation, and complications. However, ERCP findings are highly sensitive (70%–90%) and specific (90%–100%). Ductal changes may be absent or minimal in many patients with early CP (Fig. 129.2).

In the early diagnosis of CP, EUS is a useful tool. An excellent correlation exists between EUS and histologic findings. EUS findings of

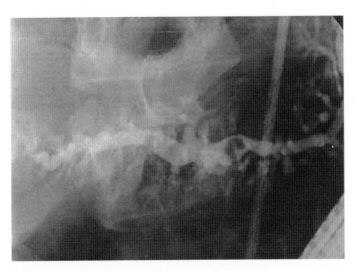

ERCP showing dilated main pancreatic duct, ductules, and intraductal calculi.

Autoimmune pancreatitis

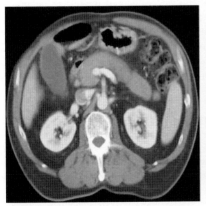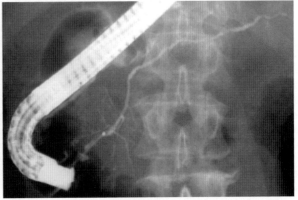

CT scan showing diffusely enlarged pancreas with delayed and thin enhancement.   ERCP showing diffusely irregular narrowing of pancreatic duct.

Fig. 129.2 Chronic and Autoimmune Pancreatitis. *CT,* Computed tomography; *ERCP,* endoscopic retrograde cholangiopancreatography. (From Chari S, Smyrk TC, Levy MJ, et al: Diagnosis of autoimmune pancreatitis: the Mayo Clinic experience, *Clin Gastroenterol Hepatol* 4:1010, 2006.)

CP are hyperechoic foci, hyperechoic strands, lobular contour, and cysts. The ductal features include dilatation, irregularity, hyperechoic margins, visible side branches, and stones. EUS quantitative elastography can also be used to quantify the degree of fibrosis and stage of CP. MRCP has generally replaced ERCP for recognizing ductal changes. Secretin-stimulated MRCP provides excellent visualization of the main duct and its side branches compared with nonstimulated MRCP.

Exocrine pancreas insufficiency occurs only when more than 90% of exocrine pancreatic function is lost. Tests to screen pancreatic exocrine functions lack sensitivity. A fecal fat estimation at 72 hours will help in establishing steatorrhea. Other stool tests for exocrine insufficiency include fecal chymotrypsin and elastase-1.

COMPLICATIONS

Obstructive jaundice in CP, as a result of CBD stenosis, is a frequent complication. The distal CBD that traverses the head of the pancreas is involved transiently in acute exacerbations of CP or permanently as a result of fibrosis of the region or by compression from a pseudocyst. Clinical manifestations are similar to those of pancreatic carcinoma and include chronic pain, jaundice, and persistent elevation of serum alkaline phosphatase levels. Ultrasonography, percutaneous transhepatic cholangiography, ERCP, MRCP, and EUS delineate the stricture and proximal dilatation of CBD and intrahepatic biliary radicles. Surgical drainage by choledochojejunostomy relieves symptoms.

Fibrosis of the head of the pancreas may involve the adjacent duodenum, causing epigastric pain, postprandial fullness, nausea, and vomiting. Diagnosis is established by performing an upper gastrointestinal series and esophagogastroduodenoscopy. Surgical treatment may be needed to relieve obstruction.

Thrombosis of the splenic vein, splenic artery aneurysm, and pseudoaneurysm are complications of CP. The splenic and portal veins may also be compressed by a pseudocyst or may be occluded by fibrosis from adjacent inflammation. A segmental form of portal hypertension, characterized by gastric and esophageal varices, may develop, and life-threatening variceal bleeding may occur.

Pancreatic ascites is a manifestation of duct disruption. Approximately 95% of the cases of pancreatic ascites are associated with CP. Unilateral and bilateral pleural effusions may occur with pancreatic ascites often the result of a leaking pseudocyst or a pleuropancreatic fistula, which can be demonstrated by MRCP or ERCP. Surgical therapy is needed.

Any form of CP (alcoholic, tropical, hereditary, or idiopathic) is associated with a high incidence of cancer of the pancreas.

MANAGEMENT

Managing CP includes treating the associated pain, diabetes, and steatorrhea. A multidisciplinary team approach is needed, with an internist coordinating treatment and gastroenterologist, psychiatrist, pancreatic surgeon, social worker, and diabetologist as consultants.

Abstinence from alcohol use is the single most important step in the management of patients with CP.

The options for pain relief are medical, nutritional, pharmacologic, endoscopic, or surgical.

An important step in the management of pain is to first exclude the treatable causes such as pseudocysts, CBD obstruction, and peptic ulcer disease. Pain relief is usually higher and deterioration of pancreatic function slower in alcohol-abstinent patients.

The method for cancer pain relief proposed by World Health organization (WHO) can be followed in the management of CP. Three-step management starts with nonopioids to weak and then to strong opioids,

according to need. In clinical practice one may start with nonsteroidal antiinflammatory drugs (NSAIDS) and then progress to strong opioids. Tricyclic antidepressants (TCAs) such as amitriptyline and nortryptaline can be used with some added benefit. Pregabalin has been shown to alleviate pain in CP. Most patients need opioid analgesics for symptom relief.

The diet should be adequate in calories, high in protein (~24% of calories), moderate in carbohydrate (46%), and low in fat (30%). Small, frequent, low-fat meals are recommended to minimize pancreatic stimulation. Hospitalization, total cessation of oral intake of food, and short-term use of peripheral parenteral nutrition (PPN) or total parenteral nutrition (TPN) may be needed in acute exacerbations. Supplementation with antioxidant vitamins may reduce the recurrence of pain. Intrajejunal feeding, preferably with medium-chain triglyceride-rich food, stimulates cholecystokinin (CCK) production less than oral feedings and is preferred over TPN.

Oral pancreatic enzyme supplements are recommended to offer pain relief. The clinical utility is very limited. CPCP *octreotide acetate,* a synthetic analog of somatostatin, administered subcutaneously, offers transient pain relief. Continuous octreotide treatment is expensive and impractical.

Types of endoscopic therapy for pain are (1) sphincterotomy, (2) internal drainage of pancreatic cysts, (3) extraction of stones from the pancreatic duct, with or without extracorporeal shock wave lithotripsy (ESWL), (4) guidewire catheter dilatation of strictures, and (5) pancreatic stents. A procedure is chosen based on the location of calculi or strictures.

The efficacy of *celiac plexus block* (CPB), either percutaneously or with surgical or EUS guidance, has not been established. CPB is associated with complications such as epidural or intraperitoneal hematomas, hypotension, gastroparesis, diarrhea, and sexual dysfunction.

Surgery is a consideration when pain is severe enough to interfere with daily life and when it cannot be managed medically. Surgery is tailored to ductal morphology, presence of an inflammatory mass in the head of the pancreas, and the expertise of the surgeon. Surgical candidates can be divided into two broad groups: those with dilated pancreatic ducts (big duct disease), who are more likely to benefit from ductal drainage, and those with small- to normal-sized ducts (small duct disease), who may need pancreatic resection or denervation.

Longitudinal or lateral *pancreaticojejunostomy* (modified Puestow procedure) is preferred when the pancreatic ducts are large enough for anastomosis.

In patients whose ducts are not dilated and in whom previous drainage failed, or in whom pathologic changes predominantly involve a particular area of the gland, resection offers good pain relief that tends to be more permanent than after pancreaticojejunostomy. In the last decade, total pancreatectomy with autologous islet cell transplantation has emerged as a promising treatment for the refractory pain of CP.

ADDITIONAL RESOURCES

Anderson MA, Akshintala V, Albers KM, et al: Mechanism, assessment and management of pain in CP: recommendations of a multidisciplinary study group, *Pancreatology* 16(1):83–94, 2016.

Apte MV, Pirola RC, Wilson JS: Pancreatic stellate cells: a starring role in normal and diseased pancreas, *Front Physiol* 3:344, 2012.

Chari ST: Diagnosis of autoimmune pancreatitis: the evolution of diagnostic criteria for a rare disease, *Clin Gastroenterol Hepatol* 15(10):1485–1488, 2017.

Conwell DL, Lee LS, Yadav D, et al: American pancreatic association practice guidelines in CP: evidence-based report on diagnostic guidelines, *Pancreas* 43(8):1143–1162, 2014.

De la Iglesia-García D, Huang W, Szatmary P, et al: Efficacy of pancreatic enzyme replacement therapy in chronic pancreatitis: systematic review and meta-analysis, *Gut* 66(8):1354–1355, 2017.

Goulden MR: The pain of CP: a persistent clinical challenge, *Br J Pain* 7(1): 8–22, 2013.

Hobbs PM, Johnson WG, Graham DY: Management of pain in CP with emphasis on exogenous pancreatic enzymes, *World J Gastrointest Pharmacol Ther* 7(3):370–386, 2016.

Majumder S, Takahashi N, Chari ST: Autoimmune pancreatitis, *Dig Dis Sci* 62(7):1762–1769, 2017.

Sheth SG, Conwell DL, Whitcomb DC, et al: Academic pancreas centers of excellence: guidance from a multidisciplinary CP working group at *PancreasFest, Pancreatology* 17(3):419–430, 2017.

Singh VK, Drewes AM: Medical management of pain in CP, *Dig Dis Sci* 62(7):1721–1728, 2017.

Yadav D, Hawes RH, Brand RE, et al: Alcohol consumption, cigarette smoking, and the risk of recurrent acute and CP, *Arch Intern Med* 169:1035–1045, 2009.

130

Pancreatic Cancer

C. S. Pitchumoni

CLINICAL PICTURE

Globally, pancreatic cancer causes more than 331,000 deaths per year, ranking as the seventh leading cause of cancer death in both sexes together. In the United States, pancreatic cancer is the fifth leading cause of cancer mortality. In 2018, approximately 55,400 individuals are expected to be diagnosed with pancreatic cancer. Because the 1-year mortality is high, approximately 44,330 will die of pancreatic cancer. In the United States, the incidence of pancreatic cancer is slightly more in men than in women (10.6 vs. 8 per 100,000) and is higher in black and Jewish populations.

Mortality and incidence rates are often identical because of the delay in diagnosis and poor prognosis. The peak incidence is in the seventh and the eighth decades of life. The increasing prevalence of obesity is a strong factor. Pancreatic cancer is asymptomatic in early stages. Later, the symptoms and signs are influenced by the location of the tumor. A tumor of the head causes early obstructive jaundice associated with dark urine and clay-colored stool (lack of bile pigment). When a tumor is located in the body or tail, jaundice is infrequent.

Almost 90% of the pancreatic cancers are moderately differentiated *adenocarcinomas* that arise from the ductular epithelium (Fig. 130.1). Most of these tumors (60%–70%) are localized in the head of the pancreas, and the rest (18%–20%) arise in the body and tail or are multifocal and infiltrate diffusely throughout the gland (20%). Tumors of the body and tail are often diagnosed at more advanced stages, carrying poor prognosis.

Acinar cell carcinoma, giant cell carcinoma, adenosquamous carcinoma, intraductal papillary mucinous tumors, cystadenocarcinoma, leiomyosarcoma, and lymphoma account for less than 10% of other pancreatic cancers. Cystic neoplasms are discussed separately.

The risk factors are listed in Box 130.1. Cigarette smoking is the greatest risk factor for pancreatic cancer. Approximately 30% of the cases are attributed to heavy smoking in terms of number of cigarettes smoked and duration of smoking. Chronic pancreatitis of any cause (alcoholic, tropical, or hereditary) is associated with high risk.

Pancreatic type of pain is the initial feature in nearly 80% of the patients. In its early stages, pancreatic cancer mimics a number of other conditions that cause epigastric or back pain. Other symptoms include weight loss, anorexia, nausea, jaundice, diarrhea, and depression. Diabetes mellitus or glucose intolerance may develop a few months to a year preceding the onset of other symptoms. Small tumors of the head or ampulla cause early obstructive jaundice or symptoms of acute recurrent pancreatitis.

Pain is frequent, as is weight loss, particularly in patients with tumors of the body and tail of the pancreas. Hematemesis and melena may occur in late stages because of the development of gastric varices resulting from splenic vein occlusion. Ascending cholangitis characterized by fever and chills may occur. A palpable, distended gallbladder, usually the result of bile duct obstruction, is termed *Courvoisier sign* or *Courvoisier gallbladder* and is seen in 25% of patients. Supraclavicular lymph node enlargement (Virchow node), periumbilical mass (Sister Mary Joseph nodule), and palpable rectovaginal or rectovesical nodularity (Blumer shelf) are signs of advanced disease (Fig. 130.2). A nonspecific sign (Trousseau sign) is the migrating thrombophlebitis that occurs in all advanced cancers and is not specific for pancreatic cancer.

Even when appropriate diagnostic tests such as computed tomography (CT) are performed early, the findings may be nondiagnostic and may require follow-up studies weeks or months later for development of more specific radiologic signs.

DIAGNOSIS

In any patient older than 50 years who has unexplained jaundice, weight loss, upper abdominal or back pain, anorexia, or idiopathic pancreatitis, the index of suspicion for pancreatic cancer should be high. New-onset diabetes mellitus without obesity or family history, particularly combined with any of these symptoms, should alert the physician to the possibility of pancreatic cancer. More than half the number of patients present with metastatic disease and have a 5-year survival of less than 2%.

Depending on tumor size and degree of histologic differentiation, the level of cancer antigen (CA) 19-9, the most widely used serum

---

BOX 130.1 Risk Factors for Pancreatic Cancer

Etiologic Associations
- Cigarette smoking
- Chronic pancreatitis
- Older age (>65 years)
- Male sex
- African Americans
- High-fat diet?
- Diabetes mellitus?
- Exposure to industrial toxins

Associated Genetic Syndromes
- Hereditary pancreatitis
- Hereditary nonpolyposis colorectal cancer (HNPCC)
- Ataxia telangiectasia
- Von Hippel-Lindau syndrome
- Peutz-Jegher syndrome
- Hereditary breast (BRCC2)/ovarian cancer
- Multiple endocrine neoplasia 1 (MEN-1) syndrome
- Familial atypical multiple mole melanoma (FAMMM) syndrome

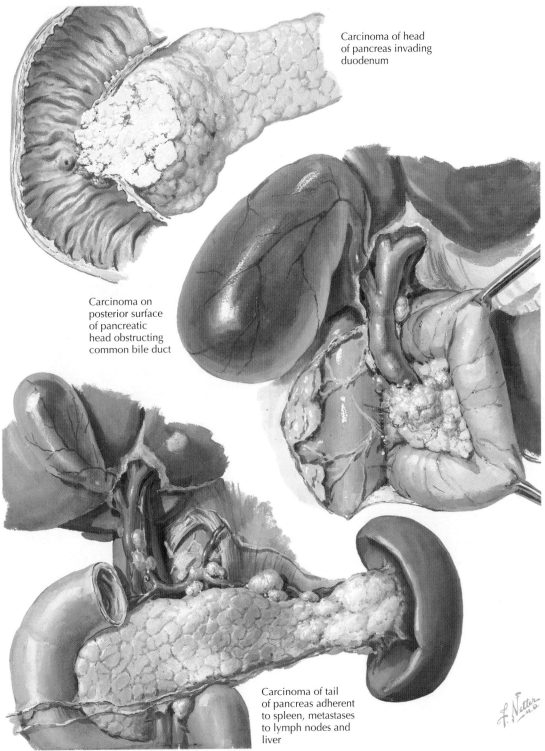

Carcinoma of head
of pancreas invading
duodenum

Carcinoma on
posterior surface
of pancreatic
head obstructing
common bile duct

Carcinoma of tail
of pancreas adherent
to spleen, metastases
to lymph nodes and
liver

Fig. 130.1 Pancreatic Cancer: Clinical Features.

marker, varies. In tumors less than 2 cm in diameter, the level may be immeasurable. Elevated CA 19-9 levels are highly correlated with the presence of pancreatic cancer. False elevations are seen in chronic pancreatitis and in benign obstructive jaundice. Macrophage inhibitory cytokine-1 (MIC-1) is a valuable tumor marker for the diagnosis of pancreatic cancer. It has a good correlation with CA 19-9. Tissue polypeptide–specific antigen is another recently described serum marker.

Improvements in imaging technology, including spiral CT, magnetic resonance imaging (MRI), positron emission tomography (PET), and endoscopic ultrasound (EUS) have helped us in identifying pancreatic cancer and staging. CT scan of the pancreas is the primary modality for diagnosis. The two concerns are early diagnosis and proper staging. The resectability is determined by absence of distant metastasis and absence of tumor involvement of major blood vessels.

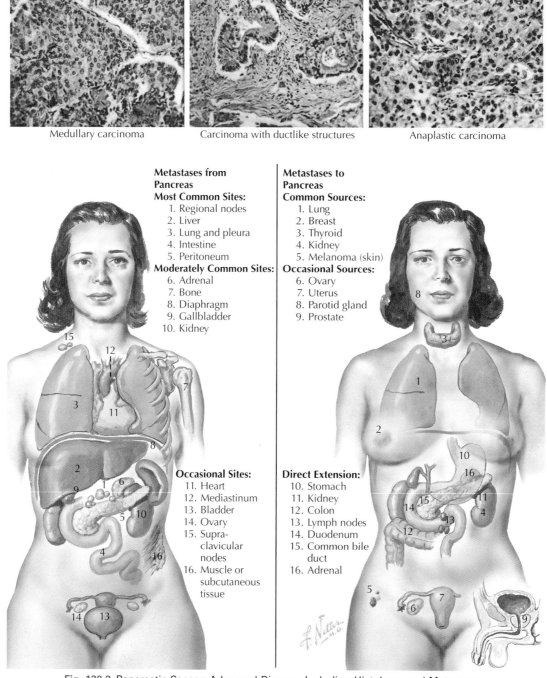

Medullary carcinoma   Carcinoma with ductlike structures   Anaplastic carcinoma

Metastases from Pancreas
Most Common Sites:
1. Regional nodes
2. Liver
3. Lung and pleura
4. Intestine
5. Peritoneum

Moderately Common Sites:
6. Adrenal
7. Bone
8. Diaphragm
9. Gallbladder
10. Kidney

Occasional Sites:
11. Heart
12. Mediastinum
13. Bladder
14. Ovary
15. Supra-clavicular nodes
16. Muscle or subcutaneous tissue

Metastases to Pancreas
Common Sources:
1. Lung
2. Breast
3. Thyroid
4. Kidney
5. Melanoma (skin)

Occasional Sources:
6. Ovary
7. Uterus
8. Parotid gland
9. Prostate

Direct Extension:
10. Stomach
11. Kidney
12. Colon
13. Lymph nodes
14. Duodenum
15. Common bile duct
16. Adrenal

Fig. 130.2 Pancreatic Cancer: Advanced Disease, Including Histology, and Metastases.

Abdominal ultrasonographic findings are suboptimal for diagnosing pancreatic cancer. Contrast-enhanced, thin-section helical CT of the pancreas helps to diagnose, evaluate the extent of the disease (sensitivity and specificity more than 80% and 95%, respectively), and assess tumor resectability. Contrast-enhanced MRI using intravenous gadolinium-diethylene triamine pentaacetic acid (DTPA) is useful for detecting small pancreatic tumors. Ductal size is best evaluated by magnetic resonance cholangiopancreatography (MRCP). The combination of findings of a mass in the head of the pancreas on cross-sectional imaging with a "double duct sign," dilated bile and pancreatic ducts suggests pancreatic cancer. Double duct sign may also occur in chronic pancreatitis with a mass in the head. Functional imaging modalities such as PET scanning are superior to conventional CT imaging. EUS is a minimally invasive technique in the evaluation of cancer resectability and the most accurate method for detecting vascular and lymph node enlargement. EUS-guided, fine-needle aspiration (FNA) allows cytologic evaluation. EUS-FNA has a high sensitivity (85%–90%) with a specificity of near 100%. Angiography has limited value.

TREATMENT AND MANAGEMENT

The principles of management of pancreatic cancer are as follows. Depending on the stage, management of pancreatic cancer includes nutritional support, surgical resection, chemotherapy, radiation therapy, endoscopic and surgical palliation of pain, and chemoradiation for unresectable cancer. Approximately 85% to 90% of pancreatic cancers are unresectable. Optimal therapy requires a multidisciplinary team approach by a medical oncologist, interventional radiologist, interventional gastroenterologist, radiotherapist, internist, and pain management specialist.

The Whipple procedure *(pancreaticoduodenectomy)* is the standard surgical procedure. The technique involves resection of the distal stomach, gallbladder, proximal jejunum, and regional lymph nodes. The mortality rate is less than 5% in expert hands. The new pylorus-preserving Whipple procedure reduces the incidence of postgastrectomy symptoms. Palliative surgery for the relief of biliary obstruction eliminates pruritus and probably has some benefit in promoting nutrition.

Current data suggest that the combination of pancreaticoduodenectomy with postoperative adjuvant *5-fluorouracil* (5-FU) and external beam radiation therapy improves the duration of survival. Chemoradiation has been suggested for patients with locally advanced unresectable pancreatic cancer to improve survival and quality of life and to downstage advanced locoregional disease to allow surgical resection. *Gemcitabine* (2′,2′-difluorodeoxycytidine; Gemzar) is a deoxycytidine analog capable of inhibiting DNA replication and repair. Gemcytabine therapy modestly prolongs survival but improves quality of life by decreasing pain and the need for opioid analgesics. FOLFRINOX is a combination of four chemotherapeutic agents (irenotecan, 5-FU, leucovorin, and oxaliplatin). FOLFRINOX improves the survival rate of metastatic cancer by a few months. External beam radiation therapy with 5-FU chemotherapy, intraoperative radiation therapy (brachytherapy or electron beam), and external beam radiation therapy with novel (radiosensitizing) chemotherapeutic agents are options. Palliation of pain using percutaneous or EUS-guided celiac ganglion block, an intraoperative approach, or thoracoscopic splanchnicectomy improves quality of life.

Many palliative procedures are available to manage obstructive jaundice. Establishing a biliary drainage by ERCP and stenting achieves more than 90% success. Percutaneous transhepatic biliary drainage is an option in candidates not suitable for ERCP.

ADDITIONAL RESOURCES

Ferlay J, Soerjomataram I, Ervik M, et al: *GLOBOCAN 2012: Estimated Cancer Incidence, Mortality and Prevalence Worldwide in 2012 v1.0.* International Agency for Research on Cancer. https://www.altmetric.com/details/21798233.

Fogel EL, Shahda S, Sandrasegaran K, et al: A multidisciplinary approach to pancreas cancer in 2016: a review, *Am J Gastroenterol* 112(4):537–554, 2017.

Howlader N, Noone AM, Krapcho M, et al: *SEER Cancer Statistics Review, 1975-2014,* National Cancer Institute. Bethesda, MD, https://seer.cancer.gov/csr/1975_2014/, based on November 2016 SEER data submission, posted to the SEER web site, April 2017.

Mettu NB, Abbruzzese JL: Clinical insights into the biology and treatment of pancreatic cancer, *J Oncol Pract* 12(1):17–23, 2016.

Pittman ME, Rao R, Hruban RH: Classification, morphology, molecular pathogenesis, and outcome of premalignant lesions of the pancreas, *Arch Pathol Lab Med* 141(12):1606–1614, 2017.

Rebours V, Boutron-Ruault M, Schnee M, et al: Risk of pancreatic adenocarcinoma in patients with hereditary pancreatitis: a national exhaustive series, *Am J Gastroenterol* 103:111–119, 2008.

Ruarus A, Vroomen L, Puijk R, et al: Locally advanced pancreatic cancer: a review of local ablative therapies, *Cancers (Basel)* 10(1):2018. pii: E16.

Tempero MA: Introduction: pancreatic adenocarcinoma: the emperor of all cancer maladies, *Cancer J* 23(6):309, 2017.

Thibodeau S, Voutsadakis IA: FOLFIRINOX chemotherapy in metastatic pancreatic cancer: a systematic review and meta-analysis of retrospective and phase II studies, *J Clin Med* 7(1):2018. pii: E7.

Yadav D, Lowenfels AB: The epidemiology of pancreatitis and pancreatic cancer, *Gastroenterology* 144(6):1252–1261, 2013.

131

Cystic Neoplasms of the Pancreas

C. S. Pitchumoni

The increasing use of abdominal imaging studies such as abdominal ultrasound, computed tomography (CT) scan, and magnetic resonance imaging (MRI) has contributed to the incidental detection of pancreatic cysts, some of which may be malignant and others premalignant or benign. Overall in asymptomatic patients, 2.5% have pancreatic cysts, and the number increases to 10% in those older than 70 years. Once detected, the clinician should not ignore the finding even in the asymptomatic patient. The topic has thus assumed tremendous importance, and various guidelines are recently proposed to manage the problem.

The three most common epithelial tumors of the pancreas are serous cystic neoplasms (SCNs), mucinous cystic neoplasm (MCNs), and intraductal papillary mucinous neoplasm (IPMN). The less frequent are the cystic endocrine, solid, and pseudopapillary tumors. Pancreatic cysts can be classified as mucinous or nonmucinous, based on the nature of the cyst content. The mucinous cysts are either malignant at the time of initial diagnosis or have a higher potential for malignant progression as compared with serous cysts.

The best imaging modalities to identify the nature of these cysts are multidetector CT and MRI. The accuracy of providing the correct histologic diagnosis by these modalities is low and ranges from 40% to 60%. Diagnostic endoscopic retrograde cholangio-pancreatography (ERCP) has very little role, but endoscopic ultrasound (EUS) plays a major role in characterizing the cysts and in performing tests in the cyst aspirate.

SEROUS CYSTIC NEOPLASM

SCNs are generally benign and accounts for 16% of resected cystic tumors of the pancreas. Malignant transformation to cystadenocarcinoma is extremely rare.

The presenting symptoms are nonspecific. Abdominal pain, fullness, palpable mass are rare features. Von Hippel-Lindau syndrome is a risk factor.

Imaging studies of the pancreas characteristically show a honeycomb appearance with central calcification scar. SCNs are usually less than 5 cm in diameter but can be as large as 25 cm.

Surgery may be indicated only in selected cases. Symptomatic cysts and a finding of rapid enlargement and presence of solid components in the cyst are considered indications for surgery. A conservative approach of surveillance imaging is recommended.

MUCINOUS CYSTIC NEOPLASM

Nearly 23% of all resected cystic tumors are MCNs. Some of the clinical features are median age of diagnosis in the late 40s and a female preponderance. More than 90% of the time the solitary tumor is located in the body or the tail of the pancreas (Fig. 131.1). Most of the patients are initially asymptomatic or have only nonspecific gastrointestinal complaints.

Pathologically the tumor shows an inner epithelial layer consisting of mucin-secreting cuboidal epithelium and an outer layer of the ovarian-like stroma. The cyst does not communicate with the pancreatic duct, and the cyst fluid is low in amylase, unlike in a pseudocyst. The cyst fluid is to be analyzed for a mucinous lesion using tumor markers such as CA 19-9, carcinoembryonic antigen (CEA), and CA 15-3. The best predictor of a mucinous lesion is an elevated CEA. Cytology is specific but insensitive. Because of high malignant potential, all MCNs are considered surgical.

INTRADUCTAL PAPILLARY MUCINOUS NEOPLASMS

Ductal dilatation from mucin production is the characteristic feature of IPMNs. There are two types of IPMN based on the degree of involvement of the main pancreatic duct, the main duct IPMN (MD-IPMN) and the branch duct IPMN (BD-IPMN).

MD-IPMN is characterized by male predominance, the age of presentation in the mid-60s, and has a malignant potential more than 40%.

The clinical presentation may be asymptomatic when incidentally discovered or with abdominal pain. Weight loss, acute pancreatitis, and diabetes mellitus are other manifestations.

Radiologically, MD-IPMN shows either segmental or diffuse dilatation of the main pancreatic duct, greater than 5 mm, with no other identifiable cause such as stricture or stones or tumor for ductal dilatation. The diagnosis of IPMN is by imaging studies, EUS, and rarely ERCP. Magnetic resonance cholangio pancreatography (MRCP) is superior to ERCP in visualizing the side branches. Pathologically IPMNs show ductal dilatation and papillary overgrowth of ductal epithelia. The histologic abnormalities range from low-, moderate-, to high-grade dysplasia.

The BD-IPMN at presentation is mostly asymptomatic and has a much less malignant potential. BD-IPMN affects one or more side branches of the pancreatic ducts and communicates with a nondilated pancreatic duct.

The management of MD-IPMNs is surgery. The treatment of BD-IPMN is controversial, especially when asymptomatic and in the elderly. The discussion here does not include details on nonneoplastic cysts (i.e., pseudocysts, congenital cysts). Table 131.1 summarizes the diagnostic approach to incidentally discovered pancreatic cysts, including pseudocysts of the pancreas.

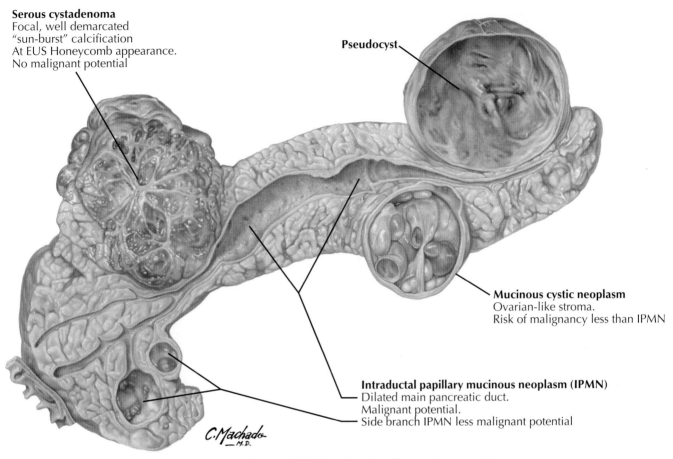

Serous cystadenoma
Focal, well demarcated
"sun-burst" calcification
At EUS Honeycomb appearance.
No malignant potential

Pseudocyst

Mucinous cystic neoplasm
Ovarian-like stroma.
Risk of malignancy less than IPMN

Intraductal papillary mucinous neoplasm (IPMN)
Dilated main pancreatic duct.
Malignant potential.
Side branch IPMN less malignant potential

C.Machado
M.D.

Fig. 131.1 Cystic Tumors. *IPMN,* Intraductal papillary mucinous neoplasm.

TABLE 131.1 Characteristics of Common Pancreatic Cysts

Parameters	Pseudocyst	IPMN (MD and BD)	MCN	SCN
Demographic	Alcohol abuse, history of pancreatitis, middle-aged men	Middle-aged and older individuals	Middle-aged women	Usually in older women
location	Common in tail, solitary small to very large in size	Common in pancreatic head, maybe incidental and multifocal	Body and tail, incidental, single lesion	Entire pancreas, many small cysts or oligo/macrocystic
CT/MRI	Usually unilocular cyst, parenchymal inflammatory changes	MD: diffuse or focal involvement of MPD; BD: cyst or cluster of cysts maybe multifocal, ductal communication	Large cysts with thick septae, peripheral calcification, wall thickening	Microcystic multiple small cyst, central fibrous scar with calcification, sometimes oligocystic
Cytology	Degenerative debris, inflammatory cells, histocytes, no epithelial cells	Colloidlike mucin stains positive, mucinous epithelial cells with varying degrees of atypia, sparsely cellular	Mucinous epithelial cells with varying degrees of atypia, colloidlike mucin, mucin stains positive	Usually acellular and nondiagnostic, small cluster of cells with bland cuboidal morphology, glycogen stain positive, mucin negative
Cyst fluid analysis	Thin, clear or brown to green, nonmucinous sometimes hemorrhagic CEA concentration very low, amylase and lipase concentrations usually high	Thick, viscous mucus, CEA concentration usually high, amylase concentration maybe high (60%), KRAS mutation (+) (80%)	Thick, viscous mucus, CEA concentration usually high, KRAS mutation (+) (14%), GNAS mutation (−)	Clear and thin, maybe hemorrhagic, CEA and amylase concentrations very low.

BD, Branch duct; *CEA,* carcinoembryonic antigen; *CT,* computed tomography; *IPMN,* intraductal papillary mucinous neoplasm; *MCN,* mucinous cystic neoplasm; *MD,* main duct; *MPD,* main pancreatic duct; *MRI,* magnetic resonance imaging; *SCN,* serous cystic neoplasm.
From Brugge WR: Diagnosis and management of cystic lesions of the pancreas, *J Gastrointest Oncol* 6(4):375-388, 2015.

ADDITIONAL RESOURCES

Basar O, Brugge WR: My treatment approach: pancreatic cysts, *Mayo Clin Proc* 92(10):1519–1531, 2017.

Bauer F: Pancreatic cystic lesions: diagnostic, management and indications for operation. Part I, *Chirurgia (Bucur)* 112(2):97–109, 2017.

Brugge WR: Diagnosis and management of cystic lesions of the pancreas, *J Gastrointest Oncol* 6(4):375–388, 2015.

Dudeja V, Allen PJ: Premalignant cystic neoplasms of the pancreas, *Semin Oncol* 42(1):70–85, 2015.

Tanaka M, Chari S, Adsay V, et al: International consensus guidelines for management of intraductal papillary mucinous neoplasms and mucinous cystic neoplasms of the pancreas, *Pancreatology* 6:17e32, 2006.

Tanaka M, Fernández-del Castillo C, Adsay V, et al: International consensus guidelines 2012 for the management of IPMN and MCN of the pancreas, *Pancreatology* 12:183e97, 2012.

Vege SS, Ziring B, Jain R, et al: American gastroenterological association institute guideline on the diagnosis and management of asymptomatic neoplastic pancreatic cysts, *Gastroenterology* 148:819e22, 2015.

132

Pancreatic Neuroendocrine Tumors (Islet Cell Tumors)

C. S. Pitchumoni

Pancreatic neuroendocrine tumors (PNETs), also known as "islet cell tumors," represent a group of rare neoplasms of the neuroendocrine cells of the gastropancreatic system (Fig. 132.1). PNETs constitute fewer than 5% of the pancreatic tumors. They may be functioning tumors producing distinct clinical syndromes based on the hormone (gastrin, insulin, and glucagon) produced, or nonfunctioning tumors (60%–90%), diagnosed because of their mass effect or malignant behavior. The incidence of PNET is increasing.

Polypeptide hormone–producing cells of the pancreatic islets (islets of Langerhans) have a common embryologic origin within the neural crest and subsequently migrate to the foregut enlargement of the pancreas. These tumors have similar histology but can be distinguished by immunohistochemistry.

PNETs constitute four familial syndromes: multiple endocrine neoplasia type 1 (MEN-1), von Hippel-Lindau syndrome (VHL), neurofibromatosis type 1, and tuberous sclerosis complex (TSC). These tumors are benign or malignant. PNETs may occur with an autosomal dominant inheritance as part of MEN-1 syndrome. MEN-1 syndrome is a disorder of three glands: parathyroid, pancreatic islets, and pituitary. MEN-2 tumors include pheochromocytoma and adenoma or hyperplasia of parathyroid glands. Insulinomas and gastrinomas are the most common functioning PNETs. Other functioning tumors are less than 3% and are vasoactive intestinal peptide–secreting tumor (VIPoma), glucagonoma, and somatostatinoma.

Clinical picture, diagnosis, and treatment of PNETs vary greatly depending on the syndrome and secretory production, as discussed under insulinoma, gastrinoma, and glucagonoma.

The diagnostic studies include serum levels of hormones in functioning PNETs. There are several tumor markers available. Chromogranin A (CgA) is an acidic glycoprotein that is produced and excreted by PNETs. Circulating CgA levels are useful markers with a high specificity and a sensitivity ranging from 27% to 81%.

Computed tomography (CT) scan of the abdomen, magnetic resonance imaging (MRI), endoscopic ultrasound (EUS), somatostatin-receptor scintigraphy (SRS, octreotide scan), positron emission tomography (PET) scan are useful. EUS is particularly helpful in detecting small lesions such as gastrinomas and insulinomas.

INSULINOMA

Insulinoma is the most common functional PNET. Almost 60% occur in middle-aged women. Insulinomas can be sporadic or familial, a component of MEN-1 syndrome. Approximately 10% of patients with insulinoma have the MEN-1 syndrome. Most of the tumors are solitary, relatively benign, less than 2.5 cm in diameter, and evenly distributed throughout the pancreas.

Fasting hypoglycemia is a common clinical manifestation of insulinoma. Headache, visual disturbances, dizziness, lightheadedness, confusion, weakness, grand mal seizures, and coma are the neuroglycopenic symptoms. Hypoglycemia-induced catecholamine response causes diaphoresis, tremulousness, palpitations, irritability, and hunger. Hypoglycemic symptoms are precipitated by fasting or exercise and respond to carbohydrate ingestion. Obesity is a consequence of hunger and increased eating.

Diagnosis

After 72 hours of supervised fasting, the patient displays the Whipple triad: (1) hypoglycemic symptoms (central nervous system, vasomotor), (2) documented hypoglycemia, and (3) relief of symptoms after glucose intake. Hypoglycemia usually develops within 24 hours of fasting. A serum insulin level of 5 mU/mL or more with concomitant plasma glucose level less than 45 mg/dL (2.5 mmol/L) indicates insulinoma. Factitious hypoglycemia is ruled out by fasting plasma levels, C-peptide, and proinsulin.

Abdominal CT, MRI, and EUS are all useful in diagnosing. Visceral angiography and indium 111–labeled octreotide nuclear imaging are other diagnostic modalities.

Treatment and Management

The goal of management is to prevent hypoglycemia through frequent small meals. Diazoxide, 100 to 150 mg every 8 hours, prevents insulin release. Other therapies include calcium channel blockers, corticosteroids, and glucagon. Octreotide therapy is useful in some patients with insulinoma.

Surgical exploration and enucleation of the tumor are needed in most patients. Insulinomas are often single and benign, and the surgical cure rate is high.

GASTRINOMA

Gastrinoma, or Zollinger-Ellison syndrome (ZES), is a rare cause of peptic ulcer disease. Tumors of the pancreatic or duodenal wall G cells are responsible for the signs and symptoms. Hyperparathyroidism is the most common associated endocrine abnormality.

Clinical Picture

Recurrent peptic ulcer, associated with secretory diarrhea, raises suspicion for ZES. Pathophysiologic effects are secondary to hypergastrinemia and hypersecretion of gastric hydrochloric acid (HCl). Severe esophagitis is thus an accompanying lesion. Precipitation of bile acids by excessive HCl and inappropriate pH for pancreatic lipase activity causes steatorrhea.

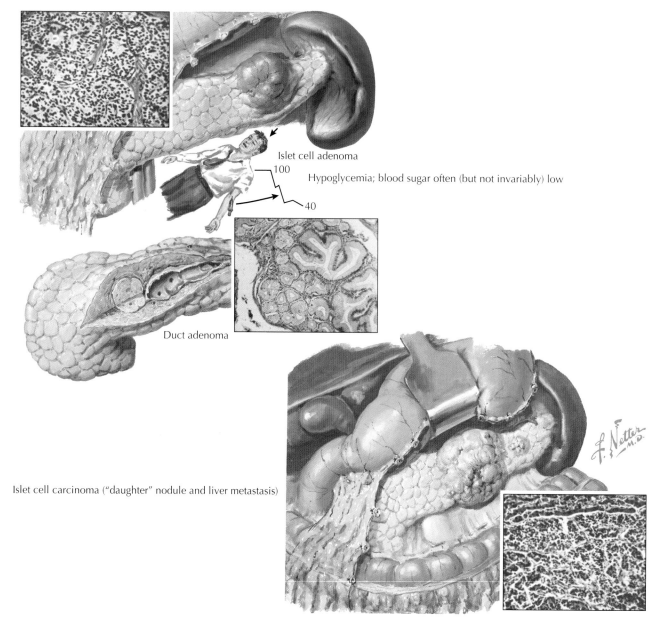

Islet cell adenoma

100

Hypoglycemia; blood sugar often (but not invariably) low

40

Duct adenoma

Islet cell carcinoma ("daughter" nodule and liver metastasis)

Fig. 132.1 Pancreatic Neuroendocrine (Islet Cell) Tumors: Adenoma and Carcinoma.

Diagnosis

Elevated plasma gastrin level (normal < 100 pg/mL; ZES > 1000 pg/mL) and basal acid output of 15 mEq/h or greater are features of gastrinoma. Other hypergastrinemic conditions include pernicious anemia (achlorhydria), atrophic gastritis, chronic renal failure, and the rare postoperative condition of retained antral syndrome after Billroth II surgery and chronic proton pump inhibitor (PPI) use. In patients with gastrinoma, intravenous injection of secretin causes a paradoxical increase in plasma/gastrin of 20 pg/mL or greater above the basal level.

EUS is currently the most sensitive and specific localization procedure with a sensitivity of 82% and a specificity of 92%. Venous sampling by angiography is not routinely indicated. It is an option for patients in whom conventional imaging fails to localize a tumor. Gastrinomas and other PNETs are visualized after injection of isotope-labeled somatostatin analogs, such as indium 111–octreotide. The sensitivity of this test is the highest ranging from 70% to 80%.

Treatment and Management

Effective control of gastric hypersecretion is possible with a proton pump inhibitor. Total gastrectomy is not recommended to deal with the complications of peptic ulcer disease. Octreotide is effective in suppressing gastrin release.

Most gastrinomas in the pancreas can be removed by enucleation, and large tumors can be removed by resective procedures. In patients with hepatic metastases, newer techniques include chemoembolization, cryotherapy, and alcohol ablation.

GLUCAGONOMA

Glucagonoma arising from pancreatic alpha cells is characterized by diabetes mellitus, severe dermatitis (necrolytic migratory erythema), neuropsychiatric symptoms, glossitis or stomatitis, diarrhea, weight loss, anemia, and venous thromboses. Hypoaminoacidemia as a result of catabolic effects of glucagon is responsible for the skin rash.

Tumors are solitary and large (>6 cm). The plasma glucagon level is greater than 500 pg/mL (normal < 100 pg/mL). CT, MRI, and EUS are helpful in the diagnosis.

Octreotide therapy reverses skin rash, reduces weight loss, and decreases diarrhea. Surgical therapy requires major pancreatic resection. Nutritional support is a major component of therapy.

VIPOMA (VASOACTIVE INTESTINAL PEPTIDE SECRETING TUMOR)

The characteristic features of VIPoma (Verner-Morrison syndrome) are watery diarrhea, hypokalemia, and achlorhydria (WDHA syndrome). Approximately 50% of the tumors are malignant, and 75% also secrete pancreatic polypeptide. Fasting plasma VIP level is greater than 500 pg/mL when the patient has diarrhea. Medical therapy includes rehydration and correction of hypokalemia. Octreotide therapy gives prompt relief from diarrhea. Tumor enucleation and partial pancreatectomy are surgical options.

ADDITIONAL RESOURCES

Amin S, Kim MK: Islet cell tumors of the pancreas, *Gastroenterol Clin North Am* 45(1):83–100, 2016.

Cloyd JM, Poultsides GA: Non-functional neuroendocrine tumors of the pancreas: advances in diagnosis and management, *World J Gastroenterol* 21(32):9512–9525, 2015.

Dromain C, Déandréis D, Scoazec JY, et al: Imaging of neuroendocrine tumors of the pancreas, *Diagn Interv Imaging* 97(12):1241–1257, 2016.

Kim MK: Endoscopic ultrasound in gastroenteropancreatic neuroendocrine tumors, *Gut Liver* 6(4):405–410, 2012.

Pea A, Hruban RH, Wood LD: Genetics of pancreatic neuroendocrine tumors: implications for the clinic, *Expert Rev Gastroenterol Hepatol* 9(11):1407–1419, 2015.

Tang LH, Basturk O, Sue JJ, Klimstra DS: A practical approach to the classification of WHO Grade 3 (G3) well-differentiated neuroendocrine tumor (WD-NET) and poorly differentiated neuroendocrine carcinoma (PD-NEC) of the pancreas, *Am J Surg Pathol* 40(9):1192–1202, 2016.

Uccella S, Sessa F, La Rosa S: Diagnostic approach to neuroendocrine neoplasms of the gastrointestinal tract and pancreas, *Turk Patoloji Derg* 31(Suppl 1):113–127, 2015.

Gallbladder and Bile Ducts

C. S. Pitchumoni

133

Anatomy and Function of the Gallbladder

C. S. Pitchumoni

The gallbladder is a pear-shaped organ, usually 10 cm (4 inches) in length and 3 to 5 cm in diameter, that is attached to the inferior surface of the liver (Fig. 133.1). Two-thirds of the gallbladder is covered by peritoneum. The fundus of the gallbladder projects beyond the liver; the body (or corpus) is in contact with the second portion of the duodenum and the colon; and the infundibulum (Hartmann pouch), located at the free edge of the lesser omentum, bulges forward toward the cystic duct. The neck is the part of the gallbladder between the body and the cystic duct.

The gallbladder has four layers: mucosa, muscularis, connective tissue, and, in most parts, serosa. Right and left hepatic ducts unite to form the 2- to 3-cm-long hepatic duct, which in turn combines with the cystic duct to form the *common bile duct* (CBD), which is 10 to 15 cm long. In approximately 85% of people, the CBD is partially or totally covered by pancreatic tissue posteriorly as it approaches the duodenum. In more than 66%, the CBD and the major pancreatic duct share a common channel, 2 to 7 mm in length, before emptying into the duodenum. The *sphincter of Oddi* (SO) is a muscular structure in the area of distal CBD, approximately 4 to 10 mm in length and mostly within the wall of the duodenum, that regulates the flow of bile and pancreatic juice.

Normally, the gallbladder has a volume capacity of approximately 30 to 60 mL. However, when it is actively reabsorbing water, sodium, chloride, and other electrolytes continuously, as much as 450 mL of secretion can be stored. The most potent stimulus for gallbladder contraction is the duodenal hormone *cholecystokinin* (CCK), but it is also stimulated by acetylcholine from vagi and the enteric nervous system. The normal bile contains 70% bile salts, 22% phospholipids, 4% cholesterol, 3% proteins, and 0.3% bilirubin, along with the electrolytes of plasma. Water and electrolytes are reabsorbed, whereas cholesterol, lecithin, and the bile salts become concentrated during fasting.

When the gallbladder contracts, the SO relaxes. The SO has variable basal pressure and phasic contractile activity that are regulated by nerves, hormones, CCK, and secretin.

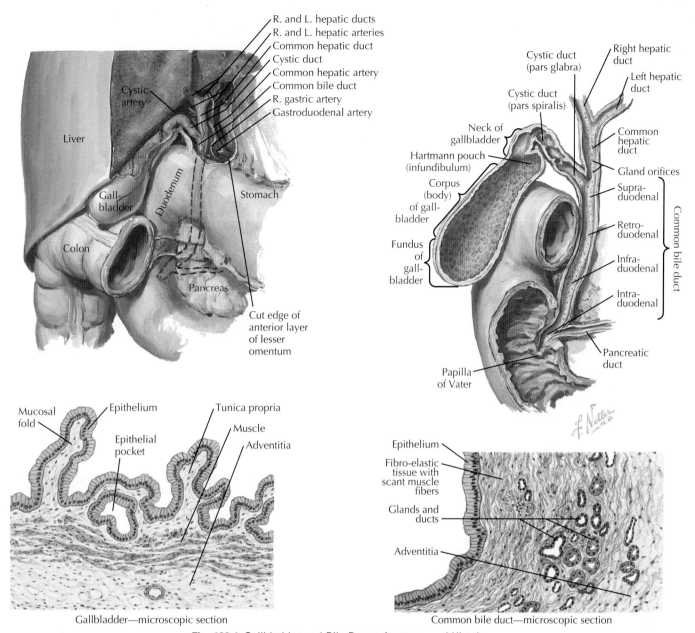

Fig. 133.1 Gallbladder and Bile Ducts: Anatomy and Histology.

ADDITIONAL RESOURCES

Afghani E, Lo SK, Covington PS, et al: Sphincter of oddi function and risk factors for dysfunction, *Front Nutr* 4:1, 2017.

134

Gallstones

C. S. Pitchumoni

EPIDEMIOLOGY OF GALLSTONE DISEASE

In the United States, an estimated 20% of adults older than 40 years of age and 30% of those older than 70 years have gallstone disease. Nearly 700,000 lap choles are performed every year. The prevalence of gallstone disease is low in Asians and Africans. The highest prevalence is in Native Americans (Pima Indians) and in Latin American populations. In white women, the prevalence is 5% to 15% in those younger than 50 years and approximately 25% in those older than 50, compared with 4% to 10% and 10% to 15%, respectively, in white men. Both generalized obesity and metabolic syndrome, the two risk factors for gallstone disease are increasing in prevalence.

More than 75% of the gallstones in the US population are *cholesterol* stones. The risk factors attributable to cholesterol stones are tabulated (Table 134.1).

TYPES OF GALLSTONES

Gallstones are divided into three major types—cholesterol, black pigment, and brown pigment—based on their composition and pathogenesis. In general, all gallstones form as a result of a change in bile composition, either an increase in the composition of a normal biliary component that exceeds its solubility or a decrease in a solubilizing component, or both (Fig. 134.1). Consequently, an insoluble substance called a *nidus* becomes supersaturated, and insoluble particles become sequestered and aggregate.

Cholesterol gallstone disease contributes to the occurrence of more than 80% of gallstones. These stones consist of pure cholesterol monohydrate crystals agglomerated by a mucin-glycoprotein matrix. Other constituents include unconjugated bilirubin and small amounts of calcium phosphate.

TABLE 134.1 Risk Factors for Cholesterol Stones

Risk Factor	Comments
Age	Uncommon before age 20 years (exception: Mexican-American girls)
Gender	Female/male ratio highest in youngest patients; narrows to 2:1 after age 50
Nationality	Highest: Scandinavia, Northern Europe, Chile, and northern parts of India Lowest: sub-Saharan Africa and Asia
Race/ethnicity	Highest: Pima Indians of southern Arizona (70% of Pima women older than 25 years), other Native American tribes, and Alaskans Lowest: American blacks
Genetic	Several genes are associated with the principal metabolic pathways involved in formation of gallstones
Family history	Higher risk in first-degree relatives of gallstone patients
Obesity	Relative risk rises sharply as degree of obesity increases; women more often affected Metabolic syndrome High body mass index (BMI) is a risk factor
Rapid active weight loss	Bile is lithogenic because of reduced bile acid secretion
Parity	Moderately elevated risk with increased parity
Diabetes mellitus	Good association in Mexican Americans Unclear association in other groups
Ileal/Crohn disease	Bile is lithogenic when ileal reabsorption is decreased
TPN	Usually, sludge and pigment stones caused by bile stasis and gallbladder distention
Medications	Estrogen therapy, oral contraceptive use, and octreotide therapy
Diet	Association with high consumption of simple sugars Low prevalence in vegetarians
Spinal cord injury	Abnormal gallbladder motility may be a factor
Miscellaneous	Celiac disease, vagotomy, and duodenal diverticula are rare associations No significant relationship with hyperlipoproteinemia

TPN, Total parenteral nutrition.

Pathogenesis of Gallstones

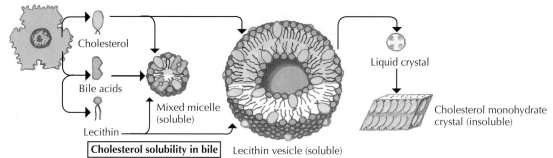

Solubility of cholesterol in bile depends on incorporation of cholesterol in bile acid–lecithin micelles and lecithin vesicles. When bile becomes saturated with cholesterol, vesicles fuse to form liposomes, or liquid crystals, from which crystals of cholesterol monohydrate nucleate.

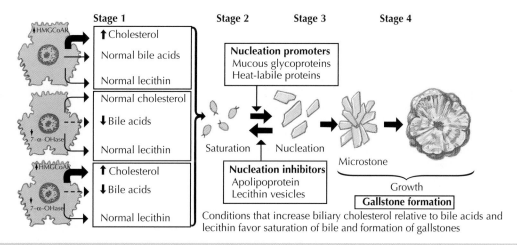

Predisposing factors

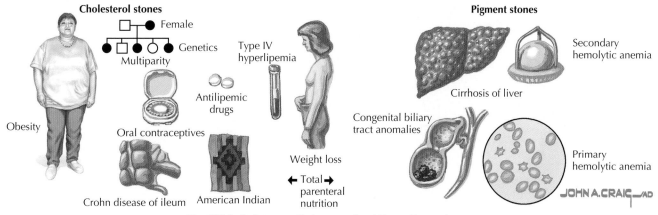

Fig. 134.1 Gallstones: Pathogenesis of Stone Formation.

The pathogenesis of cholesterol gallstones is well studied (see Fig. 134.1). Major components of bile are bile salts, phospholipids, and cholesterol. *Bile salts,* synthesized from cholesterol, constitute the two primary *bile acids,* cholic acid and chenodeoxycholic acid. *Cholesterol* is only slightly soluble in aqueous media but is made soluble through formation of mixed micelles with bile salts and *phospholipids,* mainly lecithin. The enterohepatic circulation of bile acids resulting from bile reabsorption from the terminal ileum, along with hepatic synthesis, keeps the bile acid pool physiologically optimal to maintain the cholesterol in solution.

At least four mechanisms are involved in the formation of cholesterol gallstones: (1) supersaturation of bile with cholesterol, (2) nucleation

of cholesterol monohydrate with subsequent crystallization and stone growth, (3) delayed emptying or gallbladder stasis, and (4) decreased enterohepatic circulation of bile acids. When the rate of bile acid secretion or the return of bile acid through enterohepatic circulation is decreased, as in patients with terminal ileal disease (e.g., Crohn disease), the relative cholesterol content increases, and bile becomes supersaturated *(lithogenic).* Lithogenic bile that stays within the gallbladder alters gallbladder motility and stimulates mucous secretion by the gallbladder epithelium.

Gallbladder sludge, the reversible but early stage of gallstone formation, is the suspension of precipitated bile dispersed in a viscous, mucin-rich liquid phase. Its chemical composition is mostly cholesterol monohydrate crystals, calcium bilirubinate, calcium phosphate, and calcium carbonate. Sludge may disappear, or it may progress to develop gallstones. Sludge may cause cholecystitis, pancreatitis, or biliary pain. Sludge formation is associated with pregnancy, rapid weight loss, obesity, prolonged fasting, and total parenteral nutrition (TPN) and following bariatric surgery. Intravenously administered ceftriaxone, a third-generation broad-spectrum cephalosporin, can condense and crystalize in the gallbladder to form biliary sludge.

Clinical manifestations of sludge include biliary colic, acute cholangitis, and acute pancreatitis. It is detected in the right upper quadrant on ultrasonography as low-amplitude echoes without acoustic shadowing.

Brown pigment stones are morphologically, chemically, and clinically distinct from black pigment stones. The brown pigment stone is laminated with alternating regions of brown and tan material and tends to cake when powdered. Brown pigment stones contain only small amounts of calcium phosphates and calcium carbonates. They develop in the gallbladder and in the intrahepatic and extrahepatic ducts and are associated with polymicrobial infection (e.g., *Escherichia coli*). Bacterial degradation by enzymes, primarily β-glucuronidase, deconjugates bilirubin and lecithin to free fatty acids. Brown pigment stones are mostly radiolucent. A decrease in effective bile salt micelles promotes cholesterol supersaturation. The predominant symptoms of brown pigment stone disease are jaundice, chills, fever, and abdominal pain. Cholangitis is common.

Black pigment stones are composed largely of calcium salts of unconjugated bilirubin, carbonate, and phosphate. The bilirubinate salts of black pigment stones are amorphous. Black pigment stones are clinically associated with hemolytic syndromes, cirrhosis of the liver, chronic alcoholism, malaria, TPN, and old age. Almost 50% of patients with sickle cell anemia and 15% to 40% of those with sickle cell disease have pigment stones by age 20 years.

More than 66% of black pigment stones but only 10% of cholesterol stones are radiopaque on abdominal plain films. The increased concentration of unconjugated bilirubin in the pathogenesis of black pigment stones is probably nonbacterial and nonenzymatic. Gallbladder stasis and defective acidification of gallbladder bile in an alkaline environment favor the formation of calcium phosphate and calcium carbonate. In hemolytic anemias, bilirubin levels increase 10-fold, with elevated gallbladder volume and stasis. Black pigment stones also develop in children and young adults.

ADDITIONAL RESOURCES

Agresta F, Campanile FC, Vettoretto N, et al: Laparoscopic cholecystectomy: consensus conference-based guidelines, *Langenbecks Arch Surg* 400(4): 429–453, 2015.

Camilleri M, Malhi H, Acosta A: Gastrointestinal complications of obesity, *Gastroenterology* 152(7):1656–1670, 2017.

Portincasa P, Di Ciaula A, de Bari O, et al: Management of gallstones and its related complications, *Expert Rev Gastroenterol Hepatol* 10(1):93–112, 2016.

135

Acute Cholecystitis

C. S. Pitchumoni

Acute cholecystitis is inflammation of the gallbladder after persistent obstruction of the gallbladder outlet from an impacted stone, resulting in increased gallbladder pressure, rapid distention, decreased blood supply, and gallbladder ischemia, with subsequent bacterial invasion, inflammation, and possible perforation (Fig. 135.1). Approximately 10% to 20% of patients with symptomatic gallstones develop acute cholecystitis.

CLINICAL PICTURE

Steady and severe abdominal pain over the right upper quadrant radiating to the back, the right scapula, or the right clavicular area and associated with fever, nausea, anorexia, and vomiting is the main symptom of acute cholecystitis. Physical examination reveals tenderness over the gallbladder area. As the gallbladder area is palpated, the patient is asked to take a deep breath that brings the gallbladder down to the palpating hand. At the height of inspiration, as the gallbladder touches the palpating hand, the breath is arrested with a gasp *(Murphy sign)*. The sign is not found in chronic cholecystitis. Sensitivity to Murphy sign may be diminished in elderly patients. Complications of acute cholecystitis are empyema of the gallbladder, gangrene with perforation, intraabdominal abscess, and diffuse peritonitis.

Laboratory findings include leukocytosis with a shift to the left and mildly elevated bilirubin and alkaline phosphatase levels. Serum amylase and lipase levels are normal or only mildly elevated unless there is concomitant acute pancreatitis. The differential diagnosis includes acute pancreatitis, appendicitis, acute hepatitis, peptic ulcer disease, disease of the right kidney, right-sided pneumonia, Fitz-Hugh-Curtis syndrome (gonococcal perihepatitis), liver abscess, perforated viscus, and cardiac ischemia.

DIAGNOSIS

History and physical examination followed by the basic laboratory tests including complete blood count and serum liver tests are needed in the preliminary evaluation. Abdominal ultrasound is indicated in all patients. Ultrasound examination of the right upper quadrant of the abdomen can detect gallstones with a sensitivity and specificity greater than 95%, in addition to being useful in imaging the liver, biliary ducts, and the pancreas. The findings include gallstones, sludge, lumen distention, mural thickening with a hypoechoic or anechoic zone within the thickened wall, and pericholecystic fluid. Sonographic Murphy sign is defined as the presence of maximal tenderness elicited by direct pressure of the transducer over the gallbladder. Abdominal computed tomography (CT) is needed only when the diagnosis is vague or when abscess formation or gangrene is suspected. Gallstones, sludge, gallbladder distention, mural thickening, pericholecystic fluid, and subserosal edema are major findings.

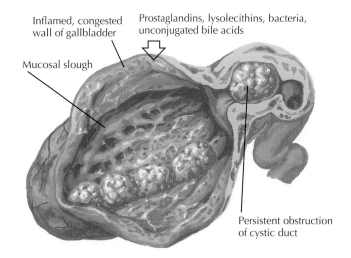

Inflamed, congested wall of gallbladder

Prostaglandins, lysolecithins, bacteria, unconjugated bile acids

Mucosal slough

Persistent obstruction of cystic duct

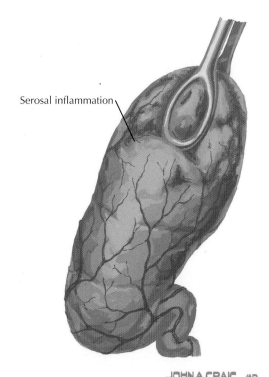

Serosal inflammation

JOHN A.CRAIG—AD

Fig. 135.1 Acute Calculous Cholecystitis.

Magnetic resonance cholangiopancreatography (MRCP), a noninvasive technique for evaluating the intrahepatic and extrahepatic bile ducts, is superior to ultrasound for detecting stones in the cystic duct. Magnetic resonance imaging (MRI) also helps in diagnosing complications of acute cholecystitis. Hepatobiliary iminodiacetic acid (HIDA) scintigraphy involves intravenous injection of a nuclear isotope to determine the patency of the cystic duct. It also demonstrates patency of the common bile duct (CBD) and ampulla. Positive HIDA testing is nonvisualization of the gallbladder with normal excretion of the isotope into the CBD and duodenum. HIDA scanning is highly sensitive (95%) and specific (90%) for acute calculous cholecystitis. In acute *acalculous* cholecystitis, HIDA findings may be falsely negative because the cystic duct remains patent. False-positive results occur when the gallbladder cannot be visualized despite an unobstructed cystic duct, such as in severe liver disease and hyperbilirubinemia, after biliary sphincterotomy, and in fasting patients receiving total parenteral nutrition (TPN) who already have a maximally full gallbladder because of prolonged lack of stimulation.

TREATMENT AND MANAGEMENT

Management of acute cholecystitis includes bowel rest, parenteral fluids and nutrition, and intravenous antibiotics. Common organisms include *Escherichia coli*, *Enterococcus*, *Klebsiella*, and *Enterobacter*. The need for antibiotics in uncomplicated cholecystitis is debatable, although in clinical practice, most patients receive antibiotics. A combination of ampicillin (2 g intravenously every 4 hours) and gentamicin (dosed according to weight and renal function) is one of the many choices for empiric treatment. β-Lactam–based therapy and fluoroquinolones are other options.

The definitive therapy for acute cholecystitis is laparoscopic *cholecystectomy*. Early laparoscopic cholecystectomy, within 72 hours of onset of symptoms, is safe and shortens the hospital stay. Laparoscopic cholecystectomy eliminates the need to incise the rectus abdominis muscle, reduces postoperative pain, and shortens hospital stay and convalescence. The risk for CBD injury is 0.2% in both laparoscopic and open surgical approaches. Patients at high risk may be treated with percutaneous cholecystostomy in association with antibiotic therapy as a temporary measure. Other complications of laparoscopic cholecystectomy include bowel and liver lacerations, bile leak, gallstone spillage and abscess formation, and major bleeding. However, the risk for most of these complications is low with the increasing experience of the surgeon.

A new era in gastrointestinal surgery involves cholecystectomy with access to the peritoneal cavity through normal anatomy, known as "natural orifice" transluminal endoscopic surgery.

ADDITIONAL RESOURCES

Guruswamy KS, Samaj K: Early versus delayed laparoscopic cholecystectomy for acute cholecystitis, *Cochrane Database Syst Rev* (4):CD005440, 2006.

Keus F, de Jong JA, Gooszen HG, et al: Laparoscopic versus small-incision cholecystectomy for patients with symptomatic cholecystolithiasis, *Cochrane Database Syst Rev* (4):CD006229, 2006.

Trowbridge RL, Rutkowski NK, Shojana KG: Does this patient have acute cholecystitis?, *JAMA* 299:80–86, 2003.

136

Cholecystitis: Complications

C. S. Pitchumoni

Gangrenous cholecystitis noted in approximately 5% of the patients with acute cholecystitis implies severe gallbladder inflammation with mural necrosis associated with an increased risk for morbidity and mortality. Computed tomography of the abdomen may show mural necrosis, gas in the wall or lumen, intramural hemorrhage, pericholecystic abscess, or absent gallbladder wall enhancement (Fig. 136.1). Although laparoscopic cholecystectomy can be performed safely by experts, percutaneous cholecystectomy followed by delayed cholecystectomy is an option.

Emphysematous cholecystitis is severe acute cholecystitis caused by a gas-forming organism such as *Clostridium perfringens, Pseudomonas, Klebsiella, and Escherichia coli* noted often in the elderly and diabetics. Perforation is a complication. Abdominal ultrasound is helpful in the

diagnosis. Contrast-enhanced computed tomography (CT) confirms the presence of gas in the gallbladder wall or lumen.

Acalculous cholecystitis refers to inflammation of the gallbladder without gallstones, seen in 2% to 15% of patients undergoing cholecystectomy. It usually occurs in critically ill adults or after trauma, burns, or major surgery in particular gastric or colorectal procedures. Other risk factors include diabetes mellitus, sepsis, prolonged fasting, acquired immunodeficiency syndrome (AIDS), and hepatic arterial chemotherapy. Its pathogenesis is attributed to the occlusion of the cystic duct by viscous bile. The prognosis is poor, and mortality is 60%. The diagnosis is made by abdominal ultrasound (US) or CT scan. The findings are a distended gallbladder with edematous wall, pericholecystic fluid and positive Murphy sign on sonography. Complications

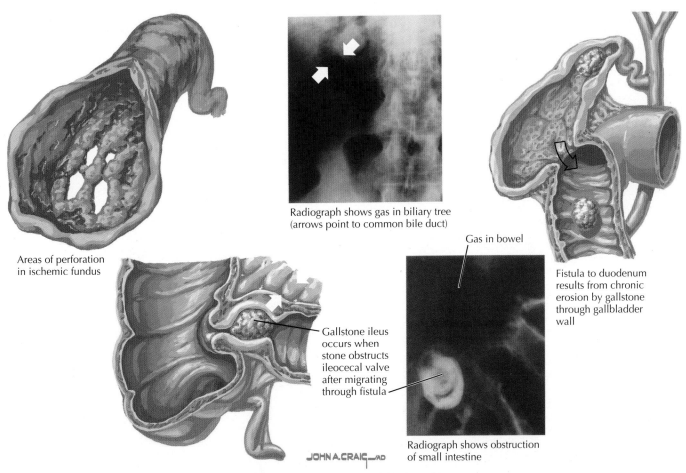

Radiograph shows gas in biliary tree (arrows point to common bile duct)

Areas of perforation in ischemic fundus

Gas in bowel

Fistula to duodenum results from chronic erosion by gallstone through gallbladder wall

Gallstone ileus occurs when stone obstructs ileocecal valve after migrating through fistula

Radiograph shows obstruction of small intestine

JOHN A. CRAIG—AD

Fig. 136.1 Complications of Cholecystitis.

include mural necrosis, gangrene, and perforation. Abdominal ultrasonography reveals gallbladder distention, mural thickening (>5 mm), pericholecystic fluid, positive sonographic Murphy sign, and emphysematous cholecystitis with gas bubbles arising in the fundus of the gallbladder (champagne sign). Percutaneous aspiration of the bile under sonographic guidance may help with the diagnosis. Percutaneous cholecystostomy is an emergency procedure required to temporize the critical illness.

Chronic cholecystitis may be secondary to repeated attacks of uncomplicated acute cholecystitis or without prior attacks (see Chapter 137). The symptoms are vague and may be only nonspecific epigastric or right upper quadrant pain. Histologically, patients have chronic inflammatory cell infiltration of the gallbladder associated with gallstones and thickening of the gallbladder wall.

Mirizzi syndrome is a rare condition in which a stone impacted in the cystic duct causes severe inflammation and may erode into the common bile duct (CBD), producing an inflammatory mass around the cholecystocholedochal fistula and obstructing the CBD. The clinical relevance is that the surgeon should not mistake the CBD for the cystic duct.

AIDS cholangiopathy is an inflammation of the biliary tract manifesting late in the course of illness most often caused by cytomegalovirus, *Cryptosporidium*, *Microsporum*, and *Mycobacterium avium*, seen when the CD4 count is less than 100 cell/mm^3. The disease has become infrequent with the advent of highly active antiretroviral therapy (HAART). The disease may manifest as papillary stenosis, sclerosing cholangitis, and extrahepatic duct strictures. The magnetic resonance cholangiopancreatography (MRCP) imaging resembles that of primary sclerosing cholangitis. Treatment of AIDS cholangiopathy is unsatisfactory. Endoscopic sphincterotomy, stricture dilatations, and stenting are options.

ADDITIONAL RESOURCES

Kim D, Iqbal SI, Ahari HK, et al: Expanding role of percutaneous cholecystostomy and interventional radiology for the management of acute cholecystitis: an analysis of 144 patients, *Diagn Interv Imaging* 99(1):15–21, 2018.

Kirkwood R, Damon L, Wang J, et al: Gangrenous cholecystitis: innovative laparoscopic techniques to facilitate subtotal fenestrating cholecystectomy when a critical view of safety cannot be achieved, *Surg Endosc* 31(12):5258–5266, 2017.

Sousa I, Fernandes A, Távora I: Emphysematous cholecystitis: imaging diagnosis of an emergent condition, *Acta Med Port* 29(11):761, 2016.

137

Chronic Cholecystitis

C. S. Pitchumoni

Cholelithiasis and cholecystitis are classified into three types based on presentation: (1) silent gallstones, in which gallstones are detected accidentally and are truly asymptomatic; (2) symptomatic gallstone disease; and (3) abdominal symptoms mimicking cholelithiasis but caused by a comorbid condition such as peptic ulcer or irritable bowel syndrome.

ASYMPTOMATIC GALLSTONE DISEASE

Approximately 15% of the adults in the United States are estimated to have gallstones. Almost 60% to 80% of the gallstones are incidentally found during routine abdominal sonography, but most patients do not have symptoms or abdominal symptoms are not from gallbladder disease. Approximately 20% of persons with silent gallstones may develop symptoms by 20 years. It is unusual to develop gallstone-related complications without first developing at least an episode of biliary pain. Symptoms develop with a rate of 1% to 4% per year. Patients with asymptomatic gallstones do not require cholecystectomy except in countries where gallbladder carcinoma is prevalent. Box 137.1 lists indications for prophylactic cholecystectomy.

Porcelain gallbladder (PGB) is a rare, asymptomatic, chronic cholecystitis characterized by intramural calcification of the gallbladder wall. PGB was once considered to be a strong indicator for cholecystectomy because of its high association with gallbladder cancer. The association

is currently felt to be a weak one. Patchy mucosal calcification carries a higher risk of cancer than does diffuse intramural calcification. Plain abdominal radiographs reveal an incidental calcified gallbladder. The incidence of gallbladder carcinoma is as high as 33%, and prophylactic cholecystectomy is warranted.

SYMPTOMATIC GALLSTONE DISEASE

Clinical Picture

Patients with symptomatic gallstones have episodic epigastric (or right upper quadrant) pain radiating to the back, right scapula, or right shoulder and lasting at least 15 to 30 minutes (Fig. 137.1). Although frequently known as "biliary colic," the term is a misnomer because generally the pain is constant and not colicky. The pain may be mild, moderate, or severe. Nonspecific symptoms such as bloating, flatulence, and heartburn are no more frequent in patients with gallstones than in the general population.

Gallstones can cause biliary colic, acute cholecystitis, obstructive jaundice by a common bile duct (CBD) stone, ascending cholangitis, and acute pancreatitis. Stones may fistulate into the duodenum from the gallbladder. *Bouveret syndrome* refers to an impacted stone in the duodenum causing obstruction. A gallstone may become impacted near the terminal ileum, leading to small bowel obstruction; in *gallstone ileus,* a supine abdominal radiograph may show air in the biliary tree. Physical examination will reveal right upper quadrant tenderness. Fever, abdominal rigidity, and rebound tenderness are signs of acute cholecystitis.

Diagnosis

A history of right upper quadrant abdominal pain requires evaluation with abdominal ultrasound, the "gold standard" for the diagnosis of gallbladder stones. The test is conducted with the patient having fasted for at least 8 hours so that the stones can be seen in a distended gallbladder, surrounded by bile. Ultrasonographic criteria constitute an echogenic focus that casts an acoustic shadow and seeks gravitational dependency. Although echogenic, *sludge* (or multiple small gallstones) does not cast an acoustic shadow. Sludge is viscous and does not seek gravitational dependency as rapidly as "gravel."

Plain films of the abdomen and oral cholecystography are seldom used to diagnose gallstone disease. Only 15% to 20% of gallstones are seen on plain films of abdomen. Computed tomography and magnetic resonance imaging are not indicated initially to diagnose gallstone disease but may be helpful to evaluate complications.

Management

Treatment of biliary colic is with analgesics. Nonsteroidal antiinflammatory drugs (NSAIDs) such as diclofenac or indomethacin in combination

---

> **BOX 137.1 Indications for Prophylactic Cholecystectomy in Patients With Silent Gallstones[a]**
>
> 1. High risk for gallbladder cancer
>   - Native American women with gallstones
>   - Solitary stone or stone burden > 3 cm
>   - Porcelain gallbladder (indication is currently questioned)
>   - Gallbladder polyps > 12 mm
> 2. Carriers of *Salmonella typhi*
> 3. Sickle cell disease (calcium bilirubinate stones)
> 4. Incidental cholecystectomy during another abdominal surgery (chronic hemolytic conditions, risk of malignancy, and bariatric surgery)
> 5. To be considered in heart transplant patients
> 6. Plan to live for long periods in remote parts of world with poor medical facilities

[a]Diabetes mellitus is not an indication for prophylactic cholecystectomy. Cholecystectomy is not performed routinely in all patients undergoing bariatric surgery.

Sudden obstruction (biliary colic)

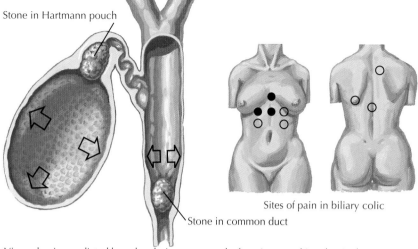

Stone in Hartmann pouch

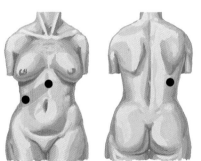

Sites of pain in biliary colic

Stone in common duct

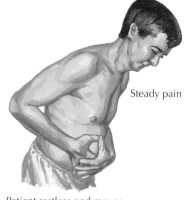

Steady pain

Patient restless and moves
about seeking position of relief

Visceral pain, mediated by splanchnic nerve, results from increased intraluminal pressure
and distention caused by sudden calculous obstruction of cystic or common duct

Persistent obstruction (acute cholecystitis)

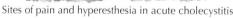

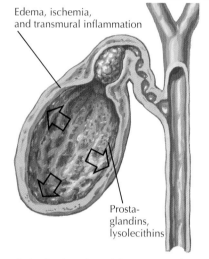

Edema, ischemia,
and transmural inflammation

Prosta-
glandins,
lysolecithins

Sites of pain and hyperesthesia in acute cholecystitis

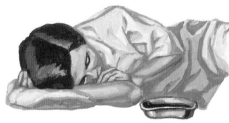

Patient lies motionless because minor movement
(even breathing) increases pain. Nausea common.

Parietal epigastric or right upper quadrant pain results from ischemia and inflammation of gallbladder
wall caused by persistent calculous obstruction of cystic duct. Prostaglandins and lysolecithins released.

JOHN A. CRAIG—AD

Fig. 137.1 Mechanisms of Biliary Pain.

with antispasmolytics are recommended. Therapy for gallstone disease
is mostly laparoscopic. Open surgery is needed in complicated cases.
Nonsurgical therapy is seldom used currently. Ursodeoxycholic acid
is advocated when lithogenic bile production is increased or microlithiasis is suspected, as in obese patients after bariatric surgery or in
patients with idiopathic pancreatitis, but has no role in symptomatic
gallstone disease.

ADDITIONAL RESOURCES

European Association for the Study of the Liver (EASL): EASL clinical
practice guidelines on the prevention, diagnosis and treatment of
gallstones, *J Hepatol* 65(1):146–181, 2016.
Khan ZS, Livingston EH, Huerta S: Reassessing the need for prophylactic
surgery in patients with porcelain gallbladder: case series and systematic
review of the literature, *Arch Surg* 146(10):1143–1147, 2011.

138

Choledocholithiasis and Cholangitis

C. S. Pitchumoni

Stones in the common bile duct (CBD) are either primary or secondary. Primary stones are formed de novo in the CBD as a result of bacterial action on phospholipid and bilirubin (see Chapter 134). Secondary stones, including cholesterol and pigment stones, are formed in the gallbladder and are passed into the CBD.

CHOLEDOCHOLITHIASIS

The prevalence of CBD stones varies depending on several factors. Along with stones in the gallbladder, choledocholithiasis is noted in 10% to 20% of patients with symptomatic gallstones. In addition, in the immediate postoperative period, almost 1% of cholecystectomy patients have a retained stone. The prevalence of concomitant CBD stones increases with advancing age. Hemolysis predisposes patients to black pigment stones. Bacterial or parasitic infection of the biliary tract, a foreign body in the duct (surgical sutures and clips), and juxtapapillary duodenal diverticula increase the prevalence of brown pigment stones. *Ascaris* infection is a rare cause of CBD stones in endemic areas. Anatomic abnormalities such as low entry of the cystic duct (<3.5 cm from ampulla) and sphincter of Oddi dysfunction predispose patients to CBD stones. Intrahepatic calcium bilirubinate stones (Oriental cholangiopathy) are noted in Japanese and Korean patients. An iatrogenic form of choledocholithiasis is the development of pigment stones (regardless of original type of gallstones) after endoscopic sphincterotomy, which permits bacterial colonization of the CBD, deconjugation of bilirubin, and formation of pigment stones.

Clinical Picture

In patients with intact gallbladder, the symptoms of choledocholithiasis and cholecystolithiasis are clinically similar, and the diagnosis of CBD stones cannot be made based solely on symptomatology. CBD stones may be asymptomatic for many years, or they may present with jaundice or with biliary colic, pancreatitis, or acute suppurative cholangitis (Fig. 138.1). "Biliary colic," a misnomer for the constant pain over the right upper quadrant, lasts for 30 minutes to several hours and is associated with nausea, vomiting, and diaphoresis but is not related to food intake. Prolonged obstruction for 4 to 5 years without therapy leads to biliary cirrhosis. Elevated serum bilirubin concentration (2 to 14 mg/dL) and elevated alkaline phosphatase levels indicate cholestasis.

Diagnosis

CBD stone is to be clinically suspected in symptomatic gallstone disease (acute cholecystitis), acute pancreatitis, and rarely in postcholecystectomy patients. Evaluation of liver enzymes (aspartate transaminase [AST], alanine aminotransferase [ALT], alkaline phosphatase [ALP]) and bilirubin is the initial step. Completely normal biochemical test results have an excellent negative predictive value. Marked elevation of AST and ALT levels occur in acute CBD obstructive disease.

Abdominal ultrasound (US) and/or computed tomography (CT) are initial diagnostic procedures. However, small bile duct stones are missed by the procedures. The predictor for CBD stone is high if there is clinical ascending cholangitis, increased CBD size on US, and bilirubin level of greater than 4 mg/dL. A nondilated CBD on US with no liver test abnormality is associated with low probability (<5%) for CBD stone. Magnetic resonance cholangiopancreatography (MRCP) is an important alternative to exclude choledocholithiasis in patients at low or intermediate risk (Fig. 138.2). MRCP has 85% to 90% sensitivity and a higher specificity. Small stones at the distal end of the CBD can be missed. Intraoperative cholangiography is an option with a high sensitivity and specificity but the added procedure prolongs the duration of surgery. Endoscopic ultrasound (EUS) is less invasive, entails no complications, and has a sensitivity and specificity of 90% to 100%. As a diagnostic modality for CBD stones, endoscopic retrograde cholangiopancreatography (ERCP) is not indicated in all cases of a suspected CBD stone. A minority of those with strong predictors of CBD stone (CBD stone in abdominal ultrasound, clinical ascending cholangitis and serum bilirubin of >4 mg/dL) require preoperative, intraoperative, or postoperative endoscopic retrograde cholangiography (ERC). Patients with intermediate predictors of CBD stone need MRCP or EUS to confirm the diagnosis and the need for endoscopic therapy. In some cases, CBD stones are diagnosed at surgery by palpation of the duct, intraoperative cholangiography, or choledochoscopy.

Management

The recommended treatment of choice is by ERC with sphincterotomy and stone extraction (Fig. 138.3). Approximately 85% to 90% of CBD stones can be removed with Dormia basket or balloon catheter. Other options available for difficult stones include lithotripsy (mechanical, shock wave, laser, and extracorporeal), and biliary stenting.

CBD stones diagnosed at laparoscopic cholecystectomy may require conversion to open surgery and CBD exploration. Advances in laparoscopic biliary surgery now allow experienced surgeons to manage CBD stones at the same time. Postoperative ERC is necessary if intraoperative removal of CBD stones is unsuccessful. Elective cholecystectomy is recommended in most patients after endoscopic clearance of CBD stones. In elderly patients with multiple comorbid conditions or with cirrhosis, surgery may be risky, and endoscopic therapy alone may be acceptable.

CHOLANGITIS

In 1877 Charcot first described *pyogenic cholangitis* in patients with right upper quadrant pain, fever, and jaundice (Charcot triad). A severe form of cholangitis includes two additional features: hypotension and mental confusion (Reynolds pentad). The absence of Charcot triad does not exclude the diagnosis, because its sensitivity is only 50% to

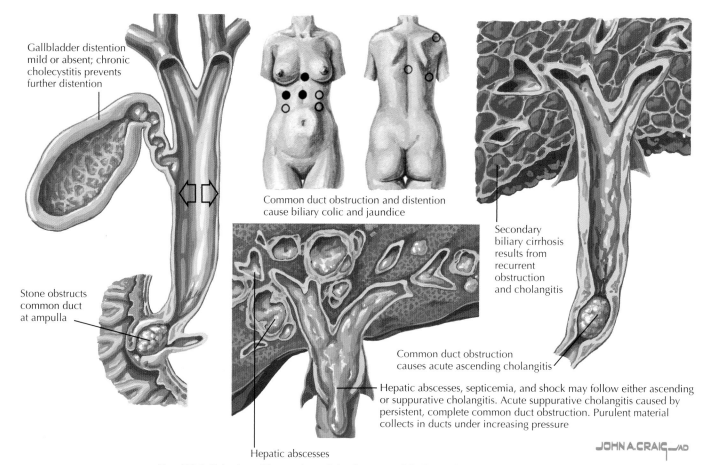

Gallbladder distention mild or absent; chronic cholecystitis prevents further distention

Common duct obstruction and distention cause biliary colic and jaundice

Secondary biliary cirrhosis results from recurrent obstruction and cholangitis

Stone obstructs common duct at ampulla

Common duct obstruction causes acute ascending cholangitis

Hepatic abscesses, septicemia, and shock may follow either ascending or suppurative cholangitis. Acute suppurative cholangitis caused by persistent, complete common duct obstruction. Purulent material collects in ducts under increasing pressure

JOHN A.CRAIG⎯AD

Hepatic abscesses

Fig. 138.1 Calculous Obstruction of the Common Bile Duct (Choledocholithiasis).

70%. In more than 80% of patients, the most important contributory cause for pyogenic cholangitis is CBD obstruction by choledocholithiasis, promoting bacterial overgrowth. Cholangitis may be secondary to malignant CBD obstruction or may be iatrogenic, caused by instrumentation (ERCP, stricture dilatation), postoperative biliary stricture, or papillary stenosis. Normally sterile bile becomes infected when local defenses are impaired. Elevated intraductal pressure decreases resistance to bacterial growth in bile, an otherwise excellent culture medium. Once cholangitis starts, infection may spread locally to the liver and to the systemic circulation, along with toxemia. Malignant obstruction, often total, is less likely to cause cholangitis, presumably because reflux of duodenal contents does not occur. The term cholangitis also includes entities other than that due to CBD stone or stricture, because, for example, cholangitis is associated with liver flukes, immunoglobulin G (IgG)4-associated disorders, and primary biliary cholangitis.

Clinical Picture

The classic picture of intermittent fever, pain, and jaundice is seen in 50% to 70% of patients with cholangitis. Shaking chills suggesting bacteremia occurs in two-thirds of patients. Cholangitis in the elderly patient may be atypical but should be suspected when there is sudden onset, mental confusion, lethargy, and delirium. Abdominal pain may be mild or even absent. Physical findings include fever, right upper quadrant tenderness, and jaundice. Rarely, hypotension and mental confusion occur, indicating a severe form of the disease. Untreated bacterial cholangitis has a poor prognosis, and even with treatment, mortality rates range from 5% to 30%.

Diagnosis

Leukocytosis and elevated serum bilirubin and alkaline phosphatase levels are characteristic. Blood culture should be performed early in the evaluation. Rarely, liver function abnormalities mimic acute hepatitis, with greatly elevated serum levels of AST and ALT. However, normal liver enzyme levels do not exclude cholangitis. Hyperamylasemia, when noted, is mild and less than three times the upper limit of normal.

The diagnosis of cholangitis is supported by abnormal laboratory values and imaging studies. Abdominal ultrasonography helps in evaluating the size of the CBD and the presence of stones. Abdominal CT may show the same findings, although less precisely, and MRCP better delineates the ductal morphology. Blood culture is usually positive for enteric organisms. Organisms that frequently cause cholangitis are *Escherichia coli*, *Klebsiella*, *Enterococcus*, *Enterobacter*, *Streptococcus*, and *Pseudomonas aeruginosa*; anaerobic bacteria are found in less than 10% of patients. Leukopenia, thrombocytopenia, coagulopathy, and renal failure suggest severe disease.

Management

Cholangitis is managed with appropriate antibiotics and aggressive fluid resuscitation. The severity of cholangitis can be graded from mild to moderate to severe (see Fig. 138.2). Presence of organ dysfunction is an important parameter of severity and requires emergency biliary decompression by endoscopic papillary large balloon dilatation with endoscopic sphincterotomy to remove CBD stones. Mechanical lithotripsy

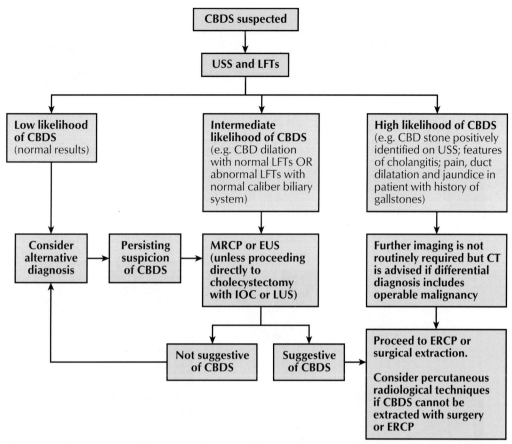

Fig. 138.2 Investigation of Suspected Common Bile Duct Stone *(CBDS)*. *CT*, Computed tomography; *ERCP*, endoscopic retrograde cholangiopancreatography; *EUS*, endoscopic ultrasound; *IOC*, intraoperative cholangiography; *LFT*, liver function test; *LUS*, laparoscopic ultrasound; *MRCP*, magnetic resonance cholangiopancreatography; *USS*, ultrasound scanning. (Reused with permission from Williams E, Beckingham I, El Sayed G, et al: Updated guideline on the management of common bile duct stones (CBDS), *Gut* 66:765-782, 2017.)

is needed in a selected few patients. The goal is to relieve the obstruction to bile flow as early as possible. A nasobiliary drainage catheter helps decompression of bile and in performing subsequent cholangiographic studies. Percutaneous transhepatic cholangiography under local anesthesia is another option. The procedure may be complicated by bile leak, biliary vascular fistula, pneumothorax, bile peritonitis, and catheter-related sepsis. Surgical exploration for ductal decompression is performed after initial management. Failure of biliary decompression indicates the need for emergency surgery.

Lap chole is to be performed prior to discharge after clinical stability is achieved with antibiotic therapy and intravenous (IV) fluid support.

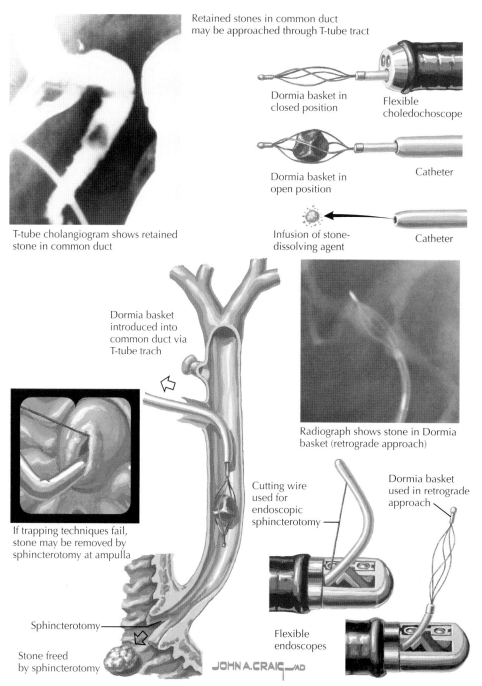

Retained stones in common duct
may be approached through T-tube tract

Dormia basket in closed position

Flexible choledochoscope

Dormia basket in open position

Catheter

Infusion of stone-dissolving agent

Catheter

T-tube cholangiogram shows retained stone in common duct

Dormia basket introduced into common duct via T-tube trach

Radiograph shows stone in Dormia basket (retrograde approach)

Cutting wire used for endoscopic sphincterotomy

Dormia basket used in retrograde approach

If trapping techniques fail, stone may be removed by sphincterotomy at ampulla

Flexible endoscopes

Sphincterotomy

Stone freed by sphincterotomy

JOHN A. CRAIG—AD

Fig. 138.3 Management of Stones.

ADDITIONAL RESOURCES

Copelan A, Kapoor BS: Choledocholithiasis: diagnosis and management, *Tech Vasc Interv Radiol* 18(4):244–255, 2015.

Fogel EL, Sherman S: ERCP for gallstone pancreatitis, *N Engl J Med* 370(2):150–157, 2014.

He H, Tan C, Wu J, et al: Accuracy of ASGE high-risk criteria in evaluation of patients with suspected common bile duct stones, *Gastrointest Endosc* 86(3):525–532, 2017.

Kiriyama S, Takada T, Strasberg SM, et al: TG13 guidelines for diagnosis and severity grading of acute cholangitis (with videos), *J Hepatobiliary Pancreat Sci* 20:24–34, 2013.

Lee SP, Roberts JR, Kuver R: The changing faces of cholangitis, *F1000 Research* 5:1409, 2016.

Maple JT, Menachem BT, Anderson MA, et al: The role of endoscopy in the evaluation of suspected choledocholithiasis, *Gastrointest Endosc* 71(1):1–9, 2010.

Williams E, Beckingham I, El Sayed G, et al: Updated guideline on the management of common bile duct stones (CBDS), *Gut* 66(5):765–782, 2017.

139

Sphincter of Oddi Dysfunction

C. S. Pitchumoni

The sphincter of Oddi (SO) is a smooth muscular structure usually 7 to 13 mm in length encircling the distal common bile duct (CBD) and the pancreatic duct (a common channel opening into the ampulla of Vater). The three functions of the SO are control of the flow of bile and pancreatic secretions into the duodenum, prevention of reflux of duodenal juice into the pancreaticobiliary system, and regulation of gall bladder function. Papillary stenosis refers to the type of SO dysfunction (SOD) related to a structural abnormality. Biliary dyskinesia is a functional blockage at the high-pressure zone attributed to spasm and/or hypertrophy or neuropathy of the sphincteric nerves. The advent of biliary manometry has contributed to a better understanding of the SO functions. The "gold standard" in evaluating SO dysfunction is manometry, which is invasive because it needs an endoscopic retrograde cholangiopancreatography (ERCP) setting.

ANATOMY AND PHYSIOLOGY

The SO is composed of a biliary and a pancreatic sphincter. The common ductal segment passes obliquely through the duodenal wall and terminates at the papilla of Vater, a small nipplelike protrusion less than 1 cm in diameter. Numerous variations are observed as the common bile and pancreatic ducts join (Figs. 139.1 and 139.2). The sphincter function is regulated by neuronal and hormonal factors.

The SO has a rich supply of nerves—intrinsic catecholamine-containing neurons, nonadrenergic noncholinergic (NANC) including substance P, vasoactive intestinal peptide (VIP), somatostatin, calcitonin gene–related peptide, met-enkephalin-like immunoreactivity, prominent galanin-like immunoreactivity, and nitric oxide—most of which play a role in SO function. Spontaneous motor activity of the SO is primarily myogenic in nature and is presumed to be regulated by interstitial cells of Cajal. During the fasting stage, SO motility is integrated with migrating motor complex, which alters the flow of bile into the duodenum. The basal pressure of SO is 15 mm Hg (3–35 mm Hg). The duodenal hormone cholecystokinin that contracts the gallbladder also relaxes the SO.

CLINICAL PICTURE

As a poorly understood benign functional disorder, SOD involves the biliary or pancreatic sphincter with varying presentations. Biliary type of pain in a patient with previous cholecystectomy is suggestive of biliary SOD which may present with or without elevated liver enzymes. However, SOD can occur even with the gallbladder intact. Pancreatic sphincter dysfunction causes intermittent acute pancreatitis, which is often considered idiopathic. Biliary SOD is classified into three categories in the Milwaukee Classification System. Type I SOD is characterized

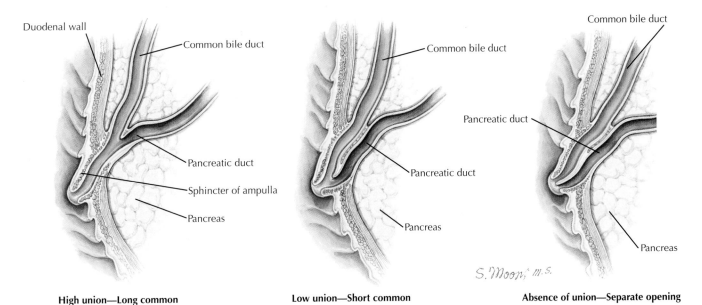

High union—Long common **Low union—Short common** **Absence of union—Separate opening**

Fig. 139.1 Variations in Ductal Anatomy in Sphincter of Oddi Dysfunction.

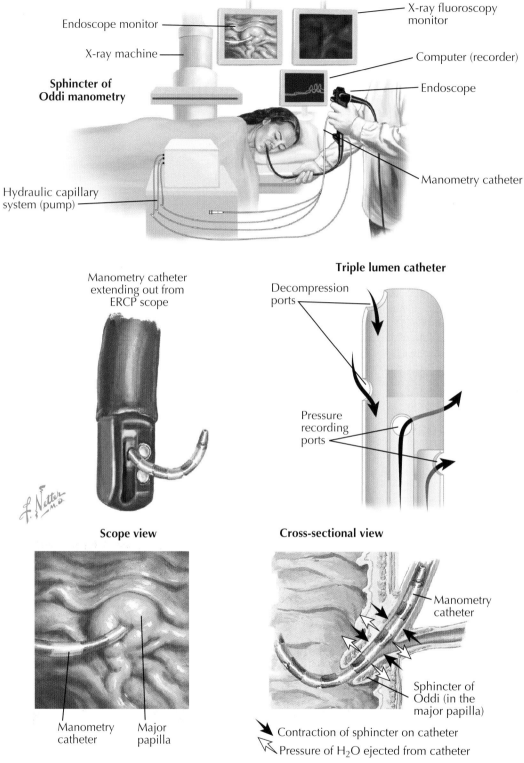

Endoscope monitor

X-ray machine

Sphincter of Oddi manometry

Hydraulic capillary system (pump)

X-ray fluoroscopy monitor

Computer (recorder)

Endoscope

Manometry catheter

Manometry catheter extending out from ERCP scope

Triple lumen catheter

Decompression ports

Pressure recording ports

Scope view

Manometry catheter

Major papilla

Cross-sectional view

Manometry catheter

Sphincter of Oddi (in the major papilla)

Contraction of sphincter on catheter

Pressure of H_2O ejected from catheter

Fig. 139.2 Sphincter of Oddi Dysfunction, Geenen's Classification, and Sphincter of Oddi Manometry: Sphincter of Oddi Dysfunction.

by biliary type of pain with elevated liver enzymes to more than 1.1 times the upper limit of normal with a dilated duct greater than 9 mm. Type II SOD is defined as biliary pain with either liver test abnormalities or bile duct dilatation. Type III SOD, defined as biliary pain without any other objective abnormality, is to be deleted. Pancreatic SOD, diagnosed much less often compared with biliary SOD, is also classified as type I, II, and III based on presence or absence of enzyme elevation and ductal dilatation.

TREATMENT

Treatment of SOD, biliary or pancreatic, is unsatisfactory and controversial. The pharmacologic agents that relax the SO, reducing its pressure and resistance, include calcium channel blockers, tricyclic antidepressants, Botox, glycerol trinitrate, and somatostatin. The endoscopic sphincterectomy is reserved only for those with a clear diagnosis of

SOD. The recent Rome IV classification of functional disorders of the gastric intestinal tract questions the existence of type III and cautions against unwarranted sphincterotomies. The role of dual (biliary and pancreatic), sphincterectomy in recurrent idiopathic acute pancreatitis is controversial.

ADDITIONAL RESOURCES

Afghani E, Lo SK, Covington PS, et al: Sphincter of oddi function and risk factors for dysfunction, *Frontiers in Nutrition* 4:1–9, 2017.

Drossman DA, Hasler WL: Rome IV-functional GI disorders: disorders of gut-brain interaction, *Gastroenterology* 150:1257–1261, 2016.

Small AJ, Kozarek RA: Sphincter of oddi dysfunction, *Gastrointest Endosc Clin N Am* 25:749–763, 2015.

Toouli J: Sphincter of oddi: function, dysfunction, and its management, *J Gastroenterol Hepatol* 24:S57–S62, 2009.

140

Periampullary Cancer

C. S. Pitchumoni

Periampullary cancers are defined as cancers arising within 2 cm of the papilla of Vater. The term "periampullary" includes a heterogenous group of neoplasms arising from the pancreas, duodenum, distal common bile duct, or structures of the ampullary complex (Fig. 140.1). On initial presentation, all these tumors have similar clinical presentation resulting in difficulty in defining the primary site of origin. However, there are fundamental genomic and molecular differences among the four subtypes. The ampullary and the duodenal periampullary tumors have a high estimated 5-year survival (45%–49%), which is better than the bile duct cancer (27%) and pancreatic cancer (18%).

The ampulla of Vater is formed by three anatomic components: the ampulla (often formed by a common channel), the intraduodenal portion of the bile duct, and the intraduodenal portion of the pancreatic duct. Among the periampullary tumors, ampullary tumor is the second most common. Ampullary cancers can be divided into intestinal or pancreaticobiliary type based on histomorphology.

CLINICAL PICTURE

Patients typically manifest symptoms early in the course of the disease, usually in the seventh decade of life, with abdominal pain, obstructive jaundice, malaise, anorexia, and weight loss. Jaundice is progressive but occasionally may be associated with cholangitis. Iron deficiency anemia as a result of chronic low-grade bleeding is a clinical association. The triad of intermittent painless jaundice, anemia, and enlarged palpable gallbladder (Courvoisier gallbladder) is seen in less than 10% of patients. The stool may be gray or silver as a result of acholic feces mixed with melena. Recurrent acute pancreatitis of no readily identifiable etiology may be the presenting feature.

Risk factors for periampullary tumors are similar to those for pancreatic cancer. Patients with familial adenomatous polyposis are predisposed to ampullary adenomas (see Chapter 100).

DIAGNOSIS

Appropriate imaging studies are contrast-enhanced computed tomography (CT), magnetic resonance imaging (MRI) of the abdomen, and magnetic resonance cholangiopancreatography (MRCP). Gastroduodenoscopy allows visualization and biopsy of the tumor. Immunohistochemical staining is useful in differentiating carcinoma form other adenomatous tissues. Endoscopic ultrasound (EUS) helps in further evaluating tumor origin and lymph node involvement and in staging. In this respect, EUS carries a higher sensitivity (93%) than MRI (63%) and dynamic computed tomography (53%). Although not pathognomonic or sensitive enough to make a diagnosis, the double duct sign of dilated pancreatic or biliary duct is seen on endoscopic retrograde cholangiopancreatography (ERCP) or MRCP examination. ERCP defines the extent, size, and gross appearance of the tumor and is useful in palliative stenting to relieve obstructive jaundice.

TREATMENT AND MANAGEMENT

Endoscopic therapy using snare resection neodymium-doped yttrium aluminum garnet (Nd:YAG) laser ablation and photodynamic therapy are available for selected cases. Pancreaticoduodenectomy with or without Whipple procedure (pylorus preservation) is the most effective treatment for periampullary carcinoma.

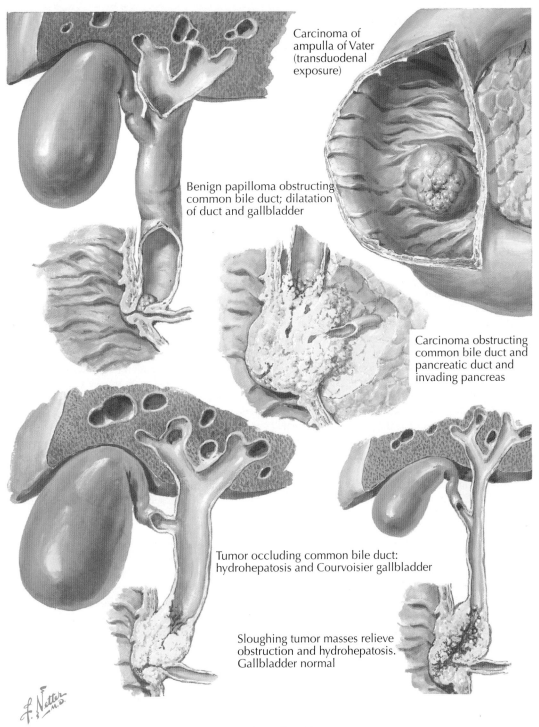

Carcinoma of ampulla of Vater (transduodenal exposure)

Benign papilloma obstructing common bile duct; dilatation of duct and gallbladder

Carcinoma obstructing common bile duct and pancreatic duct and invading pancreas

Tumor occluding common bile duct: hydrohepatosis and Courvoisier gallbladder

Sloughing tumor masses relieve obstruction and hydrohepatosis. Gallbladder normal

Fig. 140.1 Ampullary Tumors.

ADDITIONAL RESOURCES

Acharya A, Markar SR, Sodergren MH, et al: Meta-analysis of adjuvant therapy following curative surgery for periampullary adenocarcinoma, *Br J Surg* 104(7):814–822, 2017.

Chandrasegaram MD, Gill AJ, Samra J, et al: Ampullary cancer of intestinal origin and duodenal cancer—a logical clinical and therapeutic subgroup in periampullary cancer, *World J Gastrointest Oncol* 9(10): 407–415, 2017.

Feretis M, Wang T, Iype S, et al: Development of a prognostic model that predicts survival after pancreaticoduodenectomy for ampullary cancer, *Pancreas* 46(10):1314–1321, 2017.

141

Gallbladder Cancer

C. S. Pitchumoni

Although highly lethal, gallbladder cancer is extremely rare. The annual incidence in the United States is less than 7000 cases, and it is the fifth most common malignancy of the gastrointestinal (GI) tract. When the diagnosis of carcinoma of the gallbladder is incidental on routine cholecystectomy for gallstone disease, the prognosis is excellent. Incidental carcinoma of the gallbladder is noted in 1% to 3% of cholecystectomy specimens and 0.5% to 7.4% of autopsies.

Risk factors for gallbladder carcinoma include gallstones, history of chronic cholecystitis, and porcelain gallbladder (more in patchy type of porcelain gallbladder than in the diffuse type). Adenomas of the gallbladder may progress to cancer, the risk is associated with older age, single lesion, sessile shape and polyps greater than 10 mm in size. The risk is related to the size of the polyp. Polyps smaller than 1 cm seldom undergo malignant changes. Other risk factors are anomalous drainage of the pancreatic duct into the common bile duct (CBD), congenital biliary cysts, and *Salmonella* infection (chronic gallbladder infection).

In contrast to the general US population, gallbladder cancer is the most common GI malignancy in Native Americans who live in the southwest and in Mexican Americans. Worldwide, the incidence of carcinoma of the gallbladder is highest in Chile, Bolivia, and northern regions of India. The risk is higher in women and elderly populations.

Although gallstones are frequently associated with carcinoma, the incidence of carcinoma in patients with gallstone disease is extremely low. Symptomatic gallstone disease—large size of the stones (>2.5 cm) and long duration of gallstone disease (notably >40 years)—are other observed risk factors. Another risk factor for gallbladder carcinoma involves an anomalous pancreatobiliary duct junction. A strong association of *Salmonella* infection and its carrier state has been shown in many studies. Most gallbladder carcinomas are adenocarcinomas, but squamous cell tumors, mixed tumors, and adenoepidermoid tumors occasionally develop.

CLINICAL PICTURE

Most patients have nonspecific findings of right upper quadrant pain, malaise, weight loss, jaundice, anorexia, and vomiting mimicking symptomatic gallstone disease. Few patients have acute cholecystitis. At diagnosis, most patients have tumors that have invaded adjacent organs, local lymph node metastasis, or even distinct metastasis (Fig. 141.1). The 5-year survival rate is less than 5%, except when the diagnosis is incidental on routine cholecystectomy.

DIAGNOSIS

Diagnostic studies include abdominal ultrasound, computed tomography (CT), magnetic resonance imaging (MRI), and endoscopic ultrasound (EUS). Major findings are focal or diffuse mural thickening, intraluminal polypoid mass usually larger than 2 cm originating in the gallbladder wall, and most often (45%–65% of patients) a subhepatic mass replacing or obscuring the gallbladder and often invading the adjacent liver. Endoscopic retrograde cholangiopancreatography (ERCP), magnetic resonance cholangiopancreatography (MRCP), and percutaneous transhepatic cholangiography provide additional information for tumor staging and resectability. ERCP may also provide the opportunity for brush cytology and biopsy. Biochemical abnormalities indicate obstructive jaundice. Tumor markers (e.g., CEA, CA 19-9) are not helpful.

TREATMENT AND MANAGEMENT

Management is surgical, and the prognosis depends on the stage of the cancer. Most tumors at diagnosis are unresectable. If the patient is thought to have cancer, open surgery is preferred. Although simple cholecystectomy may be sufficient for T1 lesions, radical resection is needed for advanced cases. Postoperative external beam radiation therapy may reduce the rates of local recurrence. Concomitant 5-fluorouracil (5-FU), with or without mitomycin C, is part of adjuvant chemoradiotherapy. Improved survival attributed to adjuvant chemoradiotherapy has not been established. A biliary stent has been proposed as a palliative measure to relieve obstructive jaundice.

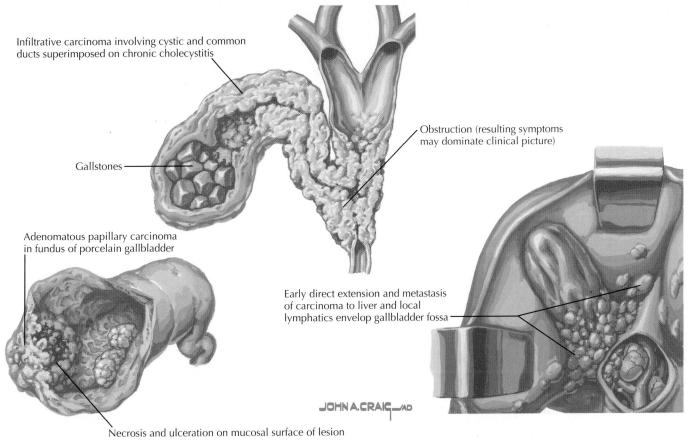

Infiltrative carcinoma involving cystic and common ducts superimposed on chronic cholecystitis

Gallstones

Obstruction (resulting symptoms may dominate clinical picture)

Adenomatous papillary carcinoma in fundus of porcelain gallbladder

Early direct extension and metastasis of carcinoma to liver and local lymphatics envelop gallbladder fossa

JOHN A.CRAIG—AD

Necrosis and ulceration on mucosal surface of lesion

Fig. 141.1 Gallbladder Cancer.

ADDITIONAL RESOURCES

Muszynska C, Lundgren L, Lindell G, et al: Predictors of incidental gallbladder cancer in patients undergoing cholecystectomy for benign gallbladder disease: results from a population-based gallstone surgery registry, *Surgery* 162(2):256–263, 2017.

Petrova E, Rückert F, Zach S, et al: Survival outcome and prognostic factors after pancreatoduodenectomy for distal bile duct carcinoma: a retrospective multicenter study, *Langenbecks Arch Surg* 402(5):831–840, 2017.

Sharma A, Sharma KL, Gupta A, et al: Gallbladder cancer epidemiology, pathogenesis and molecular genetics: recent update, *World J Gastroenterol* 23(22):3978–3998, 2017.

142

Cholangiocarcinoma

C. S. Pitchumoni

Cholangiocarcinoma (CCA) is an adenocarcinoma of the biliary tract originating from the epithelium of the intrahepatic or extrahepatic biliary duct system. Although rare in the United States, the age-adjusted rates of CCA are highest in Hispanic and Asian population and lowest in non-Hispanic white people and black people. The clinical presentation of CCA varies, depending on the location of the tumor and the level of obstruction in the biliary system (Fig. 142.1). The contemporary classification based on anatomic location includes intrahepatic (10%), perihilar (50%, including Klatskin tumor), and distal CCA (40%). Intrahepatic CCA arising from the small ducts or ductules resembles hepatoma. Some CCAs are even grouped with liver or gallbladder cancer. CCA has a dismal prognosis.

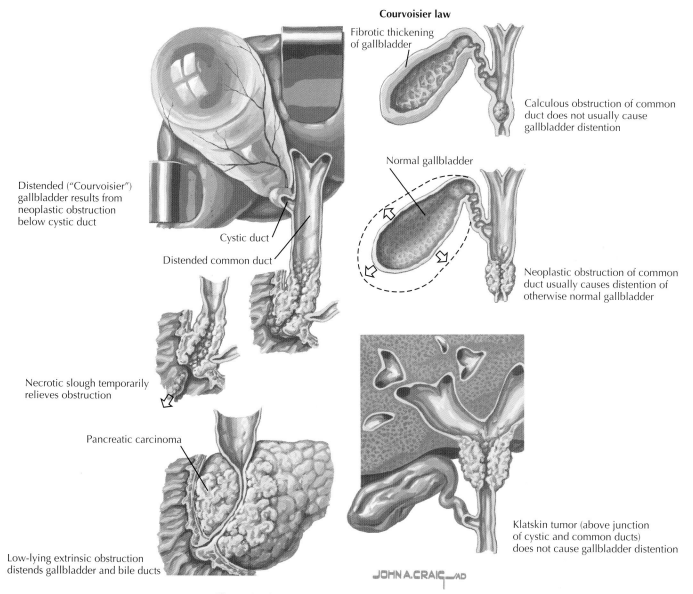

Courvoisier law

Fibrotic thickening of gallbladder

Calculous obstruction of common duct does not usually cause gallbladder distention

Normal gallbladder

Distended ("Courvoisier") gallbladder results from neoplastic obstruction below cystic duct

Cystic duct

Distended common duct

Neoplastic obstruction of common duct usually causes distention of otherwise normal gallbladder

Necrotic slough temporarily relieves obstruction

Pancreatic carcinoma

Low-lying extrinsic obstruction distends gallbladder and bile ducts

Klatskin tumor (above junction of cystic and common ducts) does not cause gallbladder distention

JOHN A. CRAIG—AD

Fig. 142.1 Neoplastic Obstruction of the Bile Ducts.

BOX 142.1 Predisposing Factors for Cholangiocarcinoma

- Primary sclerosing cholangitis
- Ulcerative colitis
- Choledochal cysts
- Caroli disease (biliary duct ectasia)
- Intrahepatic stones
- Chronic viral hepatitis (hepatitis C [HCV], hepatitis B [HBV])
- Long common channel of pancreatic and biliary duct
- Metabolic syndrome
- Infections
  - *Opisthorchis viverrini* (Thailand, Laos, Malaysia)
  - *Clonorchis sinensis* (Japan, Korea, Vietnam)
- Miscellaneous
  - Genetic polymorphism (encoding proteins participating in cell DNA repair like MTHFR, TYMS, GSTO1, and XRCC1)
  - Human immunodeficiency virus (HIV)
  - Cirrhosis of any etiology
  - Alcoholism

The major risk factor for CCA is *primary sclerosing cholangitis* (PSC), a complication of ulcerative colitis and rarely of Crohn disease. Box 142.1 lists factors predisposing to CCA. Rare conditions associated with CCA include multiple biliary papillomatosis, bile duct adenoma, and exposure to thorium dioxide, a contrast agent no longer used in radiologic studies.

CLINICAL PICTURE AND DIAGNOSIS

CCA presents classically as painless jaundice, clay-colored stools, and cola-colored urine. Pain, fatigue, malaise, and weight loss accompany advanced disease. A recently discovered entity, IgG4 disease associated cholangitis, mimics CCA because the diseases share the same clinical features. Abnormal laboratory values indicate obstructive jaundice and demonstrate elevated alkaline phosphatase, bilirubin, and γ-glutamyltransferase levels. Serum CA 19-9 levels are often elevated greater than 100 U/mL; this test is particularly useful in diagnosing CCA in PSC. Useful radiologic studies are abdominal ultrasound, computed tomography of the abdomen, magnetic resonance cholangiopancreatography, endoscopic ultrasound, and endoscopic retrograde cholangiopancreatography (ERCP). ERCP and percutaneous cholangiography are effective at assessing the location of the tumor. Spyglass evaluation of interior of bile duct represents a recent advance in the diagnostic procedure of intrabiliary pathology. Perihilar tumors, vascular invasion, lymph node metastasis, and involvement of gallbladder hepatic vein are associated with poor prognosis. A hilar location of the tumor (Klatskin tumor) has a classic cholangiographic appearance. Positron emission tomography (PET) is useful in diagnosis and staging. Brush cytology is possible during ERCP in 40% to 70% of patients. Angiography accurately shows vascular encasement and thrombosis of portal vein and hepatic artery. The differential diagnosis should include carcinoma of the head of the pancreas, gallbladder cancer, Mirizzi syndrome, and PSC.

TREATMENT AND MANAGEMENT

Treatment of CCA is unsatisfactory. The four modalities of treatment are surgical, endoscopic, chemotherapy, and radiotherapy with surgical excision is the mainstay. Radiation therapy and chemotherapy provide symptomatic relief by removing the obstruction. Endoscopic placement of plastic or metal stents is another palliative procedure. All these measures have been essentially ineffective, and the prognosis is poor.

ADDITIONAL RESOURCES

Banales JM, Cardinale V, Carpino G, et al: Expert consensus document: cholangiocarcinoma: current knowledge and future perspectives consensus statement from the European network for the study of cholangiocarcinoma (ENS-CCA), *Nat Rev Gastroenterol Hepatol* 13(5): 261–280, 2016.

Kennedy L, Hargrove L, Demieville J, et al: Recent advances in understanding cholangiocarcinoma, *F1000Res* 6:1818, 2017.

Oliveira IS, Kilcoyne A, Everett JM, et al: Cholangiocarcinoma: classification, diagnosis, staging, imaging features, and management, *Abdom Radiol (NY)* 42(6):1637–1649, 2017.

Razumilava N, Gores GJ: Cholangiocarcinoma, *Lancet* 383(9935):2168–2179, 2014.

Liver

Joseph K. Lim

Anatomy of the Liver

Kris V. Kowdley, Joseph K. Lim

TOPOGRAPHY OF THE LIVER

The liver (Greek *hepar*) is located in the upper part of the abdomen, where it occupies the right hypochondrium and the greater part of the epigastric regions (Fig. 143.1). The left lobe of the liver extends into the left hypochondrium. The liver is the largest organ of the body and weighs an average of 1300 g (800–2400 g) in women and 1500 g (800–2600 g) in men. In healthy persons, the *liver margin* extending below the thoracic cage is smooth and offers little resistance to the palpating finger. Downward displacement, enlargement, hardening, and the formation of nodes or cysts produce impressive palpatory findings. Using percussion, the examiner must consider that the lungs overlie the upper portion of the liver and that the liver, in turn, overlies the intestines and the stomach.

The projections of the liver on the body surface have added significance with liver biopsy. The projections vary depending on patient position and body build, especially the configuration of the thorax. The liver lies close to the diaphragm, and the upper pole of the right lobe projects as far as the level of the fourth intercostal space or the fifth rib; the highest point is 1 cm below the nipple, near the lateral body line. The upper limit of the left lobe projects to the upper border of the sixth rib. Here, the left tip of the liver is close to the diaphragm.

The ribs cover the greater part of the liver's right lobe, whereas a small part of its anterior surface is in contact with the anterior abdominal wall. In the *erect position,* the liver extends downward to the 10th or 11th rib in the right midaxillary line. Here the pleura projects down to the 10th rib, and the lung projects down to the 8th rib. The anterior margin of the liver crosses the costal arch in the right lateral body line, approximately on the level of the pylorus *(transpyloric line).* In the epigastrium, the thoracic cage does not cover the liver. It extends approximately three fingers below the base of the xiphoid process in the midline. Part of the left lobe is covered again by the rib cage.

Over the upper third of the right half of the liver, percussion indicates a *dull zone,* because here the diaphragm, pleura, and lung overlie the liver. Over the middle portion, percussion results in a *flat tone.* Over the lowest third of the liver, a flat tone is usually heard as well except that sometimes *intestinal resonance* is produced by gas-filled intestinal loops. The border between dullness and flatness moves on respiration and is altered by enlargement or displacement of the liver and by conditions within the thoracic cage, which change the percussive qualities of the thoracic organs. In the *horizontal position,* the projection of the liver moves a little upward, and the area of flatness appears slightly enlarged. Measurement of the span of the flat sound, best percussed in the horizontal position, allows an assessment of the size of the liver.

Projections of the liver are altered in some liver diseases (e.g., tumor infiltration, cirrhosis, syphilitic hepar lobatum) by displacement of the liver or, more often, by thoracic conditions pushing the liver downward. Subphrenic abscesses, depending on their location and size, also displace the liver downward. Ascites, excessive dilatation of the colon, and abdominal tumors may push the liver upward, and retroperitoneal tumors may move it forward. Kyphoscoliosis or "barrel chest" alters the position of the liver. In some patients, the liver is abnormally movable *(hepatoptosis),* causing peculiar palpatory findings.

SURFACES AND BED OF THE LIVER

The liver is pyramid shaped, and its apex is formed by the thin, flattened left extremity of the left lobe (Fig. 143.2). Its base is seated on the right lateral surface, which rests on the diaphragm and on the right thoracic cage, producing the *costal impressions* on this surface. Its sides are formed by the anterior, posterior, and inferior surfaces. The border between the anterior and inferior surfaces is the *anterior margin.* The liver's consistency, sharpness of edge, smoothness of surface, and movement on respiration provide clinical information. On laparotomy, the anterior margin and anterior surface are first exposed. Otherwise the hepatic surfaces are not separated by distinct margins.

The liver is covered by peritoneum except for the gallbladder bed, the hilus, adjacent parts surrounding the inferior vena cava (IVC), and a space to the right of the IVC called the *bare area,* which is in contact with the right adrenal gland *(adrenal impression)* and the right kidney *(renal impression). Peritoneal duplications,* which extend from the anterior abdominal wall and the diaphragm to the organ, form the ligaments of the liver. Although the ligaments were previously believed to maintain the liver in its position, they probably add little to its fixation, as the liver is likely kept in place by intraabdominal pressure.

The horizontal peritoneal duplication is the *coronary ligament,* the upper layer of which is exposed if the liver is pulled away from the diaphragm. The free right lateral margin of the coronary ligaments forms the *right triangular ligament,* whereas the *left triangular ligament* surrounds and merges with the left tip of the liver, the *appendix fibrosa hepatis* (fibrous appendix of liver). Over the right lobe, the space between the upper and lower layers of the coronary ligament is filled with areolar connective tissue. Below the insertion of the lower layer of the right coronary ligament, the hepatorenal space extends behind the liver.

From the middle portion of the coronary ligament originates another peritoneal duplication, the *falciform ligament,* which extends from the liver to the anterior abdominal wall between the diaphragm and the umbilicus. Its insertion on the liver divides the organ into a *right lobe* and a *left lobe.* The inferior edge of the falciform ligament is enforced to form the round ligament *(ligamentum teres),* which extends to a point at which the longitudinal fissure of the liver crosses the inferior surface. With its anterior part, this fissure separates the quadrate lobe and the left lobe *(tuber omentale)* and forms a fossa for the umbilical vein or its remnant. The fissure proceeds toward the posterior surface, creating the fossa for the ductus venosus *(ligamentum venosum* in adult life). The two fossae may be regarded as the right limb of an H-shaped

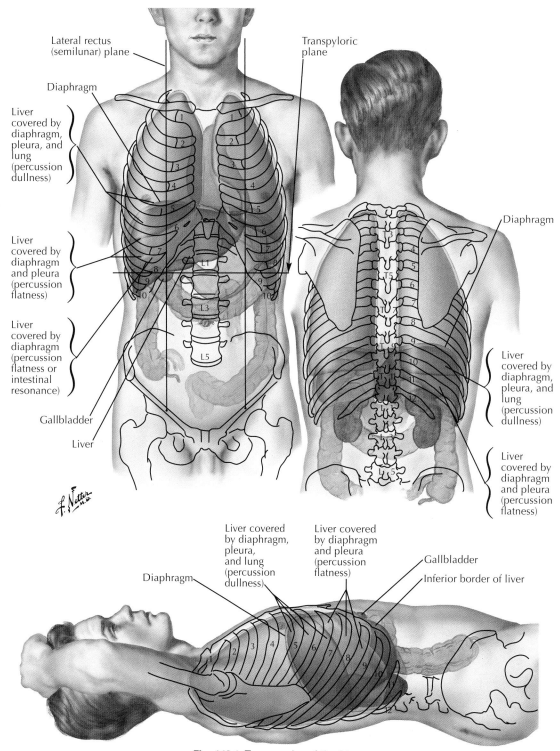

Fig. 143.1 Topography of the Liver.

pattern, characteristic of the inferior surface of the liver. The left limb is formed by the gallbladder bed and the fossa for the IVC. The horizontal limb is marked by the *porta hepatis*, which contains the common hepatic duct, hepatic artery, portal vein, lymphatics, and nerves.

The *quadrate lobe*, between the gallbladder and the fossa for the umbilical vein, is in contact with the pylorus and the first portion of the duodenum (*duodenal impression*). On the inferior and posterior surfaces lies the *caudate lobe*, between the fossa for the ligamentum venosum and the IVC; its anterior projection is the *papillary process*.

The inferior surface of the liver reveals further impressions of the organs it contacts, including the colon and right kidney (right lobe), and the esophagus and stomach (left lobe). The superior surface is related to the diaphragm and forms the domes of the liver.

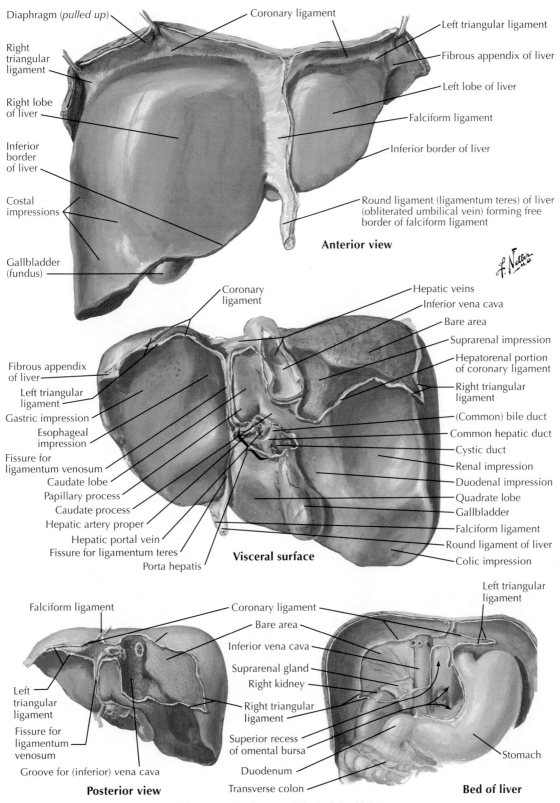

Fig. 143.2 Surfaces and Bed of the Liver.

Anterior view labels:
- Diaphragm (*pulled up*)
- Coronary ligament
- Left triangular ligament
- Fibrous appendix of liver
- Left lobe of liver
- Falciform ligament
- Inferior border of liver
- Round ligament (ligamentum teres) of liver (obliterated umbilical vein) forming free border of falciform ligament
- Right triangular ligament
- Right lobe of liver
- Inferior border of liver
- Costal impressions
- Gallbladder (fundus)

Anterior view

Visceral surface labels:
- Coronary ligament
- Hepatic veins
- Inferior vena cava
- Bare area
- Suprarenal impression
- Hepatorenal portion of coronary ligament
- Right triangular ligament
- (Common) bile duct
- Common hepatic duct
- Cystic duct
- Renal impression
- Duodenal impression
- Quadrate lobe
- Gallbladder
- Falciform ligament
- Round ligament of liver
- Colic impression
- Fibrous appendix of liver
- Left triangular ligament
- Gastric impression
- Esophageal impression
- Fissure for ligamentum venosum
- Caudate lobe
- Papillary process
- Caudate process
- Hepatic artery proper
- Hepatic portal vein
- Fissure for ligamentum teres
- Porta hepatis

Visceral surface

Posterior view labels:
- Falciform ligament
- Coronary ligament
- Left triangular ligament
- Bare area
- Inferior vena cava
- Suprarenal gland
- Right kidney
- Right triangular ligament
- Superior recess of omental bursa
- Duodenum
- Transverse colon
- Stomach
- Left triangular ligament
- Fissure for ligamentum venosum
- Groove for (inferior) vena cava

Posterior view

Bed of liver

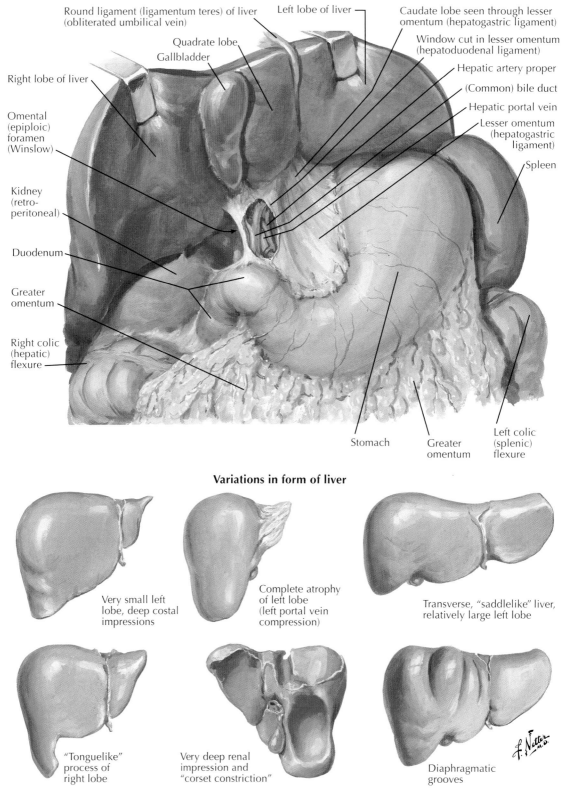

Round ligament (ligamentum teres) of liver (obliterated umbilical vein)

Left lobe of liver

Caudate lobe seen through lesser omentum (hepatogastric ligament)

Quadrate lobe

Gallbladder

Window cut in lesser omentum (hepatoduodenal ligament)

Right lobe of liver

Hepatic artery proper

(Common) bile duct

Omental (epiploic) foramen (Winslow)

Hepatic portal vein

Lesser omentum (hepatogastric ligament)

Spleen

Kidney (retro-peritoneal)

Duodenum

Greater omentum

Right colic (hepatic) flexure

Stomach

Greater omentum

Left colic (splenic) flexure

Variations in form of liver

Very small left lobe, deep costal impressions

Complete atrophy of left lobe (left portal vein compression)

Transverse, "saddlelike" liver, relatively large left lobe

"Tonguelike" process of right lobe

Very deep renal impression and "corset constriction"

Diaphragmatic grooves

Fig. 143.3 Lesser Omentum and Variations in Form of the Liver.

LESSER OMENTUM AND VARIATIONS IN FORM OF THE LIVER

If the anterior margin of the liver is lifted, the *lesser omentum* is exposed. It represents a peritoneal fold that extends from the first portion of the duodenum, lesser curvature of the stomach, and diaphragm, to the liver, where the fold inserts at the fossa of the ligamentum venosum and continues to the porta hepatis (Fig. 143.3). There, the layers are separated to accommodate the structures running to and from the hilus of the liver.

On the free right edge of the lesser omentum, the reunited peritoneal layers are enforced to form the *hepatoduodenal ligament*. The anterior boundary of the *omental foramen* (foramen of Winslow, epiploic foramen) is the entrance to the lesser abdominal cavity. The posterior wall of this cavity is formed by the IVC and the caudate lobe of the liver.

Near the right margin of the lesser omentum is the *common bile duct* (CBD), which divides into the cystic and common hepatic ducts. To the left of the CBD lies the *hepatic artery,* and behind both is the *portal vein.* The nerves and lymph vessels of the liver accompany these structures. The hilus of the liver is anteriorly limited by the quadrate lobe and posteriorly by the caudate lobe. On the right side of the hilus, the right and left hepatic ducts branch from the main hepatic duct and enter the liver. To the left of the ducts, the hepatic artery enters the liver behind the ductal branches. The forking portal vein enters posteriorly to the ductal and arterial ramifications.

The shape of the liver varies. Its great regenerative capacity and tissue plasticity permit a wide variety of forms, depending in part on pressure exerted by neighboring organs and on disease processes or vascular alterations. A greatly reduced left lobe is offset by an enlarged right lobe, which reveals conspicuous and deep costal impressions. Occasionally the left lobe is completely atrophic (see Fig. 143.3), with a wrinkled and thickened capsule and, microscopically, an impressive approximation of the portal triads, with almost no lobular parenchyma between them.

Vascular aberrations include partial obstruction of the lumen of the left branch of the portal vein by a dilated left hepatic duct or bile duct obstruction, considered the result of local nutritional deficiency, especially because the nutritional condition of the left lobe initially is poor. In other situations, associated with a transverse position of the liver, the left lobe is unduly large.

In previous centuries, the liver was frequently disfigured by laced corsets or tight belts or straps. Such physical forces may flatten and elongate the liver from above downward, with a reduction of the superior diaphragmatic surface and sometimes with tonguelike extension of the right lobe (see Fig. 143.3). In other cases, the *corset liver* is displaced and the renal impression is exaggerated. Clinical symptoms such as dyspepsia, cholelithiasis, and chlorosis have been ascribed to the corset liver, although these associations remain unproven.

Indentations on the liver produced by the ribs, diaphragmatic insertions, and costal arch are normal. In kyphoscoliosis, the rib insertions may be prominent. Parallel sagittal furrows on the hepatic convexity have been designated *diaphragmatic grooves.*

Functionally, none of these variations is currently considered significant.

CELL TYPES WITHIN THE LIVER

Major cell types unique to the liver include hepatocytes, bile duct cells, sinusoidal-lining cells (including Kupffer cells and endothelial cells), stellate cells, and immune cells (Fig. 143.4). *Hepatocytes* are the primary cell type within the liver and are responsible for a vast array of metabolic functions, including gluconeogenesis, fatty acid oxidation, synthesis of albumin and other plasma proteins, metabolism of drugs and toxins, synthesis of cholesterol, and bile acids.

Sinusoids, which are structurally different from capillaries, contain fenestrations and are of variable size, increasing from zone 1 to zone 3. Sinusoids are lined by Kupffer cells and endothelial cells. *Kupffer cells* are large macrophages unique to the liver that have phagocytic activity. These cells clear endotoxin, bacteria, and senescent red blood cells (RBCs) from the circulation and store iron from erythrocytes. Therefore the iron content of Kupffer cells is increased in conditions of increased RBC turnover, such as hemolysis or iron overload secondary to blood transfusion. By contrast, iron deposition in the liver in hereditary hemochromatosis is found primarily in periportal hepatocytes. *Endothelial*

cells in the liver express receptors for several proteins and may be crucial for the maintenance of sinusoidal blood flow by producing vasoactive substances such as endothelin-1 and nitric oxide.

Stellate cells (also called Ito cells, vitamin A–storing cells, and lipocytes) are unique to the liver and appear to play a central role in hepatic fibrogenesis and fibrinolysis. Stellate cells are transformed into fibroblasts after stimulation by cytokines, which may be released locally in response to injury. Activated stellate cells produce various types of collagen and may be responsible for the deposition of extracellular matrix. In addition, the contractility of stellate cells may be an important step in the development of portal hypertension. Stellate cells are also involved in the degradation of extracellular matrix and therefore may play a critical role in two very important hepatic pathologic processes, the development of cirrhosis and portal hypertension. Pharmacologic modulation of stellate cell activation may offer hope as future therapeutic options for the treatment of cirrhosis and portal hypertension.

The liver also contains lymphatics. The normal production of *lymph* in the liver is approximately 2 L/day, but lymph production can increase greatly in patients with cirrhosis or conditions leading to venous obstruction. Hepatic lymph has a high protein content and is collected from subendothelial *Disse* (perisinusoidal) *spaces,* adjacent to hepatic sinusoids. Hepatic lymph drains from the liver through the cisterna chyli and ultimately into the thoracic duct.

The liver also contains other immune cells, including T cells and natural killer (NK) cells, which is of particular interest because of the role of *innate liver immunity* in drug/toxin-induced liver injury.

Two distinctly different models describe current concepts of microscopic hepatic organization. The *lobule model* focuses on the hepatic vein, with the portal areas organized around the points of a pentagon (Fig. 143.5). The more complex *acinus model* is based on the functional unit of the liver being an acinus organized around terminal portal venules, bile ductules, and lymph ducts. There is axial distribution around the portal venule, with the acini clustered around the portal vein. The sinusoids, where blood leaves discrete vascular structures and freely contacts hepatocytes, radiate around the central veins (Figs. 143.6 and 143.7).

Blood enters the sinusoids from the terminal portal venules. End arterioles of the hepatic arteries also drain into the terminal portal venules. Therefore the oxygen tension (Po_2) of the blood entering the sinusoid is richest around the portal area (zone 1 of Rappaport) and lowest in the region surrounding the central vein (zone 3 of Rappaport). Po_2 is intermediate between zone 1 and zone 3 (zone 2 of Rappaport). The centrilobular region of the lobule is most susceptible to toxic, hypoxic, and ischemic injury. Classic examples include acetaminophen toxicity or hepatic artery thrombosis after orthotopic liver transplantation. Each of these zones appears to have different functions. For example, zone 1 hepatocytes play an important role in gluconeogenesis, whereas zone 3 hepatocytes are critical to lipid synthesis and glycolysis.

Bile ducts branch into smaller bile ductules that terminate in the bile canaliculus. Canaliculi are located between hepatocytes; bile drains across the bile canalicular membrane in hepatocytes into bile ductules and subsequently into bile ducts.

VESSEL AND DUCT DISTRIBUTIONS AND LIVER SEGMENTS

Intrahepatic distribution of blood vessels and bile ducts was studied on casts prepared by injecting plastic into the vascular and biliary conduits before removing tissue. Besides being valuable for the cholangiographic demonstration of the vascular apparatus in vivo, this new recognition of the liver's segmental divisions, similar to those in the

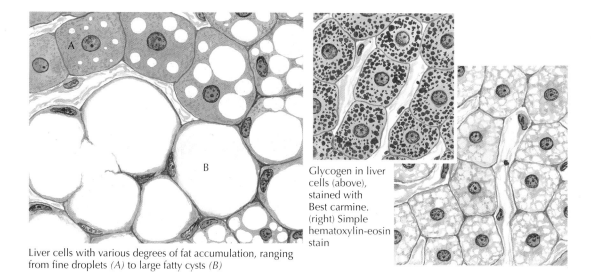

Glycogen in liver cells (above), stained with Best carmine. (right) Simple hematoxylin-eosin stain

Liver cells with various degrees of fat accumulation, ranging from fine droplets *(A)* to large fatty cysts *(B)*

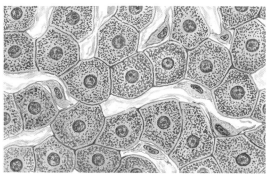

Liver cells with methyl green-pyronine stain (methyl green stains chromatin; pyronine stain cytoplasmic inclusions and nucleolus)

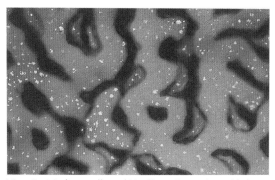

Vitamin A in liver cells and Kupffer cells made visible by fluorescence

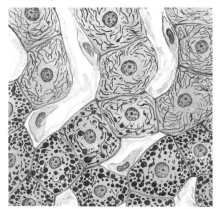

Variform mitochondria in liver cells reflecting differences in functional activity (Janus green stain)

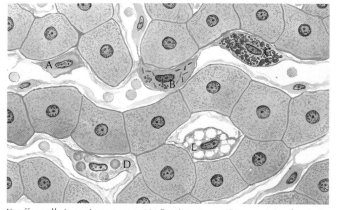

Kupffer cells in various stages. *(A)* Resting stage; *(B)* containing bacteria; *(C)* containing pigment; *(D)* containing red blood cells; *(E)* containing fat droplets

Fig. 143.4 Cell Types Within the Liver.

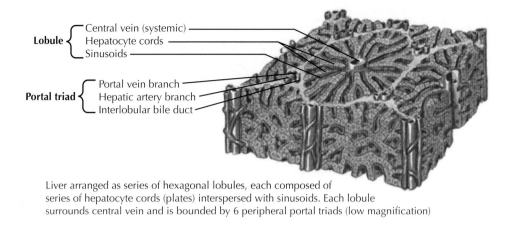

Central vein (systemic)
Hepatocyte cords
Sinusoids
Lobule

Portal vein branch
Hepatic artery branch
Interlobular bile duct
Portal triad

Liver arranged as series of hexagonal lobules, each composed of
series of hepatocyte cords (plates) interspersed with sinusoids. Each lobule
surrounds central vein and is bounded by 6 peripheral portal triads (low magnification)

Portal vein branch
Interlobular bile duct
Hepatic artery branch
Portal triad

Intercellular network
of bile canaliculi

Canaliculi formed
between tight
junctions of
adjacent
hepatocytes

Sinusoids
(fenestrated
capillaries)
border cords
of hepatocytes

JOHN A.CRAIG—AD

Hepatocyte
cord

Parts of hepatic lobule at portal triad (high magnification)

Fig. 143.5 Hepatic Architecture.

lungs, allowed partial hepatectomy or excision of single metastatic nodules.

Although the human liver, in contrast to the livers of some animals, fails to displace surface lobulation, the parallel course of the branches of the hepatic artery, portal vein, and bile ducts and the appearance of clefts in these preparations indicates a distinct lobular composition. A major lobar fissure extends obliquely downward from the fossa for the IVC to the gallbladder fossa. This does not coincide with the surface separation between the right and left lobes running along the insertion of the falciform ligament and the fossa for the ductus venosus. Through this fissure extends one of the main trunks of the hepatic vein, the

tributaries of which never follow the distribution of the other vessels but instead cross the portal vein branches in an interdigitated manner.

Each lobe of the liver is partitioned by a segmental division and is drained by a lobar bile duct of the first order (Fig. 143.8). The right division extends obliquely from the junction of the anterior and posterior surfaces downward toward the lower border of the liver and continues on the inferior surface toward the hilus, dividing the *right lobe* into anterior and posterior segments, each of which is drained by a bile duct of the second order. The left segmental cleft runs on the anterior surface along the attachments of the falciform ligament and on the visceral surface through the umbilical fossa and ductus venosus

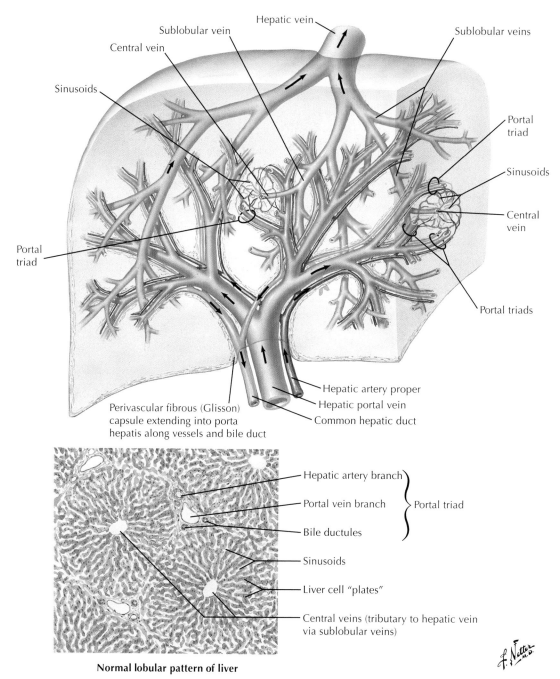

Normal lobular pattern of liver

Fig. 143.6 Vascular Ductal Relations and Liver Lobules.

fossa, extending toward the hilus. This fissure divides the *left lobe* into medial and lateral segments but is often crossed by bile ducts and vessels. The *lateral segment* corresponds to the classic descriptions of the left lobe, whereas the aspect of the *medial segment* on the visceral live surface corresponds to the quadrate lobe. The four bile ducts of the second order form those of the third order, which drain either the superior or the inferior corresponding segment. Thus the bile ducts and the accompanying vessels can be designated according to the lobes, segments, and areas to which they belong.

The anatomically distinct *caudate lobe* has a vascular arrangement that divides it into a left portion, drained by the left lobar duct, and a right portion, drained by the right lobar duct. The *caudate process,* connecting the caudate lobe with the right lobe of the liver, has a separate

net of vessels, which usually communicates with branches of the right lobar duct.

Neither the caudate lobe nor other parts of the liver provide effective communication between the right and left lobar duct systems. Intrahepatic anastomoses between intraparenchymal branches of the arteries also have not been found, but in 25% of cases, interconnections between the right and left systems exist through small extrahepatic or subcapsular anastomosing vessels.

The distribution of draining bile ducts and afferent blood vessels is schematically depicted here (Fig. 143.6), but individual variations are abundant, especially in the lateral superior vessel and ducts for the appendix fibrosa. Rudimentary bile ducts are common in this region. Segmental bile duct variation occurs more often on the right

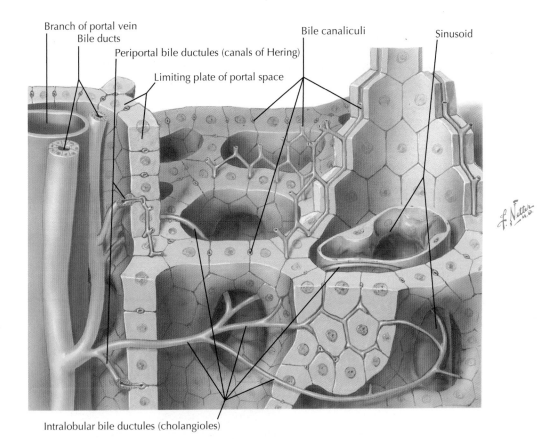

Branch of portal vein
Bile ducts
Periportal bile ductules (canals of Hering)
Limiting plate of portal space
Bile canaliculi
Sinusoid

Intralobular bile ductules (cholangioles)

Low-power section of liver

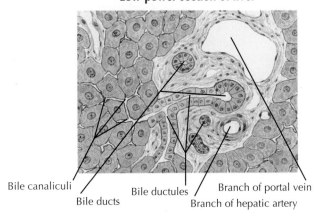

Bile canaliculi
Bile ducts
Bile ductules
Branch of portal vein
Branch of hepatic artery

Note: In the top illustration, bile canaliculi appear as structures with walls of their own. However, as shown in histologic section, boundaries of canaliculi are actually a specialization of surface membranes of adjoining liver parenchymal cells

Fig. 143.7 Intrahepatic Biliary System.

side, whereas variation in segmental arteries is more common on the left side.

ARTERIAL BLOOD SUPPLY OF THE LIVER, BILIARY SYSTEM, AND PANCREAS

Several studies, including the painstaking dissections of Michels, have revealed considerable variation in the arterial supply of the liver, biliary system, and pancreas (Figs. 143.9 and 143.10). According to the conventional description, observed in approximately 55% of examined specimens, the *celiac artery* or *celiac axis* is a short, thick trunk that originates in the aorta just below the aortic hiatus in the diaphragm.

It extends horizontally and forward above the pancreas and splits into the left gastric, hepatic, and splenic arteries. An inferior phrenic artery, usually starting from the aorta, or a dorsal pancreatic artery (see later)—otherwise departing from the splenic artery, the hepatic artery, or the aorta—may exceptionally derive from the celiac axis. The *left gastric* (or coronary) artery, the smallest of the three celiac branches, starting at the cardia, extends along the lesser curvature of the stomach to anastomose with the *right gastric* artery.

The *splenic artery*, the largest of the three celiac branches in adults, takes a somewhat tortuous course to the left, along and behind the upper border of the pancreas. At a variable distance from the spleen, it breaks into a number of terminal branches that enter the hilus of

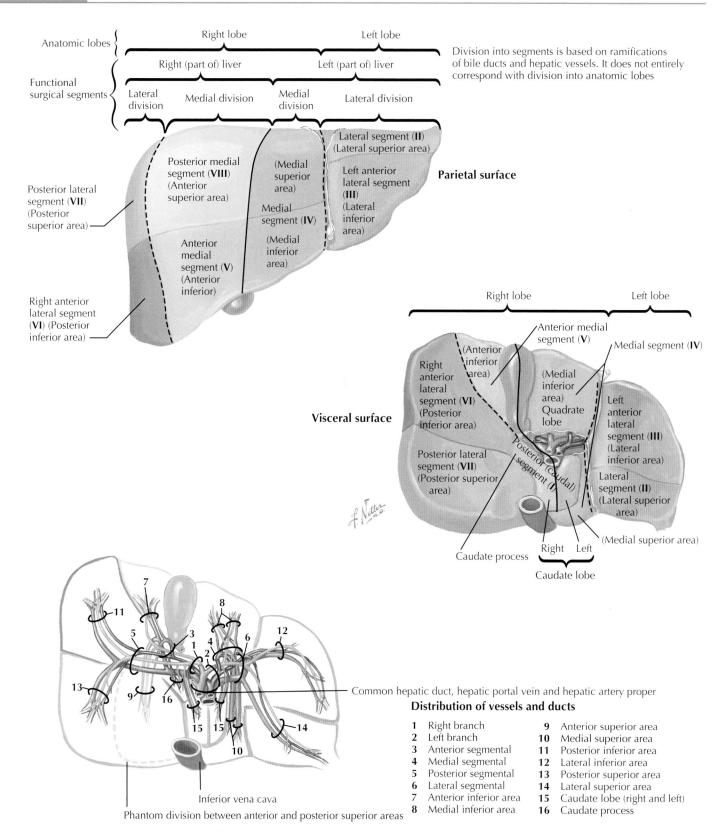

Division into segments is based on ramifications of bile ducts and hepatic vessels. It does not entirely correspond with division into anatomic lobes

Anatomic lobes { Right lobe   Left lobe

Functional surgical segments { Right (part of) liver   Left (part of) liver

Lateral division   Medial division   Medial division   Lateral division

Parietal surface

Lateral segment (**II**) (Lateral superior area)

Left anterior lateral segment (**III**) (Lateral inferior area)

Posterior medial segment (**VIII**) (Anterior superior area)

(Medial superior area)

Medial segment (**IV**) (Medial inferior area)

Anterior medial segment (**V**) (Anterior inferior)

Posterior lateral segment (**VII**) (Posterior superior area)

Right anterior lateral segment (**VI**) (Posterior inferior area)

Visceral surface

Right lobe   Left lobe

Anterior medial segment (**V**)   Medial segment (**IV**)

(Anterior inferior area)

Right anterior lateral segment (**VI**) (Posterior inferior area)

(Medial inferior area) Quadrate lobe

Left anterior lateral segment (**III**) (Lateral inferior area)

Posterior lateral segment (**VII**) (Posterior superior area)

Posterior (caudal) segment (**I**)

Lateral segment (**II**) (Lateral superior area)

(Medial superior area)

Caudate process

Right   Left

Caudate lobe

Common hepatic duct, hepatic portal vein and hepatic artery proper

Distribution of vessels and ducts

1	Right branch	**9**	Anterior superior area
2	Left branch	**10**	Medial superior area
3	Anterior segmental	**11**	Posterior inferior area
4	Medial segmental	**12**	Lateral inferior area
5	Posterior segmental	**13**	Posterior superior area
6	Lateral segmental	**14**	Lateral superior area
7	Anterior inferior area	**15**	Caudate lobe (right and left)
8	Medial inferior area	**16**	Caudate process

Inferior vena cava

Phantom division between anterior and posterior superior areas

Fig. 143.8 Vessel and Duct Distributions and Liver Segments.

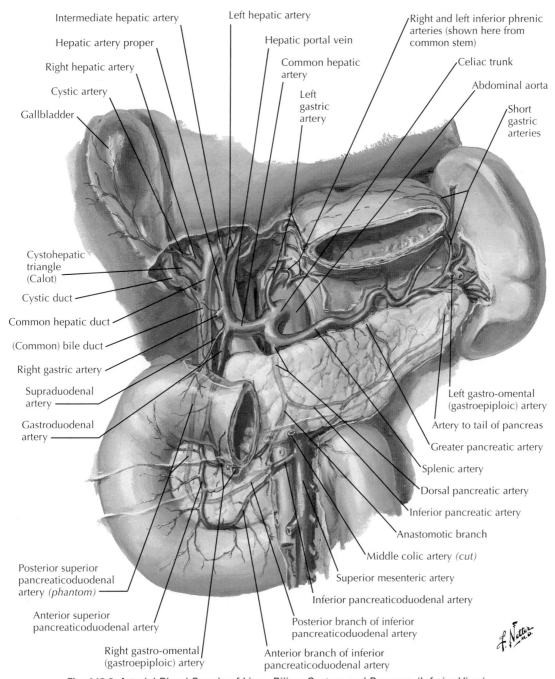

Intermediate hepatic artery

Hepatic artery proper

Right hepatic artery

Cystic artery

Gallbladder

Left hepatic artery

Hepatic portal vein

Common hepatic artery

Left gastric artery

Right and left inferior phrenic arteries (shown here from common stem)

Celiac trunk

Abdominal aorta

Short gastric arteries

Cystohepatic triangle (Calot)

Cystic duct

Common hepatic duct

(Common) bile duct

Right gastric artery

Supraduodenal artery

Gastroduodenal artery

Left gastro-omental (gastroepiploic) artery

Artery to tail of pancreas

Greater pancreatic artery

Splenic artery

Dorsal pancreatic artery

Inferior pancreatic artery

Anastomotic branch

Middle colic artery (cut)

Superior mesenteric artery

Inferior pancreaticoduodenal artery

Posterior superior pancreaticoduodenal artery (phantom)

Anterior superior pancreaticoduodenal artery

Right gastro-omental (gastroepiploic) artery

Posterior branch of inferior pancreaticoduodenal artery

Anterior branch of inferior pancreaticoduodenal artery

Fig. 143.9 Arterial Blood Supply of Liver, Biliary System and Pancreas (Inferior View).

the spleen. The *left gastroepiploic* artery and the *short gastric* arteries usually have their origins in one of these terminal branches.

The *hepatic artery,* intermediate in size, passes forward and to the right to enter the right margin of the lesser omentum, in which it ascends, lying to the left of the CBD and anterior to the portal vein. As the hepatic artery turns upward, it gives origin first to the gastroduodenal artery (see later), then usually to the supraduodenal artery, and finally to the right gastric artery. The *supraduodenal artery,* which may also originate from the right hepatic or the retroduodenal artery, descends to supply the anterior, superior, and posterior surfaces of the proximal duodenum. The right gastric artery passes to the left along the lesser curvature of the stomach to anastomose with the left gastric artery. The continuation of the hepatic artery beyond the origins of these

vessels is known as the *common hepatic artery (arteria hepatica propria).* It ascends and divides into several branches, most often the *right hepatic* and *left hepatic* arteries; the *middle hepatic* artery usually arises from the left hepatic artery. The right hepatic artery generally passes behind the common hepatic duct to enter the cystic *Calot triangle,* formed by the cystic duct, the hepatic duct, and the liver. Occasionally, however, the right hepatic artery crosses in front of the bile duct. All terminal branches of the hepatic artery enter the liver at the porta hepatis. The *cystic artery* also has many variations.

In general the arterial supply to the pancreas, CBD, and adjacent portions of the duodenum originates from branches of the gastroduodenal, superior mesenteric, and splenic arteries. The *gastroduodenal artery,* after its origin from the common hepatic artery, passes downward

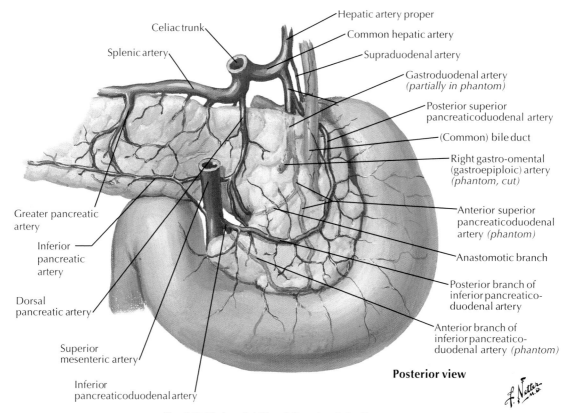

Celiac trunk

Splenic artery

Hepatic artery proper

Common hepatic artery

Supraduodenal artery

Gastroduodenal artery
(partially in phantom)

Posterior superior
pancreaticoduodenal artery

(Common) bile duct

Right gastro-omental
(gastroepiploic) artery
(phantom, cut)

Greater pancreatic
artery

Inferior
pancreatic
artery

Dorsal
pancreatic artery

Superior
mesenteric artery

Inferior
pancreaticoduodenal artery

Anterior superior
pancreaticoduodenal
artery (phantom)

Anastomotic branch

Posterior branch of
inferior pancreatico-
duodenal artery

Anterior branch of
inferior pancreatico-
duodenal artery (phantom)

Posterior view

Fig. 143.10 Arterial Blood Supply of the Pancreas.

to course behind the first portion of the duodenum and in front of the head of the pancreas. Before or immediately after passing behind the duodenum, it gives origin to the *posterosuperior pancreaticoduodenal* artery, also known as the *retroduodenal* artery. Its origin is often hidden by dense fibrous tissue; passing to the right and downward over the CBD, it gives off a branch comprising the principal blood supply of that duct. The retroduodenal artery continues downward behind the head of the pancreas and between the duodenum and CBD, finally turning to the left to unite with the posterior branch of the *inferior pancreaticoduodenal* artery, also known as the *posteroinferior pancreaticoduodenal* artery.

At the lower border of the pylorus, the gastroduodenal artery divides into a larger right gastroepiploic artery and a smaller anterosuperior pancreaticoduodenal artery. The *right gastroepiploic* enters the greater omentum to follow the greater curvature of the stomach. The *anterosuperior pancreaticoduodenal* artery continues downward on the anterior surface of the head of the pancreas as far as its lower border, where it turns upward to unite with the *anterior branch* of the inferior pancreaticoduodenal artery, also known as the *anteroinferior pancreaticoduodenal* artery. In approximately 40% of cases, no common inferior pancreaticoduodenal artery exists, and the anterior and posterior vessels originate separately from the superior mesenteric artery.

The head of the pancreas and the second and third portions of the duodenum are thus supplied by two arcades, an anterior and a posterior arch. The *posterior arch* is formed by the posterosuperior pancreaticoduodenal (retroduodenal) artery uniting with the posteroinferior pancreaticoduodenal artery. The *anterior arch* is formed by the gastroduodenal and anterosuperior pancreaticoduodenal arteries uniting with the anteroinferior pancreaticoduodenal artery. The posterior span is situated at a somewhat higher level than the anterior arch. Both give off branches that anastomose with each other through and around the pancreas, supplying that organ and the duodenum.

Branches of the splenic artery are the chief suppliers to the neck, body, and tail of the pancreas. Some of these are small twigs given off by the splenic artery as it courses along the upper border of the pancreas. Three branches, however, are usually larger than the others and have achieved the distinction of individual names. The *dorsal pancreatic* artery, also known as the *superior pancreatic* artery, although usually originating from the beginning of the splenic artery, may also arise from the hepatic or celiac artery or the aorta. It runs downward, behind, and into the pancreas, dividing into left and right branches. The left branch generally comprises the transverse pancreatic artery. The right branches constitute an anastomotic vessel to the anterior pancreatic arch and a branch to the pancreatic lingual. The *great pancreatic* artery originates from the splenic artery further to the left and passes downward, dividing into branches that anastomose with the transverse or inferior pancreatic artery. The *artery for tail of pancreas* (arteria caudae pancreatis) originates from the splenic artery or from its terminal branches at the tail of the pancreas and divides into branches that anastomose with the terminal twigs of the transverse pancreatic artery. The *transverse pancreatic* artery, usually the left branch of the dorsal pancreatic, courses behind the body and tail of the pancreas close to its lower border. It may originate from or communicate with the superior mesenteric artery.

The other branches of the splenic artery are variable terminal branches to the spleen, the left gastroepiploic artery, the short gastric arteries to the stomach fundus, and usually branches that anastomose with the left inferior phrenic artery.

HEPATIC ARTERY VARIATIONS

Variations are commonly found in the origin and course of the hepatic artery or its branches (Michels) (Fig. 143.11). These involve the right and left hepatic arteries equally and are of great

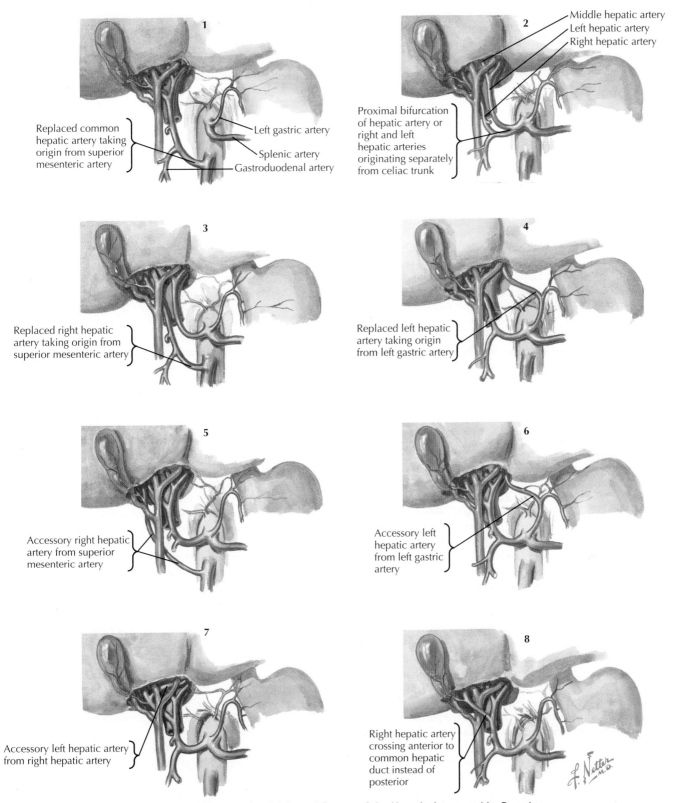

Fig. 143.11 Variations in the Origin and Course of the Hepatic Artery and Its Branches.

surgical significance due to the risk for liver necrosis upon unintended ligation.

A *replaced* hepatic artery originates from a different source than in the standard description and substitutes for the typical vessel. An *accessory* artery is a vessel additional to those originating according to standard description.

An example of replacement is the origin of the common hepatic artery from the superior mesenteric artery. The common hepatic artery passes through or behind the head of the pancreas, and its ligation during a pancreaticoduodenal resection deprives the liver of its arterial blood supply. Under these circumstances, only the left gastric and splenic arteries arise from the celiac axis.

In addition, right or left hepatic arteries may originate independently from the celiac axis or fork from a short common hepatic artery. Under these conditions, the *gastroduodenal* artery originates from the right hepatic artery and the *superior mesenteric* artery, whereas the left hepatic artery, in turn giving off the middle hepatic artery, derives from the *celiac axis*. Ligation of the replaced right hepatic artery (more common than accessory right hepatic artery)—especially where it crosses the junction of the cystic and the common ducts, as during cholecystectomy—deprives the right lobe of the liver of its blood supply. In contrast, ligation of an accessory right hepatic artery that derives from the superior mesenteric is less significant because another right hepatic artery runs its typical course. Under these circumstances, two right hepatic arteries may be found in the Calot triangle.

An aberrant left hepatic artery, originating from the *left gastric* artery, is a replaced artery in 50% of patients and an accessory in the other 50%. If replaced, only the right hepatic artery comes from the celiac axis, whereas in the presence of an accessory vessel, the common hepatic artery takes its usual course. Ligation of a replaced left hepatic artery, as during gastrectomy, endangers the blood supply to the left lobe of the liver.

An accessory left hepatic artery may also originate from the right hepatic artery. In approximately 12% of patients, the right hepatic artery, originating at its typical site of departure, crosses in front of the common hepatic duct instead of behind it; this is a variation worth remembering during exploration of the duct. The described variations are also significant in the formation of collaterals after obstruction or ligation of an artery.

Other variations shown in Fig. 143.11, but not described, are less common but should not be ignored when operating in this field.

PORTAL VEIN TRIBUTARIES AND PORTACAVAL ANASTOMOSES

The portal vein forms behind the head of the pancreas at the height of the second lumbar vertebra (L2) through a confluence of the superior mesenteric and splenic veins (Fig. 143.12). It runs behind the first portion of the duodenum and then along the right border of the lesser omentum to the hilus of the liver, where it splits into its hepatic branches. The portal vein receives the *coronary vein*, which is the continuation of the left gastric vein and the esophageal venous plexus. The coronary vein, in turn, connects with the *short gastric* veins, the *azygos* and *hemiazygos* veins, in the lower and middle parts and with various branches of the superior vena cava, such as the innominate and inferior thyroid veins in the upper part of the esophageal region. The portal vein further accepts the *pyloric* vein, which, together with the coronary and gastric veins, forms a loop. The left main branch of the portal vein admits the *paraumbilical* veins and occasionally a persisting umbilical vein.

The *superior mesenteric* vein, one of the constituents of the vena portae, originates at the root of the mesentery, mainly from the *middle colic, right colic,* and *ileocolic* veins. It further accepts the *inferior pancreaticoduodenal* vein, which runs in front of the third portion of the duodenum and the uncinate process of the pancreas. The *right gastroepiploic* vein, coming from the right aspects of the greater curvature of the stomach, enters the superior mesenteric vein before the latter unites with the splenic vein.

Splenic and inferior mesenteric veins usually have a common terminal end portion behind the body of the pancreas. The *inferior mesenteric* vein starts with the superior hemorrhoidal veins and continues in the posterior abdominal wall, receiving many tributaries, especially the *left colic* vein. The *splenic* vein begins at the hilus of the spleen and admits the *left gastroepiploic* vein, short gastric veins (both communicating with esophageal veins), and pancreatic veins, which anastomose with retroperitoneal veins and thus with the caval system.

The shortness of the main stem of the portal vein prevents complete mixing of the blood coming from its constituents, so the right extremity of the liver receives chiefly blood coming from the superior mesenteric vein. The left lobe receives blood from the coronary, inferior mesenteric, and splenic veins, whereas the left part of the right lobe, including the caudate and quadrate lobes, receives mixed blood. These "streamlines," demonstrated in animals, are not seen during portal venography, and it is uncertain whether they occur in humans. Their existence has been assumed, however, to explain the localization of tumor metastases and abscesses, and the predominance of massive necrosis in the left lobe in fulminant viral hepatitis, presumably due to loss of nutrient-rich blood from the small intestine.

Portacaval anastomoses have great clinical significance. They dilate when blood flow in the portal vein and the liver is restrained, can relieve portal hypertension, and may be lifesaving in case of acute portal hypertension. As in chronic obstruction, however, portacaval anastomoses may shunt blood from the liver, resulting in hepatic insufficiency.

Dilatation of the hemorrhoidal veins results in hemorrhoidal piles, with the danger of hemorrhage, thrombosis, and inflammation. Varicosities of the esophageal veins (less with cardiac veins of stomach) may lead to *esophageal hemorrhage,* among the most dangerous complications of portal hypertension (see Chapter 149). *Retroperitoneal varicose* portacaval anastomoses have less clinical significance. *Paraumbilical anastomoses* lead to marked dilatation of the veins in the anterior abdominal wall, which may converge toward the umbilicus to form *caput medusae.*

PORTAL VEIN VARIATIONS AND ANOMALIES

Although major anatomic variations of the portal venous system are less common than in the hepatic arterial system, minor variations of surgical importance are common and are of relevance to shunt procedures for portal hypertension (Fig. 143.13).

The length of the portal vein varies between 5.5 and 8 cm, with an average of approximately 6.5 cm; mean diameter is 1.09 cm. In cirrhosis, however, the diameter is considerably wider. It is of practical importance that in slightly more than 10% of patients, no vessel enters the main stem of the portal vein, although in most patients several veins are admitted that may be torn during the dissection for portacaval anastomoses. Severe hemorrhage may result, and their ligation may interfere with the size of the portal vein and the performance of the anastomosis.

In more than two-thirds of patients, the *gastric coronary* vein is of major significance because portal drainage from esophageal varices enters the left aspect of the portal vein. Otherwise portal drainage enters at the junction of the splenic and superior mesenteric veins, whereas in almost 25% of patients it joins the splenic vein. Under these circumstances, the *pyloric* vein may enter the portal vein stem. On its right aspect, the portal vein may admit the superior pancreaticoduodenal vein, and close to the liver the cystic vein frequently joins the right branch of the portal vein.

The usual anatomic description of the formation of the portal vein is found in only about 50% of patients. In the other half, the *inferior mesenteric* vein enters the junction of the splenic and superior mesenteric veins or joins the superior mesenteric vein.

The size of the *splenic vein,* of major importance in splenorenal shunts, averages less than 0.5 cm between the splenic hilus and the junction with the inferior mesenteric vein. As a rule the splenic vein is widened to a lesser degree in portal hypertension than the portal vein. Because the splenic vein is effectively embedded in the cephalad portion of the pancreas; the many pancreatic venous tributaries are so short that they may be easily torn during shunt procedures; therefore their ligation creates technical problems.

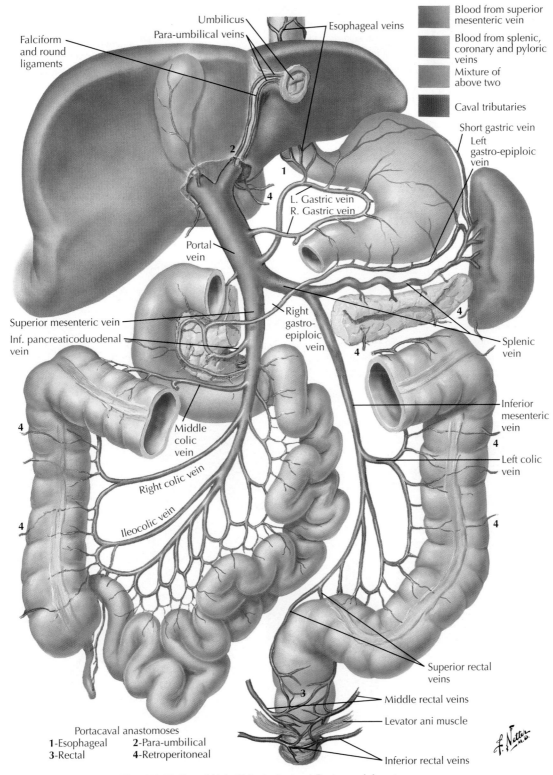

Fig. 143.12 Portal Vein Tributaries and Portacaval Anastomoses.

Among rare *congenital anomalies* of the portal vein, one of high surgical significance involves an abnormal position anterior to the head of the pancreas and the duodenum. Another rare but physiologically interesting anomaly is the entrance of the portal vein into the IVC, which suggests that the liver can function without portal vein blood and the hepatic artery can be considerably enlarged. Extremely rare is an entrance of the pulmonary vein into the portal vein, probably caused by a disturbance in early fetal development of the venous systems. Again, congenital *strictures* of the portal vein at the hilus of the liver are rare but may result in severe portal hypertension, which may not be relieved by surgical anastomoses.

Variations

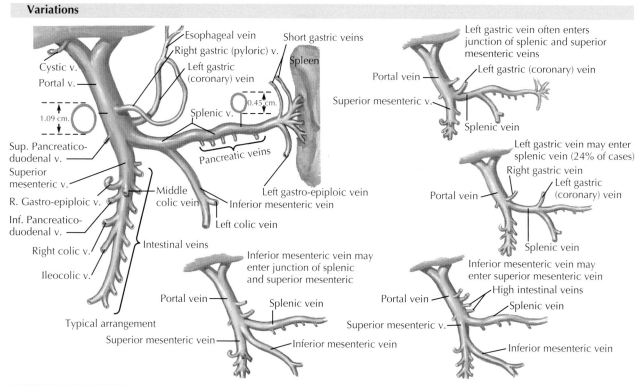

Anomalies

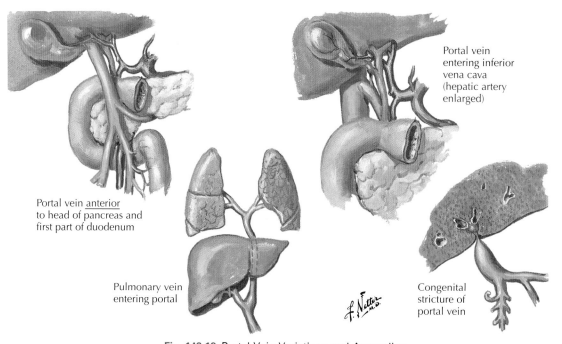

Fig. 143.13 Portal Vein Variations and Anomalies.

ADDITIONAL RESOURCES

Rappaport AM, Wanless IR: Physioanatomic considerations. In Schiff L, Schiff ER, editors: *Diseases of the liver*, ed 7, Philadelphia, 1993, Lippincott, pp 1–41.

Saxena R, Theise ND, Crawford JM: Microanatomy of the human liver-exploring the hidden interfaces, *Hepatology* 30:1339–1346, 1999.

Tabibian JH, Masyuk AI, Masyuk TV, et al: Physiology of cholangiocytes, *Compr Physiol* 3:541–565, 2013.

Teutsch HF: The modular microarchitecture of human liver, *Hepatology* 42:317–325, 2005.

Yamamoto K, Sherman I, Phillips MJ, Fisher MM: Three-dimensional observations of the hepatic arterial terminations in rat, hamster and human liver by scanning electron microscopy of microvascular casts, *Hepatology* 5:452–456, 1985.

144

Liver Function Tests

Kris V. Kowdley, Joseph K. Lim

Liver function tests (LFTs), also known as liver enzymes or liver chemistries, generally refer to a panel of serum biochemical studies used to screen for and monitor liver disease. This panel evaluates hepatic components ranging from hepatocellular necrosis and damaged hepatic synthetic capacity to the liver's ability to excrete breakdown products. LFTs also describe a battery of dynamic tests that provide real-time evaluation of liver function, generally by measuring hepatic blood flow, metabolic capacity, or excretory function.

Serum liver biochemical tests can be divided into three groups: (1) markers of hepatocellular injury, including alanine transaminase (ALT) and aspartate transaminase (AST); (2) markers of cholestasis, including alkaline phosphatase (ALP), 5′-nucleotidase, γ-glutamyltransferase (GGT), and bilirubin; and (3) markers of liver synthetic function, including serum albumin and prothrombin time (PT).

In general, the hepatocellular liver enzymes reflect the degree or severity of hepatic necroinflammation. Serum AST and ALT are found in much higher concentrations within hepatocytes than in the circulation. Therefore processes leading to necrosis or swelling of hepatocytes are associated with leakage of these enzymes into the plasma, resulting in increased concentrations. By contrast, elevated serum concentrations of the cholestatic liver enzymes (e.g., ALP) may be attributed to release from damaged hepatocytes or to induction of these enzymes by processes that damage biliary epithelia, such as bile duct obstruction by stones or cholestatic liver disease (e.g., primary biliary cirrhosis, primary sclerosing cholangitis).

Clinicians are routinely tasked with the evaluation of abnormal liver chemistries. In the context of emerging evidence for increased liver-related mortality in individuals with elevated serum ALT and validation of standardized cut-offs for normal values for liver chemistries, clinical practice guidelines currently incorporate new thresholds for normal serum ALT (29–33 IU/L in men, 19–25 IU/L in women) and standardized algorithms to facilitate an individualized approach to evaluation.

Serum concentrations of albumin and bilirubin are more appropriately described as LFTs than liver transaminases; serum *albumin* is a measure of hepatic synthetic capacity, whereas *bilirubin* level reflects the uptake, conjugation, and biliary excretion of bilirubin, a breakdown product from senescent red blood cells. *PT* is a measure of prothrombin synthesis, a vitamin K–dependent process.

The *serum bilirubin test* is the only blood test that measures the liver's excretory function, including uptake, conjugation, and biliary excretion. Other tests examine the liver's ability to perform specific metabolic functions and often involve administration of a compound, after which its metabolite can be measured in the serum, breath, or urine. These metabolic LFTs are more sensitive for hepatic dysfunction than the serum bilirubin test, but they may lack specificity. Nevertheless, these tests have proven useful in certain patients, such as those with compensated cirrhosis being considered for liver resection or surgery to decompress portal hypertension and whose hepatic functional reserve must be determined.

BREATH TESTS

Breath tests of liver function have been developed based on the principle that the rate of conversion of orally or intravenously radiolabeled carbon 14 (^{14}C), which is converted to $^{14}CO_2$ and is subsequently exhaled, can be collected and quantified as a measure of liver function. Breath tests are infrequently used in the United States, primarily because of the inconvenience of using radiolabeled ^{14}C. Other breath tests now measure galactose or caffeine clearance.

Human and animal studies have shown that the *aminopyrine breath test* is a quantitative measure of the mixed-function system. Patients with cirrhosis have a decreased clearance of aminopyrine, which correlates with a decreased rate of $^{14}CO_2$ appearance in breath, presumably because of the decreased mass of hepatic microsomal mass containing mixed-function oxidases. Aminopyrine breath test results also correlate with other markers of hepatic function, such as serum albumin and PT. The aminopyrine breath test is also helpful to determine the extent of severe hepatocellular disease, as in fulminant hepatitis, although is rarely used clinically in this context.

Recently, a *methacetin breath test* was introduced to measure flow-dependent hepatic microsomal function. The substrate, ^{13}C methacetin, is metabolized in the liver by *O*-demethylation to $^{13}CO_2$ and acetaminophen.

CLEARANCE TESTS

Indocyanine green (ICG) is a dye with a high hepatic extraction ratio. Almost all the dye is excreted unchanged in bile; there is no significant enterohepatic circulation, and levels in the serum can be measured by atomic absorption spectrophotometry. Because ICG is excreted with little metabolic activity in the liver, the ICG clearance test has been used primarily to measure hepatic blood flow using the Fick equation. The proportion of ICG retained is inversely related to liver function (i.e., higher retention correlates with decreased liver function).

Galactose clearance is reduced in patients with cirrhosis and chronic hepatitis but not in patients with biliary obstruction. However, it is unclear whether this test contributes increased sensitivity to standard LFTs, such as albumin and bilirubin.

Caffeine clearance is another test of hepatic metabolic activity and is measured by caffeine concentration in saliva. The caffeine clearance test has the advantages of noninvasive collection and avoidance of radioactivity. The main limitation is the confusion introduced by smoking, which increases caffeine clearance.

MONOETHYLGLYCINEXYLIDIDE FORMATION

Monoethylglycinexylidide (MEGX) is a first-pass metabolite of lidocaine. *Lidocaine,* when administered intravenously at a subtherapeutic dose (1 mg/kg), is rapidly cleared and metabolized by the liver to MEGX. Thus MEGX formation reflects hepatic blood flow and metabolic activity. In the early era of liver transplantation, the MEGX test engendered much enthusiasm as a useful test to determine hepatic reserve and optimal timing for liver transplantation. However, the rapid increase in demand for donor organs and the subsequent implementation of the Model for End-Stage Liver Disease (MELD) scoring systems have rendered the MEGX test less clinically relevant, except when liver resection or portosystemic shunt is considered.

Other imaging-based tests are currently under investigation as possible modalities for quantitative evaluation of liver function, including gadolinium-ethoxybenzyl-diethylenetriamiinepentaacetic acid (Gd-EOB-DTPA)-enhanced magnetic resonance imaging (MRI), or technetium-99m-galactosyl serum albumin (99m-Tc-GSA) or 99m-Tc-mebrofenin hepatobiliary scintigraphy.

ADDITIONAL RESOURCES

Afolabi P, Wright M, Wooton SA, Jackson AA: Clinical utility of 13C-liver function breath tests for assessment of hepatic function, *Dig Dis Sci* 58:33–41, 2013.

Geisel D, Ludemann L, Froling V, et al: Imaging-based evaluation of liver function: comparison of 99m-Tc-mebrofenin hepatobiliary scintigraphy and Gd-EOB-DTPA-enhanced MRI, *Eur Radiol* 25:1384–1391, 2015.

Green RM, Flamm S: AGA technical review on the evaluation of liver chemistry tests, *Gastroenterology* 123:1367–1384, 2002.

Kwo PY, Cohen SM, Lim JK: ACG Clinical Guideline: Evaluation of abnormal liver chemistries, *Am J Gastroenterol* 112:18–35, 2017.

Mallory MA, Lee SW, Kowdley KV: Abnormal liver test results on routine screening: how to evaluate, when to refer for a biopsy, *Postgrad Med* 115(3):53–56, 59–62, 66, 2004.

Pijls KE, de Vries H, Nikkessen S, et al: Critical appraisal of 13C breath tests for microsomal liver function: aminopyrine revisited, *Liver Int* 34: 487–494, 2014.

Prati D, Taioli E, Zanella A, et al: Updated definitions of healthy ranges for serum alanine aminotransferase levels, *Ann Intern Med* 137:1–10, 2002.

Pratt DS, Kaplan MM: Evaluation of abnormal liver-enzyme results in asymptomatic patients, *N Engl J Med* 342:1266–1271, 2000.

Stravitz RT, Ilan Y: Potential use of metabolic breath tests to assess liver disease and prognosis: has the time arrived for routine use in the clinic? *Liver Int* 37:328–336, 2017.

145

Prothrombin Formation

Kris V. Kowdley, Joseph K. Lim

The liver is the site of synthesis of several major proteins involved in coagulation, including factors I, II, V, VII, IX, X, XII, and XIII. The formation of factors II (prothrombin), VII, IX, and X is dependent on g-carboxylation, which is a vitamin K–dependent step.

Prothrombin time (PT) represents a valuable test for assessment of liver synthetic function.

PT is a measure of the time taken to convert prothrombin (factor II) to thrombin (activated factor II). This test is a simple yet useful measure of the body's coagulation. Causes of PT prolongation include the following (Fig. 145.1):

- Inadequate dietary intake of vitamin K, leading to decreased g-carboxylation of proteins involved in coagulation
- Inability to absorb vitamin K because of insufficient bile acid concentrations in the lumen of the intestine, such as from cholestatic liver disease or bacterial overgrowth
- Intrinsic hepatocellular dysfunction, resulting in failure to synthesize prothrombin despite adequate vitamin K stores
- Ingestion of drugs or toxins (e.g., warfarin) that interfere with prothrombin production

Parenteral administration of vitamin K may help differentiate between inadequate vitamin K stores and liver dysfunction as the cause of a prolonged PT. Usually three parenteral doses of vitamin K are sufficient to differentiate intrinsic liver disease from vitamin K deficiency. Patients with intrinsic liver disease fail to correct PT after vitamin K supplementation. This test can be particularly helpful in patients with cholestatic liver disease, in whom PT prolongation results from vitamin K deficiency and liver dysfunction.

ADDITIONAL RESOURCES

Bajaj SP, Joist JH: New insights into blood clots: implications for the use of APTT and PT as coagulation screening tests and in monitoring of anticoagulant therapy, *Semin Thromb Hemost* 25: 407–418, 1999.

Lee JH, Kweon OJ, Lee MK, et al: Clinical usefulness of international normalized ratio calibration of prothrombin time in patients with chronic liver disease, *Int J Hematol* 102:163–169, 2015.

Nilsson IM: Coagulation and fibrinolysis, *Scand J Gastroenterol Suppl* 137: 11–18, 1987.

Tripodi A, Chantarangkul V, Primignani M, et al: The international normalized ratio calibrated for cirrhosis (INRliver) normalizes prothrombin time results for model for end-stage liver disease (MELD) calculation, *Hepatology* 46:520–527, 2007.

Uotila L: The metabolic functions and mechanism of action of vitamin K, *Scand J Clin Lab Invest Suppl* 201:109–117, 1990.

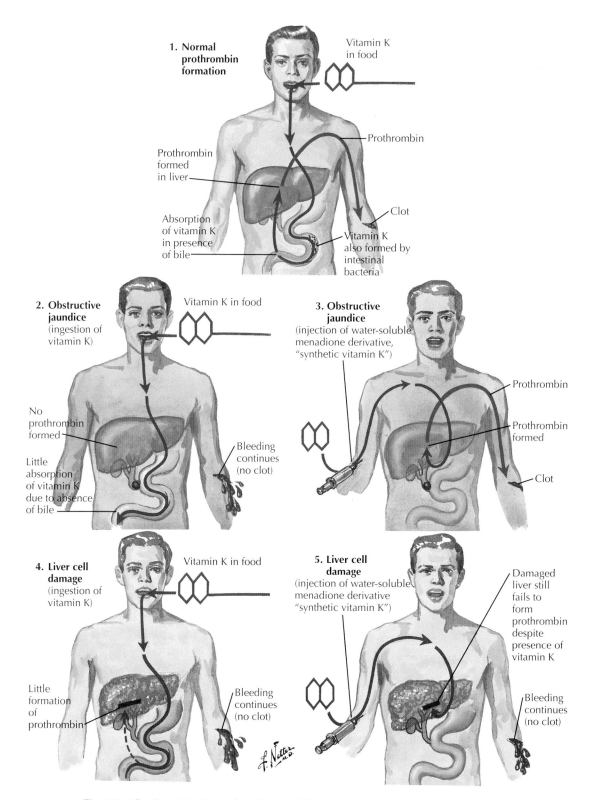

Fig. 145.1 Prothrombin Formation: Normal, Obstructive Jaundice, and Liver Cell Damage.

146

Bilirubin and Bile Acid Metabolism

Kris V. Kowdley, Joseph K. Lim

"Bilirubin and bile acid metabolism represent major functions of the liver."

Bile is secreted by the liver and serves many functions. *Hepatocytes* are the source of bile production and secrete bile through specialized receptors. The biliary route is responsible for the elimination of lipid-soluble toxins, secretion of bile acids, transport of cholesterol into the gastrointestinal (GI) tract, and absorption of fats and fat-soluble vitamins, in addition to drugs, toxins, and heavy metals. Biliary epithelial cells further modify the bile secreted by hepatocytes through the addition of water, bicarbonate, and other compounds. Bile is stored in the gallbladder, where it is concentrated and then secreted into the lumen in response to hormonal and dietary signals.

The composition of bile has been studied in detail. Its predominant components are bile acids (Figs. 146.1 and 146.2), which serve several functions, most importantly the absorption of fats and fat-soluble vitamins through the formation of *micelles,* which are formed by bile acids, cholesterol, phosphatidyl choline, and lecithin, and act as detergents.

Bile also has a critical role in the excretion of bilirubin, a breakdown product of red blood cells (RBCs). Bilirubin from senescent RBCs is conjugated by the liver through glucuronidation into bilirubin diglucuronide, thus rendering it water soluble and capable of transport in bile. Failure of the liver to conjugate or excrete bilirubin can result in retention of unconjugated bilirubin in the plasma, which in turn may cause clinical symptoms such as jaundice, scleral icterus, dark urine, and acholic stools.

Bile is important for the excretion of many organic anions and cations, including drugs and toxins, and has multiple other components, including steroid hormones, fat-soluble vitamins, cytokines such as tumor necrosis factor-α, and leukotrienes and divalent cations, most importantly *copper.* In fact, regulation of body copper stores occurs predominantly through the excretion of biliary copper. Chronic cholestatic disorders such as primary biliary cirrhosis and primary sclerosing cholangitis are often associated with excess copper accumulation in the liver. Hepatic copper content in these disorders can approach levels observed in patients with *Wilson disease,* a genetic disorder caused by a loss-of-function mutation in the *ATPB7* gene, which regulates copper excretion through the biliary tract. Copper accumulates in the liver over time, with subsequent copper overload in other organs which may result in multiorgan copper toxicity.

Bile may contain other proteins such as albumin, lysosomal enzymes, and haptoglobin and, because of the presence of secretory immunoglobulin A (sIgA) in bile, may additionally serve an important role in immune surveillance in the GI tract.

Bile flow has bile acid–dependent and bile acid–independent components. Most bile flow depends on bile acids, which appear to have varying effects on bile flow based on their physicochemical properties and other factors. By contrast, bile acid–independent bile flow generally results from an osmotic effect of anions and represents a smaller portion of bile. Improved understanding of bilirubin and hepatic organic anion/cation transport has occurred through recent investigations which have identified and cloned specific transporters (e.g., mdr2/MDR3) in mice and humans responsible for biliary secretion and transport of these compounds (Fig. 146.3). For example, MDR3 is a member of a class of proteins that confer resistance to certain chemotherapeutic agents, and its normal function is to maintain biliary phospholipid transport. Biliary phospholipids may have a cytoprotective effect in biliary epithelia against the toxic effect of bile acids on cell membranes. Creation of a knockout mouse lacking the *mdr2* gene results in chronic cholestatic liver disease, analogous to chronic cholestatic disorders such as primary biliary cirrhosis in humans.

Several nuclear receptors are activated by ligands that regulate expression of hepatobiliary transporters at a transcriptional and posttranscriptional level. These are regulated, in turn, by bile acids, drugs, hormones, and cytokines. The clinical expression of many cholestatic liver disorders may be influenced by activation of these nuclear receptors, which include farnesoid X receptor (FXR), pregnane X receptor (PXR), constitutive androstane receptor (CAR), vitamin D receptor (VDR), retinoic acid receptor (RAR), liver receptor homolog-1 receptor (LRH), peroxisome proliferator activated receptor-alpha (PPARa), and glucocorticoid receptor (GR).

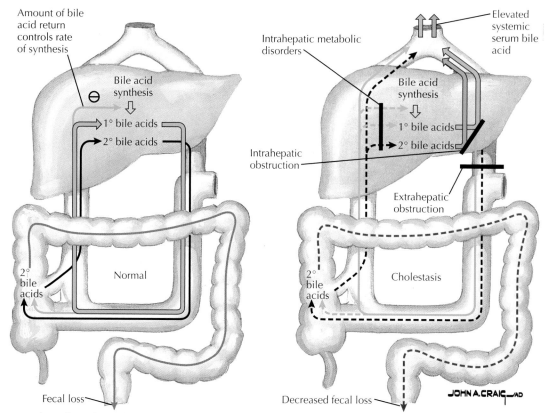

Amount of bile acid return controls rate of synthesis

Bile acid synthesis

1° bile acids

2° bile acids

Normal

2° bile acids

Fecal loss

Bile acids synthesized by liver secreted into gut, reabsorbed, and recycled through liver, with small amount lost in feces

Intrahepatic metabolic disorders

Elevated systemic serum bile acid

Bile acid synthesis

1° bile acids

2° bile acids

Intrahepatic obstruction

Extrahepatic obstruction

Cholestasis

2° bile acids

Decreased fecal loss

JOHN A. CRAIG—AD

Extrahepatic obstruction or intrahepatic disorders that affect bile synthesis, transport, absorption, or secretion result in decreased enterohepatic circulation of bile acids

Cellular mechanisms of metabolism

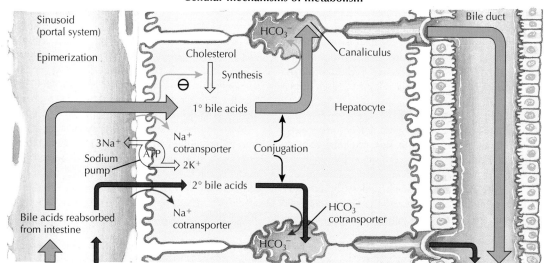

Sinusoid (portal system)

Epimerization

Cholesterol

Synthesis

1° bile acids

3Na⁺

Na⁺ cotransporter

Sodium pump   ATP   2K⁺

Conjugation

2° bile acids

Na⁺ cotransporter

Bile acids reabsorbed from intestine

HCO_3^-

Canaliculus

Hepatocyte

HCO_3^- cotransporter

HCO_3^-

Bile duct

Primary (1°) acids synthesized, conjugated, and sectreted into canaliculi. In gut, portion of bile acid is converted to secondary (2°) bile acids. Bile acids (90%) reabsorbed into portal system and returned to liver; in hepatocytes, primary forms recycled and secondary acids epimerized and excreted

Fig. 146.1 Bile Acid Circulation and Metabolism: Enterohepatic Circulation and Cellular Mechanisms of Metabolism.

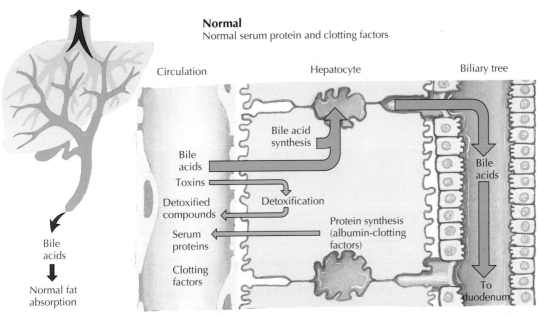

Normal
Normal serum protein and clotting factors

Hepatocytes (with polarity of transport and secretion) synthesize serum proteins and clotting factors and secrete them into bloodstream. Bile acids absorbed from circulation and secreted along with newly synthesized bile acids into biliary tree. Toxins absorbed from circulation, detoxified, and returned to circulation

Cholestasis

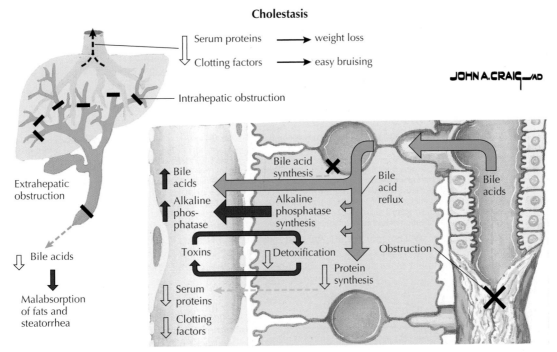

JOHN A. CRAIG AD

Obstructed bile flow and reflux of bile acids into hepatocytes result in increased synthesis and secretion of alkaline phosphatase. Resultant hepatocellular damage inhibits synthesis of proteins and clotting factors and limits detoxification

Fig. 146.2 Hepatic Protein and Bile Acid Metabolism: Normal Serum Protein and Clotting Factors and Cholestasis.

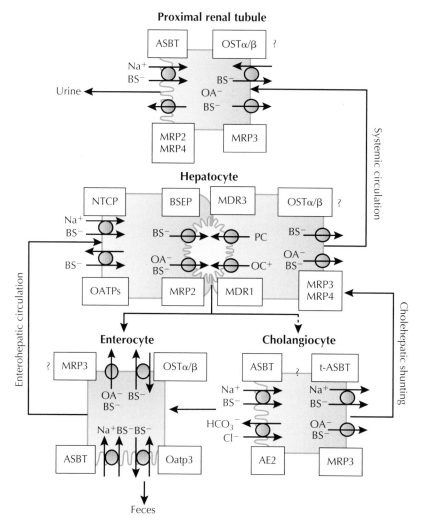

Bile acids are taken up by the hepatocytes via Na⁺, the bile canaliculus via BSEP—determining bile salt–dependent bile flow, while divalent bile acids and anionic conjugates (e.g., bilirubin diglucuronide, glutathione) are excreted via MRP2—determining bile salt–independent bile flow. MDR3 mediates the canalicular secretion of phospholipids, which form mixed micelles together with bile acids and cholesterol. MDR1 excretes the bulk of organic cations. Basolateral bile acid export pumps (e.g., MRP3, MRP4) provide alternative excretory pathway for otherwise accumulated biliary constituents. Bile composition is further modified along the biliary passage by secretion of bicarbonate via AE2 and reabsorption of bile acids via luminal ASBT. A shortcut (called "cholehepatic shunting") between cholangiocytes and hepatocytes is proposed by basolateral export of bile acids from the cholangiocytes via MRP3 and possibly t-ASBT and hepatocellular reuptake. In the terminal ileum bile acids are reabsorbed by ASBT and, to certain degrees, in rodents by Oatp3 and effluxed on the basolateral pole of enterocytes via OSTα/β and possibly to a lesser extent via MRP3 into portal circulation. Similar to the cholangiocyte and enterocyte, in the proximal renal tubules, bile acids are reabsorbed from the glomerular filtrate via ASBT to minimize bile salt loss. Possibly, renal MRP2 and MRP4 may be involved in the secretion of bile acids into the urine under cholestatic conditions.

Fig. 146.3 Hepatobiliary Transporters in Liver and Extrahepatic Tissues. (From Wagner M, Trauner M: Transcriptional regulation of hepatobiliary transport systems in health and disease: implications for a rationale approach to the treatment of intrahepatic cholestasis, *Ann Hepatol* 4(2):77-99, 2005.)

ADDITIONAL RESOURCES

Chiang JY: Bile acid metabolism and signaling, *Compr Physiol* 3:1191–1212, 2013.

Elferink RP: Understanding and controlling hepatobiliary function, *Best Pract Res Clin Gastroenterol* 16:1025–1034, 2002.

Kullak-Ublick GA, Stieger B, Hagenbuch B, Meier PJ: Hepatic transport of bile salts, *Semin Liver Dis* 20:273–292, 2000.

Oude Elferink RP, Groen AK: Mechanisms of biliary lipid secretion and their role in lipid homeostasis, *Semin Liver Dis* 20:293–305, 2000.

Tomer G, Shneider BL: Disorders of bile formation and biliary transport, *Gastroenterol Clin North Am* 32:839–855, 2003.

Trauner M, Claudel T, Fickert P, et al: Bile acids as regulators of hepatic lipid and glucose metabolism, *Dig Dis* 28:220–224, 2010.

Wagner M, Trauner M: Transcriptional regulation of hepatobiliary transport systems in health and disease: implications for a rationale approach to the treatment of intrahepatic cholestasis, *Ann Hepatol* 4(2):77–99, 2005.

147

Clinical Manifestations of Cirrhosis

Kris V. Kowdley, Joseph K. Lim

Cirrhosis is associated with a broad spectrum of clinical manifestations of cirrhosis which may manifest in many different forms (Fig. 147.1). Chills, high fever, and leukocytosis are induced by an infected extrahepatic biliary obstruction and are observed in secondary biliary cirrhosis. Peripheral neuropathy may signal the presence of malnutrition as a complication of cirrhosis. Manifestations of hepatic insufficiency are common and are the result of liver cell damage with loss of hepatic function because of the diversion of blood by extrahepatic portacaval collaterals and intrahepatic portohepatic venous anastomoses. Palpation and percussion may uncover either an enlarged or shrunken liver, although in most patients with cirrhosis, the organ is firm to palpation.

Severe jaundice is seen in only a minority of patients, although a subicteric hue is more common. Central nervous system (CNS) manifestations vary from somnolence to precomatose manifestations—reflected in flapping tremor, mental confusion, and electroencephalographic changes—to frank coma. *Bleeding diathesis* is caused by a defect in the hepatic formation of serum proteins active in the processes of blood coagulation, especially factors II (prothrombin) and VII. Capillary damage also may be important.

Fibrinogen formation is usually not decreased in cirrhosis, but it may be increased. Hypoproteinemia and compression of the inferior vena cava by ascites may explain the presence of ankle edema. Liver disease can result in anemia of the macrocytic or normochromic type, caused by hypersplenism and a nonspecific toxic effect on the bone marrow. Testicular atrophy, gynecomastia, female escutcheon, pectoral, axillary alopecia, and marked reddening of the thenar and hypothenar *(palmar erythema)* are believed to be caused by excess circulating estrogen resulting from decreased clearance by the liver. Cutaneous *spider nevi* are typically found on the upper half of the body (neck, forearm, and dorsum) but may involve the mucous membranes and consist of a central arteriole from which many small vessels radiate. Cirrhosis-associated increases in estrogenic activity may result in gynecomastia in men, and spider nevi hair loss and hirsutism in women.

Liver failure combined with the effects of portal hypertension leads to ascites, esophageal varices, and the dilatation of abdominal veins *(caput medusae)*. Leukopenia, thrombocytopenia, and anemia result from enlargement of the spleen and signs of hypersplenism. The pathogenesis and diagnosis of cirrhosis are discussed in Chapter 157.

ADDITIONAL RESOURCES

Rockey DC: The cell and molecular biology of hepatic fibrogenesis: clinical and therapeutic implications, *Clin Liver Dis* 4:319–355, 2000.

Schuppan D, Afdhal NH: Liver cirrhosis, *Lancet* 371(9615):838–851, 2008.

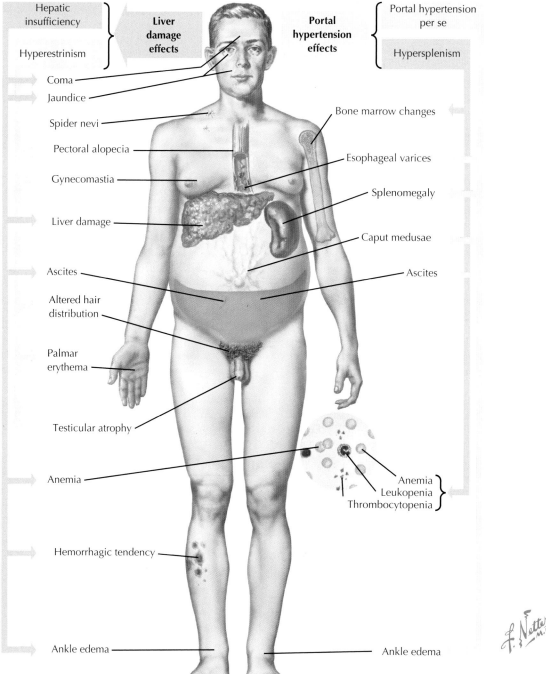

Fig. 147.1 Clinical Manifestations of Cirrhosis.

148

Physical Diagnosis of Liver Disease

Kris V. Kowdley, Joseph K. Lim

The diagnosis of chronic liver disease can be established on the basis of characteristic examination findings, which are more clinically overt in patients with cirrhosis and hepatic decompensation. Symptoms such as deepening jaundice, dark urine, light stools, and progressive increase in abdominal girth, as well as more nonspecific complaints of weakness and anorexia, may signal the presence of underlying liver disease.

Icterus, described as a yellow staining of the skin, sclerae, and mucous membranes, may be present in extrahepatic obstructive jaundice and in hepatocellular injury (Fig. 148.1). The icterus present in *prehepatic* (hemolytic) jaundice tends to be associated with a milder severity of yellow staining. In *hepatic* and *posthepatic* jaundice, the yellow staining may be more severe and associated with dark urine (often described as "coca-cola" color) and pale acholic stools. In contrast, in prehepatic jaundice, bilirubin does not appear in the urine, although both urine and feces may be dark due to increased urobilinogen. Importantly, little or no jaundice may be present in some cases of advanced liver disease.

Palpation of an enlarged or tender liver is one of the most striking indications of either primary or secondary liver disease. In patients with relaxed abdominal walls or in thin persons with low diaphragms, the liver may be palpable even in the absence of hepatic disease. In patients with biliary cirrhosis, fatty liver, or either a primary or secondary hepatic neoplasm, the liver may be profoundly enlarged and nodular. Patients with congestive heart failure (CHF) or constrictive pericarditis may also have an enlarged, tender liver. In some patients with advanced or rapidly progressing liver disease, the organ may be small and nonpalpable. An atrophic liver incapable of regeneration is often an ominous finding in patients with known hepatic disease.

Physical exam findings of splenomegaly, ascites, and caput medusae may signal the presence of portal hypertension, although the spleen may be enlarged in patients with parenchymal liver disease without portal hypertension (e.g., CHF).

Other supportive findings such as clubbing of the fingers and whitening of the nail beds may also be seen in patients with cirrhosis, although they are not specific for hepatic disease. Severe *pruritus,* with or without jaundice, often represents the signature symptom in patients with cholestatic liver disease and is often seen in patients with posthepatic jaundice, believed to result from increased concentration of bile salts in the bloodstream. Chronic cholestatic liver diseases such as primary biliary cholangitis are associated with elevated serum alkaline phosphatase and serum cholesterol.

Exam findings of presacral and ankle edema may be observed in patients with advanced liver disease as a result of decreased serum albumin and sodium retention, although may be caused by nonhepatic etiologies (e.g. CHF, renal disease, venous insufficiency), although is more likely to be hepatic in origin in patients with coexisting abdominal ascites. In addition, an intermittent febrile reaction may be observed in up to 25% of patients with cirrhosis that has been attributed to hepatic necroinflammation.

ADDITIONAL RESOURCES

Heidelbaugh JJ, Bruderly M: Cirrhosis and chronic liver failure: part I—Diagnosis and evaluation, *Am Fam Physician* 74(5):756–762, 2006.

Tsochatzis EA, Bosch J, Burroughs AK: Liver cirrhosis, *Lancet* 383:1749–1761, 2014.

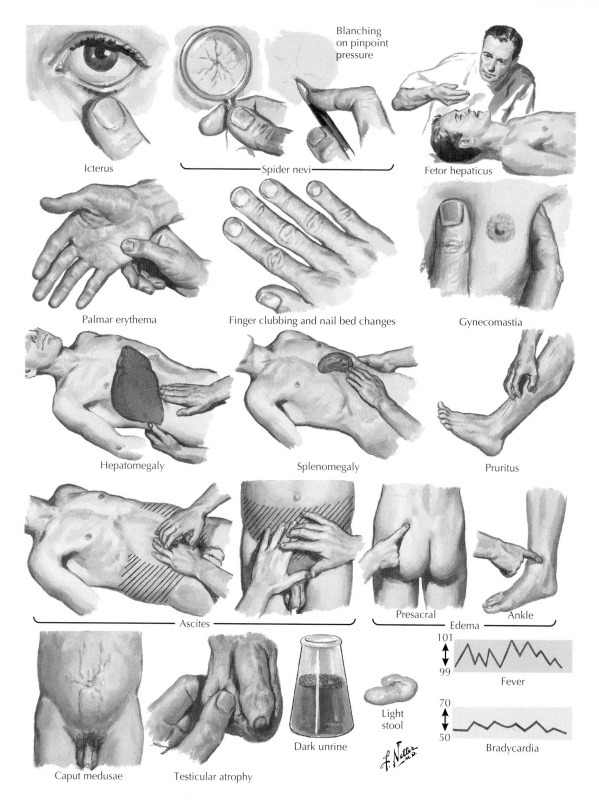

Icterus

Blanching on pinpoint pressure

Spider nevi

Fetor hepaticus

Palmar erythema

Finger clubbing and nail bed changes

Gynecomastia

Hepatomegaly

Splenomegaly

Pruritus

Ascites

Presacral

Ankle

Edema

Caput medusae

Testicular atrophy

Dark unrine

Light stool

Fever

Bradycardia

Fig. 148.1 Physical Diagnosis of Liver Disease.

149

Causes of Portal Hypertension

Kris V. Kowdley, Joseph K. Lim

Portal hypertension is the primary complication of liver cirrhosis which results in a broad spectrum of complications such as ascites, hepatic encephalopathy, and variceal hemorrhage. Portal hypertension is defined by the increase in hepatic venous pressure gradient (HVPG) greater than the normal value of approximately 5 to 6 mm Hg because of (1) blockage in the intrahepatic portal venous system, most commonly due to liver cirrhosis (sinusoidal portal hypertension); (2) impaired outflow of blood from the liver (postsinusoidal portal hypertension); or (3) increased pressure in the extrahepatic portal venous system, as from thrombosis of the portal vein (presinusoidal portal hypertension).

The *suprahepatic* (postsinusoidal) form of portal hypertension is most often caused by heart failure with passive congestion, particularly in patients with tricuspid regurgitation or constrictive pericarditis. Alternatively, this may occur due to obstruction of the main hepatic veins (Fig. 149.1), also known as *Budd-Chiari syndrome*, which is a rare condition resulting from thrombosis associated with hypercoagulable states, congenital abnormalities, or mechanical obstruction. In suprahepatic portal hypertension, the liver is typically large and tender; and associated with ascites and mild to moderate splenomegaly.

The most frequent type, *intrahepatic* (sinusoidal) portal hypertension, is most commonly caused by cirrhosis, although it may occur in the context of primary hepatic carcinoma or schistosomiasis. In intrahepatic portal hypertension, severe splenomegaly and esophageal varices are often present.

In *infrahepatic* (presinusoidal) portal hypertension, the liver is typically normal in size, but severe splenomegaly and esophageal veins may be seen. This form may occur in younger patients, most commonly due to portal vein thrombosis in context of tumors, inflammatory masses, or congenital anomalies. On rare occasions, severe portal hypertension has been observed in children without detectable anatomic alterations.

ADDITIONAL RESOURCES

Da BL, Koh C, Heller T: Noncirrhotic portal hypertension, *Curr Opin Gastroenterol* 34:140–145, 2018.

De Bruyn G, Graviss EA: A systematic review of the diagnostic accuracy of physical examination for the detection of cirrhosis, *BMC Med Inform Decis Mak* 1:6, 2001.

Hennenberg M, Trebicka J, Sauerbruch T, Heller J: Mechanisms of extrahepatic vasodilation in portal hypertension, *Gut* 57(9):1300–1314, 2008.

Khanna R, Sarin SK: Idiopathic portal hypertension and extrahepatic portal venous obstruction, *Hepatol Int* 12(Suppl 1):148–167, 2018.

McGuire BM, Bloomer JR: Complications of cirrhosis: why they occur and what to do about them, *Postgrad Med* 103:209–212, 217–218, 223–224, 1998.

Sanyal AJ, Bosch J, Blei A, Arroyo V: Portal hypertension and its complications, *Gastroenterology* 134(6):1715–1728, 2008.

Schuppan D, Afdhal NH: Liver cirrhosis, *Lancet* 371(9615):838–851, 2008.

Simpson KJ, Finlayson ND: Clinical evaluation of liver disease, *Baillieres Clin Gastroenterol* 9:639–659, 1995.

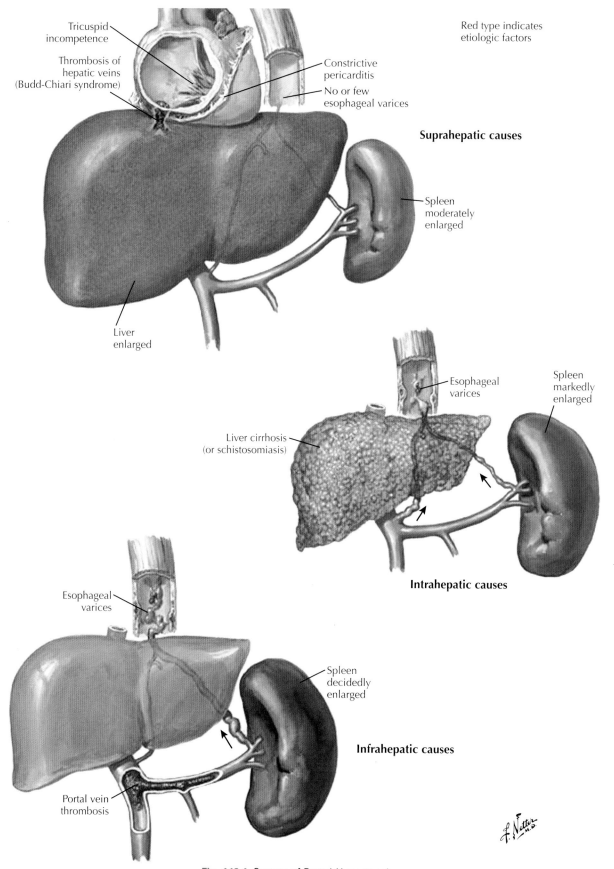

Tricuspid incompetence

Thrombosis of hepatic veins (Budd-Chiari syndrome)

Red type indicates etiologic factors

Constrictive pericarditis

No or few esophageal varices

Suprahepatic causes

Spleen moderately enlarged

Liver enlarged

Esophageal varices

Spleen markedly enlarged

Liver cirrhosis (or schistosomiasis)

Intrahepatic causes

Esophageal varices

Spleen decidedly enlarged

Infrahepatic causes

Portal vein thrombosis

Fig. 149.1 Causes of Portal Hypertension.

150

Ascites

Kris V. Kowdley, Joseph K. Lim

Ascites is one of the most common and serious complications of cirrhosis and has significant prognostic importance as a marker of hepatic decompensation and liver failure. The development of ascites is associated with a decrease in overall and liver-related survival and may be associated with related complications such as spontaneous bacterial peritonitis (SBP) and hepatorenal syndrome (HRS). The development of SBP is associated with a 2-year survival rate of 50% to 60%, particularly in patients with decompensated cirrhosis.

Ascites is defined as an accumulation of transudative fluid in the abdominal cavity which presumably emanates from the liver and possibly the peritoneum. The pathogenesis of ascites is complex and likely multifactorial (Fig. 150.1). There are several theories which may explain ascites formation. The *underfill theory* states that extravasation of fluid into the abdominal cavity results in intravascular volume depletion, leading to renal salt and water retention and increased total body volume, a process which may be exacerbated by peripheral vasodilatation which is commonly seen in cirrhosis. The *overflow theory* states that ascites in cirrhosis results from primary renal salt and water retention, with leakage of fluid into the extravascular space because of increased plasma volume. The *hepatorenal hypothesis* states that ascites results from a hepatorenal reflex signaling the kidney to increase salt and water absorption in response to changes in sinusoidal blood flow or pressure, through neuronally and hormonally mediated mechanisms.

CLINICAL PICTURE AND DIAGNOSIS

Ascites due to cirrhosis typically occurs in the context of an altered hemodynamic state marked by changes in prostaglandins, the renin-angiotensin system, atrial natriuretic peptide, alcohol dehydrogenase, and other hormones and clinically may resemble sepsis due to an increased cardiac output and decreased systemic vascular resistance, which may be further exacerbated by nitric oxide–mediated systemic vasodilation stemming from portal hypertension and portosystemic shunts.

Although ascites is commonly identified in patients with cirrhotic portal hypertension, clinicians should exclude alternative etiologies, including noncirrhotic portal hypertension (e.g., Budd-Chiari syndrome), as well as nonportal hypertensive causes of ascites (e.g., tuberculosis, pancreatitis, peritoneal carcinomatosis). Upon initial diagnosis of ascites, a paracentesis should be performed to calculate the serum/ascites albumin gradient (SAAG), which represents the difference between serum albumin and ascites albumin levels. SAAG greater than or equal to 1.1 signals the presence of portal hypertension as the underling etiology, whereas values less than 1.1 signal a nonportal hypertensive cause.

In addition to SAAG, ascitic protein levels may further distinguish etiology of ascites. Although ascites protein is characteristically low in patients with cirrhotic portal hypertension, ascites protein levels may be increased among patients with congestive heart failure (CHF) or Budd-Chiari syndrome.

Spontaneous Bacterial Peritonitis

Measuring ascitic fluid white blood cell counts can also be clinically useful to identify the presence of SBP. An ascitic fluid polymorphonuclear leukocyte (PMN) count greater than 250 is diagnostic of SBP. Although many patients will have the causative bacterial pathogen identified on ascitic fluid culture, it is now more common for SBP to be diagnosed on the basis of elevated PMN count alone with negative cultures, also known as *culture-negative neutrocytic ascites* (CNNA). Rarely, the neutrocytic response is lacking (PMN count < 250) in the presence of a positive ascitic fluid culture, which is described as *nonneutrocytic bacteriascites,* which occurs more commonly in immunocompromised patients with neutropenia.

SBP represents a serious complication of cirrhosis and is associated with significant morbidity and mortality. Although gram-negative organisms such as *Escherichia coli, Klebsiella,* and enterococcus species remain most common, gram-positive organisms are more commonly identified as causative pathogens. SBP is characteristically associated with single organisms on culture, and therefore the identification of multiple organisms should raise concern for secondary peritonitis, which may arise as a complication of surgery or from complicated diverticulitis or appendicitis.

TREATMENT AND MANAGEMENT

Ascites is most commonly managed with a combination of dietary sodium restriction, one or more diuretics, most commonly spironolactone ± furosemide, and/or therapeutic paracentesis. Although ascites is commonly managed adequately with diuretics, as the underlying cirrhosis and portal hypertension progress, a subset of patients fail to achieve adequate control despite maximal diuretic dosing up to spironolactone 400 mg daily plus furosemide 160 mg daily *(diuretic-resistant refractory ascites),* or fail to achieve adequate diuretic dosing due to adverse effects such as renal insufficiency *(diuretic-intractable refractory ascites).* These patients may require increasingly frequent therapeutic paracentesis, more often than once every 2 weeks, to achieve adequate control of volume overload secondary to abdominal ascites.

The primary treatment option for patients with refractory ascites is transjugular intrahepatic portosystemic shunt (TIPS), which is reserved for patients with refractory ascites and who do not have contraindications, due to well-established complications including renal insufficiency and hepatic encephalopathy. Peritoneovenous shunt procedures represent a largely historic surgical solution for refractory ascites, although are rarely performed due to high rates of shunt occlusion or failure, potentially severe, life-threatening infections, and disseminated intravascular coagulation (DIC)-like syndrome. Liver transplantation remains the preferred therapy for patients with refractory ascites, which itself is a

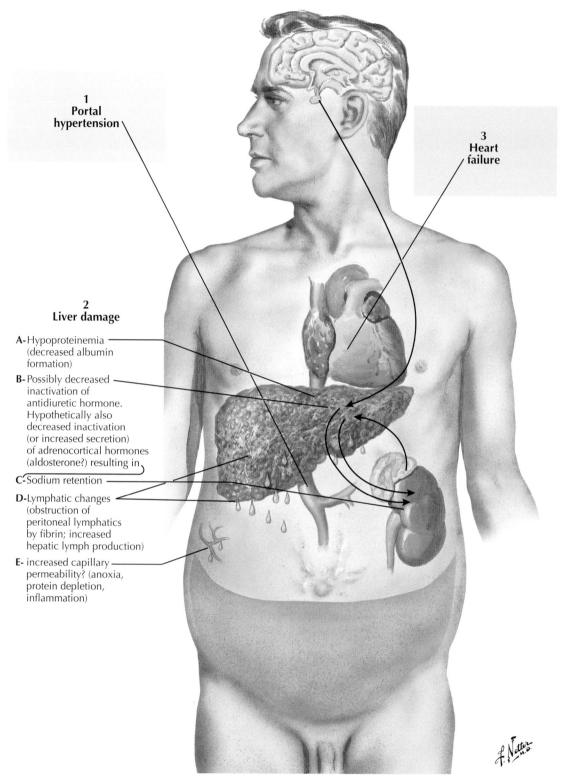

1
Portal
hypertension

3
Heart
failure

2
Liver damage

A- Hypoproteinemia
(decreased albumin
formation)

B- Possibly decreased
inactivation of
antidiuretic hormone.
Hypothetically also
decreased inactivation
(or increased secretion)
of adrenocortical hormones
(aldosterone?) resulting in

C- Sodium retention

D- Lymphatic changes
(obstruction of
peritoneal lymphatics
by fibrin; increased
hepatic lymph production)

E- increased capillary
permeability? (anoxia,
protein depletion,
inflammation)

Fig. 150.1 Causes of Ascites: Heart Failure, Portal Hypertension, and Hepatic Insufficiency.

marker for end-stage liver disease and typically associated multiple complications of portal hypertension and hepatic insufficiency.

SBP is treated with a course of antibiotics, and in cases with delayed or incomplete clinical improvement, consideration is given for surveillance paracentesis with cell count and culture to document appropriate response to treatment. After completion of an antibiotic course for a first episode of SBP, secondary prophylaxis with an oral fluoroquinolone such as norfloxacin is recommended to reduce the risk for SBP recurrence. In addition, primary prophylaxis with antibiotics is advocated in a subset of patients with severe ascites who have low total serum protein levels, which have been identified as major risk factor for the development of SBP.

ADDITIONAL RESOURCES

Garcia-Tsao G, Lim JK: Management and treatment of patients with cirrhosis and portal hypertension: recommendations from the Department of Veterans Affairs Hepatitis C Resource Center Program and the National Hepatitis C Program, *Am J Gastroenterol* 104:1802–1829, 2009.

Ge PS, Runyon BA: Treatment of patients with cirrhosis, *N Engl J Med* 375:767–777, 2016.

Ginès P, Cárdenas A: The management of ascites and hyponatremia in cirrhosis, *Semin Liver Dis* 28(1):43–58, 2008.

Ginès P, Cárdenas A, Arroyo V, Rodés J: Management of cirrhosis and ascites, *N Engl J Med* 350(16):1646–1654, 2004.

Runyon BA: Introduction to the revised American Association for the Study of Liver Diseases (AASLD) Practice Guideline: management of adult patients with ascites due to cirrhosis, *Hepatology* 57:1651–1653, 2013.

Runyon BA, AASLD Practice Guideline Committee: Management of adult patients with ascites due to cirrhosis: an update, *Hepatology* 49:2087–2107, 2009.

Tsochatzis EA, Bosch J, Burroughs AK: Liver cirrhosis, *Lancet* 383:1749–1761, 2014.

151

Hepatic Encephalopathy

Kris V. Kowdley, Joseph K. Lim

Hepatic encephalopathy (HE) is a common and debilitating complication of cirrhosis, and is characterized by cognitive impairment which occurs as the consequence of a complex series of alterations in brain functioning due to impaired liver function and portosystemic shunting. Although the pathophysiology of HE remains incompletely understood, there are several prevailing hypotheses to explain the biological origins for the distinct behavioral, cognitive, and motor changes seen in patients with chronic liver disease.

The most commonly recognized hypothesis stems from observing that increased concentrations of ammonia in the central nervous system (CNS) occur as a consequence of the failure of the cirrhotic liver to metabolize nitrogen-containing compounds, and thereby result in toxicity to neurons with associated cognitive deficits. Altered ammonia metabolism certainly plays an important role in HE, also known as *portosystemic encephalopathy* (PSE), as proven by the beneficial effects of serum ammonia reduction through pharmacotherapy on symptom improvement. However, elevated serum ammonia concentration is not necessary for PSE to occur, and there is no direct linear relationship between serum ammonia levels and symptom severity; in fact, patients with cirrhotic and noncirrhotic liver disease may have elevated serum ammonia levels in the absence of clinical PSE. Other hypotheses involve the role of other neurotransmitters such as γ-aminobutyric acid (GABA), glutamate, opiates, or GABA-induced benzodiazepine-like compounds.

A common pathway to HE is the development of early cerebral edema, astrocyte swelling, and oxidative stress in the brain which is associated with the production of reactive oxygen and nitrogen species. In addition, disruption of oscillatory networks in the brain has been demonstrated in PSE patients on magnetoencephalography and may underlie their cognitive and motor abnormalities.

There are multiple well-established risk factors which may precipitate HE, including volume depletion/dehydration, infection, gastrointestinal (GI) bleeding, constipation, electrolyte imbalance, or use of CNS depressants, particularly narcotics and benzodiazepines. GI bleeding is a particularly common cause of PSE due to the combination of nitrogen-rich blood to the gut and volume depletion.

CLINICAL PICTURE

The clinical presentation of HE can be quite variable and includes a spectrum of mental states, ranging from mild alterations (e.g., sleep/wake reversal, change in mood, and forgetfulness) to progressive degrees of lethargy, obtundation, and coma, as classified in the West Haven criteria. In the most serious stage of PSE, patients may develop a deep coma stemming from progressive cerebral edema, and eventually brainstem herniation (Fig. 151.1), which is characteristically observed in patients with acute or fulminant liver failure, although this may be seen in patients with acute on chronic liver failure.

The four grades within the West Haven criteria are summarized in Table 151.1. Grade 4 encephalopathy is associated with an increased risk for severe cerebral edema, and therefore requires close clinical monitoring in an intensive care unit.

Physical examination findings of PSE may be subtle. The most common clinical sign associated with PSE is *asterixis,* which reflects an irregular myoclonic lapse of posture with loss of muscle tone. A characteristic "flap" (see Fig. 151.1) or *"liver flap"* may be seen when patients are asked to extend their arms, dorsiflex the wrists, and spread their fingers. In patients who are unable to participate in this exam maneuver, the presence of diffuse clonus may also signal the presence of PSE. Although not universally present, the presence of a musty, fruity odor on a patient's breath, called *fetor hepaticus,* may also signal PSE.

Although the focus of the diagnosis and management of HE is on clinically overt disease, there has been increasing recognition of a subclinical form called *minimal hepatic encephalopathy,* previously described as "subclinical hepatic encephalopathy." Obvious clinical symptoms or exam findings may be lacking, although increasing data support an association between minimal HE and clinical outcomes including decreased attention span, decreased driving skill, and reduced quality of life. Lactulose therapy has been shown to improve clinical symptoms and quality of life in some patients with HE.

DIAGNOSIS

Establishing a diagnosis of HE can be challenging and requires a high index of clinical suspicion due to the wide spectrum of clinical presentations seen with this condition. In particular, during the early stages, patients may be entirely unaware of altered mental status, and initial changes may only be observed by family members who identify subtle changes in personality, irritability, or reversal of day-night cycles. In contrast, patients with more advanced stages will demonstrate obvious decreases in consciousness, with progressive lethargy, confusion, stupor, and coma.

Although not routinely performed, and not required to establish the diagnosis, electroencephalographic abnormalities may be seen, most commonly as diffuse, bilateral, high-voltage slow waves. Magnetic resonance imaging (MRI) with T1-weighted images may demonstrate increased signals in certain portions of the brain (globus pallidus). Abnormal evoked responses and abnormalities on positron emission tomography also have been noted, although are not specific to HE.

The presence, severity, and progression of PSE is of special importance in patients with acute liver failure, in whom its identification portends a poor prognosis, and may prompt the clinician to pursue referral of a patient to a liver transplant center for closer monitoring and more aggressive intervention. Patients who are otherwise eligible for liver transplantation should initiate early evaluation when admitted

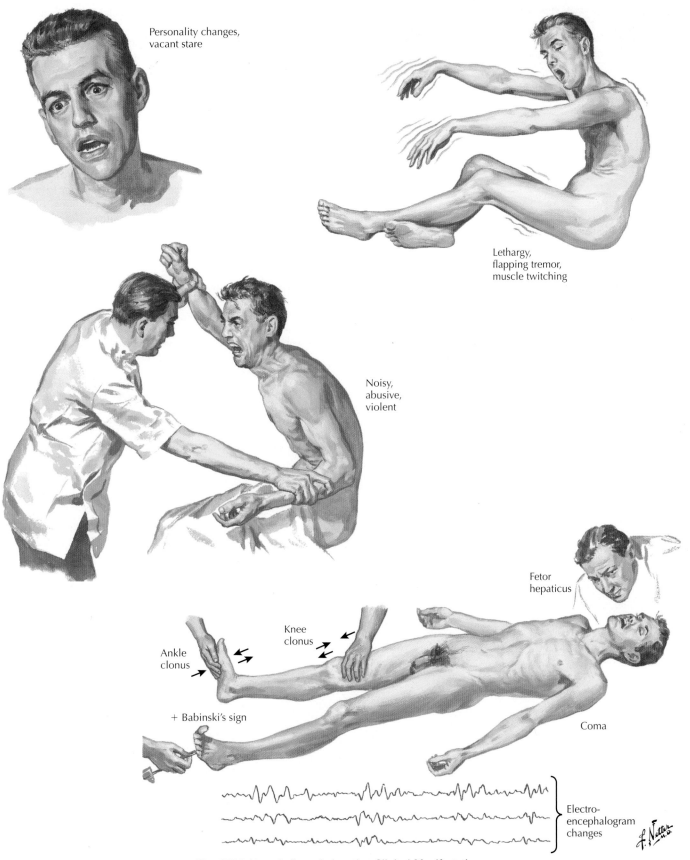

Personality changes, vacant stare

Lethargy, flapping tremor, muscle twitching

Noisy, abusive, violent

Fetor hepaticus

Knee clonus

Ankle clonus

+ Babinski's sign

Coma

Electro-encephalogram changes

Fig. 151.1 Hepatic Encephalopathy: Clinical Manifestations.

TABLE 151.1   Grading/Staging System for Hepatic Encephalopathy

Grade	Characteristics
1	Altered sleep patterns, altered mood, irritability, inability to maintain attention
2	Lethargy, altered speech, increased memory loss, dysarthria
3	Progressive stupor, decreased level of consciousness, but responsive to stimuli
4	Coma, unresponsive to painful stimuli

with signs of acute liver failure, although it is hoped that patients will demonstrate spontaneous recovery without requirement for proceeding to emergency liver transplantation.

TREATMENT AND MANAGEMENT

The primary step in the management of HE is the identification and removal of potential precipitants, such as psychoactive medications, infection, and GI bleeding. The secondary step is empiric pharmacotherapy with nonabsorbable disaccharides and antibiotics such as lactulose. Although the mechanism of action of lactulose remains uncertain, the biological rationale for the use of nonabsorbable antibiotics stems from its cathartic effect which may reduce the concentration of substrates for nitrogen formation, and possibly an increase in excretion by colonic bacteria of nitrogen or its metabolites in patients receiving lactulose. Nonabsorbable antibiotics, in particular neomycin, have also been used to treat PSE.

The most common second-line treatment for HE is rifaximin, which is a nonabsorbed derivative of rifamycin with a broad spectrum of activity, and has been used for patients who cannot tolerate, or have remained refractory to, lactulose or neomycin. Randomized controlled trials have confirmed its efficacy in secondary prevention to reduce recurrent episodes of overt HE and to increase time to rehospitalization for overt HE. There are inadequate data to support the use of rifaximin for first-line treatment, and it is typically used in combination with lactulose.

Finally, the development of HE in patients with acute liver failure should prompt the use of intracranial pressure monitoring to facilitate the management of intracranial hypertension. In addition, although protein restriction has been advocated as a treatment for HE, it is not routinely recommended due to concerns for sarcopenia and overall protein-calorie malnutrition in patients with end-stage liver disease.

ADDITIONAL RESOURCES

Amodio P: Hepatic encephalopathy: diagnosis and management, *Liver Int* 38:966–975, 2018.

Hadjihambi A, Arias N, Sheikh M, Jalan R: Hepatic encephalopathy: a critical current review, *Hepatol Int* 12(Suppl1):135–147, 2018.

Vilstrup H, Amodio P, Bajaj J, et al: Hepatic encephalopathy in chronic liver disease: 2014 practice guideline by the American association for the study of liver diseases and the European association for the study of the liver, *Hepatology* 60:715–735, 2014.

Wijdicks EF: Hepatic encephalopathy, *N Engl J Med* 375:1660–1670, 2016.

152

Hepatorenal Syndrome

Joseph K. Lim

Acute kidney injury (AKI) is a common event, occurring in approximately 20% of hospitalized patients with cirrhosis. The most common etiologies include prerenal azotemia (volume-responsive prerenal AKI), acute tubular necrosis (ATN), and hepatorenal syndrome (HRS) (functional prerenal AKI not responsive to volume repletion). Prerenal etiologies account for 60% to 70% of cases of AKI in cirrhotic patients, of which approximately one third are due to HRS. In context of progressive portal hypertension with increased splanchnic and systemic vasodilatation, decreased effective arterial volume, and activation of neurohormonal systems including the renin-angiotensin-aldosterone (RAS) system, patients with decompensated cirrhosis are uniquely susceptible to the development of AKI, experience worsening sodium and water retention, and renal vasoconstriction which overwhelms compensatory local renal vasodilator responses.

The definition of AKI in cirrhotic patients has been recently updated in alignment with Acute Kidney Injury Network (AKIN) criteria and incorporates an absolute increase in serum creatinine greater than or equal to 0.3 mg/dL or percentage increase in serum creatinine greater than or equal to 50% from baseline (stage 1), percentage increase in serum creatinine greater than or equal to 200% to 300% (stage 2), and an absolute increase in serum creatinine to greater than 4 mg/dL or percentage increase in serum creatinine to greater than 300% (stage 3). Patients who experienced a doubling of creatinine to greater than 2.5 mg/dL in less than 2 weeks in context of cirrhosis and ascites were given consideration for a diagnosis of HRS.

The updated International Ascites Club (IAC) definition of HRS includes the following criteria: (1) cirrhosis with ascites; (2) serum creatinine greater than 1.5 mg/dL; (3) no improvement of serum creatinine after at least 48 hours of diuretic withdrawal and volume expansion with albumin; (4) absence of shock; (5) no current or recent nephrotoxic drugs; (6) absence of parenchymal kidney disease as suggested by proteinuria greater than 500 mg/day, microhematuria greater than 50 red blood cells per high power field, and/or abnormal renal ultrasound.

DIAGNOSIS AND TYPES

There are two distinct forms of HRS with important differences in pathophysiology, management, and outcome (Fig. 152.1). *Type 1* HRS represents a rapidly progressive form of AKI characterized by worsening renal function and an acute rise in serum creatinine in less than 2 weeks, often precipitated by insults such as gastrointestinal bleeding and/or spontaneous bacterial peritonitis. In these patients, decreasing urine output, low serum sodium, low mean arterial pressures (MAPs), and increased plasma renin activity are observed. Type 1 HRS most commonly occurs in context of an acute deterioration of circulatory dysfunction (arterial hypotension and activation of endogenous vasoconstrictor systems), and is associated very poor prognosis.

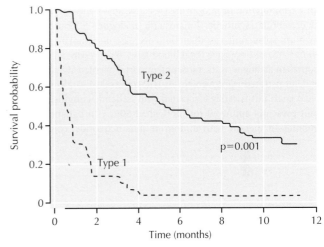

Reprinted with permission from Ginès P, Guevara M, Arroyo V, Rodés J: Hepatorenal syndrome, *Lancet* 362: 1819–1827, 2003.

Fig. 152.1 Hepatorenal Syndrome: Survival Comparison for Types 1 and 2.

In contrast, *type 2* HRS represents a more slowly progressive form which characteristically occurs in a patient with refractory ascites which is either diuretic-resistant and/or diuretic-intractable, with poor tolerability of diuretics secondary to sensitivity to renal insufficiency. Although the survival of patients with type 2 HRS is better than in patients with type 1 HRS, it remains a predictor of poorer survival among cirrhotic patients with ascites.

HRS is typically considered a diagnosis of exclusion after failure to respond to plasma volume expansion and removal of diuretics and other precipitants, but there have been increasing efforts to facilitate the diagnosis of HRS type 1 using urinary biomarkers such as neutrophil gelatinase-associated lipocalin (NGAL), although they are not presently used routinely in clinical practice. The kidney is characteristically normal on renal biopsy, as the primary defect is hemodynamic (worsening renal vasoconstriction) rather than parenchymal, although unique histologic features such as glomerular tubular reflex have been described from muscle wasting.

TREATMENT AND MANAGEMENT

The initial management of AKI in a cirrhotic patient with ascites is focused on diagnostic urine testing, a trial of plasma volume expansion, and elimination of possible precipitants. Examination of urine electrolytes and calculation of FeNa may help clarify the presence of prerenal

AKI; urine sediment evaluation may identify characteristic casts suggestive of acute tubular necrosis; renal ultrasound may help exclude postrenal causes. Patients should discontinue all diuretics, lactulose (if excess stool volume losses), vasodilators, potential nephrotoxins such as nonsteroidal antiinflammatory drugs (NSAIDs), and intravenous contrast, and undergo evaluation for coexisting infection and/or bleeding. Albumin 25% IV is administered for at minimum 48 hours at 1 g/kg for a maximum of 100 g/24 h. Diagnostic paracentesis of ascites is commonly performed to exclude spontaneous bacterial peritonitis. Therapeutic paracentesis with albumin support may be considered if tense ascites is present to decompress intraabdominal pressure, as in compartment syndrome, to augment renal blood flow.

In patients who fail to respond to plasma volume expansion for 48 hours, consideration should be given for empiric treatment of HRS with a combination of midodrine (selective alfa-1 adrenergic agonist) and octreotide (synthetic somatostatin analogue) ± albumin, which may blunt splanchnic vasodilatation, decrease neurohormonal activation of RAS, and improve renal blood flow. Terlipressin, a long-acting vasopressin analogue, is the most potent portal hypotensive agent which has demonstrated improvement in HRS reversal in randomized controlled trials but is rarely associated with ischemic complications and is not presently approved for the United States. In patients who fail combination therapy with midodrine plus octreotide, consideration may be given for intravenous vasoconstrictor therapy with norepinephrine or vasopressin. Patients with progressive renal failure in this context, and are considered candidates for liver transplantation, may be evaluated for transjugular intrahepatic portosystemic shunt (TIPS) or renal replacement therapy. These interventions are restricted to a subset of patients as a bridge to liver transplantation.

ADDITIONAL RESOURCES

Colle I, Laterre PF: Hepatorenal syndrome: the clinical impact of vasoactive therapy, *Expert Rev Gastroenterol Hepatol* 12:173–188, 2018.

Davenport A, Sheikh MF, Lamb E, et al: Acute kidney injury in acute-on-chronic liver failure: where does hepatorenal syndrome fit?, *Kidney Int* 92:1058–1070, 2017.

Gines P, Guevara M, Arroyo V, Rodes J: Hepatorenal syndrome, *Lancet* 362:1819–1827, 2003.

Nanda A, Reddy R, Safraz H, et al: Pharmacological therapies for hepatorenal syndrome: a systematic review and meta-analysis, *J Clin Gastroenterol* 52:360–367, 2018.

Piano S, Tonon M, Angeli P: Management of ascites and hepatorenal syndrome, *Hepatol Int* 12(Suppl 1):122–134, 2018.

Runyon BA: Introduction to the revised American Association for the Study of Liver Diseases Practice Guideline: management of adult patients with ascites due to cirrhosis 2012, *Hepatology* 57:1651–1653, 2013.

153

Variceal Bleeding

Kris V. Kowdley, Joseph K. Lim

Esophageal and gastric variceal bleeding represents a common and potentially life-threatening complication of cirrhosis, and occurs as a consequence of progressive portal hypertension. Patients with cirrhosis are initially categorized as having either compensated or decompensated cirrhosis, the latter defined by the development of overt hepatic decompensation events such as ascites, hepatic encephalopathy, spontaneous bacterial peritonitis, hepatic hydrothorax, or variceal hemorrhage. These complications arise predominantly from the progressive development of portal hypertension (Fig. 153.1) as part of the natural history of cirrhosis, which is defined based on measurement of hepatic venous pressure gradient (HVPG), the difference between the wedged and free hepatic venous pressure. Among patients with compensated cirrhosis, patients may have either normal portal pressure (HVPG < 5 mm Hg), mild portal hypertension (HVPG 6–9 mm Hg), or clinically significant portal hypertension (CSPH) defined as HVPG ≥10 mm Hg. It is this latter group with CSPH who are at risk for developing varices and other decompensation events such as ascites and hepatic encephalopathy.

Gastroesophageal varices (GEVs) are common and seen in approximately 50% of patients with cirrhosis, including up to 30% and 85% of patients with compensated and decompensated cirrhosis, respectively. Among patients with compensated cirrhosis, varices develop at a rate of 7% to 8% per year, of which variceal hemorrhage occurs at a rate of 10% to 15% per year. Per guidelines of the American Association for the Study of Liver Diseases (AASLD), a screening endoscopy to identify the presence of GEVs is recommended at the time of cirrhosis diagnosis. However, patients who have liver stiffness measurement (LSM) less than 20 kPa on transient elastography and normal platelet count greater than 150,000/mm³ are deemed to have a low probability (<5%) of having high-risk varices, and therefore endoscopy is not required. Patients who have no varices identified on screening endoscopy do not require further intervention, but should undergo surveillance endoscopy every 2 to 3 years. Patients with compensated cirrhosis who have small varices on screening endoscopy should undergo surveillance endoscopy every 1 to 2 years. Patients with decompensated cirrhosis with any varices, as well as patients with compensated cirrhosis with moderate or large varices, are recommended to undergo primary prophylaxis with a nonselective beta-blocker (NSBB) such as nadolol or propranolol.

DIAGNOSIS: ROLE OF ENDOSCOPY

Endoscopy is useful to identify the presence of varices in patients with cirrhosis and to distinguish high-risk features associated with an increased bleeding risk. Endoscopy is also indicated for patients with acute bleeding to identify the cause of bleeding and for therapeutic intervention. Reports indicate that 10% to 47% of liver disease and upper gastrointestinal bleeding has a nonvariceal source.

The risk for bleeding is related to the severity of liver disease using Child criteria, the presence of red wales, and the size of the varices. The simplest of several grading systems classifies varices from grades 1 to 3. *Grade 3* varices are those that occlude the lumen; *grade 1* varices disappear completely with insufflation; and *grade 2* varices are between grades 1 and 3 in size. Using these scoring systems, patients can be stratified into categories ranging from 6% to 76% risk for bleeding during 1 year of follow-up. One study concluded that varices were most likely to be found during endoscopy in patients with compensated cirrhosis when prothrombin activity was less than 70%, platelet count less than 100×10^9/L, and ultrasonographic portal vein diameter greater than 13 mm.

PRIMARY PROPHYLAXIS

Nonselective *beta-adrenergic blocking agents* (β-blockers; e.g., propranolol, nadolol) are effective in reducing the risk for a first bleed by 40% to 50% in patients with esophageal varices. Treatment with propranolol begins at 40 mg daily, and doses up to 160 mg daily may be used. Treatment is associated with lower bleed-related mortality and may improve survival.

Endoscopic sclerotherapy has been extensively studied as primary prophylaxis for variceal bleeding, with more than 1500 patients enrolled in trials. With some exceptions, however, sclerotherapy has not been effective, largely because of the high rate of adverse effects, such as pulmonary complications, fever, chest pain, and esophageal ulceration.

Portosystemic shunts are effective in primary prevention but are associated with an unacceptably high incidence of hepatic encephalopathy. A significant proportion of patients fail to tolerate β-blockers or fail to experience a reduction in portal pressure with shunt therapy. Therefore alternative therapies are needed.

Variceal band ligation has been studied as primary prevention (Fig. 153.2) and compared with β-blockers. The largest study showed reduced bleeding, from 43% in the propranolol group to 15% in the ligation group. Risk for bleeding in the propranolol group appeared unusually high, possibly because of underdosage. Band ligation does not appear to reduce overall or bleed-related mortality. Band ligation as primary prophylaxis should be reserved for patients with compensated cirrhosis with large varices or for patients with advanced liver disease with small or large varices who cannot tolerate β-blockers.

Isosorbide mononitrate at 40 mg twice daily can be used if neither ligation nor β-blocker therapy is an option.

ACUTE VARICEAL BLEEDING

Acute variceal bleeding is generally defined as visible bleeding from an esophageal varix or a gastric varix, or the presence of blood in the stomach of a patient with varices, with no other cause for bleeding. Clinically significant bleeding is defined as more than 2 U blood transfused over 24 hours, with blood pressure decreased to less than

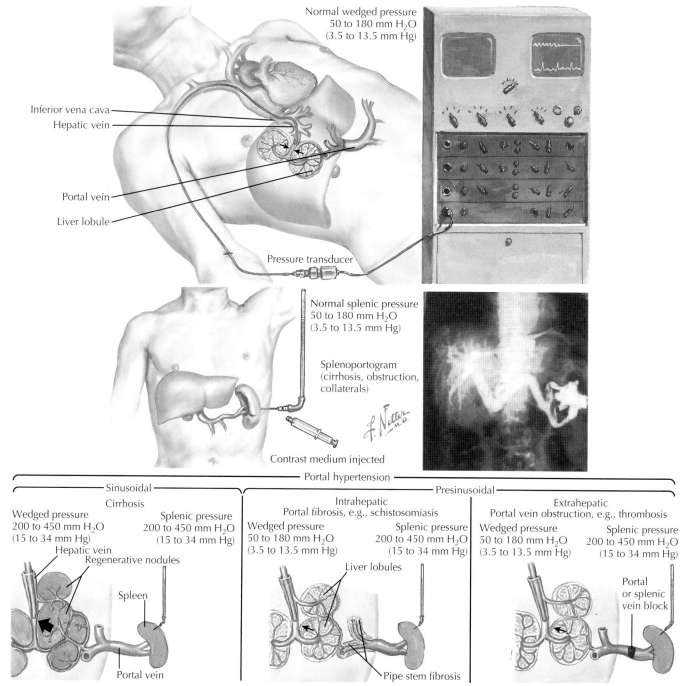

Normal wedged pressure
50 to 180 mm H₂O
(3.5 to 13.5 mm Hg)

Inferior vena cava

Hepatic vein

Portal vein

Liver lobule

Pressure transducer

Normal splenic pressure
50 to 180 mm H₂O
(3.5 to 13.5 mm Hg)

Splenoportogram
(cirrhosis, obstruction,
collaterals)

Contrast medium injected

Portal hypertension

Sinusoidal

Cirrhosis

Wedged pressure
200 to 450 mm H₂O
(15 to 34 mm Hg)

Splenic pressure
200 to 450 mm H₂O
(15 to 34 mm Hg)

Hepatic vein

Regenerative nodules

Spleen

Portal vein

Presinusoidal

Intrahepatic
Portal fibrosis, e.g., schistosomiasis

Wedged pressure
50 to 180 mm H₂O
(3.5 to 13.5 mm Hg)

Splenic pressure
200 to 450 mm H₂O
(15 to 34 mm Hg)

Liver lobules

Pipe stem fibrosis

Extrahepatic
Portal vein obstruction, e.g., thrombosis

Wedged pressure
50 to 180 mm H₂O
(3.5 to 13.5 mm Hg)

Splenic pressure
200 to 450 mm H₂O
(15 to 34 mm Hg)

Portal
or splenic
vein block

Fig. 153.1 Clinical Measurement of Portal Hypertension.

100 mm Hg or pulse rate increased to greater than 100 beats/min. Mortality associated with acute variceal bleeding is greater than 30%, and the risk is increased in patients with decompensated liver disease.

Current management of acute variceal bleeding includes pharmacologic and endoscopic therapy. Key elements of management include airway protection, early use of endoscopy, and administration of antibiotics (e.g., norfloxacin, clavulanic acid–amoxicillin) for infection prophylaxis.

Historically, vasopressin and nitroglycerin have been used as pharmacologic therapy, but this regimen is infrequently used in the United States at present. Somatostatin and its analogs (octreotide, lanreotide,

and vapreotide) are used widely. In the United States, *octreotide* is the only available agent in this category. Because of octreotide's long half-life, no loading dose is needed; a continuous infusion of 25 to 50 mg/h is the usual dose. *Terlipressin,* an analog of vasopressin used in Europe, can be given as intermittent injection and has a favorable safety profile compared with vasopressin. A Cochrane review of terlipressin for variceal hemorrhage found that terlipressin was superior to placebo and comparable to somatostatin or sclerotherapy in mortality risk. A randomized trial of terlipressin versus sclerotherapy showed the two therapies equally effective compared with placebo in controlling acute bleeding and preventing early rebleeding.

Endoscopic variceal sclerotherapy

Endoscopic variceal ligation (banding)

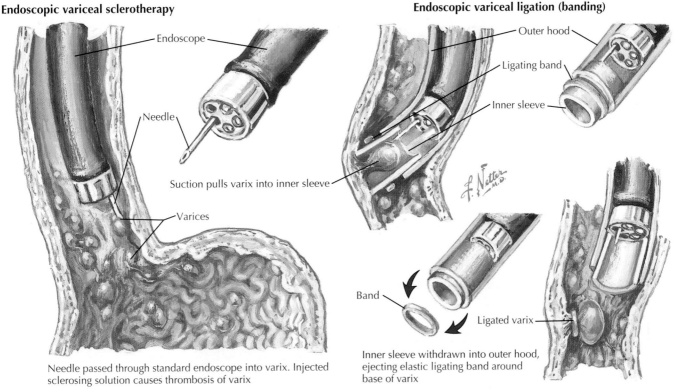

Needle passed through standard endoscope into varix. Injected sclerosing solution causes thrombosis of varix

Inner sleeve withdrawn into outer hood, ejecting elastic ligating band around base of varix

Fig. 153.2 Ligation Techniques.

Administering somatostatin analogs along with endoscopic therapy reduces transfusion requirements and is a reasonable adjunctive therapy given the low toxicity associated with these agents.

Endoscopic sclerotherapy has been used in acute variceal bleeding for two decades. A meta-analysis showed that sclerotherapy was more effective than balloon tamponade, no therapy, or vasopressin, with a 90% rate of bleeding control. However, the trials varied in type of sclerosant, technique, and follow-up. Sodium tetradecyl sulfate (15%), morrhuate sodium (5%), and ethanolamine (5%) are the most widely used sclerosants. No consensus exists as to the preferred sclerosant; variable rates of ulceration are reported with these agents.

Variceal band ligation is now the endoscopic treatment of choice because of the lower complication rate associated with this procedure (see Fig. 153.2). In one study, band ligation was shown to be equally or more effective in controlling acute bleeding than sclerotherapy and was associated with better survival. Acute rebleeding was reduced when band ligation was combined with octreotide. Although more expensive, multiband ligators should be used because of the risk for esophageal perforation associated with the overtubing necessary with the single-band ligator. The average number of bands placed ranges from 5 to 10. Patients should be treated with β-blockers or continued variceal band ligation, or a combination, for secondary prophylaxis against rebleeding.

Measuring HVPG is also predictive of early rebleeding and mortality. Patients with HVPG exceeding 20 mm Hg during the acute bleeding episode are at higher risk for early rebleeding and death at 1 year.

Therapy for Uncontrolled Bleeding

Patients whose bleeding is uncontrolled despite pharmacologic and endoscopic therapy should have a Sengstaken-Blakemore tube inserted and gastric balloon inflated. Endotracheal intubation should be strongly considered for these patients, although complications are common

(10%–30%) and severe, ranging from esophageal perforation to aspiration pneumonia. Sengstaken-Blakemore tube placement is a temporizing measure and should be instituted while evaluating the patient for transjugular intrahepatic portosystemic shunt (TIPS), referral to a liver transplantation center, or consideration for a surgical portosystemic shunt or devascularization procedure.

Shunt Procedures

Shunt surgery is best reserved for patients with controlled bleeding who have Child class A cirrhosis, patients who may fail to comply with follow-up surveillance for TIPS stenosis, and patients with portal vein thrombosis. The preferred surgical shunt is a *splenorenal* shunt because of the lower risk for encephalopathy and because this procedure does not complicate future liver transplantation (Fig. 153.3).

GASTRIC VARICES

Gastric varices are classified as *gastroesophageal varices* (GEVs) and *isolated gastric varices* (IGVs). Type 1 GEVs are present in the cardia contiguous with esophageal varices, whereas type 2 GEVs extend beyond the cardia into the fundus. Type 1 IGVs are located in the fundus, whereas type 2 IGVs are located anywhere else in the stomach or duodenum. Mortality from IGV-related bleeding, especially in the fundus, is significantly higher than that from GEV-related bleeding.

Endoscopic therapy has been used to treat bleeding gastric varices. Endoscopic therapy appears to be equally effective for GEVs as for esophageal varices. However, the success rates are much lower for IGVs, and rebleed rates are high, approaching 90% in some series. Absolute ethanol may be more effective than other sclerosing agents. Injections of cyanoacrylate and thrombin have also been used. Cyanoacrylate appears to be the more promising agent and controls acute hemorrhage in most patients, but it is associated with a high rate of rebleeding.

1 Portacaval shunt
  (end-to-side or side-to-side)
2 Splenorenal shunt
3 Splenectomy
4 Hepatic artery ligation
  (also left gastric and splenic
  artery ligation)
5 Omentopexy

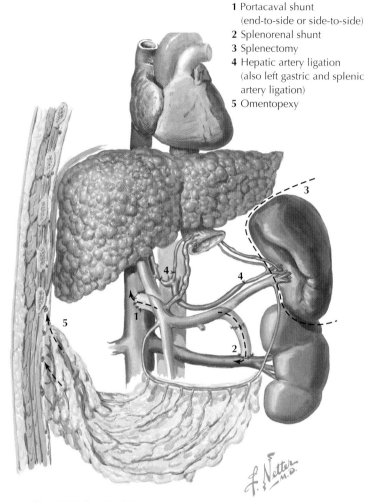

Fig. 153.3 Surgical Procedures to Relieve Portal Hypertension.

Splenic vein thrombosis should always be suspected in patients with IGV in the fundus. Angiographic or surgical splenectomy should be considered as treatment. Given the lack of effective and widely available endoscopic therapy for IGVs, especially those in the gastric fundus, TIPS is emerging as an important modality for such patients because mortality risk is low and rebleeding risk is acceptable.

ECTOPIC VARICES

Ectopic varices may form at many sites in the gastrointestinal tract, including the peritoneum, biliary tract, and genitourinary system. Ectopic varices are more common in patients with extrahepatic portal hypertension than in those with cirrhosis. Varices may also develop at enterostomy sites after abdominal surgery.

In a suggested management algorithm for patients with ectopic varices, angiographic embolization has been used with good initial control of bleeding. However, portal decompression is often necessary. Because bleeding from stomal varices can often be controlled by direct

pressure, mortality has been estimated at less than 5%, and conservative measures have been advocated rather than surgery. Injection sclerotherapy of stomal varices should be undertaken with caution because of the high risk for ulceration and tissue injury.

ADDITIONAL RESOURCES

Bosch J, Garcia-Pagan JC: Complications of cirrhosis: I—Portal hypertension, *Hepatology* 32(Suppl):141–156, 2000.

D'Amico G, Pagliaro L, Bosch J: The treatment of portal hypertension: a meta-analytic review, *Hepatology* 22:332–354, 1995.

Garcia-Pagan JC, De Gottardi A, Bosch J: The modern management of portal hypertension: primary and secondary prophylaxis of variceal bleeding in cirrhotic patients (review), *Aliment Pharmacol Ther* 28(2):178–186, 2008.

Jalan R, Hayes PC: UK guidelines on the management of variceal haemorrhage in cirrhotic patients, *Gut* 6(Suppl 3):iii1–iii15, 2000.

Vlachogiannakos J, Goulis J, Patch D, Burroughs AK: Primary prophylaxis for portal hypertensive bleeding in cirrhosis (review), *Aliment Pharmacol Ther* 14:851–860, 2000.

154

Transjugular Intrahepatic Portosystemic Shunt

Joseph K. Lim

The development of the transjugular intrahepatic portosystemic shunt (TIPS) has largely replaced surgical portocaval shunts as a definitive intervention for decompression of the portal venous system in the treatment and secondary prevention of portal hypertensive complications such as variceal hemorrhage and refractory ascites. The shunt procedure has been in clinical practice for over 30 years but did not receive strong endorsement by the American Association for the Study of Liver Diseases (AASLD) until the development of expandable metal stents covered by compounds such as polytetrafluoroethylene (PTFE) to decrease stenosis and shunt dysfunction.

The TIPS shunt procedure is generally performed by an interventional radiologist and involves placement of a catheter into the right hepatic vein through jugular vein cannulation, through which a tract is created across the hepatic vein to the portal vein, dilated, and an expanded metal stent is placed (Fig. 154.1). A technically successful TIPS shunt is one which achieves decompression of the portal vein, defined as a decrease in the hepatic venous pressure gradient (HVPG) to less than 12 mm Hg, the threshold for clinically significant portal hypertension (CSPH); a clinically successful TIPS shunt is defined by clinical resolution of complications of portal hypertension including variceal bleeding and refractory ascites. Per guidelines of the Society of Interventional Radiology, procedural units should achieve technical and clinical success in 95% and 90% of cases, respectively. Although decrease in HVPG to less than 12 mm Hg has been demonstrated to result in prevention of esophageal variceal rebleeding, optimal HVPG thresholds for resolution of gastric variceal rebleeding and refractory ascites remain less clear, although some studies have suggested a target of <8 mm Hg.

INDICATIONS, RISKS, AND CONTRAINDICATIONS

The most common indications for TIPS include acute esophagogastric variceal hemorrhage and refractory ascites, both of which are supported by controlled trial evidence. Second-line indications for which limited data are currently available include refractory hepatic hydrothorax, hepatorenal syndrome, Budd-Chiari syndrome, hepatopulmonary syndrome, portal hypertensive gastropathy, and venoocclusive disease. All patients under consideration for TIPS shunt placement should be evaluated by a gastrointestinal (GI)/hepatologist and interventional radiologist, ideally in association with a liver transplant center, and discuss the relative benefits and risks associated with the procedure. There are relatively few absolute contraindications to TIPS, including congestive heart failure, severe pulmonary hypertension (mean pulmonary pressures > 45 mm Hg), severe tricuspid regurgitation, uncontrolled sepsis, and active biliary obstruction. Relative contraindications include portal vein thrombosis, hepatic vein obstruction, large hepatomas, severe polycystic liver disease, severe coagulopathy (international normalized ratio [INR] > 5) or thrombocytopenia (platelet count < 20,000/μL), or end-stage liver disease (Child-Pugh score > 12 or Model for End-Stage

Liver Disease [MELD] score > 18), the latter of which has been associated with increased postprocedural mortality.

Prior to reaching a decision to pursue TIPS placement, patients should undergo laboratory testing for hepatic and renal function, and cross-sectional liver imaging to confirm patency of the portal venous system, and exclude liver malignancy. Although the goal of TIPS placement should be reduction of HVPG to less than 12 mm Hg, patients with gastric varices may additionally require variceal embolization which should be coordinated with an interventional radiologist. Due to increased 30-day mortality among patients with high MELD greater than 15 to 18 and serum bilirubin greater than 4.0 mg/dL, TIPS should only be placed if other options are not feasible or have previously failed, and after careful discussion of procedural risks with patients, as well as implications for liver transplantation.

COMPLICATIONS AND MONITORING

The major complications of the TIPS procedure include bleeding, TIPS dysfunction (due to occlusion, stenosis, or thrombosis), transcapsular puncture, stent migration, hemolysis, cardiopulmonary failure, and either new or worsening hepatic encephalopathy. Thrombosis of the TIPS shunt often occurs very shortly after the procedure, typically within the first 24 hours, and may stem from bile leakage into the shunt with or without an underlying hypercoagulable state. Sustaining long-term patency of the TIPS shunt has been significantly improved with the development of covered stents using polytetrafluoroethylene (PTFE). The most important adverse effect of TIPS remains encephalopathy which occurs in 20% to 30% of patients, with the highest risk observed in patients with prior encephalopathy and more advanced end-stage liver disease (MELD > 18). Patients should undergo regular TIPS surveillance with Doppler ultrasound, in addition to TIPS venography if there are imaging findings suggestive of TIPS dysfunction or worsening symptoms of portal hypertension.

One of the most common clinical complications of TIPS is hepatic encephalopathy, reported in up to 20% to 30% of patients and occasionally resulting in a comatose state. Risk factors for hepatic encephalopathy include older age, larger TIPS diameter, and advanced liver disease. Therefore TIPS should probably be avoided in patents with a previous history of recurrent severe hepatic encephalopathy.

ADDITIONAL RESOURCES

Boyer TD, Haskal ZJ: AASLD Practice Guideline: the role of transjugular intrahepatic portosystemic shunt (TIPS) in the management of portal hypertension, *Hepatology* 51:306, 2010.

Fagiuoli S, Bruno R, Debernardi Venon W, et al: Consensus conference on TIPS management: techniques, indications, contraindications, *Dig Liver Did* 49:121–137, 2017.

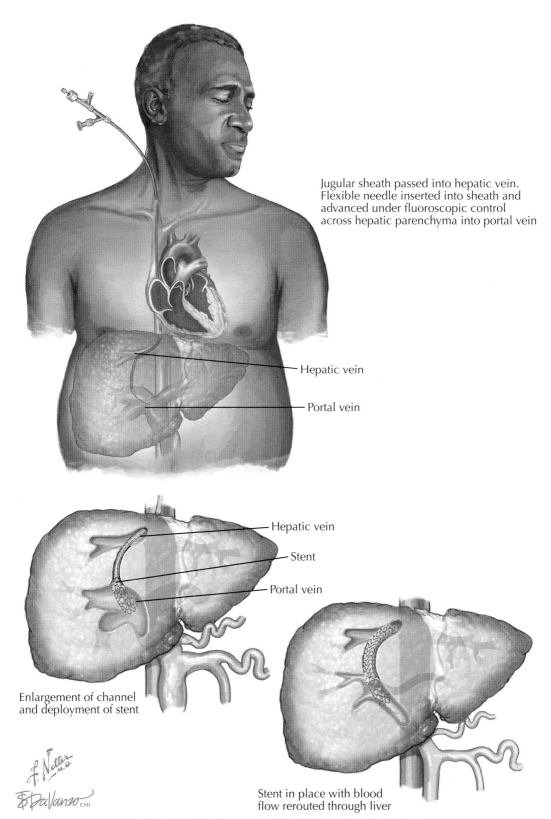

Jugular sheath passed into hepatic vein. Flexible needle inserted into sheath and advanced under fluoroscopic control across hepatic parenchyma into portal vein

Hepatic vein

Portal vein

Hepatic vein

Stent

Portal vein

Enlargement of channel and deployment of stent

Stent in place with blood flow rerouted through liver

Fig. 154.1 Transjugular Intrahepatic Portal Systemic Shunt.

Loffroy R, Estivalet L, Cherblanc V, et al: Transjugular intrahepatic portosystemic shunt for the management of acute variceal hemorrhage, *World J Gastroenterol* 19:6131–6143, 2013.

Parker R: Role of the transjugular intrahepatic portosystemic shunt in the management of portal hypertension, *Clin Liver Dis* 18:319–334, 2014.

Patidar KR, Sydnor M, Sanyal AJ: Transjugular intrahepatic portosystemic shunt, *Clin Liver Dis* 18:853–876, 2014.

Siramolpiwat S: Transjugular intrahepatic portosystemic shunts and portal hypertension-related complications, *World J Gastroenterol* 20:16996–17010, 2014.

155

Liver Biopsy

Joseph K. Lim, Kris V. Kowdley

Although significant improvement in technology has permitted an increasing role for liver imaging, serum diagnostics, and both serum and imaging-based fibrosis tools in routine clinical practice, the liver biopsy remains the gold standard assessment tool for the diagnosis and staging of acute and chronic liver disease, and may guide clinical management.

Assessment of disease activity such as in the context of autoimmune hepatitis may clarify the role of corticosteroids and/or immunosuppressive drug therapy. Identification of a pattern and zonal distribution of liver injury may help distinguish potential causes for drug-induced liver injury. Quantification of overload of iron and copper may confirm a diagnosis of hemochromatosis or Wilson disease, and guide phlebotomy or chelation therapy. Clarification of the pattern of liver injury in a liver graft posttransplant may determine the presence of acute or chronic rejection which guides treatment approach. Assessment and staging of liver fibrosis may help determine both eligibility and the appropriate regimen for the treatment of chronic hepatitis B and C infections.

TECHNIQUES

Liver biopsy can be performed percutaneously, either blindly using percussion techniques or with ultrasound (US) guidance (Fig. 155.1). US localizes an intercostal space with clear access to the liver, averting major vessels, gallbladder, and lungs. This location is marked, and the biopsy is subsequently performed at the bedside, usually in a day-surgery or ambulatory setting.

Liver biopsy can also be performed in the radiology suite under direct US or CT guidance. This technique is usually selected when biopsy is performed to study focal lesions, such as suspected hepatocellular carcinoma or adenoma. Liver biopsy can also be done using laparoscopy, although usually only when the patient is already undergoing laparoscopic surgery.

In addition to the percutaneous approach, liver biopsy can be performed using transjugular techniques, generally by interventional radiologists and for patients with a higher risk for bleeding, such as those with thrombocytopenia or coagulation abnormalities. A catheter is introduced into the right internal jugular vein and then passed into the liver through the hepatic vein. Biopsy forceps can then be used to obtain a tissue sample. The theoretic advantage of this approach is that any bleeding would occur within the vascular compartment and would be associated with a lower risk for intraabdominal bleeding.

Percutaneous liver biopsy is generally performed using local anesthesia alone, although many hepatologists have begun using a mild sedative to reduce anxiety. However, it is important that the patient be awake and alert during the performance of percutaneous liver biopsy because it is essential for patients to hold their breath, usually in the end-expiratory state. After local anesthesia with lidocaine, a trocar is used to create a tract to facilitate passage of a 16-gauge needle. A suction needle is then used to aspirate a core of liver tissue. Different types of needles are available for liver biopsy; the Klatskin needle is often used (see Fig. 155.1).

The biopsy specimen is usually placed in formalin or another fixative. A number of stains are used to evaluate the liver parenchyma. Hematoxylin and eosin stain is used to evaluate for inflammation and necrosis; trichrome stain is used to assess the presence and degree of fibrosis; and stains such as reticulin can be used to evaluate the architecture. In addition, special stains are useful to screen for specific liver diseases, such as periodic acid–Schiff with diastase for α_1-antitrypsin deficiency, Perls Prussian blue stain for iron, and a special stain for hepatitis B core antigen. Biochemical measurement of iron or copper can be performed from fresh or paraffin-embedded tissue to establish a specific diagnosis of hemochromatosis or Wilson disease, respectively.

COMPLICATIONS AND CONTRAINDICATIONS

The main risks involved in liver biopsy are pain and bleeding. Pain may be localized over the biopsy site, diffusely spread over the abdomen, or more often, referred to the right shoulder from irritation of the diaphragm. Bleeding is more serious and may result in hepatic capsular hematoma or even intraabdominal bleeding, although this is rare.

Other complications include infection, pneumothorax or hemothorax, and perforation of the gallbladder or the bile ducts. The risk for fatal complication of liver biopsy is approximately 1 in 10,000. Risk factors for complications of liver biopsy include coagulopathy and increased number of passes.

Most centers require that the patient lie on the right side for several hours after the biopsy to allow internal compression of the liver against the rib cage.

Contraindications to liver biopsy include lack of patient cooperation, bacterial cholangitis, extrahepatic bile duct obstruction, and significant coagulopathy or thrombocytopenia. Some advocate avoiding liver biopsy in patients with cystic liver lesions because of infection risk and in those with amyloidosis because of hemorrhage risk. Many experts believe that patients with large amounts of ascites should not undergo percutaneous biopsy because of the inability to compress the liver internally against the rib cage and the resulting increased risk for bleeding. However, data from controlled trials are limited to support these recommendations.

Alternate Techniques

The most important limitation of liver biopsy is *sampling variability*, especially in liver diseases with focal involvement, such as cystic fibrosis and primary sclerosing cholangitis. This has led to active investigation into other methods to assess the presence or absence of cirrhosis. Imaging techniques used include transient elastography, magnetic resonance imaging (MRI), and noninvasive serum markers of fibrogenesis (e.g.,

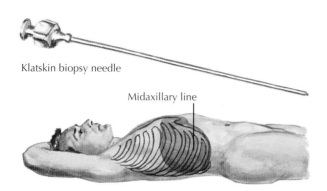

Klatskin biopsy needle

Midaxillary line

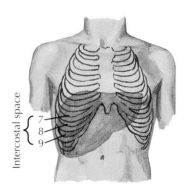

Intercostal space

7
8
9

1. Saline (1 mL) injected to expel tissue fragments from needle

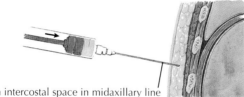

7th to 9th intercostal space in midaxillary line

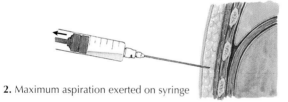

2. Maximum aspiration exerted on syringe

3. Breath held in expiration, while needle pushed to maximum depth with quick rectilinear movement without rotation; aspiration maintained

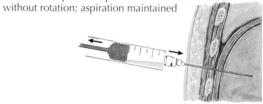

(Biopsy specimen recovered by expelling saline from syringe)

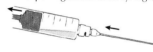

4. Needle withdrawn rapidly without rotation; aspiration maintained

Laparoscopic technique

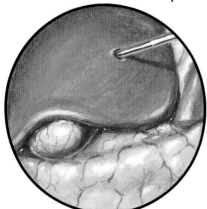

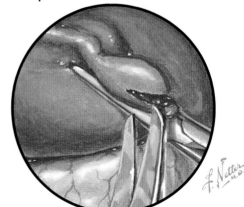

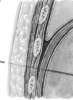

Laparoscopic needle biopsy

Laparoscopic excision biopsy

Fig. 155.1 Liver Biopsy: Percutaneous Suction and Laparoscopic Techniques.

hyaluronic acid, fragments of collagen) that may form in the liver in response to injury. Although promising, these techniques have not yet achieved sufficient positive and negative predictive value to replace liver biopsy in the clinical setting.

In the future, the combination of structural imaging studies and dynamic serum or plasma markers of fibrosis may reach sufficient reliability to replace liver biopsy in the evaluation of cirrhosis. However, liver biopsy will likely remain essential for diagnostic purposes in some patients for whom serologic testing has not established the cause of liver disease.

ADDITIONAL RESOURCES

Ble M, Procopet B, Miquel R, et al: Transjugular liver biopsy, *Clin Liver Dis* 18:767–778, 2014.

Bravo AA, Sheth SG, Chopra S: Liver biopsy, *N Engl J Med* 344:495–500, 2001.

Dezsofi A, Baumann U, Dhawan A, et al: Liver biopsy in children: position paper of the ESPGHAN Hepatology Committee, *J Pediatr Gastroenterol Nutr* 60:408–420, 2015.

Ovchinsky N, Moreira RK, Lefkowitch JH, Lavine JE: Liver biopsy in modern clinical practice: a pediatric point-of-view, *Adv Anat Pathol* 19:250–262, 2012.

Ravindran S, Hancox SH, Howlett DC: Liver biopsy: past, present, and future, *Br J Hosp Med* 77:90–95, 2016.

Rockey DC, Caldwell SH, Goodman ZD, et al: Liver biopsy, *Hepatology* 49:1017–1044, 2009.

Rustagi T, Newton E, Kar P: Percutaneous liver biopsy, *Trop Gastroenterol* 31:199–212, 2010.

Siegel CA, Silas AM, Suriawinata AA, van Leeuwen DJ: Liver biopsy 2005: when and how? *Cleve Clin J Med* 72:199–201, 2005.

Tapper EB, Lok AS: Use of liver imaging and biopsy in clinical practice, *N Engl J Med* 377:756–768, 2017.

156

Hepatic Necrosis

Joseph K. Lim, Kris V. Kowdley

Hepatic necrosis refers to any acute or chronic process which results in liver injury and eventual cell death of hepatocytes. Apoptosis represents the death of individual hepatocytes which may be a regulated physiologic process, and these individual cells undergoing apoptosis are sometimes described as *acidophilic bodies* (or "Councilman bodies"). The term *cell dropout* has also been used to describe some cases of hepatocellular necrosis. *Necrosis* implies not only the death of cells, but also the phenomena following cell death, namely, the disappearance of cells and frequently the accompanying inflammatory response. The final and irreversible stage of degeneration, hepatic necrosis, involves only the liver cells in most forms, whereas Kupffer cells and stroma remain intact. Kupffer cells respond to most types of hepatocellular degeneration and necrosis with reactive proliferation.

Although acute viral, toxic, or drug-induced hepatitis represent the most common causes of hepatocellular necrosis, any process resulting in systemic inflammation or liver-specific injury can lead to hepatic necrosis, as can insults that cause hepatic ischemia or hypoxemia. Necrosis can occur in one of several patterns:

Focal necrosis refers to involvement of single cells or a small group of cells which have been injured or have disappeared and are replaced by scavenger cells, usually neutrophilic segmented leukocytes but occasionally, especially in viral infections, histiocytes and lymphocytes (Fig. 156.1). Focal necrosis may also be the result of focal obstruction of the sinusoidal blood flow, such as by cellular debris or fibrin thrombi.

Zonal necrosis, in contrast, is characterized by its lobular distribution with involvement of a specific zone of the acinus. In *central* (or centrilobular) necrosis, the destructive process takes place around the central vein and may extend toward the periphery of the lobule. Depending on the intensity of the damage and the age of the lesions, liver cell fragments may be recognizable, or the liver cells may entirely disappear, and red blood cells (RBCs) may engorge sinusoids and tissue spaces. In more advanced stages, the framework is collapsed, and only a few scavenger cells are found mixed with Kupffer cells and RBCs. Necrosis of the liver cells in the center of the lobule is often the result of ischemia (as seen in passive congestion or shock), hypoxemia (low atmospheric pressure), or both, because this part of the hepatic lobule is most sensitive to conditions of hypoxia.

Periportal or *peripheral* necrosis indicates damage to periportal hepatocytes and in the adjoining peripheral zone of the parenchymal lobule. Inflammatory cells accumulate, often with inflammation in the portal triads. Proliferation of bile ducts and cholangiocytes is also common. Typically, periportal necrosis results from inflammation in the portal triads that extend to the peripheral zone; thus it is seen in infections involving the portal triads, in chronic biliary obstruction, and in chronic viral hepatitis. Isolated *midzonal* necrosis is rare in humans.

Extensive zonal, mainly central, necrosis often results from exposure to various poisons, toxins, or drugs but is also observed after infection or shock. Because necrosis is also produced or aggravated by cardiac failure, it is commonly difficult to distinguish contribution of each factor to primary liver cell damage. If central necrosis becomes more extensive and confluent involving more than one zone or lobule, bridges develop that connect the central zones or the portal and central zones (*bridging* necrosis). This may proceed further to almost complete loss of liver cells in a lobule (*massive* necrosis). Massive necrosis in a considerable part of the liver produces hepatic insufficiency, sometimes fatal, that historically has been termed *acute yellow atrophy* or *acute red atrophy* of the liver. The normal architecture of the liver may be difficult to recognize in massive necrosis.

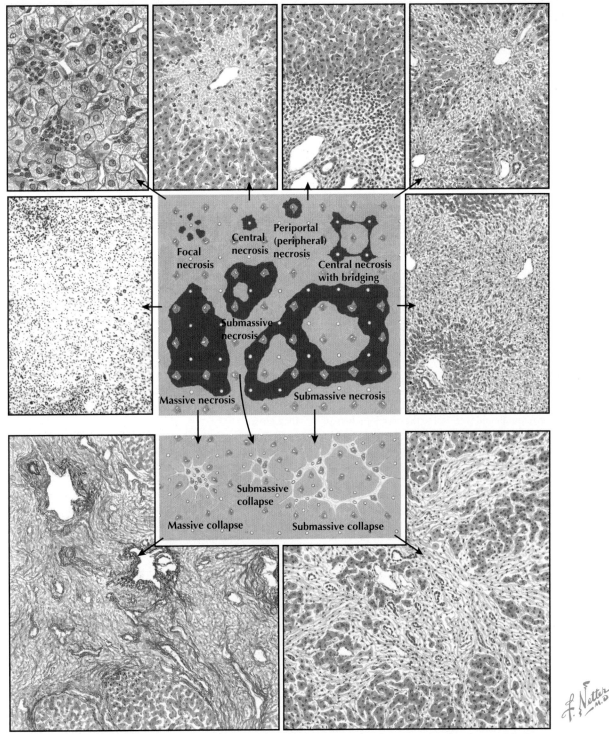

Fig. 156.1 Histologic Views of Hepatic Necrosis: Focal, Central, Submassive, Massive, and Collapse.

ADDITIONAL RESOURCES

de Oliveira da Silva B, Ramos LF, Moraes KCM: Molecular interplays in hepatic stellate cells: apoptosis, senescence, and phenotype reversion as cellular connections that modulate liver fibrosis, *Cell Biol Int* 41:946–959, 2017.

Elpek GO: Cellular and molecular mechanisms in the pathogenesis of fibrosis: an update, *World J Gastroenterol* 20:7260–7276, 2014.

Krishna M: Patterns of necrosis in liver disease, *Clin Liv Dis* 10:53–56, 2017.

Lee UE, Friedman SL: Mechanisms of hepatic fibrogenesis, *Best Pract Res Clin Gastroenterol* 25:195–206, 2011.

Seki E, Brenner DA: Recent advancement of molecular mechanisms of liver fibrosis, *J Hepatobiliary Pancreat Sci* 22:512–518, 2015.

Zhou WC, Zhang QB, Qiao L: Pathogenesis of liver cirrhosis, *World J Gastroenterol* 20:7312–7324, 2014.

157

Cirrhosis

Joseph K. Lim, Kris V. Kowdley

Liver cirrhosis is defined as the final, most advanced stage of liver fibrosis based on the Metavir, Batts-Ludwig, and Ishak histopathological staging systems.

Cirrhosis represents the end stage of any process resulting in chronic injury to the liver parenchyma. Progressive fibrosis results in the alteration of hepatic architecture and the formation of small or large nodules. The associated circulatory and hemodynamic changes may result in portal hypertension with ascites, esophageal varices, and necrosis (Figs. 157.1 and 157.2).

PATHOGENESIS

The hepatic *stellate cell*, also referred to as the *Ito cell* or *lipocyte*, is the primary storage site for retinoids and is critical to the process of hepatic fibrogenesis. On stimulation by inflammation or other noxious factors, stellate cells become contractile and are activated, demonstrating features of myofibroblasts and releasing cytokines and other inflammatory mediators. Subsequently, a deposition of extracellular matrix results in fibrosis, development of scar tissue, vascular obstruction, and sinusoidal hypertension, followed by portal hypertension and eventually hepatic failure. This dynamic process may be accelerated by the addition of hepatotoxins (e.g., alcohol, drugs) or may be decelerated by the reduction of hepatic necroinflammation through immunomodulator therapy (e.g., corticosteroids) or elimination of the inciting agent (e.g., direct antivirals for hepatitis B or C infection).

Other cells, such as fibroblasts, are also involved in the development of hepatic fibrosis. Over time, this process can result in the development of widespread scar tissue throughout the liver and ultimately leads to established cirrhosis. Cytokines that play a key role in stellate cell proliferation and activation include transforming growth factor-β, interleukins, hepatocyte growth factor, and platelet-derived growth factor. These cytokines have multiple effects; some are fibrogenetic, whereas others may promote fibrinolysis. Some are primarily proinflammatory, and others are antiinflammatory.

The progression to cirrhosis in a patient with chronic liver injury is characterized by increased deposition of extracellular matrix, ongoing inflammation, and an imbalance in favor of fibrogenetic rather than fibrinolytic pathways. The current research to identify the key mediators responsible for hepatic fibrogenesis is the first step in the development of novel antifibrotic therapies potentially capable of halting or even reversing the process leading to cirrhosis.

CLINICAL PICTURE

Clinical manifestations associated with cirrhosis are previously described in Chapter 147. The most common signs of cirrhosis include jaundice, splenomegaly, palmar erythema, and spider nevi, and the presence of overt abdominal ascites or asterixis may further signal decompensated cirrhosis or liver failure. In patients with chronic liver disease, mild or moderate thrombocytopenia may represent an early clue for advanced liver fibrosis or cirrhosis.

DIAGNOSIS

The definitive diagnosis of cirrhosis is made by liver biopsy or laparoscopy. Gross visualization of the liver by laparoscopy or surgery represents a standard approach for the diagnosis of cirrhosis. Liver biopsy is useful to establish the presence of cirrhosis, but cirrhosis cannot be entirely excluded due to small and/or fragmented biopsy specimens, or equivocal histologic findings inadequate to confirm the diagnosis.

Trichrome stain is the classic stain used to evaluate the degree or stage of fibrosis in the specimen. Most scoring systems such as Metavir and Batts-Ludwig classify biopsy specimens into four histologic stages. Generally, stages 1 and 2 represent *periportal* or *septal fibrosis,* whereas stages 3 and 4 are used to describe *bridging fibrosis* and *cirrhosis,* respectively. Some have advocated the use of additional morphometric techniques that stain collagen to better classify patients into various stages. Recent studies have examined transient elastography and magnetic resonance elastography to identify the presence of cirrhosis (see Chapter 158).

The differential diagnosis of cirrhosis includes several conditions that may have a similar histologic appearance but that are not associated with hepatic synthetic dysfunction. Some examples include focal nodular hyperplasia, nodular regenerative hyperplasia, and congenital hepatic fibrosis.

Recent research has focused on the use of noninvasive serum markers of fibrogenesis to classify patients into those with a low or high probability of cirrhosis. It is hoped that a combination of serum indices, serum fibrosis assays, and imaging-based fibrosis biomarkers may help stratify patients at low, intermediate, or high risk for cirrhosis without requiring a liver biopsy. At present, serum indices such as APRI (AST to platelet ratio index) and Fibrosis-4 score (FIB-4) (age, aspartate transaminase [AST], alanine transaminase [ALT], platelet count) are commonly used by large health organizations in population health efforts to identify patients with advanced liver fibrosis or cirrhosis. Serum fibrosis assays such as Fibrotest, Fibrospect, and Hepascore evaluate markers of fibrogenesis (e.g., hyaluronic acid, collagen types IV and VI, propeptides of various collagens, and matrix metalloproteinases) and have been validated for stratification of patients with no or mild fibrosis versus advanced liver fibrosis/cirrhosis. Imaging-based fibrosis markers using ultrasound or magnetic resonance elastography have recently emerged as viable noninvasive tools for the evaluation of liver cirrhosis for conditions such as viral hepatitis and nonalcoholic fatty liver disease.

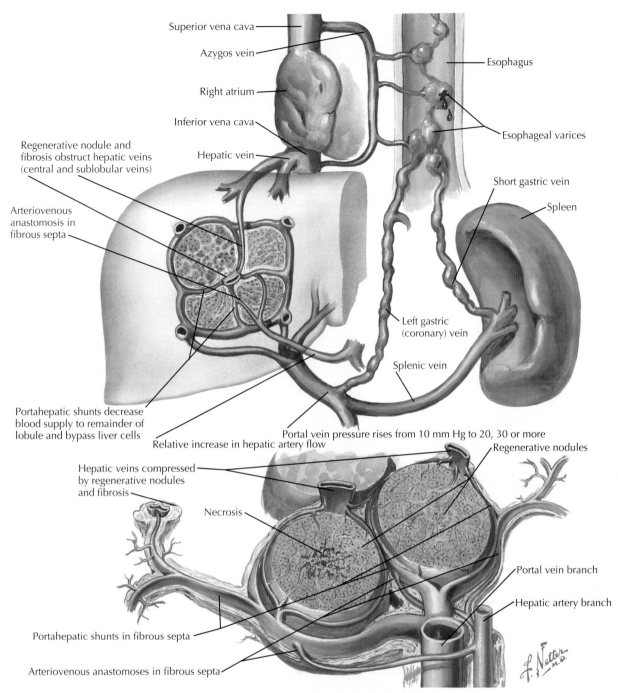

Fig. 157.1 Vascular Changes in Cirrhosis.

ADDITIONAL RESOURCES

Cardenas A, Gines P: Management of patients with cirrhosis awaiting liver transplantation, *Gut* 60:412–421, 2011.

Garcia-Tsao G, Lim JK: Management and treatment of patients with cirrhosis and portal hypertension: recommendations from the department of veterans affairs hepatitis C resource center program and the national hepatitis C program, *Am J Gastroenterol* 104:1802–1829, 2009.

Liou IW: Management of end-stage liver disease, *Med Clin North Am* 98:119–152, 2014.

Nusrat S, Khan MS, Fazili J, Madhoun MF: Cirrhosis and its complications: evidence based treatment, *World J Gastroenterol* 20:5442–5460, 2014.

Olson JC: Intensive care management of patients with cirrhosis, *Curr Treat Options Gastroenterol* 16:241–252, 2018.

Poordad FF: Presentation and complications associated with cirrhosis of the liver, *Curr Med Res Opin* 31:925–937, 2015.

Tsochatzis EA, Bosch J, Burroughs AK: Liver cirrhosis, *Lancet* 383:1749–1761, 2014.

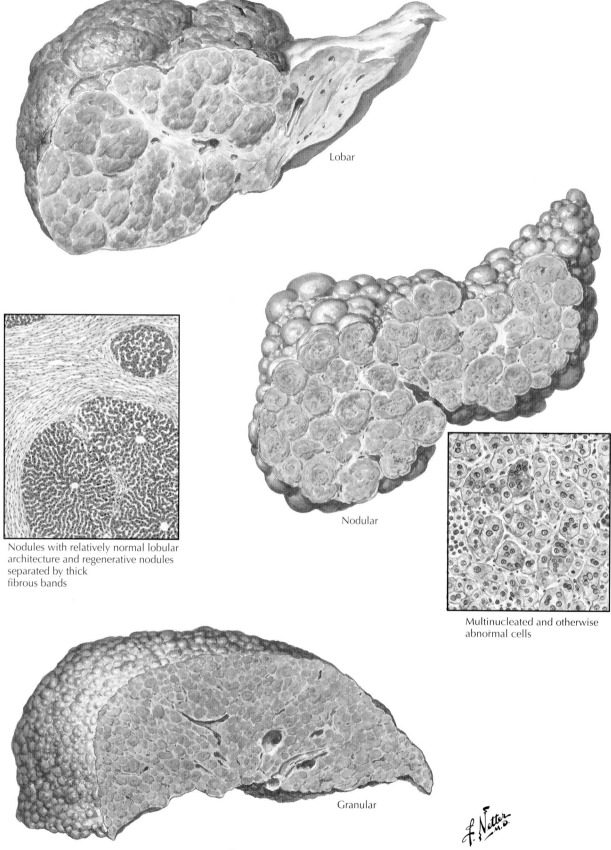

Lobar

Nodules with relatively normal lobular
architecture and regenerative nodules
separated by thick
fibrous bands

Nodular

Multinucleated and otherwise
abnormal cells

Granular

Fig. 157.2 Patterns of Cirrhosis.

158

Imaging Studies of the Liver

Joseph K. Lim, Kris V. Kowdley

The diagnosis of hepatobiliary disease frequently requires the use of imaging studies to characterize the presence of vascular and parenchymal changes which may facilitate diagnosis and management. Traditional imaging studies include abdominal ultrasonography (US), computed tomography (CT), and magnetic resonance imaging (MRI). More recent imaging techniques which incorporate liver elastography have emerged as important clinical tools to facilitate the diagnosis of liver cirrhosis, which remains an essential step in management. Several of the most commonly used techniques include vibration-controlled transient elastography (VCTE), shear wave elastography, acoustic radiation force impulse elastography (ARFI), and magnetic resonance elastography (MRE). Techniques such as VCTE are now routinely used in clinical practice, whereas others primarily used in research contexts such as MRE are now emerging as potentially important clinical tools for chronic liver diseases such as nonalcoholic fatty liver disease (NAFLD).

ABDOMINAL ULTRASONOGRAPHY

Abdominal US is often the first imaging modality used to evaluate the liver. US is easily performed, does not require intravenous (IV) access, and can provide a large amount of clinically relevant information in evaluating the liver and biliary tract. The use of Doppler technology also enables examination of the hepatic and portal venous system and the hepatic arterial flow. These latter developments have been particularly useful in the evaluation of patients after orthotopic liver transplantation and in those who have undergone placement of a transjugular intrahepatic portosystemic shunt (TIPS).

US is particularly helpful in evaluating suspected cystic lesions and in excluding the presence of dilated bile ducts. Liver cysts are often found during US and are usually asymptomatic. Based on US features, these can usually be classified as *simple cysts*. Simple cysts are anechoic and show posterior enhancement, which means there is an echogenic region behind the cystic lesion. In questionable cases, cyst aspiration can be performed to obtain cells for cytologic examination or to institute drainage if infection is a concern.

US is the most sensitive method for determining the presence of dilated bile ducts. Both intrahepatic and extrahepatic ductal dilatation can be identified, particularly in slender patients without fatty liver; thus both the presence and the level of bile duct obstruction can be identified. In patients with acute biliary obstruction (e.g., acute choledocholithiasis), however, US may not reveal dilated ducts. A number of focal liver lesions may be identified, including bacterial, fungal, and parasitic abscesses and benign and malignant lesions (e.g., hepatic adenomas, hemangiomas, hepatocellular carcinoma).

However, CT and MRI are superior to US because of the ability to administer contrast and to obtain images in various phases—arterial, portal, and hepatic venous—which can further increase the specificity of the diagnosis.

Ultrasonography is also helpful to evaluate the hepatic parenchyma. In patients with fatty liver infiltration associated with obesity, hyperlipidemia, or type 2 diabetes, diffusely increased echogenicity may be observed in the liver. Increased echogenicity of the liver is also observed in patients with cirrhosis. In addition, US may reveal features of portal hypertension, such as splenomegaly, perisplenic varices, portosystemic collaterals, and reversal of flow (hepatofugal) in the portal vein. In some patients with cirrhosis, particularly resulting from alcohol, the left lobe may be enlarged.

COMPUTED TOMOGRAPHY

CT allows visualization of the liver with the addition of contrast, which has greatly improved the ability to differentiate hypervascular from hypovascular lesions. In addition, recent advances in CT have significantly enhanced radiologic diagnosis of liver lesions. Improvements in image acquisition techniques, such as helical and spiral CT, now allow rapid imaging of the liver and the opportunity to obtain arterial and portal venous phase images with the administration of IV contrast. These techniques have made so-called four-phase CT possible, permitting imaging of the liver during noncontrast, arterial, portal venous, and hepatic venous phases. Such improvements in technique have been helpful in differentiating vascular lesions, such as cavernous hemangiomas and hepatocellular carcinoma, which usually enhances in the arterial phases and may wash out during the portal venous phase.

CT has been invaluable in the evaluation of patients before liver transplantation. In addition to increased sensitivity for the screening of hepatocellular carcinoma in patients awaiting liver transplantation, three-dimensional (3D) reconstruction of the hepatic arterial system provides the surgeon with a useful road map, which is necessary given the great variability in normal hepatic arterial anatomy (see Chapter 143).

MAGNETIC RESONANCE IMAGING

MRI has become an increasingly common approach to liver imaging. MRI has been particularly useful in patients with renal insufficiency who may be unable to receive IV contrast. In such patients, MRI with magnetic resonance (MR) angiography can be used to evaluate liver texture, assess for liver masses, and delineate vascular anatomy. In addition, T1- and T2-weighted images can improve diagnostic sensitivity. Fat emits a bright signal on T1-weighted images, which may be helpful in identifying fat or blood. Fluid and pathologic lesions may be more visible on T2-weighted images.

Ongoing research is defining the role of MR contrast agents (e.g., gadolinium), and improvements in scanning time and 3D imaging techniques have allowed better visualization of the vessels and biliary tree. The paramagnetic properties of iron can be exploited using MRI because relaxation times are inversely related to hepatic iron content

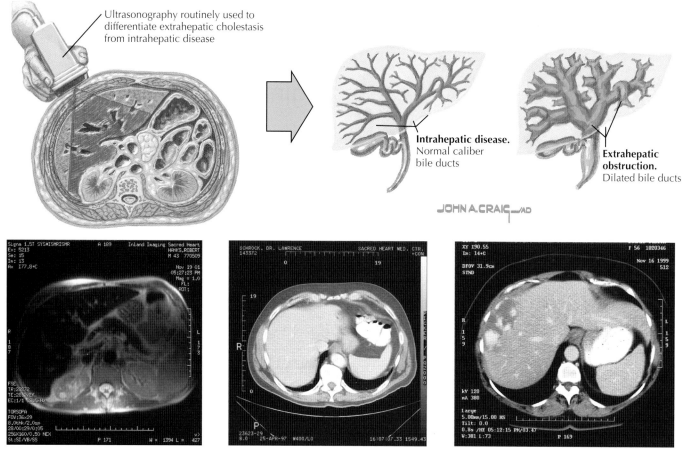

Fig. 158.1 Ultrasound, Computed Tomography, and Magnetic Resonance Imaging Studies of the Liver.

and can be quantified. Measuring hepatic iron content noninvasively will likely be possible in the near future using MRI.

CHOLANGIOPANCREATOGRAPHY

Endoscopic retrograde cholangiopancreatography (ERCP) was first introduced into clinical practice in 1968, although widespread use of this technique did not become established until the 1980s. ERCP has gradually evolved from a primarily diagnostic to a therapeutic procedure. Many therapeutic interventions are possible during ERCP, including placement of transpapillary stents to treat obstructive jaundice caused by benign or malignant strictures, bile fistulae, endoscopic sphincter-otomy to remove common bile duct stones, and endoscopic balloon dilatation for benign strictures.

The ERCP technique involves the use of a specialized side-viewing endoscope with an elevator that allows placement of a 5-French plastic catheter into the biliary tree. Once deep cannulation into the bile duct has been achieved, radiographic contrast is injected, and fluoroscopic images are obtained. Excellent visualization of all major branches of the biliary tree and the intrahepatic ducts is possible with the injection of contrast under sufficient pressure.

Additionally, ERCP is invaluable for evaluating cholestatic liver disease. It is particularly useful in assessing patients with chronic cho-lestatic liver disease in the absence of an antimitochondrial antibody. ERCP has been considered the criterion for the ruling in (or ruling out) a diagnosis of primary sclerosing cholangitis (PSC). However, the newer technique of magnetic resonance cholangiopancreatography (MRCP) is increasingly used in the diagnosis of PSC.

Representative cross-sectional imaging techniques used in evaluation of liver disease are shown in Fig. 158.1. Representative ERCP and MRCP images are shown in Fig. 158.2. ERCP is also helpful for evaluating patients with cirrhosis who have abdominal pain of suspected biliary origin, because the serum liver enzymes may not be helpful in these patients, and US may not reveal dramatic biliary dilatation. Finally, ERCP has become an indispensable modality in the management of the patient after liver transplantation, especially now that T tubes are no longer frequently used in the context of biliary duct-to-duct anastomosis.

ELASTOGRAPHY

VCTE is the most commonly used elastography method in the United States and globally, and involves application of a probe to the intercostal skin in the 9th to 11th intercostal space with acquisition of at minimum ten liver stiffness measurements to obtain a composite score between 2.5 and 75 kPa which corresponds with stage of liver fibrosis based on traditional histopathological scoring systems such as Metavir and Batts-Ludwig stages. This technique has the advantage of being noninvasive, performed in an ambulatory setting, and has been validated for the assessment of liver fibrosis across multiple liver conditions, particularly chronic hepatitis B and C infections. However, there exist several limita-tions such as increased error and technical failure with severe obesity, nonfasting state, vascular congestion, cholestasis, and significant alcohol consumption. The use of VCTE has recently been endorsed for the evaluation of liver fibrosis in gastroenterology society guidelines and may be used as an alternative to liver biopsy. *MRE* is a newer technique that estimates liver stiffness using MRI technology (Fig. 158.3) which

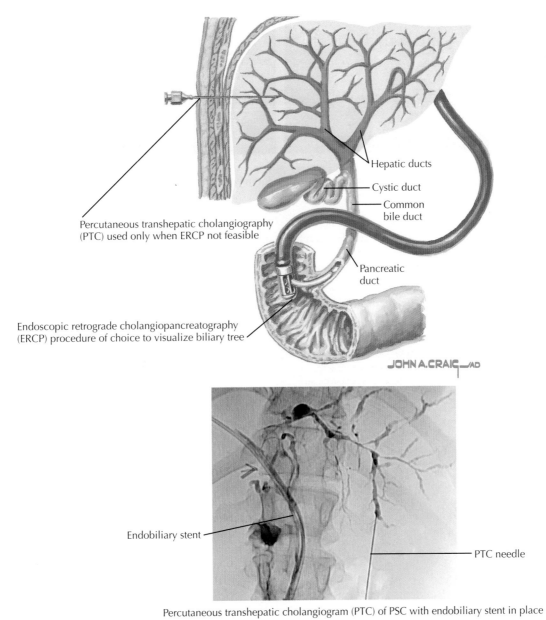

Percutaneous transhepatic cholangiography
(PTC) used only when ERCP not feasible

Hepatic ducts

Cystic duct

Common
bile duct

Pancreatic
duct

Endoscopic retrograde cholangiopancreatography
(ERCP) procedure of choice to visualize biliary tree

JOHN A.CRAIG—AD

Endobiliary stent

PTC needle

Percutaneous transhepatic cholangiogram (PTC) of PSC with endobiliary stent in place

**Fig. 158.2 Percutaneous Cholangiography and Endoscopic and Magnetic Resonance Cholangiopan-
creatography Imaging Studies of the Liver.** *PSC,* Primary sclerosing cholangitis.

Sheer Stiffness (kPa)

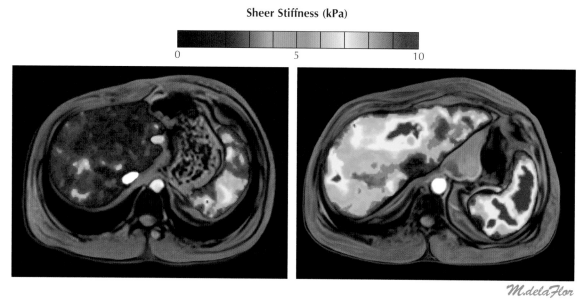

Fig. 158.3 Magnetic Resonance Elastography to Stage Hepatic Fibrosis.

overcomes several of the limitations of ultrasound-based elastography and evaluates a larger region of interest (ROI), and may represent a potentially important fibrosis assessment tool in the management of patients with NAFLD.

ADDITIONAL RESOURCES

Barr DC, Hussain HK: MR imaging in cirrhosis and hepatocellular carcinoma, *Magn Reson Imaging Clin N Am* 22:315–335, 2014.

Campos-Correia D, Cruz J, Matos AP, et al: Magnetic resonance imaging ancillary features used in Liver Imaging Reporting and Data System: an illustrative review, *World J Radiol* 10:9–23, 2018.

Castera L, Chan HL, Arrese M, et al: EASL-ALEH clinical practice guidelines: non-invasive tests for evaluation of liver disease severity and prognosis, *J Hepatol* 63:237–264, 2015.

Hennedige T, Venkatesh SK: Advances in computed tomography and magnetic resonance imaging of hepatocellular carcinoma, *World J Gastroenterol* 22:205–220, 2016.

Lim JK, Flamm SL, Singh S, Falck-Ytter YT: American Gastroenterological Association Institute guideline on the role of elastography in the evaluation of liver fibrosis, *Gastroenterology* 152:1536–1543, 2017.

Tapper EB, Lok AS: Use of liver imaging and biopsy in clinical practice, *N Engl J Med* 377:756–768, 2017.

159

Alcoholic Liver Disease

Joseph K. Lim, Kris V. Kowdley

Alcoholic liver disease remains a major primary cause of chronic liver disease in the United States and worldwide. Furthermore, alcohol is commonly implicated as a major exacerbating factor in many other liver diseases, such as hepatitis C, nonalcoholic fatty liver disease, and hemochromatosis, and therefore may play a role in a significant proportion of patients with acute and/or chronic liver disease.

Despite enormous progress in the past several decades, several key aspects of alcoholic liver disease remain unexplained, perhaps most importantly, the great variability in the relationship between quantity of alcohol consumed and risk for liver damage. However, it is generally recognized that the typical threshold level of alcohol intake associated with liver disease is 60 g daily over a 10-year period. The threshold for alcoholic liver disease is much lower among women than among men. Factors associated with this phenomenon may include the lighter body weight of women and decreased gastric alcohol dehydrogenase activity.

The pathophysiology of alcoholic liver disease is multifactorial. Numerous factors have been proposed, including genetic factors, toxic effects of alcohol, effect of prooxidant cytochromes (e.g., CYP 2E1), hypoxia, immune activation, and concomitant conditions (e.g., obesity). A key step in the metabolism of alcohol is the production of *acetaldehyde*, a hepatotoxin that mediates many steps in the evolution of hepatic necroinflammation in alcoholic liver disease. Stellate cell activation is central to the process of fibrogenesis. Over time, it can lead to the development of cirrhosis.

CLINICAL PICTURE

Clinical features of alcoholic liver disease are similar to other causes of liver disease, with some exceptions. Alcoholic liver disease is often associated with more prominent ascites in patients with otherwise-compensated liver disease. Serum liver biochemical tests may also point to a diagnosis of alcoholic liver disease because the aspartate transaminase (AST)/alanine transaminase (ALT) ratio is often greater than 2:1 and is frequently greater than 3:1.

The role of liver biopsy remains controversial in alcoholic liver disease. Some argue that biopsy should be routinely performed because occasionally, other unexpected causes of liver disease can be found in patients given a presumptive diagnosis of alcoholic liver disease (Fig. 159.1). Histologic features of alcoholic liver disease may follow one of three patterns: fatty liver (Fig. 159.2), alcoholic hepatitis, and alcoholic cirrhosis (Fig. 159.3). Frequently, all three of these findings can be found in the same patient. In addition, there may be features of ballooning degeneration of hepatocytes, Mallory (hyaline) bodies, and variable degrees of fibrosis. In contrast to patients with nonalcoholic fatty liver disease, lobular damage, Mallory bodies, periportal or bridging fibrosis, and cirrhosis are observed in a much higher proportion of patients.

DIAGNOSIS

The diagnosis of alcoholic liver disease is based on the exclusion of other causes of liver disease and the appropriate history of alcohol use. It is useful to quantify the amount of alcohol consumed by the patient on a chronic basis. The quantity of alcohol consumed in grams per day can be estimated as follows: one 12-oz can of beer, one 4-oz glass of wine, and one 1-oz shot of spirits each contain approximately 11 g of alcohol. In the assessment of alcoholic liver disease, it is also useful to identify whether the patient is tolerant of or dependent on alcohol. Several standardized questionnaires, such as CAGE (cut down, annoyance, guilt, eye opener) or research instruments such as AUDIT-C (Alcohol Use Disorders Identification Test), are widely available for this purpose. Unfortunately, reliable biomarkers for alcoholism and/or alcoholic liver disease are not available. Some tests such as gamma glutamyl transpeptidase (GGT) and carbohydrate-deficient transferrin (CDT) have been limited by low sensitivity and specificity and are not reliable for routine clinical use.

TREATMENT AND MANAGEMENT

Abstinence is the mainstay of therapy for alcoholic liver disease. Liver function can improve remarkably well after alcohol intake ceases, and is observed in nearly two-thirds of patients within 3 months of achieving sobriety. Some patients with advanced liver disease who are candidates for liver transplant recover to such a degree that liver transplantation is no longer needed, although recidivism remains a significant threat to long-term outcomes; available studies suggest that relapses to alcohol consumption occur in over 70% of patients. In addition to structured alcohol rehabilitation and relapse prevention programs, pharmacotherapy with naltrexone or acamprosate may be considered to decrease risk of relapse in patients with an established diagnosis of alcohol abuse and/or dependence.

Patients with cirrhosis are at long-term risk for hepatocellular carcinoma. Therefore screening using ultrasonography or computed tomography is appropriate among patients with established cirrhosis. Chronic alcohol consumption can also lead to increased serum transferrin–iron saturation and ferritin levels and may lead to secondary iron overload, which often mimics hemochromatosis. However, some patients with a history of heavy alcohol consumption may have hereditary hemochromatosis (see Chapter 172). Therefore serum iron studies should be obtained in all patients with a history of alcoholic liver disease, and *HFE* gene testing should be performed in patients with elevated ferritin and transferrin saturation levels greater than 45%.

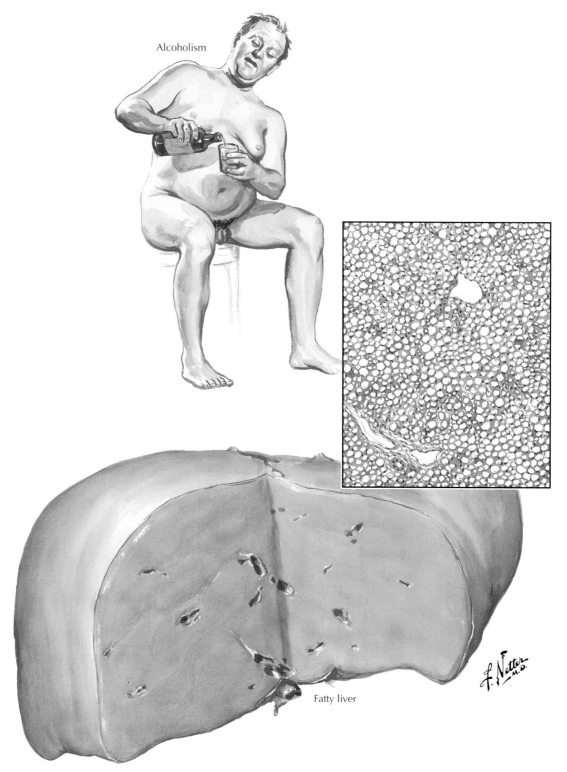

Fig. 159.1 Alcoholic Liver Disease.

COURSE AND PROGNOSIS

Long-term survival of patients with alcoholic liver disease is significantly lower than in patients with other causes of chronic liver disease, possibly as low as 7% at 10 years. Several variables may be associated with outcome in patients with alcoholic liver disease, including nutritional status, obesity, genetic factors, and concomitant use of hepatotoxic medications (e.g., acetaminophen) or infection with hepatitis C. Coexisting nonalcoholic metabolic fatty liver has recently emerged as an important cofactor for rapid disease progression in patients with alcoholic liver disease, often described as ASH (alcoholic steatohepatitis)/NASH (nonalcoholic steatohepatitis), and is currently subject to active investigation.

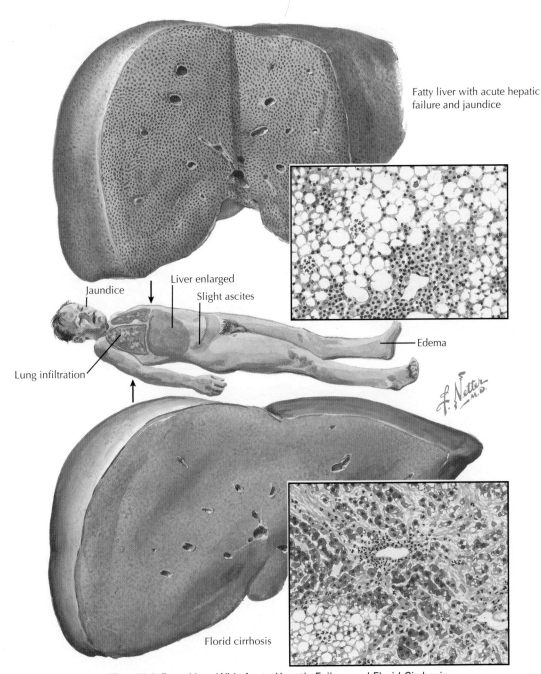

Fatty liver with acute hepatic failure and jaundice

Jaundice

Liver enlarged

Slight ascites

Edema

Lung infiltration

Florid cirrhosis

Fig. 159.2 Fatty Liver With Acute Hepatic Failure and Florid Cirrhosis.

ALCOHOLIC HEPATITIS

Alcoholic hepatitis is a potentially life-threatening complication of alcoholic liver disease. It is characterized by jaundice and moderately to markedly elevated levels of serum transaminase. Patients often have fever, right upper quadrant pain, and tender hepatomegaly. Acute cholecystitis or choledocholithiasis is often suspected because of the presence of right upper quadrant tenderness and leukocytosis. The clinical diagnosis of alcoholic hepatitis is determined by the presence of jaundice and clinical history of significant alcohol consumption up until at minimum 8 weeks prior to onset of symptoms, elevated liver enzymes (total bilirubin > 3 mg/dL, AST and ALT > 1.5 times upper limit of normal but <400 U/L, AST/ALT ratio > 1.5), and exclusion of other liver disease. A diagnostic liver biopsy is not routinely necessary for establishing a diagnosis, but should be considered in patients in whom there is uncertainty in the diagnosis; liver pathology commonly reveals a neutrophilic infiltrate accompanying steatohepatitis, with florid ballooning, degeneration of hepatocytes, and Mallory bodies.

The Maddrey's *discriminant function* has been developed to predict survival in patients with acute alcoholic hepatitis. It incorporates serum bilirubin, prothrombin time, and encephalopathy; a discriminant function ([4.6 × (prothrombin time/control [sec]) + bilirubin] > 52) or the presence of hepatic encephalopathy portend a poor prognosis in patients with acute alcoholic hepatitis. Scores ≥32 signal the presence of the

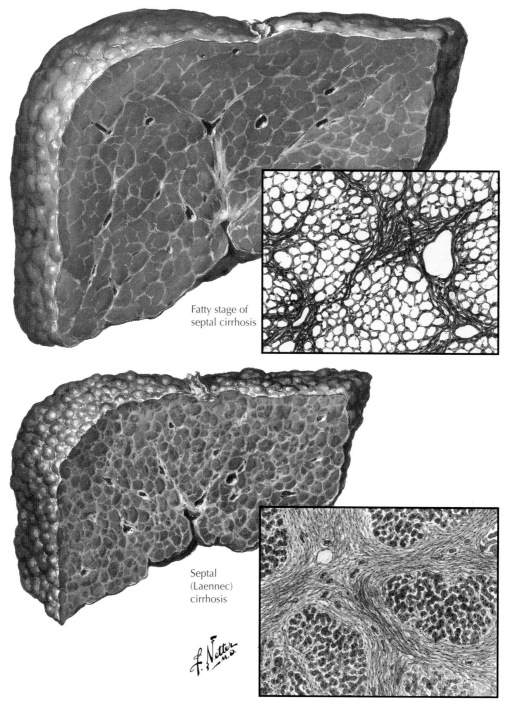

Fatty stage of septal cirrhosis

Septal (Laennec) cirrhosis

Fig. 159.3 Septal Cirrhosis.

"severe acute alcoholic hepatitis" phenotype associated with a poor prognosis, and help identify the subset of patients with alcoholic hepatitis who may warrant drug therapy. Other prognostic scoring systems currently in routine clinical use include the MELD (Model for End-Stage Liver Disease) score (poor prognosis if >20) and Glasgow Alcoholic Hepatitis score (poor prognosis if >8).

The management of severe acute alcoholic hepatitis includes a combination of treatment of nutritional deficiencies (protein-calorie, vitamin, mineral), and consideration for pharmacotherapy with corticosteroids (e.g., prednisolone) for up to 28 days in patients without contraindication to steroid use. In patients who initiate treatment with prednisolone, assessment of response to treatment should be made with the Lille score at day 7 of treatment. Nonresponders (defined as Lille score >0.45) should consider treatment discontinuation. Liver transplantation is often not possible due to center policies requiring 6 months of sobriety, although emerging evidence suggestive of favorable posttransplant outcomes in selected patients with alcoholic hepatitis signal the need for further investigation in this area.

ADDITIONAL RESOURCES

Aday AW, Mitchell MC, Casey LC: Alcoholic hepatitis: current trends in management, *Curr Opin Gastroenterol* 33:142–148, 2017.

Mitchell MC, Friedman LS, McClain CJ: Medical management of severe alcoholic hepatitis: expert review from the Clinical Practice Updates Committee of the AGA Institute, *Clin Gastroenterol Hepatol* 15:5–12, 2017.

O'Shea RS, Dasarathy S, McCullough AJ: Alcoholic liver disease: Practice Guideline of the American Association for the Study of Liver Diseases; Practice Parameters Committee of the American College of Gastroenterology, *Hepatology* 51:307–328, 2010.

Singal AK, Bataller R, Ahn J, et al: Clinical Guideline: Alcoholic liver disease, *Am J Gastroenterol* 113:175–194, 2018.

Singal AK, Louvet A, Shah VH, Kamath PS: Grand rounds: alcoholic hepatitis, *J Hepatol* 2018. [Epub ahead of print].

Singal AK, Shah VH: Therapeutic strategies for the treatment of alcoholic hepatitis, *Semin Liver Dis* 36:56–68, 2016.

160

Nonalcoholic Fatty Liver Disease and Steatohepatitis

Joseph K. Lim, Kris V. Kowdley

Nonalcoholic fatty liver disease (NAFLD) represents one of the most common causes of chronic liver disease in the United States and globally and is estimated to affect approximately 25% of the world population. The increasing prevalence of NAFLD is attributed to the concurrent rise of obesity, diabetes mellitus, hyperlipidemia, cardiovascular disease, and other manifestations of the metabolic syndrome.

The spectrum of nonalcoholic liver disease ranges from simple fatty liver, or NAFLD, to *nonalcoholic steatohepatitis* (NASH), characterized by cytolytic changes in hepatocytes, such as ballooning degeneration, Mallory (hyaline) bodies, and lobular inflammation (Fig. 160.1). It is this subset of patients with NASH who are at risk for progressive liver fibrosis, ranging from pericellular and perivenular or perisinusoidal fibrosis in zone 3 of the liver lobule to bridging fibrosis and cirrhosis. In the late stages, the fatty infiltration may disappear, leaving a picture of cirrhosis of unclear etiology, often described as *cryptogenic cirrhosis.*

Most patients with NAFLD or NASH have features of insulin resistance and may also have *syndrome X,* characterized by central or visceral obesity, type 2 diabetes, and dyslipidemia. The prevalence of NAFLD appears to be increasing rapidly, in parallel with the epidemic of obesity in Western countries. Multiple environmental factors likely play roles, including high-calorie and high-carbohydrate intake, sedentary lifestyle, and greater consumption of highly refined or processed sugars. In fact, NASH is increasingly observed in children, the population with the fastest-growing incidence of type 2 diabetes. Population-based studies suggest that the prevalence of NAFLD and NASH may be as high as 25% and 2% to 3%, respectively, in the general population. Prospective liver biopsy data from living donors in living-related liver transplantation have shown NASH in up to 25%.

The primary insult in NASH is thought to be *insulin resistance,* which may lead to increased circulating concentrations of free fatty acids. These may accumulate in the liver, leading to steatosis. A second insult, or second "hit," may lead to oxidative stress in the liver, resulting in progression to NASH. Many such possible second hits have been proposed, such as altered mitochondrial uncoupling proteins (UCP-2), cytochrome P450 2E1, excess iron, and activation of proinflammatory cytokines, such as tumor necrosis factor-α, nuclear factor kappa B, and interleukin-1, as well as other cascade pathways.

CLINICAL PICTURE

A detailed weight history should be obtained for all patients suspected to have fatty liver disease, including a history of obesity during childhood, glucose intolerance, gestational or type 2 diabetes, hypertriglyceridemia, low high-density lipoprotein level, and other disorders of lipid metabolism.

DIAGNOSIS

A diagnosis of NAFLD requires a careful and detailed history of alcohol use, potentially hepatotoxic medications, herbal supplements, and over-the-counter medications. Other factors known to cause steatohepatitis, such as jejunoileal bypass, total parenteral nutrition, and genetic or metabolic derangements, should be excluded. Severe malnutrition may also lead to NASH, manifested by *brown atrophy* of the liver (Fig. 160.2). Kwashiorkor may be associated with fatty liver disease among infants.

Steatosis and steatohepatitis are often discovered during routine medical screening. Most patients do not have symptoms. Some patients report fatigue, malaise, right upper quadrant fullness, or tenderness. Physical examination may reveal an android habitus, including central or truncal obesity and increased waist-to-hip ratio. Children with the disease are frequently obese and have *acanthosis nigricans,* a marker of insulin resistance that may be present in one-third of children and adolescents. Occasionally, patients have symptoms of advanced liver disease, including ascites, variceal bleeding, and hepatic encephalopathy.

Blood tests frequently show mild to moderate elevations of serum liver enzymes, with twofold to fivefold increases in serum aspartate transaminase (AST) and alanine transaminase (ALT). The AST/ALT ratio may be a sign of cirrhosis, but it is usually lower in patients with cirrhosis than in those with alcoholic liver disease. Fasting serum glucose and triglyceride levels may be elevated; in addition, increased levels of serum ferritin, an acute phase protein, may be present in up to 50% of patients, and increased levels of serum transferrin–iron saturation may be present in approximately 10%, although hepatic iron is not usually increased in the absence of *HFE* mutations.

Ultrasonography may reveal a so-called bright liver. Computed tomography often reveals a liver that is darker than the spleen. Magnetic resonance imaging may demonstrate fat as increased attenuation on T1-weighted images. However, noninvasive imaging modalities cannot distinguish simple steatosis from NASH. Several noninvasive serum tools have emerged which may help to identify high-risk patients requiring more specific intervention, including FIB-4 index (age, AST, ALT, platelet count) and NAFLD Fibrosis Score (NFS), which includes age, AST, ALT, platelet count, body mass index (BMI), hyperglycemia, and albumin. In addition, ultrasound-guided vibration-controlled transient elastography (Fibroscan) and magnetic resonance elastography (MRE) have emerged as useful tools for the identification of significant liver fibrosis among patients with NAFLD/NASH. Nevertheless, liver biopsy remains the "gold standard" tool for the diagnosis of NASH and should be considered in patients with NAFLD who are at increased risk for NASH and/or fibrosis, as well as for patients in whom there is a concern for alternative or coexisting etiologies for chronic liver disease.

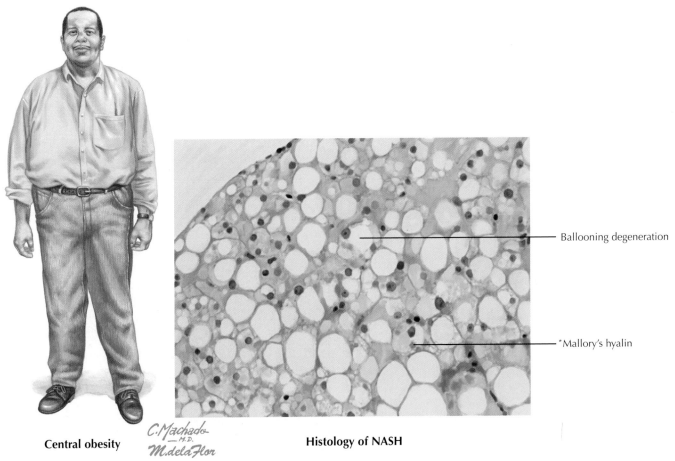

Central obesity   Histology of NASH

Ballooning degeneration

*Mallory's hyalin

Fig. 160.1 Nonalcoholic Steatohepatitis.

TREATMENT AND MANAGEMENT

Medical weight loss through diet and exercise should be encouraged and remains the first-line intervention for all patients with NAFLD. Recent studies suggest even a 7% to 10% decrease in body weight may result in histologic improvement in steatohepatitis and/or fibrosis. Pharmacologic weight loss therapy and both endoscopic and surgical bariatric procedures may be considered on a selective basis in patients with severe obesity or obesity with other manifestations of the metabolic syndrome; existing studies confirm that weight loss following bariatric surgery is associated with significant improvement in histologic and clinical outcomes related to NASH and other metabolic diseases. Exercise is an important component of a balanced weight loss regimen but alone has been demonstrated to result in improvement in NAFLD.

Specific pharmacotherapy for the treatment of NASH is currently the subject of intense investigation. There are several compounds which have demonstrated histologic benefit and are currently recommended as potential first line treatment in patients with biopsy-proven NASH, including vitamin E and pioglitazone. Due to concerns for increased risk of vascular events, malignancy, and all-cause mortality with high-dose vitamin E, it is used selectively in a subset of patients with NASH. Pioglitazone has demonstrated efficacy in histologic markers of NASH in patients with prediabetes and diabetes mellitus and can be considered in diabetic patients who otherwise meet criteria for insulin sensitizing therapy. An extensive list of investigational agents is under evaluation in phase 2 and 3 clinical trials, which provide hope for more effective treatment of NASH in the future, including several agents in phase 3 trial development targeting specific receptors important for NASH and/or fibrosis development (FXR, PPAR, CCR-2/5, and ASK-1).

ADDITIONAL RESOURCES

Chalasani N, Younossi Z, Lavine JE, et al: The diagnosis and management of nonalcoholic fatty liver disease: practice guidance from the American association for the study of liver diseases, *Hepatology* 67:328–357, 2018.

Diehl AM, Day C: Cause, pathogenesis, and treatment of nonalcoholic steatohepatitis, *N Engl J Med* 377:2063–2072, 2017.

Rinella ME: Nonalcoholic fatty liver disease: a systematic review, *JAMA* 313:226–373, 2015.

Serfaty L: Management of patients with non-alcoholic steatohepatitis (NASH) in real life, *Liver Int* 38(Suppl 1):52–55, 2018.

Wong VW, Chitturi S, Wong GL, et al: Pathogenesis and novel treatment options for non-alcoholic steatohepatitis, *Lancet Gastroenterol Hepatol* 1:56–67, 2016.

Younossi ZM, Loomba R, Rinella ME, et al: Current and future therapeutic regimens for non-alcoholic fatty liver disease (NAFLD) and non-alcoholic steatohepatitis (NASH), *Hepatology* 2017. [Epub ahead of print].

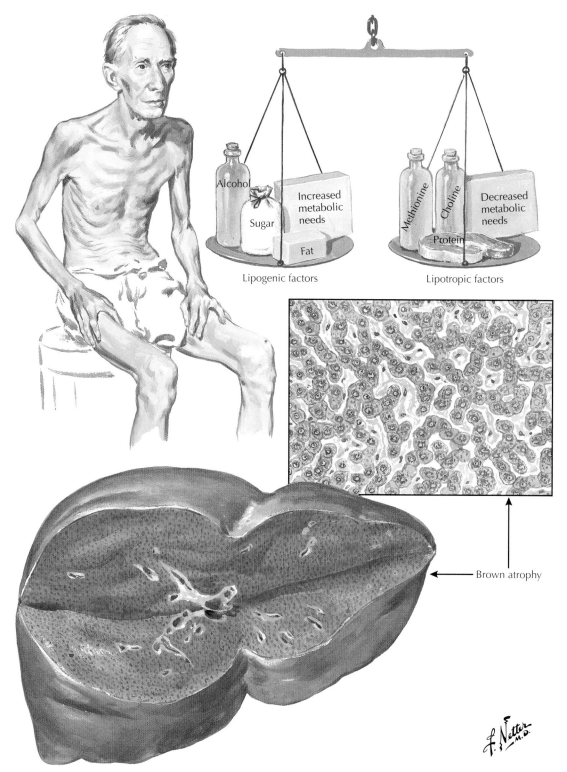

Fig. 160.2 Liver Disease Caused by Malnutrition.

161

Extrahepatic Biliary Obstruction

Joseph K. Lim, Kris V. Kowdley

Cholestatic liver disease occurs as the result of impaired bile formation and/or bile flow and is associated with clinical symptoms such as jaundice and pruritus. Extrahepatic biliary obstruction causes jaundice only if it is located between the confluence of the right and left hepatic ducts and the tip of the papilla of Vater. Obstruction of a single branch of the main hepatic duct does not produce jaundice because the unobstructed part of the liver compensates. The excretion of bile components other than bile pigments may not be as readily compensated, and serum alkaline phosphatase (ALP) or total serum cholesterol levels may be elevated in the absence of jaundice. Obstruction may be complete or incomplete; if incomplete, it is often intermittent.

Complete extrahepatic biliary obstruction is usually caused by tumors, which initially produce an incomplete obstruction but subsequently a permanent, complete occlusion (Figs. 161.1 and 161.2). Occasionally, regressive changes or hemorrhage into a tumor may result in the sloughing off of obstructive tissue, with temporary relief of a complete obstruction. This may be associated with at least chemical evidence of melena.

Intrinsic obstructive tumors are usually malignant and are represented by cancer of the biliary ducts or cancer of the papilla of Vater. Carcinoma of the pancreas (which may compress or kink the ducts), extension of carcinoma of the gallbladder, carcinomatous metastases to the hepatic lymph nodes, and other types of *extrinsic* carcinoma must invade the wall of the bile duct to produce obstruction. A tumor not fixed to the duct remains movable and cannot cause complete obstruction. For this reason, even extensive metastatic involvement of the hepatic lymph nodes, as seen in Hodgkin disease, leukemia, and reticulum cell sarcoma, seldom produces obstructive jaundice. Jaundice, if it appears in such conditions with inflammatory swelling of the hepatic lymph nodes, is almost always attributed to intrahepatic causes.

Gallstones enter the biliary ducts and due to impaction may cause initial spasm and edema. This may be associated with complete obstruction that is usually transient with rapid resolution of symptoms. However, if the stone is not expelled from the duct, incomplete obstruction persists and may result in chronic intermittent bile duct obstruction in a ball valvelike manner. In *calculous* obstruction, a short period of complete obstruction is followed by intermittent obstruction typically reflected in intermittent hyperbilirubinemia.

Strictures, whether produced by surgical injury to the biliary ducts or resulting from inflammatory lesions, may also cause biliary obstruction. Rarer causes of biliary obstruction include congenital atresia, inflammatory processes in neighboring organs (peptic ulcers, pancreatitis), duodenal diverticula, foreign bodies, and parasites.

Mechanical obstruction leads rapidly to dilatation of the biliary system above the sites of obstruction (Fig. 161.3). Obstruction of the *cystic duct* leads to dilatation of the gallbladder. If the obstruction involves the terminal portion of the cystic duct, the stone may bulge into the lumen of the common duct and produce jaundice and enlargement of the gallbladder (Mirizzi syndrome). Obstruction of the *common duct* by stones is usually associated with inflammation of the gallbladder, which may be fibrotic and does not dilate significantly. Obstruction of the duct by a tumor located near the papilla of Vater is usually associated with a normally expanding gallbladder that readily dilates and that may be palpated as a large, thin-walled cyst (Courvoisier gallbladder).

Hepatic effects of biliary obstruction, as seen on histopathology, develop more rapidly in complete than in incomplete obstruction. The first change is accumulation of bile pigment in the liver cells and Kupffer cells in the central zone of the lobule. Simultaneously, bile may amass in the form of ramified bile plugs in the dilated bile capillaries. The cytoplasm of some liver cells adjacent to the bile ductules is degenerated, and *pyknosis* (feathery degeneration) may be seen. At this stage, hyperbilirubinemia and bilirubinuria appear and serum ALP activity is elevated. Subsequently, inflammatory infiltration of the portal triads develops, with proliferation of perilobular cholangioles and periportal ducts. At this stage, ALP elevation is characteristically more prominent, and the total serum cholesterol may be elevated.

If biliary obstruction is prolonged, proliferation of the cholangioles increases, and bile casts may form even in peripheral ductules. Dilated cholangioles contain thick bile plugs, *microcalculi,* especially on the border between the lobular parenchyma and the portal triads, around which fibrosis often develops.

Although these features may be seen in intrahepatic and extrahepatic cholestasis, two features, the *extravasation of bile* and *bile infarcts,* are characteristically seen only in extrahepatic obstruction. Both appear after prolonged cholestasis when the obstruction is complete. Necroses of the epithelial lining of the interlobular bile ducts permit bile to escape into their walls, and granulation tissue appears around the golden-yellow bile in the portal triad. In circumscribed foci, the cytoplasm of liver cells is abnormal, and the bile is pigmented.

In the late stages of obstruction, secondary hepatocellular damage may be severe and may be reflected in marked abnormalities on liver function tests. In the late stages of biliary obstruction, the liver is enlarged and dark green. On the cut surface, the bile ducts appear to be severely dilated. Eventually, bands of fibrosis form and nodules regenerate, marking the beginning of cirrhosis.

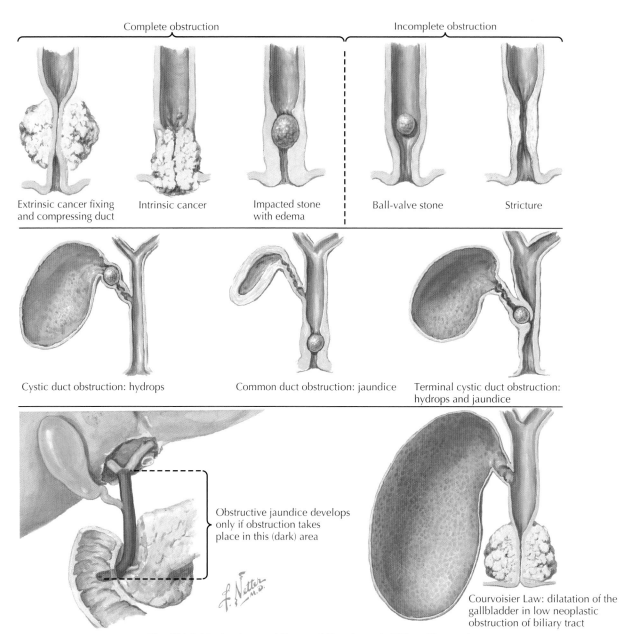

Complete obstruction

Incomplete obstruction

Extrinsic cancer fixing
and compressing duct

Intrinsic cancer

Impacted stone
with edema

Ball-valve stone

Stricture

Cystic duct obstruction: hydrops

Common duct obstruction: jaundice

Terminal cystic duct obstruction:
hydrops and jaundice

Obstructive jaundice develops
only if obstruction takes
place in this (dark) area

Courvoisier Law: dilatation of the
gallbladder in low neoplastic
obstruction of biliary tract

Fig. 161.1 Mechanism and Types of Extrahepatic Biliary Obstruction.

ADDITIONAL RESOURCES

Chazouilleres O: Novel aspects in the management of cholestatic liver disease, *Dig Dis* 34:340–346, 2016.

De Vries E, Beuers U: Management of cholestatic disease in 2017, *Liver Int* 37(Suppl 1):123–129, 2017.

Goldstein J, Levy C: Novel and emerging therapies for cholestatic liver disease, *Liver Int* 2018. [Epub ahead of print].

Gossard AA, Talwalkar JA: Cholestatic liver disease, *Med Clin North Am* 98:73–85, 2014.

Jungst C, Lammert F: Cholestatic liver disease, *Dig Dis* 31:152–154, 2013.

Nakanishi Y, Saxena R: Pathophysiology and diseases of the proximal pathways of the biliary system, *Arch Pathol Lab Med* 139:858–866, 2015.

Pollock G, Minuk GY: Diagnostic considerations for cholestatic liver disease, *J Gastroenterol Hepatol* 32:1303–1309, 2017.

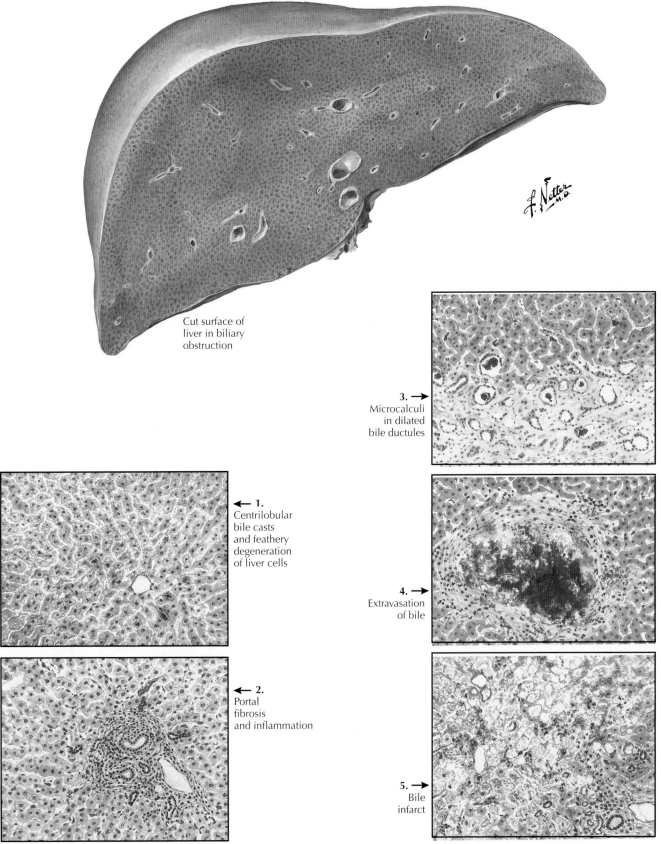

Cut surface of
liver in biliary
obstruction

3. →
Microcalculi
in dilated
bile ductules

← 1.
Centrilobular
bile casts
and feathery
degeneration
of liver cells

4. →
Extravasation
of bile

← 2.
Portal
fibrosis
and inflammation

5. →
Bile
infarct

Fig. 161.2 Liver and Histologic Stages in Extrahepatic Biliary Obstruction.

Endoscopic techniques

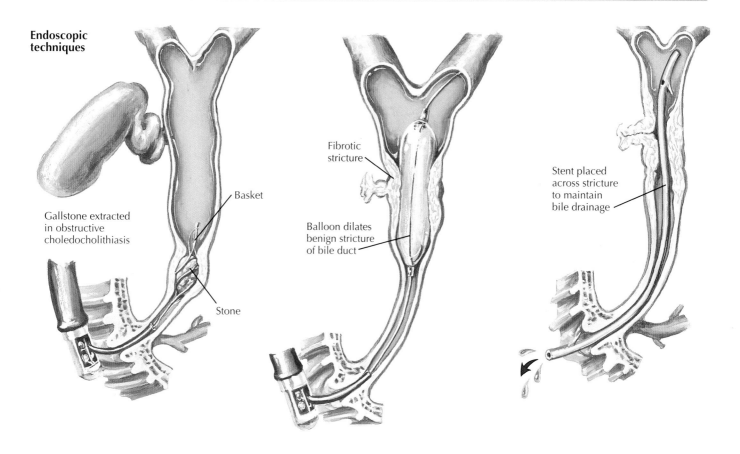

Gallstone extracted in obstructive choledocholithiasis

Basket

Stone

Fibrotic stricture

Balloon dilates benign stricture of bile duct

Stent placed across stricture to maintain bile drainage

Percutaneous (transhepatic) techniques

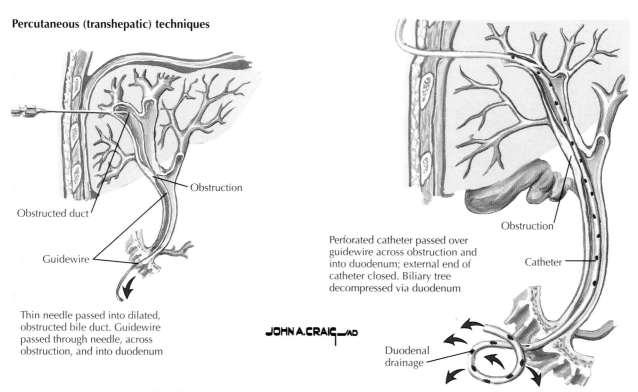

Obstructed duct

Obstruction

Guidewire

Thin needle passed into dilated, obstructed bile duct. Guidewire passed through needle, across obstruction, and into duodenum

Perforated catheter passed over guidewire across obstruction and into duodenum; external end of catheter closed. Biliary tree decompressed via duodenum

Obstruction

Catheter

Duodenal drainage

JOHN A.CRAIG—AD

Fig. 161.3 Mechanical Decompression Techniques for Biliary Obstruction.

162

Primary Biliary Cholangitis

Joseph K. Lim, Kris V. Kowdley

Primary biliary cholangitis (PBC), previously known as primary biliary cirrhosis, is a chronic cholestatic liver disorder characterized by lymphocytic cholangitis involving the small intralobular bile ducts within the liver (Figs. 162.1 and 162.2). This first step in PBC pathophysiology is followed by hepatotoxicity caused by the retention of toxic bile acids secondary to cholestasis and bile duct loss. The putative first "hit" is immunologic attack on intralobular bile ducts by activated T lymphocytes; this appears to be an autoimmune response in genetically predisposed persons. However, information is limited on the actual triggers initiating the T cell–mediated attack on bile duct cells. Although most patients with PBC have antibodies directed against the pyruvate dehydrogenase complex of mitochondria, it is unclear how this autoantibody leads to the attack of bile duct cells.

Recent data from the Fibrotic Liver Disease (FOLD) Consortium reveal that the prevalence of PBC in the United States is estimated at 29.3 per 100,000 persons, with an average age at diagnosis of 60 years, and higher prevalence in women (42.8 per 100,000 persons) and patients 60 to 70 years old (44.7 per 100,000 persons), and lower prevalence among men and African Americans. Approximately 95% of patients with PBC are women, and most are 25 to 85 years old; the diagnosis of PBC is rare in adolescents.

DIAGNOSIS

The diagnosis of PBC should be suspected in any patient with chronically elevated liver test findings in a cholestatic pattern, particularly with isolated elevation of serum alkaline phosphatase. Approximately 90% to 95% of patients are positive for the antimitochondrial antibody (AMA), which represents the serologic hallmark of the disease. However, positive AMA may be seen in 0.5% of the general population, of whom fewer than 10% will develop PBC. Conversely, approximately 5% of patients with PBC are negative for serum AMA and will require further confirmation based on characteristic clinical presentation, supportive pattern of liver injury, and histopathology. Elevated antinuclear antibody (ANA), antismooth muscle antibody (ASMA), and serum IgG (hyperglobulinemia) may also be seen. Liver biopsy in patients with PBC characteristically reveals a biliary type of chronic injury with nonsuppurative lymphocytic cholangitis, bile ductular proliferation, and variable degrees of fibrosis. Noncaseating granulomas are frequently present. Histologic stages include stage I (florid bile duct lesion), stage II (bile ductular proliferation), stage III (bridging fibrosis), and stage IV (cirrhosis) (Figs. 162.3 and 162.4). Interface hepatitis is usually absent.

Variants of PBC include the so-called autoimmune cholangiopathies or overlap syndromes. Such patients may have histologic features of PBC, but serologic findings suggest autoimmune hepatitis (antinuclear or ASMA).

The clinical presentation of PBC is highly variable and in early phases is often asymptomatic. However, fatigue and pruritus represent the most common presenting symptoms of PBC, both of which may be observed in up to 70% of patients. Other symptoms such as sicca syndrome (dry eyes and/or dry mouth), Raynaud phenomenon, and cutaneous calcinosis may also be seen.

The differential diagnosis of PBC includes any other cause of intrahepatic or extrahepatic cholestasis (Fig. 162.5). Drug-induced cholestasis is one of the most common liver diseases that may manifest in a manner similar to PBC. Increased estrogen levels due to pregnancy or oral contraceptives may also lead to intrahepatic cholestasis. Extrahepatic biliary tract obstruction is generally recognized by the identification of dilated intrahepatic or extrahepatic bile ducts on hepatobiliary imaging studies. Common causes include postoperative biliary strictures, bile duct cancer, and choledocholithiasis. Therefore it is essential to investigate and rule out biliary obstruction in any patient with acute or chronic cholestasis, particularly because cholestasis resulting from biliary obstruction may result in severe complications, and may be reversible with cholangiographic or surgical intervention. Unique histologic features of intrahepatic cholestasis caused by drugs or obstruction may help distinguish this condition from PBC in patients with atypical clinical history or negative AMA.

TREATMENT AND MANAGEMENT

Due to the underlying PBC pathophysiology of primary autoimmune-mediated bile duct injury and accumulation of toxic hydrophobic bile acids, the treatment of PBC has focused on immunosuppressive agents or drugs that reduce the toxicity associated with the retention of hydrophobic bile acids. Corticosteroids, azathioprine, cyclosporine, and other immunosuppressive therapies have been used without clear evidence of benefit.

The mainstay of therapy for PBC is *ursodeoxycholic acid* (UDCA). Multicenter randomized trials have clearly shown that UDCA slows the progression of PBC and decreases liver transplantation and mortality. Patients with moderate or severe disease appeared to derive the greatest benefit from UDCA, whereas those with mild histologic disease and well-compensated liver function (serum bilirubin < 1.4 mg/dL) did not benefit. By contrast, a US multicenter study found that patients with mild disease were most likely to benefit from UDCA; however, this study was only 2 years in duration. UDCA has been shown to improve histologic findings and possibly to reduce the severity of portal hypertension. Based on these data, UDCA was approved for the treatment of PBC at a dose of 13 to 15 mg/kg body weight daily, which appears to be superior to either low dose (5–7 mg/kg per day) or high-dose (23–25 mg/kg per day) regimens. The drug should be initiated gradually and administered in divided doses BID. Liver tests should be monitored while on therapy; approximately 20% of patients will experience normalization of liver enzymes within 2 years, and an estimated 90% of the improvement may occur within 6 to 9 months. There remain mixed findings with regard to the impact of UDCA on long-term clinical outcomes, although some recent studies suggest improvement in

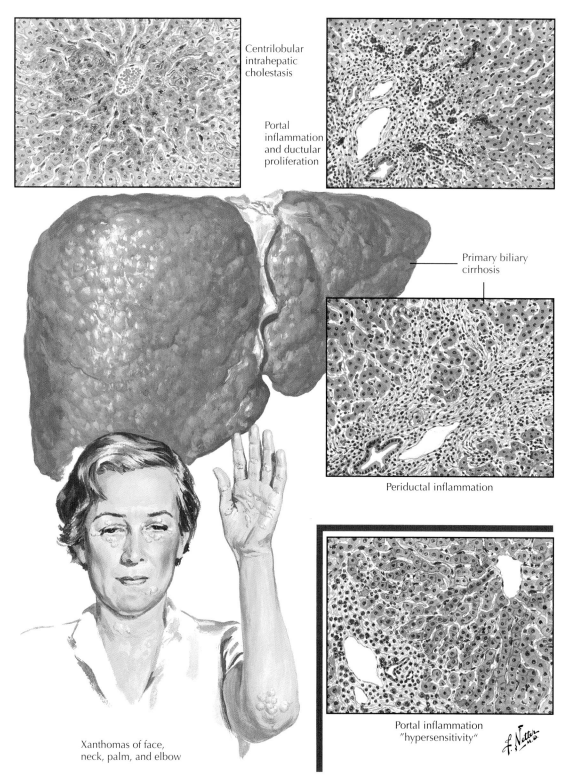

Centrilobular intrahepatic cholestasis

Portal inflammation and ductular proliferation

Primary biliary cirrhosis

Periductal inflammation

Portal inflammation "hypersensitivity"

Xanthomas of face, neck, palm, and elbow

Fig. 162.1 Pathologic Features of Primary Biliary Cirrhosis.

progression to cirrhosis, portal hypertension, and liver failure, although it does not appear to improve PBC-associated bone disease or symptoms of fatigue. Multiple scoring systems have been developed to assess response to therapy, including the Barcelona, Paris, Rotterdam, and Toronto criteria which largely focus on decrease in serum alkaline phosphatase and/or total bilirubin and liver transaminases. More recently, the GLOBE score (age, bilirubin, alkaline phosphatase, albumin, platelet count) at 1 year of UDCA therapy has demonstrated superior predictive value for transplant-free survival at 5, 10, and 15 years. For patients who fail to achieve biochemical response to UDCA after 6 to 12 months may consider salvage treatment with obeticholic acid (OCA), which has been approved by the US Food and Drug Administration (FDA) for the treatment of patients who fail to decrease serum alkaline phosphatase to less than 1.67 times upper limit of normal with UDCA. This

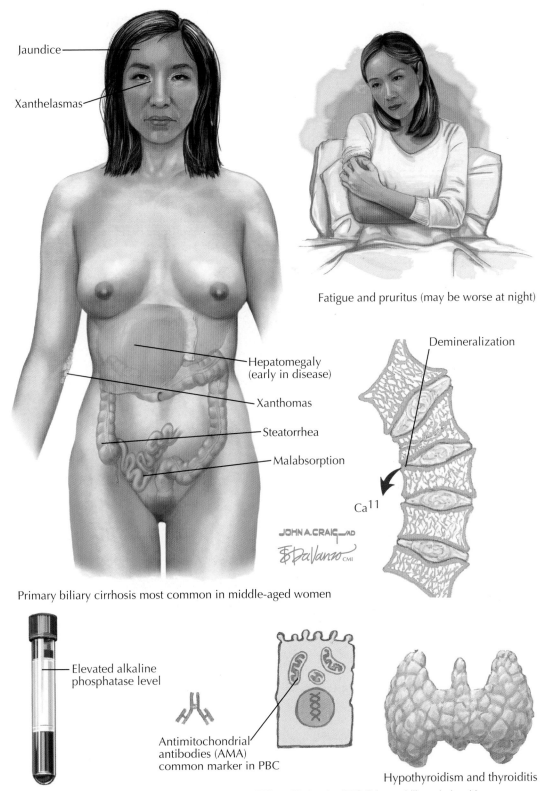

Jaundice

Xanthelasmas

Fatigue and pruritus (may be worse at night)

Demineralization

Hepatomegaly
(early in disease)

Xanthomas

Steatorrhea

Malabsorption

Ca^{11}

JOHN A.CRAIG—MD

Primary biliary cirrhosis most common in middle-aged women

Elevated alkaline
phosphatase level

Antimitochondrial
antibodies (AMA)
common marker in PBC

Hypothyroidism and thyroiditis

Fig. 162.2 Clinical Features of Primary Biliary Cirrhosis. *PBC,* Primary biliary cholangitis.

medication is dosed at 5 to 10 mg daily and requires careful monitoring due to known adverse effect of pruritus and should be used with great caution in patients with advanced liver disease in light of black box warning for severe liver events in patients with impaired liver synthetic function.

COURSE AND PROGNOSIS

Survival for patients with PBC is related to the stage of disease. Asymptomatic patients are not believed to be at increased risk for death from liver disease. Symptomatic patients are more likely to die of liver disease

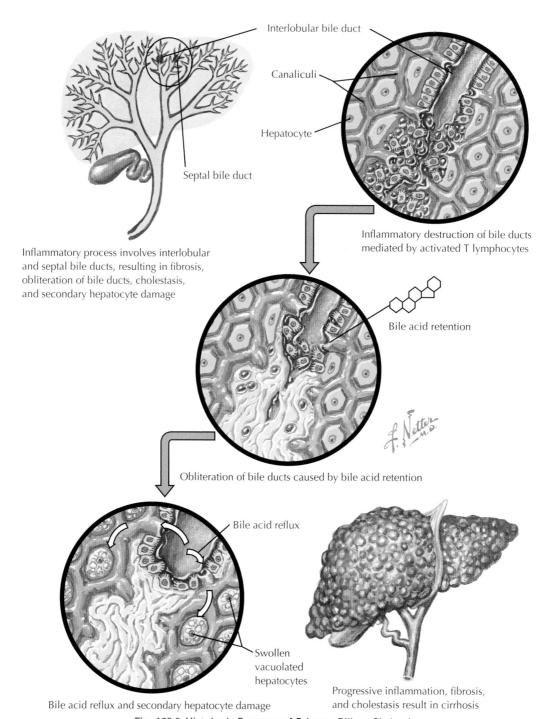

Interlobular bile duct

Canaliculi

Hepatocyte

Septal bile duct

Inflammatory process involves interlobular and septal bile ducts, resulting in fibrosis, obliteration of bile ducts, cholestasis, and secondary hepatocyte damage

Inflammatory destruction of bile ducts mediated by activated T lymphocytes

Bile acid retention

Obliteration of bile ducts caused by bile acid retention

Bile acid reflux

Swollen vacuolated hepatocytes

Bile acid reflux and secondary hepatocyte damage

Progressive inflammation, fibrosis, and cholestasis result in cirrhosis

Fig. 162.3 Histologic Features of Primary Biliary Cirrhosis.

than are control subjects. However, one study found that 90% of asymptomatic patients became symptomatic after a median follow-up of 7 years.

In addition to the GLOBE score, the *Mayo model* (serum albumin, bilirubin, prothrombin time, age, and degree of edema) has been demonstrated to predict survival for patients with and without liver transplantation and may be useful in patients with PBC-associated cirrhosis in determining the optimal time to place a patient on the liver transplantation list.

ADDITIONAL RESOURCES

Ali AH, Carey EJ, Lindor KD: Diagnosis and management of primary biliary cirrhosis, *Expert Rev Clin Immunol* 10:1667–1678, 2014.

Carey EJ, Ali AH, Lindor KD: Primary biliary cirrhosis, *Lancet* 386: 1565–1575, 2015.

Goldstein J, Levy C: Novel and emerging therapies for cholestatic liver disorders, *Liver Int* 2018. [Epub ahead of print].

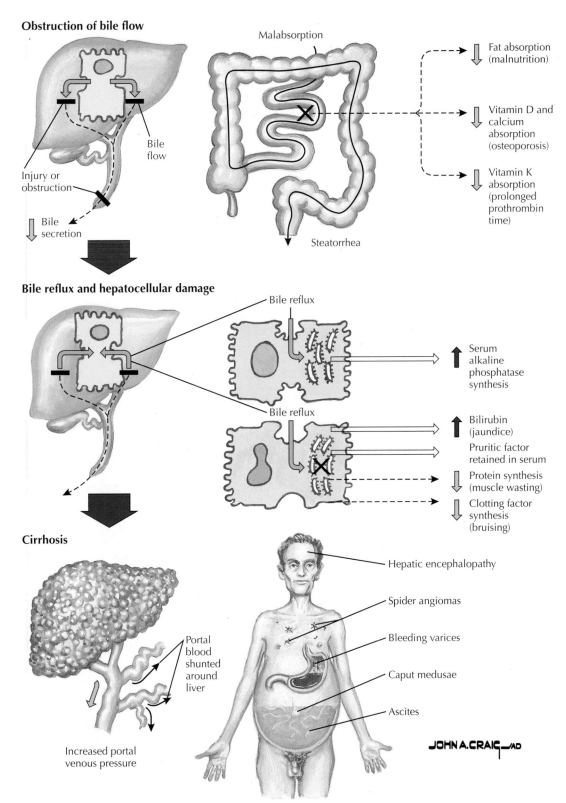

Fig. 162.4 Natural History of Cholestasis.

Hirschfield GM, Beuers U, Corpechot C, et al: EASL clinical practice guidelines: the diagnosis and management of patients with primary biliary cholangitis, *J Hepatol* 67:145–172, 2017.

Karlsen TH, Vesterhus M, Boberg KM: Review article: controversies in the management of primary biliary cirrhosis and primary sclerosing cholangitis, *Aliment Pharmacol Ther* 39:282–301, 2014.

Lindor KD, Gershwin ME, Poupon R, et al: Primary biliary cirrhosis, *Hepatology* 50:291–308, 2009.

Lu M, Li J, Haller IV, et al: Factors associated with prevalence and treatment of primary biliary cholangitis in United States health systems, *Clin Gastroenterol Hepatol* 16:1333–1341, 2018.

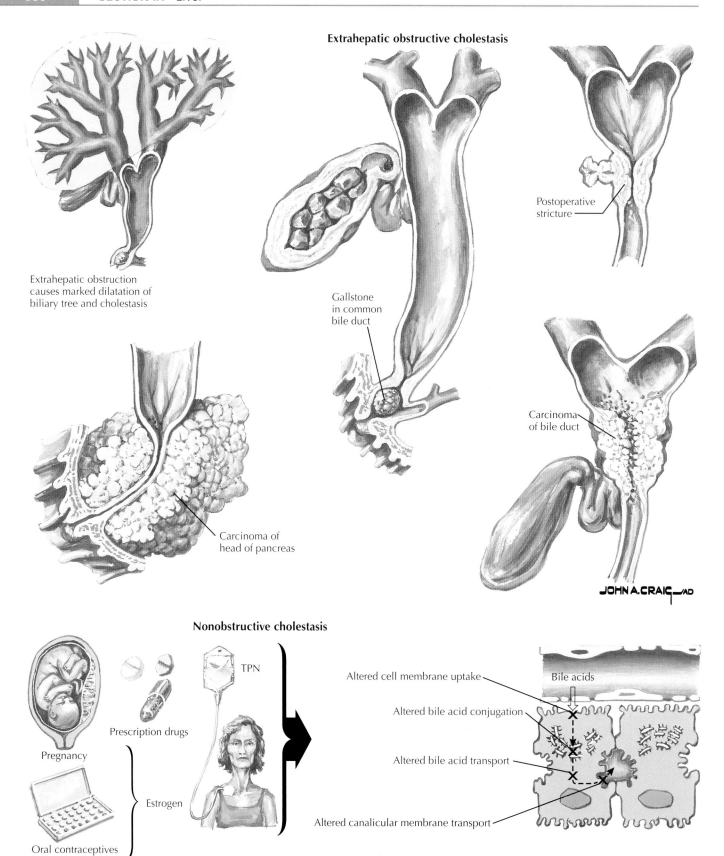

Extrahepatic obstructive cholestasis

Extrahepatic obstruction causes marked dilatation of biliary tree and cholestasis

Postoperative stricture

Gallstone in common bile duct

Carcinoma of bile duct

Carcinoma of head of pancreas

JOHN A. CRAIG—AD

Nonobstructive cholestasis

Pregnancy

Prescription drugs

TPN

Oral contraceptives

Estrogen

Bile acids

Altered cell membrane uptake

Altered bile acid conjugation

Altered bile acid transport

Altered canalicular membrane transport

Drugs, hormone changes, and other conditions can alter hepatocyte mechanisim (for bile acid uptake, conjugation transport, and excretion) causing cholestasis

Fig. 162.5 Differential Diagnosis for Primary Biliary Cirrhosis.

163

Primary Sclerosing Cholangitis

Joseph K. Lim, Kris V. Kowdley

Primary sclerosing cholangitis (PSC) represents a rare chronic, cholestatic liver disorder characterized by fibro-obliterative inflammation of the intrahepatic and extrahepatic bile duct system. Due to its strong association with inflammatory bowel disease (IBD), it is believed to have an autoimmune basis and may result in a chronic cholangiopathy with progressive fibrosis, cirrhosis, liver failure, and an increased risk for both colorectal cancer and hepatobiliary malignancies such as cholangiocarcinoma and hepatocellular carcinoma.

Several abnormalities of humoral immunity have been described in PSC, including elevated levels of serum immunoglobulin M (IgM) and IgG, as well as a high prevalence of autoantibodies, such as anti-smooth muscle antibody and antineutrophil cytoplasmic antibody. Cellular immunity is also altered in PSC. Expression of CD4 T cells in the liver is increased in PSC. One study found an antibody (colon epithelial protein [CEP]) in patients with PSC that had cross reactivity with colonic epithelial cells (Fig. 163.1).

CLINICAL PICTURE

Emerging evidence suggests genetic predisposition to PSC may influence expression of the disease, based on observations of increased prevalence among patients expressing HLA DRw52a or HLA B8, and mutations in cystic fibrosis transmembrane conductance regulator (CFTR), the cystic fibrosis gene. PSC also occurs more commonly in patients with IBD and specifically in those with *ulcerative colitis* (UC), which is observed in greater than 85% of patients with PSC and is associated with increased colonic mucosal permeability, which may promote bacterial infection of the biliary tree and chronic cholangitis.

The US and global prevalence of PSC is not clearly established, although the estimated U.S. prevalence ranges from 1 to 6 per 100,000 persons; a recent study suggested an age-adjusted point prevalence of 4.15 per 100,000 persons, with mean age at diagnosis of 44 years, with no significant difference observed between men and women. Some studies report that approximately 5% of UC patients have PSC. The estimated prevalence of UC ranges from 40 to 225 cases per 100,000; therefore 1 to 6 per 100,000 persons in the United States may have PSC. The challenge in deriving population-based estimates is the likelihood that at minimum 1 in 6 patients with PSC are asymptomatic. One study from a tertiary care referral center revealed that nearly 90% of PSC patients were found to have UC on histologic evaluation of rectal biopsy specimens, although commonly in the absence of clinical symptoms of colitis. Although two-thirds of all PSC patients are men, among patients without IBD, the male to female ratio is closer to 1:1 (Fig. 163.2).

DIAGNOSIS

The diagnosis of PSC is established on the basis of characteristic bile duct changes such as segmental dilatation and/or strictures within the intrahepatic and extrahepatic biliary tree on either magnetic resonance cholangiopancreatography (MRCP) or endoscopic retrograde cholangiopancreatography (ERCP). Percutaneous cholangiography can be considered if ERCP is unsuccessful, but it should be avoided, if possible, because of the greater technical difficulty and the increased risk for complications in the absence of intrahepatic dilatation.

Adequate filling of the intrahepatic ducts at ERCP is necessary before PSC can be excluded based on cholangiography. Cholangiography with an occlusion balloon may improve the quality of the study, but it may be associated with a higher risk for complications. Routine use of parenteral antibiotics is associated with a low rate of infectious complications in patients with PSC undergoing ERCP. A small proportion of patients with PSC may have normal findings on cholangiography due to selective involvement of smaller segmental bile ducts which may not be readily visible on standard fluoroscopic images obtained at cholangiography.

Liver biopsy is not routinely required for diagnosis but should be considered in cases of diagnostic uncertainty or to clarify stage of liver fibrosis. Classic findings of *onion skinning*, or concentric fibrosis around medium-sized bile ducts, may be identified in only 20% of histologic specimens. However, biopsy is particularly useful for determining the presence or absence of cirrhosis and thus may have important prognostic value. New noninvasive tools such as serum fibrosis assays and imaging-based elastography may soon represent viable alternatives to liver biopsy for fibrosis assessment in patients with an established diagnosis of PSC. Patients with PSC should also be considered for testing of serum IgG4 levels to exclude IgG4-associated sclerosing cholangitis.

Cholangiocarcinoma and Other Complications

The risk for cholangiocarcinoma is increased in patients with PSC (see Fig. 163.2). The true lifetime incidence of cholangiocarcinoma in PSC patients is estimated at 10% to 15%. Unfortunately, no effective screening tests are available for detecting cholangiocarcinoma early within a curative stage. Serum markers such as carcinoembryonic antigen (CEA) and cancer antigen 19-9 (CA 19-9) have been studied in PSC patients; elevated CA 19-9 level greater than 100 appears to be sensitive and specific for the diagnosis of cholangiocarcinoma in patients with PSC. Conversely, elevated serum CA 19-9 may be elevated in patients with cholangitis or cholestasis in the absence of cholangiocarcinoma. Patients with PSC are at increased risk for cholangitis, both to bile stasis associated with stricture and from obstruction caused by sludge or calculi.

TREATMENT AND MANAGEMENT

The primary treatment of PSC with dominant strictures is definitive endoscopic dilatation with or without stenting via ERCP, or alternatively percutaneous cholangiography with or without stenting if endoscopic decompression is unsuccessful or not feasible. Brush cytology and/or endoscopic biopsy should be considered in patients with a dominant

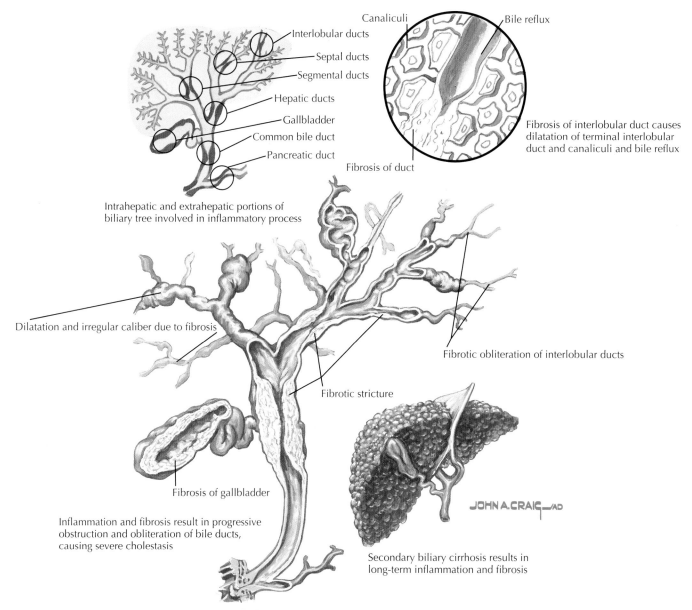

Canaliculi

Interlobular ducts

Bile reflux

Septal ducts

Segmental ducts

Hepatic ducts

Gallbladder

Common bile duct

Pancreatic duct

Fibrosis of interlobular duct causes dilatation of terminal interlobular duct and canaliculi and bile reflux

Fibrosis of duct

Intrahepatic and extrahepatic portions of biliary tree involved in inflammatory process

Dilatation and irregular caliber due to fibrosis

Fibrotic obliteration of interlobular ducts

Fibrotic stricture

Fibrosis of gallbladder

Inflammation and fibrosis result in progressive obstruction and obliteration of bile ducts, causing severe cholestasis

Secondary biliary cirrhosis results in long-term inflammation and fibrosis

JOHN A.CRAIG—AD

Fig. 163.1 Pathologic Features of Primary Sclerosing Cholangitis.

stricture to exclude a superimposed biliary malignancy. Surgical therapy represents a salvage treatment for dominant strictures if refractory to endoscopic and/or percutaneous intervention. Concurrent antibiotic therapy following decompression of biliary obstruction is commonly administered to resolve acute cholangitis; patients with recurrent or refractory cholangitis may require long-term antibiotics and consideration for liver transplantation. Several pharmacologic agents have been used to treat PSC, including corticosteroids and other immunosuppressive agents, methotrexate, and ursodeoxycholic acid (UDCA). In the largest randomized controlled trial, UDCA at 13 to 15 mg/kg per day was associated with a reduction in serum liver biochemistry values but did not improve clinical outcomes after up to 6 years of therapy. None of these agents was definitively shown to be effective in PSC. However, recent studies suggest that high-dose UDCA may be effective in PSC; 20 to 25 mg/kg per day was well tolerated and reduced serum

liver enzyme levels much more than lower doses. However, high-dose UDCA was not shown to improve survival or prevent cholangiocarcinoma in two large multicenter trials.

COURSE AND PROGNOSIS

Several studies have clearly shown that the risk for colon cancer is increased in patients with PSC and UC compared with patients with UC alone. Therefore it is appropriate for patients with UC associated with PSC to undergo annual surveillance colonoscopy with multiple biopsies every 10 cm from cecum to rectum. Patients found to have high-grade dysplasia or dysplasia associated with a mass lesion should be offered colectomy. Recent data suggest that UDCA may have a chemopreventive role in reducing the risk for dysplasia in patients with UC and PSC.

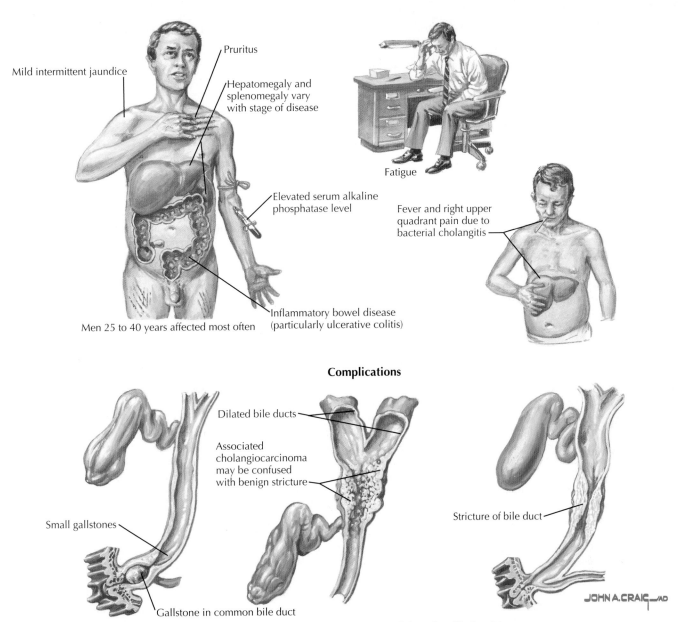

Mild intermittent jaundice

Pruritus

Hepatomegaly and splenomegaly vary with stage of disease

Fatigue

Elevated serum alkaline phosphatase level

Fever and right upper quadrant pain due to bacterial cholangitis

Men 25 to 40 years affected most often

Inflammatory bowel disease (particularly ulcerative colitis)

Complications

Dilated bile ducts

Associated cholangiocarcinoma may be confused with benign stricture

Small gallstones

Stricture of bile duct

Gallstone in common bile duct

JOHN A.CRAIG—AD

Fig. 163.2 Clinical Manifestations of Primary Sclerosing Cholangitis.

Patients with PSC are at increased risk for fat-soluble vitamin deficiency. In one study, up to 25% of PSC patients had low plasma levels of vitamin K_1 (phylloquinone, phytonadione); serum levels of the other fat-soluble vitamins (vitamin A, ^{25}[OH]-vitamin D, vitamin E) were also frequently low. Therefore it is recommended that serum levels of these vitamins be measured in patients with advanced cholestatic liver disease and that replacements be given if low levels are found. Vitamin A should be replaced with caution because of potential hepatotoxicity. Hyperlipidemia may overestimate vitamin E stores. Adjusting for plasma total lipids has been recommended when assessing vitamin E levels.

Metabolic bone disease is also more common among patients with PSC. Although osteomalacia caused by vitamin D deficiency may occasionally be found, osteoporosis is much more common.

ADDITIONAL RESOURCES

Eaton JE, Talwalkar JA, Lazaridis KN, et al: Pathogenesis of primary sclerosing cholangitis and advances in diagnosis and management, *Gastroenterology* 145:521–536, 2013.

Sedki M, Levy C: Update in the care and management of patients with primary sclerosing cholangitis, *Curr Gastroenterol Rep* 20:29, 2018.

Singh S, Talwalkar JA: Primary sclerosing cholangitis: diagnosis, prognosis, and management, *Clin Gastroenterol Hepatol* 11:898–907, 2013.

Sirpal S, Chandok N: Primary sclerosing cholangitis: diagnostic and management challenges, *Clin Exp Gastroenterol* 10:265–273, 2017.

Zein CO: Primary sclerosing cholangitis, *Clin Liver Dis* 17:211–227, 2013.

164

Autoimmune Hepatitis

Joseph K. Lim, Kris V. Kowdley

Autoimmune hepatitis (AIH) is an immune-mediated chronic liver disease believed to be initiated by the loss of tolerance to hepatocyte-specific autoantigens, which may occur spontaneously or be precipitated by antigens such as drugs, toxins, and viruses, particularly in susceptible individuals with a genetic predisposition (Fig. 164.1). AIH is characterized as a disease of young and middle-aged women, many of whom report a history of other autoimmune diseases, such as autoimmune thyroid disease, rheumatoid arthritis, psoriasis, or systemic lupus erythematosus. AIH may present in acute form, with jaundice and marked elevation of serum aminotransferases (transaminases) which signal either subfulminant or fulminant hepatitis, or alternatively as a chronic hepatitis with or without cirrhosis.

AIH may be classified as types 1, 2, and 3. Laboratory features of *type 1* include elevated liver enzymes, associated with hypergammaglobulinemia and autoantibodies at high titer (>1:120). The most common autoantibodies are antinuclear antibodies and antismooth muscle antibodies (ASMAs). *Type 2* AIH is associated with antibodies directed against LKM1 and LC-1, whereas *type 3* AIH may be associated with liver pathology revealing chronic hepatitis with an active chronic inflammatory infiltrate.

The diagnosis of AIH is established based on the presence of compatible clinical symptoms, elevated liver transaminases, increased total immunoglobulin G (IgG), and the presence of characteristic autoantibodies such as smooth muscle antibody (SMA), anti-LKM (liver-kidney-microsomal antibody), anti-SLA (soluble liver antigen antibody), or anti-LC1 (liver cytosolic antigen type 1 antibody). Liver biopsy is frequently required to confirm histologic hallmarks including plasma cell infiltration and *interface hepatitis*, which may be associated with *bridging necrosis*. The International Autoimmune Hepatitis Study Group has developed a classification system to facilitate the diagnosis of AIH based on clinical, laboratory, and histologic features which may help distinguish between negative, probable, or definite diagnosis of AIH. Similar to other autoimmune liver disorders, overlap syndromes which involve features of other conditions such as primary biliary cholangitis (PBC) and primary sclerosing cholangitis (PSC) may be observed.

Immunosuppressive drug therapy for management of AIH should be administered in patients who present with markedly elevated liver transaminases (serum aspartate aminotransferase [AST] or alanine aminotransferase [ALT] > 10× upper limit of normal) or levels > 5× upper limit of normal in tandem with elevated serum IgG > 2× upper limit of normal, and/or characteristic histologic features on liver biopsy with evidence of bridging or multilobular necrosis. Corticosteroids remain the primary immunosuppressive medication of choice, although consideration may be given for combination therapy with other agents such as 6-mercaptopurine or azathioprine as steroid-sparing therapies with the aim to initiate a slow taper of corticosteroid dose once remission has been achieved. Although multiple approaches to drug therapy have been adopted in clinical practice, a commonly recommended regimen includes initiation of prednisone at 30 mg daily in combination with azathioprine 50 mg daily. Patients should be counseled regarding the adverse effect profile of these agents, and blood thiopurine methyltransferase (TPMT) activity should be assessed in patients with cytopenia prior to or during the course of azathioprine treatment. Second-line therapies in patients who fail or are intolerant of these corticosteroids and/or 6-mercaptopurine (6-MP)/azathioprine include cyclosporine, tacrolimus, and mycophenolate.

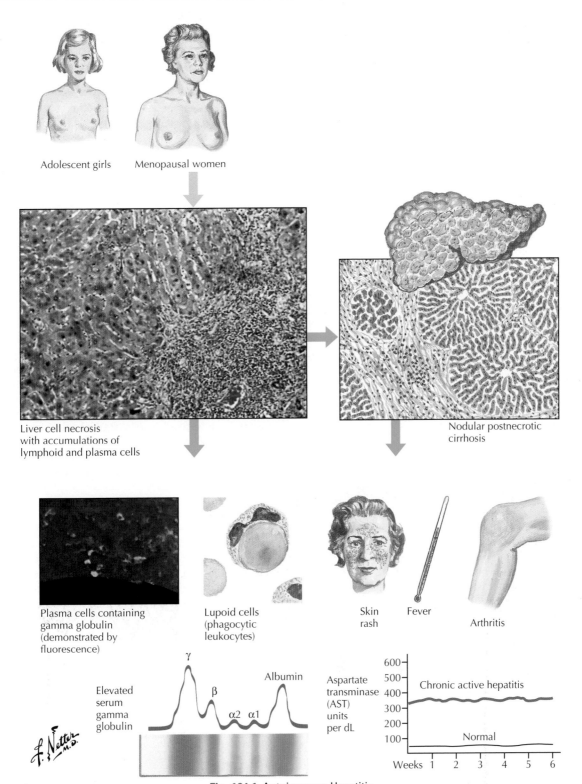

Fig. 164.1 Autoimmune Hepatitis.

ADDITIONAL RESOURCES

Czaja AJ: Diagnosis and management of autoimmune hepatitis, *Clin Liver Dis* 19:57–79, 2015.

Czaja AJ: Diagnosis and management of autoimmune hepatitis: current status and future directions, *Gut Liver* 10:177–203, 2016.

Czaja AJ: Review article: the management of autoimmune hepatitis beyond consensus guidelines, *Aliment Pharmacol Ther* 38:343–364, 2013.

Lohse AW, Chazouilleres O, Dalekos G, et al: EASL clinical practice guidelines: autoimmune hepatitis, *J Hepatol* 63:971–1004, 2015.

Manns MP, Czaja AJ, Gorham JD, et al: Diagnosis and management of autoimmune hepatitis, *Hepatology* 51:2193–2213, 2010.

Schmeltzer PA, Russo MW: Clinical narrative: autoimmune hepatitis, *Am J Gastroenterol* 2018. [Epub ahead of print].

165

Acute Viral Hepatitis (Hepatitis A, D, E)

Joseph K. Lim, Kris V. Kowdley

Acute hepatitis with a predominant hepatocellular pattern of liver injury may occur as a consequence of a diverse spectrum of etiologies, including both nonhepatotrophic and hepatotrophic viruses. Among the latter group, hepatitis A, hepatitis B, and hepatitis E infections are the most common source for acute viral hepatitis. Acute hepatitis D infection may also occur rarely in context of coexisting acute hepatitis B infection or as a superinfection in patients with chronic hepatitis B infection. Other viruses associated with acute viral hepatitis include cytomegalovirus (CMV), herpes simplex virus (HSV), and Epstein-Barr virus (EBV), which are less often associated with icteric hepatitis.

HEPATITIS A

Hepatitis A virus (HAV) is phylogenetically distinct from the other hepatitis viruses and belongs to a new genus described as *Hepatovirus*. HAV is a nonenveloped virus capable of surviving in a variety of external environments, such as dried feces and live oysters, for a prolonged time, and it can withstand relatively warm temperatures. Major modes of transmission are fecal-oral and person to person and through contaminated food and water. The incubation period is generally 1 to 2 weeks. Viral shedding in the stool often occurs before symptoms develop. Recent outbreaks of acute hepatitis A in major US cities, including San Diego and Salt Lake City in 2017 to 2018, have raised attention of public health agencies to this source of acute viral hepatitis.

The typical course of acute HAV and other viral hepatitis infections is shown in Figs. 165.1 to 165.3.

Clinical Picture

Acute HAV infection may present clinically in a manner similar to any other form of acute hepatitis. Moderate to marked elevation of serum transaminases (aminotransferases) may be present. The likelihood of jaundice increases with increasing length of exposure. Neonates and children are often asymptomatic. In fact, in many areas of the developing world, a large proportion of the population appears to have been previously exposed to HAV, based on the presence of positive anti-HAV antibody.

Several clinical patterns of HAV infection may be recognized. Acute infection may be completely asymptomatic, especially in very young patients. Many patients have symptomatic acute *icteric* hepatitis and may have all the characteristic symptoms, such as fatigue, lethargy, nausea, abdominal pain, and anorexia. Occasionally, a *cholestatic* variant may be observed, with prolonged jaundice and a highly cholestatic pattern of liver test abnormalities. *Relapsing* hepatitis has been reported in some patients, with apparent remissions and relapses that may last several months. Cholestasis and relapsing hepatitis do not increase mortality risk. In a small subset of patients, *fulminant* hepatitis may occur, necessitating urgent liver transplantation. Aplastic anemia is another rare but serious complication of acute HAV.

The incidence of these serious complications is less than 5%. Mortality risk in patients older than 50 is significantly greater than among younger patients. Chronic hepatitis is not observed among patients with acute HAV infection.

Diagnosis and Management

The diagnosis of acute HAV is established with the detection of immunoglobulin M (IgM) anti-HAV antibody in the serum. IgM anti-HAV antibody appears early in the course of infection and disappears after approximately 4 to 5 months, after which immunoglobulin G (IgG) antibody appears in the serum. IgG anti-HAV antibody is usually detectable years after infection and presumably confers lifelong immunity.

Vaccination against HAV is now widely available. In addition to its necessity for travel to areas where HAV is endemic, vaccination is recommended for all patients with chronic liver disease or immunosuppression and for homosexual men. Serum immunoglobulin injections are used for postexposure prophylaxis and should be given within 2 weeks of exposure.

HEPATITIS D

Hepatitis D virus (HDV) is a defective ribonucleic acid (RNA) virus that requires the presence of hepatitis B surface antigen (HBsAg) for infectivity. The most common modes of transmission are *coinfection* with HBV in acute infection or *superinfection* in a chronic HBV patient. In Western countries, HDV is observed predominantly in patients who are intravenous (IV) drug users and those who have had multiple blood transfusions. Acute coinfection of HDV is associated with an increased risk of fulminant hepatitis, whereas HDV superinfection in the patient with chronic HBV infection may accelerate HBV progression.

Three common HDV genotypes (1–3) have been described. Interferon therapy has been used with limited success in patients with chronic HDV infection. New investigational therapies, including those focused on oral prenylation inhibitors and oral entry inhibitors, are currently under investigation for treatment of HDV infection.

HEPATITIS E

Hepatitis E virus (HEV) is a nonenveloped RNA virus transmitted through the fecal-oral route. Large epidemics have been attributed to HEV in southeast and central Asia, the Middle East, Africa, and Mexico. Outbreaks in Mexico make this form of acute viral hepatitis clinically relevant in the United States.

Hepatitis E may be more common in developed countries than previously estimated, and HEV may be transmitted from other animals, particularly pigs. The common modes of transmission in endemic countries is usually contaminated water or water supply, although vertical transmission has been associated with acute, severe hepatitis in

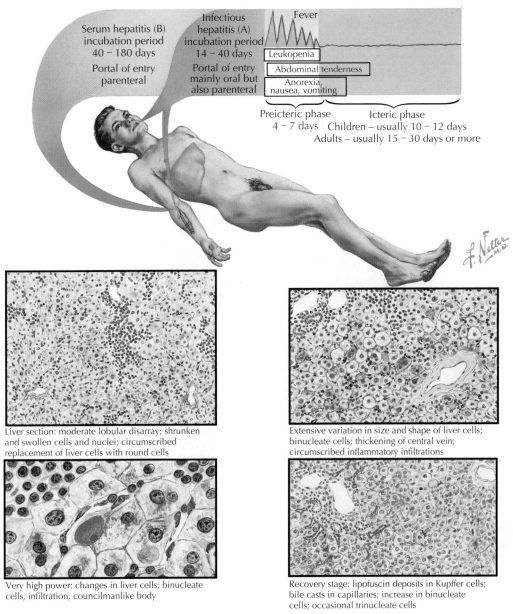

Fig. 165.1 Viral Hepatitis: Acute Form.

neonates in the presence of HEV RNA. The incubation period may be as short as 2 weeks, but the average is 6 weeks. Viral shedding begins 1 week before the onset of symptoms and last 2 to 3 weeks.

Clinical Picture

The clinical features of HEV infection are distinct. Some have reported that gastrointestinal symptoms such as diarrhea are more common than with other causes of acute viral hepatitis. Young adults appear to be at greatest risk for clinical disease. The case-fatality ratio is particularly high among pregnant women, especially in the third trimester, with mortality rates as high as 25%. As with HAV infection, chronic

disease does not occur, and HEV patients who recover do not develop chronic liver disease.

Diagnosis and Management

The diagnosis of HEV is made by detecting anti-HEV antibody in the serum. As with HAV, there is initially an IgM antibody to HEV that disappears over 4 to 5 months and is replaced by IgG antibody. Measuring HEV RNA in serum is possible and may be helpful early in the course of infection or in immunosuppressed persons. No vaccines against HEV are available; therefore the best form of prevention is to avoid possibly contaminated water.

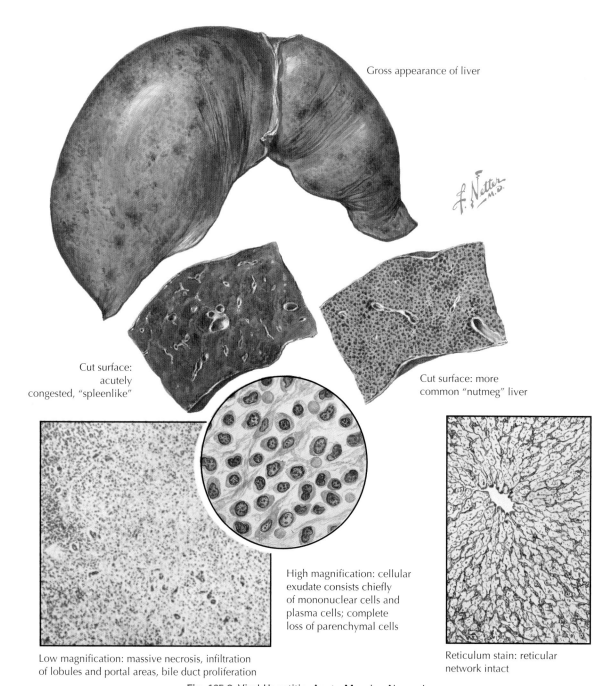

Gross appearance of liver

Cut surface: acutely congested, "spleenlike"

Cut surface: more common "nutmeg" liver

High magnification: cellular exudate consists chiefly of mononuclear cells and plasma cells; complete loss of parenchymal cells

Low magnification: massive necrosis, infiltration of lobules and portal areas, bile duct proliferation

Reticulum stain: reticular network intact

Fig. 165.2 Viral Hepatitis: Acute Massive Necrosis.

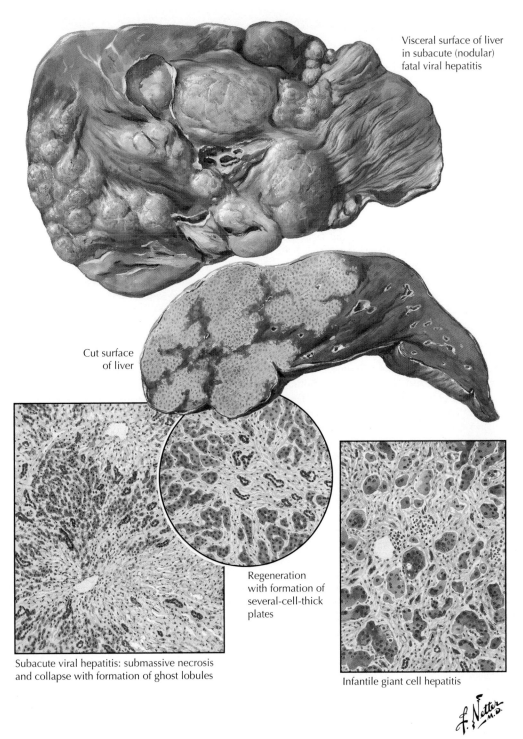

Visceral surface of liver in subacute (nodular) fatal viral hepatitis

Cut surface of liver

Regeneration with formation of several-cell-thick plates

Subacute viral hepatitis: submassive necrosis and collapse with formation of ghost lobules

Infantile giant cell hepatitis

Fig. 165.3 Viral Hepatitis: Subacute Fatal Form.

ADDITIONAL RESOURCES

Alves VAF: Acute viral hepatitis: beyond A, B, and C, *Surg Pathol Clin* 11:251–266, 2018.

Cullen JM, Lemon SM: Comparative pathology of hepatitis A virus and hepatitis E virus infection, *Cold Spring Harb Perspect Med* 2018. [Epub ahead of print].

Elazar M, Koh C, Glenn JS: Hepatitis delta infection—current and new treatment options, *Best Pract Res Clin Gastroenterol* 31:321–327, 2017.

Horvatits T, Ozga AK, Westholter D, et al: Hepatitis E seroprevalence in the Americas: a systematic review and meta-analysis, *Liver Int* 2018. [Epub ahead of print].

Kamar N, Dalton HR, Abravanel F, Izopet J: Hepatitis E virus infection, *Clin Microbiol Rev* 27:116–138, 2014.

Mohsen W, Lew MT: Hepatitis A to E: what's new?, *Intern Med J* 47:380–389, 2017.

Ponde RAA: The serological markers of acute infection with hepatitis A, B, C, D, E, and G viruses revisited, *Arch Virol* 162:3587–3602, 2017.

Von Wulffen M, Westholter D, Lutgehetmann M, Pischke S: Hepatitis E: still waters run deep, *J Clin Transl Hepatol* 6:40–47, 2018.

Hepatitis B

Joseph K. Lim, Kris V. Kowdley

Hepatitis B virus (HBV) is an enveloped, double-strand DNA virus within the Hepadnavirus family that can cause acute and chronic hepatitis. In certain populations, including Southeast Asians, Alaskan natives, and sub-Saharan Africans, in areas where HBV is highly endemic, the prevalence of chronic hepatitis B is as high as 20%. In these populations, the virus is transmitted primarily through the maternal-neonatal route, and infection usually develops during infancy or early childhood. Most infected persons exposed through maternofetal transmission acquire chronic infection. In parts of the world with low endemicity, including the United States, Canada, and Western Europe, HBV transmission occurs primarily through sexual contact in early adulthood. In this population, the clearance of hepatitis B surface antigen (HBsAg) and the development of immunity to HBV follow episodes of acute HBV infection. Fewer than 5% of these patients acquire chronic hepatitis B. However, a small proportion of patients with acute hepatitis B develops fulminant hepatitis and must undergo emergency liver transplantation. The updated 2016 estimate of global burden of chronic HBV infection is estimated at 292 million persons.

CLINICAL PICTURE

The clinical features of acute hepatitis B are variable in presentation. Initial infection may be asymptomatic, although it may transition to an icteric phase marked by overt jaundice and scleral icterus. Patients with neonatally acquired infection may have a long immunotolerant phase in the first several decades of life associated with high levels of HBV viremia but normal liver enzyme levels and minimal changes on biopsy. However, over time these patients may transition to an immunoactive phase, also known as immune clearance phase, which is marked by high HBV DNA, significantly elevated liver transaminases, and active necroinflammatory changes on biopsy, and may additionally be associated with clinical symptoms. These patients typically transition to an inactive phase in which the HBV DNA may be low or undetectable and associated with normal liver enzymes and minimal inflammation on biopsy. The majority of these patients may remain within this inactive phase long term, although a subset may experience reactivation of the virus infection, which occurs spontaneously or in context of immunosuppressive drug therapy. These reactivation flares are marked by elevated liver function tests (LFTs) and HBV DNA which may be associated with fulminant hepatitis.

The major long-term sequelae of chronic HBV infection include cirrhosis and hepatocellular carcinoma (HCC). Unlike most etiologies of chronic liver disease, HBV infection may be associated with HCC in the absence of significant liver fibrosis or cirrhosis and occur at any phase of infection; global epidemiology figures confirm that HBV represents the second leading carcinogen, after tobacco, due to its relationship with HCC. The risk for HCC is greatest in patients infected early in life, with ongoing viral replication, and in particular in patients with cirrhosis. Current guidelines recommend routine HCC surveillance in patients with chronic HBV infection who are at increased risk, including African patients age 20 years or older, Asian males age 40 years or older, Asian females age 50 years or older, patients with cirrhosis, and patients with a family history of HCC.

Extrahepatic Manifestations

Several extrahepatic manifestations of chronic hepatitis B have been reported, including vasculitis (particularly polyarteritis nodosa), glomerulonephritis, and essential mixed cryoglobulinemia. Furthermore, chronic HBV has been associated with several nonliver malignancies, most notably B-cell lymphoma.

DIAGNOSIS

The diagnosis of chronic hepatitis B infection is most commonly established on the basis of a positive HBsAg, which represents the initial screening test of choice. Testing for hepatitis B core antibody (HBcAb) and hepatitis B surface antibody (HBsAb) further clarifies prior exposure and immunity to HBV, respectively. Due to a mutation in the HBsAg, a rare subtype of chronic HBV infection is characterized by negative HBsAg, positive HBcAb, and positive HBV DNA, also known as chronic occult hepatitis B infection. Patients who are confirmed to have chronic HBV require regular laboratory surveillance with HBV viral load (quantitative HBV DNA), liver enzymes, and clarification of hepatitis B envelope antigen (HBeAg) and hepatitis B envelope antibody (HBeAb), as well as consideration for testing for HBV genotype. Patients with chronic HBV should be tested for hepatitis A virus (HAV) total antibody (Ab) to confirm immunity, as well as consideration for hepatitis C virus (HCV) Ab, human immunodeficiency virus (HIV) Ab, and hepatitis delta virus (HDV) Ab to exclude viral coinfections. However, the three-test panel of HBsAg, HBcAb, and HBsAb represents the initial diagnostic step of choice for chronic HBV infection (Fig. 166.1).

The term *chronic hepatitis B* refers to patients who are chronically infected (i.e., HBsAg positive ≥6 months). Chronic hepatitis B with evidence of persistent HBV DNA in the serum is described as *replicative* ("chronic active hepatitis"), whereas chronic hepatitis B that is persistently HBV DNA negative (very low levels in serum using polymerase chain reaction [PCR]-based assay) is classified as *nonreplicative* ("carrier hepatitis"). Patients with HBV DNA levels greater than 2000 IU/mL have replicative disease, although this cut-off level is arbitrary. The role of the HBeAg is to classify patients who are in the replicative phase as patients with a *wild-type* (HBeAg positive) or *precore mutant* profile. Most patients with high levels of HBV DNA in the blood but without measurable levels of HBeAg are thought to have a precore mutant variant of HBV (associated with stop codon in precore region

Acute Hepatitis B Virus Infection with Recovery Typical Serologic Course

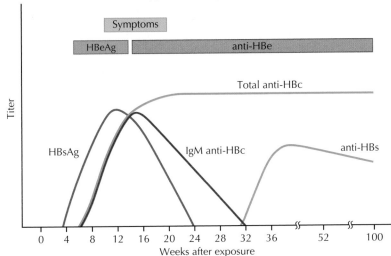

Fig. 166.1 Typical Serologic Course of Acute Hepatitis B With Recovery. *HBc,* Hepatitis B core; *HBe,* hepatitis B envelope; *HBeAg,* hepatitis B envelope antigen; *HBs,* hepatitis B surface; *HBsAg,* hepatitis B surface antigen.

Note: Serologic markers of HBV infection vary depending on whether the infection is acute or chronic.

The first serologic marker to appear following acute infection is HBsAg, which can be detected as early as 1 or 2 weeks and as late as 11 or 12 weeks (mode, 30-60 days) after exposure to HBV. In persons who recover, HBsAg is no longer detectable in serum after an average period of about 3 months. HBeAg is generally detectable in patients with acute infection; the presence of HBeAg in serum correlates with higer titers of HBV and greater infectivity. A diagnosis of acute HBV infection can be made based on the detection of IgM class antibody to hepatitis B core antigen (IgM anti-HBc) in serum; IgM anti-HBc is generally detectable at the time of clinical onset and declines to sub-detectable levels within 6 months. IgG anti-HBc persists indefinitely as a marker of past infection. Anti-HBs becomes detectable during convalescence after the disappearance of HBsAg in patients who do not progress to chronic infection. The presence of anti-HBs following acute infection generally indicates recovery and immunity from reinfection.

Source: Centers for Disease Control.

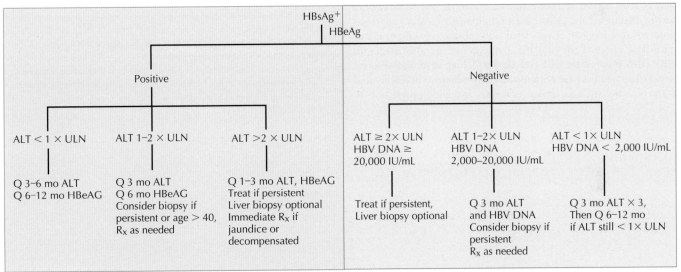

Fig. 166.2 Management of Chronic Hepatitis B Virus. *ALT,* Alanine aminotransferase; *HBeAg,* hepatitis B envelope antigen; *HBsAg,* hepatitis B surface antigen; *HBV,* hepatitis B virus; *ULN,* upper limit of normal.

of genome) and thus an inability to transcribe and translate the e protein. Alternatively, patients with HBeAg-negative chronic hepatitis B may have mutations in the basal core promoter, which downregulates eAg production.

Histologic findings in chronic HBV may resemble any other type of chronic hepatitis, with features of hepatic necroinflammation, interface hepatitis, and variable amounts of fibrosis. Unique to HBV may be the finding of ground-glass hepatocytes, which represent HBsAg. Histologic scoring systems used to grade and stage chronic hepatitis B include the Knodell Histologic Activity Index and the Batts-Ludwig, Ishak, and Meta-analysis of Histological Data in Viral Hepatitis (METAVIR) systems. Noninvasive fibrosis assessment tools including serum indices (e.g., APRI, FIB-4), serum assays (e.g., FibroTest/FibroSure, Hepascore), and imaging-based elastography (e.g., vibration-controlled transient elastography, shear wave elastography, magnetic resonance elastography) are now commonly used in place of liver biopsy for identification of patients with significant liver fibrosis to guide management.

TREATMENT AND MANAGEMENT

The primary goals of treatment for patients with chronic hepatitis B is to suppress viral replication, enable seroconversion from the HBeAg-positive to the HBeAb-positive state, normalize serum liver enzymes, and improve or stabilize histology (Fig. 166.2). Eight treatments are currently approved by the US Food and Drug Administration (FDA) for chronic hepatitis B: interferon-α (IFN-α), pegylated IFN alpha-2a (PEG-IFN), lamivudine, adefovir, entecavir, telbivudine, tenofovir disiproxil fumarate (TDF), and tenofovir alafenamide fumarate (TAF).

IFN-α is administered subcutaneously at 5 million units daily or 10 million units three times a week. PEG-IFN is administered at 180 mg subcutaneously once a week for 48 weeks. The advantages of IFN therapy include the finite duration of therapy, lack of resistance, and small possibility of HBsAg loss. However, IFN is associated with many adverse effects, such as flulike symptoms, depression, anemia, rashes, and autoimmune phenomena. Furthermore, patients frequently experience a "flare" of hepatitis during IFN therapy, which is often poorly tolerated in patients with cirrhosis, in whom IFN should be avoided.

There are three first line treatment options in current guidelines of the American Association for the Study of Liver Diseases (AASLD), European Association for the Study of the Liver (EASL), US Treatment Algorithm, and Asian American Treatment Recommendations, including PEG-IFN, entecavir, and tenofovir. *Tenofovir* and *entecavir* are potent oral agents with much lower resistance profiles and are safe and effective for long-term therapy. *Entecavir* is an oral nucleoside analogue which is associated with high efficacy, including an estimated 67% of HBeAg-positive patients achieving viral suppression to undetectable HBV DNA levels within 1 year of therapy and very low resistance rates of 1.7% up to 6 years. Tenofovir is an oral nucleotide analogue which is also associated with high efficacy, including an estimated 76% of HBeAg-positive patients achieving viral suppression to undetectable HBV DNA levels within 1 year and 0% resistance up to 6 years of therapy. The original analogue of TDF has been associated with low rates of renal toxicity and bone mineral density decline which require careful monitoring and patient selection, although a recently approved prodrug analogue, TAF, is associated with substantially lower rates of renal/bone effects. Both entecavir and tenofovir are associated with HBV DNA suppression rates exceeding 90% long term, and observational cohort studies have demonstrated improvements in biochemical markers, histology, and clinical outcomes including progression to cirrhosis, liver failure, and risk for HCC. Other historical antivirals for HBV are rarely used at this time, including lamivudine, adefovir, and telbivudine, which are associated with higher rates of drug resistance and/or adverse effects. Importantly, none of the oral antivirals are aimed at viral eradication and are routinely required for chronic treatment of indefinite duration; novel investigational agents currently in development (e.g., RNA interference, core/capsid inhibitors, core protein allosteric modifiers, immunomodulators) are focused on functional cure with HBsAg loss and HBsAb seroconversion.

Liver transplantation has been performed for end-stage liver disease caused by hepatitis B. Early reports suggested a high rate of recurrence of hepatitis and associated graft failure and decreased survival. The use of high-dose parenteral hepatitis B immune globulin and, more recently, the addition of antiviral therapy have greatly reduced the risk for recurrent hepatitis and improved graft and patient survival.

ADDITIONAL RESOURCES

Feld J, Janssen HL, Abbas Z, et al: World gastroenterology organisation global guideline hepatitis B, *J Clin Gastroenterol* 50:691–703, 2016.

Lampertico P, Agarwal K, Berg T, et al: EASL 2017 clinical practice guidelines on the management of hepatitis B virus infection, *J Hepatol* 67:370–398, 2017.

Martin P, Lau DT, Nguyen MH, et al: A treatment algorithm for the management of chronic hepatitis B virus infection in the United States; 2015 update, *Clin Gastroenterol Hepatol* 13:2071–2087, 2015.

Sundaram V, Kowdley K: Management of chronic hepatitis B infection, *BMJ* 351:h4263, 2015.

Tang LSY, Covert E, Wilson E, Kottilil S: Chronic hepatitis B infection: a review, *JAMA* 319:1802–1813, 2018.

Terrault NA, Lok ASF, McMahon BJ, et al: Update on prevention, diagnosis, and treatment of chronic hepatitis B: AASLD 2018 hepatitis B guidance, *Hepatology* 67:1560–1599, 2018.

167

Hepatitis C

Joseph K. Lim

Chronic hepatitis C virus (HCV) infection is a common bloodborne disease, affecting an estimated 3 to 5 million persons in the United States and more than 71 million persons worldwide. It was first recognized as a transfusion-associated hepatitis virus in the 1970s and described as non-A, non-B hepatitis (NANBH) until the virus was identified in 1989, ultimately leading to the initial development of antibody assays in 1992 for the diagnosis of HCV infection.

The most common routes of transmission of HCV are bloodborne, including injection or intranasal drug use, tattoo exposures, needlestick injuries, or blood transfusions, although sexual transmission may rarely occur, particularly among men who have sex with men (MSM). Acute hepatitis C infection is often asymptomatic and is associated with a very low rate of fulminant hepatitis/liver failure, estimated at 0.1%. The vast majority of patients (60%–85%) will then transition to chronic infection, although some patients may experience spontaneous immunologic clearance with resolution of infection. Chronic HCV infection is associated with substantial morbidity and mortality due to the risk for long-term progression to cirrhosis, liver failure, and liver cancer, which most commonly occur over the courses of several decades of infection, although cofactors for disease progression such as fatty liver, human immunodeficiency virus (HIV), and alcohol may contribute to faster disease progression.

CLINICAL PICTURE

Chronic HCV infection is frequently indolent in nature without detectable clinical symptoms, and a subset may have persistently normal liver enzymes in the presence of histologic inflammation and fibrosis. As such, identification of HCV requires a high index of clinical suspicion in patients with risk factors. Patients should undergo testing for genotype, as well as assessment of coinfection with HBV and/or HIV, as well as immunization for both hepatitis A virus (HAV) and hepatitis B virus (HBV). Assessment of liver fibrosis represents an essential step in the management of patients with chronic HCV infection. Although liver biopsy remains the "gold standard" test, noninvasive biomarkers including serum indices (e.g., APRI, FIB-4), serum assays (e.g., FibroTest, Hepascore), and imaging-based elastography (e.g., vibration-controlled transient elastography [VCTE], acoustic radiation force impulse imaging [ARFI], magnetic resonance elastography [MRE]) have emerged as important tools which obvious histologic examination in most patients. Approximately 20% to 25% of patients experience progression to cirrhosis within 20 years of infection, although a subset of patients may have an indolent course without progression to cirrhosis even after 40 to 60 years of infection. The risk for hepatocellular carcinoma (HCC) is estimated at 1% to 5% per year after 20 years of infection or 1% to 4% per year in patients with cirrhosis (Fig. 167.1).

DIAGNOSIS

Chronic hepatitis C should be considered in any patient with risk factors for acquisition (e.g., blood transfusions before 1992, injection drug use, tattoos or skin piercings, hemodialysis, multiple sex partners) and individuals with elevated liver enzymes (alanine aminotransferase [ALT], aspartate aminotransferase [AST]). Studies have revealed that more than three-quarters of US patients with HCV were born between the years 1945 and 1965 (also known as "baby boomers"), in whom routine screening is now recommended by the Centers for Disease Control and Prevention (CDC) and US Preventive Services Task Force (USPSTF).

The most widely used diagnostic test for hepatitis C is a second- or third-generation *enzyme-linked immunosorbent assay* (ELISA), which has high sensitivity estimated at 92% to 95% and positive predictive value of 25% to 60%. False-positive results may occur, although they are less common with new generation assays; false-negative results are uncommon, although they have been observed in patients with HIV/AIDS, in whom HCV RNA may be required to exclude HCV in patients with multiple risk factors for infection. *Recombinant immunoblot assay* has historically been used to confirm ELISA results, although it has recently been discontinued, and therefore chronic infection is confirmed with positive HCV RNA. The timing of diagnostic testing influences likelihood of identifying HCV infection. HCV RNA is the first test to identify HCV within serum, typically within the first 1 to 3 weeks, whereas HCV antibody may appear only after 1 to 3 months, and serum ALT elevation may occur in the second or third month after initial infection.

TREATMENT AND MANAGEMENT

The treatment of chronic hepatitis C infection has been transformed since 2013 with the advent of oral direct-acting antivirals (DAAs), which have formed a new standard of care in place of historical interferon-based regimens, which were associated with significant toxicity and low efficacy. Oral DAA regimens are composed of the combination of two or three distinct classes of antivirals, including NS3/4A protease inhibitors, NS5A inhibitors, and NS5B nucleoside or nonnucleoside polymerase inhibitors. First-line oral DAA regimens include sofosbuvir/ledipasvir, grazoprevir/elbasvir, glecaprevir/pibrentasvir, and sofosbuvir/velpatasvir, the latter two of which are pangenotypic, having activity against all six HCV genotypes. These regimens are associated with very high rates of viral eradication, exceeding 90%, defined as a sustained virologic response (SVR) with undetectable HCV RNA for 12 weeks following the end of treatment. Salvage regimens for patients who have failed oral DAA regimens such as sofosbuvir/ledipasvir, grazoprevir/elbasvir, and sofosbuvir/velpatasvir may be eligible for retreatment with triple

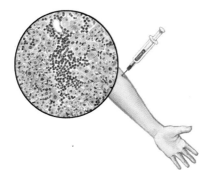

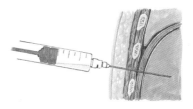

Most patients with HCV have abnormal liver (ALT, AST) findings.

Liver biopsy plays an important role in diagnosis and prognosis.

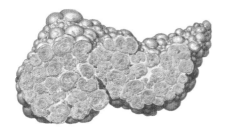

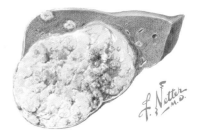

Twenty percent of patients develop cirrhosis by 20 years of age.

The risk for hepatocellular carcinoma is estimated to be 1% to 5% per year after 20 years of disease or 1% to 4% per year in patients with cirrhosis.

Fig. 167.1 Clinical Picture of Hepatitis C Infection. *HCV,* Hepatitis C virus.

combination therapy with sofosbuvir/velpatasvir/voxilaprevir per American Association for the Study of Liver Disease (AASLD)/Infectious Diseases Society of America (IDSA) guidelines.

SVR is associated with significant clinical benefits, including a decrease in risk for progression to cirrhosis, hepatic decompensation, HCC, and both liver-related and all-cause mortality. More recent data suggest that a series of extrahepatic manifestations such as cryoglobulinemic vasculitis, membranoproliferative glomerulonephritis (MPGN), and porphyria cutanea tarda (PCT) may improve in some patients. Nevertheless, a subset of patients who experience SVR remain at long-term risk for progression to cirrhosis and liver cancer and require ongoing HCC surveillance imaging, particularly if the patient has risk factors for ongoing liver injury such as alcohol consumption or fatty liver disease.

ADDITIONAL RESOURCES

Chung RT, Davis GL, Jensen DM, et al: Hepatitis C guidance: AASLD-IDSA recommendations for testing, managing, and treating adults infected with hepatitis C virus, *Hepatology* 62:932–954, 2015.

Falade-Nwulia O, Suarez-Cuervo C, Nelson DR, et al: Oral direct-acting agent therapy for hepatitis C virus infection: a systematic review, *Ann Intern Med* 166:637–648, 2017.

Omata M, Kanda T, Wei L, et al: APASL consensus statements and recommendations for hepatitis C prevention, epidemiology, and laboratory testing, *Hepatol Int* 10:681–701, 2016.

Pawlotsky JM, Negro F, Aghemo A, et al: EASL recommendations on treatment of hepatitis C 2018, *J Hepatol* 2018. [Epub ahead of print].

Webster DP, Klenerman P, Dusheiko GM: Hepatitis C, *Lancet* 385:1124–1135, 2015.

168

Hepatitis Caused by Other Viruses

Joseph K. Lim, Kris V. Kowdley

INFECTIOUS MONONUCLEOSIS

Epstein-Barr virus (EBV) is the causative pathogen for infectious mononucleosis and has been associated with a number of diseases involving B cells, including Burkitt lymphoma, nasopharyngeal carcinoma, and posttransplantation lymphoproliferative disorder.

Acute clinical features of infectious mononucleosis include fever, lymphadenopathy, severe pharyngitis, and atypical lymphocytosis (Fig. 168.1). Results of the heterophil antibody test are usually positive. Hepatic involvement resembles other causes of nonfatal acute viral hepatitis, and characteristic hepatosplenomegaly may be present in approximately 20% of patients. Serious complications include splenic rupture, meningitis, and pericarditis. Acute jaundice, fulminant hepatitis, and liver failure are rare.

Liver histology findings are often similar to those in other forms of acute hepatitis. Features such as portal and lobular inflammation, hepatocellular necrosis and acidophilic bodies, sinusoidal infiltration by monocytes, and atypical lymphocytes have been described.

The diagnosis of EBV infection is most commonly established by serologic testing for the heterophil antibody, agglutinating sheep cells, and both immunoglobulin M (IgM) and IgG antibody to EBV. However, the presence of antibody may indicate prior exposure rather than acute infection, given the ubiquitous nature of EBV, and heterophil antibody may be negative early in infection; both of these represent important challenges to establishing a diagnosis of acute EBV infection. Direct measurement of EBV viral DNA may be useful in immunosuppressed patients, in whom antiviral prophylaxis is being considered.

Posttransplantation lymphoproliferative disorder is a serious complication that typically requires both a reduction in immunosuppression dosing, and directed chemotherapy. EBV infection has also been associated with malignant transformation of lymphocytes, resulting in virally associated lymphomas.

YELLOW FEVER

Yellow fever is a rare cause of illness observed in US travelers to endemic regions of tropical/subtropical Africa and South America. It is a condition produced by a *Flavivirus* transmitted through the bit of infected mosquitoes, and virus levels may be present in the blood within the first 3 days of the disease. The *urban* form is transmitted from person to person by the female mosquito, *Aedes aegypti* (in jungle climates, white monkeys may also serve as intermediate hosts). Mosquitoes becomes infective approximately 12 days after it has fed on infected blood. In humans, a self-limited disease develops after an incubation period of 3 to 6 days, most characteristically headache, backache, photophobia, and gastrointestinal symptoms; however, a subset of patients may develop a severe toxic condition marked by acute jaundice, high fever, tachycardia, jaundice, and altered mental status, all of which may progress to oliguria and multiorgan failure. This *toxic* form is associated with a high mortality rate. When the liver is involved, the liver becomes yellow and enlarged. Liver biopsy in these patients reveal characteristic hepatocellular degeneration with fatty metamorphosis and midzonal necrosis, as well as Councilman bodies. More recent public health efforts to eradicate the *Aedes* mosquito and implement live, attenuated vaccination has helped to decrease incidence rates of yellow fever.

CYTOMEGALOVIRUS INFECTION

Cytomegalovirus (CMV) is a member of the herpes virus family which can produce a range of diseases, depending on patient age, mode of exposure, and level of immune competence. The virus is ubiquitous and is associated with high rates of seropositivity which increases with age.

Although most infections are asymptomatic, *CMV hepatitis* can be associated with significant morbidity in the neonatal period and is accompanied by jaundice, hepatosplenomegaly, central nervous system (CNS) involvement, and hemolytic anemia. In contrast, in adults, CMV may cause a nonspecific pattern of acute hepatitis which is indistinguishable from other causes of hepatitis. CMV viremia and associated disease are important clinical issues in transplantation. The virus can be transmitted with the graft, and therefore a CMV-negative patient who receives a CMV-positive organ graft is at very high risk for CMV disease for which routine surveillance and prophylactic therapy is commonly indicated.

The histologic features of CMV disease are characteristic and consist of cytomegalic cells with inclusion bodies. The diagnosis of CMV is most commonly made with a combination of serologic tests and direct measurement of serum virus levels by polymerase chain reaction (PCR)-based techniques. Several antiviral drugs are commonly used for the treatment of CMV infection, most commonly ganciclovir.

HERPESVIRUSES AND ADENOVIRUS

There are several other causes of acute nonhepatotropic viral hepatitis, including herpes viruses and adenovirus, both of which can rarely result in severe hepatitis, particularly in immunocompromised populations, in whom acute hepatitis may be fatal. *Herpes simplex hepatitis* has also been reported in pregnant women.

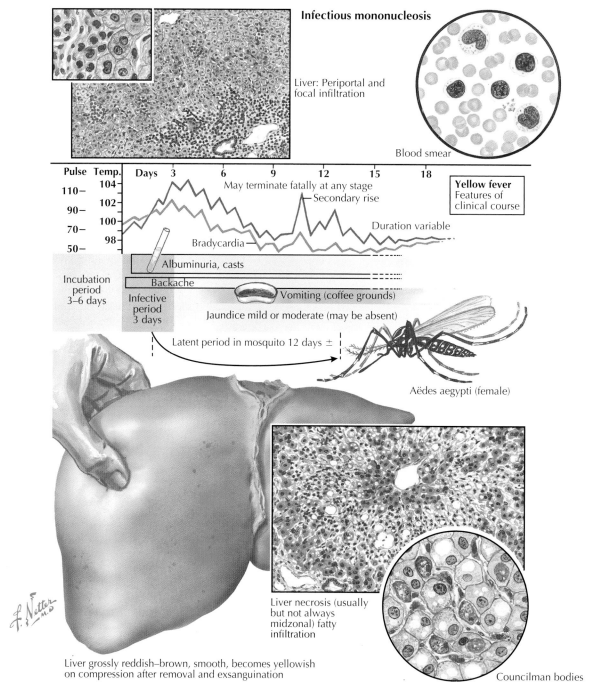

Infectious mononucleosis

Liver: Periportal and focal infiltration

Blood smear

Yellow fever
Features of clinical course

May terminate fatally at any stage

Secondary rise

Duration variable

Bradycardia

Albuminuria, casts

Backache

Vomiting (coffee grounds)

Jaundice mild or moderate (may be absent)

Incubation period 3–6 days

Infective period 3 days

Latent period in mosquito 12 days ±

Aëdes aegypti (female)

Liver necrosis (usually but not always midzonal) fatty infiltration

Liver grossly reddish–brown, smooth, becomes yellowish on compression after removal and exsanguination

Councilman bodies

Fig. 168.1 Hepatitis Caused by Other Viruses: Infectious Mononucleosis and Yellow Fever.

ADDITIONAL RESOURCES

Alves VAF: Acute viral hepatitis: beyond A, B, and C, *Surg Pathol Clin* 11:251–266, 2018.

Gupta P, Suryadevara M, Das A: Cytomegalovirus-induced hepatitis in an immunocompetent patient, *Am J Case Rep* 15:447–449, 2014.

Nam H, Nilles KM, Levitsky J, Ison MG: Donor derived viral infections in liver transplantation, *Transplantation* 2018 Jul 3 [Epub ahead of print].

Salva I, Silva IV, Cunha F: Epstein-Barr virus-associated cholestatic hepatitis, *BMJ Case Rep* 2013 Dec 16; pii:bcr2013202213.

Shaukat A, Tsai HT, Rutherford R, Anania FA: Epstein-Barr virus induced hepatitis: an important cause of cholestasis, *Hepatol Res* 33:24–26, 2005.

Yadav SK, Saigal S, Choudhary NS, et al: Cytomegalovirus infection in liver transplant recipients: current approach to diagnosis and management, *J Clin Exp Hepatol* 7:144–151, 2017.

169

Hepatotoxicity

Joseph K. Lim, Kris V. Kowdley

Drug-induced liver injury (DILI), also described as hepatotoxicity due to medications, is a common and potentially serious cause of acute and chronic liver disease. Many drugs have the capacity to cause hepatotoxicity (Fig. 169.1). In addition, a growing list of over-the-counter medications, supplements, and herbal remedies have been associated with liver injury. Hepatotoxicity may be acute or chronic; occasionally, they can result in severe acute hepatitis or fulminant hepatitis/liver failure requiring emergency liver transplantation, whereas in other cases it may result in chronic liver disease and liver cirrhosis.

CLASSIFICATION

DILI has been classified as idiosyncratic or intrinsic. *Idiosyncratic* drug reactions are not predictable, can occur with different amounts of exposure, and are highly variable in clinical presentation. Age, gender, and genetic factors may influence drug metabolism and immune response, as may dietary factors such as protein and alcohol intake. *Intrinsic* hepatotoxicity is generally a feature of agents that are inherently hepatotoxic or that produce toxic metabolites which can lead to liver injury.

Intrinsic Hepatotoxicity

Intrinsic hepatotoxins may cause liver injury through the production of free radicals or toxic metabolites. This type of hepatotoxicity is characteristically dose related and common among exposed persons, although many variables may influence the development of intrinsic hepatotoxicity. The agent may be directly toxic to cell membranes leading to hepatocellular necrosis; occasionally, there may be accompanying steatosis or cholestasis. In some cases, the toxic agent is produced in context of metabolism in the liver. The classic example of an intrinsic hepatotoxin is *carbon tetrachloride* (CCl_4), which is converted to a toxic metabolite that results in lipid peroxidation, thus causing damage to cell membranes (Fig. 169.2).

Idiosyncratic Hepatotoxicity

Idiosyncratic hepatotoxins may cause hepatotoxicity through the unpredictable production of toxic metabolites or by induction of an autoimmune process that subsequently causes liver injury. In contrast to intrinsic hepatotoxicity, only a minority of exposed persons develop liver injury.

CLINICAL PICTURE AND DIAGNOSIS

The clinical features of drug-induced hepatotoxicity can be highly variable, ranging from asymptomatic elevation of serum liver enzymes to fulminant liver failure. Although many drugs induced acute, reversible liver injury, some drugs are associated with chronic liver disease. The pattern of serum liver biochemistry elevation often reveals the type of liver injury. Some drugs produce a predominantly hepatocellular pattern, marked by increased alanine transaminase (ALT) and aspartate transaminase (AST) levels, whereas other agents produce a cholestatic pattern of liver injury, marked by predominant elevations of serum alkaline phosphatase (ALP) and γ-glutamyltransferase (GGT), with less prominent increases in serum AST and ALT.

Some drug reactions also produce unique patterns of liver enzyme elevation. For example, *acetaminophen* hepatotoxicity is more commonly observed in patients with chronic alcoholism in whom ingestion may be as little as 6 g. This pattern of hepatotoxicity likely is related to the increased production of a toxic intermediate of acetaminophen resulting from upregulation of cytochrome P450 enzymes through chronic alcohol use and its reduced clearance due to glutathione depletion. Serum AST is often strikingly elevated (5000–10,000 IU/L) and is characteristically increased several times compared with serum ALT.

Other hepatotoxic drugs can produce clinical, biochemical, and serologic patterns identical to those of idiopathic chronic autoimmune hepatitis, including evidence of positive antinuclear antibody and elevated plasma globulins; the classic example is *methyldopa*. This form of hepatotoxicity may clinically present as pruritus, which is more common with drugs associated with a cholestatic injury pattern, and may be prolonged in duration (weeks to months) and challenging to manage. Some drugs or toxins may be associated with the development of portal hypertension, including sinusoidal (alcohol), presinusoidal (nodular regenerative hyperplasia), and postsinusoidal (hepatic venoocclusive disease caused by alkylating agents as conditioning regimens for hematopoietic cell transplantation or pyrrolidine alkaloids) forms.

Histologic Patterns

Both drug-induced and toxin-induced liver injury can result in several patterns of histologic injury. Acute, severe liver injury may lead to massive hepatocellular necrosis in a diffuse zone 1 (periportal) or zone 3 (centrilobular) pattern, and there may be features of an allergic response, such as eosinophilia, as well as diffuse macrovesicular or microvesicular steatosis. Classic examples of drugs which cause microvesicular steatosis include *tetracycline* and *valproic acid*. A pattern of fatty liver and inflammation similar to nonalcoholic or alcoholic steatohepatitis can be caused by several medications, with *amiodarone* as a classic example.

Patients with chronic drug-induced liver disease may have clinical features of *chronic hepatitis*, with portal inflammatory infiltrates, or *interface hepatitis* (piecemeal necrosis). Vascular diseases may manifest with sinusoidal dilatation, venous thrombi, or peliosis. Cholestatic liver disease may be acute or chronic and may have features of hepatocellular

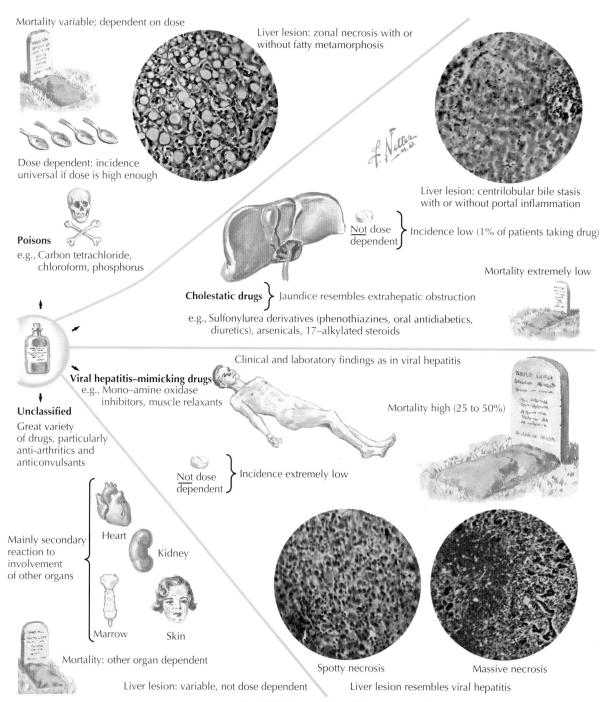

Mortality variable; dependent on dose

Liver lesion: zonal necrosis with or without fatty metamorphosis

Dose dependent: incidence universal if dose is high enough

Liver lesion: centrilobular bile stasis with or without portal inflammation

Poisons
e.g., Carbon tetrachloride, chloroform, phosphorus

Not dose dependent } Incidence low (1% of patients taking drug)

Mortality extremely low

Cholestatic drugs } Jaundice resembles extrahepatic obstruction

e.g., Sulfonylurea derivatives (phenothiazines, oral antidiabetics, diuretics), arsenicals, 17–alkylated steroids

Clinical and laboratory findings as in viral hepatitis

Viral hepatitis–mimicking drugs
e.g., Mono–amine oxidase inhibitors, muscle relaxants

Unclassified
Great variety of drugs, particularly anti-arthritics and anticonvulsants

Mortality high (25 to 50%)

Not dose dependent } Incidence extremely low

Mainly secondary reaction to involvement of other organs

Heart

Kidney

Marrow   Skin

Mortality: other organ dependent

Liver lesion: variable, not dose dependent

Spotty necrosis

Massive necrosis

Liver lesion resembles viral hepatitis

Fig. 169.1 Drug-Induced Hepatic Injuries.

damage (e.g., sulfa-containing compounds) or cholestatic injury without necroinflammatory changes (e.g., anabolic steroids).

Industrial and Household Hepatotoxins

Many chemical agents used in industrial and household products are solvents capable of causing liver injury. Occasional outbreaks of hepatotoxicity have been reported with these agents, most notably hydrocarbons and dimethylformamide (DMF), although these are increasingly rare.

Benign and Malignant Neoplasms

Several drugs have been associated with the development of liver tumors with chronic exposure. Oral contraceptive use has been implicated in focal nodular hyperplasia and nodular regenerative hyperplasia, which is believed to stem from chronic stimulation of estrogen receptors in the liver. Of greater concern is the association between drugs such as thorium dioxide (Thorotrast), vinyl chloride, and aflatoxins with malignant neoplasms such as hepatocellular carcinoma.

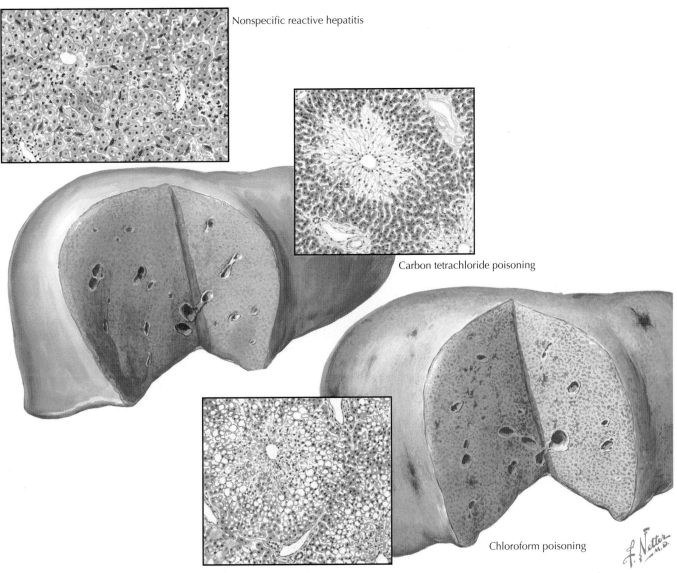

Nonspecific reactive hepatitis

Carbon tetrachloride poisoning

Chloroform poisoning

Fig. 169.2 Hepatotoxicity: Gross and Histologic Findings.

ADDITIONAL RESOURCES

Chalasani NP, Hayashi PH, Bonkovsky HL, et al: ACG Clinical Guideline: the diagnosis and management of idiosyncratic drug-induced liver injury, *Am J Gastroenterol* 109:950–966, 2014.

Davern TJ: Drug-induced liver disease, *Clin Liver Dis* 16:231–245, 2012.

Lewis JH: The art and science of diagnosing and managing drug-induced liver injury in 2015 and beyond, *Clin Gastroenterol Hepatol* 13:2173–2189, 2015.

Navarro VJ, Khan I, Bjornsson E, et al: Liver injury from herbal and dietary supplements, *Hepatology* 65:363–373, 2017.

Yamashita YI, Imai K, Mima K, et al: Idiosyncratic drug-induced liver injury: a short review, *Hepatol Commun* 1:494–500, 2017.

170

Disorders of Bilirubin Transport

Joseph K. Lim, Kris V. Kowdley

Disorders of bilirubin transport represent uncommon but clinically significant diseases which characteristically present in newborns and children. Bilirubin is a breakdown product of *heme,* which is derived from red blood cells (RBCs). Heme is initially cleaved by heme oxygenase into *biliverdin,* which is subsequently converted to bilirubin. In the circulation, bilirubin is bound to *albumin.* Bilirubin is then taken up by the liver and conjugated through glucuronidation into bilirubin monoglucuronide or diglucuronide, which is mediated by a group of enzymes called uridine diphosphate glucuronyltransferase (UGT), of which UGT1A1 is the key isoform responsible for bilirubin glucuronidation. This step enables the nonpolar bilirubin to be converted into a water-soluble form that can be excreted in bile (Fig. 170.1).

Unconjugated hyperbilirubinemia is common in the early neonatal period and is generally benign. Serum bilirubin levels that are primarily unconjugated may rise to 6 mg/dL and, in a minority of patients, may rise threefold or fourfold, which may be toxic in the neonatal period. *Kernicterus* is the term used to describe encephalopathy associated with high levels of unconjugated hyperbilirubinemia in the neonatal period. Factors associated with increased risk for neurotoxicity from bilirubin include the use of drugs that displace albumin from bilirubin, thereby increasing the exposure of free bilirubin to brain tissue. Clinical features of kernicterus include lack of muscle tone, abnormal reflexes, and possible progression to atony and death. Patients who recover from acute bilirubin toxicity may suffer long-term sequelae, including hearing impairment from cochlear damage, cerebellar abnormalities, and varying degrees of mental impairment. The mechanism behind bilirubin neurotoxicity may include impairment of DNA and RNA synthesis and protein and carbohydrate metabolism.

Disorders of bilirubin are typically classified as those resulting from increased production, decreased hepatic uptake, decreased hepatic conjugation, or decreased biliary excretion. These are discussed briefly in the following text.

Increased bilirubin production most often results from increased RBC turnover, as observed in hemolytic conditions. ABO incompatibility was a common cause of neonatal hemolysis before anti-Rh immunoglobulin was used to treat affected mothers. Other common hemolytic conditions including hereditary spherocytosis and sickle cell disease, which may lead to increased serum bilirubin levels, particularly within the neonatal period. Rarely, serum bilirubin levels may rise to greater than 3 to 5 mg/dL in persons with normal liver function but experience unconjugated hyperbilirubinemia when the liver's capacity to transport conjugated bilirubin is overwhelmed.

Decreased hepatic conjugation is most commonly the result of inherited disorders of bilirubin conjugation caused by mutations in the bilirubin-UGT1A1 enzyme, resulting in varying levels of deficiencies in its activity. *Crigler-Najjar syndrome* type 1 is defined by the presence of minimal to no activity of this enzyme and is characterized by severe, indirect hyperbilirubinemia and a high incidence of kernicterus. The syndrome represents a rare autosomal recessive disorder most commonly found in consanguineous families. Phototherapy, plasmapheresis, and orthotopic liver transplantation have been used to treat this life-threatening disorder. Crigler-Najjar syndrome *type 2* is a milder form of hepatic bilirubin-UGT deficiency marked by elevated serum bilirubin levels but few clinically significant sequelae. A third form is the *Gilbert syndrome,* a common condition which results in a mild decrease in enzyme activity and is associated with a modest elevation of serum bilirubin level (≤3 mg/dL), although it may rarely increase to greater than 3 mg/dL in patients who are fasting or under stress. The responsible mutation found in the promoter region of the gene encoding UGT1A1, which results in reduced production of bilirubin-UGT. The prevalence of the homozygous form of the variant promoter mutation is estimated at 9% in Western populations.

In contrast, *Rotor syndrome* and *Dubin-Johnson syndrome* are inherited disorders that lead to predominantly *conjugated* hyperbilirubinemia. Despite the presence of jaundice, pruritus is notably absent in these patients because bile acid transport is not impaired. Dubin-Johnson syndrome is marked by the development of a dark, heavily pigmented liver, whereas the liver appears normal in Rotor syndrome. The two conditions can be differentiated using oral cholecystography, through which the gallbladder is visualized in Rotor syndrome but not in Dubin-Johnson syndrome. In addition, the pattern of urinary coproporphyrin excretion can help to distinguish the two disorders, because excretion is increased in Rotor syndrome (2.5–5 times normal) with coproporphyrin representing the predominant form; by contrast, in Dubin-Johnson syndrome, coproporphyrin is also predominant, but the excretion of urinary coproporphyrin is normal. Both conditions have a relatively benign clinical course and are not associated with life-threatening complications. The molecular basis of these disorders has recently been characterized; conjugated bilirubin is secreted into the biliary canaliculus from the hepatocyte by the multidrug-resistant–related protein (MRP-2), also known as canalicular multispecific organic anion transporter (cMOAT). Mutations in this gene appear to be responsible for Dubin-Johnson syndrome, whereas the molecular defect in Rotor syndrome is unknown, although suspected to have an underlying autosomal recessive form of inheritance.

ADDITIONAL RESOURCES

Cvorovic J, Passamonti S: Membrane transporters for bilirubin and its conjugates: a systematic review, *Front Pharmacol* 8:887, 2017.

Erlinger S, Arias IM, Dhumeaux D: Inherited disorders of bilirubin transport and conjugation: new insights into molecular mechanisms and consequences, *Gastroenterology* 146:1625–1638, 2014.

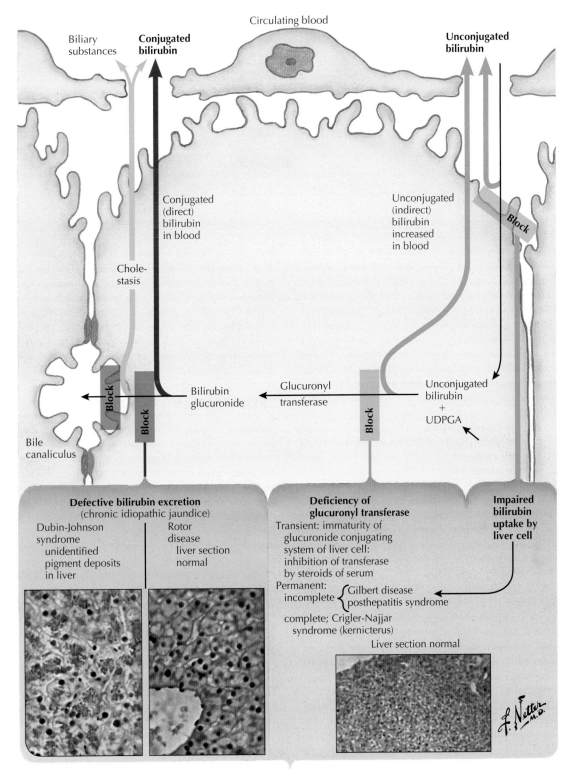

Fig. 170.1 Congenital and Familial Hyperbilirubinemia.

Fujiwara R, Haag M, Schaeffeler E, et al: Systemic regulation of bilirubin homeostasis: potential benefits or hyperbilirubinemia, *Hepatology* 67:1609–1619, 2018.

Keppler D: The roles of MRP2, MRP3, OATP1B1, and OATP1B3 in conjugated hyperbilirubinemia, *Drug Metab Dispos* 42:561–565, 2014.

Memon N, Weinberger BI, Hegyi T, Aleksunes LM: Inherited disorders of bilirubin clearance, *Pediatr Res* 79:378–386, 2016.

Sticova E, Jirsa M: New insights in bilirubin metabolism and their clinical implications, *World J Gastroenterol* 19:6398–6407, 2013.

Strassburg CP: Hyperbilirubinemia syndromes (Gilbert-Meulengracht, Crigler-Najjar, Dubin-Johnson, and Rotor syndrome), *Best Pract Res Clin Gastroenterol* 24:555–571, 2010.

α₁-Antitrypsin Deficiency

Joseph K. Lim, Kris V. Kowdley

α$_1$-Antitrypsin (α$_1$-AT) deficiency is a rare inherited liver disorder associated with both chronic liver disease and chronic obstructive pulmonary disease (COPD) with emphysema. It is recognized as the most common genetic liver disease in infants and children and may cause cirrhosis and end-stage liver disease in adults. α$_1$-AT is a serine protease inhibitor which is highly expressed in hepatocytes and secreted into blood where it inhibits trypsin, neutrophil elastase, collagenase, and chymotrypsin. The inhibition of neutrophil elastase blocks connective tissue degradation and results in protein misfolding (ZZ products), defective export, and development of insoluble aggregates within hepatocyte endoplasmic reticulum, ultimately resulting in liver cell death, inflammation, regeneration, and liver fibrosis. This deficiency affects approximately 2% of the US population and 1 in 1600 to 2800 live births in the United States and northern Europe.

α$_1$-AT deficiency is an autosomal dominant disorder, and the most common form occurs in patients with a homozygous variant of A1AT gene (SERPINA1), which results in Glu342Lys substitution in gene products (PIZZ). Approximately 2% of the US population is heterozygous for the Z allele, and 0.5% of the US population is homozygous for the Z allele. The overall prevalence of α$_1$-AT deficiency is estimated at 1 in 2000 persons, affecting approximately 1 in 1600 to 2800 live births in the United States and northern Europe. The disorder is notable for a bimodal clinical presentation (childhood and old age), whereas the lung disease form of α$_1$-AT deficiency typically presents in middle age.

CLINICAL PICTURE

Persistent jaundice in the newborn is the most common presenting symptom of α$_1$-AT deficiency. However, liver disease caused by α$_1$-AT may not be diagnosed until adolescence or early adulthood, when it may present as abdominal pain, hepatomegaly, or variceal hemorrhage. In adults, α$_1$-AT deficiency may present as emphysema, chronic hepatitis, cryptogenic cirrhosis, hepatocellular cancer, or complications of portal hypertension. Liver disease from α$_1$-AT in adults progresses slowly and is associated with a high risk for hepatocellular carcinoma in the presence of cirrhosis.

DIAGNOSIS

Per the guidelines of the American College of Gastroenterology and Alpha-1 Foundation, patients with persistently elevated serum aspartate aminotransferase (AST) or alanine aminotransferase (ALT) or unexplained chronic liver disease should be tested for α$_1$-AT deficiency with the *α$_1$-AT phenotype*. Most patients with chronic liver disease are either homozygous for PiZZ or compound heterozygous for SZ (PiSZ). Serum α$_1$-AT levels are typically 10% to 15% of normal in PiZZ patients but may be transiently normal in context of infection or other conditions due to elevations in acute phase reactants such as α$_1$-AT. Liver biopsy reveals characteristic periodic acid-Schiff stain (PAS)+ diastase-resistant globules within hepatocytes that represent the retained protein. Some studies suggest that PiMZ heterozygotes may rarely develop liver disease in the presence of other liver disease such as viral hepatitis or autoimmune hepatitis.

TREATMENT AND PROGNOSIS

Siblings of affected patients with α$_1$-AT deficiency should be screened for the disorder due to an increased risk. Liver biopsy is not routinely required but may exclude other etiologies and assess stage of liver fibrosis. No treatment is currently available for α$_1$-AT liver disease, because augmentation therapy has not been demonstrated to be effective. Orthotopic liver transplantation remains the only proven therapy for liver disease associated with α$_1$-AT deficiency among those who progress to cirrhosis and is associated with 65% long-term survival rate. Patients should be considered for referral to a pulmonology specialist for pulmonary function testing, and tobacco cessation should be advised. Possible future therapy in research development is focused on strategies such as decreasing accumulation of polymerized α$_1$-AT by stimulating its autophagy in hepatocytes.

ADDITIONAL RESOURCES

Clark VC: Liver transplantation in alpha-1 antitrypsin deficiency, *Clin Liver Dis* 21:355–365, 2017.

Mitchell EL, Khan Z: Liver disease in alpha-1 antitrypsin deficiency: current approaches and future directions, *Curr Pathobiol Rep* 5:243–252, 2017.

Sandhaus RA, Turino G, Brantly ML, et al: The diagnosis and management of alpha-1 antitrypsin deficiency in the adult, *Chronic Obstr Pulm Dis* 3:668–682, 2016.

Schonfeld EA, Brown RS Jr: Genetic testing in liver disease: what to order, in whom, and when, *Clin Liver Dis* 21:673–686, 2017.

Silverman EK, Sandhaus RA: Clinical practice: alpha-1 antitrypsin deficiency, *N Engl J Med* 360:2749–2757, 2009.

Townsend SA, Edgar RG, Eillis PR, et al: Systematic review: the natural history of alpha-1 antitrypsin deficiency, and associated liver disease, *Aliment Pharmacol Ther* 47:877–885, 2018.

172

Hereditary Hemochromatosis

Joseph K. Lim, Kris V. Kowdley

Hereditary hemochromatosis (HH) represents one of several primary iron overload disorders, such as aceruloplasminemia, ahypotransferrinemia, H-ferritin–associated iron overload, and African iron overload syndrome, and should be distinguished from secondary iron overload disorders such as dietary or parenteral iron overload, chronic liver disease, and iron-loading anemias (e.g., thalassemia minor, aplastic anemia), as well as other conditions such as ineffective erythropoiesis and porphyria cutanea tarda.

HH represents a spectrum of inherited disorders associated with parenchymal iron deposition in multiple organ systems caused by the excessive absorption of iron from a normal diet (Fig. 172.1). Iron deposition occurs in multiple organs, including the liver, heart, pancreas, skin, joints, and anterior pituitary gland. The long-term consequences include cirrhosis and hepatocellular carcinoma, diabetes mellitus, cardiomyopathy, "bronze diabetes" with hyperpigmentation of the skin and impaired glucose tolerance, arthropathy involving the metacarpophalangeal (MCP) joints, and hypogonadotropic hypogonadism.

The term "hereditary hemochromatosis" is typically used to indicate *human factors engineering (HFE)-associated hereditary hemochromatosis,* a disorder found predominantly in white populations. Initially described by Trousseau in 1865, and linked to the human leukocyte antigen (HLA)-A haplotype by Simon in the mid-1970s, the HFE hemochromatosis gene was discovered in 1996. Two common mutations were initially described, the *C282Y mutation,* indicating a cysteine-to-tyrosine substitution at amino acid 282, and the *H63D mutation,* a histidine-to-aspartate substitution at amino acid 63. Type 1 HFE-associated HH is classified as type 1a (C282T homozygosity), type 1b (compound C282T/H63D heterozygosity), or type 1c (other HFE genotypes such as S65C). Other forms of HH are less common and include type 2 HH (juvenile HH involving either hemojuvelin or hepcidin mutations), type 3 HH (TfR2 mutation-associated HH), and type 4 HH (ferroportin-associated HH). Table 172.1 lists common mutations in the *HFE* gene with their clinical interpretations.

HH is the most common genetic liver disease among persons of northern European descent, with an estimated prevalence of 1:200 to 1:500. The highest allelic frequency for the C282Y mutation is observed in northern Europe (6.4%–9.5%). An estimated 10% of the general U.S. population carries a single HFE mutation, whereas 0.5% are estimated to have a homozygous HFE mutation (1 in 200). However, the penetrance is low, with only 1% of C282Y homozygotes developing end-organ damage. Importantly, the development of clinically relevant iron overload is influenced by genetic and environmental factors such as alcohol, diabetes, exogenous iron intake, blood loss, celiac disease, and vitamin C intake.

The body iron stores in the human are regulated through gastrointestinal (GI) absorption. This is accomplished by variable expression of different iron transporters in response to physiologic signals in small intestinal crypt cells. In iron deficiency, iron absorption in the proximal small intestine is upregulated, characterized by increased expression or activity of DMT1 (mucosal iron transporter), ferroportin (FPN1), basolateral iron transporter, and transferrin receptor, and by decreased mucosal ferritin content. A similar pattern was found in some patients with HH, suggesting that the crypt cell senses a state of iron deficiency. Recent studies have revealed that a novel antimicrobial peptide produced in the liver called *hepcidin* appears to have an inhibitory effect on iron absorption. Patients with *HFE*-associated HH have inappropriately low hepcidin levels compared with healthy subjects, suggesting that the *HFE* mutation may lead to decreased efficiency in signaling hepatic iron content to crypt or intestinal absorptive cells, resulting in greater iron absorption.

CLINICAL PICTURE

Most patients with HH are asymptomatic in the early stages of disease, and therefore the identification of HH occurs through family screening or the recognition of abnormalities in liver enzymes and iron panel testing. Nonspecific symptoms may also be observed, including fatigue, generalized weakness, lethargy, apathy, and weight loss. With more progressive iron overload, organ-specific symptoms may emerge, including abdominal pain (hepatomegaly), arthralgias (arthritis), diabetes (pancreas), congestive heart failure and arrhythmias (heart), and amenorrhea/impotence (cirrhosis). Later signs typically do not develop until significant iron accumulation has occurred, most commonly in middle to late adulthood. Physical examination findings may be lacking but may indicate hepatomegaly, splenomegaly, chondrocalcinosis, congestive heart failure, increased pigmentation, and testicular atrophy.

DIAGNOSIS

The 2011 American Association for the Study of Liver Disease (AASLD) and 2017 American College of Gastroenterology (ACG) guidelines recommend that all patients with abnormal liver chemistries in the absence of acute hepatitis or evidence of liver disease should be tested for HH with a serum test panel including serum iron, transferrin saturation, and serum ferritin. Among patients with elevated serum iron and transferrin saturation greater than 45%, consideration should be given for *HFE* genotype testing. Individuals with C282Y homozygosity or C282Y/H63D heterozygosity associated with ferritin greater than 1000 or elevated liver enzymes may require liver biopsy for histopathology and calculation of the hepatic iron concentration (HIC), whereas those with ferritin less than 1000 and normal liver enzymes may proceed directly to therapeutic phlebotomy.

HFE Genetic Testing

An estimated 65% to 100% of patients with typical phenotypic HH are homozygous for C282Y. Compound heterozygosity (C282Y/H63D)

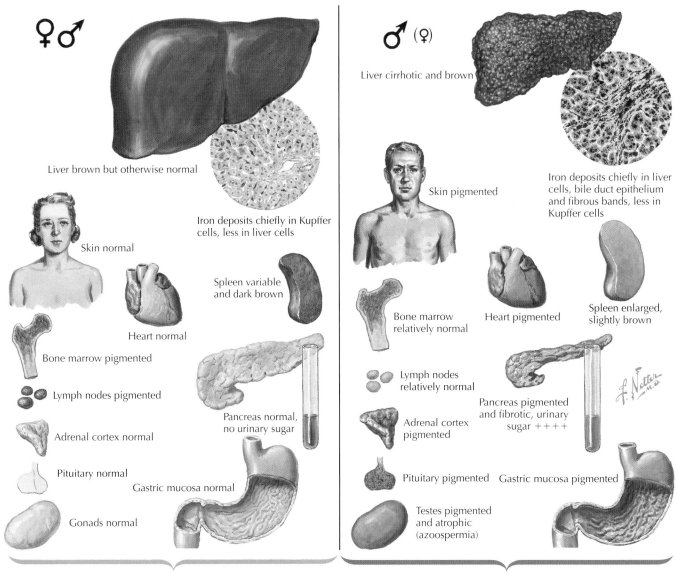

Fig. 172.1 Secondary Iron Overload and Hereditary Hemochromatosis.

TABLE 172.1 *HFE* Gene Testing in Hereditary Hemochromatosis	
Genetic Test Result	**Clinical Significance**
C282Y homozygous mutation	Greatly increased risk for iron overload.
C282Y heterozygous mutation	Usually not associated with iron overload; serum transferrin—iron saturation may be elevated.
C282Y/H63D compound heterozygous mutation	Moderately increased risk for iron overload.
H63D homozygous mutation	Increased serum iron levels but no increased risk for iron overload.
H63D heterozygous mutation	Not associated with iron overload.

occurs in approximately 5% of patients who have clinical evidence of HH, although the degree of iron overload appears to be lower. Persons who are heterozygous for the C282Y mutation typically do not develop iron overload in the absence of other liver diseases such as chronic hepatitis C infection or alcoholic liver disease. Therefore HH is defined only by the C282Y homozygous and C282Y/H63D heterozygous genotypes. Liver biopsy is generally not required in most patients for diagnosis but may be needed to quantify iron overload and assess for the presence of cirrhosis to guide clinical management.

Histologic features characteristic of HH include increased iron in hepatocytes and bile duct cells, with a paucity of iron in Kupffer cells, and a greater density of iron staining in periportal hepatocytes than around the central veins. Measuring the HIC may help to guide management with phlebotomy and/or chelation therapy.

TREATMENT AND MANAGEMENT

Phlebotomy remains the first line intervention for the treatment of HH, is viewed as safe and inexpensive, and is clearly indicated in patients with evidence of iron overload and end-organ disease. However, the role of phlebotomy in patients without end-organ disease is less certain, although it should ideally be performed before symptoms develop. Weekly phlebotomy of 500 mL whole blood is generally well tolerated and is continued until iron depletion is confirmed by serum ferritin less than 50 ng/mL and evidence of mild anemia. Studies have demonstrated that cardiac function may improve if phlebotomy is initiated before dilated cardiomyopathy develops, although phlebotomy does not appear to resolve joint symptoms in patients with HH-associated arthritis. Iron and vitamin C supplementation should be avoided in the diet. Iron chelation is generally reserved for patients with dyserythropoietic syndromes or chronic hemolytic anemia. Orthotopic liver transplantation remains an option for patients with advanced liver disease or hepatocellular carcinoma, although outcomes after orthotopic liver transplantation have been reported to be lower than other indications, which is hypothesized to stem from a higher risk of posttransplant infectious and cardiac complications. Iron reduction therapy before and after transplantation may improve posttransplant outcomes. Future therapies are focused on novel targets such as hepcidin modulation using short interfering ribonucleic acid (siRNA) and antisense oligonucleotides and offer hope for more directed therapies.

ADDITIONAL RESOURCES

Bacon BR, Adams PC, Kowdley KV, et al: Diagnosis and management of hemochromatosis: 2011 practice guideline by the American Association for the study of liver diseases, *Hepatology* 54:328–343, 2011.

Mohamed M, Phillips J: Hereditary haemochromatosis, *BMJ* 353:i3128, 2016.

Pietrangelo A, Deugnier Y, Dooley J, et al: EASL clinical practice guideline for HFE hemochromatosis, *J Hepatol* 53:3–22, 2010.

Powell LW, Seckington RC, Deugnier Y: Haemochromatosis, *Lancet* 388:706–716, 2016.

Richardson KJ, McNamee AP, Simmonds MJ: Haemochromatosis: pathophysiology and the red blood cell, *Clin Hemorheol Microcirc* 69:295–304, 2018.

Salgia RJ, Brown K: Diagnosis and management of hereditary hemochromatosis, *Clin Liver Dis* 19:187–198, 2015.

Liver Disease in Pregnancy

Joseph K. Lim, Kris V. Kowdley

Liver disease in pregnancy presents unique challenges to the clinician and requires careful and timely assessment. In addition to unique changes in the clinical course of chronic liver diseases (e.g., hepatitis B) which may occur during the course of pregnancy and at the time of delivery, a series of liver conditions unique to pregnancy have been described, including hyperemesis gravidarum, intrahepatic cholestasis of pregnancy (ICP), HELLP syndrome, and acute fatty liver of pregnancy (AFLP).

Hyperemesis gravidarum is characterized by severe nausea and vomiting during the first trimester of pregnancy. Its incidence is 0.35% to 0.8% of pregnancies, is rare to observe after 20 weeks of gestation, and may occasionally be accompanied by hyperthyroidism of uncertain etiology. In severe cases, hospitalization for intravenous hydration and antiemetic therapy may be required, and as many as 50% of patients may have abnormal results on liver function tests, which rarely reach levels greater than 1000 IU/L. Alternative etiologies such as viral hepatitis, gastric outlet obstruction, and gastroenteritis should be excluded. Treatment is limited to supportive care including hydration and antiemetics, including promethazine, ondansetron, and droperidol.

INTRAHEPATIC CHOLESTASIS OF PREGNANCY

ICP is an uncommon disorder of unknown etiology that typically develops during the second trimester and is associated with premature delivery and fetal death. The prevalence is reported to be 0.7% (United States) to 6.5% (Chile). The pathogenesis is unknown but believed to be related to genetic and hormonal factors, and patients with ICP appear to be more sensitive to the cholestatic effects of estrogen. The predominant clinical symptoms include severe pruritus and jaundice. The pruritus typically involves the palms and soles but may additionally affect the trunk and extremities. Jaundice often develops 1 to 4 weeks after the onset of pruritus in 20% to 60% of patients. Serum liver enzymes are commonly elevated and suggest either a hepatocellular, cholestatic, or mixed pattern of liver injury. Serum bile acid levels are also elevated and represent a more specific finding which signals the presence of ICP. Liver biopsy reveals bland cholestasis with bile plugs predominantly in zone 3 (central vein region) and intact portal tracts. However, liver biopsy is generally not needed for diagnosis.

The management of ICP is guided by the clinical symptoms. Early delivery at 36 weeks of gestation has been advocated for severe cases (if fetal lungs are mature) or alternatively 38 weeks for less severe cases. Cholestyramine (with vitamin K supplementation) can be used but may exacerbate fat malabsorption; ursodeoxycholic acid (UDCA) therapy represents an alternative therapeutic option. Clinical and biochemical abnormalities usually resolve a few weeks after delivery. Patients are at risk for recurrence with subsequent pregnancies or with oral contraceptive use.

HELLP SYNDROME

The HELLP acronym stands for *h*emolysis, *e*levated *l*iver tests, and *l*ow *p*latelet levels and represents a unique disorder which characteristically develops during the third trimester of pregnancy. The incidence is 0.17% to 0.85% of all live births. The mean age of the mother is 25 years (range, 14–40 years) and HELLP is usually diagnosed at 32 to 34 weeks of gestation (range, 22–40 weeks). HELLP syndrome is associated with preeclampsia, which is a common syndrome (5%–10% of pregnancies) manifested by hypertension, proteinuria, and edema.

Patients with HELLP may be asymptomatic, but the most common presenting complaint is abdominal pain; in some cases the diagnosis is made after delivery. Severe cases may be associated with renal failure or seizures (eclampsia) (Fig. 173.1). The HELLP syndrome is marked by the presence of abnormal liver enzymes, with serum aspartate transaminase (AST) levels which may range as high as 6000 U/L (mean, 250 U/L). Prothrombin time (PT) is generally normal, except in patients with severe hemolysis and/or disseminated intravascular coagulation (DIC). Peripheral blood smear reveals evidence of hemolysis with schistocytes and burr cells. Serum haptoglobin should be measured if the peripheral smear does not reveal obvious hemolysis. The complete blood count (CBC) often reveals thrombocytopenia with platelet count less than 100,000/μL, although this represents a nonspecific finding because gestational thrombocytopenia may occur in up to 8% of uncomplicated pregnancies. Notably, women with gestational thrombocytopenia are at seven times greater risk for HELLP syndrome. Liver biopsies are not routinely required to establish a diagnosis of HELLP, but pathology typically reveals fibrin deposition and hemorrhage localized to the periportal areas. The differential diagnosis includes viral hepatitis, hemolytic uremic syndrome, thrombocytopenic purpura, and AFLP.

HELLP syndrome is associated with several important complications of pregnancy, including DIC, placental abruption, renal failure, ascites, pulmonary/cerebral edema, acute respiratory distress syndrome (ARDS), and hepatic rupture. The most serious complication of HELLP syndrome is hepatic infarction, characterized by abdominal pain, fever, and marked elevation of transaminases (>5000 U/L), often accompanied by subcapsular hematoma or intraperitoneal hemorrhage which increases risk for maternal and fetal death, and may require immediate surgical intervention. Mothers who experience HELLP syndrome may additionally be at increased risk for recurrent HELLP syndrome with subsequent pregnancies. Overall maternal mortality in HELLP syndrome is estimated as high as 8%, whereas fetal mortality may be as high as 35% to 37%, with the highest risk observed in cases of rupture of hepatic hematoma, which is associated with fetal and maternal mortality rates greater than 50%.

Prompt delivery with careful fetal monitoring by an expert in high-risk obstetrics is the treatment of choice for HELLP syndrome. Clinical

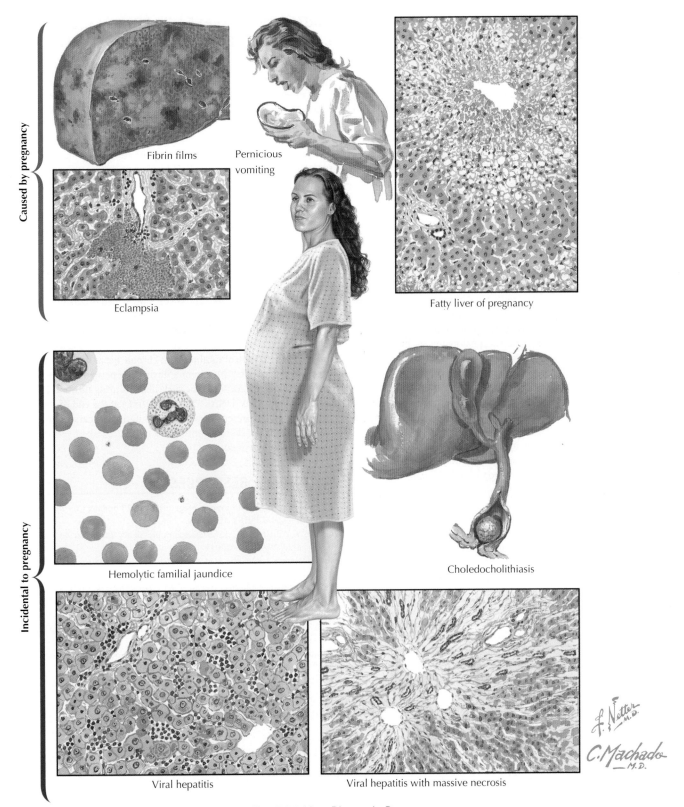

Caused by pregnancy

Fibrin films

Pernicious vomiting

Eclampsia

Fatty liver of pregnancy

Incidental to pregnancy

Hemolytic familial jaundice

Choledocholithiasis

Viral hepatitis

Viral hepatitis with massive necrosis

Fig. 173.1 Liver Disease in Pregnancy.

features of HELLP syndrome resolve within several days following delivery in most cases, although plasmapheresis may be required in patients with worsening thrombocytopenia after delivery. Liver enzymes generally return to normal after 3 to 5 days. Fortunately, infants who survive HELLP syndrome are observed to have clinical outcomes comparable with other infants of similar gestational age.

ACUTE FATTY LIVER OF PREGNANCY

AFLP is a rare condition, with an estimated incidence of 1:13,000 to 1:16,000 deliveries, and is associated with significant hepatic dysfunction, including elevated liver enzymes, prolongation of PT, hyperammonemia, and hypoglycemia. Patients typically present with clinical manifestations of AFLP during the third trimester of pregnancy, and in its most severe form may manifest as fulminant hepatic failure.

Patients with severe AFLP may have nonspecific symptoms such as malaise, fatigue, anorexia, headache, nausea, and vomiting, although they may be initially asymptomatic and incidentally detected by elevation of liver enzymes. More specific findings may be seen in some patients, including right upper quadrant pain (mimic acute cholecystitis or reflux esophagitis), polydipsia, pruritus, and jaundice. The disease may rapidly worsen within days of initial presentation with signs of acute liver failure, including hepatic encephalopathy, ascites, edema, and renal insufficiency. Clinical signs of preeclampsia such as hypertension or proteinuria may be present in greater than 50% of patients.

Laboratory testing may reveal elevated liver transaminases, which is more commonly less than 1000 IU/mL, although higher levels can rarely be observed. Marked jaundice and hyperbilirubinemia may develop, with serum bilirubin levels as high as 40 mg/dL. Extrahepatic complications have been reported, including upper gastrointestinal (GI) bleeding, renal dysfunction, DIC, severe hypoglycemia, and pancreatitis.

Liver biopsy remains the "gold standard" for diagnosis of AFLP, although is not routinely required in clinical practice. Pathology findings include vacuolization of hepatocytes and pallor in the central zone regions and characteristic microvesicular steatosis. The differential diagnosis includes acute viral hepatitis, acute toxic or drug-induced hepatitis, HELLP syndrome, drug-induced fatty liver, and biliary tract disorders.

AFLP should be considered a medical and obstetric emergency due to the potential for fulminant liver failure, which in severe cases may require urgent liver transplantation. At the time of diagnosis, patients should be promptly admitted to a liver failure unit at a transplantation center, if available, for better monitoring. Prompt delivery of the fetus is essential, and early diagnosis and management remains critical to minimize the severity of disease and the need for liver transplantation.

ACUTE LIVER DISEASE NOT SPECIFICALLY CAUSED BY PREGNANCY: VIRAL HEPATITIS

Viral hepatitis likely represents the most common liver disease during pregnancy, when hepatitis A, B, and E may all develop. *Hepatitis E* is a particularly important viral infection to identify during pregnancy due to a high case-fatality rate up to 20%, particularly if infection occurs during the third trimester. Most cases of acute hepatitis E are described among patients in the Indian subcontinent, northern Africa, and Mexico and are often characterized by the presence of predominant GI symptoms such as diarrhea. As such, it is prudent to caution pregnant women against travel to endemic areas and especially during the second and third trimesters.

Clinical features of acute *hepatitis A* infection during pregnancy are similar to those of other patients, although hepatitis A during late pregnancy may be associated with an increased risk for premature delivery; however, transmission of hepatitis A virus (HAV) to the fetus is not commonly observed.

The major concern with exposure to *hepatitis B* virus (HBV) during pregnancy is the maternofetal transmission, which occurs in more than 90% of pregnancies in the absence of prophylaxis. The administration of immune globulin and the first of three vaccination shots immediately following delivery may decrease this risk to less than 5% to 10%. Furthermore, up to 20% of mothers with chronic hepatitis B infection may experience flares of HBV viremia during the peripartum period and therefore require close virologic surveillance during this time. Mothers with very high HBV DNA (>200,000 IU/mL) at the end of the second trimester may represent candidates for antiviral therapy during the third trimester for disease control and to reduce risk of vertical transmission during delivery.

ADDITIONAL RESOURCES

Bacq Y: Liver diseases unique to pregnancy: a 2010 update, *Clin Res Hepatol Gastroenterol* 35:182–193, 2011.

Geenes V, Williamson C: Liver disease in pregnancy, *Best Pract Res Clin Obstet Gynaecol* 29:612–624, 2015.

Joshi D, James A, Quaglia A, et al: Liver disease in pregnancy, *Lancet* 375: 594–605, 2010.

Su GL: Pregnancy and liver disease, *Curr Gastroenterol Rep* 10:15–21, 2008.

Than NN, Neuberger J: Liver abnormalities in pregnancy, *Best Pract Res Clin Gastroenterol* 27:565–575, 2013.

Tran TT, Ahn J, Reau NS: ACG clinical guideline: liver disease and pregnancy, *Am J Gastroenterol* 111:176–194, 2016.

Westbrook RH, Dusheiko G, Williamson C: Pregnancy and liver disease, *J Hepatol* 64:933–945, 2016.

174

Benign Liver Tumors

Joseph K. Lim, Kris V. Kowdley

Liver tumors are commonly identified on diagnostic and screening imaging studies of the abdomen and require careful interpretation to distinguish between benign and malignant disease. Although malignant liver tumors such as hepatocellular carcinoma are described elsewhere (see Chapter 177), benign liver tumors represent one of the leading indications for consultation by gastroenterology specialist. Several nonmalignant conditions may result in the formation of nodular liver lesions (Fig. 174.1). These include regenerative nodules that develop as part of the liver's response to injury in patients with cirrhosis, including common benign nodular lesions such as focal nodular hyperplasia (FNH) and nodular regenerative hyperplasia (NRH).

FOCAL NODULAR HYPERPLASIA

FNH is a benign liver condition which has also been called hepatic hamartoma, focal cirrhosis, and hepatic pseudotumor. Most commonly observed in women between 30 and 50 years of age, patients with FNH frequently report a history of oral contraceptive (OC) use. Often an incidental finding identified on abdominal imaging or in context of evaluation of abnormal liver enzymes, most patients are asymptomatic. The pattern of liver injury is variable but may include elevation of serum alkaline phosphatase (ALP) and γ-glutamyltransferase (GGT) in a minority of patients. Patients may present with symptoms of abdominal pain, and physical examination may reveal hepatomegaly or a palpable mass over the right upper quadrant. Most patients with FNH have solitary lesions, which often measure 3 to 5 cm, and without a capsule. Most lesions are subcapsular, although FNH can be present in any location within the liver.

Liver biopsy can be helpful in confirming a radiologic diagnosis of FNH. The histopathology of the liver in FNH is characteristic with normal hepatocytes surrounded by a central area of fibrosis ("central scar") and nodules of liver parenchyma surround this central scar, often with aberrant blood vessels. FNH may not be clearly identified on abdominal ultrasonography and may require cross-sectional imaging. Computed tomography (CT) may reveal a hypervascular lesion with enhancement during the arterial phase and the characteristic central scar during the portal venous phase. Magnetic resonance imaging (MRI) with contrast reveals hypervascularity and central scar, which has high specificity for the diagnosis of FNH. Sulfur colloid scintigraphy has historically been used to differentiate FNH from adenomas and other hypervascular lesions because the presence of Kupffer cells in FNH is marked by uptake by the lesion, whereas adenomas appear "cold" on scintigraphy; due to overlap of findings with adenoma, this test is not reliable alone to confirm the diagnosis of FNH. MRI now represents the most commonly used modality to establish the presence of FNH and may commonly obviate the need for confirmatory liver biopsy.

NODULAR REGENERATIVE HYPERPLASIA

NRH is used to describe a condition in which regenerative nodules are observed in patients without cirrhosis. The pattern of hepatic fibrosis surrounding these regenerative nodules is distinct from that observed in patients with cirrhosis. In contrast to FNH, NRH typically occurs in older persons and is associated with various rheumatologic conditions. NRH is usually asymptomatic, but the large regenerative nodules may lead to compression of the portal vein and ultimately portal hypertension and its complications, including variceal bleeding. NRH should be considered as an underlying diagnosis in patients with rheumatologic or autoimmune conditions who present with signs of complications of portal hypertension, particularly those with preserved hepatic synthetic function and lack features of cirrhosis. *Felty syndrome,* a condition associated with rheumatoid arthritis, is characterized by NRH and leukopenia because of hypersplenism.

The diagnosis of NRH is generally confirmed on liver biopsy. Historically, wedge biopsy specimens obtained during surgery were obtained to establish the diagnosis because radiologic features of NRH are nonspecific. Patients with bleeding from portal hypertension may benefit from endoscopic therapy such as band ligation. In patients with normal liver synthetic function and recurrent variceal bleeding, a splenorenal shunt may be considered.

HEPATIC ADENOMA

Hepatic adenomas (HAs) are typically observed in young women, typically with a history of OC use. Approximately half of affected patients experience symptoms such as abdominal mass or abdominal pain. Liver biopsy is helpful in confirming the diagnosis and reveals classic histologic features, including normal-appearing hepatocytes with a paucity of bile ductular cells or normal liver lobules, and are often associated with the presence of a capsule.

Clinical complications of HA include hemorrhage and malignant transformation into hepatocellular carcinoma. The risk for hemorrhage is increased with growing lesion size, and therefore surgical resection is recommended for biopsy-proven adenomas that are large or symptomatic. Liver scintigraphy may be used to differentiate adenomas from FNH because adenomas generally do not contain Kupffer cells and therefore may be "cold."

CAVERNOUS HEMANGIOMA

Cavernous hemangiomas are the most commonly identified nonmalignant liver tumors. Their prevalence has been estimated at 5% to 20% and are more common in women possibly due to OC use, due to the

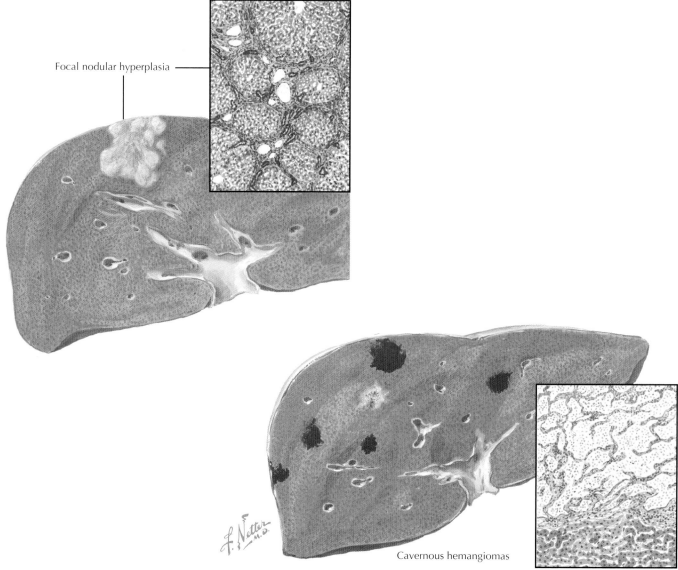

Focal nodular hyperplasia

Cavernous hemangiomas

Fig. 174.1 Nodular Liver Lesions: Focal Nodular Hyperplasia and Cavernous Hemangioma.

observation that some cavernous hemangiomas are sensitive to estrogen. The diagnosis of cavernous hemangioma often represents an incidental finding on abdominal imaging and is commonly asymptomatic. However, large lesions may be associated with abdominal pain, and hemorrhage from rupture of the hemangioma represents a rare but very serious complication. Occasionally, large cavernous hemangiomas are associated with disseminated intravascular coagulation, which is also known as *Kasabach-Merritt syndrome.*

The diagnosis of cavernous hemangioma can be established on radiologic imaging. Both CT and MRI reveal characteristic findings such as "puddling" of contrast within the tumor and increased intensity of signal during T2-weighted imaging. The management of cavernous hemangiomas is typically conservative monitoring due to a minimal risk for malignant transformation. Surgery or angiographic emboliza-tion may be considered in symptomatic patients and those with evidence of bleeding. OC use should be discontinued in women with a diagnosis of a cavernous hemangioma. Liver transplantation has been rarely performed for very large high-risk cavernous hemangiomas associated with consumptive coagulopathy.

ADDITIONAL RESOURCES

Belghiti J, Cauchy F, Paradis V, Vilgrain V: Diagnosis and management of solid benign liver lesions, *Nat Rev Gastroenterol Heaptol* 11:737–749, 2014.

Bonder A, Afdhal N: Evaluation of liver lesions, *Clin Liver Dis* 16:271–283, 2012.

Buell JF, Tranchart H, Cannon R, Dagher I: Management of benign hepatic tumors, *Surg Clin North Am* 90:719–735, 2010.

Chiche L, Adam JP: Diagnosis and management of benign liver tumors, *Semin Liver Dis* 33:236–247, 2013.

Margonis GA, Ejaz A, Spolverato G, et al: Benign solid tumors of the liver: management in the modern era, *J Gastrointest Surg* 19:1157–1168, 2015.

Marrero JA, Ahn J, Reddy KR: ACG clinical guideline: the diagnosis and management of focal liver lesions, *Am J Gastroenterol* 109:1328–1347, 2014.

Paradis V: Benign liver tumors: an update, *Clin Liver Dis* 14:719–729, 2010.

175

Granulomatous Liver Diseases

Joseph K. Lim, Kris V. Kowdley

Granulomatous liver diseases are a common finding which may be precipitated by infectious microbes or in response to systemic inflammatory or autoimmune processes. Granulomatous hepatitis may occasionally be idiopathic in origin in context of a fever of unknown origin. Granulomas of the liver are believed to originate from macrophages that are transformed into epithelioid cells after stimulation by antigens and may be composed of multinucleated giant cells. Granulomas are further classified into caseating and noncaseating granulomas, which may help distinguish between etiologic agents such as tuberculosis (which are often associated with *caseating* granulomas) and autoimmune or inflammatory processes (which are associated with *noncaseating* granulomas).

INFECTIOUS PROCESSES

The most common organisms associated with granulomas are bacteria such as *Mycobacterium tuberculosis* (MTB), *Mycobacterium avium-intracellulare* (MAI), brucellosis, listeriosis, and tularemia. Other infections associated with granuloma development include schistosomiasis, leishmaniasis, and visceral larva migrans. Rickettsial diseases, viruses (e.g., cytomegalovirus), and protozoal infections less commonly may be associated with granulomas.

Hepatic Tuberculosis

Primary hepatic tuberculosis may occur in the extremely rare congenital form, but it is usually secondary to *miliary tuberculosis* (Fig. 175.1). The most frequent lesion is the small miliary granuloma (tubercle), which may be scattered over the liver in all forms of active organ tuberculosis. Granuloma formation begins with a focal proliferation of Kupffer cells, which form small histiocytic nodules located throughout the parenchyma. Subsequently, liver cells surrounded by the histiocytes become necrotic, and in some cases, smaller or larger foci of hepatocellular necrosis with minimal mesenchymal reaction develop. In the nodules, some cells become larger and develop into epithelioid cells, the nuclei of which can divide without division of the cytoplasm, resulting in large giant cells (Langerhans). A lymphocytic infiltrate can be seen on the periphery of the granuloma. As the tubercle enlarges, central caseation necrosis may develop. Eventually, the histiocytes may transform into fibroblasts and form a capsule around the tubercle. Finally, the entire lesion becomes transformed into a nodule of collagenous connective tissue.

Acid-fast bacilli (AFB) are usually not seen in the scar, and tubercle bacilli are also difficult to culture from liver biopsy specimens. In addition, the morphologic picture of the tubercles is nonspecific because other granulomatous diseases may produce similar lesions in the wall of the central vein. Tuberculous granulomas are spread throughout the lobule, frequently close to the portal triads where they tend to coalescence.

In miliary tuberculosis (TB), the tubercles are densely spread, as readily seen on gross inspection, and they appear as white, pinhead-sized nodules best recognized through the capsule on inspection of the inferior surface of the left lobe. Hepatic miliary TB may precede pulmonary involvement, or the lungs may remain unaffected. Fever may be prolonged, and chest x-ray findings may be negative; the diagnosis is typically confirmed by liver biopsy.

Q Fever

Q fever is caused by *Coxiella burnetii*, a rickettsial organism that frequently infects cattle and other farm animals through oral or parenteral routes. Typical clinical features include fever, pulmonary infiltrates, and flulike symptoms.

SYSTEMIC AUTOIMMUNE OR IDIOPATHIC DISEASES

Granulomas can also be found in a variety of liver diseases localized to the liver or systemic diseases with liver involvement such as from autoimmune or idiopathic diseases. The most common systemic disease associated with liver granulomas is *sarcoidosis* (Fig. 175.2). This is a relatively common disease of unknown etiology, although dysregulation of the immune system is believed to play a role. Liver involvement in sarcoidosis is often manifested by abnormal liver enzymes in a cholestatic pattern, with a predominant elevation of serum alkaline phosphatase (ALP). Many patients are asymptomatic, although pruritus and fatigue represent the most common presenting symptoms. The diagnosis is confirmed by an elevated serum angiotensin-converting enzyme (ACE) level, especially in the presence of mediastinal lymphadenopathy or other supportive evidence.

Idiopathic granulomatous hepatitis is an unusual disorder characterized by high fever and florid granulomatous infiltration in the liver. Liver biopsy is frequently useful in these patients who present with elevated ALP level and a fever of unknown origin to exclude other etiologies.

OTHER CONDITIONS CHARACTERIZED BY GRANULOMAS

Hepatic granulomas similar to those in tuberculosis and sarcoidosis can be seen in many other conditions. In *brucellosis*, granulomas are irregularly spaced throughout the liver, vary in size and degree of development, and are accompanied by focal necrosis and portal inflammation (see Fig. 175.2). In *histoplasmosis*, granulomas that resemble tubercles occur together with a diffuse proliferation of the Kupffer cells, the cytoplasm of which may be loaded with the fungus *Histoplasma capsulatum*. In

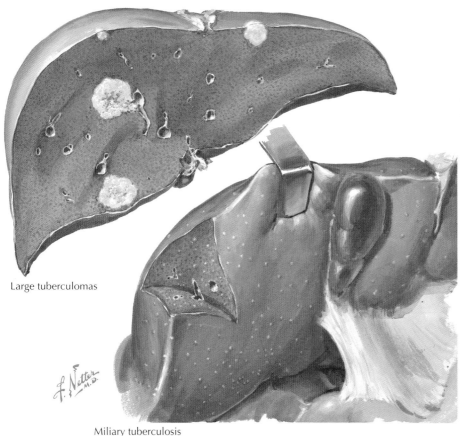

Large tuberculomas

Miliary tuberculosis

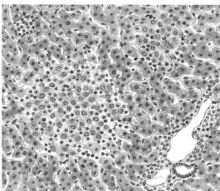

Acute miliary granulomas (soft tubercle – chiefly histiocytes)

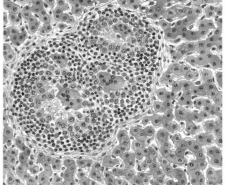

Subacute conglomerate tubercle (giant cells, caseation, histiocytes, surrounded by lymphocytes and fibrosis)

Fig. 175.1 Granulomatous Liver Diseases: Gross and Histologic Appearance.

other fungal diseases, such as *blastomycosis* or *coccidioidomycosis,* nonspecific reactive hepatitis occurs more frequently than granulomas in the liver. Tularemia, leprosy, and beryllium poisoning are less commonly associated with hepatic granulomas.

Primary biliary cholangitis (PBC) is often characterized by multiple, small, noncaseating granulomas (see Chapter 162), which are primarily located in the periportal regions, whereas they may be found throughout the hepatic lobule with drug-induced or infectious etiologies.

DIAGNOSIS

Careful assessment including detailed medical history and physical examination of the patient with hepatic granulomas is warranted because many infectious causes can be identified based on thorough history taking alone, with particular attention to travel history, medication history, occupational history, social history (e.g., drug abuse), and sexual history, as well as the presence of other systemic disorders, immunosuppression, or autoimmunity.

TREATMENT AND MANAGEMENT

The management of granulomatous liver diseases is focused on treating the underlying cause. Discontinuation of offending drugs, such as allopurinol or phenylbutazone, treatment of causative infections with antimicrobials, and corticosteroids for idiopathic granulomatous hepatitis may be considered.

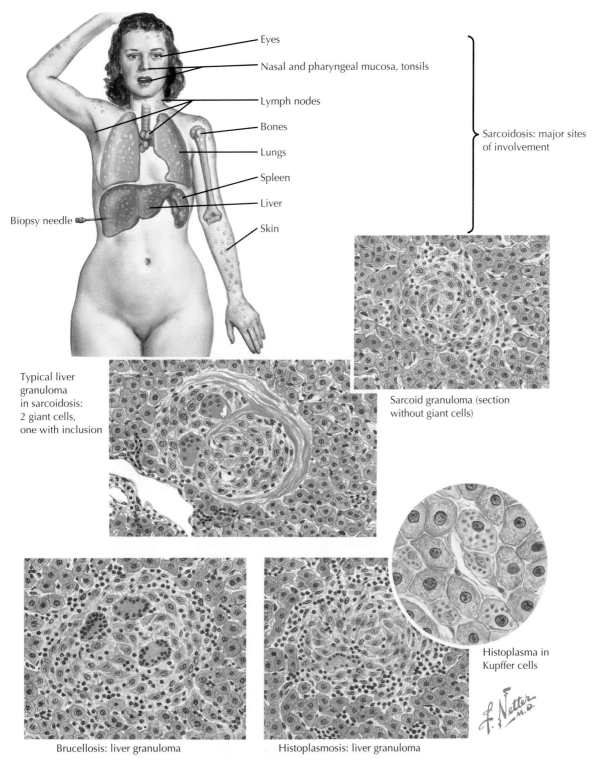

Eyes

Nasal and pharyngeal mucosa, tonsils

Lymph nodes

Bones

Lungs

Spleen

Liver

Skin

Biopsy needle

Sarcoidosis: major sites of involvement

Typical liver granuloma in sarcoidosis: 2 giant cells, one with inclusion

Sarcoid granuloma (section without giant cells)

Histoplasma in Kupffer cells

Brucellosis: liver granuloma

Histoplasmosis: liver granuloma

Fig. 175.2 Sarcoidosis Sites and Histology of Liver Granulomas.

ADDITIONAL RESOURCES

Bhardwaj SS, Saxena R, Kwo PY: Granulomatous liver disease, *Curr Gastroenterol Rep* 11:42–49, 2009.

Coash M, Forouhar F, Wu CH, Wu GY: Granulomatous liver diseases: a review, *J Formos Med Assoc* 111:3–13, 2012.

Flamm SL: Granulomatous liver disease, *Clin Liver Dis* 16:387–396, 2012.

Lagana SM, Moreira RK, Lefkowitch JH: Hepatic granulomas: pathogenesis and differential diagnosis, *Clin Liver Dis* 14:605–617, 2010.

Lamps LW: Hepatic granulomas: a review with emphasis on infectious causes, *Arch Pathol Lab Med* 139:867–875, 2015.

Tadros M, Forouhar F, Wu GY: Hepatic sarcoidosis, *J Clin Transl Hepatol* 1:87–93, 2013.

176

Wilson Disease

Joseph K. Lim, Kris V. Kowdley

Wilson disease (WD) is a rare primary copper overload disorder which was first described in 1912 by the neurologist Samuel Kinnier Wilson as "progressive lenticular degeneration" associated with cirrhosis. However, it was not until 1948 that WD was recognized as a disorder of *copper* metabolism resulting in excess copper accumulation in the liver, central nervous system, and other organs.

WD is an autosomal recessive disorder with an estimated incidence in most populations of approximately 1 in 30,000. Gene frequency varies between 0.3% and 0.7%, leading to an estimated heterozygous carrier rate of 1 in 90. WD affects men and women equally, occurs in all races, and is predominantly diagnosed in the second and third decades (majority are age 5–35 years).

The ATP7B gene mutation associated with Wilson disease *(WND)* has been mapped to chromosome 13 (13q 14.3). The gene is expressed primarily in the liver, kidney, and placenta but has also been found in other organs. The gene product is a P-type adenosine triphosphatase (ATPase), which transports copper into bile which incorporates it into ceruloplasmin. Up to 60 mutations within the *WND* locus have been identified, although fewer than half are thought to have clinical significance. A specific mutation, His 1069Gln, appears more common in WD patients of European descent, although this mutation is present in only 15% to 25% of all patients with WD. Due to the genetic heterogeneity, genetic testing is not routinely useful for a diagnosis of WD in probands, although can be used to identify affected family members once a proband has received a diagnosis.

Impaired biliary excretion of copper appears to be central to the pathogenesis of WD. Body copper stores are normally regulated through biliary excretion. The *WND* gene product is believed to be responsible for transporting copper from hepatocytes into the biliary system, which may be impaired in WD patients, although it is unclear how the defect in ATP7B alters this pathway.

CLINICAL PICTURE

WD is characterized by a variable clinical presentation, although neuropsychiatric or hepatic symptoms often represent the most common initial or presenting complaints (Fig. 176.1). Although the genetic defect is present at birth, clinical symptoms rarely develop before 5 years. Age at presentation may correlate with the organ system involved. The average age for hepatic symptoms is 10 to 14 years but appears to be later for neurologic symptoms, typically 19 to 22 years; later presentation after age 40 is less common.

Neuropsychiatric manifestations are typically seen in adolescents or young adults and are often the presenting complaint in symptomatic patients. Psychiatric symptoms include depression, mood disorders, and personality changes. The most common neurologic manifestations are tremor, drooling, hypertonicity, choreoathetosis, and parkinsonian-like findings (e.g. micrographia). Less common manifestations due to extrahepatic copper deposition include osteopenia, distal renal tubular acidosis, arrhythmias, congestive heart failure, glucose intolerance, and amenorrhea.

DIAGNOSIS

The 2017 American College of Gastroenterology (ACG) guideline recommends that all patients with persistently elevated serum aspartate aminotransferase (AST) or alanine aminotransferase (ALT), especially in patients younger than age 55 years, should undergo screening for WD with serum ceruloplasmin testing. If low, confirmatory testing with 24-hour urinary copper and slit-lamp eye exam should be pursued. The 2008 American Association for the Study of Liver Diseases (AASLD) guideline recommends that all patients age 3 to 55 years with liver abnormalities of uncertain cause and, with clinical suspicion for WD, should undergo testing with serum ceruloplasmin, 24-hour urine copper, and slit-lamp eye exam. If all three tests are abnormal, the diagnosis of WD can be made without need for liver biopsy. However, if only one or two of these criteria are met, liver biopsy is recommended to confirm the diagnosis of WD on the basis of compatible histopathology findings and dry copper weight greater than 250 µg/g. Patients with dry weight 50 to 250 µg/g may require further genetic testing for ATP7B mutations to confirm the diagnosis. Dry weight less than 50 µg/g is helpful to confirm the absence of WD. The presence of Kayser-Fleischer rings on slit-lamp exam is observed in only 50% of cases, and normal serum ceruloplasmin alone should not preclude evaluation for WD if other clinical features are present.

WD-associated mutations may be feasible in the near future.

TREATMENT AND MANAGEMENT

Patients who are diagnosed with WD should be counseled to eliminate copper-rich foods from their diet, including shellfish, organ meats, nuts, dried fruit, chocolate, and beans. WD screening should be recommended for first-degree relatives due to increased risk. Neurologic evaluation and brain magnetic resonance imaging (MRI) should be considered prior to treatment in patients with neurologic WD. Mutation analysis may also be pursued in patients in whom the diagnosis is difficult to establish based on clinical testing. Ultimately, the goals of WD therapy include removing excess body copper and preventing reaccumulation. Copper-chelating agents such as D-*penicillamine* and *trientine* represent first-line therapy. Trientine is increasingly preferred as a primary option because of the adverse effect profile of D-penicillamine. *Zinc acetate* (Galzin) acts to induce metallothionein, which blocks copper absorption in the small intestine, and has emerged as a commonly used maintenance treatment. *Ammonium tetrathiomolybdate* is an oral agent that binds to plasma copper and inhibits intestinal absorption and has been used as an alternative therapeutic option for neurologic WD.

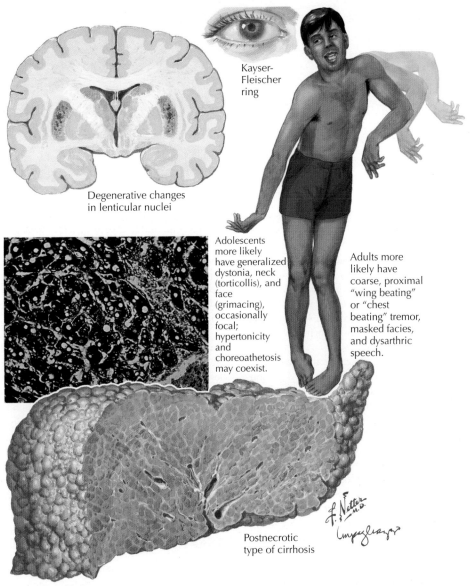

Kayser-
Fleischer
ring

Degenerative changes
in lenticular nuclei

Adolescents
more likely
have generalized
dystonia, neck
(torticollis), and
face
(grimacing),
occasionally
focal;
hypertonicity
and
choreoathetosis
may coexist.

Adults more
likely have
coarse, proximal
"wing beating"
or "chest
beating" tremor,
masked facies,
and dysarthric
speech.

Postnecrotic
type of cirrhosis

Fig. 176.1 Wilson Disease.

Liver transplantation is an effective life-saving measure for patients who have either acute or fulminant hepatitis due to WD, or progressive chronic disease despite chelation therapy, and is associated with excellent posttransplantation outcomes. Because the primary defect resides within the liver, transplantation is considered curative for WD.

ADDITIONAL RESOURCES

Ferenci P, Czlonkowska A, Stremmel W, et al: EASL clinical practice guidelines: Wilson's disease, *J Hepatol* 56:671–685, 2012.

Joshi D, Gupta N, Samyn M, et al: The management of childhood liver diseases in adulthood, *J Hepatol* 66:6313–6644, 2017.

Kathawala M, Hirschfield GM: Insights into the management of Wilson's disease, *Therap Adv Gastroenterol* 10:889–905, 2017.

Liu J, Luan J, Zhou X, et al: Epidemiology, diagnosis, and treatment of Wilson's disease, *Intractable Rare Dis Res* 6:249–255, 2017.

Ranucci G, Polishchuck R, Iorio R: Wilson's disease: prospective developments towards new therapies, *World J Gastroenterol* 23:5451–5456, 2017.

Roberts EA, Schilsky ML: Diagnosis and treatment of Wilson disease: an update, *Hepatology* 47:2089–2111, 2008.

Schilsky ML: Wilson disease: diagnosis, treatment, and follow-up, *Clin Liver Dis* 21:755–767, 2017.

Schonfeld EA, Brown RS Jr: Genetic testing in liver disease: what to order, in whom, and when, *Clin Liver Dis* 21:673–686, 2017.

177

Hepatocellular Carcinoma

Joseph K. Lim, Kris V. Kowdley

Hepatocellular carcinoma (HCC) represents one of the most important and life-threatening complications of chronic liver disease. The 5-year survival of patients with HCC remains sobering despite significant advances in the epidemiology, diagnosis, and management of this disease. The epidemiology of HCC in the United States reveals an ongoing increase in HCC incidence and incidence-based mortality. Although chronic hepatitis B virus (HBV) infection represents the most common risk factor globally, for which HBV is considered the #2 carcinogen after tobacco, other major risk factors include chronic hepatitis C infection (stage 3 or 4) and cirrhosis of any cause.

Unlike other solid organ malignancies, imaging criteria alone can confirm a diagnosis of HCC, and liver biopsy is not required for confirmation. However, the histologic features of HCC are similar to other malignancies, with increased nuclear/cytoplasmic ratios and multiple mitotic figures (Fig. 177.1). HCC has also been classified from "very well differentiated" to "poorly differentiated" cancer. Some types may be associated with extensive scar formation and are called *scirrhous* form. Other types may form structures similar to glands (*pseudoglandular* form). Staging of HCC is important for predicting prognosis and directing therapy, and several classification methods have been adopted globally, although the Barcelona Clinic Liver Cancer (BCLC) staging system is most commonly used in the United States.

CLINICAL PICTURE

Most cases of HCC are asymptomatic and require imaging surveillance for its detection. However, the diagnosis of HCC should be suspected in any patient with evidence of acute or subacute decompensation of chronic liver disease or increased abdominal pain, particularly over the right upper quadrant. Examination findings such as a firm or "rock-hard" mass, or a vascular bruit may be present given the highly vascular nature of this tumor. Clinicians should also evaluate for associated paraneoplastic phenomena.

DIAGNOSIS

Unlike other solid organ malignancies, the diagnosis of HCC can be established based on characteristic imaging findings in the absence of tissue confirmation. HCC should be suspected in a patient with high serum a-*fetoprotein* (AFP) level and/or a mass lesion seen on ultrasonography (US) or computed tomography (CT). Serum AFP has been widely used to screen for HCC in populations at risk, and in patients with cirrhosis who have AFP levels greater than 300 ng/mL, the diagnosis is likely. However, AFP may be elevated in the context of chronic liver disease alone and is not produced by 30% of liver cancers; therefore it is not sufficiently sensitive or specific for a diagnosis of HCC. In this context, serum AFP is not recommended to be used alone for HCC screening in guidelines of the American Association for the Study of Liver Diseases (AASLD) or European Association for the Study of the Liver (EASL) but may be considered as an optional test to be considered with other diagnostic criteria.

Ultrasound is a useful screening test for patients with cirrhosis and formally recommended as first line imaging study for HCC surveillance by AASLD guidelines. However, a significant proportion of nodular lesions found on US may represent regenerative nodules rather than HCCs. Triphasic CT or MRI permits rapid acquisition of liver images at various stages of contrast injection (noncontrast, hepatic arterial phase, portal venous phase), has dramatically improved the ability to diagnose HCC, and differentiates HCC nodules from regenerative nodules. However, the main disadvantage of CT screening is the cumulative risk of ionizing radiation and contrast-induced nephrotoxicity. Characteristic features of arterial phase enhancement with venous phase washout, particularly in context of a pseudocapsule, may be adequate to confirm a diagnosis of HCC.

TREATMENT AND MANAGEMENT

The treatment of HCC has evolved rapidly over the past several years. Although resection was historically viewed as the only therapeutic option associated with favorable long-term survival, several options are now considered potentially curative, including resection, radiofrequency ablation, and liver transplantation, the latter of which should be considered in all patients with HCC and cirrhosis. Patients who meet Milan criteria (single HCC lesion 2–5 cm or up to 3 HCC lesions each <3 cm) are potentially eligible for transplant listing and may qualify for special prioritization under United Network for Organ Sharing (UNOS) policy. Transarterial chemoembolization (bland or with chemotherapy beads), radioembolization, and chemotherapy represent increasingly common therapeutic options for nonoperative candidates and individuals either awaiting or ineligible for liver transplantation. *Sorafenib* is an oral multikinase inhibitor which represents a first-line chemotherapy for advanced HCC beyond Milan criteria and which demonstrated a small improvement for survival. Recently, two new agents have been approved for second-line chemotherapy for advanced HCC, including multikinase inhibitors regorafenib and lenvatinib, and checkpoint inhibitor (PD-1) nivolumab.

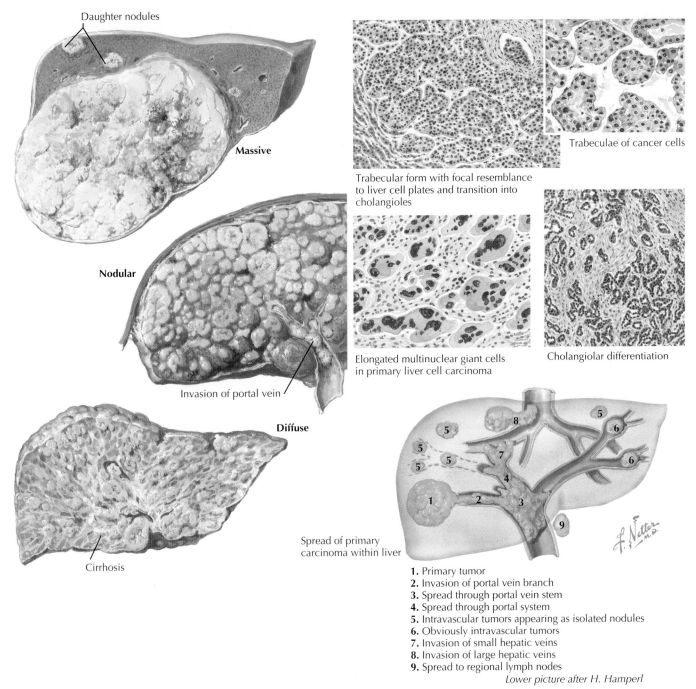

Daughter nodules

Massive

Nodular

Invasion of portal vein

Diffuse

Cirrhosis

Trabecular form with focal resemblance to liver cell plates and transition into cholangioles

Trabeculae of cancer cells

Elongated multinuclear giant cells in primary liver cell carcinoma

Cholangiolar differentiation

Spread of primary carcinoma within liver

1. Primary tumor
2. Invasion of portal vein branch
3. Spread through portal vein stem
4. Spread through portal system
5. Intravascular tumors appearing as isolated nodules
6. Obviously intravascular tumors
7. Invasion of small hepatic veins
8. Invasion of large hepatic veins
9. Spread to regional lymph nodes

Lower picture after H. Hamperl

Fig. 177.1 Hepatocellular Carcinoma: Gross and Histologic Features and Spread of Primary Carcinoma Within the Liver.

ADDITIONAL RESOURCES

Bruix J, Han KH, Gores G, et al: Liver cancer: approaching a personalized care, *J Hepatol* 62(1 Suppl 1):S144–S156, 2015.

Daher S, Massarwa M, Benson AA, Khoury T: Current and future treatment of hepatocellular carcinoma: an updated comprehensive review, *J Clin Transl Hepatol* 6:69–78, 2018.

Galle PR, Forner A, Llovet JM, et al: EASL clinical practice guidelines: management of hepatocellular carcinoma, *J Hepatol* 69:182–236, 2018.

Heimbach JK, Kulik LM, Finn RS, et al: AASLD guidelines for the treatment of hepatocellular carcinoma, *Hepatology* 67:358–380, 2018.

Llovet JM, Zucman-Rossi J, Pikarsky E, et al: Hepatocellular carcinoma, *Nat Rev Dis Primers* 2:16018, 2016.

Njei B, Rotman Y, Ditah I, Lim JK: Emerging trends in hepatocellular carcinoma incidence and mortality, *Hepatology* 61:191–199, 2015.

Padhya KT, Marrero JA, Singal AG: Recent advances in the treatment of hepatocellular carcinoma, *Curr Opin Gastroenterol* 29:285–292, 2013.

178

Liver Transplantation

Joseph K. Lim, Kris V. Kowdley

Liver transplantation represents the most important lifesaving measure for patients with cirrhosis and liver failure and has evolved from an experimental procedure in the 1970s to a widely accepted and highly effective therapy at present. The success of liver transplantation has resulted in severe mismatch between supply and demand for donor organs, and resulting need for priority allocation systems, as well as emergence of live-donor transplantation, in which a portion of the liver from a related or beneficent living donor is transplanted into a recipient.

The major indications for liver transplantation remain acute/fulminant liver failure, hepatocellular carcinoma (HCC), and end-stage liver disease (ESLD) (Figs. 178.1 and 178.2), although rarely other metabolic diseases, large benign tumors, and severe refractory pruritus from cholestatic liver disease are considered on an individual basis. Although chronic hepatitis C virus (HCV) infection and alcoholic liver disease have represented the most common etiologies of liver disease among patients requiring transplantation, nonalcoholic fatty liver disease (NAFLD)/nonalcoholic steatohepatitis (NASH) has emerged as a quickly rising indication, is expected to become the #1 indication for liver transplantation in 2020, and in fact already represents the leading etiology in adult recipients younger than 50 years.

The process of selection and assignment of organ priority for liver transplantation is managed by the United Network for Organ Sharing (UNOS), a national nonprofit organization that administers organ procurement and allocation with funding from the US government through the Organ Procurement and Transplantation Network (OPTN).

Major complications of chronic ESLD that should prompt referral to a liver transplantation center include evidence of overt hepatic decompensation, such as ascites, variceal bleeding, spontaneous bacterial peritonitis (SBP), or suspected hepatorenal syndrome. Known or suspected HCC within Milan criteria represents another common indication for liver transplantation, although some centers will consider larger tumors after they have been downsized with locoregional therapies such as radiofrequency ablation (RFA) or transarterial chemoembolization (TACE) using alternative staging systems such as the University of California at San Francisco (UCSF) criteria.

Severe allocation systems have been implemented for prioritization due to scarcity of cadaveric donor livers relative to ongoing demand in the United States. Although this was historically performed based on Child-Pugh-Turcotte scoring, which incorporated serum albumin, bilirubin, prothrombin time (PT), and presence or absence of encephalopathy and ascites, recent modeling studies have established the role of the Model for End-stage Liver Disease (MELD) score as a superior predictor of short-term mortality in patients awaiting liver transplantation. In addition to MELD variables such as total bilirubin, international normalized ratio (INR), and creatinine, serum sodium appears to further augment the predictive accuracy of short-term mortality, thus resulting in the *MELD-Na score,* which is accepted as the preferred allocation tool in the United States. The dynamic range of MELD scoring is 6 to 40, with a minimum score of 15 viewed as a minimum threshold for transplant listing. Significant regional differences in MELD score at time of transplantation currently exist, prompting ongoing discussions regarding further revisions in national organ allocation policies. Furthermore, due to the observation of rising proportion of transplanted organs being allocated for treatment of HCC in patients with low native MELD scores, recent policies have been implemented to decrease application of exception points until after a period of observation to verify HCC tumor biology and response to resection or locoregional therapy.

These systems do not apply to patients with acute fulminant liver failure, as occurs in acute viral or drug-induced hepatitis or in severe acute Wilson disease. Patients in this category are assigned the highest priority for transplantation (status 1A) and are eligible to receive a donor organ both from the local and UNOS regions and the national network without consideration of MELD score.

Detailed and thorough pretransplantation evaluation is conducted to identify any concurrent medical conditions which might preclude liver transplantation, including a detailed psychosocial assessment, with special emphasis on adequate social support, need for counseling or recovery, support programs to maintain alcohol or substance abstinence (in patients with history of abuse), vaccinations, and detailed serologic and radiologic evaluation. Human leukocyte antigen (HLA) haplotyping and detailed immunologic assessment are not routinely required.

Posttransplantation immunosuppression regimens include tacrolimus or cyclosporine, azathioprine or mycophenolate mofetil, with or without corticosteroids. In addition, many transplantation programs consider the use of antagonists to interleukin-2 as induction therapy to prevent early rejection. Outcomes after liver transplantation are typically excellent among patients who undergo transplantation for chronic liver disease, with more than 95% of patients surviving surgery, and 1-year survival rates exceeding 80% in most established programs. Factors associated with lower survival post transplantation include fulminant liver failure, age older than 60 years, and renal failure requiring concomitant renal transplantation.

Long-term outcomes are strongly influenced by the underlying disease. Conditions such as hemochromatosis, hepatitis B, and HCC are associated with lower long-term survival; chronic HCV and alcoholic liver disease are associated with intermediate survival; and autoimmune liver diseases such as autoimmune hepatitis, primary biliary cholangitis, and primary sclerosing cholangitis are associated with excellent long-term survival (85%). Improved selection of HCC patients and new antiviral therapies for chronic HCV have been associated with improved posttransplant outcomes in these patients.

Ongoing developments to maximize organ supply continue, including the use of split-liver transplantation, in which portions of one liver are transplanted into more than one recipient, and live-donor liver transplantation, in which a portion of the liver is removed from a living or beneficent donor is transplanted into a recipient. These procedures have rapidly become alternative means of liver replacement therapy

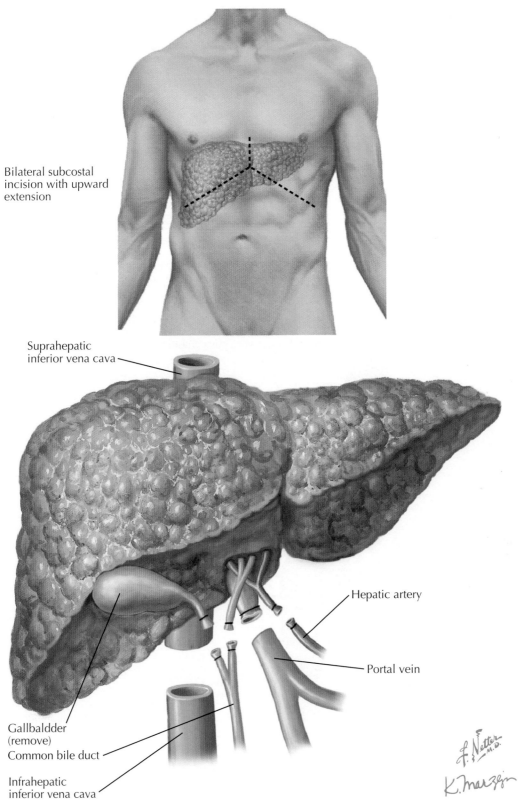

Bilateral subcostal incision with upward extension

Suprahepatic inferior vena cava

Hepatic artery

Portal vein

Gallbaldder (remove)

Common bile duct

Infrahepatic inferior vena cava

Fig. 178.1 Liver Transplantation.

Indications

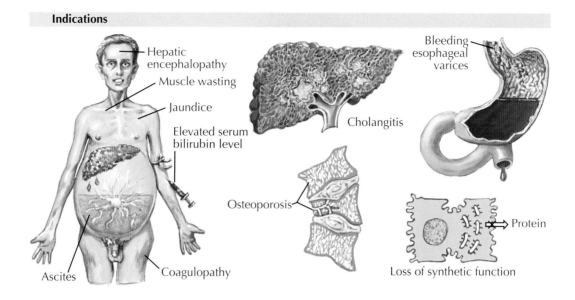

Hepatic
encephalopathy

Muscle wasting

Jaundice

Elevated serum
bilirubin level

Ascites

Coagulopathy

Cholangitis

Osteoporosis

Bleeding
esophageal
varices

Protein

Loss of synthetic function

Technique

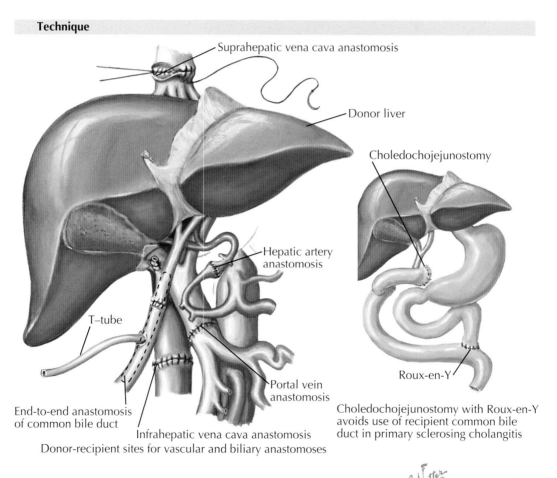

Suprahepatic vena cava anastomosis

Donor liver

Choledochojejunostomy

Hepatic artery
anastomosis

T–tube

Portal vein
anastomosis

Roux-en-Y

End-to-end anastomosis
of common bile duct

Infrahepatic vena cava anastomosis

Donor-recipient sites for vascular and biliary anastomoses

Choledochojejunostomy with Roux-en-Y
avoids use of recipient common bile
duct in primary sclerosing cholangitis

Fig. 178.2 Liver Transplantation (Continued).

and represent lifesaving treatments for many patients, particularly those with HCC and ESLD. However, important ethical and psychosocial issues surround live-donor liver transplantation and require careful consideration.

The long-term care of the liver transplant recipient requires a multidisciplinary approach. In addition to monitoring for rejection of the allograft, patients require surveillance for long-term risks such as malignancy, opportunistic infections, osteoporosis, diabetes, hypertension, atherosclerosis, viral reactivation (e.g., hepatitis B virus), and renal insufficiency.

ADDITIONAL RESOURCES

Bhat M, Al-Busafi S, Deschenes M, Ghali P: Care of the liver transplant patient, *Can J Gastroenterol Hepatol* 28:213–219, 2014.

Chascsa DM, Vargas HE: The gastroenterologist's guide to the management of the post-liver transplant patient, *Am J Gastroenterol* 2018. [Epub ahead of print].

European Association for the Study of the Liver: EASL clinical practice guidelines: liver transplantation, *J Hepatol* 64:433–485, 2016.

Koffron A, Stein JA: Liver transplantation: indications, pretransplant evaluation, surgery, and posttransplant complications, *Med Clin North Am* 92:861–868, 2008.

Lucey MR, Terrault N, Ojo L, et al: Long-term management of the successful adult liver transplant: 2012 practice guideline by the American association for the study of liver diseases and the American society of transplantation, *Liver Transpl* 19:3–26, 2013.

Martin P, DiMartini A, Feng S, et al: Evaluation for liver transplantation in adults: 2013 practice guideline by the American association for the study of liver diseases and the American society of transplantation, *Hepatology* 59:1144–1165, 2014.

179

Other Infections of the Liver: Amebiasis, Spirochetes, Actinomycosis, Echinococcus, Schistosomiasis

Joseph K. Lim, Kris V. Kowdley

SYSTEMIC

Amebiasis may be complicated by the development of an *amebic liver abscess* (Fig. 179.1). *Entamoeba histolytica* (also known as *E. histolytica*) represents the most common parasite identified in amebic liver abscess and is a commensal organism which can result in an invasive amebiasis associated with systemic illness, including fever, nausea, and diarrhea. Symptoms of amebic liver abscess include right upper quadrant pain, fever, nonproductive cough, anorexia, nausea, vomiting, and diarrhea. *E. histolytica* is transmitted primarily through feces in contaminated water and presumably enters the liver via the portal vein. Young men age 20 to 40 years are most often affected.

Amebic liver abscesses are most commonly solitary and found in the right lobe of the liver, although multiple lesions may be present. The initial diagnosis is typically established by ultrasonography or computed tomography, although it requires confirmation by antiamebic antibodies using indirect hemagglutination and enzyme-linked immunosorbent assays. Antibody test findings may be negative very early after initial infection but will remain positive for several months following infection.

The most serious complications of amebic abscesses include spread by rupture or fistulization into the chest, resulting in either pulmonary or hepatopulmonary abscess, hepatobronchial fistula, or hematogenous dissemination into the brain or other organ systems. Abdominal ultrasonography is generally adequate for the identification of amebic abscesses and reveals a hypoechoic lesion. Percutaneous aspiration should be considered if there is concern about rupture or spread to adjacent organs. Stool tests to detect *E. histolytica* may not be helpful because intestinal amebiasis may not be initially present in patients with an amebic liver abscess. Treatment with metronidazole or dehydroemetine is recommended, although tinidazole, ornidazole, and nitazoxanide may also be effective for amebic liver abscess. After the liver abscess is resolved, treatment for luminal infection is also recommended, even if the stool is negative for *E. histolytica*.

SPIROCHETAL INFECTIONS

Spirochetal infections are associated with significant potential morbidity and require a high index of suspicion for their diagnosis. *Weil syndrome*, also historically called infectious jaundice or spirochetal jaundice, is a severe form of leptospirosis caused by *Leptospira icterohaemorrhagiae* (Fig. 179.2). The disease has global impact, and the most common carriers include wild rats, dogs, and to a lesser degree, mice. These animals excrete leptospiras with the urine into stagnant water, where the organisms may survive for months. Human infection takes place either through skin abrasions or through the mouth.

Weil syndrome varies in severity. After an incubation period (6–12 days), high fever, headaches, abdominal pain, prostration, muscle pain, and conjunctivitis appear. At this stage, leptospiral organisms can be demonstrated in the blood or cerebrospinal fluid. Approximately 10 days later, the fever subsides and a toxic stage develops in which renal manifestations (sometimes progressing to renal failure), meningitis, myocardial damage, dermal and conjunctival petechiae, epistaxis, and skin rashes are conspicuous. Liver involvement occurs in approximately 50% of patients. In this period, leptospiras are more readily found in urine than in blood. The fever may recur. After the third week, a slow convalescence begins, and serum antibody findings become positive.

Despite the frequency of hepatic involvement in the patient with spirochetal jaundice, the liver shows nonspecific histologic changes such as centrilobular necrosis, a portal inflammatory infiltrate, and swollen Kupffer cells. The degree of jaundice is often out of proportion to the liver dysfunction, partly because of hemolysis. Initial management is primarily supportive, including treatment of bleeding and renal failure. Death resulting from liver failure is rare. Antibiotics are effective only if given early in the course of Weil syndrome.

Liver disease caused by *syphilis* is now infrequently observed because of improvements in early diagnosis and the availability of effective therapy. Moreover, many cases of hepatic disease in persons with syphilis may be caused by hepatitis B or C. The liver lesion now recognized to be specifically caused by secondary syphilis is the scar formed after extensive specific coagulation necrosis (gumma), which leads to focal loss of hepatic tissue. The resultant irregular deformation of the liver frequently causes bizarre shapes and is designated *hepar lobatum*. However, occasionally, deformation with enlargement of the left lobe and shrinkage of the right lobe causes unusual findings on liver palpation. Rarely, fresh yellow gummatous areas are found in the depths of the scars. Formerly, the now almost-extinct "brimstone" liver was frequently found in deeply jaundiced newborns as a characteristic of congenital syphilis, together with other syphilitic manifestations. Microscopic features are small miliary necroses (gummata), diffuse interstitial hepatitis, separated and distorted liver cell plates, increased interlobular connective tissue with intense inflammation, and demonstration of numerous spirochetes using a silver stain.

Lyme disease, a tick-borne disease caused by the spirochete *Borrelia burgdorferi*, can also be associated with elevated liver transaminases, in addition to myositis, fever, and splenic involvement.

ACTINOMYCOSIS

Actinomycosis is an infection caused by an anaerobic fungus, *Actinomyces bovis*, which is found on many plants and as a harmful saprophyte in the oral cavity, especially in peridental structures and on the tonsils. The

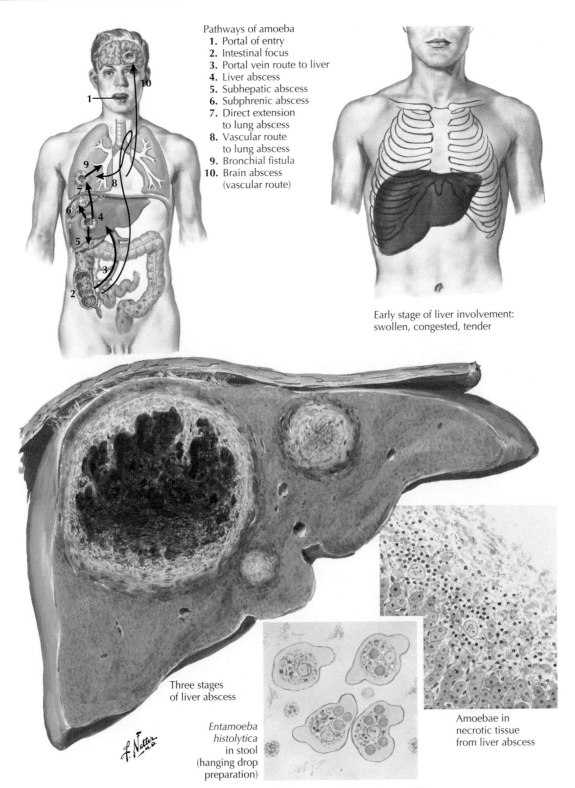

Pathways of amoeba
  1. Portal of entry
  2. Intestinal focus
  3. Portal vein route to liver
  4. Liver abscess
  5. Subhepatic abscess
  6. Subphrenic abscess
  7. Direct extension
     to lung abscess
  8. Vascular route
     to lung abscess
  9. Bronchial fistula
  10. Brain abscess
     (vascular route)

Early stage of liver involvement:
swollen, congested, tender

Three stages
of liver abscess

Entamoeba histolytica
in stool
(hanging drop
preparation)

Amoebae in
necrotic tissue
from liver abscess

Fig. 179.1 Hepatic Amebiasis: Pathways and Liver Abscess Stages.

fungus, on rare occasions, enters the deeper tissues through a break in the mucosa or skin and produces suppuration. Typical initial localizations of the abscesses are the jaws, lungs, cecum, and appendix. From the primary localization, the suppuration may spread through the vicinity.

Characteristically, actinomycotic abscesses do not respect the natural borders of the organs; they extend in all directions in the form of fistulae, which frequently extend from any original site to the body surface. Fistulous tracts are multiple, and the skin surface and the surfaces of involved organs assume a characteristic honeycomb appearance. Only rarely does the actinomycotic infection spread by the hematogenous route, through which metastatic abscesses and endocarditis may develop.

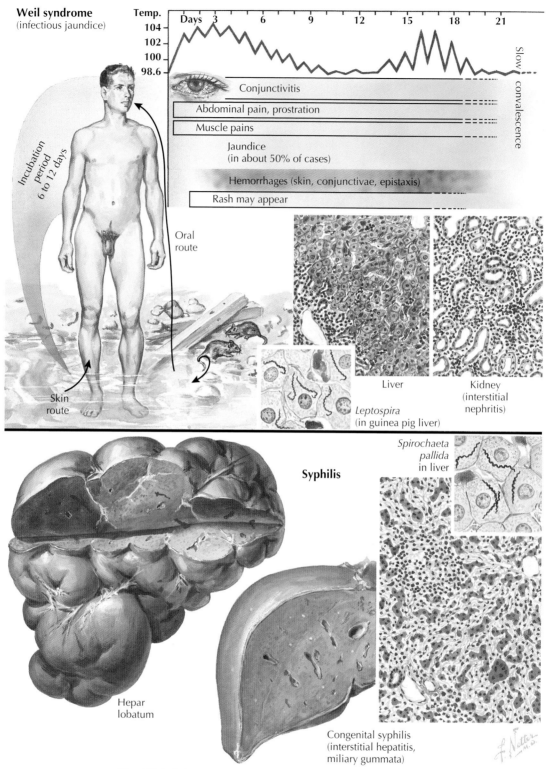

Weil syndrome
(infectious jaundice)

Temp.
104
102
100
98.6

Days 3 6 9 12 15 18 21

Slow convalescence

Conjunctivitis

Abdominal pain, prostration

Muscle pains

Jaundice
(in about 50% of cases)

Hemorrhages (skin, conjunctivae, epistaxis)

Rash may appear

Incubation period 6 to 12 days

Oral route

Skin route

Leptospira
(in guinea pig liver)

Liver

Kidney
(interstitial nephritis)

Spirochaeta pallida in liver

Syphilis

Hepar lobatum

Congenital syphilis
(interstitial hepatitis, miliary gummata)

Fig. 179.2 Spirochetal Infections: Weil Syndrome and Syphilis.

The liver is rarely the site of actinomycotic abscesses, because the primary focus is usually in the proximal colon or appendix. The liver is reached either by direct spread or through the portal vein. The *liver abscess* may also be a complication of a pulmonary actinomycosis, which may manifest as a combined *pneumopleurohepatic abscess* (Fig. 179.3). Actinomycosis and amebiasis are the main causes for hepatobronchial

fistulae. Again, the liver usually does not become involved by the hematogenous route, and in cases of isolated hepatic actinomycosis, the original site of the infection may not be identified.

The smaller liver abscess represents a yellow focus, not sharply limited, that clearly reveals its development from the coalescence of even smaller abscesses. Central portions exhibit multiple, partially communicating

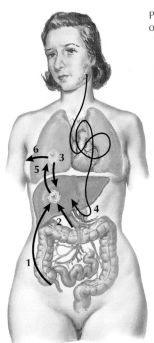

Possible routes
of dissemination
1. Directly from gut
   (appendix) to liver
2. Via portal vein
3. Extension from lung
   to liver
4. Hematogenous
   route to liver
5. Extension from
   liver to lung
6. Cutaneous
   fistula

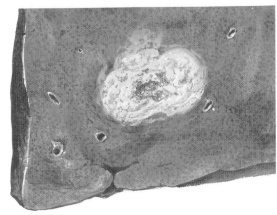

Relatively small actinomycotic abscess

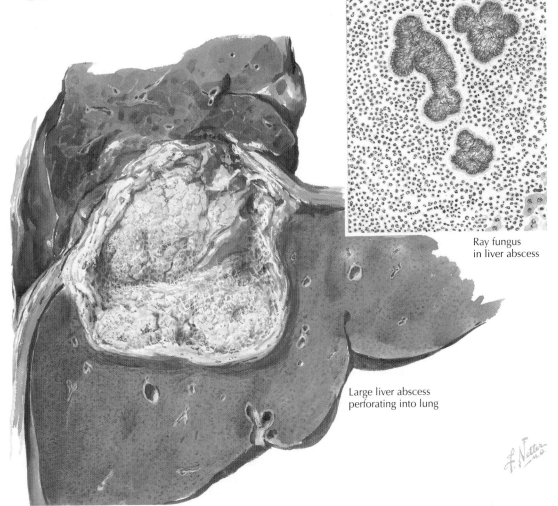

Ray fungus
in liver abscess

Large liver abscess
perforating into lung

Fig. 179.3 Actinomycosis.

cavities of different size. In the pus are small, yellow granules (sulfur granules) that consist of concentric, moderately basophilic branching filaments with eosinophilic clubbed endings; the arrangement of these filaments, best seen in tissue sections, accounts for the name *ray fungus*. In cultures, the fungus grows in short, single-branched forms, simulating diphtheria bacilli, and in branching filaments. The ray fungus is surrounded by leukocytes that, in turn, are engulfed by granulation tissue earmarked by many fat-containing foam cells. This fat accumulation accounts for the bright yellow of the lesion.

The abscess grows by direct distention until it involves the hepatic capsule, with resultant subdiaphragmatic, subhepatic, or perinephritic perihepatitis. Eventually, perforation into the surrounding viscus or skin takes place. Diffuse peritonitis is rare. An extremely shaggy wall characterizes the large abscess cavity resulting from the expansion of the smaller lesion. Secondary infection by pyogenic bacteria is a particularly dangerous complication.

Clinically, *hepatic actinomycosis* is a toxic wasting condition associated with fever, anemia, and leukocytosis. The liver is enlarged and tender, and abdominal pain develops. Ascites and jaundice are rare; involvement of the surrounding organs and multiple cutaneous fistulae contribute to the clinical picture. Hepatic function tests reveal no characteristic alterations except for manifestations of a space-occupying lesion. The prognosis may be poor due to the high risk for suppuration and spread to other organs. Combined therapy with surgical intervention and antibiotics is often required.

ECHINOCOCCOSIS (HYDATID DISEASE)

Hydatid disease remains a common and important infection in endemic countries predominantly in sheep-raising regions. *Taenia echinococcus* or *Echinococcus granulosus* is a tapeworm only 5 mm long in the adult stage. It lives in the small intestine of dogs and other canines that have been infected by ingestion of scolices-containing viscera of other animals, mainly sheep (Fig. 179.4). In the canine intestine, the scolices develop into the adult *Taenia*, a piriform head with four suckers and numerous hooklets, a short neck, and only a few segments, of which the terminal (proglottis) releases the ova.

The ova are ingested by the larval or intermediate host (sheep, cattle, and hogs) but also by humans, mostly children. In the intestinal tract of the host, the larvae hatch from the egg and migrate into the liver and, much less often, into lungs, brain, and other organs, where the larvae develop into a cyst with an outer laminated and inner germinal layer, around which forms a capsule of collagenous tissue. From the cells of the germinal layer evolve embryonal scolices, either directly or after invaginations (brood capsules) form, and eventually become endogenous *daughter cysts*.

With successive invaginations and generations of cysts, the original unilocular main cyst is eventually filled by hundreds of daughter cysts of varying size. The main cyst grows through the years, initially symptomless, until it becomes 20 cm (8 inches) or larger in diameter. Daughter cysts are often discharged from the wall and float in the lumen containing the hydatid fluid. The fluid also contains the *hydatid sand* in which the scolices may be microscopically recognized. Daughter cysts may be seen as outpouchings on the wall of the main cyst or in the surrounding hepatic tissue and, occasionally, implanted in the peritoneal lining of the mesentery. When this asexual production of scolices in the cysts eventually stops, the capsule invades the cyst. The inner surface, formerly granular, becomes smooth; the wall becomes fibrotic and sometimes calcified, and thus radiographically visible. Inflammatory reactions in the vicinity of the cyst are rare.

Echinococcosis has its highest incidence in sheep-raising countries. Three types have been identified, caused by *E. granulosus*, *E. multilocu-*

laris, and *E. vogeli*. Hydatid disease is most often associated with *E. granulosus*, which may be seen worldwide. *E. multilocularis* is most frequently observed in the Northern Hemisphere and is associated with alveolar hydatid disease.

Many hydatid infections are asymptomatic, and the cysts are mostly incidental findings during liver imaging studies. Clinical symptoms are caused by complications, most often, rupture of the cysts. Hydatid fluid entering the circulation can produce allergic manifestations and, rarely, anaphylactic shock. Rupture of daughter cysts into bile ducts or compression of the bile duct can lead to jaundice. Secondary bacterial infection of cysts causes fever and chills. Serum indirect hemagglutination test findings are usually positive.

The first-line treatment remains *albendazole*, a benzimidazole drug. However, resection using open or laparoscopic approaches has been described, and ultrasonographic percutaneous drainage is being increasingly used in combination with antimicrobial therapy. Care is taken to avoid spillage of the cyst contents because this can lead to systemic allergic reactions and possibly anaphylaxis.

SCHISTOSOMIASIS

Schistosomiasis remains a rare but clinically important parasitic infection within endemic regions of the world, particularly in South America. *Schistosoma* is a genus of trematode parasites or blood flukes, of which *Schistosoma mansoni*, *Schistosoma japonicum*, and *Schistosoma haematobium* are of importance in human pathology. *S. mansoni* is found mainly in Africa, parts of South America, and Puerto Rico, from where, with increasing emigration, it is imported to the United States. *S. japonicum* is common in the Far East. *S. haematobium* is found in Africa, especially Egypt, and in endemic foci in southern Europe and Asia. The life cycles of the three species are similar, but *S. haematobium* predominantly involves the vessels of the urinary bladder. Eggs of *S. mansoni* and *S. japonicum* are excreted with the feces of human carriers; those of *S. haematobium* are excreted with the urine.

The eggs of *S. mansoni*, approximately 140 mm long, exhibit a characteristic lateral spine (Fig. 179.5). They hatch when they fall into fresh water. The larvae, or *miracidia*, survive only a few hours, unless they can attach themselves to snails, which they penetrate. In the snail's digestive gland, the larvae pass through several stages (sporocysts) and develop into *cercariae*, which, having left the snail, propel themselves with a forked tail. They are most active in shallow water exposed to sunlight, where they may attach themselves to wading or swimming humans, whose unbroken skin or mucous membranes they enter. They eventually reach the extrahepatic tributaries and the intrahepatic branches of the portal vein, where they grow to full sexual maturity, depositing the fertilized eggs. Some eggs are extruded through the vascular wall into the intestinal lumen, where they pass with the feces, maintaining the life cycle. Other eggs are carried into the smallest portal radicles in the liver, where they are responsible for the clinical manifestations of *hepatic schistosomiasis*.

Very shortly after infestation and during migration, localized or generalized skin reactions occur, accompanied by pruritus (swimmer's itch) and fever. The liver becomes enlarged. In the peripheral blood, granulocytosis and eosinophilia (14,000–20,000 cells) are found. Within approximately 6 weeks, symptoms may entirely subside, whereas in other patients, an acute toxic stage may develop. This stage is characterized by constant or intermittent fever, mild gastrointestinal discomfort to severe abdominal pain, nausea, vomiting, and occasionally persistent cough. The liver becomes large and tender, and splenomegaly develops.

In some patients after a variable interval, chronic colitis, mesenteric lymphadenitis, and pulmonary fibrosis may develop. However, the most

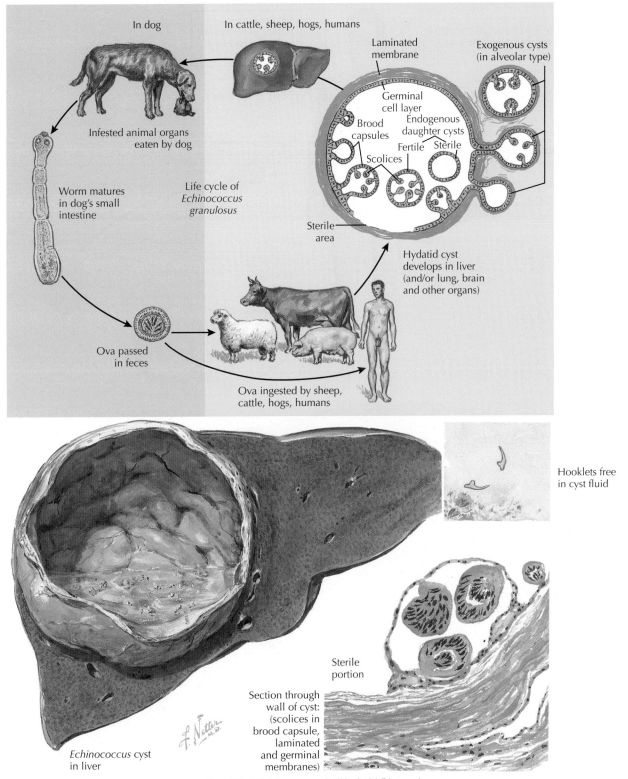

Fig. 179.4 Echinococcosis (Hydatid Disease).

dangerous manifestations occur in the portal system, where worms and ova obstruct portal venous blood flow, resulting in portal hypertension. The ova adhere to the lining endothelium, which grows over them. First, an inflammatory reaction develops, followed eventually by granuloma formation, with fibroblasts, epithelioid cells, and even giant cells. The ovum becomes necrotic, frequently calcified, and may entirely disappear, whereas the fibrosing *pseudotubercle* persists.

Liver biopsy is not routinely required but reveals distinct pathologic findings. Granulomas are readily demonstrated on histopathology, and their etiology can frequently be established by demonstrating the ova or their remnants. If the changes to the hepatic parenchyma become severe, *pipestem cirrhosis* develops. More frequently, however, the cirrhosis is similar to other forms of cirrhosis, probably because of concomitant hepatitis C infection or alcoholic liver disease.

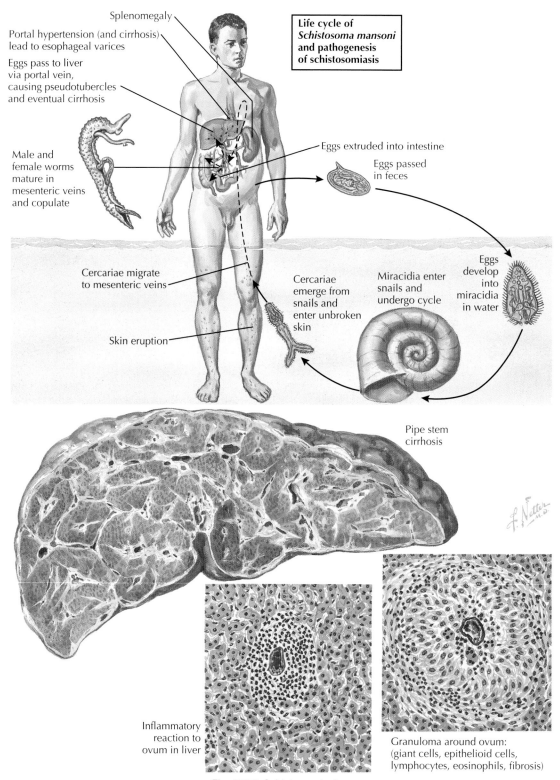

Splenomegaly

Portal hypertension (and cirrhosis) lead to esophageal varices

Eggs pass to liver via portal vein, causing pseudotubercles and eventual cirrhosis

Male and female worms mature in mesenteric veins and copulate

Cercariae migrate to mesenteric veins

Skin eruption

Life cycle of *Schistosoma mansoni* and pathogenesis of schistosomiasis

Eggs extruded into intestine

Eggs passed in feces

Cercariae emerge from snails and enter unbroken skin

Miracidia enter snails and undergo cycle

Eggs develop into miracidia in water

Pipe stem cirrhosis

Inflammatory reaction to ovum in liver

Granuloma around ovum: (giant cells, epithelioid cells, lymphocytes, eosinophils, fibrosis)

Fig. 179.5 Schistosomiasis.

ADDITIONAL RESOURCES

Avila F, Santos V, Massinha P, et al: Hepatic actinomycosis, *GE Port J Gastroenterol* 22:19–23, 2015.

Bica I, Hamer DH, Stadecker MJ: Hepatic schistosomiasis, *Infect Dis Clin North Am* 14:583–604, 2000.

Gomez I, Gavara C, Lopez-Andujar R, et al: Review of the treatment of liver hyatid cysts, *World J Gastroenterol* 21:124–131, 2015.

Gryseels B: Schistosomiasis, *Infect Dis Clin North Am* 26:383–397, 2012.

Mohidin B, Green SF, Duggineni S: Amoebic liver abscess, *QJM* 2018. [Epub ahead of print].

Sahay S, McKelvy BJ: Actinomycosis preentinh as recurrent hepatic abscesses, *Am J Med* 130:e21–e22, 2017.

180

Vascular Disorders of the Liver

Joseph K. Lim, Kris V. Kowdley

Secondary liver disease stemming from vascular pathology related to heart failure, portal vein obstruction, and Budd-Chiari syndrome represents clinically important conditions associated with significant morbidity and impairment of health-related quality of life.

THE LIVER IN HEART FAILURE

Heart failure represents one of the more common etiologies for passive congestion of the liver, which may be associated with significant clinical sequelae. Importantly, the severity of passive liver congestion does not correlate directly with the degree of hepatic involvement.

In *acute* passive congestion, the liver is significantly enlarged, the capsule is tense, the anterior edge is blunt, and on the cut surface, lobular markings are much more distinct than usual (Fig. 180.1). On closer inspection, the zones around the central veins appear dark red and depressed, distinct from the intermediate and peripheral zones, which may exhibit a yellow hue caused by fatty metamorphosis. The hepatic veins are extremely dilated, the liver cells in the central zone have disappeared, and both the sinusoids and tissue spaces are crowded with red blood cells, as are the dilated branches of the hepatic veins. Central necrosis is more marked on autopsy rather than on biopsy specimens.

Therefore *central necrosis* in a patient with heart failure may represent a terminal or a preterminal event in end-stage or severe heart failure. Occasionally, only a small rim of parenchyma is preserved on the periphery of hepatic lobules in cases of severe acute cardiac failure, such as rupture of a chorda tendinea. Clinically, the liver is very large and exquisitely tender, particularly in the gallbladder region.

In *chronic* passive congestion, the liver appears smaller than in the acute stages and smaller compared with normal. The surface is irregular and may be finely granular, whereas the capsule often is thickened and covered by organized fibrin. The liver may be diffusely fibrotic, and regenerative nodules may be present. The hepatic veins appear wider than in acute stages, and fibrosis may initially surround the central veins, leading to a "reverse lobular" pattern.

With progressive liver disease, bridging fibrosis may develop between central veins and portal areas, leading to established cirrhosis. True *cardiac cirrhosis* is the result of severe and usually long-standing passive congestion, as occurs in severe tricuspid insufficiency or constrictive pericarditis. In *cardiac hepatic fibrosis*, the tender liver appears relatively small, and jaundice and ascites may be present.

Patients with severe acute left ventricular heart failure may also develop acute ischemic hepatitis, characterized by high serum transaminase levels similar to those seen with *shock liver*, and may be associated with hypotension or hypoxemia. Jaundice and tender hepatomegaly may also develop. Some patients may have evidence of synthetic dysfunction with hepatic encephalopathy. Liver biopsy is not routinely required for diagnosis but may reveal centrilobular necrosis, which may be severe and lead to necrosis of hepatocytes in central areas, sinusoidal congestion, and a neutrophilic inflammatory infiltrate.

PORTAL VEIN OBSTRUCTION

Most cases of portal vein thrombosis are associated with underlying cirrhosis, malignancy, or pancreatitis. An acute decrease in systemic blood pressure may also lead to portal venous obstruction (Fig. 180.2). In the absence of a known cause, many cases of portal vein thrombosis may occur in association with hypercoagulable states such as polycythemia vera. Sudden, complete obstruction of the portal vein and its branches by a thrombus may lead, in rare cases, to a clinically dramatic picture dominated by hematemesis, melena with diarrhea, rapidly developing ascites, abdominal pain, peritonitis, ileus, and rapid coma and death. However, many of these patients also have associated thrombosis of the superior mesenteric vein. Jaundice is characteristically uncommon. Precipitating factors include splenectomy or other procedures involving the portal system. Portal vein thrombosis may also develop in patients during the course of cirrhosis or as a complicating feature of hepatocellular carcinoma with extrahepatic spread.

In *acute* portal vein thrombosis, the wall of the small intestine may also show changes, including edema and hemorrhage. The spleen is generally enlarged, but in patients without history of cirrhosis, the liver may be unremarkable. The thrombosis may originate from the portal vein itself or may extend into it from a splenic or a mesenteric vein thrombus or distally from thrombi in the intrahepatic branches of the portal vein.

A more gradual decrease in the portal circulation is well tolerated, possibly because of the development of collaterals. The thrombosis may result in cordlike shrinkage of the portal vein or a spongy cavernous transformation caused by recanalization of the thrombus itself. The liver shows minimal changes in isolated portal vein thrombosis, and jaundice is usually absent. The main complication, variceal bleeding, is generally better tolerated than in patients with cirrhosis. Ascites may be present.

Extrahepatic portal vein obstruction is common in developing countries, particularly India, and is a common cause of noncirrhotic portal hypertension. It is associated with extensive collateral circulation around the portal vein, leading to formation of ectopic varices in the peribiliary and peripancreatic regions. Variceal hemorrhage is the most common complication.

Treatment of portal vein obstruction focuses on managing the complications of portal hypertension. In patients without an underlying history of cirrhosis, a workup for a hypercoagulable state is indicated. Endoscopic therapy is effective for patients with variceal bleeding, and portal decompression is appropriate for patients with preserved hepatic synthetic function. Transjugular intrahepatic portosystemic shunt (TIPS) has been used in some patients with portal venous obstruction, especially when the acute portal vein thrombosis is associated with Budd-Chiari syndrome.

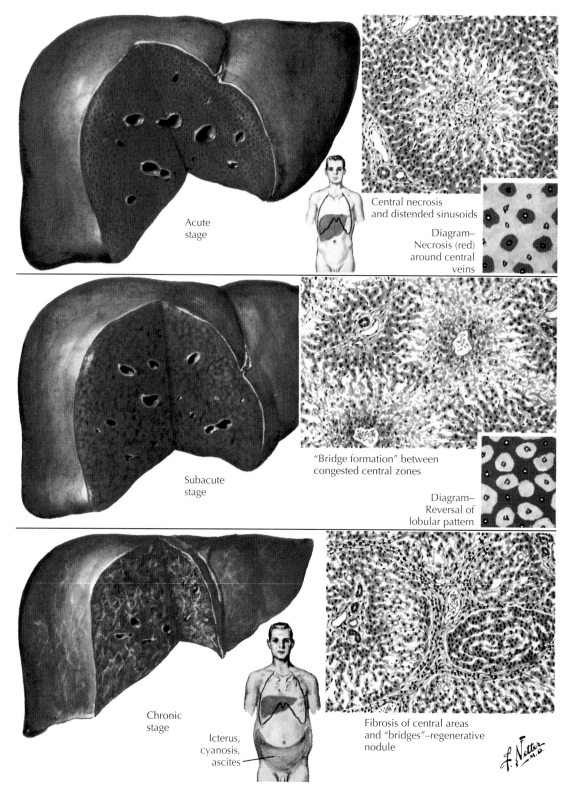

Acute
stage

Central necrosis
and distended sinusoids

Diagram–
Necrosis (red)
around central
veins

Subacute
stage

"Bridge formation" between
congested central zones

Diagram–
Reversal of
lobular pattern

Chronic
stage

Icterus,
cyanosis,
ascites

Fibrosis of central areas
and "bridges"–regenerative
nodule

Fig. 180.1 The Liver in Heart Failure: Cardiac Liver and Shock.

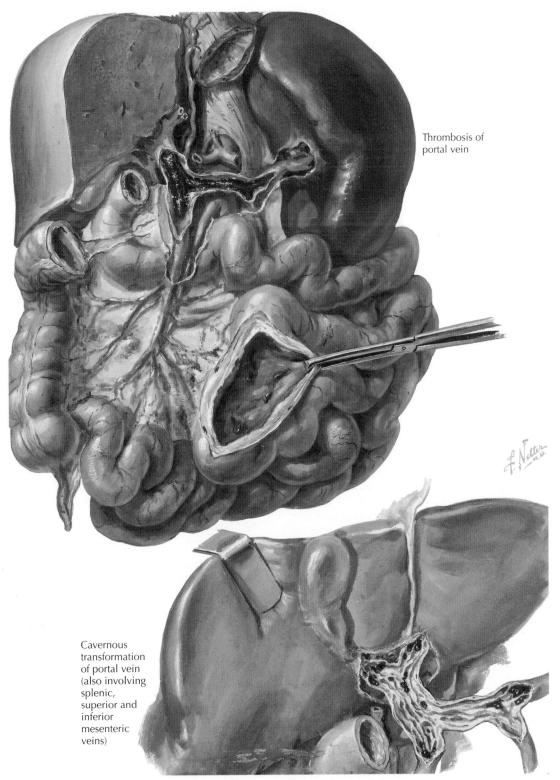

Thrombosis of portal vein

Cavernous transformation of portal vein (also involving splenic, superior and inferior mesenteric veins)

Fig. 180.2 Portal Venous Obstruction.

BUDD-CHIARI SYNDROME

Budd-Chiari syndrome is characterized by clinical features associated with hepatic venous outflow obstruction. Although this term is generally used to describe a specific entity, namely, hepatic venous obstruction associated with acute or chronic thrombosis, the level of outflow obstruction in the liver may be in any location from the suprahepatic cava to the right atrium.

Clinical Picture

Most cases of Budd-Chiari syndrome are observed in patients with hypercoagulable states. Acute or chronic outflow obstruction at the level of the hepatic vein results in portal hypertension and may lead to necrosis caused by decreased perfusion from impaired inflow into the sinusoids through the portal vein. Portal vein thrombosis may develop and may exacerbate this ischemic process.

Patients with Budd-Chiari syndrome may also have acute hepatic venous obstruction from thrombosis. This presentation may be associated with the development of rapidly worsening liver failure and may represent a medical emergency. Acute thrombosis develops suddenly in the hepatic veins, with inadequate time for the development of collaterals to decompress the portal hypertension. The clinical presentation may vary depending on the chronicity of the thrombotic process and the formation of portosystemic collaterals. Clinical manifestations of Budd-Chiari syndrome may include tender hepatomegaly, ascites, jaundice, and coagulopathy. Hepatic encephalopathy and liver failure are ominous signs.

Diagnosis

Radiologic diagnosis using abdominal sonography and duplex examination of the hepatic veins is extremely sensitive and can be diagnostic in many patients. Direct venography using the transjugular technique can be used to confirm the diagnosis. In addition, transjugular liver biopsy can be performed to determine the presence or absence of cirrhosis. Often, computed tomography shows a prominent caudate lobe, which drains uniquely and directly into the vena cava, thus perhaps avoiding atrophy in classic cases of Budd-Chiari syndrome. In some patients, the prominent caudate lobe is mistaken for a mass on imaging studies.

The differential diagnosis of Budd-Chiari syndrome includes any cause of hepatic outflow obstruction, such as heart failure, severe tricuspid insufficiency, or constrictive pericarditis. Physical examination and cardiac echocardiography can usually differentiate these causes. Hepatic venoocclusive disease may have similar features on liver biopsy, but in Budd-Chiari syndrome, the hepatic veins are usually visualized and patent, and histopathology is marked by centrilobular hemorrhage, congestion, and organized thrombi in advanced cases. The most common cause of a hypercoagulable state leading to Budd-Chiari syndrome is *polycythemia vera*, although other causes include protein C, protein S, and antithrombin III deficiency, among other rarer etiologies such as paroxysmal nocturnal hemoglobinuria (PNH).

Treatment and Management

Management of Budd-Chiari syndrome is focused on decompression of portal hypertension in acute cases and in patients without cirrhosis. Surgical decompression and TIPS have been used with success. Medical therapy with thrombolytic agents may be helpful for patients with acute thrombosis. Liver transplantation is an option for patients with cirrhosis or with acute liver failure and if previous therapies have failed. Although there is concern about recurrent thrombosis after liver transplantation, limited studies suggest favorable long-term outcomes. However, long-term anticoagulation is often required after liver transplantation, which may be associated with an increased risk for bleeding complications.

ADDITIONAL RESOURCES

Basit SA, STone CD, Gish R: Portal vein thrombosis, *Clin Liver Dis* 19:199–221, 2015.

DeLeve LD, Valla DC, Garcia-Tsao G: Vascular disorders of the liver, *Hepatology* 49:1729–1764, 2009.

Harding DJ, Perera MT, Chen F, et al: Portal vein thrombosis in cirrhosis: controversies and latest developments, *World J Gastroenterol* 21:6769–6784, 2015.

Loudin M, Ahn J: Portal vein thrombosis in cirrhosis, *J Clin Gastroenterol* 51:579–585, 2017.

Martens P, Nevens F: Budd-chiari syndrome, *United European Gastroenterol J* 3:489–500, 2015.

Plessier A, Rautou PE, Valla DC: Management of hepatic vascular diseases, *J Hepatol* 56(Suppl 1):S24–S38, 2012.

Valla DC: Budd-chiari syndrome/hepatic venous outflow tract obstruction, *Hepatol Int* 12(Suppl 1):168–180, 2018.

Valla DC, Cazals-Hatem D: Vascular liver diseases on the clinical side: definitions and diagnosis, new concepts, *Virchows Arch* 2018. [Epub ahead of print].

181

Bile Duct Cancer

Joseph K. Lim, Kris V. Kowdley

Bile duct cancer, also called *cholangiocarcinoma* (CCA), refers to malignancies arising from the epithelia of biliary ductal cells. The incidence of CCA is low, estimated at 8 per 1 million population. Major risk factors for bile duct cancer include primary sclerosing cholangitis (PSC), *Clonorchis sinensis* infection, *Opisthorchis viverrini* infection, older age, exposure to thorium dioxide (Thorotrast), congenital bile duct abnormalities (e.g., Caroli disease), and prior biliary-enteric drainage procedures. Among patients with PSC, the annual risk for CCA is estimated at 2%, with 10-year cumulative incidence ranging between 6% and 11% and 30-year cumulative incidence of 20%; of CCA cases diagnosed in patients with PSC, a striking 30% are identified within the first year of PSC diagnosis.

CCAs are generally classified as hilar, intrahepatic, and distal. *Hilar CCA* is the most common form, accounting for 50% to 60% of cases (Figs. 181.1 and 181.2). Most CCAs are adenocarcinomas, although different histologic patterns may be seen and may reveal an intense desmoplastic reaction around the tumor, facilitating tissue acquisition for diagnosis through endoscopic retrograde cholangiopancreatography (ERCP) or percutaneous cholangiography.

The diagnosis of CCA is notoriously difficult to establish early in the disease course, largely due to local or distant spread which has occurred by the time of clinical presentation, most commonly jaundice or biliary dilatation/strictures. Other clinical manifestations may include fever from associated cholangitis, weight loss, and abdominal pain. The symptom of jaundice is more common in patients with distal CCA, whereas abdominal pain is more common among patients with the peripheral or intrahepatic forms of CCA.

ERCP represents the ideal method to establish the diagnosis of CCA because it provides radiographic evidence suggestive of possible bile duct cancer and permits tissue confirmation by selective bile duct biopsies. Several serum markers such as cancer antigen (CA) 19-9, carcinoembryonic antigen (CEA), and CA 125 may be elevated, although they are nonspecific and both high and normal levels may be observed in the presence of malignancy. However, very high serum levels of CA 19-9 (>100) in patients with PSC has excellent predictive value for CCA, particularly in patients without concurrent cholangitis.

The prognosis for patients with CCA is commonly poor due to late stage of presentation, with an average 5-year survival of approximately 10%. Surgical resection for cure remains the best hope for long-term survival, but a small minority are candidates at the time of diagnosis. For patients with unresectable disease, palliative decompression of malignant strictures using plastic or metal stents can decrease risk for bacterial cholangitis and relieve symptoms of pruritus.

Liver transplantation is not routinely performed for patients with hilar CCA due to the high risk for recurrent malignancy and poor long-term survival. However, carefully selected patients with early-stage PSC may be considered on an individual basis because long-term survival may be feasible in conjunction with adjuvant or neoadjuvant therapy. Gemcitabine has been approved for oncologic treatment of CCA and is frequently used in combination with other agents such as cisplatin or oxaliplatin. Other drugs that have been used for CCA include 5-fluorouracil (5-FU), capecitabine, and paclitaxel with limited success, and ongoing investigation for novel therapies for hilar CCA are needed.

ADDITIONAL RESOURCES

Blechacz B, Komuta M, Roskams T, Gores GJ: Clinical diagnosis and staging of cholangiocarcinoma, *Nat Rev Gastroenterol Hepatol* 8:512–522, 2011.

Bridgewater J, Galle PR, Khan SA, et al: Guidelines for the diagnosis and management of intrahepatic cholangiocarcinoma, *J Hepatol* 60:1268–1289, 2014.

Esnaola NF, Meyer JE, Karachristos A, et al: Evaluation and management of intrahepatic and extrahepatic cholangiocarcinoma, *Cancer* 122:1349–1369, 2016.

Razumilava N, Gores GJ: Cholangiocarcinoma, *Lancet* 383:2168–2179, 2014.

Rizvi S, Gores GJ: Pathogenesis, diagnosis, and management of cholangiocarcinoma, *Gastroenterology* 145:1215–1229, 2013.

Zhu AX: Future directions in the treatment of cholangiocarcinoma, *Best Pract Res Clin Gastroenterol* 29:355–361, 2015.

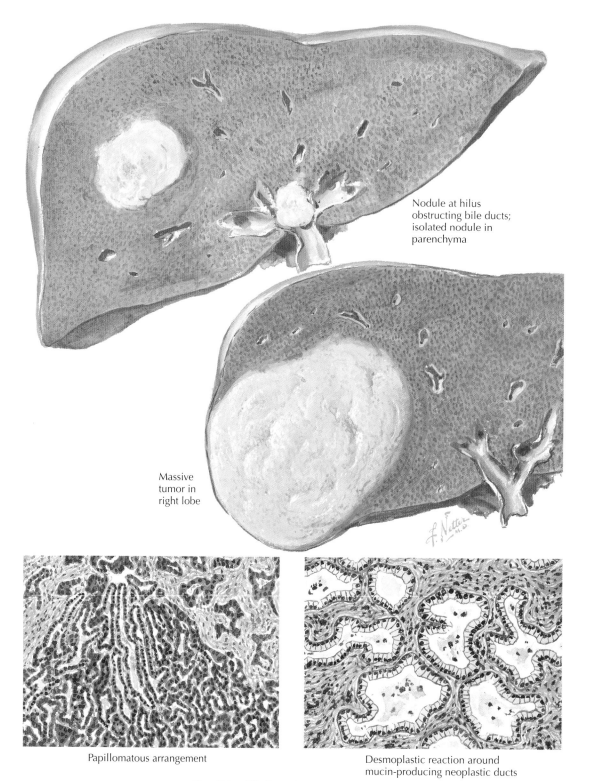

Nodule at hilus
obstructing bile ducts;
isolated nodule in
parenchyma

Massive
tumor in
right lobe

Papillomatous arrangement

Desmoplastic reaction around
mucin-producing neoplastic ducts

Fig. 181.1 Bile Duct Carcinoma of Liver.

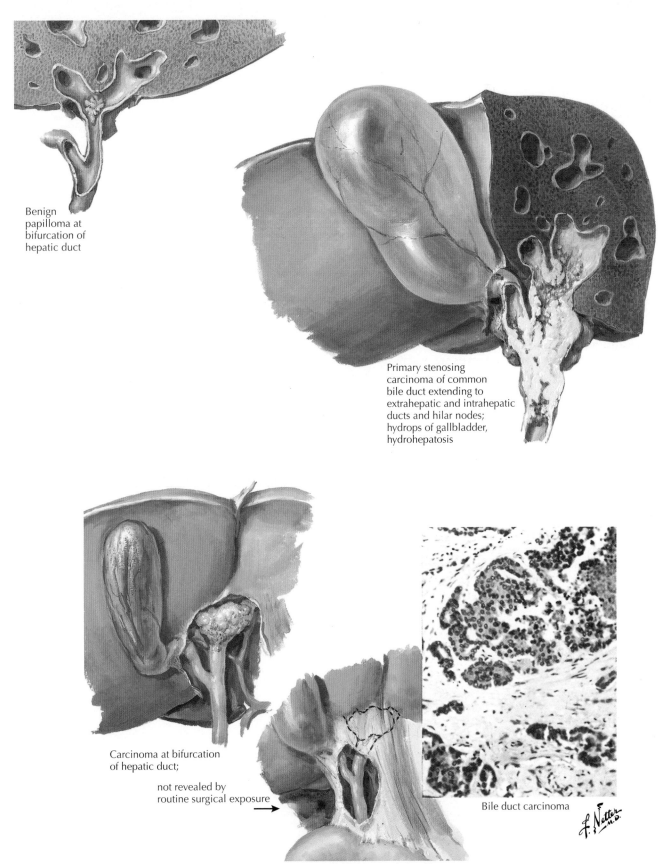

Benign
papilloma at
bifurcation of
hepatic duct

Primary stenosing
carcinoma of common
bile duct extending to
extrahepatic and intrahepatic
ducts and hilar nodes;
hydrops of gallbladder,
hydrohepatosis

Carcinoma at bifurcation
of hepatic duct;

not revealed by
routine surgical exposure →

Bile duct carcinoma

Fig. 181.2 Bile Duct Cancer: Benign Papilloma and Carcinomas.

182

Metastatic Cancer

Joseph K. Lim, Kris V. Kowdley

Although the focus of oncologic investigation of the liver is centered on primary liver malignancies such as hepatocellular carcinoma and cholangiocarcinoma, secondary liver malignancies far outnumber primary malignancies in the United States. One of the most common sites of primary malignancy from which carcinoma metastasizes to the liver is the gastrointestinal (GI) tract, particularly colon cancer. Other common primary cancers that metastasize to the liver include stomach, esophagus, pancreas, and gallbladder. Other non-GI cancers such as malignant melanoma (particularly ocular melanoma) and primary lung cancer may also spread to the liver. Liver metastases are typically detected through abdominal computed tomography (CT), magnetic resonance imaging (MRI), or other cross-sectional imaging during cancer staging or surveillance (Fig. 182.1).

Colon cancer is the most common primary GI tract tumor associated with metastases to the liver. Isolated liver metastases may occur years after the primary colon malignancy has been treated, and therefore long-term CT surveillance is recommended to identify evidence of hepatic involvement. Directed treatment for hepatic metastases from primary colon cancer includes surgical resection in patients with potentially resectable metastases (mets) with either neoadjuvant or postoperative chemotherapy. First line chemotherapy regimens include FOLFOX (oxaliplatin plus fluorouracil and leucovorin), FOLFIRI (irinotecan plus fluorouracil and leucovorin), and XELOX (oxaliplatin plus capecitabine). The addition of targeted agents such as bevacizumab have demonstrated the potential to augment tumor response and survival. Second line treatment of metastatic colorectal cancer such as cetuximab or panitumumab (if tumor does not have RAS or BRAF V600E mutation) or immune checkpoint inhibitors such as nivolumab or pembrolizumab (if mismatch repair–deficient mutation) may be considered. Long-term remissions and cures have been described after resection of isolated liver metastases from colorectal cancer with or without chemotherapy.

Neuroendocrine tumors also frequently spread to the liver and may be functionally active and produce a variety of hormones which have clinical and biochemical effects. Islet cell tumors, glucagonomas, insulinomas, and carcinoid tumors which produce vasoactive intestinal peptide (VIP) may lead to clinical symptoms that are hormone specific. Surgical resection and antihormonal therapies such as octreotide have been recommended for the management of neuroendocrine tumors. Other tumors involving the liver include mesenchymal cell tumors (e.g., GI stromal tumors) and adenocarcinomas from unknown primary sites.

ADDITIONAL RESOURCES

Akgul O, Cetinkaya E, Ersoz S, Tez M: Role of surgery in colorectal cancer liver metastases, *World J Gastroenterol* 20:6113–6122, 2014.

Machairas N, Prodromidou A, Molmenti E, et al: Management of liver metastases from gastrointestinal stromal tumors: where do we stand?, *J Gastrointest Oncol* 8:1100–1108, 2017.

Schwarz C, Kaczirek K, Bodingbauer M: Liver resection for noncolorectal metastases, *Eur Surg* 50:113–116, 2018.

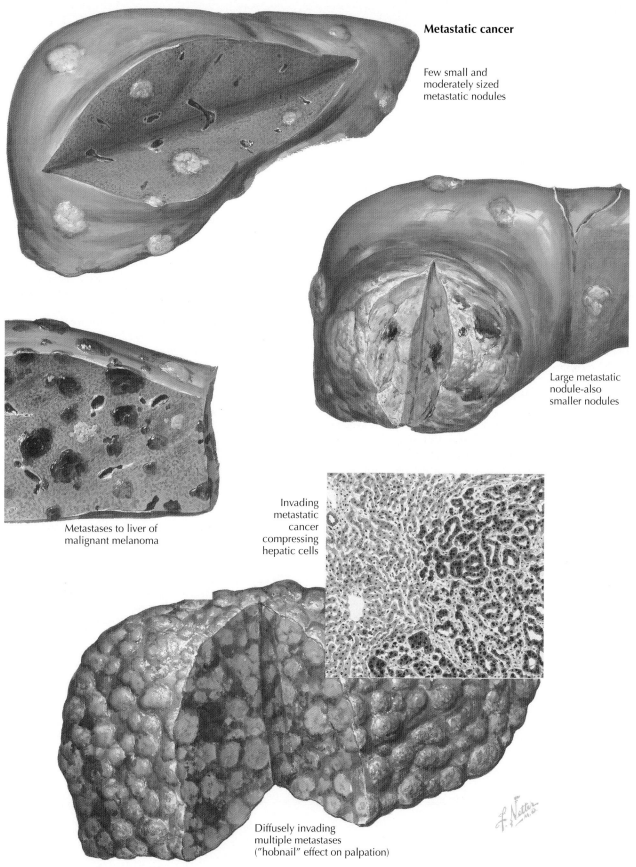

Metastatic cancer

Few small and moderately sized metastatic nodules

Large metastatic nodule–also smaller nodules

Metastases to liver of malignant melanoma

Invading metastatic cancer compressing hepatic cells

Diffusely invading multiple metastases ("hobnail" effect on palpation)

Fig. 182.1 Metastatic Liver Cancer.

183

Hepatic Trauma

Joseph K. Lim, Kris V. Kowdley

Trauma to the liver represents a common secondary complication to both penetrating and blunt abdominal trauma injuries, likely due to its size, location, and fixation within the abdomen. Only the brain is more commonly involved in blunt trauma injuries.

Bullet and stab wounds penetrate to various depths and produce an intrahepatic canal with a ragged wall and a lumen filled with blood. In more than one-quarter of penetrating thoraco-abdominal wounds, the liver is injured, resulting in either *ruptures* or *laceration,* which may vary in size and number (Fig. 183.1). Blunt trauma usually results from motor vehicle accidents or falls, through which the liver may be lacerated by broken ribs or crushed by the impact of the thoracic cage and resisting spine. The internal stress of countercoup effects during a blunt injury may cause both subcapsular and central lacerations, although if the impact is mild the injury may be limited to a subcapsular hematoma.

Rupture of the liver capsule from blunt injury is more likely to occur if the liver has become more friable or if capsular tension has increased because of the formation of an abscess, cyst, infections (e.g., malaria), viral hepatitis, or fatty infiltration. In contrast to the spleen, true spontaneous ruptures of a minimally damaged liver are likely very rare and have been reported in context of postprandial hyperemia, pregnancy, and amyloidosis.

Subcapsular hematomas and small lacerations or ruptures typically heal without clinical sequelae except for a white or pigmented subcapsular scar. However, loss of blood into the peritoneal cavity may be associated with peritoneal irritation, and rarely hematomas may become infected, leading to the development of complicated intrahepatic, subphrenic, or subhepatic abscesses, hepatic cysts, and/or biliary fistulae. Portal vein thrombosis and arterial aneurysms represent rare complications.

Severe lacerations or rupture of the liver are associated with substantial morbidity and mortality, particularly as a consequence of military injury. Severe hemorrhage of the liver associated with early death may occur due to unique factors such as thin hepatic vein wall thickness, highly vascular nature of the liver, and intrinsic anticoagulant properties of bile. Late mortality may be influenced by bile peritonitis and multiorgan failure including acute kidney injury with hepatorenal syndrome. Detached liver tissue pieces appear to be better tolerated within the peritoneal cavity and may be organically attached in the lateral gutter (see Fig. 183.1).

Laboratory findings in patients who experience hepatic trauma are often remarkably normal because liver enzymes are rarely elevated unless accompanied by ischemic hepatitis. Jaundice and associated hyperbilirubinemia are rare and occur primarily if there is associated rupture of the gallbladder and/or bile ducts or as the result of liver abscesses or traumatic cholangitis, as in the case of obstruction of the biliary ducts from foreign bodies (e.g., bullets).

ADDITIONAL RESOURCES

Boese CK, Hackl M, Muller LP, et al: Nonoperative management of blunt hepatic trauma: a systematic review, *J Trauma Acute Care Surg* 79:654–660, 2015.

Cirocchi R, Trastulli S, Pressi E, et al: Non-operative management versus operative management in high-grade blunt hepatic injury, *Cochrane Database Syst Rev* (8):CD010989, 2015.

Mebert RV, Schnuriger B, Candinas D, Haltmeier T: Follow-up imaging in patients with blunt splenic or hepatic injury managed nonperatively, *Am Surg* 84:208–214, 2018.

Melloul E, Denys A, Demartines N: Management of severe blunt hepatic injury in the era of computed tomography and transarterial embolization: a systematic review and critical appraisal of the literature, *J Trauma Acute Care Surg* 79:468–474, 2015.

Li M, Yu WK, Wang XB, et al: Non-operative management of isolated liver trauma, *Hepatobiliary Pancreat Dis Int* 13:545–550, 2014.

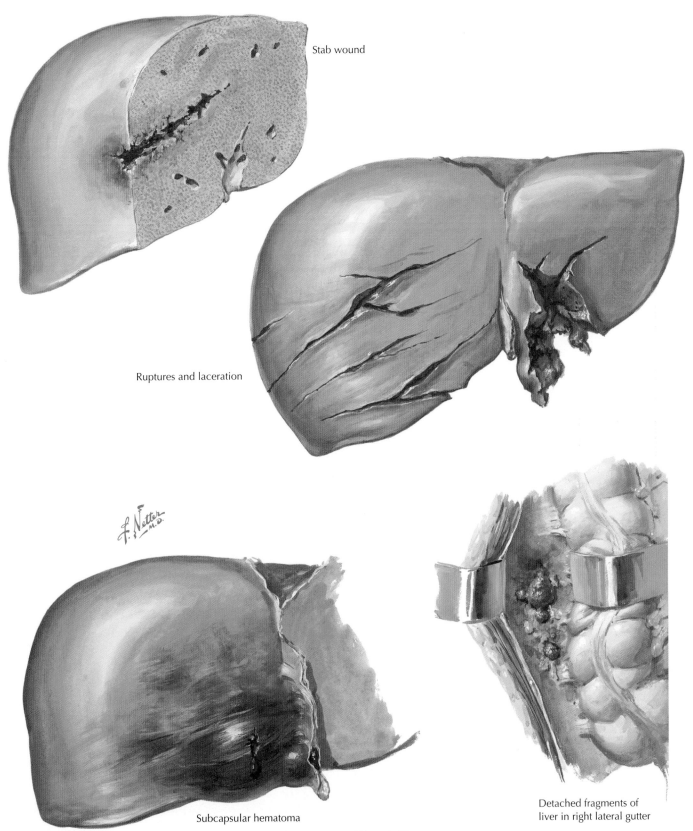

Stab wound

Ruptures and laceration

Subcapsular hematoma

Detached fragments of
liver in right lateral gutter

Fig. 183.1 Types of Hepatic Trauma.

Nutrition and Gastrointestinal Disease

James S. Scolapio

184

Dietary and Nutritional Assessment

James S. Scolapio

Clinical history, including dietary history, laboratory values, and anthropometric measurements, remains the standard for assessing patients' nutritional status. No single laboratory test or piece of clinical information provides a definitive diagnosis of "malnutrition." For example, an isolated finding of low serum albumin does not necessarily imply the patient is malnourished. Knowledge of the patient's underlying disease process is fundamental to understanding and diagnosing malnutrition.

Assessment begins with screening and identifying persons at risk for malnutrition. For hospital patients, the Joint Commission on Accreditation of Healthcare Organizations requires nutritional screening within 24 hours of the hospitalization. A registered dietitian usually performs this initial screening. Dietary risk factors are easy to identify and provide clues that a patient may be malnourished. These risk factors include inadequate quantity and quality of food intake, presence of chronic disease, history of alcohol abuse, increased nutrient losses from diarrhea, increased nutrient requirements from infection and burns, and various psychosocial factors. A *24-hour diet recall* is one method to determine the dietary intake of a patient. Accuracy of the recall depends greatly on the patient's memory, and family members often need to be interviewed. Written *food diaries* and *calorie counting* are other methods used to collect information regarding food intake.

Nutritional assessment should also include anthropometric measurements, typically body weight, height, skinfold thickness, and *midarm muscle circumference* (MAMC). Body weight is one of the most useful nutritional parameters to monitor in patients who are ill. Unintentional weight loss greater than 20% over less than 6 months is associated with *protein-energy malnutrition* (PEM) and functional abnormalities in most patients. *Body mass index* (BMI), calculated as weight (kg) divided by height (m^2), is used to characterize patients who have PEM or who are obese. Although all experts may not accept consistent BMI ranges, the normal BMI range is considered to be 18 to 25 (Table 184.1).

Measuring *skinfold thickness* is one of the easiest methods to estimate body fat stores. Measuring body fat requires a skinfold *caliper*. The *triceps skinfold* (TSF) thickness is representative of total body fat stores. Skinfold represents a double layer of subcutaneous tissue, including a small and relatively constant amount of skin and variable amounts of adipose tissue. For arm measurements, the most important factor is to use the midpoint of the upper arm and the same arm for repeat measurements. A thickness of less than 3 mm suggests severe depletion of fat. A TSF thickness greater than 8 mm is usually considered to represent adequate stores.

The MAMC is a method to estimate skeletal muscle mass. A tape measure is used to determine the upper arm circumference at the same arm location used in the TSF thickness. The MAMC is calculated using the following equation:

$$\text{MAMC (cm)} = \text{Upper arm circumference (cm)} \\ - [0.314 \times \text{TSF thickness (mm)}]$$ (Eq. 184.1)

An MAMC less than 15 cm (6 inches) is considered severely depleted muscle reserve, and an MAMC greater than 21 cm is considered to represent adequate reserve.

A number of laboratory tests can be used to obtain information about a patient's nutritional status; however, none is specific for malnutrition. Assessing *nitrogen balance* is perhaps the best test for balance of food intake and total losses. Unfortunately, accurate nitrogen collection is cumbersome and requires an experienced laboratory. Difficulty in obtaining a complete 24-hour collection of urine and feces poses another potential clinical limitation of this test. Although low *serum albumin* level may be a marker of increased morbidity and mortality, serum levels can also be altered by the retention of extracellular fluid and the acute stress response. Therefore serum albumin is not usually a true marker of PEM. Other laboratory tests that may be used to evaluate malnutrition and potential etiologies include a 72-hour fecal fat collection, creatinine-height index, total lymphocyte count, total iron-binding capacity, and isolated vitamin, mineral, and trace element deficiencies.

Subjective global assessment (SGA) has become an accepted method for evaluating the degree of malnutrition (http://nutritioncareincanada.ca/sites/default/uploads/files/SGA%20Tool%20EN%20BKWT_2017.pdf [Accessed May 2018]). SGA provides a combination of the patient's medical history and physical findings. No laboratory testing is used. Studies have shown a good correlation between SGA score and more sophisticated laboratory tests. Specific questions from the medical history include amount of weight loss over the preceding 6 months, changes in dietary intake, gastrointestinal symptoms that may account for reduced food intake or malabsorption, the patient's functional status (bedridden or full capacity), and the stress response of the patient's underlying illness. Physical findings are scored as normal (0), mild (1+), or severe (3+) and include the degree of subcutaneous fat and muscle loss. Based

TABLE 184.1	Body Mass Index
Grade	**Body Mass Index**
Obesity	
III	>40
II	30–40
I	25–29.9
Normal	>18.5 to <25
Protein-Energy Malnutrition	
I	17.0–18.4
II	16.0–16.9
III	<16

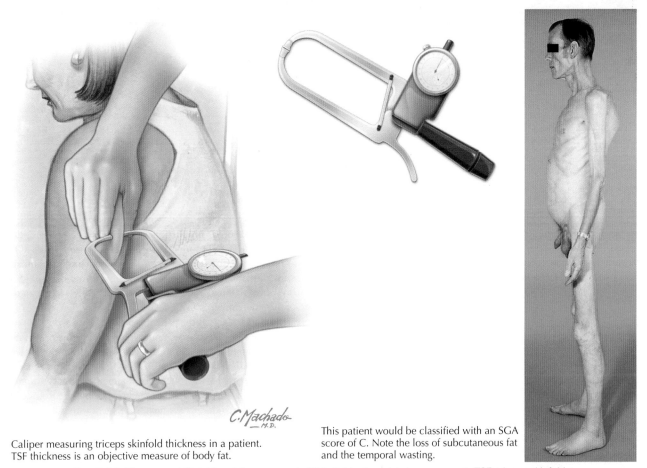

Caliper measuring triceps skinfold thickness in a patient. TSF thickness is an objective measure of body fat.

This patient would be classified with an SGA score of C. Note the loss of subcutaneous fat and the temporal wasting.

Fig. 184.1 Dietary and Nutritional Assessment. *SGA,* Subjective global assessment; *TSF,* triceps skinfold. (From Forbes CD, Jackson WF: *A color atlas and text of clinical medicine,* St Louis, 1993, Mosby.)

on medical history and physical findings, patients are ranked in one of three categories: *A,* good nutrition; *B,* moderate malnutrition; or *C,* severe malnutrition. Patients with C scores demonstrate obvious physical signs of malnutrition and an overall loss of at least 10% of their usual weight (Fig. 184.1).

ADDITIONAL RESOURCES

Detsky AS, McLaughlin JR, Baker JP, et al: What is subjective global assessment of nutritional status?, *JPEN J Parenter Enteral Nutr* 11:8–13, 1987.

Morgan SL, Weinsier RL: *Fundamentals of clinical nutrition,* ed 2, St Louis, 1998, Mosby–Year Book.

Macronutrients and Energy

James S. Scolapio

Energy requirements can be measured at bedside by indirect calorimetry or can be estimated using the Harris-Benedict equation. An estimate of *resting energy expenditure* (REE) can be derived from standard regression formulas based on various population studies. The most common formula used is the *Harris-Benedict equation*, as follows:

$$\text{Women (kcal/day)} = 655.10 + (9.46 \times \text{Weight, kg})$$
$$+ (1.86 \times \text{Height, cm}) - (4.68 \times \text{Age, yr})$$

(Eq. 185.1)

$$\text{Men (kcal/day)} = 66.47 + (13.75 \times \text{Weight, kg})$$
$$+ (5 \times \text{Height, cm}) - (6.76 \times \text{Age, yr})$$

(Eq. 185.2)

This regression equation was derived from studies on healthy subjects at rest and was not designed to address the stress and hypercatabolism seen in many disease states. Stress factors have been developed for certain clinical situations. The *stress factor* for patients after elective surgery is 1.2 times the resting REE and 1.5 times the REE for burn patients.

A reasonable correlation seems to exist between the measured REE by indirect calorimetry and that predicted from the Harris-Benedict equation. For most hospital patients, caloric needs are approximately REE × 1.2 to 1.5. *Indirect calorimetry* is based on the principle that energy expenditure is proportional to oxygen (O_2) consumption and carbon dioxide (CO_2) production. The *respiratory quotient* (RQ) is the ratio of CO_2 produced and O_2 consumed and provides information on substrate use. Each of the three major substrates has *n* RQ: 1.0 for carbohydrate, 0.8 for protein, and 0.7 for fat. An RQ less than 0.7 suggests that the patient is using fat as the primary fuel, whereas an RQ greater than 1.0 suggests the patient is being overfed with carbohydrate.

Nutrition substrates or macronutrients include protein, carbohydrate, and fat. The appropriate mix of substrate depends on the clinical state and the desired goals. In general, 1.0 to 1.5 g/kg/day of *protein*, 30% of total calories as *lipid* (fat), and the remaining substrate as *carbohydrate* is a desirable combination. In some circumstances, the substrate mixture may need modification. For example, in a patient with pulmonary disease and CO_2 retention for whom carbohydrates impose a greater demand on the respiratory system, carbohydrate intake should be minimized. Higher protein requirements are common in trauma and burn patients.

ADDITIONAL RESOURCES

Morgan SL, Weinsier RL: *Fundamentals of clinical nutrition*, ed 2, St Louis, 1998, Mosby–Year Book.

Micronutrient and Vitamin Deficiency

James S. Scolapio

Various vitamins and trace elements may be deficient in patients with gastrointestinal disease, who may present clinically with abnormal physical and laboratory findings (Table 186.1). The best guide to determine the dietary adequacy of vitamins and minerals is the US *recommended daily allowance* (RDA).

Fat-soluble vitamin (e.g., A, D, E, K) deficiency can result in significant fat malabsorption, as occurs in short bowel syndrome, celiac disease, and chronic pancreatitis (Fig. 186.1). *Water-soluble vitamin* (e.g., niacin, thiamine) deficiency is less common in malabsorptive states and tends to occur more often in patients with poor dietary habits, as in chronic alcohol abuse. Vitamin B_{12} deficiency can occur after total gastrectomy, with terminal ileal disease, and with greater than 100 cm resection of the terminal ileum (Fig. 186.2).

Inorganic trace elements are essential for health and include iron, chromium, manganese, copper, zinc, and selenium. A deficiency of any of these trace elements may also result in abnormal clinical and laboratory findings (see Fig. 186.2).

TABLE 186.1 Vitamins and Trace Elements: Dietary Sources and Deficiencies

Vitamin	Dietary Source	Deficiency
Thiamine (B_1)	Cereals, grains, pork, legumes, wheat grain seeds, nuts	Wernicke-Korsakoff encephalopathy, high-output congestive heart failure, lactic acidosis, peripheral neuropathy, nystagmus
Niacin	Red meat, liver, milk, eggs, corn	Pellagra, dermatitis, diarrhea, dementia, stomatitis, Hartnup disease
Cobalamin (B_{12})	Meat, eggs, dairy	Megaloblastic anemia, subacute combined degeneration of spinal cord, pernicious anemia, progressive neuropathy
Folic acid	Yeast, liver, vegetables, fruits, nuts	Pancytopenia, megaloblastic anemia, glossitis, stomatitis
Ascorbic acid	Citrus fruit, tomatoes, green vegetables, peppers	Perifollicular hyperkeratosis (scurvy), hemorrhage
Biotin	Milk products, eggs, liver	Scaly dermatitis, alopecia, lethargy, hypotonia, lactic acidosis
Vitamin A	Fish oils, liver, egg yolk, fortified dairy products, carotenoids, green leafy vegetables	Night blindness, xerosis, Bitot spots, hyperkeratosis of skin
Vitamin D	Fortified milk, breads, fatty fish	Osteomalacia, rickets, reduced serum calcium
Vitamin E	Whole wheat, vegetable oils	Hemolytic anemia, spinocerebellar degeneration, neuropathy, ophthalmoplegia
Vitamin K	Green leafy vegetables, dairy products, cereals	Bleeding, increased prothrombin time
Iron	Red meat, fish, oysters, dried beans, fortified breads and cereals	Hypochromic microcytic anemia, cheilosis, weakness
Zinc	Shellfish, meat, eggs	Acrodermatitis enteropathica, diarrhea, apathy, impaired growth, hair loss, skin rash, dysgeusia, reduced wound healing
Copper	Liver, legumes, shellfish, nuts, seeds, whole grains	Microcytic hypochromic anemia, leukopenia, neutropenia, osteoporosis, Menkes syndrome
Chromium	Brewer's yeast, vegetable oils, liver, cereals	Glucose intolerance, peripheral neuropathy, metabolic encephalopathy
Selenium	Meat, poultry, fish, cereal, grains, seafood	Dilated cardiomyopathy, myositis, weakness, white nails, Keshan disease

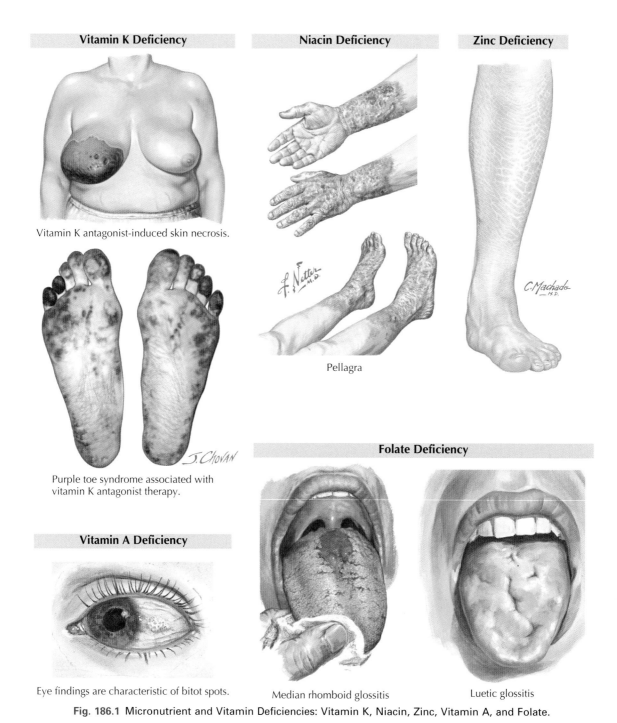

Vitamin K Deficiency

Vitamin K antagonist-induced skin necrosis.

Purple toe syndrome associated with vitamin K antagonist therapy.

Vitamin A Deficiency

Eye findings are characteristic of bitot spots.

Niacin Deficiency

Pellagra

Zinc Deficiency

Folate Deficiency

Median rhomboid glossitis

Luetic glossitis

Fig. 186.1 Micronutrient and Vitamin Deficiencies: Vitamin K, Niacin, Zinc, Vitamin A, and Folate.

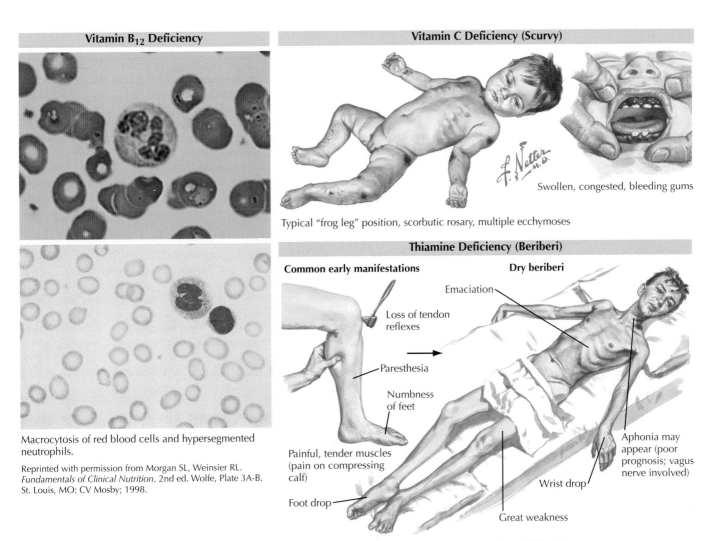

Vitamin B₁₂ Deficiency

Macrocytosis of red blood cells and hypersegmented neutrophils.

Reprinted with permission from Morgan SL, Weinsier RL. *Fundamentals of Clinical Nutrition*. 2nd ed. Wolfe, Plate 3A-B. St. Louis, MO: CV Mosby; 1998.

Vitamin C Deficiency (Scurvy)

Swollen, congested, bleeding gums

Typical "frog leg" position, scorbutic rosary, multiple ecchymoses

Thiamine Deficiency (Beriberi)

Common early manifestations

Loss of tendon reflexes

Paresthesia

Numbness of feet

Painful, tender muscles (pain on compressing calf)

Foot drop

Dry beriberi

Emaciation

Aphonia may appear (poor prognosis; vagus nerve involved)

Wrist drop

Great weakness

Fig. 186.2 Micronutrient and Vitamin Deficiencies: Vitamin B₁₂, Vitamin C, and Thiamine.

Enteral Nutrition

James S. Scolapio

Clinical guidelines for nutrition support, including enteral nutrition, have been published by the American Society of Parenteral and Enteral Nutrition.

For patients unable to take in sufficient calories by mouth for more than 10 to 14 days, *total enteral nutrition* (TEN), or tube feeding, is the preferred route to provide nutritional support. Compared with total parenteral nutrition (TPN), enteral feeding is associated with fewer infectious complications and is less expensive. Access for TEN can be through the nasal route or by a percutaneously placed gastric or small-bowel tube. In patients who require TEN for less than 4 weeks, the nasal route is preferred. Using a nasal tube beyond 4 weeks may cause significant nasal irritation and is uncomfortable for many patients.

A nasogastric or nasojejunal tube can usually be placed at beside. Nasojejunal tube placement may require the assistance of endoscopy or fluoroscopy by interventional radiology. Usually, a soft, 10- to 12-French-diameter tube should be used. Tubes smaller than 10-French tend to become occluded, and tubes larger than 12-French are uncomfortable for most patients. Although limited studies are available, the current literature suggests that placing a nasal or a percutaneous jejunal tube may reduce the risk for aspiration compared with gastric tubes. Therefore any patient at risk for gastric aspiration should have a feeding tube placed postpylorically, preferably beyond the ligament of Treitz. Similarly, any patient who has gastric dysmotility or is at increased risk for gastric reflux should have a percutaneous jejunal tube rather than a percutaneous gastric tube.

If tubes are placed at bedside without endoscopy or fluoroscopy, tube position should be confirmed with abdominal radiography. Data regarding the use of promotility agents to enhance the placement of feeding tubes are inconclusive.

With gastric feeding, the enteral formula can be given by gravity or by continuous pump feeding. Data comparing the two methods regarding gastric aspiration risk are inconclusive but suggest that risk may be reduced with pump feeding. When feeding into the small intestine, pump feeding is encouraged. Gravity feeding into the small intestine has been associated with bloating and diarrhea.

Feeding should be initiated at a rate of 20 to 25 mL/h and should be advanced every 12 hours in 20-mL increments until the goal rate is reached. Gastric *residual volumes* (RVs) should be checked in gastric-fed patients. A RV greater than 200 to 400 mL 2 hours after the last feeding indicates delayed gastric emptying and increases the risk for gastric aspiration. The patient must be carefully assessed and examined to determine whether it is appropriate to continue with feeding. Adding blue dye or methylene blue to the enteral formula should no longer be used as a marker of aspiration because deaths have been reported in patients with sepsis. Other complications of tube feeding besides aspiration include diarrhea, nasal ulceration, and hyperglycemia. Metabolic complications with TEN are less common than in patients receiving TPN.

Various enteral formulas are available for clinical use and hospitals usually have a set formulary. Most enteral formulas contain 1.0 kcal/mL. Defined formulas, including elemental, semielemental, disease-modifying, and immune-enhancing formulas, are specific for disease states. In general, data are limited regarding their clinical benefit compared with the standard polymeric formula. For example, immune-enhancing formulas have not been shown to improve mortality rates compared with traditional formulas.

Long-term enteral feeding is usually given in the home through a percutaneous endoscopic gastrostomy tube. The most common indications are neurologic disease, such as cerebrovascular accident (stroke), and after radiation therapy for head and neck cancer. Medicare and most insurance companies require that enteral feeding will be needed for at least 3 months and the patient will be unable to take sufficient calories by the oral route.

ADDITIONAL RESOURCES

A.S.P.E.N Board of Directors, Clinical Guideline Task Force: Guidelines for the use of parenteral and enteral nutrition in adult and pediatric patients, *JPEN J Parenter Enteral Nutr* 26(1 Suppl):1SA–138SA, 2002.

Bankhead R, Boullata J, Brantley S, et al: Enteral nutrition practice recommendations, *JPEN J Parenter Enteral Nutr* 33:122–167, 2009.

Dietary Fiber

James S. Scolapio

Dietary fiber is the *nonstarch polysaccharide* part of plant foods that is poorly digested by human enzymes. In the latter half of the 20th century, physicians and scientists began to understand the importance of dietary fiber in maintaining health and dietary fiber deficiencies in causing disease. Cleave first noted the increased sugar intake that resulted from decreased dietary fiber intake. Epidemiologists and gastroenterologists such as Burkett, Trowell, Painter, Walker, Heaten, and Eastwood then began to stress the importance of dietary fiber in maintaining normal gastrointestinal (GI) function and in preventing disease.

CHEMISTRY AND PROPERTIES

Food chemists analyzed plant foods first for crude fiber content, then began to correlate fiber content with various parts of plants. Because dietary fibers are extremely complex chemical compounds, it has been difficult for food scientists to decide on simple methods to identify their components in all foods. However, understanding the properties of fiber in the GI tract has facilitated making the distinction between soluble and insoluble fibers. In Englyst's classic method, after extraction, substances can be broken down as *soluble, insoluble,* and *cellulose,* which constitute the nonstarch polysaccharide component. Some resistant starch is left over from the chemical process.

Components in the plant cell walls are cellulose, noncellulose polysaccharides (soluble and insoluble), lignin, waxes, protein, and ash. Major classes of *noncellulose polysaccharide* are rhamnogalacturonans, arabinogalactans, β-glucans, xylans, mannans, and xyloglucans. Gums and mucilages develop but are not strictly part of the plant cell walls; they are complex heteroglycans with branch structures. Bacterial fermentation clearly shows that bacterial enzymes almost completely ferment soluble fibers but poorly ferment insoluble fibers or cellulose.

PHYSICAL PROPERTIES

Important physical properties of dietary fiber and its components are particle size and polysaccharides. Depending on how food is cooked or processed, *particle size* will be large or greatly reduced. In some cases, reduction in size can completely disrupt the plant cell wall. Therefore particle size is important in determining some of the properties discussed here.

Polysaccharides may be hydrophilic and may have a definite water-holding capacity. This varies with the food, and certainly, cellulose is limited to swelling property, which depends on polysaccharide type. Some polysaccharides are able to form gels, and some can become extremely viscous. These properties affect nutrient ion absorption, although the gels are completely fermented by bacterial action, freeing any substances that are trapped.

The water-holding property of insoluble fibers is particularly important for maintaining larger, softer stool. Insoluble fibers are poorly fermented by bacteria. Hence this water-holding property is helpful in maintaining a larger stool bulk throughout the colon.

Ion Binding

Uronic acid–containing polysaccharides and the lignin components of dietary fiber have acidic functional groups that react with ions. Calcium, iron, and zinc can be bound, but they are readily freed. Similarly, bile salts can be bound. This appears to be an extremely dynamic process that may not necessarily interfere with absorption but may actually enhance it by bringing a particular substance to the site in the intestine where it is best absorbed.

FIBER INTAKE

The intake of dietary fiber varies greatly from society to society and within societies. Studies indicate that people from underdeveloped countries, such as Asia and Africa, eat as much as 60 to 80 g of dietary fiber daily, given that the main component of their diet is cereal fiber. In Western societies, the consumption is generally 5 to 10 g of dietary fiber daily. This great variation is attributed to selectivity and lifestyle. Diets are becoming more balanced worldwide as knowledge of the benefits of dietary fiber increases.

EFFECT ON THE GASTROINTESTINAL TRACT

Dietary fiber has specific effects on the GI tract. It should be remembered that *soluble* fiber may have different effects than *insoluble* fiber but that most foods are mixed. Because fiber enters into the dynamics of intraluminal microecology, its effects vary with the fluid, pH, and lumen contents of other substances. Nevertheless, overall dietary fiber may slow gastric emptying, may have an inhibitory effect on pancreatic enzyme activity, and depending on the nutrients and particular foods involved, may slow absorption from the small intestine.

Fibers vary in their ability to slow oral-to-fecal transit time. It is a complicated interface, but guar gum can delay hydrogen-to-breath time, whereas bran and gum tragacanth have lesser effects. Pectin and cellulose seem to have no effect. However, when treating constipation, it is important knowing that transit time and bulk are increased. Pectin has been clearly shown to decrease the absorption of cholesterol.

COLON AS A FERMENTER

Bacterial flora of the distal ileum and colon ferment various fibers at various rates. The matrix that exists in the colon, with its vast bacterial population of aerobes and anaerobes, ferments soluble fibers at a 10-fold greater rate than it ferments insoluble fibers. It also produces short-chain fatty acids that are pivotal for the health of the colon and for the control of cholesterol metabolism through the enterohepatic circulation. *Butyric acid* is the main fuel of colonocytes; *acetic acid* is the building block for cholesterol; and *propionic acid* appears to have some controlling mechanism on cholesterol development. These short-chain fatty acids are produced in the colon and are absorbed through the enterohepatic circulation, if not directly used for fuel by colonocytes.

Depending on the amount of dietary fiber eaten, stool size varies greatly. In general, an 8- to 10-g diet produces approximately 100 mL of stool, whereas a 25- to 30-g diet produces as much as 300 mL of stool. Eventually, the amount of short-chain fatty acid produced will vary. Furthermore, if the dietary fiber intake is heavy in soluble fiber, such as from fruits and vegetables or psyllium seed, the bacterial flora will increase and flourish and will be larger than if the dietary fiber consists of cellulose and insoluble fibers from bran. In the latter case, the stool volume might still be large, but this results from the water-holding property of insoluble fiber rather than increased bacterial flora.

EFFECT ON DISEASE

It is now well accepted that dietary fiber ameliorates constipation and diarrhea (see Chapters 111 and 136). In addition, colon diverticula are less common in those who eat high-fiber diets, and diverticular formation may be prevented in susceptible subjects. Diverticular disease may develop in persons who eat low-fiber diets for decades. It is recommended that the patient with diverticular disease maintain a high-fiber diet.

When acute diverticulitis develops, physicians usually restrict the amount of dietary fiber the patient can consume until the episodes have been resolved.

USE AND TREATMENT

Treatment and prevention of colonic polyps, colonic cancer, coronary artery disease, and stroke have remained extremely controversial. A meta-analysis has revealed conflicting results. However, some large national studies reveal that subjects on high-fiber diets experience less polyp formation and fewer coronary artery diseases. Consequently, most clinicians recommend a high-fiber diet to prevent diverticulosis of the colon, polyp formation, and atherosclerotic disease. This is a controversial issue, and the literature substantiates both positions.

Recent studies also indicate that subjects who eat high-fiber diets tend to experience less morbid obesity. Naturally, these subjects eat less fat and sugar; thus their high-fiber diet decreases their nutrient energy intake.

The therapeutic recommendation for the intake of dietary fiber is 20 to 35 g daily, depending on the meal size and caloric intake. Some recommend approximately 10 to 12 g per 1000 calories. The recommendation also states that broad types of dietary fiber should be consumed and that the intake should include a mixture of soluble and insoluble fiber.

Table 188.1 lists the dietary fiber content of the most common foods. A daily high-fiber cereal plus three to five portions (depending on size) of fruits or vegetables will usually satisfy the body's need for soluble and insoluble fiber. Dietitians and clinicians usually recommend five portions of fruits, vegetables, or grains, averaging 4 to 5 g each, and thus meeting the necessary requirement of 20 to 35 g daily.

TABLE 188.1 **Dietary Fiber Food Sources**				
	Serving Size	**Soluble Fiber Content per Serving (g)**	**Insoluble Fiber Content per Serving (g)**	**Total Fiber Content per Serving (g)**
Vegetables (Cooked, Unless Otherwise Noted)				
Asparagus	¾ cup	0.8	2.3	3.1
Bean sprouts, raw	½ cup	0.3	1.3	1.6
Beans				
Green	½ cup	0.5	1.6	2.1
Kidney	½ cup	2.5	3.3	5.8
Lima	½ cup	1.1	3.2	4.4
Pinto	½ cup	2.3	3.3	5.3
White	½ cup	1.4	3.6	5.0
Broccoli	½ cup	0.9	1.1	2.0
Brussels sprouts	½ cup	1.6	2.3	3.9
Cabbage	½ cup	0.9	1.1	2.0
Carrots	7 inch	1.1	1.2	2.3
Cauliflower	½ cup	0.4	0.6	1.0
Celery, raw	½ cup	0.4	0.9	1.3
Corn, kernels	½ cup	1.7	2.2	3.9
Eggplant	½ cup	0.8	1.2	2.0
Kale	½ cup	1.4	1.4	2.8
Lettuce, raw	½ cup	0.1	0.2	0.3
Okra	½ cup	1.0	3.1	4.1
Onions, raw	½ cup	0.8	1.8	2.6
Peas	½ cup	0.4	2.8	3.2
Potatoes				
Sweet, baked	½ large	0.7	1.0	1.7
White, baked	½ medium	1.0	1.0	1.9
Radishes, raw	5 medium	0.1	0.5	0.6

TABLE 188.1   Dietary Fiber Food Sources—cont'd

	Serving Size	Soluble Fiber Content per Serving (g)	Insoluble Fiber Content per Serving (g)	Total Fiber Content per Serving (g)
Squash				
Acorn	½ cup	0.5	3.8	4.3
Zucchini	½ cup	1.3	1.4	2.7
Tomato, raw	1 medium	0.2	0.6	0.8
Turnip	½ cup	0.8	0.9	1.7
Zucchini	½ cup	0.5	0.7	1.2
Fruits (raw)				
Apple, with skin	1	0.8	2.0	2.8
Apricots	2	0.7	0.8	1.5
Avocado	⅛ fresh	0.5	0.7	1.2
Banana	½ medium	0.3	0.7	1.0
Blackberries	½ cup	0.7	3.9	4.5
Cherries	10	0.3	0.9	1.2
Figs	1½	1.1	1.2	2.3
Grapefruit	½ medium	0.6	1.1	1.7
Grapes	12	0.1	0.4	0.5
Melon, cantaloupe	1 cup	0.3	0.8	1.1
Orange	1 small	0.3	0.9	1.2
Peach	1 medium	0.6	1.0	1.6
Pear	½ medium	0.5	2.0	2.5
Pineapple	½ cup	0.3	0.9	1.2
Plums	3 small	0.7	1.1	1.8
Raspberries	¾ cup	0.4	6.4	6.8
Strawberries	¾ cup	0.7	1.3	2.0
Grain Products				
Bread				
Bagel, plain	½	0.3	0.4	0.7
French	1 slice	0.3	0.7	1.0
Rye	1 slice	0.3	0.6	0.9
White enriched	1 slice	0.3	0.3	0.5
Whole wheat	1 slice	0.3	1.2	1.4
Cereal				
All-Bran (100%)	⅓ cup	1.7	7.0	8.6
Corn flakes	1 cup	0.2	0.3	0.4
Shredded wheat	1 biscuit	0.4	2.4	2.8
Fiber one	½ cup	0.8	11.1	11.9
Raisin bran	¾ cup	0.9	4.4	5.3
Oatmeal (oats)	⅓ cup	1.4	1.3	2.7
Crackers				
Graham	2 squares	0.5	2.3	2.8
Saltine	6 crackers	0.3	0.4	0.7
Rice				
Brown	½ cup	0.2	2.2	2.4
White	½ cup	0.01	0.09	0.1
Spaghetti	½ cup	0.3	0.5	0.8
Nuts				
Almonds	1 tbsp	0.1	1.0	1.1
Peanuts, roasted	10	0.2	0.4	0.6

ADDITIONAL RESOURCES

Bazzano LA, He J, Ogden LG, et al: Fruit and vegetable intake and risk of cardiovascular disease in U.S. adults: the first national health and nutrition examination survey epidemiologic follow-up study, *Am J Clin Nutr* 76:13–19, 2002.

Cleave TL: *The saccharine disease*, New Canaan, Conn, 1975, Keats Publishing.

Holscher HD: Dietary fiber and prebiotics and the gastrointestinal microbiota, *Gut Microbes* 8:1–42, 2017.

Slattery ML, Curtin KP, Edwards SL, Schaffer DM: Plant foods, fiber, and rectal cancer, *Am J Clin Nutr* 79:274–281, 2004.

Trowell H, Burkett D, Heaton K: *Dietary fibre, fibre-depleted foods and disease*, London, 1985, Academic Press.

Parenteral Nutrition

James S. Scolapio

Parenteral nutrition, or *total parenteral nutrition* (TPN), is indicated for patients who are unable to take in sufficient calories by the oral route for more than 10 to 14 days and for whom total enteral nutrition (TEN) is not possible (e.g., intestinal obstruction, severe malabsorption). Contraindications for TPN include a functional gastrointestinal (GI) tract, intended use less than 3 days, and imminent death from the underlying disease. Although patients usually prefer TPN to a nasogastric feeding tube, TPN is associated with a higher risk of infection from catheter sepsis and other metabolic complications.

Access for parenteral nutrition can be through a peripheral vein, if the dextrose concentration will be less than 5%, or through a central vein if the dextrose concentration will be greater than 5%. Administering a dextrose concentration greater than 5% through a peripheral vein can result in thrombophlebitis. When administering *central* parenteral nutrition, direct subclavian vein placement has traditionally been the method of placement. However, a peripherally inserted central catheter inserted through the brachial vein and advanced to the superior vena cava is the preferred method because it averts the risk for pneumothorax associated with the placement of subclavian lines. Before infusion is initiated, proper insertion of the catheter tip in the superior vena cava should be confirmed by chest radiograph.

TPN is usually given as a 2-L, 3-in-1 (3:1) solution containing carbohydrate, protein, and lipid mixed together. Intravenous lipid is typically used to supply 20% to 40% of daily calories. Energy and protein requirements should be calculated as described in Chapter 265. TPN volume should be reduced in patients with congestive heart failure, significant renal disease, and fluid overload. The TPN formula also contains electrolytes, multivitamins, and trace elements.

Infusion rate should be based on a 24-hour period. The patient should be started on half the rate (40 mL/h) for the first 24 hours; this can be increased to full rate (80 mL/h) if tolerated by the patient. Serum electrolyte levels should be checked at least twice a week while the patient receives TPN in the hospital. Blood glucose levels should also be monitored closely while the patient receives TPN. If blood glucose levels are higher than 200 mg/dL, regular insulin may need to be added to the TPN solution to maintain glucose levels lower than 200 mg/dL, because hyperglycemia is a risk factor for infection. A sliding scale of regular insulin will also suffice without having to add insulin to the TPN solution. Serum triglyceride levels should be checked at least weekly to prevent serum levels from exceeding 500 mg/dL.

The most common complication of TPN is *catheter sepsis*. Nursing staff must follow strict sterile catheter techniques. To prevent bacterial contamination of the solution, the TPN solution should not be kept at room temperature longer than 24 hours, and an in-line filter should always be used. Tapering the TPN infusion by 50% for 30 to 60 minutes before discontinuing it helps to prevent symptomatic hypoglycemia.

When TPN is used in the home, it is referred to as *home parenteral nutrition.* Indications for home parenteral nutrition include short bowel syndrome, severe radiation enteritis, distal intestinal fistula, and mechanical intestinal obstruction when surgery is not immediately possible. Medicare will not reimburse patients with a functioning GI tract or in whom TPN will be required for less than 3 months. A certificate of medical necessity must be completed before hospital discharge, documenting that the TPN will be required for at least 3 months. Hospital case managers should be directly involved in arranging hospital discharge, ensuring all criteria are met for insurance reimbursement.

Home parenteral nutrition is associated with complications that must be recognized and addressed appropriately. These include catheter infection, liver disease, and metabolic bone disease. Multiple trace elements, which include manganese, copper, chromium, selenium, and zinc, should be checked at least every 6 months. Cholestatic liver disease increases the risk for manganese and copper toxicity because these two trace elements are excreted primarily through the hepatobiliary system.

ADDITIONAL RESOURCES

A.S.P.E.N Board of Directors, Clinical Guideline Task Force: Guidelines for the use of parenteral and enteral nutrition in adult and pediatric patients, *JPEN J Parenter Enteral Nutr* 26(1 Suppl):1SA–138SA, 2002.

A.S.P.E.N Clinical Guidelines: Parenteral nutrition ordering, Order review, Compounding, Labeling, and Dispensing, *JPEN J Parenter Enteral Nutr* 38: 334–377, 2014.

Scolapio JS, Fleming CR, Kelly DG, et al: Survival of home parenteral nutrition–treated patients: 20 years of experience at the Mayo Clinic, *Mayo Clin Proc* 74:217–222, 1999.

Malnutrition

James S. Scolapio

Malnutrition can be classified as primary or secondary. *Primary malnutrition* is caused by inadequate food supply, which is common in many countries in the developing world but less common in the United States. *Secondary malnutrition* results from an underlying chronic disease process. Anorexia nervosa is an example of a condition causing secondary malnutrition (Fig. 190.1).

Patients with gastrointestinal disease are most predisposed to secondary malnutrition because of reduced oral intake of food, intestinal obstruction, altered absorption, and digestion of nutrients. *Malnutrition,* which can be defined as unintentional weight loss of more than 10% of usual body weight over 3 months, may occur in hospital patients. Malnutrition has been associated with increased infections, impaired wound healing, increased postoperative complications, longer hospital stay, and higher mortality. Dietary energy and protein deficiencies usually occur together, although one form may predominate.

Kwashiorkor is the term used when severe protein deficiency is the primary cause of malnutrition, and *marasmus* is the term used when severe energy or calorie deficiency is the primary cause of the malnutrition (Fig. 190.2). *Marasmic kwashiorkor* is the term used to describe the combination of chronic energy and protein deficiency. *Protein-energy malnutrition* (PEM) and *protein-calorie malnutrition* are more common terms for malnutrition. A body mass index (BMI) less than 16 represents severe PEM. Worldwide, socioeconomic and environmental factors are leading causes of PEM.

The diagnosis of marasmus includes a clinical history of inadequate calorie intake, usually from a chronic illness, and physical findings of

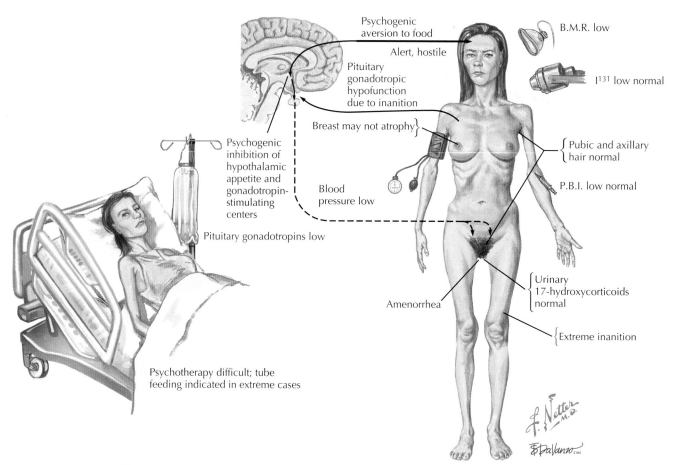

Fig. 190.1 Eating Disorders: Anorexia Nervosa and Bulimia. *B.M.R.,* Basal metabolic rate.

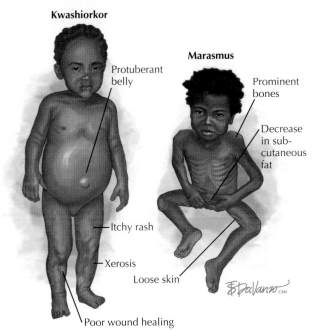

Kwashiorkor

Protuberant belly

Marasmus

Prominent bones

Decrease in sub-cutaneous fat

Itchy rash

Xerosis

Loose skin

Poor wound healing

Fig. 190.2 Kwashiorkor and Marasmus.

severe wasting of muscle and subcutaneous fat. Patients with marasmus frequently are at 60% of their expected weight for height, and children often have greatly impaired longitudinal growth. Hair thinning and hair loss with dry, flaky skin are also common. Diminished skinfold thickness and reduced midarm muscle circumference and temporal wasting illustrate the loss of fat and skeletal muscle, respectively, in these patients. Serum albumin levels are usually normal in patients with marasmus.

Diagnostic features of kwashiorkor include pitting edema of the feet and legs, skin ulceration, and epidermal sloughing. In contrast to marasmus, kwashiorkor occurs in the United States predominantly in patients with acute, highly metabolic illness, such as trauma and burns. Subcutaneous fat and muscle mass are often preserved, although careful inspection usually reveals more muscle wasting. Delayed wound healing, skin breakdown, and infection are also common. The abdomen may protrude because of an edematous stomach and intestinal loops. The most common biochemical findings in kwashiorkor are reduced serum albumin level, lymphopenia, and anemia.

Treating PEM requires replacing fluids, macronutrients, and micronutrients. Caution must be used to avoid rapid repletion and when reintroducing feeding in patients with severe PEM. Refeeding should be done slowly to prevent *refeeding syndrome*. Rapid refeeding with oral, enteral, or parenteral nutrition can result in acute decreases in serum phosphorus, potassium, and magnesium levels, resulting in cardiac arrhythmia and death. Acute thiamine deficiency is also a potential concern during refeeding in patients with severe PEM.

ADDITIONAL RESOURCES

Shils ME: *Modern nutrition in health and disease*, ed 9, Baltimore, 1999, Williams & Wilkins.

Surgical Treatment of Obesity

Rishabh Shah, Garrett Wegerif, James S. Scolapio, Samuel Szomstein, Emanuele Lo Menzo, Raul J. Rosenthal

DEMOGRAPHICS

Obesity has reached epidemic proportions in the United States. The number of obese persons increased by 34% from 2000 to 2016. Nearly 40% of adults and 18% of children are now obese. In Hispanic and black populations, the prevalence is near 50% for adults. Worldwide, the number of overweight people has increased to approximately 38%, with 500 million now obese.

Patients with a body mass index (BMI) between 25 and 29.9 are considered overweight, and a BMI greater than 30 is considered obese. Other factors, such as fat distribution and weight gain, modify the risk within each BMI category. One of the etiologies of obesity derives by the ingestion of more calories than are expended, so excess calories are stored as fat. However, genetic and environmental factors contribute to obesity. The marked increase in obesity in the past 20 years cannot be attributed to genetic factors alone and are most likely caused by changes in the environment.

Obesity is responsible for at least 30 other diseases. Type 2 diabetes (T2DM) is associated with severe obesity in 20% of patients. Hypertension, hyperlipidemia, obstructive sleep apnea (OSA), hypoventilation, asthma, gastroesophageal reflux disease (GERD), coronary artery disease (CAD), chronic heart failure (CHF), cerebrovascular accident (CVA, stroke), nonalcoholic steatohepatitis (NASH), low back pain, degenerative joint disease (DJD), pseudotumor cerebri, urinary stress incontinence, and polycystic ovary syndrome (PCOS) are all associated with obesity. Furthermore, as released by the Office of Disease Control, approximately 40% of cancers are associated with obesity and 55% of those in obese females. The most common type of cancers that are associated with obese patients are esophagus, uterus, breast, prostate, liver, and kidney. Patients are also prone to ventral and incisional hernias. Severely obese people are at risk for mental disorders, including depression and anxiety, as well as eating disorders.

Even the fat distribution in the body plays a role in the prevalence of comorbidities. In fact, persons with increased abdominal fat are at increased risk for diabetes, hypertension, hyperlipidemia, and ischemic heart disease (metabolic syndrome) compared with those with increased gluteal and femoral fat (Fig. 191.1).

As a result, the increased BMI translates to a decreased life span. Severely obese women are twice as likely to die as those of normal weight. The increase in prevalence of obesity worldwide and its growing effect on related medical diseases and mortality have empowered both medical and surgical efforts to combat this growing epidemic.

Among the different potential and popular treatments for obesity are diets, behavioral modifications, and physical activity. *Dietary modification* should encourage patients to eat three meals daily, to avoid snacking between meals, to avoid energy-dense and high-fat foods, and to increase the intake of fruits and vegetables. *Physical activity* is also important for overall health for cardiovascular benefits but is not helpful in achieving meaningful weight loss without reduction of caloric intake.

The next level of treatment includes pharmacotherapy because it can help selected patients to achieve *and* maintain weight loss. Patients receiving pharmacotherapy for obesity should also be involved in efforts to change their lifestyles, including developing the habits of healthy eating and adequate exercise. Weight loss is usually 3 to 5 kg over placebo, but the weight tends to be regained once the medications are discontinued.

Surgery is the most effective approach for achieving weight loss in the extremely obese patient (BMI ≥ 40). Indications for surgery include BMI greater than 40 or BMI between 35 and 40 and severe obesity-related diseases, such as diabetes and OSA. Serious psychiatric disorders are absolute contraindications for surgery. Of the various types of obesity surgery, the *gastric bypass* procedure, also known as the Roux-en-Y, and the sleeve gastrectomy (SG), are the most popular.

INDICATIONS

Surgical therapy focuses on those with a BMI of 35 kg/m^2 or greater, although evidence now indicates that obese individuals with BMI lower than 35 may benefit from surgery as well, especially if they have T2DM.

Body mass index is the most practical and widely used measure of an individual's size. It is calculated by dividing the patient's weight in kilograms by the height in meters squared (kg/m^2). In adults, BMI is categorized as follows:

- Underweight less than 18.5 kg/m^2
- Normal weight 18.5 to 24.9 kg/m^2
- Overweight 25 to 29.9 kg/m^2
- Class I obesity 30 to 34.9 kg/m^2
- Class II obesity 35 to 39.9 kg/m^2
- Class III obesity 40 to 49.9 kg/m^2 (severely, extremely, or morbidly obese)
- Class IV obesity ≥50 kg/m^2 ("super-obese")

Bariatric surgery should be considered for patients who have failed medical management, such as dieting, exercise, and drug therapy. According to the National Institutes of Health, candidates for surgery should have a BMI greater than 40 or BMI greater than 35 and major comorbidity, such as T2DM, OSA, obesity-related cardiomyopathy, or DJD. Currently, patients with BMI greater than 30 (or as low as 27.5 in Asian population) with poorly controlled hyperglycemia should also be considered for bariatric surgery. The American Diabetes Association has also published similar guidelines in 2017. Patients must have tried to lose weight by medical methods, must be motivated, and must be informed about the procedure and potential consequences. They must also be an acceptable surgical risk.

Patients who may not be considered for surgery include those with unstable CAD, severe pulmonary disease, portal hypertension, or active substance abuse, as well as those unable to carry out the necessary

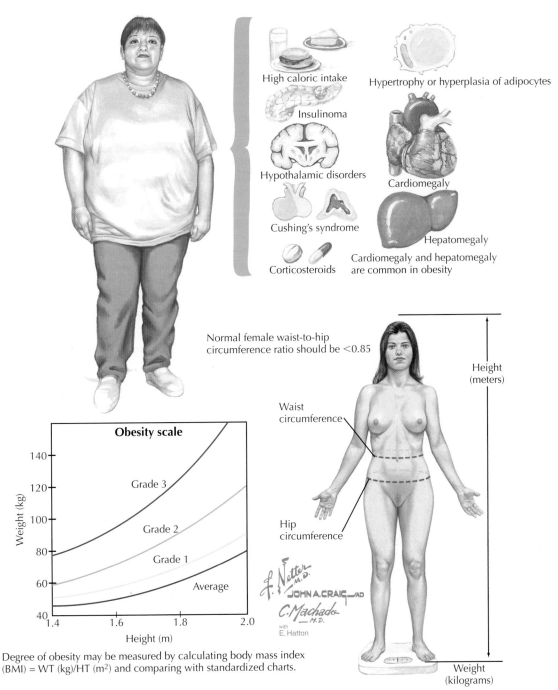

High caloric intake

Hypertrophy or hyperplasia of adipocytes

Insulinoma

Hypothalamic disorders

Cardiomegaly

Cushing's syndrome

Hepatomegaly

Corticosteroids

Cardiomegaly and hepatomegaly
are common in obesity

Normal female waist-to-hip
circumference ratio should be <0.85

Height
(meters)

Waist
circumference

Hip
circumference

Obesity scale

Grade 3

Grade 2

Grade 1

Average

Weight (kg)

140

120

100

80

60

40

1.4   1.6   1.8   2.0

Height (m)

Weight
(kilograms)

Degree of obesity may be measured by calculating body mass index
(BMI) = WT (kg)/HT (m^2) and comparing with standardized charts.

Fig. 191.1 Obesity

postsurgical lifestyle changes. Contraindications also include untreated major depression or psychosis, active binge eating, or severe coagulopathy. Bariatric surgery has proven to be effective, safe, and beneficial in those older than 65 or younger than 18 years of age. These age limits that were considered in the past as a contraindication are now being relaxed as long-term positive outcome data in both populations are reported.

PREPARATION

Before surgical intervention, patients must attend an educational seminar and interact with former surgical patients. They receive a tutorial on the procedure, are evaluated by a psychiatric therapist, and meet with

a nutritionist. Many patients will need to have sleep apnea ruled out if they have high BMI or severe symptoms. Cardiac and pulmonary evaluations are performed to assess the risk of anesthesia. Patients undergoing gastric bypass and SG are evaluated by upper endoscopy because, after the gastric pouch is created and the stomach is divided, access to the stomach is extremely difficult. In addition, the presence of Barrett esophagus is considered a relative contraindication in patients who are selected for SG. The preoperative endoscopic evaluation can recognize other important, acute and chronic pathologies such as hiatal hernias, masses, and ulcers. Patients also undergo blood testing for thyroid disease, liver disease, and T2DM. Postoperatively, patients are encouraged to follow up with nutrition and psychiatric support groups.

TYPES OF BARIATRIC PROCEDURES

Historically, the bariatric surgical procedures were classified according to their malabsorptive or restrictive mechanism. The *restrictive* procedures limit caloric intake by creating a small stomach pouch, ranging from virtual in the adjustable gastric band and to a long narrow gastric tube in the gastric sleeve. Weight loss depends on a decrease in caloric intake and therefore is more gradual.

The primary mechanism of *malabsorptive* procedures is to create rapidly emptying and diverting pathways for food and digestive substances so that they meet distally within the small-bowel lumen and therefore have a smaller length of absorptive surface area in which to interact. In addition, the rapid emptying of undigested food to the distal small bowel will stimulate incretins that participate in the remission of diabetes. The biliopancreatic diversion (BPD) and duodenal switch are examples of malabsorptive procedures. The Roux-en-Y gastric bypass (RYGB) combines features of both restriction and malabsorption with the creation of a small stomach pouch and a 25% to 30% functional small-bowel bypass. However, more modern classifications take into account other potential mechanisms of action of the bariatric procedures, such as modification of enterohormones, alterations in the complex brain-gut-pancreas-visceral fat axis, modification of bile salts, and modifications to the gut flora.

The trend now is toward minimally invasive approaches to bariatric surgery; studies show better cost effectiveness and safety than with open procedures (Fig. 191.2).

Restrictive Surgery

The *SG* was historically the first part of the BPD procedure, and in recent years the procedure has been separated into two stages to lower the mortality rates seen in higher-BMI patients undergoing BPD. Since then, SG has gained support as a purely restrictive, stand-alone procedure, and currently comprises close to 70% of all bariatric surgeries performed in the United States. SG entails the creation of a stomach tube from cardia to antrum that involves removal of the fundus and body of the stomach along the greater curvature. The antrum is left intact. Weight loss occurs from restriction due to a smaller stomach and anorexia from which the ghrelin-producing cells have been removed. Patients experience approximately 30% to 60% excess weight loss (EWL) in 1 year. Patients who reach a plateau or who regain weight may opt for conversion to a laparoscopic RYGB.

The *intragastric balloon* is an endoscopically placed temporary solution for weight loss in obese patients. The soft balloon is inserted in the stomach and inflated with saline. The distended device fills the stomach and induces satiety while causing restriction. Intragastric balloon placement has the disadvantages of nausea, vomiting, abdominal pain, ulceration, and balloon migration, as well as its temporary effect, because it has to be removed or replaced after 6 months.

Laparoscopic adjustable gastric banding (LAGB) is a purely restrictive procedure that separates a micropouch from the remainder of the stomach. The band is composed of (1) a silicone band with a balloon inner tube that wraps around the stomach, (2) a port that lies under the skin on the rectus muscle for access, and (3) tubing to connect the two. The band is accessed 4 to 6 weeks after surgery by inserting a needle and syringe into the port and injecting or withdrawing fluid. In this manner, the balloon increases in diameter, and the aperture between the two stomach compartments becomes smaller as the patient undergoes more restriction.

The LAGB was widely used because of easy placement, quick recovery and same-day discharge or 1-day hospital stay, and lower complication rate. Advantages of the LAGB include no stapling of bowel, 0% to 0.5% mortality with adjustability, and minimal nutritional complications.

The band is potentially reversible because it can be completely removed; however, often, chronic changes at the esophagogastric junction persist even after removal. The adjustable band which initially replaced the vertical banded gastroplasty (VBG), another purely restrictive operation, has now almost completely been abandoned in favor of the SG. This is mostly due to high rates of removal of conversion to other procedures secondary to poor long-term weight loss, as well as significant complications such as band erosion or prolapse.

The *vertical banded gastroplasty* is a purely restrictive procedure in which the upper cardia of the stomach is separated by a vertical staple line from the remainder of the stomach. The outlet is then encircled with a mesh or a band. The outlet aperture is not adjustable. Further eating may result in vomiting if the pouch is not allowed to empty. Weight loss occurs because of decreased caloric intake of solid food. *Excess weight loss* is as much as 66% at 2 years and 55% at 9 years. The ability to consume high-calorie liquid meals and sweets and gradually increased pouch capacity caused by overeating are major disadvantages. The VBG has become antiquated because it combines the disadvantages of a higher complication rate and the inability to adjust the band. The rate of revision ranges from 20% to 56% and mainly results from staple line disruption, stomal stenosis, band erosion, band disruption, pouch dilatation, vomiting, and GERD.

Malabsorptive Surgery

Biliopancreatic diversion was developed because of poor results with jejunoileal bypass; many patients developed kidney problems and liver failure. The BPD involves a partial gastrectomy that is anastomosed distally to the ileum. There is a long segment of Roux limb and a short common channel where the food and biliopancreatic juices meet to allow for absorption. The process results in significant malabsorption and 72% EWL at up to 18 years postoperatively. The procedure is now performed laparoscopically with similar results. Disadvantages of BPD include mortality of 1% and high incidence of protein malnutrition, anemia, diarrhea, and stomal ulceration.

The BPD with duodenal switch (BPD/DS) is a BPD that differs by creating a partial SG with preservation of the pylorus. A Roux limb with a short common channel is also created. The BPD/DS has been recommended for patients with supermorbid obesity (BMI > 50). Unfortunately, the high mortality rate has led to the development of a staged procedure, with the gastric sleeve done first, then BPD later if more weight loss is necessary. BPD/DS results in less stomal ulceration and diarrhea than BPD and can be performed laparoscopically. It is not performed routinely because of high morbidity and mortality.

Mixed Procedures

The *Roux-en-Y gastric bypass* was once the most common surgical procedure for weight loss in the United States. Developed in 1967 by Mason and Ito, it included a partial gastrectomy and loop gastrojejunostomy. It was originally performed after the observation that patients lost weight after ulcer surgery. The procedure was modified by Griffin in 1977 to include a Roux-en-Y. The first laparoscopic bypass was performed by Wittgrove in 1994. Laparoscopy has a lower incidence of incisional hernia and wound infection, a faster recovery, and more rapid return to work than open surgery. It is safely performed by well-trained and experienced surgeons.

Weight loss after gastric bypass is mostly attributed to restriction but also to malabsorption. It has better weight loss averages than the purely restrictive procedures. The bypass is composed of a 30-mL gastric pouch separated from the gastric remnant and restricting food intake and emptying. The pouch is connected by a stoma to the small bowel, creating a Roux-en-Y segment. The remnant stomach and duodenum empty gastric acid, pancreatic enzymes, and bile through a 30-cm to

Gastric stapling (vertical banded gastroplasty)

Gastric bypass (Roux-en-Y)

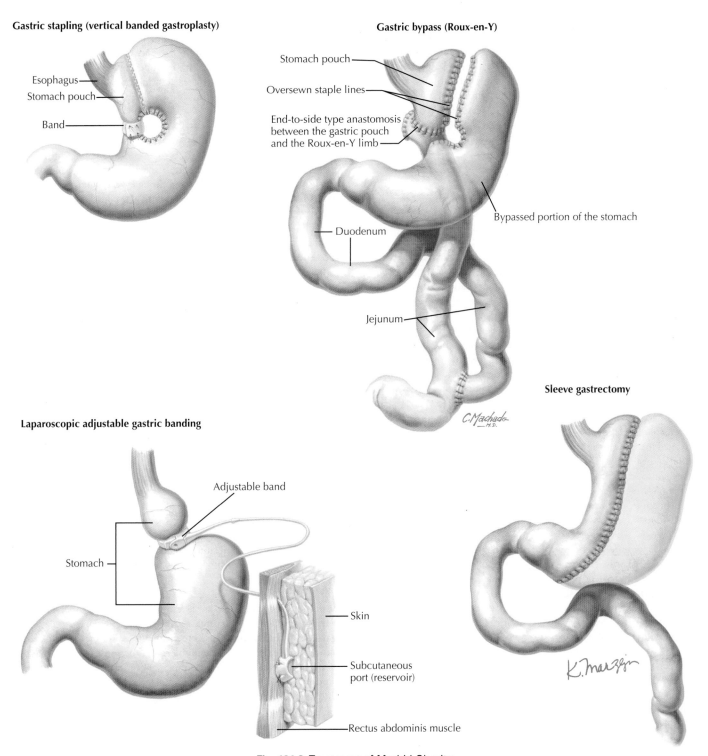

Esophagus

Stomach pouch

Band

Stomach pouch

Oversewn staple lines

End-to-side type anastomosis
between the gastric pouch
and the Roux-en-Y limb

Bypassed portion of the stomach

Duodenum

Jejunum

C. Machado
M.D.

Sleeve gastrectomy

Laparoscopic adjustable gastric banding

Adjustable band

Stomach

Skin

Subcutaneous
port (reservoir)

Rectus abdominis muscle

K. Marzžęn

Fig. 191.2 Treatment of Morbid Obesity

50-cm biliopancreatic limb, which is connected to the "food" or Roux-en-Y limb at 75 to 150 cm distally. At this location, significant digestion begins. A short Roux limb will not add the benefit of malabsorption, although limbs longer than 200 cm in long-limb bypass may lead to decreased absorption of vitamins and nutrients and complications of malnutrition.

The gastrojejunostomy may cause "dumping," which results in rapid emptying of concentrated contents into the small bowel and symptoms of lightheadedness, nausea, diaphoresis, abdominal pain, and diarrhea. Some patients develop a negative conditioning response when eating concentrated foods to prevent this response. Ghrelin is a peptide hormone secreted in the stomach and duodenum that stimulates people to eat. Its response to eating is inhibited by the gastric bypass and the SG. Recent evidence suggests that an exaggerated response of peptide-yy may also contribute to loss of appetite.

Early weight loss is rapid but reaches a plateau after 18 months, after which patients tend to gain weight if behavior modification is not instituted. Long-term studies include open techniques with a larger gastric pouch and range from 50% to 60% EWL for up to 16 years postoperatively. Most recent EWL is currently 70% to 80% with the laparoscopic technique and a 30-mL gastric pouch. After bypass, overall comorbidity is reduced as much as 96%. T2DM is resolved or improved in 83% to 98%, hypertension in 52% to 92%, GERD in 88% to 98%, OSA in 86% to 93%, dyslipidemia in 70% to 96%, and osteoarthritis in 93% of patients.

COURSE AND PROGNOSIS

Surgery is the most effective option in attempting to reverse the effects of comorbidities and improve quality of life and extend life expectancy. Evidence shows that bariatric surgery is effective in improving and resolving medical problems. Additional benefits include reduced medication costs and fewer lost workdays. However, bariatric surgery is also associated with significant perioperative complications and mortality.

It is now believed and documented by extensive peer reviewed literature that bariatric surgery is the best treatment for T2DM. In the late 2000s, the previously named American Society for Bariatric Surgery changed their name to American Society of Metabolic and Bariatric Surgery (ASMBS) to account for the emerging field of metabolic surgery, which includes treatment of diabetes, hypertension, and hyperlipidemia. Evidence suggests that T2DM improvement and resolution may occur in restrictive procedures directly related to the amount of EWL. A recently published randomized control trial comparing bariatric surgery versus intensive medical therapy showed both SG and gastric bypass outperformed medical therapy in improving glycated hemoglobin and obviation of insulin use. Malabsorptive procedures may involve another mechanism that changes the body's response to gastrointestinal (GI) hormones, such as incretins, glucagon-like peptide, and glucose-dependent insulinotrophic polypeptide.

Two meta-analyses reported that mean overall percent of EWL was 61% to 64%, which varied according to procedure. Mortality at 30 days was 0.1% for purely restrictive procedures, 0.5% for gastric bypass, and 1.1% for BPD or DS. Diabetes completely resolved in 77% and resolved or improved in 86% of patients. Hyperlipidemia improved in 70% or more of patients. Hypertension resolved in 62% and resolved or improved in 79% of patients. OSA resolved in 86% and resolved or improved in 84% of patients. Greater weight loss occurred with gastric bypass compared with gastroplasty. Laparoscopic surgery resulted in less wound complications than open surgery.

Two studies reported a 29% reduction in mortality after bariatric surgery and a 40% reduction in mortality from all causes. Deaths from diabetes decreased by 92%, from CAD by 56%, and from cancer by 60%. However, accidental death and suicide increased in incidence. A population study reported that obese surgical patients had a lower overall mortality rate of 0.7% versus 6.2% in the nonsurgical group.

Guidelines for the current accreditation program under the ASMBS include integrated preoperative/postoperative care with nutritional, behavioral, and medical programs and a commitment to report data to ASMBS Quality Improvement Program.

The obesity epidemic must be reversed with a global effort to alter eating behavior and promote exercise. Until then, surgery will remain the most viable option to treat morbid obesity and related comorbidities.

MANAGEMENT OF COMPLICATIONS

Bariatric surgery is an elective procedure for the high-risk obese population. Despite great improvements in surgical technique and postoperative care, the morbidity is still approximately 30% with bariatric surgery. These patients have an *increased inflammatory response,* making them prone to overwhelming shock in the presence of complications. Patient monitoring is essential in the first postoperative days because small changes in vital signs can be the earliest indication of complications. Often, when the patient develops clear signs of sepsis, the complication has already developed.

Another clear sign that must be monitored in the postoperative patient is persistent *tachycardia.* A heart rate greater than 120 beats/min in the bariatric patient is a concern, even if the patient otherwise appears stable. Tachycardia is the most sensitive sign of a pulmonary embolism (PE), bleeding, or an anastomotic leak. It is not specific but can be present in up to 72% of patients with complications and is often the first sign to appear. All patients with postoperative tachycardia should be monitored until the cause is elucidated and resolved.

Laparoscopic sleeve gastrectomy (LSG) is the most common bariatric procedure performed in the United States, and *Roux-en-Y gastric bypass* has the highest complication rate because of its complexity.

This chapter discusses complications of bariatric surgery that include those specific to RYGB LSG. *Laparoscopic adjustable gastric band* will also be covered. Early complications include bleeding, anastomotic leak, deep venous thrombosis (DVT), and PE. Late complications include anastomotic stricture, marginal ulcer, gastrogastric fistula (GGF), bowel obstruction, metabolic disorders (Fig. 191.3).

Early Complications
Bleeding

Bleeding is a complication inherent to any surgical procedure; its incidence may be slightly increased in the bariatric population because of the rigorous DVT prophylactic regimen. In our experience, postoperative hemorrhage is seen in 4% of patients. The bleeding is intraluminal in 60% of bleeding cases and intraperitoneal in 40%. Postoperative bleeding can be diagnosed by clinical signs of tachycardia, hypotension, increased drain output, and decreased hemoglobin level or collection on computed tomography (CT) scan. The most common site of intraluminal bleeding is at the anastomotic level. Bleeding can be successfully managed with observation supported by blood transfusion in 75% of patients; 25% of our bleeding patients required reexploration.

Anastomotic Leak

Anastomotic leak is the second leading cause of death (after PE) following gastric bypass (bariatric) surgery. Leak occurs in 2% of patients regardless of the technique used to create the anastomosis, with most leaks occurring on day 3. As with bleeding, the most common site of leak is at the anastomotic level, with a higher prevalence at the gastrojejunostomy, followed by the jejunojejunostomy, the gastric pouch, and finally the gastric remnant.

Early detection of anastomotic leaks is vital to successful management. The most sensitive sign of leak is persistent tachycardia (72% of patients); left shoulder pain, abdominal pain, and fever are not as sensitive. GI studies and CT scan can detect leaks in only 30% and 56% of cases, respectively. Because of the lack of specificity in clinical presentation and imaging studies, surgical exploration should be part of the diagnostic algorithm. Approximately 60% of patients will require surgical intervention. Patients who achieve good drainage through the original drains placed and show no signs of sepsis may be treated conservatively with strict nothing-by-mouth (*nil per os,* NPO) status, total parenteral nutrition, and intravenous (IV) antibiotics. Patients with signs of sepsis should undergo diagnostic laparoscopy, abdominal washout, and drain placement. Any attempt to redo the anastomosis is strongly discouraged because of the increased risk of anastomotic breakdown in the presence of inflammation.

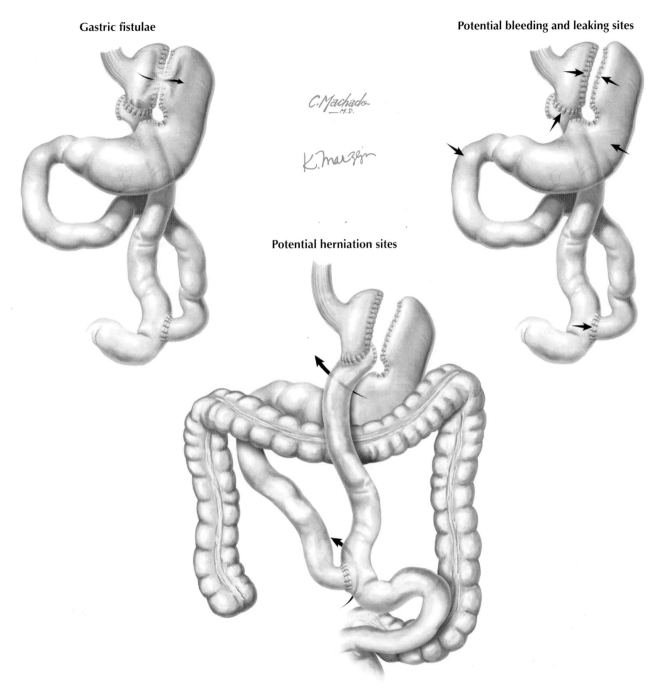

Gastric fistulae

Potential bleeding and leaking sites

Potential herniation sites

Fig. 191.3 Complications of Bariatric Surgery

Leaks are also a potential complication after LSG, seen in 0.8% of cases. Most leaks are located at the most proximal part of the staple line by the gastroesophageal (GE) junction. They can be classified according to chronicity from time of surgery.

	Time From Surgery
Acute	<7 days
Early	7 days to 6 weeks
Late	6 weeks to 12 weeks
Chronic	>12 weeks

Acute and early leaks can be treated with endoscopic means or surgical washout and wide drainage. Late and chronic leaks do best with gastrectomy and esophagojejunostomy, or Roux limb jejunal anastomosis at the leak site.

Pulmonary Embolism and Deep Venous Thrombosis

PE is the leading cause of death after bariatric surgery. The incidence of PE after RYGB is 0.41%. Risk factors for PE and DVT development are older than 50 years of age, postoperative anastomotic leak, smoking, and previous DVT/PE. All patients undergoing RYGB should receive subcutaneous heparin before and after surgery, as well as compression stockings and early ambulation. Low-molecular-weight heparin should be avoided the first 48 hours postoperatively because of an increased incidence of bleeding. Patients with a previous history of PE/DVT, pulmonary hypertension, or lymphedema or with severely impaired ambulation should be considered for prophylactic placement of an inferior vena cava (IVC) filter.

Late Complications
Stricture
The incidence and severity of stricture varies based on the type of procedure.

For gastric bypass, anastomotic stricture, mainly at the level of the gastrojejunostomy, is a relatively common complication, seen in 1.6% to 20% of bariatric patients. Symptoms usually start 3 weeks after surgery. Patients present with nausea, vomiting, and inability to progress to solid foods. Diagnostic studies should include upper GI series and upper endoscopy.

Management of stricture consists of serial endoscopic balloon dilatations (usually up to three), separated by 2-week intervals. Initial dilatations should not exceed 8 mm because of the risk of perforation (2.2%); subsequent dilatations can be increased up to 18 mm. The patient with perforation will complain of abdominal pain and distention, and a plain abdominal film will reveal free air under the diaphragm. These perforations can be treated conservatively with IV antibiotics and NPO status if the patient is asymptomatic. Alternatively, if the patient shows any sign of sepsis, or if a large extravasation of contrast is seen on radiographic studies, diagnostic laparoscopy and drain placement are essential. Failed weight loss after dilatation is not seen in patients on long-term follow-up.

The incidence of stricture is much lower after LSG (0.7%), but it is still a potential complication. Patients will present with excessive nausea, vomiting, and dehydration. An upper GI study is diagnostic. Most strictures will resolve after endoscopic balloon dilatation, but surgical interventions, such as, partial resection, and conversion to RYGB may be necessary with a long stricture not amenable to dilatation.

Marginal Ulcer
Marginal ulceration after gastric bypass is diagnosed in 1% to 16% of patients. Predisposing factors are active smoking and preoperative *Helicobacter pylori* infection. Patients usually present with midepigastric pain and/or upper GI bleeding. Upper endoscopy is diagnostic. In most cases, ulceration is seen at the jejunal mucosa of the gastrojejunostomy and mucosal erythema of the gastric pouch. Most bleeding ulcers respond to endoscopic therapy. Patients should take proton pump inhibitors (PPIs) and sucralfate for 2 months. Smoking cessation is mandatory.

Gastrogastric Fistula
GGF is a challenging late complication, with an incidence of approximately 1%. The vast majority of GGFs are symptomatic at diagnosis. Symptoms consist of moderate to severe epigastric pain, nausea, and vomiting, with GI bleeding in fewer cases. CT may show oral contrast in the gastric remnant, but this finding is of low specificity because contrast may reflux from the biliopancreatic limb. The most sensitive test is a barium swallow with position changes (erect, supine, left lateral, and right lateral decubitus); esophagogastroduodenoscopy (EGD) may be diagnostic in some cases.

The GGF may resolve after medical treatment, so the presence of GGF is not an indication for prompt surgery. The surgical management of symptomatic GGF after medical failure consists of laparoscopic partial remnant gastrectomy with or without trimming of the gastric pouch, fistulous tract, or both, while leaving the gastrojejunostomy intact.

Because remnant gastrectomy may be associated with a high complication rate, surgical treatment should be offered to patients with intractable disabling symptoms, evidence of anastomotic leak, or peritonitis.

Bowel Obstruction
Severe bowel obstruction (SBO) after laparoscopic RYGB has many causes, usually iatrogenic etiologies resulting from narrow anastomoses, tight closure of mesenteric defects, mesenteric or intramural hematomas, anastomotic leaks, incarcerated ventral hernias, internal hernias, and adhesions. Patients may develop symptoms in the immediate postoperative period up to years after surgery. The incidence of SBO varies from 0.4% to 7.45%. With the adoption of the laparoscopic approach, postoperative SBO secondary to adhesions and incisional hernias has been reduced. However, a higher incidence of SBO caused by internal hernias is seen, compared with the open procedure, if the retrocolic retrogastric route is chosen to advance the alimentary limb. Internal herniation can occur at the jejunojejunostomy, Petersen space, or the transverse mesocolonic defect after a retrocolic approach.

If internal herniation is suspected, the patient must be taken to the operating room as soon as possible to reduce the herniation and prevent intestinal necrosis. Most SBO cases can be approached laparoscopically, but the conversion rate is higher due to loss of working space because of distended bowel. Procedures include lysis of adhesions, closure of mesenteric defects, and reconstruction of the jejunojejunostomy.

Metabolic Complications
Nutritional deficiencies are rare in purely restrictive procedures such as LAGB or LSG, unless the patient has significant changes in eating habits or complications. Macronutrient deficiency or protein-calorie malnutrition can be found in up to 5% of gastric bypass patients, and its prevalence is directly proportional to the length of the alimentary limb. Most of these patients can be managed by nutritional consult and guidance. Micronutrient deficiencies include vitamins, minerals, trace metals, and electrolytes, all of which are absorbed at specific sites in the small intestine. The bypassing of these sites and the reduction in the small intestine's absorptive capacity can lead to deficiencies. The most common deficiencies associated with RYGB are iron, vitamin B_{12}, calcium, and vitamin D. Complications of these deficiencies range from anemia to irreversible encephalopathy. All patients undergoing gastric bypass should be instructed to take nutritional supplements for the rest of their lives. Follow-up with annual testing of vitamin levels is mandatory.

When nutritional consult and vitamin supplements do not correct the patient's nutritional deficiencies, parenteral nutrition should be started, with consideration of revision or reversal of the bypass.

ADDITIONAL RESOURCES

Adams TD, Gress RE, Smith SC, et al: Long-term mortality after gastric bypass surgery, *N Engl J Med* 357:753, 2007.

Angrisani L, et al: Bariatric surgery and endoluminal procedures: IFSO worldwide survey 2014, *Obes Surg* 27(9):2279–2289, 2017.

Ballesta C, Berindoague R, Cabrera M, et al: Management of anastomotic leaks after laparoscopic Roux-en-Y gastric bypass, *Obes Surg* 18(6):623–630, 2008.

Belachew M, Legrand M, Vincenti VV, et al: Laparoscopic placement of adjustable silicone gastric band in the treatment of morbid obesity: how to do it, *Obes Surg* 5:66, 1995.

Buchwald H, Avidor Y, Braunwald E, et al: Bariatric surgery: a systematic review and meta-analysis, *JAMA* 292:2004, 1724.

Carrodeguas L, Szomstein S, Soto F, et al: Management of gastrogastric fistulas after divided Roux-en-Y gastric bypass surgery for morbid obesity: analysis of 1,292 consecutive patients and review of literature, *Surg Obes Relat Dis* 1(5):467–474, 2005.

Chevallier JM, Zinzindohoué F, Douard R, et al: Complications after laparoscopic adjustable gastric banding for morbid obesity: experience with 1,000 patients over 7 years, *Obes Surg* 14(3):407–414, 2004.

Cho M, Kaidar-Person O, Szomstein S, Rosenthal RJ: Laparoscopic remnant gastrectomy: a novel approach to gastrogastric fistula after Roux-en-Y gastric bypass for morbid obesity, *J Am Coll Surg* 204(4):617–624, 2007.

Christou NV, Sampalis JS, Liberman M, et al: Surgery decreases long-term mortality, morbidity, and health care use in morbidly obese patients, *Ann Surg* 240:416, 2004.

Cummings DE, Weigle DS, Frayo RS, et al: Plasma ghrelin levels after diet-induced weight loss or gastric bypass surgery, *N Engl J Med* 346:1623–1630, 2002.

DeMaria EJ: Bariatric surgery for morbid obesity, *N Engl J Med* 356:2176–2183, 2007.

Dixon JB, O'Brien PE, Playfair J, et al: Adjustable gastric banding and conventional therapy for type 2 diabetes, *JAMA* 299:316, 2008.

Filho AJ, Kondo W, Nassif LS, et al: Gastrogastric fistula: a possible complication of Roux-en-Y gastric bypass, *J Soc Laparoendosc Surg* 10(3):326–333, 2006.

Frezza EE, Reddy S, Gee LL, Wachtel MS: Complications after sleeve gastrectomy for morbid obesity, *Obes Surg* 19(6):684–687, 2009.

Glenny AM, O'Meara S, Melville A, Wilson C: The treatment and prevention of obesity: a systemic review of the literature, *Int J Obes Relat Metab Disord* 21:715–737, 1997.

Gonzalez R, Haines K, Nelson LG, et al: Predictive factors of thromboembolic events in patients undergoing Roux-en-Y gastric bypass, *Surg Obes Relat Dis* 2(1):30–35, 2006.

Gonzalez R, Sarr MG, Smith CD, et al: Diagnosis and contemporary management of anastomotic leaks after gastric bypass for obesity, *J Am Coll Surg* 204(1):47–55, 2007.

Gumbs AA, Duffy AJ, Bell RL: Incidence and management of marginal ulceration after laparoscopic Roux-Y gastric bypass, *Surg Obes Relat Dis* 2(4):460–463, 2006.

Hales CM, et al: Prevalence of obesity among adults and youths: United States 2015-2016, *NCHS Data Brief* No. 288, October 2017.

Hess DS, Hess DW: Biliopancreatic diversion with a duodenal switch, *Obes Surg* 8:267, 1998.

Jones SB, Jones DB: *Obesity surgery: patient safety and best practices*, Woodbury, Conn, 2009, Cine-Med, pp 33–34.

Kothari SN, Lambert PJ, Mathiason MA: A comparison of thromboembolic and bleeding events following laparoscopic gastric bypass in patients treated with prophylactic regimens of unfractionated heparin or enoxaparin, *Am J Surg* 194(6):709–711, 2007.

Lalor PF, Tucker ON, Szomstein S, Rosenthal RJ: Complications after laparoscopic sleeve gastrectomy, *Surg Obes Relat Dis* 4(1):33–38, 2008.

Lo Menzo E, Szomstein S, Rosenthal R: Reoperative bariatric surgery, *ASMBS Textbook of Bariatric Surgery*, Springer, 2014.

Ma C, et al: Effects of weight loss interventions for adults who are obese on mortality, cardiovascular disease, and cancer: systematic review and meta-analysis, *BMJ* 359:2017.

Martin K, Mani M, Mani A: New targets to treat obesity and the metabolic syndrome, *Eur J Pharmacol* 763:64–74, 2015.

Mehran A, Szomstein S, Zundel N, Rosenthal R: Management of acute bleeding after laparoscopic Roux-en-Y gastric bypass, *Obes Surg* 13(6):842–847, 2003.

National Institutes of Health: Gastrointestinal surgery for severe obesity: consensus development conference panel, *Ann Intern Med* 115:956, 1991.

Ogden CL, Yanovski SZ, Carroll MD, Flegal KM: The epidemiology of obesity, *Gastroenterology* 132:2087–2102, 2007.

Podnos YD, Jimenez JC, Wilson SE, et al: Complications after laparoscopic gastric bypass: a review of 3464 cases, *Arch Surg* 138(9):957–961, 2003.

Poitou Bernert C, Ciangura C, Coupaye M, et al: Nutritional deficiency after gastric bypass: diagnosis, prevention and treatment, *Diabetes Metab* 33(1):13–24, 2007.

Pories WJ, Swanson MS, MacDonald KG, et al: Who would have thought it? An operation proves to be the most effective therapy for adult-onset diabetes mellitus, *Ann Surg* 222:339, 1995.

Rasmussen JJ, Fuller W, Ali MR: Marginal ulceration after laparoscopic gastric bypass: an analysis of predisposing factors in 260 patients, *Surg Endosc* 21(7):1090–1094, 2007.

Regan JP, Inabnet WB, Gagner M, Pomp A: Early experience with two-stage laparoscopic Roux-en-Y gastric bypass as an alternative in the super-super obese patient, *Obes Surg* 13:861, 2003.

Rogula T, Yenumula PR, Schauer PR: A complication of Roux-en-Y gastric bypass: intestinal obstruction, *Surg Endosc* 21(11):1914–1918, 2007.

Roman S, Napoleon B, Mion F, et al: Intragastric balloon for "non-morbid" obesity: a retrospective evaluation of tolerance and efficacy, *Obes Surg* 14:539, 2004.

Rosenthal RJ, Szomstein S, Kennedy CI, et al: Laparoscopic surgery for morbid obesity: 1,001 consecutive bariatric operations performed at the bariatric institute, Cleveland clinic Florida, *Obes Surg* 16(2):119–124, 2006.

Sasson M, et al: Comparison between major and minor surgical procedures for the treatment of chronic staple line disruption after laparoscopic sleeve gastrectomy, *Surg Obes Relat Dis* 12(5):969–975, 2016.

Schauer PR, et al: Bariatric surgery versus intensive medical therapy for diabetes—5 year outcomes, *N Engl J Med* 376(7):641–651, 2017.

Schauer P, Ikramuddin S, Hamad G, Gourash W: The learning curve for laparoscopic Roux-en-Y gastric bypass is 100 cases, *Surg Endosc* 17:212, 2003.

Scopinaro N, Gianetta E, Adami GF, et al: Biliopancreatic diversion for obesity at eighteen years, *Surgery* 119:261, 1996.

Seidel JC, Halberstadt J: The global burden of obesity and the challenges of prevention, *Ann Nutr Metab* 66:7–12, 2015.

Sjostrom L, Narbro K, Sjostrom CD, et al: Effects of bariatric surgery on mortality in Swedish obese subjects, *N Engl J Med* 357:741, 2007.

Suter M, Jayet C, Jayet A: Vertical banded gastroplasty: long-term results comparing three different techniques, *Obes Surg* 10:41, 2000.

Telem DA, et al: Updated panel report: best practices for the surgical treatment of obesity, *Surgical Endoscopy* epub March 2018.

Tucker ON, Escalante-Tattersfield T, Szomstein S, Rosenthal RJ: The ABC system: a simplified classification system for small bowel obstruction after laparoscopic Roux-en-Y gastric bypass, *Obes Surg* 17(12):1549–1554, 2007.

Ukleja A, Afonso BB, Pimentel R, et al: Outcome of endoscopic balloon dilation of strictures after laparoscopic gastric bypass, *Surg Endosc* 22(8):1746–1750, 2008.

US Department of Health and Human Services: *Statistics related to overweight and obesity*, Bethesda, Md, 2008, Weight Control Information Network (WIN). http://www.win.niddk.nih.gov/publications/PDFs/stat904z.pdf.

Gastrointestinal Diseases Related to Nutrition

James S. Scolapio

PANCREATITIS

Acute pancreatitis is an example of a disease process possibly affected by method of feeding (total parenteral nutrition [TPN] versus total enteral nutrition [TEN]). In a prospective study of 54 patients with acute mild pancreatitis, catheter sepsis was 10 times higher in the TPN group than in control subjects who received intravenous fluids only. In the same study, pneumothorax occurred only in the TPN group, and length of hospital stay was longer in the TPN group. This study suggests a significant risk associated with giving TPN to patients with mild pancreatitis.

Based on recent recommendations from the American Society of Parenteral and Enteral Nutrition, patients with mild pancreatitis, who typically resume eating within 7 to 10 days of leaving the hospital, should not receive TEN or TPN unless they have lost significant weight, defined as greater than 10% of usual weight, in the previous 6 months. A study compared complications in 38 patients with severe acute pancreatitis treated with either TEN or TPN. Septic complications, hyperglycemia, peripancreatic necrosis, and cost were all greater in those patients who had received TPN. Mortality rate was similar in the two groups.

Another prospective study of 34 patients with severe pancreatitis compared outcomes with TEN and TPN and found that multiorgan failure, abdominal sepsis, and mortality were greater in the TPN group. In addition, markers of disease severity—including C-reactive protein, Acute Physiology and Chronic Health Evaluation II score, and immunoglobulin M endotoxin—were all higher in patients receiving TPN. Although bacterial translocation was not formally evaluated, TEN might have reduced bacterial translocation compared with TPN, explaining why outcomes were better with TEN. Another study of 156 patients with pancreatitis reported that hypocaloric feeding with TEN resulted in fewer septic and metabolic complications than TPN feeding. More than 50% of the TPN patients were hyperglycemic versus only 15% of TEN patients. Despite fewer complications in the TEN group, mortality rates were the same in both groups. Current data support the superiority of TEN over TPN in managing patients with acute severe pancreatitis.

In patients with chronic pancreatitis, the cause of malnutrition is multifactorial, including fear of postprandial abdominal pain (sitophobia), steatorrhea, anorexia, and often coexistent alcoholism. Steatorrhea and azotorrhea (fecal protein loss) occur when lipase and trypsin secretion are reduced by 90%. Nutritional management first begins with appropriate management of a patient's abdominal pain. Analgesics should be given at least 30 minutes before meals to prevent postprandial exacerbation of pain. Meta-analysis failed to show a beneficial effect of exogenous pancreatic enzyme replacement in relieving abdominal pain. Treatment of exocrine insufficiency focuses on giving adequate pancreatic enzymes. The minimal dose of lipase required is 28,000 IU/meal. Enzymes should be given with meals to ensure adequate mixing with food. Weight maintenance, symptomatic improvement of diarrhea, and decreased

72-hour fecal fat excretion are the goals of therapy. Dietary fat intake should not be restricted. Fat-soluble vitamins and vitamin B_{12} should be replaced if necessary.

INFLAMMATORY BOWEL DISEASE

The outcomes of TEN and TPN have also been evaluated in patients with inflammatory bowel disease (IBD). Whether the combination of complete bowel rest and TPN can be used successfully as primary therapy in patients with acute IBD with or without other medical therapy is controversial.

The literature suggests that patients with Crohn *enteritis* might achieve clinical remission with the combination of bowel rest and TPN. Indirect evidence, however, suggests that TPN is less effective than steroid therapy in active Crohn disease. Results suggest that nothing by mouth and TPN for 3 to 6 weeks results in a clinical response rate of 64% in patients with acute Crohn disease. In most of these studies, however, prednisone was given simultaneously with TPN, making it difficult to discern whether the positive effects observed resulted completely from bowel rest and TPN or from the combined effects of prednisone and TPN. Data also suggest that administering TEN with an elemental peptide-based or polymeric formula for 3 to 6 weeks results in a remission rate of approximately 68%, which is similar to the remission rate reported with TPN and bowel rest. The positive benefit is most likely related to the lipid composition of the enteral formulas. Monounsaturated fatty acid (oleic acid), which is present in most enteral formulas, is not a precursor to inflammatory mediators (arachidonic acid and eicosanoic synthesis), which may explain the beneficial effect observed.

On the other hand, current literature suggests that patients with Crohn colitis and idiopathic ulcerative colitis do not respond any better to TPN and bowel rest (with or without prednisone) than patients treated with prednisone and oral diet. In these studies, TPN resulted in 10% more complications than enteral feeding. Complications included pneumothorax from central catheter placement, catheter sepsis, and various metabolic complications. Enteral feedings using elemental formulas appear to have limited benefit in Crohn colitis and idiopathic ulcerative colitis. Therefore surgery should not be delayed for TPN or TEN in patients with refractory colitis. Indications for bowel rest and TPN include patients with mechanical bowel obstruction, distal small bowel fistula, and toxic megacolon who are not judged to be surgical candidates and who have been without food for 10 to 14 days.

LIVER DISEASE

Cirrhosis is perhaps one of the best examples of protein-calorie malnutrition. Poor dietary intake and altered substrate metabolism are the primary reasons for malnutrition in this group of patients. Malnutrition has a negative impact on survival.

Oral dietary therapy is the mainstay of nutritional treatment. Although nasogastric feeding tubes can be safely placed in most patients, use beyond 4 weeks is difficult because of nasal discomfort and risk for bleeding from thrombocytopenia and impaired coagulation. Gastrostomy feeding tubes cannot be safely placed in patients with ascites given the risk for peritonitis. In most patients except those with refractory hepatic encephalopathy, protein intake should not be restricted and should provide 1.5 g/kg per day of total calories. Vegetable protein is better tolerated than animal protein because it produces fewer aromatic amino acids, thought to be the responsible mediators of hepatic encephalopathy.

Branched-chain amino acids may be helpful in select patients with refractory disease. Fat-soluble vitamin levels should be checked and augmented if they are low. Concentration levels of serum vitamin A may not reflect hepatic vitamin A concentrations; therefore replacement should be administered with caution given the risk for vitamin A toxicity to the liver.

Orthotopic liver transplantation is the principal treatment for malnutrition in patients with cirrhosis. Within 4 months of transplantation, increased muscle mass and improved functional status are clinically evident.

SHORT BOWEL SYNDROME

Short bowel syndrome is a collection of signs and symptoms used to describe the nutritional and metabolic consequences after major resection of the small intestine. In adults, resection for Crohn disease and intestinal infarction are the primary reasons for short bowel syndrome.

Diarrhea, fluid and electrolyte losses, and weight loss characterize short bowel syndrome. Patients with less than 100 to 150 cm of remaining small intestine often require TPN for survival. Patients with enough remaining colon and 50 cm or more of residual small bowel can usually survive on an oral diet without TPN. After surgical resection, the remaining intestine undergoes a process of adaptation, including structural and functional changes that tend to maximize nutrient and fluid absorption. Changes include villus cell hyperplasia and increased brush border enzyme activity. These changes can occur up to 1 year after intestinal resection.

Dietary management of short bowel syndrome depends on whether a patient has retained part of the colon. The patient who has retained colon benefits from a diet high in complex carbohydrates and low in fat. The colon can convert complex carbohydrates to short-chain fatty acids (acetate, propionate, butyrate). The production of short-chain fatty acids stimulates sodium and water absorption and provides additional calories for intestinal absorption. Oxalate should be restricted in the diets of patients with short bowel syndrome and partial colon because oxalate is absorbed principally from the colon, resulting in oxalate nephropathy. Vitamin B_{12} should be replaced if more than 100 cm of a patient's terminal ileum has been resected or if it is severely diseased.

Patients with large volumes of diarrhea (2 L/day) should be administered antimotility agents to reduce the amount of volume loss. Oral rehydration solutions are also beneficial for some patients with short bowel syndrome. Octreotide should be reserved for patients with high stool output despite the use of antimotility agents and oral rehydration therapy. Exogenous trophic factors—including growth hormone, glutamine, and glucagon-like peptide-2 (GLP-2)—have been used to increase nutrient absorption in patients with short bowel syndrome. Teduglutide, an analog of naturally occurring GLP-2, was approved by the US Food and Drug Administration (FDA) in 2012 for the treatment of select patients. Parenteral nutrition remains the treatment of choice for the patient with refractory disease who cannot survive on an oral diet alone. Small-bowel transplantation is indicated for patients with recurrent line sepsis, lack of venous access, and progressive TPN-induced liver disease.

ADDITIONAL RESOURCES

ASPEN Board of Directors: Clinical guideline task force: guidelines for the use of parenteral and enteral nutrition in adult and pediatric patients, *JPEN J Parenter Enteral Nutr* 26(Suppl 1):1SA–138SA, 2002.

Cagir B, Geibel J: Short-bowel syndrome treatment and management—medical therapy, *Medscape* 1–3, 2017.

Forbes A, Escher J, Hebuterne X: ESPEN guideline: clinical nutrition in inflammatory bowel disease, *Clin Nutr* 36:321–347, 2017.

Gianott L, Meier R, Lobo DN: ESPEN guidelines on parenteral nutrition: pancreas, *Clin Nutr* 28:428–435, 2009.

McClave SA, Chang WK, Dhaliwal R, Heyland DK: Nutrition support in acute pancreatitis: a systemic review of the literature, *JPEN J Parenter Enteral Nutr* 30:143–156, 2006.

Pironi L, Arends J, Bozzetti F: ESPEN guidelines on chronic intestinal failure in adults, *Clin Nutr* 35:247–307, 2016.

Scolapio JS, Raimondo M, Lankisch M: Nutritional support in pancreatitis, *Scand J Gastroenterol* 35:1010–1015, 2000.

Scolapio JS, Ukleja A: Short-bowel syndrome, *Curr Opin Clin Nutr Metab Care* 1:391–394, 1998.

Shuja A, Malespin M, Scolapio J: Nutritional considerations in liver disease, *Gastroenterol Clin North Am* 47:243–252, 2018.

INDEX

A

Abdomen
  acute, 173f
  acute peritonitis, 170–172, 174f
    diagnosis, 171–172
  benign paroxysmal peritonitis (familial
      Mediterranean fever), 173–175, 176f
    clinical picture, 173–174
    diagnosis, 174–175
    treatment, 175
  chronic peritonitis: peritoneal tuberculosis,
      172–173, 175f
  region and planes, 164–165, 166f
Abdominal abscess, 196–200
  indications, 198–200
    relevant anatomy, 198
    technique, 199
    types of incisions, 199–200, 199f–200f
  laparoscopic access, 197–198, 198f
  open exploratory laparotomy approach, 198
  robotic access, 196–197
Abdominal actinomycosis, 402–403, 403f
Abdominal aorta, 171f–172f, 497f
Abdominal discomfort
  in ascariasis, 413
  in fish tapeworm infection, 421–422
Abdominal distention
  in cecal volvulus, 321
  in chronic intestinal pseudo-obstruction, 236
  in congenital intestinal anomalies, 225
  in gastroparesis, 113
  in malabsorption, 253f
  in sigmoid volvulus, 321
  in trichuriasis, 409
  in Whipple disease, 256f
Abdominal esophagus, 2, 4f
  blood supply of, 5, 7f
  histology of, 13f
Abdominal mass
  in abdominal actinomycosis, 402
  in hepatic adenoma, 589
  in hepatocellular carcinoma, 596
  in pancreatic cancer, 450–451
  in small intestine intussusception, 268
Abdominal pain
  in acute cholecystitis, 465
  in acute pancreatitis, 439
  in amebiasis, 404
  in α1-antitrypsin deficiency, 582
  in appendicitis, 325
  in cecal volvulus, 321
  in cholangiocarcinoma, 613
  in choledocholithiasis, 471
  in Crohn disease, 342
  in diverticulitis, 329
  in dwarf tapeworm infection, 423
  in eosinophilic gastroenteritis, 266
  in familial adenomatous polyposis, 363
  in focal nodular hyperplasia, 589
  in fructose intolerance, 246, 246f
  in gastritis, 132

Abdominal pain (Continued)
  in gastroesophageal reflux disease, 49
  in gastrointestinal tuberculosis, 399
  in gastroparesis, 113
  in hepatic adenoma, 589
  in hepatitis A, 566
  in hepatocellular carcinoma, 596
  in hereditary hemochromatosis, 583
  in intestinal obstruction, 233
  in irritable bowel syndrome, 239, 240f
  in lymphogranuloma venereum, 377–379
  in malignant small bowel tumor, 273
  in microscopic colitis, 354
  in peptic ulcer perforation, 138
  in periampullary carcinoma, 478
  in pork tapeworm infection, 420
  in schistosomiasis, 606
  in sigmoid volvulus, 321
  in small intestine intussusception, 268
  in spirochetal infections, 602
  in strongyloidiasis, 415
  in trichinosis, 424
  in trichuriasis, 409
  in typhoid fever, 387
  in Whipple disease, 255, 256f
Abdominal radiographs, in intestinal obstruction,
    233
Abdominal ultrasonography
  in choledocholithiasis, 471
  in gallbladder stones, 469
  in gangrenous cholecystitis, 467–468
  in liver, 539, 540f
  in symptomatic gallstone disease, 469
Abdominal wall
  abdominal cavity hernias, 187–195
  anatomy, 164–169
  anterior, 165f
  anterolateral, 164
  congenital abnormalities, 169, 169f
  liver and, 487
  and viscera, 171f
Aberrant left hepatic artery, 499f, 500
Abscess
  actinomycotic, 603–604, 605f
  in amebiasis, 602, 603f
  anorectal, 374–376, 375f
  appendiceal, 324, 324f
  in Crohn disease, 348
  hepatic
    in abdominal actinomycosis, 402, 403f
    amebic, 404
  lymphogranuloma venereum-related, 377–379
  pneumopleurohepatic, 604
  subphrenic, 487
Absorption, large intestine, 291–293, 292f
Acalculous cholecystitis, 466–468
Acanthosis nigricans, 548
Accessory hemiazygos vein, 7–8, 8f
Accessory left hepatic artery, 500
Acetaldehyde, 543
Acetic acid, 291, 629–630
Achalasia, 69–72, 70f
  pneumatic dilatation for, 144
  in pulsion diverticula, 31–32
Acholic stool, 302
Acid hypersecretion, in peptic ulcer disease, 137

"Acid rebound", 99
Acid reflux
  in Barrett's esophagus, 57–58
  in esophagitis, 53
  in gastroesophageal reflux disease, 49
Acid reflux test, 50
Acid-induced esophagitis, 53
Acidophilic bodies, 534
Acinar cell carcinoma, 448
Acinar cells, 431
Acini, 429f–430f
Acinus model of hepatic organization, 491, 494f
Acquired immunodeficiency syndrome (AIDS),
    384
Acquired megacolon, 319
Actinomyces, esophageal ulcer and, 54
Actinomyces bovis, 602–603
Actinomyces israelii, 402
Actinomycosis
  abdominal, 402–403, 403f
  liver, 602–608, 605f
Actinomycotic abscess, 603–604, 605f
Acute abdomen, 229
Acute acalculous cholecystitis, 466
Acute appendicitis, 324, 324f
Acute cholecystitis, 465–466, 465f, 470f
Acute diarrhea, 248
Acute esophagitis, 53–54, 53f
Acute fatty liver of pregnancy (AFLP), 587f, 588
Acute gastric ulcers, 132–134, 133f
Acute gastritis, 129, 132–134, 133f
Acute kidney injury (AKI), 523
Acute massive necrosis, in acute viral hepatitis,
    568f
Acute pancreatitis, 438–442
  clinical picture of, 439
  complications of, 441–442
  diagnosis of, 439
  etiologic associations for, 438b
  etiology of, 438–439
  imaging procedures for, 439, 440f
  intraabdominal complications of, 441–442,
      442f
  severity of, 438t
  sphincter of Oddi dysfunction and, 475–477
  systemic complications of, 441
  treatment and management for, 440–441
Acute perforation, in peptic ulcer disease, 138
Acute peritonitis, 170–172, 174f
  diagnosis, 171–172
Acute portal vein thrombosis, 609
Acute red atrophy of liver, 534
Acute variceal bleeding, 45, 525–527
Acute viral hepatitis, 566–569, 567f–569f
  hepatic necrosis and, 534
Acute yellow atrophy of liver, 534
Adalimumab, 352, 353t
Adefovir, for hepatitis B, 571
Adenocarcinoma
  colon, 358f
    Crohn disease and, 348
  duodenum, 154, 155f
  esophageal, 78, 79f
  gastric, 151, 152f
    after subtotal gastrectomy, 159–160
  small bowel, 272–273, 272f

Page numbers followed by "f" indicate figures,
"t" indicate tables, and "b" indicate boxes.

646